PHARMACEUTICAL
BIOTECHNOLOGY

PHARMACEUTICAL BIOTECHNOLOGY

Dr. S.P. Vyas
Ph.D. (Pharmaceutics)
Fellow of Commonwealth Academic Staff, U.K. (London)
Professor, Department of Pharmaceutical Sciences,
Dr. Harisingh Gour University,
Sagar - 470 003 (M.P.)

Dr. V.K. Dixit
Ph.D. (Pharmacognosy)
Professor & Head, Department of Pharmaceutical Sciences,
Dr. Harisingh Gour University,
Sagar - 470 003 (M.P.)

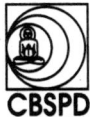

CBSPD

CBS Publishers & Distributors Pvt Ltd

New Delhi • Bengaluru • Chennai • Kochi • Kolkata • Lucknow • Mumbai
Gujarat • Hyderabad • Jharkhand • Nagpur • Patna • Pune • Uttarakhand

PHARMACEUTICAL BIOTECHNOLOGY

ISBN: 978-81-239-0614-0

Copyright © Authors and Publisher

First Edition: 1998

Reprint: 1999, 2001, 2002, 2003 (Twice), 2004, 2005, 2006, 2007, 2008, 2009, 2010, 2011, 2012, 2016, 2018, 2019, 2020, 2021, 2023, **2026**

Published by **Satish Kumar Jain** and produced by **Varun Jain** for

CBS Publishers & Distributors Pvt Ltd

4819/XI Prahlad Street, 24 Ansari Road, Daryaganj, New Delhi 110 002, India
Ph: 011-23289259, 23266838

Website: www.cbspd.com
e-mail: delhi@cbspd.com

Corporate Office: 204 FIE, Industrial Area, Patparganj, Delhi 110 092
Ph: 011-4934 4934   Fax: 011-4934 4935   e-mail: publishing@cbspd.com; publicity@cbspd.com

Branches

- **Bengaluru:** Seema House 2975, 17th Cross, K.R. Road, Banasankari 2nd Stage, Bengaluru 560 070, Karnataka, India
  Ph: +91-80-26771678/79   Fax: +91-80-26771680   e-mail: bangalore@cbspd.com

- **Chennai:** 18/8B, Subbarayan Street, Shenoy Nagar, Chennai 600 030, Tamil Nadu, India
  Ph: +91-44-42032115, 26681266   e-mail: chennai@cbspd.com

- **Kochi:** 42/1325, 1326, Power House Road, opposite KSEB, Power House, Ernakulam 682 018, Kochi, Kerala, India
  Ph: +91-484-4059061–65   Fax: +91-484-4059065   e-mail: kochi@cbspd.com

- **Kolkata:** 147, Hind Ceramics Compound, 1st Floor, Nilgunj Road, Belghoria, Kolkata 700 056, West Bengal, India
  Ph: +91-33-25633055–56   e-mail: kolkata@cbspd.com

- **Lucknow:** Basement, Khushnuma Complex, 7-Meerabai Marg (behind Jawahar Bhawan), Lucknow 226 001, UP, India
  Ph: +91-522-4000032   e-mail: tiwari.lucknow@cbspd.com

- **Mumbai:** PWD Shed. Gala No. 25/26, Ramchandra Bhatt Marg, Next to JJ Hospital Gate No. 2, Opposite Union Bank of India Noorbaug Mumbai 400 009, Maharashtra, India
  Ph: +91-22-66661680/89   e-mail: mumbai@cbspd.com

Representatives

- Gujarat   • Hyderabad   • Jharkhand   • Nagpur   • Patna   • Pune   • Uttarakhand

For trade terms please contact customercare@cbspd.com

For general enquiries please contact info@cbspd.com

Printed at: Chaman Enterprises, Daryaganj, Delhi, India

DEDICATED TO

Sir Harisingh Gour,

Founder Vice Chancellor of University of Saugar, Sagar, 1946

A symbol of inspiration, strength of character, and academic excellence

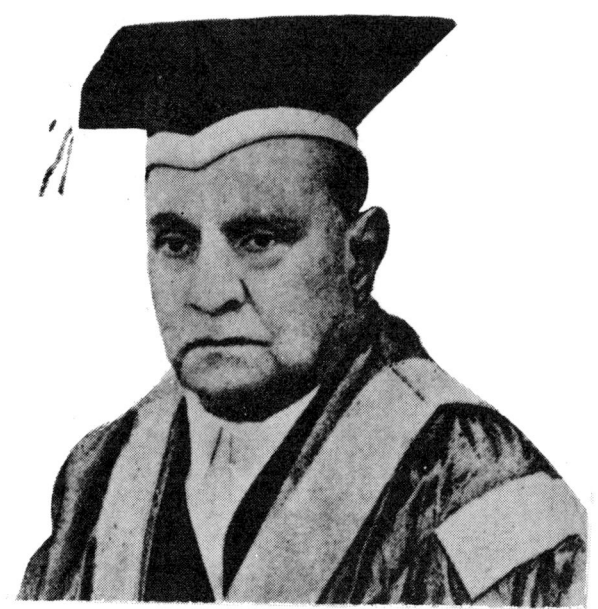

PREFACE

The progress in the field of Biotechnology has been spectacular as substantial technical and scientific growth in basic sciences has widened its horizons. The recent advances in the field of basic genetics have opened up new vistas, potentials and possibilities. Highly proliferating genetic engineering, concept of bio-cellular synthesis units for tailored novel molecules, bioprostheses, immobilization, gene cloning for organ culture, monoclonal antibodies as piloting modules in targeted drug delivery, have become a reality now. Similarly, single cell protein as food and nutrient substitutes, probiotics, gene therapy for genetic diseases, therapeutic recombinant proteins *ex vivo* expression, superovulation and subsequent foddering in surrogate mothers has ushered in an era of new found realities. These developments and allied discoveries aroused a lot of interest in the health care sector. The biotechnological products have already gained nearly 10% share of the pharmaceutical market of united states. It is expected that this sector (Pharmaceutical Biotechnology) will attain a two fold expansion by the turn of this century, and will certainly surpass the computer industry in size, significance and growth. Rapidly expanding population has increased the demand of newer diagnostics and super class novel therapeutics.

At present, the need of diagnostics is mostly met by imports, primarily due to lack of awareness and interest in indigenous developments in this field at the academic as well as industrial level. Our competence or experience in the field of diagnostics and biotechnological therapeutics is insignificant. Impending changes (as in patent law and post GATT scenario), not only necessitate but turn it to be an imperative, that we should strengthen our biotech base; so that indigenous technology can be developed. The foreseen problems have been appreciated, and as a result AICTE, DBT and other government agencies have made recommendations for the inclusion of pharmaceutical biotechnology as one of the core course component of pharmacy education, with the intention that it should broadly be accepted and developed in to a specialized field at post-graduate level. Since we are teaching biotechnology for last many years, we have realized that adequate subject matter on biotechnology is scattered and hence there is a need to compile it systematically. The present venture is an attempt in this direction. We hope the material incorporated in this book in a consolidated, concise, comprehensive and conceivable form will prove to be useful to the students, academicians and industrial scientists.

The present text is a concerted effort where the existing examples have been used to exemplify phenomenological aspects of the biotechnological process, with the help of figures, microphotographs and schematics. An attempt has been made to make the contents more adoptable and illustrative. With well adherent propensity towards pharmaceuticals, the fundamental aspects have been elaborated for their pharmaceutical applications. Embedded prospects and possible potentials not only acquaint readers, but also help in conceiving research problems. The book has been prepared keeping in view the requirements of students who offer Pharmaceutical Biotechnology at under-graduate and post-graduate levels. We sincerely hope that this maiden attempt shall receive the attention of readers.

Chapter 1 is introductory in nature. Chapters 2 to 6 provide basic information about enzymes, their production, immobilization technology and its application and fermentation from general considerations to industrial applications. The process of immobilization has been discussed in the light of its classical applications, in novel drug delivery design, diagnostic testing, stabilization of biotechnological pharmaceuticals and analysis. Chapters 7 and 8 deal with *ex vivo* cell and culture technology, pertaining to plant and animals, and its applications in pharmaceutical biosynthesis, trait improvement, organ culture methods, single cell proteins etc. Chapter 9 dwells upon the basic genetics to prime up the existing familiarity and knowledge in this rapidly expanding science. Chapter 10 presents recombinant DNA technology where gene engineering, cloning and expression as well as various other applications have been discussed. On the basis of information provided in earlier chapters, chapters 11 of this book sums up the modes, mechanisms and means of gene therapy. Chapter 12 and 13 provide information on basic immunology, hybridoma technology, monoclonal antibodies, their manufacturing and applications. With the advent in contemporary research, the vaccination concept has undergone various dimensional changes which have been taken up in chapter 14 'Current Trends in Vaccines'. The level of complexity and set of challenges encountered in protein and peptide delivery have been discussed and various approaches including site specific modification, site directed delivery and newer trends and horizons in safe and effective administration of biotechnological products have been presented in chapter 15. The book acquires its completion with the presentation of chapter 16, which projects applications of biotechnological concepts in targeted drug delivery concepts at the molecular and cellular levels. Various strategies for selective drug targeting with special reference to engineered liposomal constructs have also been discussed. We sincerely hope that the contents shall evince a genuine interest in academic portals. The references and suggested readings at the end of each chapter are highly selective. A few research papers have also been added to the list. The emphasis has been placed on reviews and source book. In lieu of parsimony in building library collections relatively narrow but highly selective selection of sources has been employed.

An attempt has been made to bring out this volume up to the satisfaction of the readers. However, comments in any form are welcome.

We are grateful to Prof. G. Gregoriadis, Head , CDDR, The school of Pharmacy, University of London, whose continual encouragement and valuable suggestions have helped us to bring out this text. We also wish to place on record encouragement received from our worthy Vice Chancellor, Shri Shiv Kumar Shrivastava. We would be failing in our duty if we do not acknowledge the invaluable contribution of our group of leading scientists comprising of Mr. Vikas Jaitely, Mr. Parijat Kanaujia, Mr. N. Venkatesan, Mr. R. Srinivasan, Miss Preeti Venugopalan and Mr. Vaibhav Sihorkar in presentation of book. We express our heartfelt thanks to Prof. S. Sivaraman and Dr. D.V. Kohli for their great help in proof reading of the manuscript.

We thankfully acknowledge suggestions from Dr. Amarjeet Singh, Vice President, Panacea Biotech Ltd., New Delhi, and Dr. Himadri Sen Vice President, Ranbaxy Labs, Gurgaon.

We are highly indebted to our family members; Mrs. Vasundra Vyas, Miss Veena, Master Himanshu, Miss Sonal and Anchal and Mrs. Suman Dixit, Master Parth and Miss Prathu for their immeasurable support and patience observed during the hours devoted to the manuscript. Friends and many well wishers have helped in our attempt to produce this book on Pharmaceutical Biotechnology. We gratefully acknowledge the same.

January 22, 1998   S. P. VYAS
Sagar - 470 003,   V.K. DIXIT

CONTENTS

INTRODUCTION AND HISTORICAL PERSPECTIVE

1.1. BIOTECHNOLOGY : AN INTRODUCTION

Occasional developments in basic and biosciences lead our knowledge to be much more application oriented with great potential for further innovation. The developments which revolutionized 'biosciences' could be sporadic but certainly imparted great wealth to the more specialized discipline; referred to as **biotechnology**. The domain of biotechnology thus integrates most modern and highly specific technologies on one hand and traditional fermentation processes which our ancestors developed and practiced thousands of years ago, on the other. The use of fermentation technology in the preparation of medicinal agents can well be traced long back especially in the Indian system of medicine 'The Ayurveda' particularly has ever been engaged in the utilization of the fermented products as medicaments. However, the interest in the subject has been generated in the last few decades. Before going into an in-depth study of the subject it is necessary to know its evolution.

Biology is the science of living creatures. There is a great diversity in life starting from the simplest virus to the complex human being. But the basis of all organisms is the tendency towards organization leading to diverse forms. So the similarity between a man and bacteria is at the cellular level only. Further understanding of chemistry throws light on the atoms and molecules which are basically the same in the living and non living, just differing in the type and diversity of organization. Attempts have been made to postulate the theory of life using some fundamentals of biological and chemical sciences leading to the subject called **Biosciences**. Fundamental Biosciences account for the relationship between life and matter either through vitalism (that life is made possible by some force that is neither chemical nor physical) or mechanism (that life can be explained entirely in chemical or physical terms). However, the study is fast leading to newer conclusions.

Fundamental biosciences deal with the study of living systems in a wider perspective (Fig.1.1). Enormous research and the newer information drawn there from have led to revolutionary developments in the field of industrial and applied biosciences. It has led newer perspectives of biology (growing with a multitude) and an increase in scientific knowledge. This knowledge of biological sciences offered to better industrial and therapeutic success and has been referred to as **applied biosciences**. This is the area where man has over powered other biological communities for a better living.

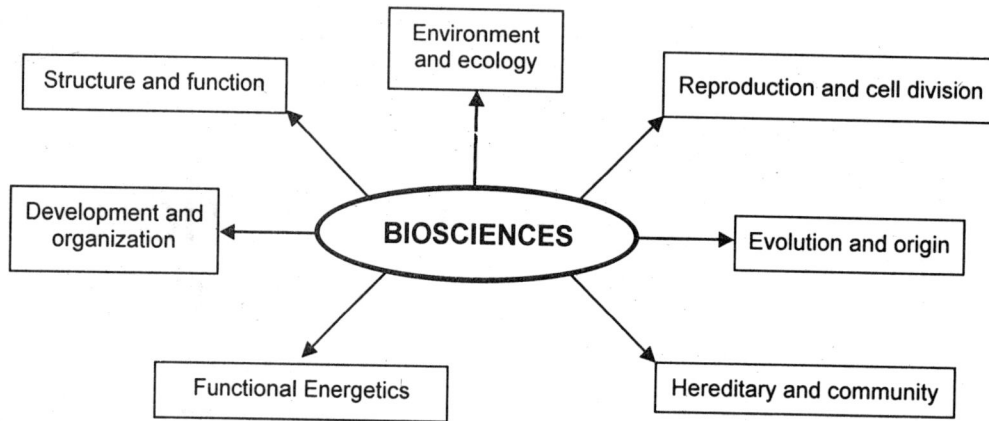

Fig. 1.1 : Biosciences a wider field and perspective

Applied biosciences cover the aspect of production and detection of newer therapeutics viz., antibiotics, peptides, better agricultural science, conservation of living resources, etc. (Fig.1.2). Therefore it could be said that fundamental biosciences have been developed to form applied biosciences for better living and building a good economic status.

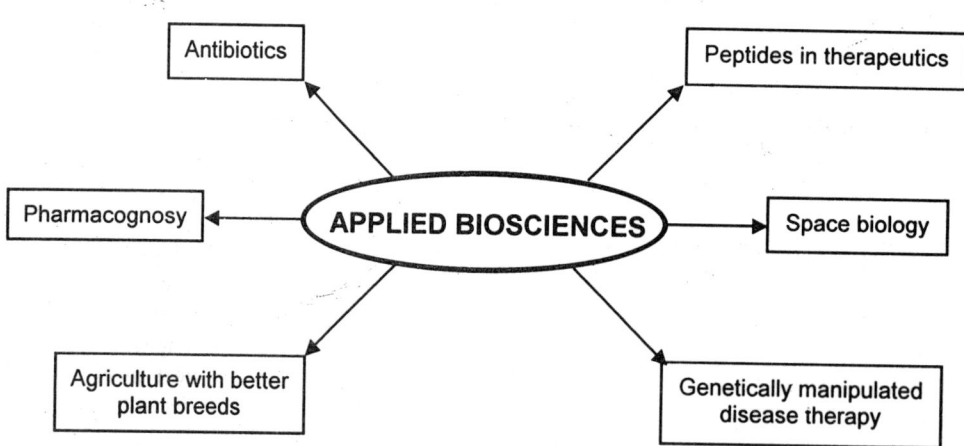

Fig. 1.2 : Applied biosciences in building a newer status of life

With advances in biosciences particularly in the fields of microbiology, molecular biology and biochemistry utilizing better instrumental facilities, a newer branch of biology has emerged as *Biotechnology*. It is referred to as a link between the biological (life) sciences, physical sciences, chemical sciences and technological achievement, commonly referred to as the '*clever*' science of biology. The word biotechnology was coined in mid 1970's as a mixture of '*biological technology*' so as to differentiate from biomedical engineering and biochemical engineering. One of the most recently quoted definitions of biotechnology is "*the application of scientific and engineering principles to the process of materials by biological agents to provide better goods and services"*. But the terminology looks a bit vague. Another frequently quoted definition of biotechnology is *"the application of biological organisms, systems and processes for manufacturing and service industry"*. Still all aspects of the subjects are not clarified. Hence, biotechnology could be represented as a mixture of various biological sciences for better services in field of medicine and agriculture (Fig.1.3). Biotechnology has been identified and experimented upon as a science of techniques which makes use of biological systems interalia. In a real sense it could be presented as an alloy of many disciplines influenced by various parental sciences.

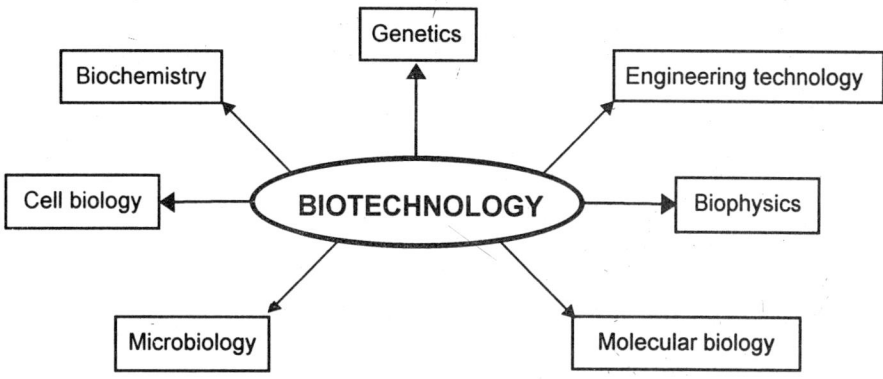

Fig. 1.3 : Various basic biological disciplines involved in the origin of biotechnology

The advances in the field of biotechnology have altogether influenced many fields of applied sciences. This has led to the introduction of many branches of biotechnology as agriculture biotechnology, medical biotechnology, engineering biotechnology, pharmaceutical biotechnology, textile biotechnology, paper bio-technology etc. Each of these branches could be defined as follows:

Agriculture biotechnology: The field of agricultural sciences in which the production of newer variety of high yielding, pest and disease resistant, and cost effective agricultural plants are developed by using the biotechnology based concepts of mutagenesis, rDNA technology and gene cloning.

Medical biotechnology: The area of medical sciences which utilizes the diagnostic aids like the AIDS detection kits, glucose measuring kits etc., and attempts for correction of some hereditary disorders by gene incorporation utilizing the basic concepts of biotechnology is termed as medical biotechnology. The production of artificial organs like the liver and kidney are the emerging fields of the subject.

Engineering biotechnology: The utilization of biotech based enzyme sensors for chemical process monitoring, utilization of some genetically modified strains of microbes as an aid in the chemical synthesis, degeneration of the industrial wastes by some cloned bacteria are grouped together and referred as engineering biotechnology.

Biomedical Engineering: Preparation of some artificial organs as an option or replacement alternative for the vital organs lost due to accident or birth disorders utilizing the biotechnological concepts like polymer engineering, enzyme immobilization etc. is known as biomedical engineering.

Textile and Paper Biotechnology: The application of the concepts of biotechnology as the polymer engineering, production of some special microbe strains, as well as process monitoring using biotech based sensors in production of special fibers is termed as textile biotechnology. The same implies for the paper biotechnology. Furthermore, the immobilization of the enzymes being utilized for the production can further support in the cost effective production of better quality textile and paper.

Environmental biotechnology: The destruction of the wastes from industrial, urban or other sources utilizing specially cloned micro-organisms is a major application that is a part of deals with environmental biotechnology. It also uses the techniques for the purification of the waste water as well as the industrial wastes, safe to be discharged into the rivers or sea.

Mining and Metal Biotechnology: This is a field which has been undergoing expansion during this decade. It utilizes the concept that there are some groups of micro-organisms which erode the surface of the metals; *Thiobacillus ferroxidans* oxidizes sulfur and iron present in the soil, *Leptospirillum ferroxidans, T. organoparpus* degrade pyrates (FeS_2) and Chalcopyrite ($CuFeS_2$). This branch deals with the isolation of the micro-organisms which are capable of affecting these types of degradation and utilizes them in the isolation and purification of the metals and minerals.

Leather Biotechnology: Leather industry is based on the tanning of the skin from the animals using various enzyme systems. The development in the field of enzyme immobilization technology has offered the advantage for the automation of the technology and more cost effective treatment of the leather.

Pharmaceutical Biotechnology: It is a major branch of biotechnology undergoing fast development. The concepts based on biotechnology, in the production of the therapeutic proteins and hormones, fermentation products like the antibiotics, specially designed vaccines or drug design using the receptor hypothesis, gene correction, drug delivery to specific tissues (targeted delivery), production control using the biosensors, artificial bioprostheses, standardization of chemotherapeutic agents and the diagnostic aids using the gene cloning technology, recombinant DNA technology, enzyme immobilization, monoclonal antibodies and mutagenesis have been exploited and attempted for possible use. Furthermore, all the fields of medical biotechnology have to be linked with the pharmaceutical biotechnology in order to attain the approvals from FDA.

The last few decades have witnessed some revolutionary advancements in biological sciences which have dramatically affected the future of design and development of pharmaceuticals in an unprecedented manner. The concept of molecular biology and biotechnology has altogether changed the scenario of pharmaceutical developments. Emergence of DNA cloning technology, known commonly as recombinant DNA (rDNA) technology and the methodologies for production of monoclonal antibodies called hybridoma technology, are the counter pieces of revolution, which are the outcome of decades of continual basic research directed towards molecular biology, cell biology and immunology. Similar developments in the field of biological sciences, commonly referred as 'biotechnology', have facilitated the development, designing, discovery, as well as production of drug(s). Not only drugs but also the technology for better therapeutics and diagnostics have been put forth.

Some major advancements in the field of pharmaceuticals in the last few decades have come forth as a result of extensive research and advancement in pharmacology, analytical chemistry, synthetic organic chemistry, biochemistry and drug delivery. The field of biotechnology has thus an attractive opportunity for maximum developments. It is 10 years now after FDA approval was granted for the first biotechnological product, recombinant human insulin; over 100 products derived from biotechnological principles have progressed to the stage of clinical use or human trials. Over the next 10 years, the global sale for biotechnology based products is expected to approximate $30 billion per annum. It is therefore abundantly clear that the practice of pharmacy has been and will continue to be, strongly influenced by the field of biotechnology and the practicing pharmacist should surely understand the concepts now being created. Some milestones in the history of pharmaceutical biotechnology are listed in table 1.1.

The production of enzyme or hormone based pharmaceuticals has been revolutionized by the recombinant DNA technology. Consider the case of insulin; since its discovery in 1921 by Banting and Best, many animals have been sacrificed so as to achieve very small quantities of the protein. However, since 1986 the recombinant production process has overtaken the markets. The human genetic coding for proinsulin is inserted in *Escherichia coli* cells, which were then grown by fermentation to produce proinsulin. The connecting peptide was further cleaved and converted enzymatically from proinsulin to human insulin. Currently the product is being manufactured by Eli-Lilly and company. The recombinant DNA technology offered many added advantages like production of non-immunogenic, more effective, cheaper products, sparing animal life too.

It has been a subject of debate for years as to how to define pharmaceutical biotechnology as well as how to justify the nomenclature. It was evolved out of vigorous discussion, that as pharmaceutical aspects of chemistry and analysis were respectively accepted as pharmaceutical chemistry or pharmaceutical analysis, it appears to be appropriate to accept the name for the field that encompasses pharmaceutical aspects of biotechnology as pharmaceutical biotechnology. Obviously the products which occur naturally and of microbiological or biological origin having applicable potential in pharmaceutical industry in human therapeutics, in disease diagnosis as well as clinical monitoring of patients may largely be covered under the discipline of pharmaceutical biotechnology. Obviously, the major areas which could be considered include antibodies as microbial secondary metabolites, monoclonal antibodies, genetic engineering and related products, enzyme products, microbial steroid conversion, recombinant vaccine, single cell proteins, animal and plant cell cultures for production of pharmaceuticals, immunomodulators, blood products, tissue banks, protein hydrolysates, and glandular products. Furthermore, other products which too belong to biologicals may include sera, diagnostic agents, organic acids, vitamins, nucleotides, oligonucleotides, antisense, plasma expanders, alkaloids, sutures and ligatures and other microbiological products used in diagnostic and biological assays.

Table 1.1 : Milestones in biotechnology

(The unprecedented development and growth of biotechnology has been an outcome of some of the following mentioned successive, discrete milestone discoveries and events in basic biological research)*.

S. No.	Milestone	Scientist and Year
1.	Proposed double helix model for 3 dimensional structure of DNA after X-ray diffraction data	R.E. Franklin and M. H. Wilkins; J.D Watson and F.H. Crick, 1952-1953
2.	Cleavage of DNA by restriction endonucleases	W. Arber, 1962; M. Meselson and R. Yuan, 1968
3.	Determination of genetic code	M. Nirenberg, S. Ochoa and P. Heder, 1966; H.G. Khorana, 1966
4.	Identification of DNA ligase	M. Gellert, 1967
5.	DNA cloning techniques	H.W. Boyer, S. Cohen and P. Berg 1971-1972
6.	Emergence of rDNA technology	Bordon Conference on Nucleic acids, June 1973
7.	Hybridoma creation	C. Milstein and G. Kohler, 1976
8.	Guidelines issued by Recombinant Advisory Committee (RAC)	1976
9.	DNA sequencing technology	F. Sangar, 1977; W. Gilbert, 1977
10.	US approval of first diagnostic kit using monoclonal antibody technology (MAb)	Anti-C3d Bioclone: Orthro diagnostics 1981
11.	US approval for first pharmaceutical product derived from DNA technology [Human Insulin (Humulin)]	Genetech and Eli Lilly and Co. 1982)

*Huber, B.E., FASEB, 3(1), 1989, 5

A concept central to pharmaceutical development is the postulation of the presence of 'receptor substances' in biological systems to which drugs would bind with specificity, thus eliciting their responses. Receptor concept has been propounded by Ehrlich from his studies of antigen-antibody interaction and binding of dye to cells. Earlier developments in drug discovery were based upon hypothetical receptor mediated drug action since methods for isolation of receptors were not established.

The new technological advancements of recombinant DNA and monoclonal antibody technology address the receptor site of the drug selectively and enable scientists to have real understanding of mode of the drug action mechanism. The ability to obtain detailed structure of receptors and the molecular ligands using biological analysis of the gene sequence, production of receptors in large quantities for structural analysis and development of specific antibody reagents to analyze their presence in organs and tissues have opened new vistas for newer drug development and for modification of old drug entities.

The recombinant DNA technology may be appreciated as a milestone which has led to a qualitative and quantitative growth in research in the field during this century. Some of the products originating from genetic engineering are clotting factor, colony stimulating factors, dismutases, erythropoietins, MAbs, recombinant soluble CD4, tumor necrosis factor and tissue plasminogen. Using monoclonal antibodies a variety of diagnostic kits have been developed. Some of the classical advents include: ovarian cancer detecting test, and kits for detection of tumor in stomach and intestine as well as kits for pregnancy testing. The diagnostic kits developed are of greater precision, accuracy and reproducibility. Similarly, immunoradiometric assay kits for measurement of interferon or other autocoids are interesting examples of biotechnological development which have significantly contributed towards diagnostic pharmaceuticals. The hybridoma technology which provided pivotal base for monoclonal antibody production is one of the important inventions in biotechnology on which what we call modern pharmaceutical biotechnology mainly depends upon. The most important utilization of the hybridoma based antibodies is their specific utilization in the target oriented therapy so as to attain cell specific delivery of the drugs like anticancer and anti-HIV drugs etc.

Enzyme related products which nearly count two dozen are employed in therapeutics and preventive medicine. The therapeutic values are mainly classified to be as clotting factor, digestive aids, antithrombolytic agents, diffusive enzymes, anti-inflammatory enzymes and some specifically designed or aimed enzymes (e.g. urokinase, chymotrypsin, penicillinase, glucocerbrosidase, streptokinase, etc.). One of the various functions of an enzyme is biochemical conversion which has been greatly exploited for the conversion of racemic DL-amino acids to biologically active α-amino acids tyrosine to L-dopa, etc. Similarly the steroidal conversion where the conversion products are of pharmaceutical importance, have been reported using free and immobilized enzyme systems as well as immobilized microbial cells.

Effect of most of the drugs is through interaction with molecular constituents of cells. Amongst these nucleic acids, mainly DNAs are the receptors for a variety of chemotherapeutic agents used in the treatment of cancer. In the wake of the detailed understanding of gene expression provided by molecular biological tools, newer therapeutic approaches of targeting to nucleic acids are under development. An analysis of cellular carbohydrates, which are often linked to proteins, promises newer opportunities for drug development. This area named as '**glycobiology**' could be identified as one of the recent developments in biotechnology. In a very similar direction, an in depth knowledge of cell biology has revealed the importance of lipids and lipid conjugates in cellular functioning. These molecules play a vital and structural role in anchoring proteins to membranes. Lipids and lipid derivatives are involved as intracellular effectors in the pathways of transduction of extracellular signals.

The most beneficial part of biotechnology is the ability to produce therapeutically active proteins and peptides. Use of therapeutically active proteins and peptides predates the developments in pharmaceutical biotechnology. For instance antihaemophilic factor VIII, immunoglobulin fraction isolated from human sources were well established prior to the advent of recombinant DNA techniques. But due to reasons of safety and low production rates they could not be adopted and exploited as therapeutics. Recombinant materials revolutionized the production of peptides. Now they can be produced in large quantities.

Proteins and peptide based drugs have been extensively utilized in replacement therapies in cases where the patient is unable to produce the required protein in sufficient quantities as in the case of insulin in Type I diabetics. The case of subunit and peptide vaccines represent the class which has been utilized for their improved therapeutic potential due to their ability to produce large quantities of proteins with directed changes in primary sequences. The development of the recombinant based protein products is increasing day by day like growth hormone, interferons, interleukines, cytokines. It could well be concluded that the field of professional pharmacy is being affected significantly by biotechnology.

1.2. PHARMACIST AND BIOTECHNOLOGY: A NEWER RESPONSIBILITY

The introduction of biotechnology based products has introduced newer responsibilities to be realized by the pharmacist. Throughout, the history, pharmacy has successfully adapted to the changes within the pharmaceutical industry and medicine. Now the biotechnology revolution has presented pharmacy with a unique challenge. If they are to meet these new challenges successfully, pharmacists must continue to fulfill their existing responsibilities while developing additional roles.

Evaluating the new products is one way that pharmacy can adapt itself to the changing medical environment. Although new biotechnology products are often assumed to be better than the standard therapeutics, in some cases the existing therapies may be equally efficacious and less expensive for the patient and the health care systems. For example, alteplase is considerably more expensive than other fibrinolytic compounds but may be no more effective. Pharmacists should promote sound scientific judgment in selecting new agents for formulary inclusion.

Recent advances in understanding of the immune system, genetics, recombinant DNA, hybridomas, and monoclonal antibodies have led to a rapid increase in the number of biotechnological products. Substantial investments by government agencies in basic biotechnology research and applied industrial research have resulted in the development of at least 81 biotechnology drugs and vaccines for human use (1990). The new products offer promise for the treatment of a wide variety of disorders in virtually every medical subspecialty, including oncology, hematology, cardiology, immunology, and endocrinology. As the knowledge base for biotechnology continues to expand, future research may shift its focus from treating disease to preventing it through gene therapy and the development of genetically engineered vaccines, and other pharmaceuticals.

The rapid expansion in the field of biotechnology products has presented new opportunities for the pharmacist while creating a new set of responsibilities. These responsibilities provide new opportunities for the pharmacist so as to develop newer skills and expand their role in clinical pharmacy services, clinical research, drug distribution and drug information. However, to retain responsibility for the dispensing of the new biotechnology products pharmacists must keep abreast of innovation in this area, including the development of the new drug-delivery systems and expanding contemporary pharmacy services, to fulfill the unique demands .imposed by the new products.

The most developing field of biotechnology in which the pharmacist has to work extensively is the unique drug and drug delivery systems. They are a complex and a newer variety of the pharmaceutical agents with which the pharmacist must become familiar. Further complicating the picture is the fact that many of the new biotechnology products are proteins that are targeted towards the specific uses. Most of them also have very short half life and may require unique delivery systems because simple oral administration is generally not possible.

Strategies for drug delivery currently being explored, include encapsulating the drug in the coating(s) that protects it until absorption can occur, combining the drug with the biodegradable polymer, enclosing the drug in the liposomes or other vesicular carriers or red blood cells before directing the drug to the specific site and then modifying the surface so as to achieve the targetability, designing transdermal and nasal delivery systems, delivering the agents as prodrugs that undergo biotransformation *in vivo*, combining the drug with the monoclonal antibodies that will attach to a specific target providing the proteins and the other therapeutic hormones in a deterred environment so as to protect from the lytic system(s) of the body. Other approaches focus on a variety of controlled drug release systems or implantable drug pumps.

Not only the specialized delivery system but also the development of the artificial organs and the blood purification systems is offering newer responsibility to be shouldered by the pharmacist especially in undertaking the clinical trials. The artificial liver developed by the encapsulation of the hepatocytes and bypassing the diseased liver by a blood circuit offers a major challenge for the pharmacist. Furthermore, the development of the blood purification systems based on the *ex-vivo* separation of the plasma from the cells and its purification and reconstitution has offered a further responsibility to the pharmacist. Hence it could be stated that although the development in the field of the pharmaceutical biotechnology has led to a number of products into the market it has also led to a major challenge for the pharmacist to tackle. The newer responsibility has made the understanding of the subject more desirable and vital in the modern pharmaceutical scenario.

1.3. BIOTECHNOLOGY AND INDUSTRY

In essence, biotechnology may be defined as the collection of industrial processes that involve the use of biological systems. As compared to pharmaceutical drug development, the history of industrial biotechnology is quite short. In chronological order, after the discovery of genetic engineering and monoclonal antibody related technologies, their commercialization began in 1970's. Small biotech concerns entered the area, whereas large capital concerns were slow to take up biologically oriented drug discovery program., Genetech was the first biotech based concern to be launched by Eli-Lilly in early 80's. Since then many concerns have been formed. At present, a high proportion of international biotechnological efforts are concentrated mainly in the US. In 1992 'Genetic Engineering-The News Guide to Biotechnology Companies', 737 companies from 25 countries have been listed, out of them, 547 are from the US. A more recent report puts the number of biotechnology based companies in the US to be 742 with a majority of these focusing on the development of therapeutic agents.

The impact of biotechnology on the pharmaceutical industry is changing quickly. 'Traditional biotechnology', in the form of antibiotic production is still much more valuable in commercial terms than the 'modern biotechnology' involving genetic engineering. The antibiotic market is worth $10 billion annually or about 5% of the total pharmaceutical market. By contrast the total sales from the much heralded revolution, through therapeutic proteins still lags well behind any one small molecule blockbuster. However, there are several areas where molecular biology and genetic engineering are influencing drug discovery and drug development. In particular, the techniques have provided humanized antibodies, new insight into the disease mechanism and novel functional assays including cloned and expressed human receptors and transgenic mice.

Initially, small biotech concerns of early 80's focused their major efforts on improved production of therapeutically active proteins such as insulin, factor VIII and human growth hormone. However, after the discovery of Interferon, an antiviral protein for its anticancer activity, major interest of pharmaceutical biotechnology has shifted. Further, the major attention seems to shift towards the other less established natural proteins which were available in small quantities such as clot-dissolving protein, cell growth factors, tissue plasminogen activator, etc. With the involvement of multinational pharmaceutical concerns in the development of therapeutic proteins more funds could be localized and with their previous experience in clinical trial based studies, some major breakthroughs could be anticipated. Since this brought into existence a newer class of drugs, the Food and Drug Administration (FDA) and other approving authorities had to enforce and enact some newer laws and regulations in order to take care of the safety of such products. As a source of guidance to biotech industry, several 'points to consider' include documents dealing with different aspects of biological drug approval process have been published by FDA in the US.

Within such a short period of time, the pharmaceutical drug discovery, drug production and drug delivery aspects have been revolutionized so much that every major pharmaceutical concern has some in-house research efforts in biotechnology and many have gained access to select technologies through alliances with or ownership of smaller biotechnology companies. It could now be said that 'biotechnology is an integral part of pharmaceutical R&D'. The early years of biotechnology offered some dazzling challenges and high prospects for financial investments. Although initial expectations have been somewhat unfulfilled, about 100 'biotech' drugs are at various stages of clinical development and over a dozen have won FDA approval. Broadly they could be grouped as blood products, immunotherapeutics, infectious disease products. Table 1.2 mentions some of the biotechnologically derived products which have obtained FDA approval. There are still hundreds which are in some phase of clinical trials and some others have been forwarded for approval. Some of these products are listed in table 1.3 separately.

After considering all the factors it would be fair to state that biotechnology in the last few decades has become a part of pharmaceutical development. The recent decade in particular has seen some unprecedented developments in this field. Further, the developments will have an impact on the practice of medicine and on the pharmaceutical industry. Although this impact at present is unpredictable, exciting pathway are bound to open up carrying us into the twenty-first century.

Table 1.2 : Biotechnological drugs and vaccines tested and approved until 1992

S. No.	Generic Name	Product Name	Company	Approval Date
1.	Human insulin	Humulin	Eli Lilly	Oct., 1982
2.	Sometrem	Protropin	Genetech	Oct., 1985
3.	DigoxinImmune Fab	Digibind	Burroughs Wellcome	April, 1986
4.	Muromonab CD3	Orthoclone OKT3	Ortho Biotech	June 1986
5.	Interferon-α-2b	Intron A	Schering-Plough	June 1986
6.	Interferon-α-2a	Roferon-A	Hoffmann-La-Roche	June 1986
7.	Hepatitis-B-vaccine	Recombivax HB	Merk	July 1986
8.	Somatotropin	Humatrope	Eli Lilly	March 1987
9.	Alteplase	Activase	Genetech	Nov., 1987
10.	Heamophilus-B-conjugate vaccine	Hib Titer	Praxis Biologics	Dec., 1988
11.	Epoietin-α	Epogen	Amgen	June 1989
12.	Hepatitis-B-vaccine	Engerix-B	SmithKline Beecham	Sept., 1989
13.	Interferon-α-n3	Alferon N	Interferon Sciences	Oct., 1989
14.	Interferon-γ-Ib	Actimmune	Genetech	Dec., 1990
15.	Filgrastim	Neupogen	Amgen	Feb., 1991
16.	Epoitin-α	Procrit	Ortho Biotech	Feb., 1991
17.	Sargramostim	Prokin	Hoechst-Roussel	March 1991
18.	Sargramostim	Leukin	Immunex	March 1991
19.	Aldesleukin	Proleukin	Cetus	June, 1992

1.4. GMP COMPLIANCE AND BIO-PHARMACEUTICAL FACILITIES

Recent years have witnessed an explosive growth in the biotechnology industry in the area of development and manufacture of a variety of new products. Most of the interest has been focused on the development of biopharmaceutical products such as vaccines, therapeutic proteins and monoclonal antibodies.

The development activity has reached a point where companies are commercializing their products. Being the most developed country, in USA alone companies such as Genetech, Amgen, Centocor and others have brought products into the market. Some other companies have contracted with them around the globe for designing and construction of manufacturing facilities for these products in compliance with the FDA and cGMP. Most of the biopharmaceuticals being developed are derived from the application of recombinant DNA technology. For regulatory purpose, most of these products are classified as **biologicals**. It is important to recognize that United States FDA has two main regulatory groups with the responsibilities for different therapeutic products.

In most of the countries of the world and especially in Indian based concerns the regulatory considerations applicable are very similar to those in the FDA of United States. The Center for Drug Evaluation and Research (CDER) is concerned with the traditional products that are produced by fermentation or organic synthesis and which are readily characterized with well defined analytical methods. These include antibiotics, analgesics, anti-inflammatory agents, etc. Most of the recombinant therapeutic products with the exception of insulin are regulated by the Center for Biologics Evaluation and Research (CBER). Traditionally, CBER was responsible for the regulation of vaccines, blood products and other natural products. CBER has framed strict rules of compliance in their regulations for biotechnological products because of their distinctiveness from chemical drugs.

Biologicals differ from the pure chemical drugs in the following respects:
1. They are derived from living organisms
2. These products are typically complex biochemical mixtures
3. Biologicals are usually difficult to assay and quantify

Table 1.3 : Biotechnological products which have been in process of approval until 1992

S.No	Product Name	Company	US Development Status
1.	Superoxide dismutase	Bio-Technology General, Bristol Mayers	Phase II
2.	PEG-SOD (Superoxide dsmutase)	Sterling Drugs, Enzon	Phase II/III
3.	Morgens srile pwder (Epoietin-β)	Genitics Institute, Chugai-Upjohn	Application submitted
4.	Eprex	Ortho-Pharmaceuticals	In Human clinical trials
5.	Prourokinase	Collaborative research, Sandoz	Phase II/III
6.	Tissue pasminogen activator	Genetics Institute, Wellcome Biotechnology	Phase II/III Application pending
7.	Nupogen (Granulocyte/ colony stimulating factor)	Amgen	Phase III
8.	Granulocyte macrophage/ colony stimulating factor	Amgen	Phase II/III
9.	KoGENate (Factor VIII)	Cutter Biologicals	Application submitted
10.	Recombinant factor VIII	Bexter Healthcare, Genetics Institute	Phase I
11.	Mono-IX (Factor IX)	Rhone Poulene Rorer	Application submitted
12.	Insulin like growth factor I	Chiron, Ciba-Geigy	Phase I
13.	Norditropin (Somatotropin)	Novo Nordisk	Application submitted
14.	Saizen (Somatotropin)	Senoro Laboritories	Application submitted
15.	Bio tropin	Genetech	Application submitted
16.	VaxSyn® HIV-1	MicroGeneSys	In clinical trials
17.	HIVAC-le vaccine	Bristol Mayer/Oncogen	Phase I
18.	Alferon Gel (interferon-α-2b)	Busch Biotech	Application submitted
19.	Betaseron (interferon-β)	Berlex Laboratories	Phase III
20.	Centoxin (HA-1A Mab)	Centocor	Application submitted
21.	E5 (Mab)	Pfizer, Xoma	Application submitted
22.	XomaZymase-CD5 Plus (Mab)	Xoma	Application submitted
23.	Orthozyme CD5 (muromonab CD5-RTA)	Ortho Biotech	Application submitted
24.	DNase (rh DNase)	Genetech	Phase III

4. In many instances the correlation of the assays with biological and clinical activity is difficult
5. These products are usually susceptible to damage from heat and/or shear stress.
6. The loss of configuration is difficult to control
7. These products are susceptible to contamination from many sources.

Due to these differences and CBER's past experience with vaccines and blood products, their regulatory approach differs form CDER in two major ways; first, product approval strategies and second, in the application of GMP's to all stages of the manufacturing even to the earliest stages of cell culture maintenance and inoculum scale-up. Because of the GMP and licensing requirements, the design of the manufacturing unit and facilities is very important. Plant design and layout is crucial for effective control of people and material flow facilities. The design and the specifications of the materials for plant process and utility systems are critical for reproducible processing, prevention of .the product contamination and effective clean-in-place capabilities. Finally, the entire facilities must be validated.

According to the GMP considerations the major requirements are:

1. the use of recombinant organisms requires the identification of the contaminant level tolerable and identification of those processing areas requiring corrective measures;
2. the layout of the work areas which address the need to protect the product from contamination during processing;
3. the particular requirement of the bulk production including culture maintenance, media and the buffer preparation, inoculum scale up, fermentation, product recovery and purification and the finishing aspects which include operation such as formulation, filling and packaging.

The US regulatory requirements for architectural consideration for the biopharmaceutical building are presented in 21CFR, parts 210, 211 and 212. The specific intent of these regulations is to provide broad guidelines without detailed specifications for the designing facilities. In this way the technological improvement can be incorporated without the need to rewrite the regulations. In the case of biopharmaceuticals the FDA is particularly interested in the details of the facility layout. The flow of people and material through the facility is as important as the traditional mass and energy balance the process. Integration of the building design with the process system is highly imperative.

SUGGESTED READINGS

Anon. **Commercial biotechnology : An international analysis,** (1984) Washington, DC, Office of Technology Assessment, OTA-BA-218.

Bailey, J.E., (1991) *Towards a science of metabolic engineering,* **Science,** 252, 1668-1674.

Blakebrough, N. (Ed.), (1967/68) *Biochemical and Biological Engineering,* **Science,** Vol-I and II, Academic Press, London, New York.

Burril, G. S, (1991) **Biotech: A changing environment,** Mary Knn. Liebert., New York.

Dibner, M.D. and Timmermanns, P.B., (1986) *Biotechnology and the pharmaceutical industry: new cardiovascular drugs,* **Hypertension,** 8, 965-970

Edward, H. J., (1989) *Recombinant human erythropoietin,* **American Journal of Hospital Pharmacy,** 46, Suppl 2, S20-S23.

Ehrilich, P.R. and Wilson, E.O., (1991) *Biodiversity studies: Science and policy,* **Science,** 253, 758-762.

Gage, L.P., (1986) *Biopharmaceuticals : drugs of the future,* **American Journal of Pharmaceutical Education,** 50, 368-370

Guttermann, J., (1988) *Overview of advances in the use of biological proteins in human cancer,* **Semin. Oncol.,** 15, 2-6.

Hodgson, J., (1991) **Biotechnology,** 10, 863-866.

Huber, B.E., (1989) **FASEB,** 3 (1), 5

Lehninger, A.L. (1970), Biochemistry, Worth Publishers, New York.

Marx, J.L. (Ed), (1989) **A revolution in Biotechnology,** Cambridge University Press, Cambridge.

Mary-Jose, T., (1989) *Human insulin: DNA technology's first drug,* **American Journal of Hospital Pharmacy,** 46, Suppl. 2, S9-S10.

Mossinghof, G.J., (1989) **Biotechnology Medicine,** Pharmaceutical manufacture association.

Mossinghoff, G.J. (1988), **Charting biotechnology based pharmaceuticals : a record number of products are in the US research pipeline,** Biotech Product Development, 7, 1-5

Shamel, R. D. (1990), **Biotechnology: What in the store of 1990's,** Consult. Resh. Corp., Mensleft, Spring.

Smith, G., (1969) *An Introduction to Industrial Mycology,* 6th Ed, Edward Arnold, London.

Stewart, C.F. and Fleming, R.L. (1989), *Biotechnology products : New opportunities and responsibilities for the pharmacist,* **American Journal of Hospital Pharmacy,** 46, Suppl 2, S4-S8.

Swaminathan, M.S., (Ed.) (1991) **Biotechnology in Agriculture: A Dialogue,** Macmillan, Madras

Wiseman, A., (1983), **Principles of Biotechnology,** Chapman and Hall, New York.

Young, F.E., (1988), The care and feeding of new biotechnology, **Gene,** 62, 1-5 (Editorial)

ENZYMES

2.1. INTRODUCTION AND HISTORICAL BACKGROUND

Cell, the basic building block of living systems effectively functions, utilizing enzymes, the biocatalyst, which are remarkable in their catalytic efficiency, and substrate as well as reaction specificity. Enzymes have extraordinary catalytic power and high degree of specificity for their substrate. They are functional units of cell metabolism. All the chemical reactions occurring in plants, micro-organisms and animals proceed at a measurable rate as a direct consequence of enzymatic catalysis.

Much of the history of biochemistry in a way is the history of enzyme research. Biological catalysis has been known for nearly 150 years. In 1837 Berzelius recognized that there were naturally occurring 'ferments' which promoted chemical reactions. Catalysis in biological systems was first recognized in the early 1800's from the studies of the digestion of meat by secretion of the stomach and the conversion of starch into sugar by saliva and various plant extracts. In 1850's Louis Pasteur concluded that fermentation of sugar into alcohol by yeast is catalyzed by '*ferments*'. He also postulated that these ferments are inseparable from the structure of yeast. These ferments were later named as *enzymes* (in yeast). The major landmark in the history of enzymes came in 1897 when Edward Buchner extracted the soluble active form from yeast cells and set of enzymes that catalyses the fermentation of sugar to alcohol. Emul Fischer carried out the first systematic studies on enzyme specificity in the early twentieth century. In 1926 James Sumner isolated *urease* in pure crystalline form from Jack beans. He also established the protein nature of urease. In 1930, John Northrop and his colleagues crystallized pepsin and trypsin and found them to be proteins.

During the succeeding half century enzymology has developed at apace (Table 2.1). The significant developments during this fruitful period are: elucidation of major metabolic pathways, for example glycolysis and tricarboxylic acid cycle, discovery of various biochemical events of digestion, muscular contraction, endocrine function, coagulation and their roles in the maintenance, control and integration of complex metabolic processes, kinetic frameworks to rationalize the observations of enzyme action and inhibition and development of procedures designed to analyze the structures of functionally sensitive proteins.

After this, intensive research started on the enzymes, enzyme catalyzed reactions, and enzymes involved in cell metabolism. Today some 2000 different enzymes have been identified each of which catalyzing a different chemical reaction. More recently, attention has increasingly been directed to the application of the enzymes. The high efficiency of enzymes make them potentially valuable catalyst in industry and their specificity of action is providing benefits in clinical medicine.

Table 2.1 : Chronology of enzyme studies

Name	Year	Work
Payen and Persoz	1833	Alcohol precipitation of thermolabile 'diastase' from malt
Berzelius	1835	Concept of catalysis
Berzelius	1837	Recognition of biological catalysis
Pasture	1850	Fermentation of sugar into alcohol by yeast
Wilhelmy	1850	Quantitative evaluation of the rates of sucrose inversion
Kuhne	1878	Investigations of trypsin catalyzed reactions and introduction of word 'enzyme'
Fischer	1894-5	'Lock and Key' hypothesis of enzyme specificity
Bertrand	1896-7	Coenzyme or Coferment (now known as cofactors)
Buchner	1897	Extraction of soluble active form of enzyme from yeast cells
Duclaux	1898	Nomenclature- substrate plus suffix 'ase'
Henri	1901-3	General procedures for the derivation of kinetic rate laws, principle of enzyme-substrate complex
Harden and Young	1906	Coezymase (NAD)
Michaelis and Menten	1913	Extension of the kinetic theory of enzyme catalysis
Briggs and Haldane	1925	Derivation of enzyme rate equations using the steady-state approximation
Sumner	1926	Crystallization of urease
Northrop and Kunitz	1930-3	Crystallization of proteolytic enzymes
Cori and Cori	1937-9	Muscle phosphorylase
Beadle and Tatum	1940	'One gene one enzyme' hypothesis
Chances	1943	Spectroscopic techniques
Koshland	1953	'Induced fit' hypothesis
Umbarger Yates Pardee	1956	Control of enzyme activity through feedback inhibition
Sutherland	1956	Cyclic AMP adenyl cyclase
Anfinsen	1956-8	Amino acid sequence determines folding pattern and activity of ribonuclease
Jacob Monod and Changeux	1961	Allosterism
Phillips Johnson and North	1965	Three-dimensional structure of lysozyme obtained at 1.5A resolution

2.2. NATURE OF ENZYMES

Enzymes are defined as soluble, colloidal, organic catalysts which are produced by living cells, but are capable of acting independently of the cells. Enzymes behave as catalyst in small quantities relative to the concentration of their substrates. The total amount of substrate transformed per mass of enzyme is often very large. All enzymes are proteinaceous in nature without any exception and exhibit all properties of the protein. Disruption of characteristic folding of polypeptide chains of a native enzyme protein by extreme temperature or extreme pH or by treatment with other denaturing agents, results in to the total loss of catalytic activity. Thus primary, secondary, tertiary and quaternary structures of enzyme proteins are necessary for their catalytic activity. Their catalytic activity depends mainly upon the integrity of their structure as proteins. Enzymes have molecular weights ranging from about 12,000 to over 1 million. Furthermore, some enzymes consist only of polypeptides and contain two chemical groups other than amino acid residues, e.g. pancreatic ribonuclease.

Many enzymes require a specific, heat stable, low molecular weight organic molecule, a coenzyme. Furthermore, some enzymes require both a coenzyme and one or more metal ions for activity. A complete catalytically active enzyme consisting of the protein part together with the bound coenzyme or metal is known as **holoenzyme**. The protein part of an enzyme is referred to as **apoenzyme**. A coenzyme may bind covalently or noncovalently to the apoenzyme. In some enzymes the coenzyme or metal ion is only loosely and transiently bound to the protein but in others it is tightly and permanently bound, in which it is called a **prosthetic group**.

Prosthetic group denotes a covalently bound coenzyme. Coenzymes and metal ions are stable on heating, whereas the protein part of an enzyme (apoenzyme), is denatured by heat.

$$\begin{array}{ccc}\text{Holoenzyme} = & \text{Apoenzyme} + & \text{Prosthetic group} \\ \text{(Total enzyme)} & \text{(Protein)} & \text{(Non-protein)}\end{array}$$

Prosthetic groups may be categorized functionally into two major classes, *coenzymes* and *cofactors*. The first may be considered biosynthetically related to the vitamins. For example, the coenzyme nicotinamide adenine dinucleotide (NAD) important for cellular energy metabolism incorporates the vitamin niacin into its chemical make up. In addition coenzyme may be regarded as co-substrate, undergoing a chemical trans-formation during the enzyme reaction (NAD is reduced to NADH) reversal of which requires a separate enzyme, possibly from different cellular location. They may therefore travel intracellularly between apo-enzymes and by transferring chemical groupings integrate several metabolic processes.

Table 2.2 provides the list of the more common coenzymes and their functions. By comparison, cofactors, for example pyridoxal phosphate or hem groups, remain with one enzyme molecule and in conjunction complete a cycle of a chemical change brought about by one enzyme turnover.

Table 2.2 : Coenzymes used in transfer of specific atoms or functional groups

Coenzyme	Entity transferred
Biocytin	CO_2
Coenzyme A	Acyl groups
Flavin adenine dinucleotide	Hydrogen atoms (electrons)
3'-Deoxyadenorylcohalamine (coenzyme B_{12})	H atoms and alkyl groups
Nicotinamide adenine dinucleotide	Hydrogen atoms (electrons)
Pyridoxal phosphate	Amino groups
Tetrahydrofolate	Other one carbon groups
Thyamin pyrophosphate	Aldehydes

Other enzymes, for example carboxypeptidase require metal ions as cofactors, the divalent cations Mg^{2+}, Zn^{2+}, Mn^{2+} being most common; these are often termed as enzyme *activators*. Table 2.3. lists various enzymes and their respective co-factors.

Table 2.3 : Some enzymes and their cofactors

Enzyme	Cofactors	Enzyme	Cofactors
Arginase	Mn^{++}	Alcohol dehydrogenase	Zn^{++}
Carbonic anhydrase	Zn^{++}	Catalase	Fe^{++} or Fe^{+++}
Cytochrome oxidase	Cu^{++}	Cytochrome oxidase	Fe^{++} or Fe^{+++}
DNA polymerase	Zn^{++}	Glutathione peroxidase	Se
Glucose 6-phosphatase	Mg^{++}	Hexokinase	Mg^{++}
Nitrate reductase	Mo	Peroxidase	Fe^{++} or Fe^{+++}
Pyruvate kinase	K^+ and Mg^{++}	Urease	Ni^{++}

2.3. STRUCTURE OF ENZYMES

All enzymes act as catalysts and only small quantities, relative to the concentrations of their substrate are needed to significantly increase the rate of chemical reactions, while they themselves undergo no net change. Like all true catalysts, an enzyme does not change the final equilibrium position of a reaction, which is thermodynamically determined, and only the *rate* of attainment of equilibrium of a feasible reaction is increased. In addition to their catalytic properties, enzymes exhibit the chemical and physical behavior of proteins, their electrolytic behaviors, solubility, electrophoretic properties and chemical reactivities. The catalytic activity of enzymes depend on the L-α-amino acid sequence and peptide bonds constituting the protein molecule (Fig. 2.1). Enzymes differ considerably from traditional chemical catalysts such as hydrogen ions, heavy metals or metal oxides. These are most effective in organic solvents, at very high temperatures or at extreme pH values; enzymes operate most efficiently under very mild conditions. Departure in terms of deviation from homogenous aqueous solutions, physiological pH and temperature rapidly destroys their activities, but under normal conditions the increase in rate is rarely matched by their non-protein counterparts.

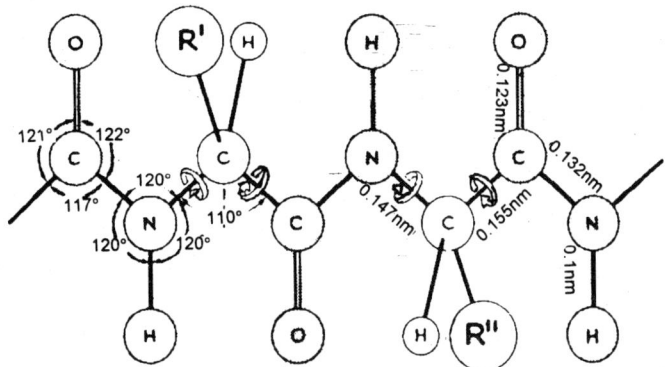

Fig. 2.1 : Polypeptidic backbone of an enzyme

The linear chain of amino acid residues joined by peptide bonds, which constitute a protein molecule is called the *primary structure*. Localized folding of the primary structure is referred as *secondary structure* and the overall folding of the molecule is entitled *tertiary structure*. The agglomeration of the several folded chains is known as *quaternary structure*.

2.3.1. Primary and secondary structures

Three dimensional analysis of the amino acid sequence of hen's egg white lysozyme have illustrated several features inherent to primary structure. These are:

1. Molecules derived from the same source have similar order of amino acid residues and appear to be random with no obvious predictability.
2. Even though many enzymes are intramolecularly crosslinked through disulfide bridges of cysteine, no branching occurs.

Present evidences give an indication that few of the amino acids are superfluous and most are 'functional', i.e., most co-operatively determine the higher orders of structural organization and hence the catalytic activity. On comparing the primary structures of enzymes performing similar functions, extensive structural homo-logies were observed in their sequence, particularly in the patterns of their non-polar residues. For example, pancreatic juice contains five inactive precursors (zymogens) viz. chymotrypsinogen A, B and C, trypsinogen and proelastase, all of which are activated to the respective proteases by proteolytic cleavage.

The overall folding of the amino acid sequence to give the functional enzyme appears to be unorganized, but on minute observation, it can be seen that regions are organized into structures of definable symmetry (Fig.2.2). For instance, residues 24-34 and 41-54 are folded into elements of secondary structure, α-helix and β-sheet respectively. These are named after the corresponding structures of the α- and β-keratins that were obtained by X-ray diffraction data of crystalline short polypeptides. The peptide bond was found to be shorter than the 0.14nm of a single carbon-nitrogen bond by approximately 0.001nm, and also had more double bond character. Rotation around this bond is restricted at normal temperatures, causing the peptide bond and the two adjacent α-carbon atoms to lie in one plane, with the carbonyl oxygen and amino hydrogen in the energy minimum of a *trans* configuration, as illustrated in figure 2.1. Rotation can then only occur around those bonds close to the α-carbon atoms, and the possible types of stable structure which maximize the number of hydrogen bonds, are restricted to the α-helix and β-plated sheet.

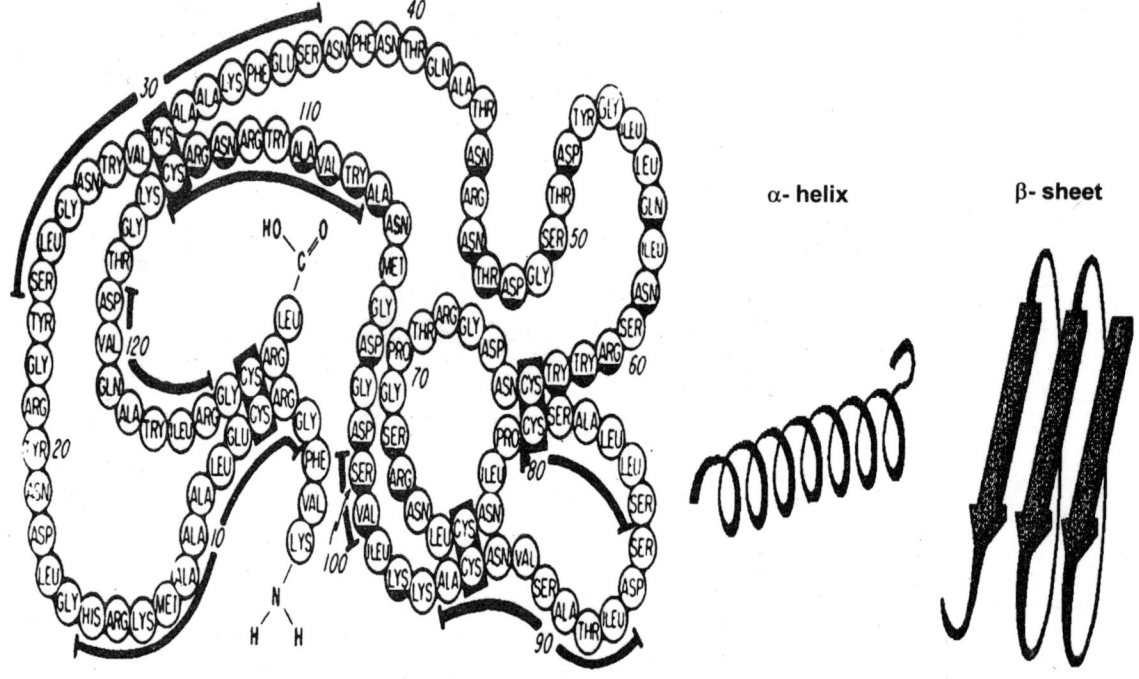

α- helix   β- sheet

Fig. 2.2 : Primary structure of lysozyme

2.3.2. Tertiary structure

The overall folding of the polypeptide chain, which includes the organized secondary structure as well as random stretches, is attributed to the tertiary structure (Fig. 2.3). At present one of the most reliable and powerful methods to determine the three dimensional structure of a protein, and in combination with the primary sequence, for portraying the relative stereochemical positions of the atoms is X-ray crystallography. X-rays are utilized because their wavelength and molecular dimensions in the protein crystal are of the same order of size.

The enzymes listed in table 2.4 that catalyze dissimilar reactions have been found to possess unique tertiary structures, but several generalizations can be afforded due to the accumulated atomic details. In spite of the regional flexibility, all the compactly folded molecules have very little space inside to accommodate even small water molecules. This interior mainly consists of hydrophobic side chains (of leucine, phenylalanine, tryptophan, valine, etc.) and is surrounded by the polar amino acids (arginine, aspartic acid, etc.). The enzyme involved in catalyzing similar reaction types and possessing homology in their primary structures, especially in the sequence of their non-polar residues (the aggregation of which provides the driving force for protein folding) also possess three-dimensional homology. For instance, all the members of the serine proteases family have tertiary conformations with a common hydrophobic core.

A second type of localized three-dimensional homology, that is not evident from amino acid sequence data, has been observed with enzymes binding similar cofactors. For example, tertiary structures of dogfish-muscle lactate DH (dehydrogenase), horse-liver alcohol DH and lobster and *B. stearothermophilus* glyceraldehyde-3-phosphate DH, all of which require NADH as coenzymes, can be divided into separate domains, i.e., polypeptide regions associated with particular functions. The two domains being : a catalytic domain which is structurally unique to each individual enzyme and a coenzyme binding domain whose construction is remarkably similar to all. The coenzyme binding domain is comprised of six parallel strands of β-plated sheet and four α-helices, and these are found arranged in the sequence β-α-β along the primary structure. The continuous amino acid sequences constituting the domain are however not located identically in the overall primary structures.

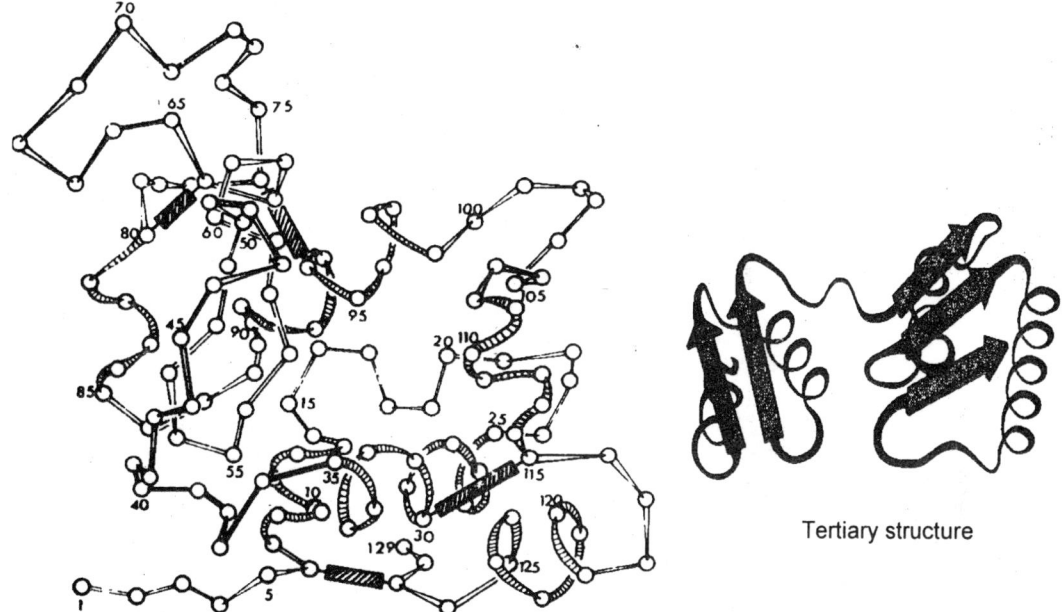

Fig. 2.3 : Main chain conformation of hen's egg white lysozyme in tertiary structure

Tertiary structure

Table 2.4 : X-ray crystallography of enzymes

Enzyme	Source	Molecular Weight	Resolution(Å)
Adenyl kinase	Porcine muscle	22,000	3
Alcohol dehydrogenase	Horse liver	80,000	2.9
Aspartate transcarbamoylase	*E. coli*	3,10,000	5.5
Carbonic anhydrase B	Human erythrocytes	30,000	2.2
Carbonic anhydrase C	Human erythrocytes	30,000	2
α-Chymotrypsin	Bovine pancreas	3,600	2, 2.8
Elastase	Porcine	25,900	3.5
Hexokinase	Yeast	51,000	2.3
Lysozyme	BacteriophageT[4]	18,800	2.5
	Hen's egg white	14,600	2
	Human	14,500	2.5
Papain	Papaya latex	23,000	2.8
Protease	*Rhizopus chinensis*	35,000	5.5
Pyruvate kinase	Cat muscle	2,40,000	6
Ribonuclease A	Bovine	13,600	2
Ribonuclease S	Bovine	13,600	2
Superoxide dismutase	Bovine	16,000	3, 5.5
β-Trypsin	Bovine pancreas	24,000	1.8, 2.7

2.3.3. Quaternary structure

Enzymes from intracellular origin generally also possess quaternary structure, which is an agglomeration of several units of tertiary structure. In these enzymes each of the contributing tertiary structure is termed a *subunit* or *monomer* and the complete complex as an *oligomer,* and a dimer, trimer, tetramer, etc. depending on the number of subunits it contains (Fig. 2.4). Oligomeric proteins are classified as *homologous* (containing identical subunits) and *heterologous* (containing different subunits). Quaternary structure cannot be stabilized by covalent bonds, on the contrary the subunits associate through combinations of the weaker forces.

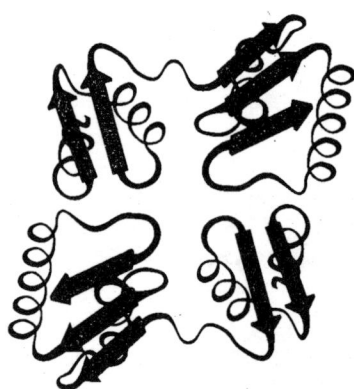

Fig. 2.4 : Schematic representation of the quaternary structure of enzymes

2.4. CLASSIFICATION AND NOMENCLATURE

The purpose of classification is to identify and emphasize relationship and similarities among enzymes in a precise and concise manner. Early attempts to devise a system of nomenclature for enzymes produced a series of ambiguous and generally uninformative names such as emulsin, ptyalin and zymase. Enzymes were later named for the substrate on which they acted by adding the suffix **-ase**. Thus enzymes that split starch (amylon) were termed amylase; those that split fat (lipos), lipase; and those that acted on proteins, proteases. Groups of enzymes were designated as oxidizes, glycosidases, dehydrogenases, decarboxylases, etc.

Recent studies on the mechanism of enzyme catalyzed reactions have led to a more rationalized classification of enzymes where reaction types and reaction mechanisms form the basis. This classification system is known as International Union of Biochemistry (IUB) system of enzyme classification. The major features of IUB System of classification of enzymes are as follow:

Reactions (and the enzymes catalyzing them) are divided into 6 major classes, each with 4-13 subclasses. These six major classes are listed below, together with examples of some important subclasses.

The enzyme name consists of two parts. The first is the name of substrate(s). The second ending in -ase, indicates the type of reaction catalyzed.

Additional information to clarify the nature of the reaction, may follow in parentheses. For example, the enzyme catalyzing the following reaction known as the maleic enzyme, is designated as 1.1.1.37 L-malate : NAD oxidoreductase.

$$\text{Malate} + NAD^+ = \text{Pyruvate} + CO_2 + NADH + H^+$$

Each enzyme has a systemic code number (E.C.) This number characterizes the reaction type as to class (first digit), subclass (second digit), and subsubclass (third digit). The fourth digit is for the particular enzyme name. Thus, E.C.2.7.1.1. denotes class 2 (a transferase), subclass 7 (transfer of phosphate), subsubclass 1(an alcohol function as phosphate acceptor). The final digit denotes the enzyme, hexokinase, or ATP:D-hexose-6-phosphotransferase, an enzyme catalyzing phosphate transfer from ATP to the hydroxyl group on carbon 6 of glucose.

The 6 major classes of enzymes with some examples are given below.

1. Oxidoreductases : Enzymes catalyzing oxidation-reduction between two substrates, S and S'.

$$S_{\text{ reduced}} + S'_{\text{ oxidized}} = S_{\text{ oxidized}} + S'_{\text{ reduced}}$$

This important class includes the enzymes formerly known either as dehydrogenases or as oxidizes. Enzymes of this class catalyze the oxidoreduction of CH-OH, CH-CH, C=O, CH-NH$_2$ groups. Subclasses of this class includes:

1.1. Enzymes acting on the CH-OH groups as electron aonor

      1.1.1.1. Alcohol : NAD oxidoreductase [alcohol dehydrogenase]

$$\text{Alcohol} + NAD^+ = \text{aldehyde or ketone} + NADH + H^+$$

1.4. Enzymes acting on the CH-NH$_2$ group as electron donor

1.4.1.3. L-Glutamate: NAD(P) oxidoreductase (deaminating)[glutamic dehydrogenase of animal liver]
NAD(P) means that either NAD or NADP acts as the electron acceptor.

$$\text{L-Glutamate} + H_2O + NAD(P)H + H^+ = \alpha\text{-ketoglutarate} + NH_4 + NAD(P)H + H^+$$

1.9. Enzyme acting on the haeme groups of electron donors

1.9.3.1. Cytochrome C : O$_2$ oxidoreductase [cytochrome oxidase]

$$\text{4 Reduced cytochrome C} + 4H^+ = \text{4 Oxidized cytochrome C} + 2H_2O$$

1.11. Enzyme acting on H$_2$O$_2$ as electron acceptor

1.11.1.6. H$_2$O$_2$: H$_2$O$_2$ oxidoreductase [catalase]

$$H_2O_2 + H_2O_2 = O_2 + 2H_2O$$

2. Transferase : Enzymes catalyzing a transfer of a group, G (other than hydrogen), between a pair of substrates S and S'.

$$S\text{-}G + S' = S'\text{-}G + S$$

The enzymes belonging to this class mainly catalyze the transfer of one carbon groups, aldehyde or ketone residues, and acyl, alkyl, glycosyl, phosphorous or sulfur containing groups. Some important subclasses of transferases include:

2.3. Acetyltransferases

2.3.1.6. Acetyl Co-A : choline O-acetyltransferase[choline acetyltransferase]
Acetyl Co-A + choline = Co-A + O-acetylcholine

2.4. Glycosyltransferases

2.4.1.1. α-1,4-Glucan:orthophosphate glycosyl transferase [phosphorylase]

$$(\alpha\text{-}1,4\text{-Glucosyl})_n + \text{orthophosphate} = (\alpha\text{-}1,4\text{-Glucosyl})_{n-1} + (\alpha\text{-D-glucose-1-phosphate})$$

2.7. Enzyme catalyzing transfer of phosphorous containing groups

2.7.1.1. ATP:D-hexose-6-phosphotransferase [hexokinase]
ATP + D-hexose = ADP = D-hexose-6-phosphate

3. Hydrolases : Enzyme catalyzing the hydrolysis of ester, ether, peptides, glycosyl, acid-anhydride, C-C, C-halide, or P-N bonds. For example hydrolysis of an acylcholine:

$$\text{An acylcholine} + H_2O = \text{choline} + \text{an acid}$$

3.1. Enzyme acting on ester bonds

3.1.1.8. Acylcholine acid hydrolase [pseudocholinesterase]

3.2. Enzyme acting on glycosyl compounds

3.2.1.23. β-D-galactoside galactohydrolase [β-galactosidase]

$$\text{A } \beta\text{-D galactoside} + H_2O = \text{an alcohol} + \text{D-galactose}$$

3.4. Enzymes acting on peptide bonds: The classical names (pepsin, plasmin, rennin, chymotrypsin) have been largely retained due to overlapping and dubious specificity which makes systematic nomenclature impractical.

4. Lyases : Enzyme that catalyses the removal of groups from substrates by mechanisms other than hydrolysis, leaving double bonds. Includes enzymes acting on C-C, C-O, C-N, C-S, and C-halide bond. Important subgroups are :

4.1.2. Aldehyde - lyases

4.1.2.7. Ketose-1-phosphate aldehyde-lyase [aldolase]
A ketose-1-phosphate = dihydroxyacetone phosphate + an aldehyde

4.2. Carbon-oxygen lyases

4.2.1.2. L-Malate hydrolyase [fumerase]
L-Malate = fumerate + H$_2$O

5. Isomerase : All enzymes catalyzing interconversion of optical, geometric, or positional isomers are the examples of this class. Some sub classes are:

Table 2.5 : Example of enzymes from six major classes

Major class	Enzyme	Reaction description	Example of reaction catalysed	Coenzyme involved
Oxido-reductase	Lactate dehydrogenase	Oxidation of the secondary alcohol L-lactate to pyruvate a ketone	$HO-C-H + NAD^{\oplus} \rightleftharpoons C=O + NADH + H^{\oplus}$ (L-Lactate → Pyruvate)	NAD+ (Nicotanimide adenine dinucleotide)
Transferase	Alanine transaminase (Alanine transferase)	Transfer of an amino group	L-Alanine + α-Ketoglutarate ⇌ Pyruvate + L-Glutamate	Pyridoxal phosphate
Hydrolase	Trypsin	Hydrolysis of Lys-Y (or Arg-Y)peptide bonds when Y≠Pro	Lysine residue within polypeptide chain + $H_2O \rightarrow$ C-terminal lysine polypeptide fragment + New N-terminal polypeptide	None
Lyase	Pyruvate decarboxylase	Decarboxylation of pyruvate	Pyruvate → Acetaldehyde + Carbon dioxide ($O=C=O$)	Thiamine pyrophosphate
Isomerase	Alanine racemase	Interconversion of D and L isomers of alanine	L-Alanine ⇌ D-Alanine	Pyridoxl phosphate
Ligase	Glutamine synthetase	ATP-dependent synthesis of L-glutamine	L-Glutamate + ATP + $NH_4^{\oplus} \longrightarrow$ L-Glutamine + ADP + P_i	ATP

5.1. Racemases and epimerases
      5.1.1.1. Alanine racemase
           L-Alanine = D-alanine

5.2. Cis-trans isomerase
      5.2.1.3. All trans-retinene 11-*cis-trans* isomerase [retinene isomerase]

           All *trans*-retinene = 11-*cis-trans* retinene

5.3. Enzymes catalyzing interconversion of aldose and ketoses
      5.3.1.1. D-Glyceraldehyde-3-phosphate ketol isomerase [triosephosphate isomerase]
           D-Glyceraldehyde-3-phosphate = dihydroxyacetone phosphate

6. Ligases (Ligare = 'to bind') : Enzymes catalyzing the linkage together of compounds coupled to breaking of a pyrophosphate bond in ATP or a similar compound. Included are the enzymes catalyzing reactions forming C-O, C-S, C-N, and C-C bonds. Representative subclasses are:

6.2. Enzymes catalyzing formation of C-S bonds
      6.2.1.4. Succinate: CoA ligases (GDP) [succinic thiokinase]
           GTP + succinate + CoA = GDP + P_i + succinyl-CoA

6.3. Enzymes catalyzing formation of C-N bonds
      6.3.1.2. L-Glutamate: ammonia ligase (ADP) [glutamine synthetase]
           ATP + L-glutamate + NH_4^+ = ADP + orthophosphate + L-glutamine

6.4. Enzymes catalyzing formation of C-C bonds
      6.4.1.2. Acetyl -CoA : CO_2. ligases (ADP) [acetyl CoA carboxylase]
           ATP + acetyl-CoA + CO_2 = ADP + P_i + malonyl-CoA

2.5. FACTORS AFFECTING ENZYME ACTION

An enzyme is a catalyst and it greatly enhances the rate of specific chemical reaction. They cannot change the equilibrium of a reaction, i.e., an enzyme accelerates the forward and backward reaction by precisely the same factor . Enzymes accelerate the attainment of equilibrium but do not shift their position. A chemical reaction of substrate S to form product P goes through a transition state S* that has a higher free energy than either S or P.

$$S \xrightarrow{\text{K}} S^* \xrightarrow{\text{V}} P$$
    Substrate   Transition   Product
                  state

The transition state is the most seldom occupied species along the reaction pathway because it has the highest free energy. The activation energy of a reaction is the amount of energy in calories required to bring all the molecules in 1 M of a substance at a given temperature to the transition state at the top of the energy barrier, i.e., the Gibb's free energy of activation [G*] which is equal to the difference in free energy between the transition state and the substrate (Fig. 2.5). The rate of any chemical reaction is therefore proportional to the concentration of the transition state of species, which depends on G* because it is in equilibrium units.

There are two general ways in which the rate of a chemical reaction can be increased:
1. By increasing the temperature which increases the concentration of transition state species
2. By adding catalyst: Catalysts accelerate chemical reactions by finding a lower 'pass' over the energy barrier. The catalyst [C], combines transiently with the reactant [A] to produces a new complex [CA] whose transition state has a much lower energy of activation than the transition state of [A] reactant molecule in uncatalyzed state (Fig. 2.5). The [CA] complex then reacts to form the product [P], releasing the free catalyst, which can then combine with another molecule of [A] to repeat the cycle.

2.5.1. Effect of substrate concentration

The effect of varying the substrate concentration on the initial rate of an enzyme catalyzed reaction when enzyme concentration is held constant, could be followed in the figure 2.6. At very low concentration of substrate the rate of reaction is very slow, but increases with an increase in substrate concentration. The rate of enzyme catalyzed reaction however does not increase beyond a certain concentration of the substrate. No matter how high the substrate concentration is raised beyond this point, the reaction rate will tend to approach but never reach a plateau. At this plateau, called the maximum rate (V_{max}), the enzyme is 'saturated' with its substrate and can function no faster.

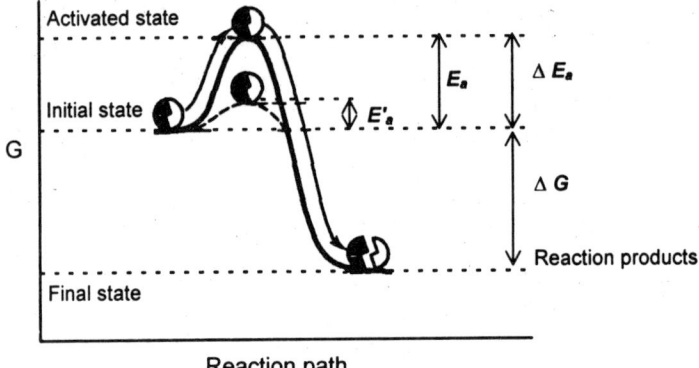

Fig. 2.5 : Energy curve for catalyzed and uncatalyzed reactions

This saturation effect is exhibited by nearly all enzymes. It led Victor Henri to the conclusion (in 1903) that an enzyme combines with its substrate molecule to form an enzyme substrate complex.

$$E + S \longrightarrow ES$$

The ES complex then breaks down through a second reversible reaction, which is slower to yield the reaction product P and the free enzyme E.

$$ES \longrightarrow E + P$$

Since the second reaction is the rate limiting step, the overall rate of the enzyme catalyzed reaction must be proportional to the concentration of the enzyme-substrate complex. At any given point of time in an enzyme catalyzed reaction the enzyme exists in two forms, the free or uncombined form [E] and the combined or complexed form [ES]. The rate of the catalyzed reaction is maximum when virtually all of the enzyme is present as the [ES] complex and the concentration of free enzyme [E] vanishes to lowest. This condition may possibly exist at a very high concentration of the substrate.

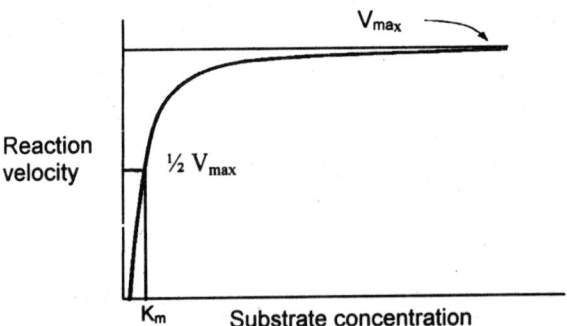

Fig. 2.6 : Effect of substrate concentration on rate of enzyme catalyzed reaction

2.5.1.1. The Michaelis-Menten equation

Mathematical relationship between rate of reaction and substrate concentration has been discussed by Michaelis and Menten. Many enzymes show the typical hyperbolic curve (Fig. 2.6) relating the reaction velocity to the substrate concentration with a gradual approach to saturation of enzyme with substrate. There are two cardinal points in such plots.

1. K_m - the substrate concentration giving half maximum velocity.
2. V_{max} - maximum velocity toward which the rate approaches at infinitely high substrate concentration.

Michaelis and Menten suggested that much additional informations can be derived from the hyperbolic saturation curves of enzymes when they are translated into a simple mathematical form. The Michaelis and Menten equation is basically an algebraic expression of the hyperbolic curves in which the important terms are substrate concentration[S], initial velocity (V_o), V_{max} and K_m. According to early views of Henri and of Michaelis and Menten, it may be assumed that the substrate [S], combines with the enzyme, to form the complex [ES], according to the reversible reaction.

$$E + S \underset{k_2}{\overset{k_1}{\rightleftharpoons}} ES \qquad \text{---(2.1)}$$

k_1 the velocity constant characteristic for the reaction that leads to the formation of ES
k_2 the characteristics for the dissociation of ES

The next step involves the formation of product P and the generation of free enzyme

$$ES \xrightarrow{k_3} P + E \qquad \text{---(2.2)}$$

Then [E_t] represents the total enzyme concentration (the sum of free and combined enzyme). [ES] is the concentration of the enzyme-substrate complex {[E_t]-[ES]} represents the concentration of free or uncombined enzyme [S], the substrate concentration, is ordinarily far greater than [Et], so that the amount of [S] bound by [E] at any given time is negligible compared with the total concentration S

The rate of formation of [ES] in reaction (2.1) is assessed by following equation

Rate of formation = k_1 {[conc. of free enzyme]}[conc. of substrate]

$$= k_1 \{[E_t]-[Es]\} [S] \qquad \text{----(2.3)}$$

where k_1 is the rate constant of reactions (2.1). The rate of formation of ES from E+P by reversible reaction (2.2) is very small and may thus be neglected.

The rate of breakdown of ES in reactions (2.1) & (2.2)

Rate of breakdown = k_2 [ES] + k_3 [ES] \qquad ---(2.4)

in which k_2 and k_3 are the rate constants for the reverse reaction (2.1) and the forward direction of reaction (2), respectively.

When the rate of formation of [ES] equals the rate of breakdown, and the [ES] concentration remains to be constant, such state of reaction is referred as steady state.

Rate of formation of [ES] = rate of breakdown of [ES]

$k_1\{[E_t]-[ES]\} [S] = k_2 [ES] + k_3[ES]$ \qquad ---(2.5)

$k_1 [E_t] [S] - k_1 [S] [ES] = k_2 [ES] + k_3 [ES]$

$k_1 [E_t] [S] = [ES] \{k_1 [S] + k_2 + k_3\}$

therefore, $\qquad [ES] = \dfrac{k_1 [E_t] [S]}{\{k_1[S] + k_2 + k_3\}}$

$$[ES] = \dfrac{[E_t] [S]}{[S] + \dfrac{k_2 + k_3}{k_1}} \qquad \text{---(2.6)}$$

The initial velocity, according to the Michaelis and Menten theory, is determined by the rate of breakdown of [ES] in reaction (2.2), where rate constant is k_2. Thus we have

$V_o = k_3 [ES]$

$[ES] = \dfrac{V_o}{k_3}$

Replacing the value of [ES] in equation (2.6)

$$\frac{V_o}{k_3} = \frac{[E_t]\,[S]}{\dfrac{[S] + k_2 + k_3}{k_1}}$$

$$V_o = \frac{k_3[E_t]\,[S]}{\dfrac{[S] + k_2 + k_3}{k_1}} \qquad\qquad\text{-----(2.7)}$$

If $\dfrac{k_2 + k_3}{k_1} = K_m$ - Michaelis Menten constant and $V_{max} = k_3\,[E_t]$ is the rate when all the available [E] is presented as [ES]

$$V_o = \frac{V_{max}\,[S]}{[S] + K_m} \qquad\qquad\text{----(2.8)}$$

This was proposed by Michaelis-Menten as an equation for a one-substrate enzyme catalyzed reaction. This equation presents a quantitative relationship between the initial velocity V_o, the maximum velocity V_{max} and initial substrate concentration all related through the Michaelis-Menten constant.

When the initial reaction rate is exactly one-half the maximum velocity, i.e., when $V_o = 1/2\ V_{max}$, then the Michaelis Menten equation could be written as :

$$\frac{1}{2} = \frac{[S]}{K_m + [S]} \qquad\qquad\text{-----(2.9)}$$

$K_m + [S] = 2[S]$ or
$K_m = [S]$ \qquad (when V_o is exactly $1/2\ V_{max}$)

2.5.1.2. Transformed Michaelis-Menten equation

The double reciprocal plot : The Michaelis-Menten equation can be algebraically transformed into other forms that are more useful in graphical processing of experimental data. One common transformation is derived simply by taking the reciprocal of both sides of the Michaelis-Menten equation (Eq. 2.8) to give the transformed Michaelis-Menten equation (Eq. 2.10) which is known as the **Lineweaver-Burk equation**.

$$\frac{1}{V_o} = \frac{K_m + [S]}{V_{max}\,[S]}$$

$$\frac{1}{V_o} = \frac{K_m}{V_{max}} + \frac{1}{V_{max}} \qquad\qquad\text{----(2.10)}$$

For enzymes obeying the Michaelis-Menten relationship exactly, a plot of $1/V_o$ against $1/[S]$ yields a straight line (Fig. 2.7). This line will have a slope of K_m/V_{max} and intercept of $1/V_{max}$ on the $1/V_o$ axis and an intercept of $-1/K_m$ on the $1/[S]$ axis. The plot is known as **Lineweaver-Burk plot or double reciprocal plot** (Fig. 2.7). This plot has the great advantage of allowing more accurate determination of V_{max} which can only be approximated from a simple plot of V_o vs [S]. The double reciprocal plot of enzyme catalyzed reactions rate data are very useful in analyzing enzyme inhibition. The Michaelis-Menten equation is basic to all aspects of the kinetics of enzyme action. If K_m and V_{max} are known then the reaction rate of an enzyme at any given concentration of its substrate can be easily calculated. Table 2.6 lists various enzymes, their Michaelis-Menten constants and pH optima along with their sources.

Most enzymatic reactions including those with two or more participating substrates can quantitatively be analyzed by employing the Michaelis-Menten theory. This fact has constituted strong evidence, that enzymes catalyze reactions by combining temporarily and transiently with their substrate, thus lowering the activation energy of the overall reaction. The formation of enzyme-substrate complex can often be detected directly by physico-chemical methods, e.g., by characteristic changes in the absorption spectrum of the enzyme when its substrate is added. The Michaelis-Menten parameters K_m and V_{max} are valuable and important indices of a particular enzyme/substrate system and thus their accurate numeric evaluation is essential. Although they can be obtained directly from the hyperbolic dependence of V_o and [S].

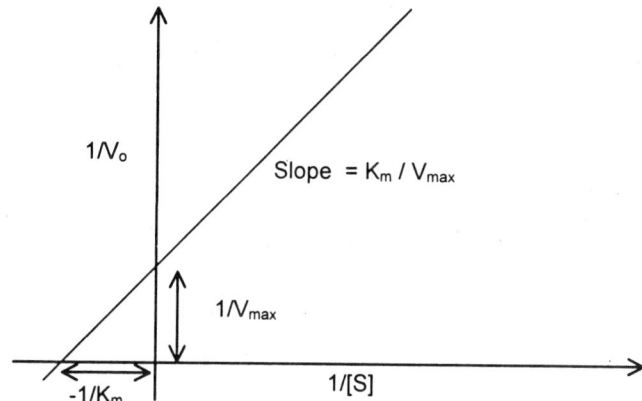

Fig. 2.7 : Lineweaver-Burk plot

1. It is not always possible to use sufficient quantities of the substrate to enable determination of the V_{max}.

2. Even if the substrate is highly water soluble, the resulting environmental changes, formation of non-productive substrate-enzyme complexes or salt effect may invalidate the results obtained.

3. The evaluation of these constants depends upon a few points only in the middle and the high ends of the substrate range and it is obviously sounder practice to use as much of the experimental data as possible. For these reasons Lineweaver-Bruk plot is preferred.

Table 2.6 : pH optima and Michaelis constants for some enzymes

Enzyme	Source	Substrate	pH Optimum	K_m
Amylase	Saliva and pancreas	Starch	6.0-7.0	0.8-0.25%
Carboxylase	Yeast	α-Keto acids	4.8	0.01M for pyruvic acid
Catalase	Liver	H_2O_2	6.3-9.5	0.025M
Dipeptidase	Intestine	Dipeptides	7.3-8.1	0.02-0.07 M for glycyl-leucine
Lipase	Pancreas	Ethyl butyrate	7.0	>0.03 M in phosphate buffer
Phosphatase	Bone	Glycero-phosphate	5.5	0.09 M
Pepsin	Stomach	Various proteins	1.5-2.5	4.5 % for ovalbumin
Saccharase	Mammalian intestine	Sucrose	6.2	0.02 M
Urease	Soybean	Urea	7.2-7.9 ca.	0.025 M

2.5.2. Concentration of enzyme

The rate of an enzyme catalyzed reaction measured during initiation is directly proportional to the concentration of enzyme. The initial rate of a reaction is the rate measured when almost no substrate has been reacted to form the product and permits the reverse reaction to occur. The enzyme [E] combines with substrate [S] forming an **enzyme-substrate complex [ES]**, which decomposes to form a product, [P], and free enzyme.

$$E + S \rightleftharpoons ES \rightleftharpoons E + P \qquad \text{---(2.11)}$$
$$\text{or}$$
$$E + S \rightleftharpoons E + P \qquad \text{---(2.12)}$$

Rate of forward reaction : $Rate_1 = k_1 [E] [S]$ ---(2.13)

Rate of backward reaction : $Rate_2 = k_2 [E] [P]$ ---(2.14) where k_1 and k_2 are the rate constants for the forward and backward reaction respectively.

The overall equilibrium constant $K_{eq} = \dfrac{k_1}{k_2} = \dfrac{[E]\,[P]}{[E]\,[S]} = \dfrac{[P]}{[S]}$ ---(2.15)

The enzyme concentration thus has no effect on the equilibrium constant. Impure pepsin and trypsin show reaction velocities more nearly proportional to the square root of the enzyme concentration. Northrop demonstrated that highly purified pepsin, within limits, does digest protein at a rate that is almost proportional to its concentration. In the presence of increased concentration of reaction products this linear relationship may not hold.

2.5.3. Concentration of reaction products

The addition of products of enzyme reaction to a system containing purified enzyme destroys the linear relationship between enzyme concentration and reaction rate. Thus if peptic digestion products are added to a system in which purified pepsin is hydrolyzing protein, the rate of reaction is similar to the rate obtained with a crude pepsin preparation. Addition of either glucose or fructose inhibits the hydrolysis of 2% sucrose by yeast invertase. This could be due to formation of a more stable complex of enzyme and reaction products than of enzyme and substrate, which obstructs the active centers of a certain proportion of the enzyme molecules. It is also assumed that, in the presence of high concentrations of reaction products some resynthesis by enzyme may occur; that would result in an apparent decrease in the rate of decomposition.

2.5.4. pH

The activity of an enzyme is determined usually by the pH of the system in which it operates. Each enzyme has an optimum pH i.e., a $[H^+]$ concentration at which the enzyme reacts at maximum level. The optimum pH changes with; varying conditions of time, temperature, concentration of substrate, or other factors. Moderate pH changes affect the ionic state of the enzyme and frequently that of substrate also. When enzyme activity is measured at several pH values, optimal activity is generally observed between pH 5.0 and 9.0. However, a few enzymes, e.g., pepsin, are active well outside this range.

The pH-activity curve is bell-shaped (Fig. 2.8) and is governed by the following factors:

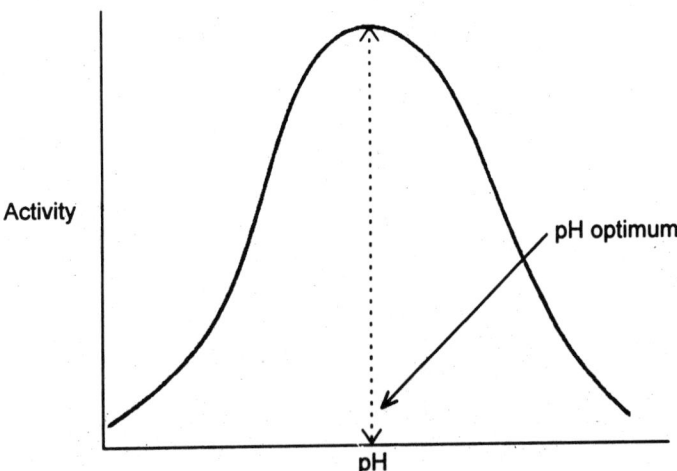

Fig. 2.8 : Effect of pH on the activity of the enzyme

1. Denaturation of enzyme at extremely high or low pH values.
2. Effect on the charged state of substrate or enzyme.

In the case of an enzyme, the charge changes may affect activity either by changing structure or by changing the charge on an amino acid residue that is functional in substrate-binding or catalysis. If a negatively charged enzyme [E⁻] reacts with a positively charged substrate [S⁺] then at low pH values [E⁻], will get protonated and would lose its negative charge. Similarly, at very high pH values, [S⁺] will ionize to lose its positive charge. Since the only forms that will interact are [S⁺] and [E⁻], extreme pH values will lower the reaction velocity as shown in figure 2.8 (bell shaped curve of pH-enzyme activity). Only the area under the curve for both [E] and [S] in the appropriate ionic state, and the maximal concentration of [E] and [S] are correctly charged at X. The result is the bell-shaped pH-activity curve.

2.5.5. Temperature

Chemical reactions, both catalyzed and noncatalyzed proceed at a faster rate as the reaction temperature is increased. This is true of enzymatically catalyzed reactions. In general only up to 50°C. Above this temperature heat denaturation of enzymes starts. In a few exceptional cases, the speed of reaction slows and ceases at or around temperature 70°C to 80°C. The exact ratio by which the velocity changes for a 10°C rise is the Q_{10}, or temperature coefficient. The velocity (V_o) of many biologic reactions roughly doubles with a 10°C rise in temperature(Q_{10} =2), and is halved if the temperature is decreased by 10°C. The Q_{10} values for few enzymes are listed in table 2.7.

Table 2.7 : Q_{10} values for some enzymes

Enzyme	Q_{10} value
Catalase	2.3 (0-10°), 2.19 (10-20°)
Urease	1.81 (20-30°), 1.90 (30-40°)
Maltase (Yeast)	1.90 (10-20°), 1.44 (20-30°), 1.28 (30-40°)
Succinic oxidase	2.0 (30-40°), 2.1 (40-50°)
Invertase	1.76 (15-25°), 1.62 (25-35°)

When the rate of enzyme-catalyzed reaction is measured at several temperatures, the results shown in figure 2.9 come to be typical. For most enzymes, optimal temperature approximates those of the environment of the cell. For the warm blooded organism i.e., man, this is 37°C. The optimal temperature for the digestive enzymes of the gastro-intestinal tract to operate maximally is around 40°C. Certain plant enzymes may have optimum temperature as high as 60°C.

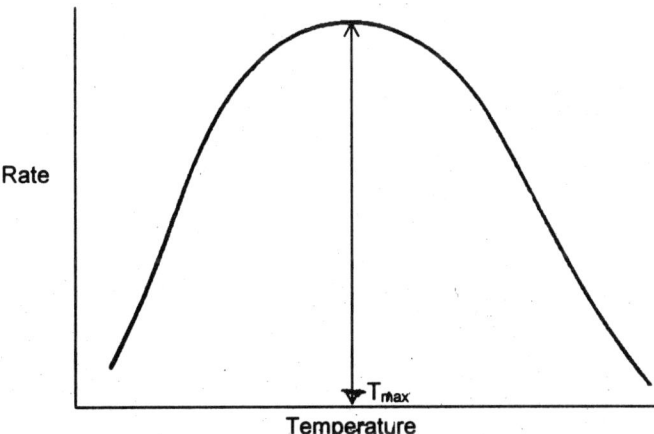

Fig. 2.9 : Effect of temperature on the rate of the enzyme catalyzed reaction

The increase in the rate below optimal temperature results from the increased kinetic energy of the reacting molecules. As the temperature is raised still further, the kinetic energy of the enzyme molecule becomes so high that it exceeds the energy barrier in order to break the secondary bonds that hold the enzyme in its native or catalytically active form. However, simultaneously there is a loss of secondary and tertiary structures and a parallel loss of biological activity.

2.5.6. Time

For an enzyme catalyzed reaction, an optimum pH or an optimum temperature can not be independent of time. For example the optimum temperature of many enzymes from warm blooded animals is approximately 37°C only if the time is measured in hours; if time is measured in days, the optimum temperature may be much lower; further, if the time is measured in minutes, perhaps the optimum temperature could be as high as 70°C or above.

2.5.7. State of oxidation of enzyme

Enzymes containing sulfhydryl groups are activated by certain reducing agents and inactivated by aeration or other mild oxidizing treatments. Representative examples of this class are papain, urease and succinic dehydrogenase. Glutathione, cysteine, hydrogen sulfide, and HCN activate these enzymes. Such activation might be accounted for the removal of inactivating heavy metal ions. Recent studies suggested that actual reduction of disulfide linkage (-S-S-) in the enzyme molecules to sulfhydryl (-SH) groups may be responsible for the activation.

2.5.8. Activators

Many ions and molecules have the capacity to activate some enzymes. Metals ions are activators of a number of enzymes (Table 2.3). Pepsin (as proenzyme pepsinogen) is activated by H^+ to form the active enzyme. Many reducing agents (cysteine, glutathione) act as enzyme activators of enzyme containing sulfhydryl groups. Enzyme themselves activate other enzymes or proenzymes; e.g., enterokinase activates trypsinogen to form active trypsin. Trypsinogen, pepsinogen and chymotrypsinogen, are such enzymes known as *zymogens*.

2.5.8.1. Zymogen activation

Zymogen activation involves the hydrolysis of uniquely located peptide bond in the zymogen molecule. In bovine and porcine trypsinogen the primary activation involves the hydrolysis (by trypsin) of a lysyl-isoleucine bond which liberates an amino terminal hexapeptide in the bovine (Val-Asp$_4$-Lys) and an amino terminal octapeptide (Phe-Pro-Thr-Asp$_4$-Lys) in the porcine variety, with the subsequent liberation of active enzyme in either of case. Another zymogen activation involves the procarboxypeptidase A which occurs in the pancreas in two forms which can be easily separated into larger form (S6) of molecular weight 87,000 and the smaller (S3) form of molecular weight 64,000. Activation of the S6 form with trypsin led to fractions with different catalytic activities; one fraction was an endopeptidase and the other a carboxypeptidase.

2.6. MODE OF ENZYME ACTION

Mode of enzyme action involves the nature of the enzyme substrate interaction responsible for the reaction specificity of the biologic catalysts. The Michaelis-Menten theory of enzyme action provides the basis for much of the present research on mechanism of enzyme action. This theory, the enzyme-substrate complex theory, assumes combination of enzyme and substrate in phase one (sometimes known as transition phase) of the enzyme activity and liberation of enzyme and the products of the catalysis in phase two of the reaction:

Enzyme + Substrate $\rightleftharpoons$ Enzyme-Substrate complex $\rightleftharpoons$ Enzyme + Product

One key factor of enzyme to act as catalyst is their ability to bind effectively one or (more frequently) both reactants in a bimolecular reaction with an accompanying increase in local reactants concentration and hence in local reaction rate. Enzymes are both extremely efficient and highly selective catalysts. To understand these distinctive properties of enzymes, the concept of 'active' or 'catalytic site' must be introduced.

2.6.1. The catalytic site

The region of an enzyme concerned with substrate binding and catalysis is termed as **active site**. The large size of proteins relative to substrates led to the concept that a restricted region of the enzyme is concerned with the catalysis. This region, ' the catalytic site', has been recognized from three dimensional models of enzymes that suggest that a far greater portion of the protein interacts with the substrate than was formerly supposed. Different models of the catalytic sites have been proposed so far, the most relevant models are discussed here.

2.6.1.1. The lock and key or template model

Many properties of enzymes can be explained in terms of the rigid 'lock and key' model of an active site. The model of a catalytic site proposed by Emil Fischer visualized interaction between substrate and enzyme in terms "**lock and key**" analogy. This lock and key, or rigid template, model (Fig. 2.10), is still useful for understanding certain properties of enzymes. The ordered binding of two or more substrates can be explained by this model. It states that the enzymatic specificity lies in a strict conformity of the substrate with the active center of enzyme.

According to Fischer, the enzyme is a rigid structure whose active center is a replica of the substrate. The enzymatic reaction is feasible if the substrate matches the active center as the key fits into the lock. If the substrate ('key') becomes slightly modified, it no longer fits the active center ('lock'), and no reaction takes place. The Fischer's hypothesis is rather attractive since it provides a simple explanation of the specificity of enzymatic action.

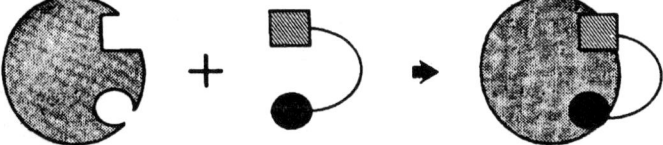

Fig. 2.10 : Formation of enzyme substrate complex according to lock and key mode

2.6.1.2. The 'Induced fit' model

In the induced fit model of a catalytic site, the substrate induces a conformational change in the enzyme that creates the catalytic site. Koshland found an unfortunate feature of Fischer's model in the form of rigidity of the catalytic site and gave a more general model ,i.e., 'induced fit' model. This model has considerable experimental support. In the Fischer model, the catalytic site is presumed to be oriented and preshaped to fit the substrate but in the Koshland model, the substrate induces a conformational change in the enzyme (Fig. 2.11). Changes in tertiary or quaternary structure of the relatively large enzyme molecule thus can exert mechanical leverage on the substrate.

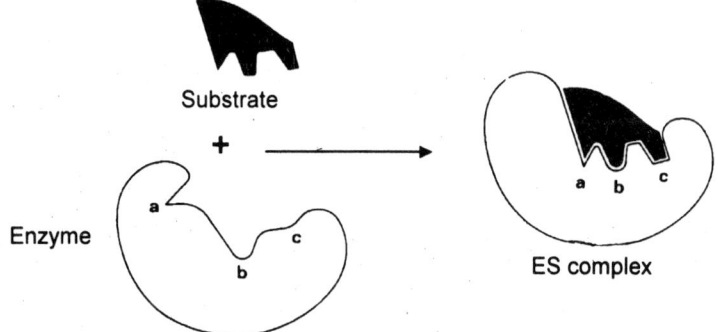

Fig. 2.11 : Enzyme substrate interaction according to 'Induced fit model'

This concept may explain why enzymes are proteins and thus much larger than most substrate molecules. The conformational changes align amino acid residues or other groups on the enzyme in the correct spatial orientation for substrate binding, catalysis, or both.

2.6.2. Proximity and orientation

Mutual orientation of reactants is a very specific property of enzymes enabling them to accelerate the conversion (to increase the reactivity of substrates) by a few orders of magnitude. The contact site of the enzyme active center binds specifically the substrate, providing thereby for their mutual orientation and approach so as to facilitate the intervention of catalytic groups. The formation of enzyme substrate complex may take place in such a way that the susceptible bond is in a close proximity to the catalytic group and also is precisely oriented, thus greatly increases the probability that the ES complex will enter the transition state (Fig. 2.12).

Orientation of two or more molecules, incapable of realization via chaotic collisions in an aqueous medium or on the surface of an inorganic catalyst, favors a drastic increase in the reaction rate. An ordered arrangement of substrates leads to a drop in entropy and, consequently, to diminution of the activation energy.

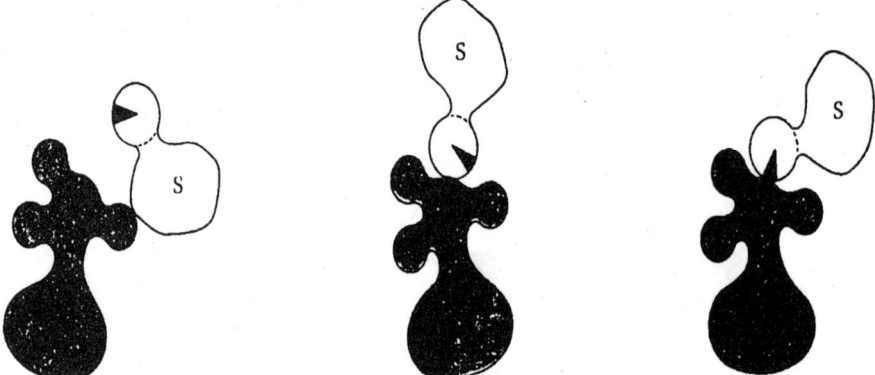

Fig. 2.12 : Diagrammatic representation of proximity and orientation

2.6.3. General acid-base catalysis

The active site of an enzyme possesses functional groups of specific amino acid residues capable of acting both as an acid (good proton donors) and as a base (good proton acceptors). When the substrate is anchored at the active site, its molecule becomes liable to the influence of electrophilic and nucleophilic groups of the catalytic site, which results in an electron density redistribution in the substrate molecule regions accessible to attack by acid base groups. Such general-acid or general-base groups are powerful catalysts for many organic reactions in aqueous systems. Histidine exhibits clearly defined acid-base properties. Blocking of the histidine residue entails the enzyme inactivation. The acid-base catalysis is typical of hydrolases, lyases and isomerases.

a. Some proton-donating groups

$-COO$

$-NH_2$

$-S^-$

b. Some proton-accepting groups

$-COOH$

$-^+NH_3$

$-SH$

2.6.4. Covalent catalysis

Covalent catalysis is observed in the enzymes capable of forming covalent bonds between the substance and the catalytic group of the active site. Some enzymes react with their substrates to form very unstable, covalently joined enzyme-substrate complexes, which undergo further reaction to form the products much more readily than the uncatalyzed reaction. Some of the enzymes exhibiting a covalent catalytic behavior are listed in table 2.8. Most enzymes are capable of a simultaneous involvement in the above mechanisms, which provides for their high catalytic activity.

Table 2.8 : Some of the enzymes exhibiting covalent catalytic behavior

Enzyme	Reactive group	Typical covalent enzyme-substrate intermediate
Chymotrypsin, trypsin, thrombin, esterase	Serine $HO\text{-}CH_2\text{-}CH\text{-}$	Acylserine
Phosphoglucomutase, alkaline phosphatase	Serine $HO\text{-}CH_2\text{-}CH\text{-}$	Phosphorylserine
Glyceraldehyde-3-phosphate dehydrogenase papain	Cysteine $HS\text{-}CH_2\text{-}CH\text{-}$	Acylcysteine

2.7. MECHANISM OF ENZYME ACTION

Hummel and Kalnitzky interpreted enzyme mechanism to mean the characterization of the sequential transition states undergone by the enzyme-substrate complex during catalysis. In the present chapter we will consider the nature of the enzyme-substrate interaction responsible for the reaction specificity of these biologic catalysts and various proposed models for the catalytic site.

The molecular events that accompany conversion of substrate to products can elaborate upon the subject matter of the mechanism of enzyme action. The Michaelis-Menten theory of enzyme action is the basis of much of the present research on mechanisms. In this chapter a detailed description of catalysis by the proteolytic enzyme chymotrypsin is used to illustrate the principle of catalysis that is applied to enzymes in general.

2.7.1. Mechanism of catalysis by chymotrypsin

2.7.1.1. The "intermediary enzymology" of chymotrypsin

Like many other proteases, chymotrypsin also catalyses the hydrolysis of certain esters. The molecular events in catalysis are termed "intermediary enzymology. Chymotrypsin catalyses hydrolysis of peptide bonds in which the carboxyl group is contributed by an aromatic amino acid (Phy, Try, or Trp) or by one with a bulky nonpolar R group (Met). The synthetic substrate *p*-nitrophenyl acetate facilitates colorimetric analysis of chymotrypsin activity because hydrolysis to *p*-nitrophenol which in alkali, converts into the chromophore anionic form S.

2.7.1.2. "Stop flow" kinetics reveals the intermediary enzymology of chymotrypsin

The kinetics of chymotrypsin of *p*-nitrophenylacetate can be studied in a "stop-flow" apparatus. The method utiizes substrate quantities of enzymes and measures the events in the first few milliseconds. The salient features of the slow flow kinetics of chymotrypsin are:

A. Release of *p*-nitrophenyl anion with chymotrypsin. Hydrolysis of *p*-nitrophenylacetate takes place in two distinct phases:
  (i) a burst phase characterized by rapid liberation of anion; and
  (ii) a subsequent 'steady state' phase, slower release of additional anion.

B. The slow step in catalysis by chymotrypsin is hydrolysis of the chymotrypsin-acetate (CT-Ac) complex. Once ail the available chymotrypsin has been converted to CT-Ac, no further release of *p*-nitrophenyl acetate anion can occur until more free chymotrypsin is liberated by the slow, hydrolytic removal of acetate anion from the CT-Ac complex. The free chymotrypsin then is available for further formation of chymotrypsin-*p*-

nitrophenyl acetate complex (CT-PNP) and CT-Ac complexes with attended release of PNP. Formation and decay of the enzyme-substrate complex, based on the Michaelis-Menten kinetics can be represented as :

$$CT + PNP \longrightarrow CT\text{-}PNP \longrightarrow CT\text{-}Ac \longrightarrow CT$$
$$\downarrow \qquad\qquad \downarrow \qquad\qquad \downarrow$$
$$Phenol \qquad\qquad H_2O \qquad\qquad Ac^-$$

CT = Chymotrypsin, PNP = *p*-nitrophenyl acetate, CT-PNP = Chymotrypsin-*p*-nitrophenyl acetate complex, CT-Ac = Chymotrypsin- Acetate complex

Formation of CT-PNP and CT-Ac complex is fast relative to the hydrolysis of CT-Ac complex.

C. A 'charge relay network' functions as a proton shuttle during catalysis by chymotrypsin. The charge relay network of chymotrypsin involves 3 aminoacyl residues that are far apart in a primary structural sense but within a tertiary structural sense; while most of the charged residues of chymotrypsin are at the surface of the molecule, those of the charge relay network are 'buried' in the otherwise nonpolar interior of the molecule. These charge relay residues trigger sequential proton shifts that shuttle protons in the reverse direction. An analogous series of proton shifts is believed to accompany the hydrolysis of physiologic chymotrypsin substrate such as a peptide.

2.7.1.3. Role of selective proteolysis in creation of the catalytic sites of enzymes

Certain proteins are manufactured and secreted in the form of inactive precursor proteins known as proproteins. When the proteins are enzymes, the proteins are termed as ***proezymes*** or ***zymogens***. Conversion of a proprotein to the mature protein involves selective proteolysis. This converts the proproteins by one or more successive proteolytic clips, to a form in which the characteristic activity of the mature protein (its enzymatic activity) is expressed. Examples include the hormone insulin (proinsulin), the digestive enzyme chymotrypsin (chymotrypsinogen) and several factors of the blood clotting and of the blood clot dissolution cascades and the connective tissue protein collagen (procollagen). The conversion of prochymotrypsin (Pro-CT), a 2,4,5-aminoacyl residue polypeptide, to the active enzyme α-chymotrypsin involves 3 proteolytic clips and the formation of an active intermediate known as π-chymotrypsin (π-CT) and subsequently to the mature catalytically active enzyme α-chymotrypsin (α-CT).

2.7.1.4. Ordered and random binding of specific enzyme

Most enzymes catalyze a reaction between two or more substrates, yielding one or more products. The order in which an enzyme binds its substrate may be random or ordered. Many require coenzymes proceeded by 'Ping-Pong' mechanism (so termed because the enzyme alternates between forms E and E').

While a coenzyme frequently may be regarded as a second substrate, certain coenzymes (e.g., pyridoxal phosphate) are covalently bonded to the enzyme or bound noncovalently so tightly that dissociation rarely occurs (e.g., thiamine pyrophosphate). In these cases the enzyme-coenzyme complex is regarded as the enzyme.

2.7.1.5. Enzyme as general acid or general base catalysis

Once the substrate has been bound at the catalytic site, the charged (or chargeable) functional groups of the side chains of nearby aminoacyl residues may participate in catalysis by functioning as acidic or basic catalysts. There are two broad categories of acid-base catalysis by enzymes: **general** and **specific** (acid or base) catalysis. Reactions whose rates vary in response to changes in H^+ or H_3O^+ concentration but are independent of the concentrations of the other acids or bases present in the solution are said to be subjected to specific acid or specific base catalysis. Reactions whose rates are responsive to all the acids (proton donors) or bases (proton acceptor) present in solution are said to be subjected to general acid or general base catalysis.

To determine whether a given enzyme-catalyzed reaction is a general or specific acid or base catalysis, the rate of reaction is measured under two set of conditions: (1) at various pH values but at a constant buffer concentration, and (2) at constant pH values but at various buffer concentrations. In this context, if the rate of the reaction changes as a function of pH at constant buffer concentration, the reaction is said to be specific base/acid catalyzed if the pH is above/below 7.0 If the reaction rate at a constant pH increases as the buffer concentration increases, the reaction is said to be subjected to general base/acid catalysis, if the pH is above/below 7.0.

2.7.1.6. Metal ion participation in mechanism of action

Over 25% of all enzymes contain tightly bound metal ions or require them for activity. The role of these metal ions is studied by x-ray crystallography, magnetic resonance imaging (MRI), and electron spin resonance (ESR). **Metallozymes** contain a definite quantity of functional metal ion that is retained throughout purification. Metal-activated enzyme binds metals less tightly but requires added metals.

For ternary complexes of the catalytic site (Enz), a metal ion (M), and substrate (S) that exhibit 1:1:1 stiochiometry, 4 types of complexes are possible :

Enz--S--M   M--Enz--S
Substrate-bridge complex   Enzyme-bridge complex
Enz--M--S   M
Simple metal-bridge complex   Enz $<$ | Cyclic metal-bridge complex
                                                                        S

All 4 complexes are possible for metal activated enzyme. Metallozymes cannot form the EnzSM complex, because they exist as EnzM. Three generalization can be stated :

1. Most of the kinases (ATP:phosphotransferases) form substrate-bridge complexes of the type Enzyme-nucleotide-M.
2. Phosphotransferases (phosphoenolpyruvate or pyruvate used as substrate), enzymes catalyzing other reactions of phosphoenolpyruvate and carboxylases form metal bridge complexes (Enz-M-S).
3. A given enzyme may form one type of bridge complex with one substrate and a different type with another.

Metal ions may participate in each of the 4 mechanisms by which the enzymes are known to accelerate the rates of chemical reaction :

1. General acid-base catalysis
2. Covalent catalysis
3. Approximation of reactants, and
4. Induction of strain in the enzyme or substrate

The metal ions most commonly used in enzymatic catalysis are Mn^{2+}, Ca^{2+} and Mg^{2+}. Iron and manganese are used in haeme protein. Metal ions are Lewis acids and can share an electron pair, forming a sigma bond. Metal ions may be considered as 'super acids' since they exist in neutral solution. Metal ions can also accept electrons via sigma or pi bonds to activate electrophiles or nucleophiles. By donating electrons, metals can activate nucleophiles or act as nucleophiles themselves. The co-ordination sphere of a metal may bring together enzyme and substrate or form chelate-producing distortion in either, the enzyme or substrate. A metal ion may also mask a nucleophile and thus prevent an otherwise likely side reaction.

2.8. ENZYME INHIBITION

The normal state of living matter is a delicately balanced, spatially and temporally coordinated organization. If a substance causes an adverse effect on this balance it is usually termed a poison, alternatively if it redresses a pathologic imbalance it is regarded as a drug. Both may be enzyme inhibitors. An enzyme inhibition decreases the activity of an enzyme without significantly disrupting its three-dimensional macromolecular structure. Inhibition is therefore distinct from denaturation and is the result of a specific action by a reagent directed or transmitted to the active site region. Studies of enzymes can yield much information about :

1. The substrate specificity of enzymes
2. The nature of functional group at the active site
3. Mechanism of the catalytic activity.

4. Usefulness in elucidating metabolic pathways in cells
5. Some drugs, useful in medicine appear to function because they can inhibit certain enzymes in malfunctioning cells.

The pharmacological action of drugs is based largely on enzyme inhibition. Common examples are found in the action of the sulfonamides and other antibiotics. In the great majority of cases, the enzyme (or coenzyme) inhibited is not known. The development of nerve gases, insecticides and herbicides (weed killer) is based on enzyme inhibition studies.

There are two major types of enzyme inhibition;
1. Irreversible
2. Reversible

2.8.1. Irreversible inhibition

Irreversible inhibitors are those which combine with or destroy a functional group on the enzyme molecule that is necessary for its catalytic activity. An irreversible inhibitor dissociates very slowly from its target enzyme because it becomes very tightly bound to the enzyme, either covalently or non covalently. Chemical modification is particularly valuable for probing the physico-chemical character of an enzyme and for determining the nature and reactivity of its constituent amino acids. It is therefore an important part of the investigation of proteins that have yet to be crystallized and of membrane bound proteins.

Modification of the enzyme can indicate the position of the active site and which of several possible amino acids are essential to its function. In addition the preparation of derivatives for peptide sequencing, the production of isomorphous heavy atom derivatives for X-ray analysis and crosslinking stabilization of the enzyme depends on the application of modifying reagents. These reagents can be divided into groups and site selective types.

2.8.1.1. Group specific reagents

There are several methods of determination for the groups essential to enzymatic activity. One most widely used method is differential labeling. Group selective modification of the enzyme is generally performed in the presence of a substrate analog, to protect the active site. The protector is then removed and the enzyme again exposed to the modifier. If the activity is retained by the substrate protected enzyme but lost when deprotected, then the group tested for activity is presumed to be present at or near the active site. If prior to the second treatment, both inhibitor and excess reagent are removed and the latter replaced by radioactivity labeled modificant, the active site will be specifically tagged. Table 2.9 gives a representative list of the more selective reagents.

Table 2.9 : Chemical modification of amino acid side chains

Amino Acid	Reagent
Arginine	Nitromalondialdehyde, phenylglyoxal
Aspartic acid/ Glutamic acid	Triethyloxonium fluoroborate, water soluble carbodiimide plus glycine methyl ester
Cysteine/ Cystine	Phosphorothioate, performic acid; 5,5'-dithiobis(2-nitrobenzoic acid); p-chloromercurybenzoate
Histidine	Iodoacetamide, diazonium-1 H-tetrazole
Lysine	Methyl acetimidate maleic anhydride
Methionine	Hydrogen peroxide, β-propiolactone
Tryptophan	Iodine, N-bromosuccinimide

These methods have several drawbacks. First is the lack of absolute specificity shown by a modifier for a given functional group. Alkyl halide preferentially reactive with lysine and α-amino groups, will also modify cysteine and threonine. This leads to considerable complication in the isolation procedures and in the interpretation of labeling patterns. Another drawback is that a lack of reactivity cannot be taken as an evidence for the absence of a functional group. Neighboring residues may either sterically hinder reagent approach to a 'buried' group or restrict formation of the transition state for reaction even though the residue may be initially accessible.

2.8.1.2. Site specific modification

There are four types of compounds which specifically modify active sites: (a) substrate, (b) pseudosubstrate, (c) affinity labels, and (d) 'suicide' or 'k_{cat}' inhibitor.

2.8.1.2.1. Substrate

The substrate is the almost perfect site-specific reagent but the bonds formed in the Michaelis complex are often labile and transitory making isolation of an enzyme bound species almost impossible. In certain cases however it has proven possible to trap an intermediate in the enzyme reaction. Reasonable mechanisms proposed for acetoacetate decarboxylase catalyzed decarboxylation and class I aldolase catalyzed reactions envisage initial schiff base formation between the incoming substrate and an amino group in the enzyme:

$$E-NH_2 + R_1R_2-C=O \longrightarrow E-N=CR_1R_2 \longrightarrow E-NH^+=CR_1R_2$$

Dihydroxyacetone phosphate $R_1 = -CH_2-O-PO_3H_2$, $\quad R_2 = -CH_2-OH$

Acetoacetate $\quad\quad\quad\quad\quad R_1 = -CH_2-O-CH_3$, $\quad\quad R_2 = -CO_2H$

In the presence of their substrates both enzymes were inhibited by sodium borohydride which was found to reduce the imines to the stable secondary amines $E-NH-CHR_1R_2$. The carbon-nitrogen single bonds, being resistant to the catalytic action of the enzymes and the protein degradative and sequencing procedures, permitted the isolation and identification of active site sequences.

Another example is iodoacetamide, which can react with sulfhydral (-SH) groups of essential cysteine residues or with the imidazole group of essential histidine residues. With the help of such inhibitors the hydroxyl group of serine, the thiol group of cysteine and the imidazole group of histidine have been identified as participating in the catalytic activity of different classes of enzymes

2.8.1.2.2. Pseudosubstrates

The pseudosubstrates possess certain characteristics which are common with the actual enzyme substrate. The designation pseudosubstrate has been particularly applied to di-isopropyl fluorophosphate (DFP) and its analogues. Di-isopropyl fluorophosphate (DFP), also known as Di-iso-propyl phosphofluoridate (DIPF), one of these agents, reacts with hydroxyl group of an essential serine residue at the active site of enzyme acetylcholine-esterase to form a catalytically inactive derivative. These organohalophosphates react rapidly and irreversibly with enzymes trypsin, chymotrypsin, thrombin and acetylcholinesterase. In each case the reaction is stoichiometric, resulting in the loss of a single active site serine residue.

Acetylcholine catalyses the hydrolysis of acetylcholine, a neurotransmitter functioning in certain portions of the nervous system (Fig. 2.13). Acetylcholine is released by a stimulated nerve cell into the synapse, with another nerve cell. Once the acetylcholine has been secreted into the synapse, it binds to receptor sites on the next nerve cell, causing the latter to propagate the nerve impulse. Before a second impulse can be transmitted through a synapse, the Ach secreted after the first impulse must be hydrolyzed by the acetylcholinesterase to acetate and choline which have no transmitter activity.

Animals treated with DFP, become paralyzed in certain functions because of failure of nerve impulses to be transmitted properly. This has led to the development of **malathion** and other insecticides that are relatively nontoxic for human and animals. Malathion is inactivated and is degraded by higher animals into products that are believed to be harmless to them, but it is converted by enzymes of insects into an active inhibitor of their Acetylcholine esterase (Fig. 2.14).

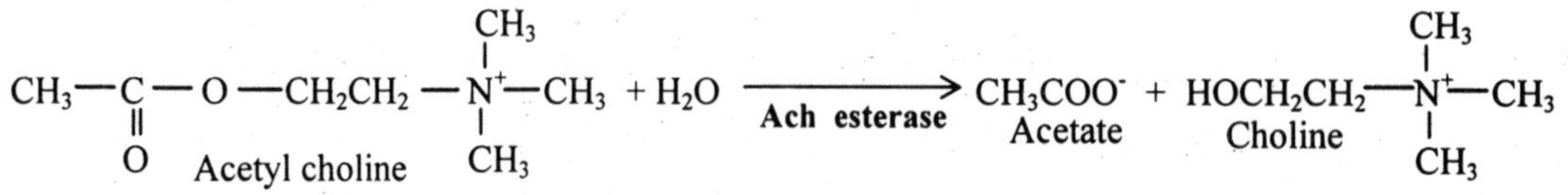

$$CH_3-\underset{\underset{O}{\|}}{C}-O-CH_2CH_2-\underset{\underset{CH_3}{|}}{\overset{\overset{CH_3}{|}}{N^+}}-CH_3 + H_2O \xrightarrow{\text{Ach esterase}} CH_3COO^- + HOCH_2CH_2-\underset{\underset{CH_3}{|}}{\overset{\overset{CH_3}{|}}{N^+}}-CH_3$$

Acetyl choline   Acetate   Choline

Fig. 2.13 : Normal activity of Acetylcholine

DFP has been found to inhibit a whole class of enzymes, many of them capable of catalyzing hydrolysis of peptide or ester linkages. They include not only acetylcholinehydrase but also trypsin, chymotrypsin, elastase, phosphoglycomutase and cocconase. All the DFP inhibited enzymes have an essential serine residue in their active site, which participates in their catalytic activity.

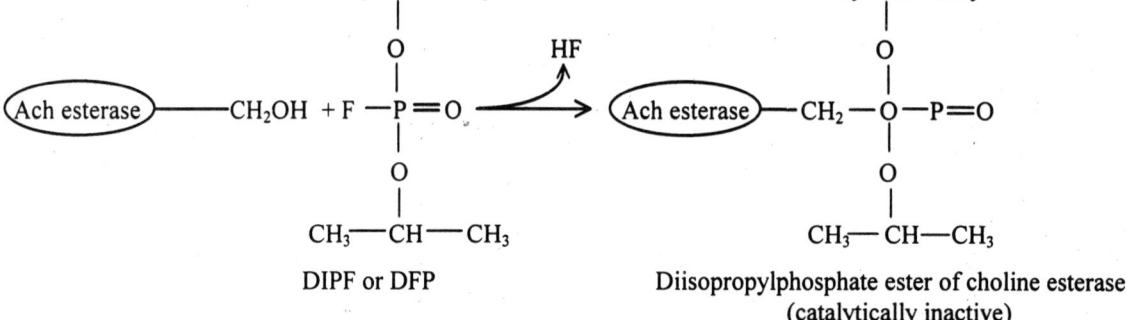

DIPF or DFP   Diisopropylphosphate ester of choline esterase
                               (catalytically inactive)

Fig. 2.14 : Effect of DIPF on the activity of acetylcholine esterase

2.8.1.2.3. Affinity labels

Reversible binding is unable to provide good information concerning the active site. A more fruitful approach reported by Schoellman and Shaw suggested the synthesis of substrate analog possessing molecular requisites complementary to the active site and in addition have incorporated chemically reactive groupings. By mimicking the substrate, they argued, such molecules would be held at high concentrations in the sites and once in position the reactive group(s) would then form irreversible covalent attachment to amino acid side chains in their vicinities. Hence, such compounds are designated as *affinity labels*. Various enzymes and their affinity labels are listed in table 2.10.

Table 2.10 : Various affinity labels

Enzyme	Reagent	Residue modified
Carboxypeptidase B	α-N-Bromoacetyl-D-arginine	Glutamate
	Bromoacetyl-p-aminobenzylsuccinate	Methionine
α-Chymotrypsin	Tosyl-L-phenylalanine chloromethyl ketone (TPCK)	Histidine 57
	Glycidol phenyl ether	Methionine 192
	Phenylmethanesulphonyl fluoride	Serine 195
Fumerase	Bromomesaconate	Methionine, histidine
β-Galactosidase	N-Bromoacetyl-β-D-galactosylamine	Methionine
Lactate dehydrogenase	3-Bromoacetylpyridine	Cysteine, histidine
Lysozyme	2',3'-Epoxypropyl-β-D-(N-actylglucosamine)₂	Aspartate 52
RNA polymerase	5-Formyl-uridine-5'-triphosphate	Lysine
Triose phosphate isomerase	Glycidol phosphate	Glutamate

An example of affinity label is the chloromethyl ketone of tosylphenylalanine (TPCK) as a possible affinity label for chymotrypsin.

$$CH_3 - C_6H_4 - SO_2 - HN - CH - CO - CH_2 - Cl$$
$$|$$
$$CH_2C_6H_5$$

Tosyl-L-phenylalanine chloromethyl ketone(TPCK)

The specificity requirement is fulfilled by incorporation of large aromatic benzyl group because chymotrypsin preferentially cleaves peptide bonds adjacent to phenylalanine, tryptophan and tyrosine. The enzyme-inhibitor complex is probably stabilized by hydrogen bond formation between the ketone and the active site serine. The proteases irreversibly and rapidly inactivated by TPCK, amino acid analysis indicated that one histidine molecule had been modified.

2.8.1.2.4. 'Suicide' or 'k-cat' inhibitors

This term was coined first by Abeles and Maycock and then by Rando. The two main characteristics of this type of irreversible inhibitor are (i) non-reactivity of the precursor before it interacts with the enzyme active site and (ii) activation and subsequent inhibition catalyzed by the same active site residues as those responsible for substrate transformation. This second characteristic thus adds an extra dimension to the specificity of inhibition, in that the catalytic reactivity of the enzyme is employed to effect its modification. Such compounds can therefore be regarded as catalytic inhibitors as opposed to affinity labels or transition-state analogs whose selectivity reside in their binding powers. Suicide inhibitors can then provide additional evidence on the mechanism of an enzymatic reaction.

The postulated intermediary catalytic formation of activated double bonds causing the observed inhibition is a common feature of suicide inhibitors, and the selectivity opens up a fascinating approach to the design of pharmacologically active agents. For example, pargyline, currently employed clinically in antihypertension therapy inhibits monoamine oxidase stoichiometrically via enzymatic formation of a relatively stable flavin-allene adduct (Fig. 2.15). Once formed the electrophilic allene is in a favorable position to attack any adjacent nucleophile and thus inactivates the enzyme.

The natural antibiotic, rhizobitoxine $NH_2-CH(CH_2OH)-CH_2-O-CH:CH-CH(NH_2)CO_2H$ which resembles the substrate cystathionine $NH_2-CH(CO_2H)-CH_2-S-CH_2-CH(NH_2)CO_2H$ of bacterial β-cystathionine, irreversibly prevents its cleavage into homocysteine and pyruvate probably also by acting as a suicide inhibitor.

$$C_6H_5-CH_2-N(CH_3)CH_2-C:CH$$

Pargyline

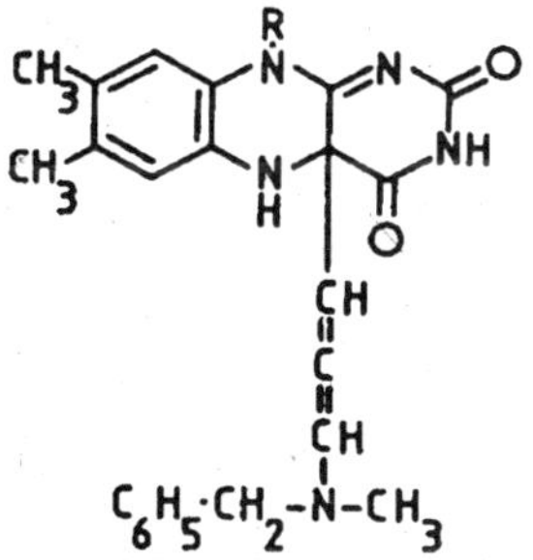

Fig. 2.15 : Structure of pargyline and Flavin-allene adduct

Penicillin irreversibly inactivates a key enzyme responsible for bacterial cell-wall synthesis. Penicillin consists of a thiazolidine ring fused to a β-lactam ring, to which a variable R group is attached by a peptide bond. In benzyl penicillin, R is a benzyl group. The β-lactam ring is very labile and this property is closely tied to the antibiotic action of penicillin.

Penicillin interferes with the synthesis of the bacterial cell wall. The cell wall macromolecule, called as peptidoglycan consists of linear polysaccharide chains that are cross linked by short peptides. The enormous bag shaped peptidoglycan confers the mechanical support and prevents bacteria from bursting due to high internal osmotic pressure (Fig. 2.16).

In 1965, James Park and Jackstorming deduced that penicillin blocks the last step in cell wall synthesis namely the cross-linking of different peptidoglycan strands. This cross-linking reaction is catalyzed by glycopeptide transpeptidase. Penicillin inhibits the cross-linking transpeptidase.

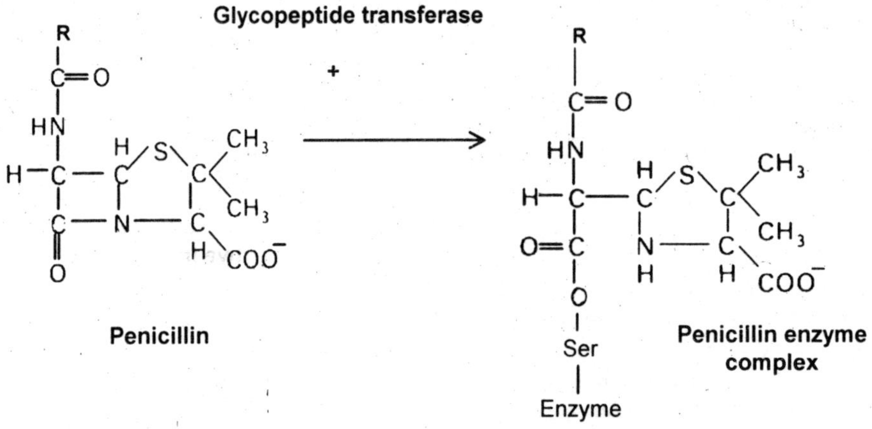

Fig. 2.16 : Inhibition of glycopeptide transpeptidase by penicillin

2.8.2. Reversible inhibition

Reversible inhibition is characterized by a rapid dissociation of the enzyme inhibitor complex. In this type of inhibition, the enzyme can bind with the substrate, forming an [ES] complex. Reversible inhibitors of enzymes have also provided much important information on enzyme structure in regard to the active site present on different enzymes.

There are two types of reversible inhibition

1. Competitive and
2. Non-competitive

2.8.2.1. Competitive inhibition

A competitive inhibitor competes with the substrate for binding to the active site but, once bound, can not be transformed by the enzyme. In competitive inhibition, the enzyme can bind substrate (forming an [ES] complex) or inhibitor (EI complex) but not both at a time (ESI). Competitive inhibitors resemble the substrate and bind to the active site of the enzyme preventing the substrate from binding to the same active site. A competitive inhibitor diminishes the rate of catalysis by reducing the proportion of enzyme molecules bound to a substrate. Competitive inhibition can be reversed or relieved by increasing the substrate concentration. For example. if an enzyme is 50% inhibited at a given concentration of the substrate and competitive inhibitor, we can diminish the per cent inhibition by raising the substrate concentration.

Competitive inhibitors usually resemble the normal substrate in three-dimensional structure. Because of this resemblance the competitive inhibitor 'tricks' the enzyme in binding to it. Competitive inhibition can be quantitatively analyzed by the Michaelis-Menten theory. The competitive inhibitor [I] simply combines reversibly with the enzyme to form [EI] complex. However, the inhibitor [I] cannot be attacked by the enzyme to form new reaction products.

$$E + I \rightleftharpoons EI$$

The classic example of competitive inhibition is the action of malonate on succinate dehydrogenase, a member of the group of enzymes catalyzing the citric acid cycle. This enzyme catalyses the removal of two hydrogen atoms from succinate one from each of the two methylene ($-CH_2-$) groups.

Succinate dehydrogenase is inhibited by malonate, which resembles succinate in having two ionized carboxyl groups at pH 7.0, but differs in having only three carbon atoms. Malonate occupies the active site, keeping the enzyme away from acting on its normal substrate. The reversibility of the inhibition by malonic acid is shown by the fact that increasing the succinate concentration will reduce the extent of inhibition by a given concentration of malonate (Fig. 2.17).

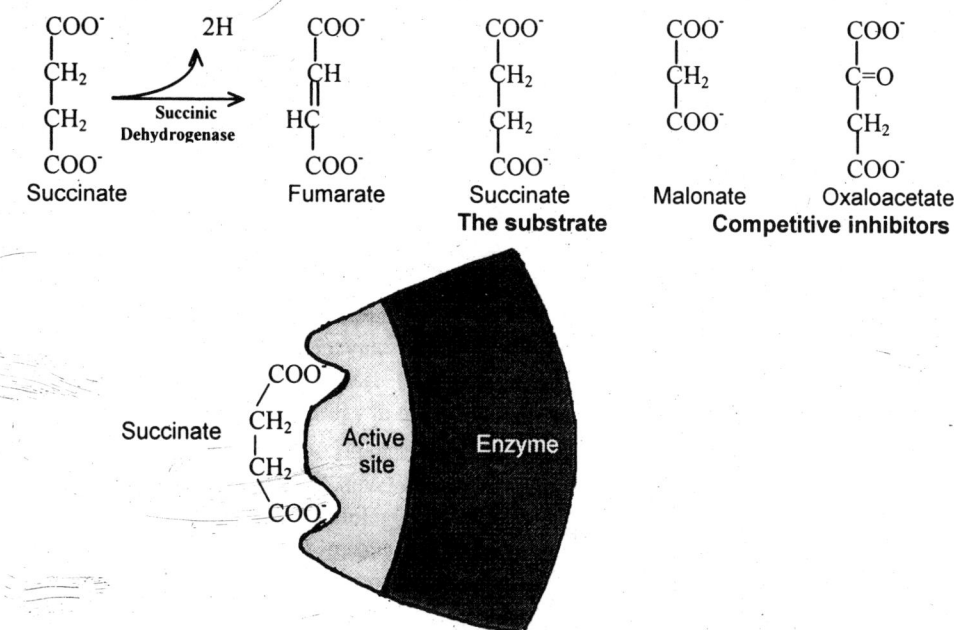

Fig. 2.17 : Succinate dehydrogenase reaction and its competitive inhibition

Ethanol is used therapeutically as a competitive inhibitor to treat Ethylene glycol poisoning. Ethylene glycol itself is not lethal but the harm is accounted for oxalic acid, an oxidation product of ethylene glycol. Kidneys are severely damaged by the deposition of oxalate crystals. Ethylene glycol is oxidized to an aldehyde by the action of enzyme alcohol dehydrogenase. This reaction can be effectively inhibited by administering an intoxicating dose of ethanol (Fig 2.18). Ethanol is a competing substrate for alcohol dehydrogenase and therefore it blocks the oxidation of ethylene glycol to aldehyde products. The ethylene glycol is then excreted harmlessly. Ethanol is also used as a competing substrate for treating methanol poisoning.

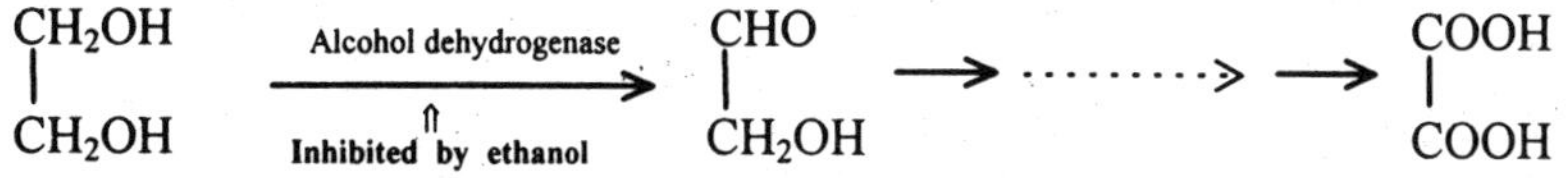

$$\underset{\overset{|}{CH_2OH}}{CH_2OH} \quad \xrightarrow[\text{Inhibited by ethanol}]{\text{Alcohol dehydrogenase}} \quad \underset{\overset{|}{CH_2OH}}{CHO} \quad \longrightarrow \cdots\cdots\cdots\rightarrow \quad \underset{\overset{|}{COOH}}{COOH}$$

Fig. 2.18 : Enzymatic conversion of ethylene glycol to oxalic acid is competitively inhibited by ethanol

In gout, uric acid accumulates in tissues and causes symptoms of gout. Uric acid is formed by oxidation of hypoxanthine by xanthine oxidase. Allopurinol, which has a structural resemblance to hypoxanthine, by competitive inhibition decreases the formation of uric acid (Fig. 2.19). Allopurinol also inhibits the enzymatic oxidation of mercaptopurine, which is used as an antineoplastic antimetabolite.

Monoamine oxidase (MAO) oxidizes pressor amines like adrenaline and noradrenaline. Ephedrine and amphetamine which have similar structure as adrenaline and noradrenaline inhibit monoamine oxidase and thus prolong the action of the pressor amines.

The sulfonamides and sulfones act as antibacterial by competitively inhibiting the incorporation of PABA to form dihydropteroic acid. Similarly trimethoprim is an inhibitor of folate reductase needed to convert dihydrofolic acid (FAH_2) into tetrahydrofolic acid (FAH_4) in bacteria.

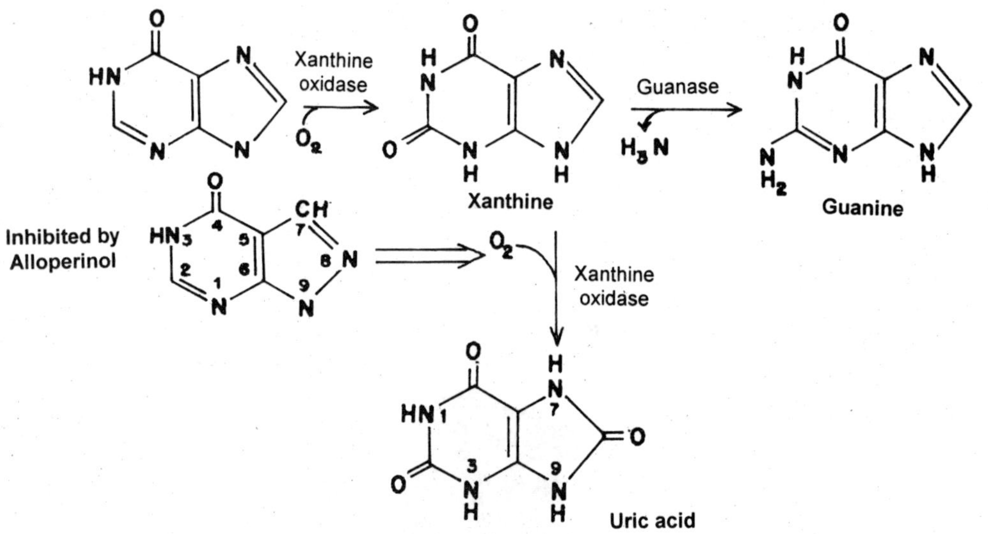

Fig. 2.19: Inhibition of conversion of xanthine to uric acid by allopurinol

In the chemotherapy of malaria tetrahydrofolate synthesis inhibitors are widely used e.g., pyrimethamine, chloroguanide, cycloguanil, trimethoprim, sulfadoxine, sulfadiazine, 4,4'-diaminodiphenylsulfone (DDS) etc. Malarial dihydrofolate reductase is structurally different from mammalian dihydrofolate reductase and is 2,000 times more sensitive to the antimalarial drugs. The malarial protozoa is unable to use pyrimidine nucleoside of host and therefore must synthesize its own, which requires the folinic acid and other tetrahydrofolic acid cofactors. Thus any drug that inhibits the synthesis of dihyrofolic acid in malarial protozoa or selectively inhibits the dihydrofolate reductase of malarial protozoa in turn, will inhibit the growth and kill the protozoa. The biguanides (chloroguanide), diamino-pyrimidines (pyrimethamine) and dihydrotriazines (cyloguanil) are selective inhibitors of malarial protozoa.

Guanosine ······ *p*-Aminobenzoic acid ······> Dihydropteroic acid

⇑

Inhibited by
Sulfonamide, sulfones

Dihydrofolic acid (FAH_2) ——— / ······ Folate reductase ——> / ······> Tetrahydrofolic acid (FAH_4)

⇑

Inhibited by Trimethoprim

········> In Bacteria

——> In Human

2.8.2.2. Noncompetitive inhibition

In non-competitive inhibition, which is a reversible process, the inhibitor substrate can bind simultaneously to an enzyme molecule. In non-competitive inhibition, the inhibitor binds at a site on the enzyme other than the substrate binding site, altering the conformation of the enzyme molecule so that reversible alteration followed by inactivation of the catalytic site results. The binding sites of substrate and inhibitor do not overlap. Non-competitive inhibition, in contrast with competitive inhibition, cannot be circumvented by increasing the substrate concentration (Fig. 2.20). Non-competitive inhibitors bind reversibly to both, the free enzyme and the ES complex to form the inactive complexes EI and ESI:

$$E + I \rightleftharpoons EI$$

$$ES + I \rightleftharpoons ESI$$

for which there are two inhibitor constants:

$$K_I^{ES} = \frac{[E]\,[I]}{[EI]} \qquad\qquad K_I^{ES} = \frac{[ES]\,[I]}{[ESI]}$$

which may or may not be equal.

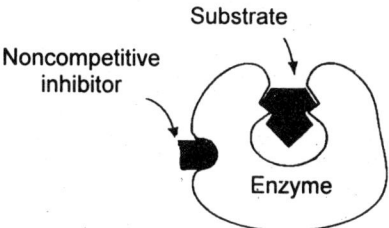

Fig. 2.20 : Noncompetitive inhibition

The most important non-competitive inhibition is given by reagents that can combine reversibly with some functional group of the enzyme (outside the active site) that is essential for maintaining the catalytically active three dimensional conformation of the enzyme molecule. Some enzymes possessing -SH group are non-competitively inhibited by heavy metal ions. Some enzymes that require metal ions for activity are inhibited noncompetitively by agents capable of binding the essential metal. For example, the chelating agent EDTA reversibly binds Mg^{++} and other bivalent cations and thus non-competitively inhibits some enzymes requiring such ions for activity.

Noncompetitive inhibitors are exemplified by cyanides which are capable of strongly binding with the trivalent iron forming part of the catalytic moiety of hemin enzyme, cytochrome oxidase. Blocking of this enzyme switches the respiratory chain off, and the cell can no longer exist. Heavy metal ions and their organic compounds belong to noncompetitive inhibitors of enzymes and due to this reason they are very toxic in nature (mercury, lead, arsenic, etc.). For example they can block the S-H groups that make part of the catalytic site of an enzyme (Fig. 2.21). The complex enzyme-inhibitor can add a substrate, but subsequently no conversion of the substrate occurs, since the catalytic site of enzyme remain blocked.

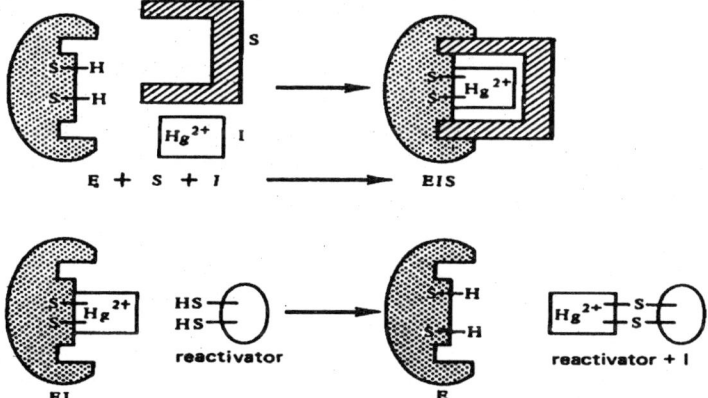

Fig. 2.21 : Action of noncompetitive inhibitor (mercury ions) and mechanism for reactivation of an enzyme blocked by noncmpetitive inhibitor.

2.8.3. Kinetics of competitive and non-competitive inhibition

Competitive and non-competitive inhibitions are kinetically distinguishable by the use of double reciprocal plot. In competitive inhibition, the intercept of the plot of 1/V vs 1/[S] is the same in the presence and absence of inhibitor, although the slope is different (Fig. 2.22).

$$E + I \rightleftharpoons EI$$

$$ES + I \rightleftharpoons ESI$$

This reflects the fact that V_{max} is not altered by a competitive inhibitor. Competitive inhibition can be overcome by a sufficiently high concentration of substrate. At a sufficiently high concentration, virtually all the active sites are occupied by substrate and the enzyme turns to be fully operative. The increase in the slope of the plot indicates the strength of binding of competitive inhibitor.

In the presence of a competitive inhibitor:

$$\frac{1}{V_o} = \frac{1}{V_{max}} + \frac{K_m}{V_{max}} \frac{(K_i + [I])}{Ki} \frac{1}{[S]} \qquad \text{---(2.16)}$$

in which [I] is the concentration of inhibitor and K_i is the dissociation constant of [EI] complex.

$$E + I \rightleftharpoons EI$$

$$K_i = \frac{[E][I]}{[EI]} \qquad \text{---(2.17)}$$

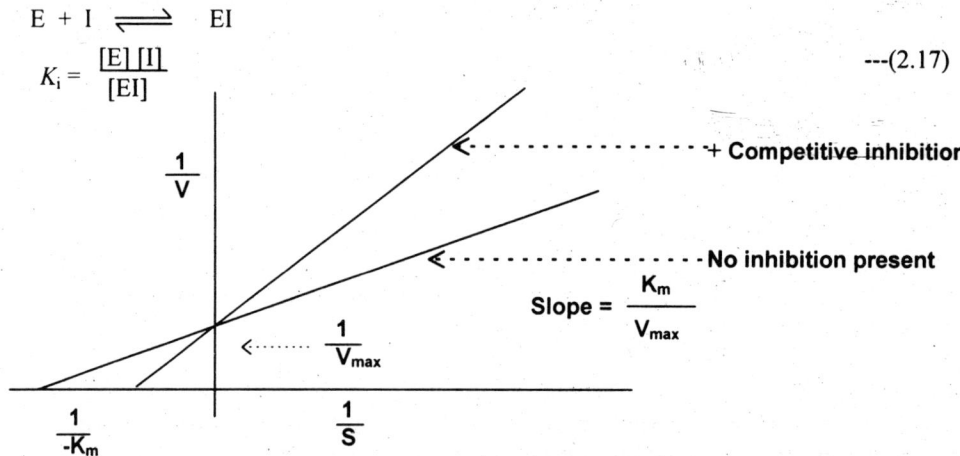

Fig. 2.22 : A Lineweaver-Burk plot of enzyme kinetics in the presence and absence of competitive inhibitor.

The slope of curve is increased by the factor $(1 + [I]/K_i)$ in the presence of a competitive inhibitor.

In noncompetitive inhibition V_{max} is decreased to V'_{max}, and so intercept on the vertical axis is increased. The new slope which is equal to K_m/V'_{max} is larger by the same factor (Fig. 2.23). In contrast with V_{max}, and K_m are not affected by this kind of inhibition.

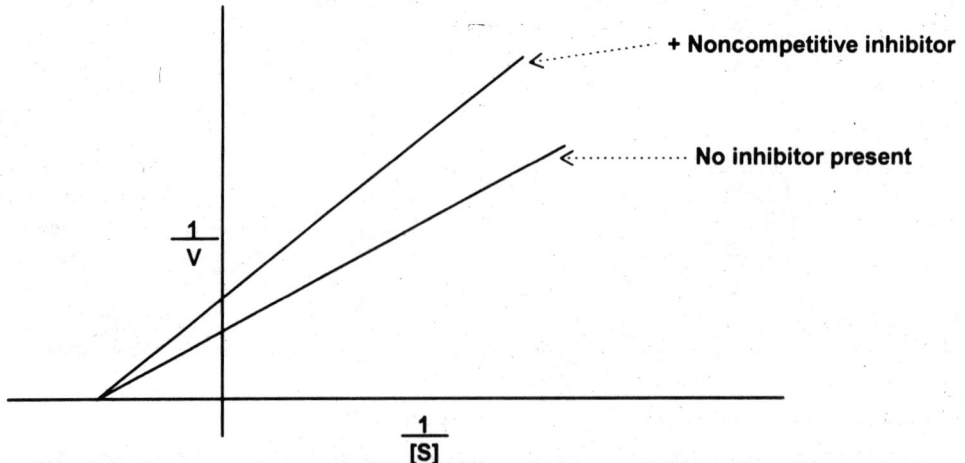

Fig. 2.23 : A Lineweaver-Burk plot of enzyme kinetics in the presence and absence of noncompetitive inhibitor.

Non-competitive inhibition cannot be overcome by increasing the substrate concentration. The maximum velocity in the presence of a non-competitive inhibitor V'_{max} is given by:

$$V'_{max} = \frac{V_{max}}{1 + [I]/K_i}$$

---(2.18)

2.9. REGULATION OF ENZYME ACTIVITY

The net flow of carbon through any enzyme catalyzed reaction might be influenced by
1. Changing the absolute quantity of enzyme present
2. Altering the pool size of reactants other than enzyme, and
3. Altering the catalytic efficiency of enzyme.

2.9.1. Regulation of enzyme quantity

Regulation of enzyme quantity is determined by the net balance between enzyme synthesis and enzyme degradation. The enzyme level in a cell can be changed by either increasing its rate of synthesis or by either decreasing its rate of degradation or combination of both. The net result will be an increased enzyme level. The enzyme quantity at a particular time in a particular cell can be affected by various factors outlined below :
1. Genetic basis - Increased rate of enzyme synthesis
2. Induction - Increased rate of enzyme synthesis
3. Repression and depression - Decreased rate of enzyme degradation

2.9.1.1. Control of enzyme synthesis
2.9.1.1.1. Genetic basis

An enzyme that is protein in nature is essentially expressed by its respective gene contained in master genome. The expression typically remains to be the same as discussed for protein synthesis later in this book. The structure of enzyme is determined by the trinucleotide code contained in RNA that is attached to polyribosomes. The ribosomal RNA contains anticodon for the tRNA-amino acid complex. Thus serves as adapter molecule. The mRNA contains codon component of gene whereas tRNA bears anticodon to mRNA. The primary structure of an enzyme is dictated by the trinucleotide (triplet) code of necessary RNA attached to polyribosomes and by the matching bases of a transfer RNA-amino acid complex. The sequence of purine and pyrimidine bases of the messenger RNA is in turn dictated by a complementary base sequence that is part of a master DNA template or gene in the nucleus of the cell. Information for protein synthesis stored in DNA, thus determines a cell's ability to synthesize a particular enzyme. One gene generally codes for one polypeptide, and two genes for a protein containing two dissimilar polypeptides. It has been suggested that proteins of the bacteriophage ϕX 174 are coded not for a single protein, however they are coded for two different polypeptides. For example, the sequence GAAUAGA is read both as GAA-UAG and AAU-AGA.

Mutational changes alter the DNA code and result in to the synthesis of a protein molecule with a modified primary structure. In some cases, this may result in altered structures at higher levels of organization also. If the mutation results in change which is not lethal, the modified genetic information is transmitted to the progeny of the cell. As a result, there frequently arises a transmissible metabolic defect, which occurs at the step formerly catalyzed by the new defective enzyme. Many human genetic diseases are known in which one enzyme or another is either totally inactive or is otherwise defective in the catalytic or regulatory functions. In such diseases (Table 2.11) the defective enzyme molecule may contain one or more wrong amino acids in its polypeptide chain(s) as a result of a mutation of the DNA coding for it.

2.9.1.1.2. Induction

The rate of enzyme synthesis can be induced by various molecules which act as inducers. For a molecule to be metabolized or for an inducer to act, it must first enter the cell. In some cases, a specific transport system or **permease** is needed. The permease itself may be inducible. Permeases share many properties in common with enzymes and appear to perform functions analogous to the cytochromes in electron transport insofar as they appear to transport substrates without causing a net change in substrate structure.

Table 2.11 : Some human genetic disease with specific defective enzyme

Disease	Defective enzyme
Albinism	Tyrosine 3-monooxygenase
Alkeptoneuria	Homgentisate 12-dioxygenase
Galactosemia	Galactose 1-phosphate uridylyl transferase
Homocysteinuria	Cystathionine β-synthase
Phenylketoneuria	Phenylalanine 4-monooxygenase
Tay-Sachs disease	Hexosaminidase A

The phenomenon of enzyme induction is explained with the help of the example of *Escherichia coli* (*E. coli*). *E. coli* grown on glucose does not ferment lactose, due to the absence both of a specific permease for a β-galactoside (lactose) and of the enzyme β-galactosidase, which hydrolyses lactose to glucose and galactose. If lactose or certain other β-galactosidase are induced then the culture can ferment lactose. Although, in general inducers serve as substrates for the enzymes or permeases, they induce compounds structurally similar to the substrate which may be inducers but not substrates. They are termed as **gratutious inducers**.

Variations in induction patterns in bacteria also occur at the genetic level where the structured genes which specify a group of catabolic enzymes comprise of an operon, all the enzymes expressed by operon are induced by a single inducer. This phenomenon is termed as co-ordinate induction.

2.9.1.1.3. Repression and depression

Presence of specific amino acids in the culture media curtails the synthesis of amino acid by bacteria via **repression**. A small molecule such as histidine or leucine, acting as a co-repressor, can ultimately block the synthesis of the enzymes involved in its own biosynthesis. In *Salmonella* species, addition of histidine, and addition of leucine represses synthesis of the first three enzymes unique to leucine biosynthesis. In both cases, these biosynthetic enzymes comprised of operons; co-ordinate repression occurs following addition of the end products histidine or leucine. However, this mode is not general for all biosynthetic pathways since the genetic information specifying the structure of biosynthetic enzymes may be organized into more than one operon. Following removal or exhaustion of an essential biosynthetic intermediate from the medium, the genetic information coding for the biosynthesis of enzymes is again expressed. This constitutes, what is termed **depression**, may be co-ordinate or non-coordinate.

2.9.1.2. Enzyme turnover

The combined processes of enzyme synthesis and degradation constitute enzyme turnover. While turnover occurs both in bacteria and mammals, the enzyme levels are regulated on this basis. **Schoenheimer's classical work** suggests that body proteins are in a state of 'dynamic equilibrium', a concept extended to other body constituents, including lipids and nucleic acids. In man and other animals, the regulation of intracellular levels of enzymes thus involves regulation of both enzyme synthesis and of enzyme degradation.

There is now considerable evidence that enzyme levels in mammalian tissues may be altered by a wide range of physiologic, hormonal or dietary manipulations. Glucocorticoids increase the concentration of tyrosine transaminase by stimulating its rate of synthesis. Insulin and glucagon despite their mutually antagonistic physiologic effects, both independently increase the rate of synthesis by 4 to 5 folds. Similarly, the activity of 8-aminolevullinate synthase, is increased as much as 50 fold by drugs which produce experimental prophyria, and this effect is blocked by glucose.

2.9.2. Availability of reactants

Kinetic and regulatory properties of enzymes have value with respect to insights into physiological processes in intact cells, tissues and organisms. The localization of specific metabolic processes in the cytosol or within specific cellular organelles permits regulation of these processes. The extensive compartmentation of metabolic processes has potential for a sophisticated and finely tuned regulation of metabolism. The translocation of essential metabolites across compartmental barriers may be achieved via shuttle mechanisms. In general, these shuttle mechanisms involve conversion of the material to be translocated in to a form permeable to the compartmental barrier. This is followed by transport and conversion back to the original form on the other side of the barrier. Consequently, these interconversions require, for example, cytosolic and mitochondrial forms of the same catalytic activity.

2.9.2.1. Effective concentrations of substrates and coenzymes

The mean cellular concentrations of a substrate; coenzyme or metal ion do not have any significant relationship with respect to the *in vivo* enzyme activity. However, the concentration of essential metabolites in the neighborhood of the enzyme in question is of importance. Measuring this metabolite concentration within the cellular compartments is however of little importance. The total concentration of 2,3-diphosphoglycerate, in erythrocytes is extremely high, although the concentration of free diphosphoglycerate is probably comparable to that of other tissues. This is due to the binding of diphosphoglycerate with hemoglobin.

A more sophisticated kinetic approach for *in vivo* situation employs an equation of the Michaelis-Menten form, but assumes steady state kinetics: where S_f, is the concentration of free substrate but it does not hold for macromolecular complexes.

$$V = \frac{K E_t S_f}{K_m + S_f} \qquad\qquad --- (2.19)$$

2.9.2.2. Compartmentation of enzyme and enzyme system

In eukaryotic cells, different enzymes and enzyme systems are segregated into the various organelles and intracellular structures. This facilitates regulation of various processes independently. Table 2.12 lists the intracellular distribution of some important enzymes and metabolic sequences in a model mammalian cell.

Table 2.12 : Compartmentation of some major enzymes and metabolic processes

Cell structure	Enzyme
Plasma membrane	Amino acid transport systems, Na^+-K^+ATPase
Cytosol	Glycolysis, glyconeogenesis and glycogenesis, HMP pathway fatty acid synthesis, purine and pyrimidine catabolism, amino acyl-tRNA synthetase
Mitochondria	Tricarboxylic acid cycle, electron transport and oxidative phosphorylation, fatty acid oxidation, urea synthesis
Nucleus	DNA and RNA synthesis
Endoplasmic reticulum (Rough and Smooth)	Protein synthesis, steroid synthesis, glycosylation, detoxification
Lysosomes	Hydrolases
Golgi apparatus	Glycosyl transferases, glucose-5-phosphatase, formation of plasma membrane and secretery vesicles
Peroxizomes	Catalase, D-amino oxidase, urate oxidase

Some processes such as urea biosynthesis and gluconeogenesis, depend on the interplay of reactions occurring in more than one compartment. A further extension of spatial organization occurs in multicellular organisms in which different tissues have their distinctive metabolic characteristics that are subjected to control in response to special needs of the organism.

2.9.2.3. Role of metal ions

Bacterial glutamine synthetase offers well documented example of metal ion regulated enzyme activity. In the absence of metal ions *E. coli* glutamine synthetase assumes a relaxed configuration that is catalytically inactive.

Addition of Mg^{2+} or Mn^{2+} converts the synthetase to the active 'tightened' form. In addition to metal ion regulated these conformational changes, adenylation of the synthetase causes a complete change in divalent cation specificity. Another example is carbonic anhydrase which requires zinc ion for its activity. Removal of zinc from carbonic anhydrase leads to the loss of activity. Furthermore, no other ion has been found to replace zinc from the enzyme. Some other similar enzymes are listed in table 2.2 which require metal ion for their activity.

2.9.2.4. Macromolecular complexes

Organization of enzymes catalyzing a protected sequence of metabolic reactions is a macromolecular complex series that co-ordinates the activities of the enzymes concernes and channelises intermediates along a chosen metabolic pathway. Appropriate alignment of the enzymes can facilitate transfer of product from one enzyme to other enzyme without prior equilibration and without the metabolic pool formation of the intermediates. This permits a finer level of metabolic control than is possible without the isolated component of the complex.

Conformational changes in one component of the complex may be transmitted by protein-protein interaction to other enzyme of the complex. Amplification of regulatory effects is thus readily achieved. Consider the case of the combined dehydrogenation and decarboxylation of pyruvate to acetyl-CoA isomer, there is a segmental action of three different enzymes of pyruvate dehydrogenase complex viz. pyruvate dehydrogenase E1, dehydrolipoyl transacetylase E2, dihydrolipoyl dehydrogenase together working with five different coenzymes thyamine pyrophosphate (TPP), flavin adenine dinucleotide (FAD), coenzyme A (CoA), nicotinamide dinucleotide (NAD) and lipoic acid. These enzymes and coenzymes are organized into a multienzyme cluster.

2.9.3. Regulation of catalytic efficiency

Changes in the enzyme activity that occur independence of the quantity of enzyme present, can be designated as effects on catalytic efficiency. In cell metabolism, groups of enzymes work together in sequential chain or systems to carry out a given metabolic process, such as the conversion of glucose into lactic acid in skeletal muscles or the synthesis of an amino acid from simpler precursors. In such enzyme systems the reaction product of the first enzyme becomes the substrate of the next and so on.

In each enzyme system there is at least one enzyme, the **pacemaker** that sets the rate of the overall reaction because it catalyses the slowest or rate-limiting step. Such pacemaker enzymes not only have a catalytic function but also have capabilities of increasing or decreasing their catalytic activity in response to certain signals. These pacemaker enzymes, whose activity is modulated through various types of molecular signals, are called **regulatory enzymes**. There are two major classes of regulatory enzymes: allosteric or noncovalently regulated enzymes (described elsewhere) and covalently regulated enzymes.

2.9.3.1. Cascade system or covalent modification

The catalytic properties of some enzymes are markedly altered by the covalent attachment of some small groups. Enzyme activity is regulated by cyclic interconversion of enzyme into two forms modified form and unmodified form. The interconversions brought about by a "converting enzyme" which together with the two forms of the enzyme (modified and unmodified) constitutes a cascade system.

In many of these enzymes, the modification involves phosphorylation of the enzyme at a -OH group of serine, threonine or tyrosine. Such cascade systems include liver phosphorylase, glycogen synthetase, etc. The converter enzymes are usually protein kinases and themselves exist in an inactive form and require to be activated by substances like cyclic AMP. The production of cyclic AMP is in turn regulated by an enzyme *adenyl cyclase* under hormonal control.

Regulatory enzyme glycogen phosphorylase of muscle and liver catalyses the reaction :

$$(\text{Glucose})_n + \text{Phosphate} \longrightarrow (\text{Glucose})_{n-1} + \text{glucose-1-phosphate}$$

Glycogen Shortened glycogen chain

The glucose-1-phosphate so formed is then broken down into lactic acid in the muscles or into free glucose in the liver.

The enzyme glycogen phosphorylase occurs in two forms:
1. The active form phosphorylase *a*, and
2. The relatively inactive form phosphorylase *b*.

Phosphorylase *a* has two polypetide chain subunits, each with one specific serine residue in its sequence that is phosphorylated at its hydroxyl group. These serine phosphate residues are required for maximum activity of the enzyme. The phosphate group can be hydrolytically removed from phosphorylase-*a* by an enzyme called phosphorylase phosphatase.

$$\text{Phosphorylase } \boldsymbol{a} + 2H_2O \xrightarrow{\hspace{4cm}} \text{Phosphorylase } \boldsymbol{b} + 2Pi$$
$$\text{(More active)} \hspace{6cm} \text{(Less active)}$$

Thus the active form of glucagon phosphorylase is converted into the relatively inactive form due to the cleavage of the two covalent bonds between the phosphoric acid and the two specific serine residues in the enzyme. Phosphorylase *b* can intern be reactivated i.e., covalently transformed back into active phosphorylase *a* by another enzyme phosphorylase kinase. The enzyme catalyses the transfer of phosphate groups from ATP to the hydroalkyl groups of the specific serine residue in phosphorylase *b* (Fig. 2.24).

$$2ATP + \text{Phosphorylase } \boldsymbol{b} \xrightarrow{\hspace{4cm}} 2ADP + \text{Phosphorylase } \boldsymbol{a}$$
$$\text{(less active)} \hspace{6cm} \text{(more active)}$$

The breakdown of glycogen in skeletal muscles and in the liver is regulated by alteration in the ratio of the active and inactive forms of enzyme.

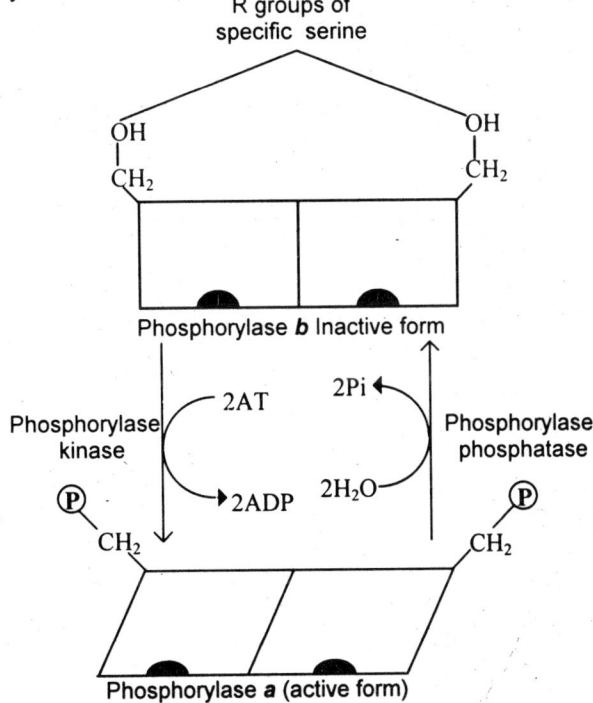

Fig. 2.24 : Regulation of Glycogen phosphorylase by covalent modification

2.9.3.2. Isoenzymes (multiple form)

Many enzymes occur in more than one molecular forms in the same species, at the same time or even in the same cell. In such cases the different forms of the enzymes may catalyze the same reaction, however they have different kinetic properties and different sequence of amino acids. These could be very well distinguished and separated by the application of appropriate procedures. These multiple forms of enzymes are named as **isoenzymes** or **isozymes**.

Isoenzymes are physically distinct forms having the same catalytic activity, thus they catalyze the same reaction. Medical interest in isoenzyme was stimulated by the discovery in 1957 that human serum contained several lactate dehydrogenates isoenzymes and that their relative proportions that change significantly in certain pathologic conditions. Lactate dehydrogenase catalyses the reversible oxidation of lactate to pyruvate.

$$\text{Lactate} + NAD^+ \rightleftharpoons \text{Pyruvate} + NADH + H^+$$

Lactate dehydrogenase occurs in animal tissue as five different isoenzymes separable by electrophoresis at pH 8.6, using a starch agar or a polyacrylamide gel supporting medium. The isoenzymes have different charges at this pH and migrate to 5 regions of the electrophoretogram. Isoenzymes are then identified by enzyme catalyzed reduction of a colorless dye to a specific colored form. All the lactate dehydrogenase isoenzymes contain four polypeptide chains, each of molecular weight 33,500, but the five isoenzymes contain varying ratio of two kinds of polypeptides which differ in composition and sequence. The active lactate dehydrogenase molecule consists of 4 subunits of 2 types, A chains (also designated as M) and B chains (also designated as H). Only the tetrameric molecule possesses catalytic activity. In skeletal muscle the lactate dehydrogenase isoenzyme that predominates contains four A chains, and in heart the predominately isoenzyme contains four B chains. In other tissues it exists as a mixture of five possible forms, which may be designated as AAAA, AAAB, AABB, ABBB and BBBB.

2.9.3.1. Proenzymes

Regulation of the activity of the enzymes could be achieved by the synthesis of the enzyme in a catalytically inactive or proenzyme forms. Conversion of the proenzyme to the active enzyme is catalyzed either by proteolytic enzymes or by hydrogen ions. Various proenzymes and their respective enzymes are listed in table 2.13.

Table 2.13 : Various proenzymes and their enzymes

Proenzyme		Enzyme
Pepsinogen	$\xrightarrow{\text{H+ or pepsin}}$	Pepsin
Trypsinogen	$\xrightarrow{\text{Trypsin or enterokinase}}$	Trypsin
Chymotrypsinogen	$\xrightarrow{\text{Trypsin}}$	Chymotrypsin
Procarboxypeptidase	$\xrightarrow{\text{Trypsin}}$	Carboxypeptidase

Similarly, conversion of fibrinogen to fibrin involves limited proteolysis catalyzed by thrombin. Under normal physiologic conditions, thrombin exists as the inactive precursor of prothrombin. These involve a cascade of activation reactions, many of which are based on proteolysis. Limited proteolysis is thus one of the key regulatory factor in the complex process of blood coagulation.

2.10. ALLOSTERIC ENZYMES

Allosteric term is derived from Greek 'allo' means other and 'stereos' means space or site. Allosteric enzymes are those having other sites. The properties of allosteric enzymes are significantly different from those of simple nonregulatory enzymes and they include:

1. Like all enzymes allosteric enzymes have catalytic sites which bind the substrate and transform it but they also have one or more regulatory or allosteric sites for binding the regulating metabolites which are called the **effectors** or **modulators**. The allosteric enzymes are specific in regard to their modulators as the catalytic

sites are specific for the substrate (Fig. 2.25). Many allosteric enzymes have the substrate binding site and the modulator binding site on different subunits, which are referred as the catalytic [C] and regulation [R] subunits respectively. Binding of the positive modulator M to its specific site on the regulatory subunit is communicated to the catalytic subunit through a conformational change rendering the catalytic subunit active and capable of binding the substrate S with high affinity. On dissociation of the modulator M from the regulatory subunit the enzyme reverts to its inactive or less active form. The enzyme is specific for its substrate, whereas the allosteric site is specific for its modulator.

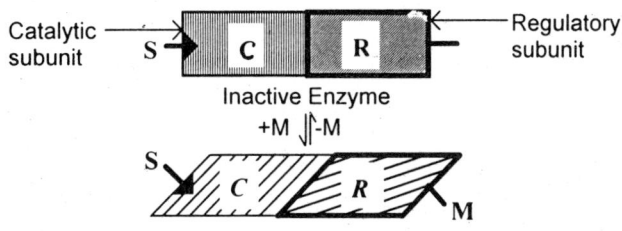

Fig. 2.25 : Activation of allosteric enzyme by conformational change

2. Allosteric enzyme molecules are generally larger and more complex than those of simple enzymes. Most of them have two or more polypeptide chains or subunits.
3. Allosteric enzymes usually show significant deviation from classical Michaelis-Menten theory.
4. They are inhibited by the end product of multienzyme system.
5. Treatment with mercurials, urea, proteolytic enzymes, high or low pH, etc. may produce loss of feedback control with retention of catalytic activity.
6. Many allosteric effectors confer enhanced resistance to heat denaturation of the allosteric enzyme.
7. Unlike most enzymes, regulatory enzymes undergo reversible inactivation at 0°C.
8. All known allosteric enzymes possess tertiary, and in some cases also quaternary structure.

In some multienzyme systems the first or regulatory enzyme, is inhibited by the end product of the multienzyme reaction process. When the concentration of the end product of such a metabolic sequence increases above its normal steady state concentration, indicating that it is being produced in an excess of the cell's needs, the end product of the sequence acts as a specific inhibitor of the first, or regulatory enzyme of the sequence. The whole enzyme system thus slows down to reduce the rate of end product formation. This is known as *feedback inhibition* mechanism.

A classical example of this type of inhibition is the conversion of L-threonine to L-isoleucine using bacterial enzyme system. In this sequence of five enzymes, the first, threonine dehydrogenase, is inhibited by isoleucine, the end product of enzyme reaction. No other enzyme of this sequence gets inhibited by isoleucine, nor the intermediates in this sequence of reaction, are inhibitory to the threonine dehydrogenase. This inhibition is reversible, when the isoleucine concentration decreases, the activity of threonine dehydrogenase increases (Fig. 2.26). The binding of isoleucine to the regulatory site of threonine dehydrogenase is noncovalent thus it is readily reversible.

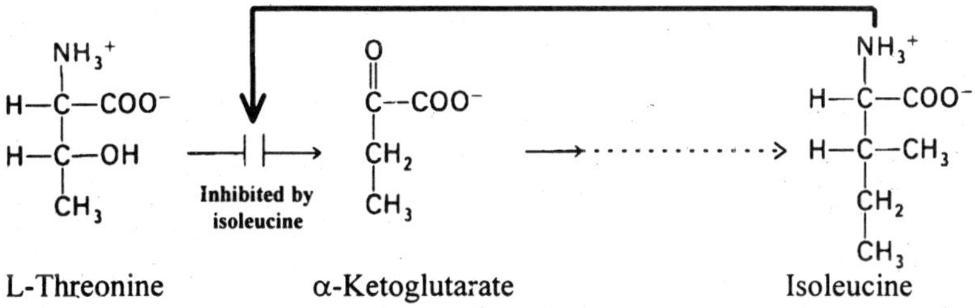

L-Threonine   α-Ketoglutarate   Isoleucine

Fig. 2.26 : Feedback inhibition of conversion of L-threonine to isoleucine

2.10.1. Effect of modulators

Allosteric enzymes may be inhibited or stimulated by their modulators. When the allosteric site is occupied by a specific inhibitory or negative modulator, which happens when the modulator concentration in the cell rises as a result the enzyme undergoes a change to a less active or inactive form, in other words it is 'turned off'. When the inhibitory modulator leaves the allosteric site with decreasing modulator concentration in the cell, the enzyme is switched back to its active or 'on' form. The negative modulator is generally the end product of the enzyme reaction. This type of allosteric enzymes are known as **heterotropic enzymes**.

There are also allosteric enzymes which are stimulated by their modulator molecules. In this case the stimulatory or positive modulator is not the end product of the enzymes reaction sequence but some other metabolite that serves as the molecular signal to the enzyme to speed up the catalytic activity. The stimulatory modulation of this type is often brought about by the substrate molecule itself. Allosteric enzyme belonging to **homotropic class** (because the substrate and modulator are identical), involve two or more steps for substrate binding, particularly when modulator is other than the substrate (heterotropic).

Some allosteric enzymes may have two or more modulators, may be opposite in effect, so that one or more modulators of the enzyme are stimulatory likewise one or more may be inhibitory. In these, more complex enzyme reactions, each modulator has its own specific allosteric site, which when occupied, signals the enzyme either to speed up its catalytic action or slow it down (Fig. 2.27).

Hemoglobin is an allosteric protein. Once the first haem-polypeptide subunit of a hemoglobin molecule binds an oxygen molecule, it communicates this information to the remaining subunits, which respond by greatly increasing their oxygen affinity. Such communication amongst the four haem-polypeptide subunits of hemoglobin, is the result of co-operative interaction between the subunits. Because binding of one molecule of oxygen increases the probability that further molecules of oxygen will be bound to the remaining subunits, so this is known as **positive co-operativity**.

Fig. 2.27 : Linear pattern of allosteric modulation showing stimulatory and inhibitory regulations

Aspartate transcarbamoylase is feed back inhibited by cytidine-s-triphosphate (CTP), the final product of the pyrimidine pathway. Pryimidine biosynthesis begins with the formation of N-carbamoyl-aspartate from aspartate and carbamoyl phosphate. The reaction is catalyzed by aspartate transcarbamoylase (ATCase). The enzyme ATCase is feed back inhibited by the final product of the synthesis cytidine-s-triphosphate (CTP) (Fig. 2.28).

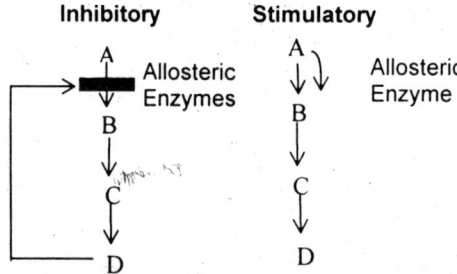

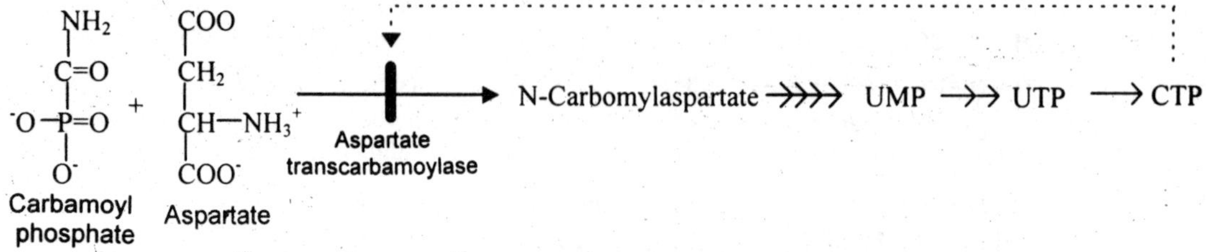

Fig. 2.28 : Feedback inhibition of aspartate transcarbomylase by CTP

The binding of carbamoyl phosphate and aspartate is co-operative as reflected in sigmoidal dependence of reaction velocity on substrate concentration. Co-operative binding seems to switch on the synthesis of N-carbamoylaspartate, over a narrow range of concentration of substrates. The regulation of the rate of pyrimidine nucleotide synthesis operates through the enzyme aspartate trancarbamoylase which catalyses the first reaction of the sequence. This enzyme is inhibited by cytidine-s-triphosphate (CTP) the end product of this sequence of reactions.

The ATCase molecule consists of six catalytic subunits and six regulatory subunits. The catalytic subunits bind the substrate molecules and the allosteric subunits bind the allosteric inhibitor CTP. The entire ATCase molecule, as well as its subunits, exist in two conformations, active and inactive. When the regulatory subunits are unoccupied, the enzyme is maximally active. However, when CTP accumulates it is bound to the regulatory subunits to cause a change in their conformation. This change is transmitted to the catalytic subunits which then transform to an inactive conformation. The presence of ATP prevents the changes induced by CTP (Fig. 2.29).

2.10.2. Model for allosteric enzymes

Two models have been proposed to explain the mechanism of regulation of allosteric enzymes :
1. Concerted model proposed by Monod-Wyman-Changeua and
2. Sequential model proposed by Koshland, Nemethy and Filmer.

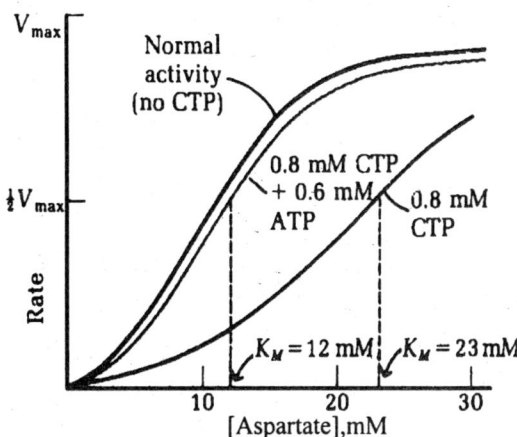

Fig. 2.29 : Effect of various modulator on the catalytic activity of aspartate transcarbamoylase

2.10.2.1. The Monod-Wyman-Changeua (MWC) concerted model

The simple model explain the sigmoid binding curve by assuming:
1. Allosteric enzymes are oligomeric, composed of definite numbers of protomeric subunits.
2. Each protomer exists in two conformational states in equilibrium, a relaxed (R) form with a higher affinity for substrate and a tense (T) form with a lower affinity which is predominant form when unliganded, and
3. The conformational change from T (represented by □) to R (represented by O) occurs with conservation of symmetry, i.e., all subunits in each state have the same conformation and the same intrinsic ligand affinity.

According to this model, the binding of one molecule enhances the rate of binding of other substrate molecules as a result of binding site interaction in which conversion from one state to another is concerted with all subunits underlying a simultaneous transition. For an allosteric dimer the substrate binding can be represented as shown in figure 2.30.

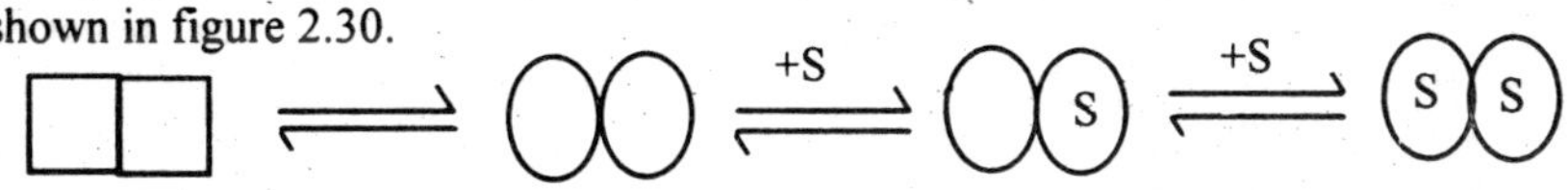

Fig. 2.30 : Representation of substrate binding to an allosteric dimer

It is also proposed that substrate molecules have higher affinity to bind with the relaxed state than with the tense state. Formation of RS will reduce the R-state concentration of enzyme, but since this state is in equilibrium with the T-form some of this will be relaxed. If initially very little of the R-state is present i.e., if the ratio T/R of the unliganded species is large, the relative amount of the T-state converted to the R-state on substrate binding will also be large, however if the enzyme already exists predominately in the relaxed state the relative amount of conformational change will be small. The ratio T/R is called the *allosteric constant* (L). Greater is the numerical value of L, the greater is the degree of the co-operativity between subunits and if the L is small so that essentially all the enzyme is in the R-state then there will be no co-operative subunit interaction.

This model is able to explain the theoretical curves based on the allosteric constant (L), the dissociation constant (K_R) for substrate binding to the tense state, which is suitable for the hemoglobin oxygen binding. This model have limitation that only positive and negative co-operativity is predicted. This model can be applied to symmetrical enzymes only.

2.10.2.2. The Koshland-Nemethy-Filmer (KNF) sequential model

This model makes four assumptions :
1. There are only two conformational state (R and T) accessible to any subunit.
2. Only one unliganded conformational state exists for an enzyme.
3. The association of a ligand molecule with one subunit induces a conformational change in that subunit which is transmitted to adjacent unfilled subunits so altering their ligand association.
4. The conformational change elicited by the binding of substrate in one subunit can decrease the substrate-binding affinity of other subunits in the same enzyme molecule.

The binding process in an allosteric enzyme according to this model is shown in figure 2.31 where K_1 and K_2 are association constants.

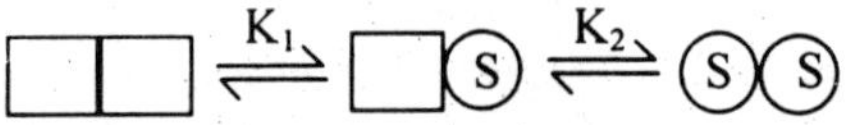

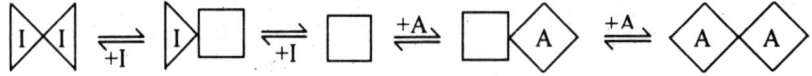

Fig. 2.31 : Binding of substrate to an allosteric dimmer according to the sequential model

Each subunit can exist in two conformational states, □ and O; binding of the substrate to a subunit changes its conformation, in this case from □ to O. The result of this conformational change is an alteration in the specificity and strength of the intersubunits contacts. They could facilitate subsequent substrate binding, to elicit positive co-operativity.

This model can also be extended to the association of inhibitors and activators (Fig. 2.32).

Fig. 2.32. : Binding of activators and inhibitors

The differences between this and concerted model are:
1. It does not assumes an equilibrium between R and T forms in the absence of substrate;
2. The involvement of mixed intermediate formed as a consequence of the subunits undergoing conformational changes in sequence; and
3. Negative co-operativity can be accounted for, since the model assumes that symmetry is not conserved on ligand binding, the conformational transitions each subunit undergoes depends on the energy of activation.

2.10.3. Kinetics of allosteric enzymes

Allosteric enzymes usually differ from classical Michaelis Menten relationship between substrate concentration and reaction rate, because their rate is dependent on enzyme modulator whether it is inhibitory or stimulatory in nature. Many allosteric enzymes, especially homologous exhibit a sigmoid curve (Fig. 2.33.A) relating initial velocity to substrate concentration, as compared to the rectangular hyperbola yielded by the Michaelis-Menten relationship. The sigmoid curve implies the binding of the first substrate molecule to the enzyme, supports the binding of the subsequent substrate molecules to the other substrate molecules or the enzyme as well as other molecule to the other substrate sites e.g., binding of oxygen to hemoglobin enhances the binding of subsequent oxygen molecules. Such sigmoid curves are examples of positive co-operativity. This accounts for the sigmoid rather than hyperbolic increase in the rate of enzyme activity on increasing the substrate concentration (Fig. 2.33 A). In some types of allosteric enzymes, binding one substrate molecules decreases the binding of subsequent substrate molecules. This is an example of negative co-operativity. This results in a flattened plot of initial reaction velocity versus substrate concentration. A small change in substrate concentration is ineffective and saturation is achieved more slowly as compared to non regulatory or positive co-operative enzymes (Fig. 2.33 B).

Homotropic allosteric enzyme has multiple binding sites for its substrate and acts co-operatively, so that the binding of one molecule of the substrate greatly enhances the binding of subsequent substrate molecules. In case of heterotropic enzymes, where the modulator is some metabolite other than the substrate itself, the shape of curve is related to whether the modulator is positive (stimulatory) or negative (inhibitory). If the modulator is positive, it may cause the substrate saturation curve to become more hyperbolic, with a decrease in $K_{0.5}$ but no change in V_{max}, thus resulting into an increased rate at a fixed substrate concentration (Fig. 2.33B). Other allosteric enzymes respond to a stimulatory modulator by an increase in V_{max}, with little change in $K_{0.5}$ (Fig. 2.33 C). If the modulator is negative or inhibitory, the substrate saturation curve may become more sigmoid, with an increase in $K_{0.5}$ (Fig. 2.33B). Allosteric enzymes therefore show different types of responses in their substrate activity curves because some have inhibitory modulators, some have stimulatory modulators, and some have both.

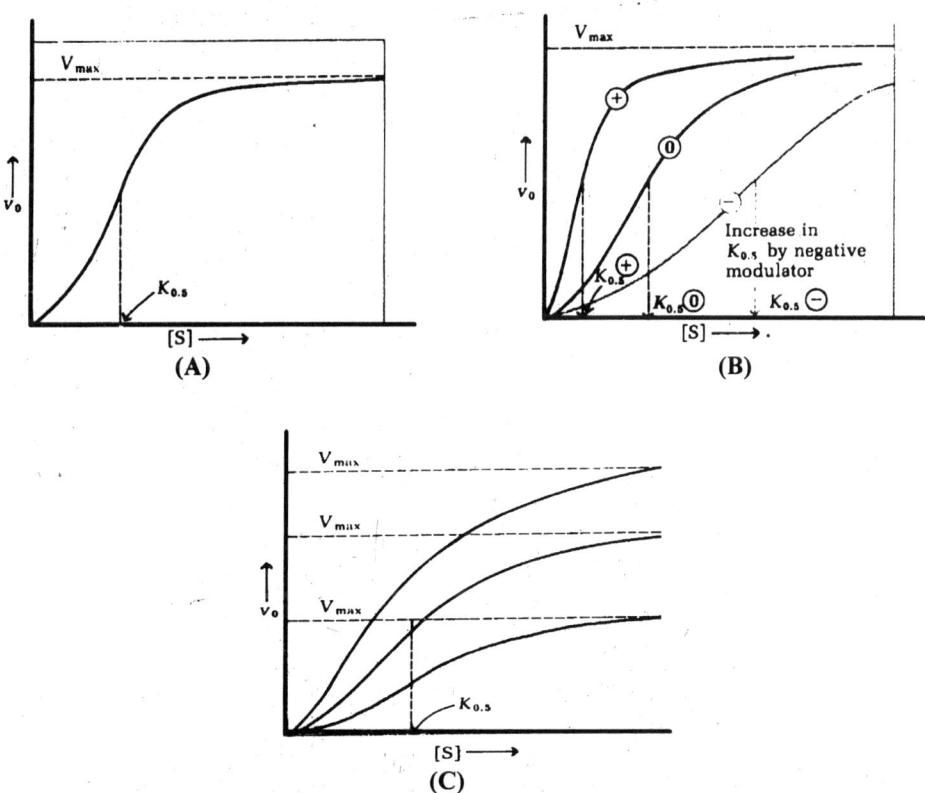

Fig. 2.33 : Double reciprocal plot for allosteric enzymes
A. Sigmoid curve given by homotropic enzymes
B. Effect of positive (+), negative (-) and no modulator (O) on an allosteric enzyme
C. A rare type of modulation in which V_{max} is modulated but $K_{0.5}$ is not changed

2.11. PHARMACEUTICAL APPLICATIONS

2.11.1. Diagnostic applications

The assay of enzyme levels in the extracellular body fluids (blood plasma and serum, urine, digestive juices, amniotic fluid and cerebrospinal fluid) are important aids to the clinical diagnosis and management of diseases. Although the majority of enzyme catalyzed reactions take place within living cells, whenever an energy imbalance occurs in the cells as a result of exposure to infective agents, bacterial toxins, etc., enzymes 'leak' out through the membranes into the circulation. This causes their fluid level to be raised above the normal cellular level. Measurement of the type, extent and duration of these raised enzyme activities can then provide information about the identity of the damaged cell and indicate the degree of injury. Enzyme assay can make significant contribution to the diagnosis of diseases because a minute change in enzyme concentration can be easily measured. Measurement of the changes in enzyme level therefore offer a greater degree of organ and disease differentiation as compared to other possible clinico-chemical parameters such as albumin or gamma globulin.

Now a days, the diagnostic specificity of enzyme tests is such that they are restricted mainly to confirming diagnosis providing data to be weighed with other clinical evidences due to lack of disease specific enzymes. Table 2.14 lists some diagnostically important enzymes which are most frequently assayed in clinical laboratories.

Table 2.14 : Diagnostically important enzymes

Enzyme and abbreviation	Tissue source*	Reaction
Acetylcholinesterase ACHE	BE	Acetylcholine to acetate and choline
Acid phosphatase SP	Pr E	Phosphate monoester to alcohol and Pi (pH 8-10)
Alanine aminotransferase GPT (AAT)	L	Alanine to gultamate
Alkaline phosphatase AP	BILPIK	Phosphate monoester to alcohol and Pi (pH 8-10)
α-Amylase	Pa S	Starch to maltose
Aspartate aminotransferase GOT (AST)	HLMKB	Aspartate to glutamate
Cholinesterase CHE	L	Acylcholine to fatty acid and choline
Chymotrypsin CT	PA	Proteins to polypeptides
Creatine lipase CPK	MHB	Creatine to creatine phosphate
Fructose-biphosphate aldolase ALD	MH	Fructose-1,6-biphosphate to triose phosphate
γ-Glutamyl transferase GGT	KL	γ-Glutamyl peptide to γ-glutamylamino acid
Hydroxybutyrate dehydrogenase HBD (LD1)	H	2-Hydroxybutyrate to 2-oxybutyrate
Isocitrate dehydrogenase ICD	L	Isocitrate to oxoglutarate
Lactate dehydrogenase LD	HLMK	Lactate to pyruvate
5'-Nucleosidase 5.N	Ht Pa	5'-Ribonucleotide to ribonucleoside
Ornithine carbamoyltransferase OCT	L	Carbamoyl-P to Citrulline
Triacylglycerol lipase	Pa	Triacylglycerol to diacylglycerol and fatty acid

* *B, brain; E, erythrocytes; H, heart muscle; Ht, hepatobiliary tract; I, intestinal mucosa; K, kidney; L, liver; M, skeletal muscle; Pa, pancreas; Pl, placenta; Pr, prostate gland; S, saliva.*

2.11.1.1. Enzyme in the diagnosis of liver and biliary system disorders

Liver diseases were among the first to which serum enzyme tests were applied. They have proved to be most successful due to the large size of the organ and wide variety and abundance of enzymes. The liver-function enzymes GOT, GPT and AP are assayed, to determine the site and nature of liver disease LD, GGT, OCT and CHE are also monitored. Various enzymes used in the diagnosis of liver diseases along with their respective level are listed in table 2.15.

2.11.1.2. Enzyme in heart disease

No single enzyme has yet been found entirely specific for myocardial damage and a combination of results from assays of CPK, GOT and HBD, each of which have been shown to be elevated in more than 90% of cases; is used for diagnostic purposes. The elevated enzyme activities in serum after acute myocardial infarction is shown in figure 2.34.

Table 2.15 : Liver diseases and enzymes used to diagnosis

Disease	Enzyme used	Enzyme level
Acute hepatitis	GOT and GPT	20 to 50 times of normal level
Chronic hepatitis and cirrhosis	All liver transaminases	3 to 12 fold than normal level and inflammation of the liver
Fatty liver	GPT	2 fold than normal
Solvent poisoning of liver	GOT GPT LD	GOT:GPT:LD 6500:3000:10000 (U/ml)
Hepatobiliary disease (obstructive jaundice)	GOT and GPT	5 to 10 fold

The level of CPK starts rising after three to four hours of the initial onset of pain, followed in order by GOT and AST (HBD) which appear after an elapse of approximately eight hours. The maximum level reached in same sequence, CPK after 24 hours, LD 1 after 36 hours and AST after about two days. The rise in enzyme levels is fairly moderate, AST and CPK rise four to ten fold above their respective normal levels and LD 1 approximately five fold higher than normal.

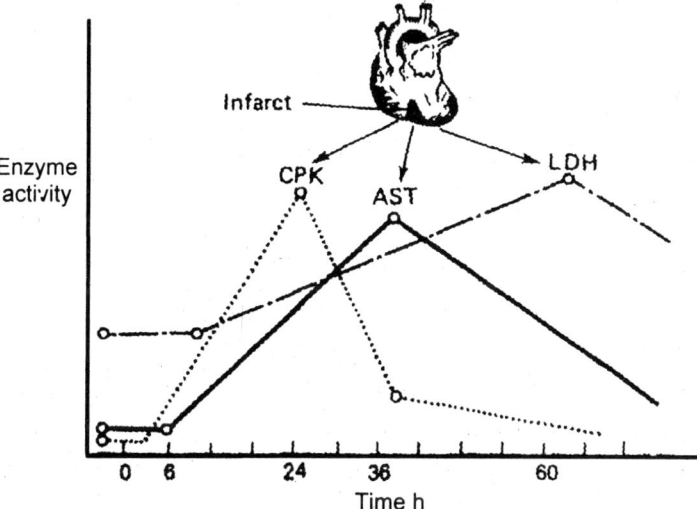

Fig. 2.34 : Serum enzyme activities after myocardial infarction

2.11.1.3. Diagnosis of muscle disease

Skeletal muscle disorders include the diseases of the muscle fibers (myopathies) or of the muscle nerves (neurogenic disorders). In myopathies CPJ, LD, ALD, GOT and GPT levels are raised. In the case of neurogenic diseases and hereditary diseases, CPK is occasionally raised (2 to 3 fold). Damage to the muscle may be due to extensive muscular exercise, drugs, physical trauma, inflammatory diseases, microbial infection or metabolic dysfunction or it may be genetically predisposed. In muscular disorders the level of CPK is elevated in serum with the highest frequency and is assayed in the diagnosis of these disorders.

2.11.2. Enzymes in therapeutics

Many enzymes are used as therapeutic agents now a days, due to some of their specific characteristics which are as following :

1. They are specific to their substrates;

2. they are capable of producing the desired effect without eliciting any side reaction;

3. they are water soluble; and
4. they are highly efficient in biological environment.

Enzymes as therapeutic agents also have drawbacks which limit their applications. The large molecular structure and high molecular weight excludes them from the intracellular domains. They are highly antigenic because of their proteinaceous nature. They are rapidly cleared from blood plasma. Extensive purification from pyrogens and toxins is necessary for parenteral enzymes which increases the cost. Table 2.16 lists some therapeutically important enzymes.

2.11.2.1. Enzyme therapy of neoplastic disease

The enzyme therapy of cancer is based on the principle of depriving the abnormal cells of their essential metabolic precursor (amino acids, nucleic acid and folates). Several enzymes have been tested for and proved suitable as antitumor agents. L-asparaginase, L-arginase, carboxypeptidase G (folate depletion), L-glutaminase, L-methioninase, L-phenylalanine ammonia lyase, L-serine dehydratase, L-tyrosinase and xanthine oxidase have been tested for their anticancer activity.

Table 2.16 : Therapeutically important enzymes

Enzyme preparation	Source	Therapeutic application
Asparaginase (amidase)	E. coli, guinea pig serum	Cytotoxic agents
Bromelain (protease)	Ananas comosus	Inflammation, oedema
Chymotrypsin (protease)	Bovine pancreas	Inflammation oedema ophthalmology and upper respiratory tract diseases
Deoxyribonuclease (DNA hydrolysis)	Bovine pancreas	Reduces viscosity of pulmonary secretions
Dextranase (Dextran hydrolysis)	Penicillum funiculosum	Dental plaque restriction
Diastase (Starch hydrolysis)	Malt	Amylaceous dyspepsia
Galactosidase (Lactose hydrolysis)	Aspergillus niger	Inherited β-galalctosidase deficiency
Hyaluronidase (Mucopolysaccharide hydrolysis)	Animal testes	Increase absorption rate, increase effectiveness of local anesthetics
Pancreatin	Animal pancreas	Pancreatitis
Papain (Protease)	Carica papaya	Dyspepsia and gastritis
Penicillinase	Bacillus cereus	Penicillin allergy
Plasmin (Protease)	Plasminogen	Thrombotic disorders anticoagulation
Streptodornase (DNA-ase)	Streptococci	Depolymerization of DNA in purulent exudates
Streptokinase (Protease)	Streptococci	Thromboemolic diseases
Trypsin (Protease)	Animal pancreas	Cleaning necrotic tissue
Tissue plasminogen activator (Protease)	Recombinant DNA tech.	Thromboemolic diseases
Urokinase (Protease)	Human urine	Thromboemolic diseases

L-Asparaginase is the most extensively studied enzyme. It is used in the treatment of three neoplastic diseases, acute lymphoblastic leukemia, leukemic lymphosarcoma and myeloblastic leukemia. It deprives the tumor cells of their nutritional asparagine supply. Asparagine is required by the cell for protein synthesis and impaired protein synthesis is probably responsible for the immunosuppression and toxic effects of asparaginase therapy.

$$\text{L-Asparagine} + \text{PPi} + \text{AMP} \xrightleftharpoons{\text{Asparaginase}} \text{L-Aspartate} + \text{NH}_3 + \text{ATP}$$

The future of enzyme therapy in cancer is very bright but the problems of antigenicity and short circulation time remain to be overcome.

2.11.2.2. Enzymes as thrombolytic agents

The fibrinolytic system dissolves intravascular clots as a result of the action of plasmin, a nonspecific protease that digests fibrin. Plasminogen is an inactive precursor of plasmin and is converted to plasmin by cleavage of a single peptide bond. Plasmin digests fibrin clots and other plasmin proteins including several coagulation factors. Therapy with thrombolytic enzymes tend to digest fibrin clots of vascular injury.

The general clinical use of enzyme is the promotion of thrombolysis. The rationale of enzymatic fibrinolysis relies on the supposition that increasing the levels of circulating proteases should more rapidly dissolve the blood clot or preformed thrombus.

Currently, two types of enzyme are used, one with direct and general proteolytic activity such as plasmin or trypsin and other which increases the level of native plasmin such as plasminogen activator. Clinical evidence supports the second alternative. Promotion of natural lysis utilizes the avalanche effect of the cascade, and does not require a prior infusion to neutralize circulating anti-proteases and lastly it is more specific. Two lysokinase plasminogen activators have been used as thrombolytic agents; streptokinase and urokinase.

2.11.2.3. In digestive disorders and inflammations

Enzymes have been used over many years to supplement enzyme deficiencies of the pancreas and small intestine. Pancreatin (obtained from alcoholic extract of animal pancreas) is administered buccally to enhance the enzymatic digestion of starch and proteins in patients with pancreatic cyst and pancreatitis. Pancreatin along with lipase is used to treat patients with fatty stools.

Hydrolytic enzymes e.g., papain and extracts from fungi *Aspergillus niger* and *A. oryzae* are used to increase absorption from the small intestine. These extracts containing amylases and proteases along with cellulases assist the degradation of the indigestible fibbers of cabbages etc., and so reducing dyspepsia and flatulence.

Micro-organisms are used as large scale sources of therapeutic enzymes. *Saccharomyces cerevisiae, S. fragilis, Bacillus subtilis* and two *Aspergillus* species are recommended safe by FDA (USA) for oral administration. β-Galactosidase (from *A. oryzae*) is used by the patients suffering from inherited intestinal disease lactose deficiency. Children with this genetic disorder are unable to digest milk lactose. β-Galacto-sidase catalyses the conversion of lactose to glucose and galactose which are readily absorbed by the intestine. Penicillinase (from *Bacillus subtilis*) is used to treat hypersensitivity reaction caused by penicillin antibiotic. The enzyme catalyzes the hydrolysis of penicillin to penicillanic acid, which is nonimmunogenic.

Microbial and plant hydrolases are also used to reduce inflammation and oedema. Thrombin, trypsin, chymotrypsin, papain, streptokinase, streptodornase, and serrapeptidase have been subjected to clinical trials. They are administered orally and have significant proteolytic activity in the serum. Streptodornase has shown pain relieving action on systemic injection. The preparations have also been used to clean dirty wounds and necrotic tissue and to remove debris from second and third degree burns.

2.12. PRODUCTION OF ENZYMES

2.12.1. Source and location of enzymes

All living cells produce enzymes. They are obtained from plant tissues, animal tissues, and micro-organisms. The quantities of enzymes produced on a industrial scale from plants and animal sources are considerable, but microbial enzymes have become increasingly important for both technical and economic reasons. Enzymes from plant tissues require large quantities of plant material and quantity of enzyme obtained is very small. Animal enzymes are by products of meat industry. Micro-organisms have achieved considerable importance during the last three decades. Microbial enzymes are not subjected to any of the production and supply limitations of plant and animal enzymes. The production capacity of microbial enzymes may be expanded and furthermore, the types of enzymes available from micro-organisms are almost unlimited. The microbes offer following advantages over other sources of enzymes:

1. The growth of micro-organism is very fast and they can be grown on medium containing cheap raw material.
2. The genetic engineering and manipulations of microbial cell are possible in the laboratory to increase the yield of enzymes.
3. Large amounts of enzymes can be produced from microbes.

4. **Animal** sacrifice can be prevented.

In a living cell (plant or animal), mitochondrias have highly organized structure and contain a large number of enzymes, for example, glutamate dehydrogenase. The granular microsomes, lysosomes and ribosomes also contain important enzymes. For example, the ribosomes are the site of protein biosynthesis and lysosomes contain many hydrolases. The soluble portion of the cytoplasm contains enzymes responsible for glycolysis. In the bacterial cell some structures of plant and animal cells are not present. Outside the nucleus, the cell is filled with a granular cytoplasm. Enzymes are present in the granules, the soluble cytoplasm and in or adsorbed on the cell membrane.

2.12.2. Selection of micro-organism

Selection of micro-organism for the enzyme production is made on the following basis:

1. The micro-organisms should produce extracellular enzymes, because their isolation and separation is simple and far less expensive, but only hydrolases have been reported to occur extracellularly.
2. The organisms must give high yields of enzymes.
3. The fermentation time should be less.
4. Strain must not produce byproducts which inhibit the growth of micro-organisms.
5. The organisms must be non pathogenic.
6. The organisms must grow on cheap raw material.
7. The organisms must adjust themselves to the physical and chemical properties of the culture medium such as temperature, pH, the availability of substrates, etc.

At the present time, generally two genera, namely *Aspergillus* and *Bacillus* are used for the industrial production of enzymes.

2.12.3. Fermentation media

The production media must contain sources for carbon, nitrogen, energy, minerals, macronutrients, micro-nutrients and growth factors in the case of auxotropic micro-organisms. If inducible enzyme is to be produced, the inducer should be added to the medium. Sometimes, coenzymes act as an inducer or constituents of the media may have an induction effect. Products of the enzyme-catalyzed reactions may also act as inductors. Fermentation of catabolic enzyme is inhibited by the direct or indirect effect of products on their activity, e.g., production of proteases in *Bacillus* species by amino acids. Various sources of carbon, nitrogen and other growth substances are summarized in table 2.17.

Table 2.17 : Constituents of fermentation media and their sources

Constituents	Various sources
Source of carbon and energy	Cereal meal, soybean meal, potato starch, wheat or rice bran, molasses.
Source of nitrogen	Fish meal, gelatin, casein, soybean meal, bran, distillers' solubles peptones.
Source substances and trace elements	Yeast extract, corn steep liquor, plant oil, meal of oil-bearing seeds bran.

2.12.4. Fermentation

There are several procedures available for fermentation, however, for the production of enzymes only three methods are used :1. Submerged culture, 2. Solid-substrate culture and, 3. Deep bed cultivation.

2.12.4.1. Submerged culture

In submerged cultures, the production usually takes place in mechanically stirred bioreactors of capacities 20,000 to 1,00,000 liters batch fermentation. Generally the main fermentation lasts for 50 to 200 hours depending upon the enzyme and micro-organism used. Continuous fermentation have only limited use because of difficulty in sterilization of the nutrient media, and instability of highly mutated production strains. On industrial scale, continuous fermentation has been used for the production of glucose isomerase.

The total yield of enzyme depends upon the rate of enzyme synthesis during different growth phases. In an inducible system with catabolic repression, a maximum enzyme synthesis is frequently obtained in stationary phase, when the micro-organism has fallen to zero. Now a days, the operation is carried out in a two stage cascade, in which the high concentration of cell mass is first produced and then the production of enzyme is carried out in a second reactor under different conditions. Furthermore, the effect of nutrient media, pH, temperature, partial pressure of oxygen and aeration must be taken into account. The yield of extracellular enzymes can be increased by the addition of surfactants.

After completion of fermentation the ferment is cooled and the cell mass is separated. Extracellular enzymes are found in the culture filtrate and thus biomass is discarded but with intracellular enzymes the biomass contains the enzymes and thus culture filtrate is discarded.

2.12.4.2. Solid-substrate culture (surface culture)

In this process, the micro-organism is cultivated on a solid substrate enriched with a high concentration of nutrients, micronutrients and minerals and having a large surface area, e.g., cereal meal, wheat bran and/or rice bran. This method is adapted for the extraction of enzymes from fungi, such as *Penicillium*, *Aspergillus*, etc. The moisture content of the medium is low which inhibits the growth of bacteria. There are two processes available for growth of fungi namely, drum process and tray process.

In drum process horizontally rotating drums are used for the cultivation of fungi. In tray process, the fungi are cultivated in trays of size 2 X 40 cm. The substrate is spread in the form of a thin layer of 1 to 10 cm thickness. The micro-organisms (in the form of spores) are inoculated and then the trays are incubated in an air-conditioned room. Recently a process known as high-heap process has been used in which a continuous stream of air is forced through the nutrient substrate. This ensures supply of oxygen as well as removal of heat of reaction. The growth phase extends upto 1 to 7 days.

After completion of growth and fermentation, the fungi are homogenized and dried (moisture content 10% to 15%). The homogenized powder can be used directly or the fungal mycelium is extracted with water and further purified before use.

2.12.4.3. Deep-bed cultivation

In this method the micro-organisms are cultivated in rectangular vessels of dimensions 18 X 200 inch. The nutrient medium is added into the vessels upto a height of 2 feet. Cereal meal, wheat bran, rice bran, soybean meal, potato flakes, etc. are used as medium. The medium is sterilized and then inoculated with organism. The temperature of the culture vessel is maintained to enhance the growth of organism. After completion of growth, the microbes are used in the extraction of enzymes.

2.12.5. Extraction of enzymes

Extraction refers to the liberation of enzymes from cells or cellular constituents. Extraction is started by mechanical, physical, chemical, or a combination of these methods to disrupt the cell wall or membrane. For extraction of either intra- or extra-cellular enzymes, it may be necessary to modify the nature of liquid medium to complete the dissociation. Certain enzymes require the presence of a cofactor, lipid or carbohydrates to maintain their activity during the extraction.

2.12.5.1. Disintegration of animal and plant tissues

Most animal enzymes are localized in the particular organ or in muscles. These organs are minced in a vertical cutter mixer after removal of fat. Freezing the animal tissue often assists grinding and avoids blockage by wet tissue. Frozen meat grinders are used for this purpose. The ground tissues are then passed through a colloid mill which produces maximum cell disintegration.

Grinding of plant tissues has classically been concerned with dried tissues such as seeds which contain less enzymes than green tissues. For grinding of green tissues, the plant material is macerated by grinding in hammer mill or some other chopper mills, and the marc is pressed. Lytic enzymes are also used to disrupt the cell wall.

2.12.5.2. Disruption of microbial cells

Microbial cells produce both extracellular and intracellular enzymes. The extracellular enzymes do not require cell disruption but the release of intracellular enzymes from micro-organisms however requires a more vigorous method of cell breakage. The various methods of microbial cell disruption are represented in figure 2.35.

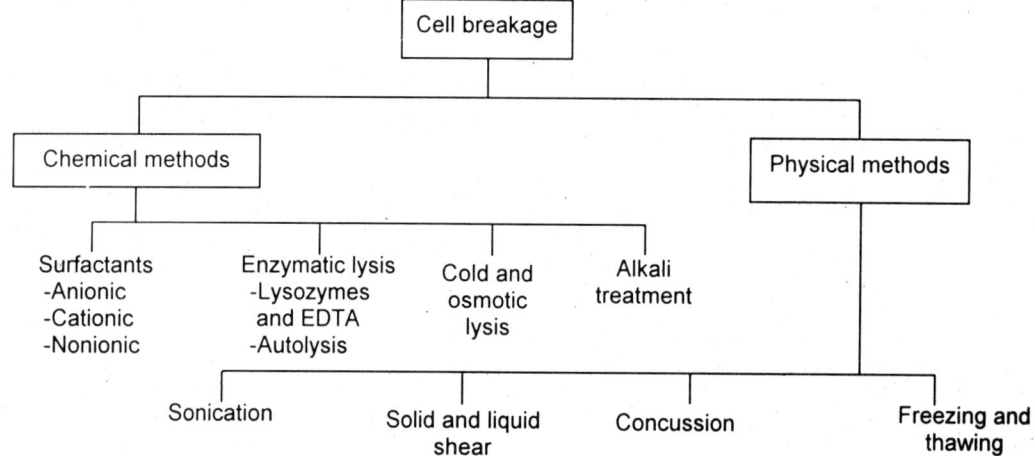

Fig. 2.35 : Various methods of microbial cell disruption

2.12.5.2.1. Disruption by chemical methods

A. Surfactants : Ionic (cationic and anionic) and nonionic surfactants are used to lyse microbial cells. Surfactants have the capability to solubilize the microbial cell wall. Commonly used surfactants are sodium dodecyl sulfate, cetyl triethyl ammonium bromide, triton X-100 , various tweens, etc.

B. Enzymatic lysis : In large scale operations autolysis is the most commonly used technique for the extraction of enzymes. A suspension of cells is maintained at elevated temperature (23 to 37°C) for several hours. After cooling, the cell extract is collected by centrifugation. This method is used in the extraction of transaldolase from frozen *Candida utilis*, invertase from baker's yeast, glucose-6-phosphate dehydrogenase from yeast, etc. Autolysis is used for the extraction of intracellular enzymes. The method has risk of thermal denaturation of enzymes or its destruction by cellular proteases.

Microbial cell lysis can also be carried out by using lysozymes such as egg white lysozyme. Lysozyme hydrolyses the glycosidic bonds in the glycopeptide component of bacterial cell wall. In the presence of EDTA the cells usually lysed releasing intracellular enzymes.

C. Cold and osmotic shock : A rapid reduction of temperature from normal growth temperature to 0°C results in loss of viability in micro-organisms, ATP, and 260 nm absorbing material from the cells. This technique is not applicable for large scale production, because cell suspensions with a density greater than 10^8/ml show little or no effect of osmotic shock and bacteria are more susceptible to cold shock

Disruption of cell by osmotic shock involves following steps :
1. Washing of bacteria to remove growth medium by a buffer solution.
2. Resuspending the washed cells in a 20 % buffered sucrose solution and,

3. Removal of cell by centrifugation.

The paste is then suspended in water and sudden increase in osmotic pressure inside the cells causes the release of cell constituents.

D. Alkali treatment : A sudden increase in pH will cause the lysis of bacterial cell wall. This procedure is used in the large scale extraction of L-asparaginase from *Erwinica chrysantheme*. The usefulness of this method depends upon the pH stability of the desired enzyme. If the desired enzyme is inactivated by alkaline pH, then this method is not applicable.

2.12.5.2.2. Disruption by physical methods

A. Sonication : Ultrasonic waves are used frequently for cell lysis on small and laboratory scales. The ultrasonic or sonic waves traveling through a liquid are consisted of alternate compression and rarefaction. If a wave is high enough in amplitude, then cavity is produced, as a result of the making and breaking of bubbles. These bubbles or cavities make many cycles producing high local pressure of about 20,000 atmospheres. The mechanical shocks are felt at a distance of a few microns. Ultrasonic waves have been used successfully in a number of extraction procedures. It is used especially in the extraction of enzymes and proteins at small scale.

B. Freezing and thawing : The effects of freezing and thawing are similar to those observed during cold and osmotic shock. In addition to the difference in osmotic pressure between intra-and extra-cellular fluids, the intra- and extra-cellular crystal formation further damages the cell wall. 10 % of the total soluble protein release has been estimated during the process of disruption.

C. Solid and liquid shear : In solid shear, frozen (-20°C) microbial paste is placed in a cylindrical hole (0.1 to 1mm in diameter) in a metal block and a tight fitting plunger is then inserted. 1,000 to 4,000 atmospheric pressure is applied at the top of this plunger. A very high percentage of cells are ruptured by this method.

In liquid shear, the microbial suspension is passed through a narrow orifice at pressure up to 40,000 psi. Sometimes French Press is also used for this purpose. Cells undergo disruption due to extreme shear during passage through the orifice. Over 90 % of cell breakage was found with baker's yeast after a single passage at 20,000 psi.

D. Concussion : Microbial cells can be disrupted by bombardment with hard particles such as glass beads. Several types of mills are used for this purpose such as agitator bead mill, ball mill, colloidal mill, etc.

2.12.5.3. Aqueous and solvent extraction

Disruption of microbial cells does not necessarily lead to breakdown of molecular complexes with other cell components such as lipids, nucleic acids, and carbohydrates. The liquid extraction of the enzyme from insoluble particles can provide a tool for the fractionation in which extractants of increasing eluting power are employed.

There are two general methods of extraction of enzyme from broken cells:

1. Extract all possible materials under mild conditions using salt solution as solvent in which most of the enzymes are stable.

2. Selective extraction of enzymes utilizing the differential solubility of enzymes in different solvents. In this method the first extraction is performed using a solvent in which only a few enzymes are soluble and then repeating with other solvents in which other enzymes are soluble.

Comminuted microbial cells are extracted batchwise in stirred jacketed vessels. The particle size determines not only the rate of extraction, but also the amount of extract which gets adsorbed on the particle surface. With a given quantity of extracting fluid the use of many fractions of the liquid leads to a more nearly complete removal of the desired solute than does the use of the entire liquid in a single extraction. Further improvements in extraction efficiency may be obtained through arranging the staged extraction in countercurrent continuous flow. After extraction of enzymes, the spent solids are removed by filtration, centrifugation or sedimentation. Some examples of combination of solvents used in the extraction of enzymes are listed in table 2.18.

2.12.6. Purification of enzymes

2.12.6.1. Removal of lipids

Removal of lipids is usually accomplished as early as possible because they interfere with the separation of proteins. The classical method of lipid removal is to make an acetone powder of the ground cells. In this method, the ground cells are mixed with cold acetone (-10°C). This is repeated with acetone at 0°C and finally with acetone at 20°C. The procedure primarily removes water and some lipid. The lipid is removed later with petroleum ether or ether at room temperature.

Table 2.18 : Some enzymes and the solvent for extraction

Enzyme	Source	Solvent
Fungal lipase	Fungi	Water
Glycerol phosphate dehydrogenase (GPDH)	Rabbit muscle	1mM disodium EDTA containing 2mM 2-mercaptoethanol
Cholesterol esterase	Pancreas	Dil.H_2SO_4 in the presence of protease inhibitor

Other methods of lipid removal are the extraction of lipids from solutions of enzymes in 20-50 % v/v n-butanol at 0°C, and lipid extraction using various gases under supercritical conditions. In the later method liquid CO_2 is most commonly used for the removal of lipids from biological materials.

2.12.6.2. Removal of nucleic acids

Purification of intracellular enzymes and to a less extent animal enzymes is complicated by the presence of nucleic acid. Nucleic acid can be precipitated by high molecular weight polyvalent cations such as protamine sulfate, cetyl triethyl ammonium bromide, streptomycin sulfate and polyethyleneimine. These polyvalent cations form a complex between negatively charged phosphate residues of the nucleic acid molecules and positively charged groups of precipitants. The resulting complex is then separated by centrifugation.

2.12.6.3 Purification by differential solubility

This is the most commonly used method for enzyme purification. It is based on precipitation of the active enzyme or other proteins and soluble substances.

2.12.6.3.1. Salting out

In this procedure, the precipitation of proteins is accomplished by high concentration of neutral salts. The most frequently used salts are ammonium sulfate and sodium sulfate. Ammonium sulfate is inexpensive and is highly soluble (767g/lit.) which permits salting out of practically all protein.

2.12.6.3.2. Temperature and pH

Most proteins exhibit increased solubility with temperature elevation. The differential stability of enzymes at high temperatures is quite significant and selective heat denaturation is commonly used on industrial scale. Thus, by controlled heating of extracts, inert protein materials may be denatured. This procedure is used in the purification of α-amylase, ribonuclease, adenyl kinase, cholesterol esterase and glutamate dehydrogenase.

Alteration of pH is also used as a method of fractional precipitation. The different proportions of basic and acidic groups of different enzymes lead to wide range of pH values at which enzymes exhibit isoelectric zero net charge characteristics. The principal difficulty in using differential pH precipitation is the pH stability of desired enzymes which is limited.

2.12.6.3.3. Organic solvent

Organic solvents are used in fractional precipitation of proteins based on their dielectric constants. When an organic solvent is added to the aqueous solution of enzyme, the dielectric constant of the solution is decreased hence the solubility of enzyme is decreased. However, since enzymes have their internal hydrophobic amino acid residues and are relatively loosely folded, an alternative on adding the organic solvent is for the molecule to refold into a new and inactive form is with hydrophobic residues exposed on the surface. The danger of refolding and consequently denaturation is greater as temperature increases. This leads to a requirement for low temperature, often below 0°C and fractionation with organic precipitants

Various organic solvents used in the protein purification are methanol, ethanol, isopropyl alcohol and acetone. Ethanol has been the most commonly and widely used organic solvent due to its acceptability in food and pharmaceutical industry.

2.12.6.3.4. Nonionic polymers and multiphase systems

High molecular weight polymers such as dextrans and polyethylene glycols (PEG) have been used in the isolation of biological material in three ways :

1. For the concentration of biological component including viruses by dialysis and by liquid-liquid extraction in the aqueous two phase mixtures.

2. As a stabilizer on a particular component in solution, and

3. As a precipitant which causes the formation of a solid protein phase.

Two phase systems can be used to separate enzymes from cell homogenates and at the same time achieve a certain degree of purification. Dextran-PEG two phase system has been used in the production of commercial intracellular food enzymes.

2.12.6.3.5. Crystallization

After extraction and purification it may be possible to crystallize the enzyme. The first crystals of enzyme may contain a number of other proteins. Crystallization and recrystallization are more effective procedures in enzyme purification. The most widely used method of crystallization is from ammonium sulfate solutions. In this method the salt is added to a concentrated enzyme solution until a slight turbidity appears. It is then allowed to stand while the salt concentration is increased by:

1. Adding a strong solution of the salt dropwise at long intervals;

2. through a fine capillary;

3. through a dialysis membrane; or

4. the solution may simply be allowed to evaporate slowly.

Crystallization may be initiated by changing pH or temperature at constant salt concentration. Glycerol phosphate dehydrogenase, pyruvate kinase, lactate dehydrogenase, urease and glutamate dehydrogenase have been purified using crystallization.

2.12.6.4. Purification by chromatographic methods

Purification of enzymes by differential solubility is concerned with enzyme recovery with little purification. The purification of enzymes is brought about by various chromatographic techniques based on the differential migration of enzymes. The various chromatographic methods used for enzyme purification are adsorption, ion exchange, gel and affinity chromatography.

2.12.6.4.1. Adsorption chromatography

The earliest chromatographic purifications were accomplished by using inorganic substances that adsorbed the biochemicals by VanderWaal's forces and steric interaction. The most widely used adsorbent in enzyme purification is calcium phosphate gel, especially crystalline form hydroxyapatite (HA). The calcium and phosphate ions on the surface of HA crystals form bonds with charged groups of proteins. Acidic and neutral proteins bind to calcium sites on HA. The elution of acidic and neutral proteins is generally achieved with low concentrations of phosphate buffers of pH 6.8. Basic proteins bind to phosphate group on HA crystals. Alkaline phosphatase from bacteria was purified using HA. Amino transferases from *E. coli* were also purified with 6 fold in specific activity.

2.12.6.4.2. Ion exchange chromatography

Ion exchange chromatography can be defined as the separation of one species from another, applied to the mobile phase, by the differential binding and release of these solutes to the fixed charges of the ion exchanger. Almost all enzymes are polar in nature and can be charged. Ion exchange chromatography is the most generally used among all the available chromatographic techniques for enzyme purification. Ion exchange chromatography of enzymes usually employs derivatives of cellulose, agarose, dextrans or resins. The cross-linked matrix of agarose is commonly used in the purification of bioactive enzymes and pharmaceuticals because of its following properties :

1. stable bed volume;
2. high capacity, flow rate and resolving power;
3. good chemical stability between pH 3 to 10;
4. good thermal stability upto 70°C which makes it suitable for autoclaving.

The anion exchangers most commonly used are diethylaminoethyl cellulose, triethylamino cellulose and triethanolamine coupled to cellulose through glycerol and polyglycerol chain mixed groups (ECTEOLA cellulose). The cation exchangers used are carboxymethyl cellulose, sulfoethyl cellulose, acrylic acid resin, phospho cellulose, etc.

Fractionation of enzymes by ion exchange chromatography can be performed on a column or by a batch method. Enzymes whose isoelectric points are well removed from neutral pH are generally more easily purified using batch method. L-Asparaginase which has an isoelectric point of 6.8, a 100 fold purification is possible using carboxymethyl cellulose batch column. The batch method is also useful in removing nucleic acids from enzymes.

2.12.6.4.3. Gel filtration chromatography

This technique is also known as permeation, molecular sieve, molecular exclusion, restricted diffusional or steric chromatography. In gel filtration chromatography, the separation of proteins is brought about on the basis of their molecular size. The sample is applied on the surface of a column of appropriate porous beads of the hydrated gel and solvent is percolated through the column. The fractionation of proteins depends on the molecular size to enter pores. The molecules too large to penetrate porous structure of the beads, are excluded and passed through in the void volume of the column. Smaller molecules which can enter porous beads, move more slowly through the column, since they spend a proportion of their time in the beads. Therefore, molecules are eluted in order of decreasing molecular size.

There are three available gel filtration media for enzyme purification:
1. Partially cross-linked dextrans (Sephadex) with a fractionation range up to 2,50,000 daltons.
2. Cross-linked granulated polyacrylamide gels with a fractionation range up to 400,000 daltons.
3. Granulated agarose gel (Sepharose) with a fractionation range up to 50,000 to 40,000,000 daltons.

For large scale purification, gels of allyl dextran cross-linked with N,N-methylene bis acrylamide (Sepharoyl) are ideally suited. Alkaline phosphatase and restriction endonucleases have been purified by using 25 X 80 cm. column of Ultrogel Ac and Sepharcyl S-200 respectively.

2.12.6.4.4. Affinity chromatography

This method depends upon specific interaction between the analyte and a complementary group which is covalently bound to the column packing. A solution containing macromolecules to be purified is passed through a column containing an insoluble polymer or gel to which a specific competitive inhibitor or other ligands have been covalently attached. Proteins not exhibiting appreciable affinity for the ligand will pass unretarded through the column, whereas those which recognize the ligand will be retarded with an extent related to the affinity constant under the experimental conditions. The specifically retained proteins can then be eluted by washing the ligand-protein complex with a solution of displacing agent such as an inhibitor or by changing the pH or ionic strength of the elution solvent to favor dissociation.

The insoluble supports for enzyme purification by affinity chromatography are hydrophilic cellulose derivatives, polystyrene gels, cross-linked dextrans, beaded agarose, glass beads and polyacrylamide gels. A number of chemical derivatives of agarose and polyacrylamide have been prepared for enzyme purification. Affinity matrices used for enzyme purification fall into two categories :

1. Those which are specific for the desired enzyme by the specificity of the ligand such as substrate, substrate analogs, inhibitors or antibody of the enzyme, and

2. Those which will interact with a related group of enzymes because of an immobilized general ligand such as cofactors (5'-AMP, 2',5'-ADP, NAD^+ and others) which is specific for a class of enzymes and hydrocarbon ligands or dyes, which will interact with a large number of different enzymes.

The total cost of enzyme isolation can be reduced by the introduction of an affinity step. Tissue plasminogen activator (t-PA) from cultures of human kidney cells has been purified by using α-benzylsulfonyl-p-amino-Sepharose.

2.12.6.4.5. Electrophoresis and ultracentrifugation

Electrophoretic purification is based on the mobility of proteins when placed in an electrical field. This technique is capable of highest resolution of enzymes employing physico-chemical separation. This method is now largely used as a tool for separation of isoenzymes and other enzymes related for diagnostic purposes. Generally free-boundary electrophoresis, zone electrophoresis on supports such as paper, starch, and cellulose powder, electrophoresis in agarose and acrylamide gels, and isoelectric focusing are the techniques frequently used for laboratory scale enzyme purification and characterization.

Recently, an industrial scale continuous electrophoretic separator has been developed in UK. The unit can draw as many as 29 separate fractions in potential applications as isolation and purification of high value pharmaceutical enzymes and other proteins. Proteins in solution have the tendency to sediment at high centrifugal force, so it is possible to separate a protein from a mixture by centrifugation. Better separation of proteins has been achieved by density gradient centrifugation where sucrose or glycerol is used as density gradient. With more sophisticated continuous flow utracentrifugation whole cells, viruses and subcellular components can be separated.

2.12.7. Finishing operations

Finishing operations such as enzyme desalting, concentration, purity control and storage are of greater importance.

2.12.7.1. Desalting

Excessive amounts of inorganic salts must be removed from enzyme products. The salts present in one enzyme may be inhibitory to the other enzymes present in clinical diagnostic reagents. Furthermore, desalting may be essential at intermediate stages of enzyme isolation, for example, prior to ion exchange adsorption. The simplest and oldest method of salt removal is dialysis. The principle function of dialysis is to remove small molecules such as salts from larger ones, especially enzymes to be purified. Mixed bed ion exchange, classical method of removing small ions, has been applied to some of the robust enzymes. Mixed bed cation and anion exchange resins are used to remove both positive and negative ions.

2.12.7.2. Concentration of enzymes

After extraction both intracellular and extracellular enzymes are obtained as dilute solution and must be further concentrated before further use. On small scale, precipitation and adsorption are used to concentrate the enzymes. On industrial scale ultrafiltration has been used.

2.12.7.2.1. Ultrafiltration

Ultrafiltration is used to separate macromolecules and colloidal particles by he use of a membrane. Hydraulic pressure is used as driving force for solvent molecules to pass through the membrane while the microporous membrane prevents the passage of large solute molecules. Membranes with exclusion limits of 2,000 to 3,00,000 daltons are available for ultrafiltration. Ultrafiltration (molecular weight cut offs between 500 and 300,000) can remove small molecules.

The enzyme solution is fed into a cell fitted with a membrane which retains the selected protein while being permeable to solvent and small molecules. Positive pressure applies to the solution or negative pressure to the collecting chamber, acts as driving force that causes the flow of solvent and small solute molecules across the membrane. Large volumes can be reduce to a few milliliters in only one or two hours.

Diafiltration is a useful method of removing salts and other low molecular weight contaminants from dilute enzyme solution. In this method the water is fed to the ultrafilter cell so that molecules other than water are effectively removed from the system.

2.12.7.2.2. Drying

The methods of drying that have been developed for food and pharmaceuticals apply effectively to the enzymes. The extracellular enzymes in food industry are frequently used as dried free flowing powders. The drying of enzymes largely depends upon the thermal stability of enzymes. The more robust enzymes may be vacuum dried or spray dried while the delicate ones are freeze-dried or spray dried. The spray drying is widely used for extracellular bacterial enzymes while most intracellular enzymes are dried by freeze-drying process.

2.12.7.2.3. Vacuum evaporation

In the production of extracellular enzymes, the diluted enzyme solution is concentrated under vacuum at temperatures below 40°C. The equipment which has been used in the concentration of fruit juices may be used for the industrial scale concentration of enzymes at reduced temperature. In a typical application an enzyme solution was concentrated in two stages from 8% or 12% to 35% solids, then to 65 % solids.

2.12.7.3. Storage

Good storage properties are of paramount importance in industrial production of enzymes. Loss of activity on storage will be a loss of product in its purest and most expensive form. All enzymes have limited shelf life due to inherent active-conformation liability in the minority of molecules present in high energy states, at that temperature at any given time. This inherent loss can be delayed by cross-linking, immobilization or by using enzyme stabilizers such as sugars, certain ions and cofactors.

Majority of enzyme products are marketed as dry powders, a few enzymes are available in a liquid or a suspension form. These products generally contain compounds which reduce the loss of enzyme activity on storage, which prevents microbial growth, enzyme stabilizers and cofactors. Compounds generally used for these purposes are glycols, propylene glycol, ethylene glycol, sorbitol, mannitol, thiol, reducing agents, sodium chloride, salts of organic hydroxy acids and other salts of buffers, sodium benzoate, and esters of parahydroxy benzoic acid. Recently compounds such as gelatin, dextrans, partially hydrolysed collagen, gum arabic, albumin, polyamines, poly-L-lysine and glycerol monoethers are used as stabilizers.

Enzyme containers should be kept sealed to prevent the escape of a stabilizing atmosphere and also to maintain the low moisture content (below 50%) of the solid product. The storage temperature should be low but not freezing because freezing may cause denaturation of certain enzymes.

2.13. INDUSTRIAL ENZYMES

Of about 3,000 enzymes known today only a few are industrially exploited. These are mainly extracellular hydrolytic enzymes which degrade naturally occurring polymers such as starch, proteins, pectins and cellulose.

2.13.1. Bacterial α- amylases

Bacterial and fungal α-amylases are enzymes which have been manufactured industrially on a large scale. Bacterial α-amylase is an endoenzyme that cleaves α-1,4 bonds in amylose and amylopectin, leading to a rapid fall in the viscosity of gelatinized starch solution (endohydrolysis of starch also known as liquefaction of starch).

The end product recovered following the action of α-amylase are dextrans together with small quantities of glucose and maltose. Native starch is exposed to previous hydration (gelatinization of starch) before it is to be reacted by amylases. The α-amylase from *Bacillus amyloliquefaciens* is active upto 90°C and this high temperature. stability (for gelatinization purpose) has been exploited on the industrial scale. *Bacillus licheniformis* has also been used industrially for the production of α-amylases. α-Amylases are metallo-proteins, stabilized by Ca^{++} and inhibited by chelate forming agents. The activity and stability of the α-amylase from *B. licheniformis* is less dependent on the calcium content of solution as compared to the α-amylase from the *B. amylolequefaciens*. Maximum activity has shown by both enzymes at pH 6.5 to 7.

The fermentation of bacterial amylases is accomplished in submerged culture at neutral pH and at temperature between 30 to 40°C. Cereal meal and starch rich medium are used along with an organic source of nitrogen. After 10 to 20 hours, formation of α-amylase starts and continues for another 100 hours. pH of the medium must be below 6 during the fermentation to prevent the denaturation of α-amylase. The α-amylase is accompanied by other extracellular enzymes. *Bacillus licheniformis* produces a serine protease, while *B. amyloliquefaciens* produces, a neutral protease along with hemicellulase and β-glucanase.

The liquefaction of starch with α-amylase is carried out in a continuous or batch reactor. The extent of the desired hydrolysis of the starch is determined by the intended later use. Surface sizing of paper, manufacturing of coating compounds and paints require a colloidal starch solution with a final viscosity. Limited degradation of starch is brought about by α-amylase to achieve that particular viscosity. In the production of glucose syrup the α-amylase is used in the first step of enzymatic degradation yielding a mixture of glucose and fructose with high fructose content. In the production of dextrans degradation of starch is required as far as 10 dextrose equivalents (dextrose equivalents give the reducing power as a percentage of that of dextrose). The increasing production of alcohol as a fuel from starch-containing raw material is opening greater possibilities of use for α-amylases and glucoamylases.

2.13.2. Fungal α-amylases

Fungal α-amylases are mainly obtained from Aspergillus species (*A. niger, A. oryzae*). They greatly differ from the bacterial amylases by their lower deactivation temperature, low optimum pH (pH 4-5) and high saccharifying action. They are less suitable for the liquefaction of starch than bacterial α-amylases. The production of fungal α-amylase is carried out in solid-substrate culture and sometimes in submerged culture with selected strains of *Aspergillus*. Fermentation medium used remains the same as in the case of bacterial α-amylases but the concentration of glucose inhibits the formation of amylase, therefore the concentration of glucose in the fermentation media must be controlled and kept low. In solid-substrate culture other fungal enzymes are produced. The protease content is higher when produced by solid-substrate culture as compared to α-amylase produced by submerged culture. The amount of glucoamylase is low in both methods.

Fungal α-amylases are used in the manufacture of baked products where this enzyme is added to amylase-poor flour to shorten and standardize the proof time of dough. They are also used in the production of maltose-rich syrups and various areas of the foodstuffs industry.

2.13.3. Bacterial proteases

Bulk of the bacterial proteases are produced from *Bacillus licheniformis*. The bacteria is cultivated in a fermentation medium enriched by protein and protein hydrolysate. The pH of media is adjusted to neutral and temperature is kept between 30 to 40°C. Addition of carbohydrates in position increases the yield of enzyme. The production begins when the culture passes into the stationary phase (after 10 to 20 hours) and takes place at an approximately constant rate for many hours so long as protein is still present in the medium. Starch hydrolysate are degraded and assimilated by *B. licheniformis*, but at the end of the fermentation the serine protease is practically the only protein in the culture suspension.

Proteases can also be produced by fermentation of *B. amyloquefaciens* but the yield of protease is high in the case of *B. licheniformis* (10% or more of the protein added to the medium). The culture supernatant contains other enzymes especially large amount of α-amylase in the case of *B. amyloliquefaciens*. Proteases obtained from above two species are known as subtilisins and from *B. amyloliquefaciens* is known as alkaline protease. Nowadays serine proteases have been obtained from all lophilic species of *Bacillus*. These proteases have a better pH stability (upto pH 12) as compared to *Subtilisins* (pH 8 to 11).

The bulk of the alkaline proteases is used as additives to detergents in the form of granulates, prills or marumerizer pellets. Proteases increase the quality of cleansing power of detergent as well as facilitate the removal of protein containing soils such as blood; egg yolk, chocolate and increase the detachment of the soil from the fibers. The stability of subtilisins is independent of metal ions, hence complexing additives in detergents such as EDTA or tripolyphosphates do not greatly interfere. Today about 80% of the detergents in the market contain enzyme in concentration about 0.015 to 0.025%. The high alkali resistance of alkaline proteases make them suitable for leather industry, for the dehairing (nuding) of skins and to reduce softening times. They show better stability in detergents when the complexing agent EDTA or tripolyphosphate is replaced by citrate or gluconate.

2.13.4. Fungal proteases

Fungal proteases are produced from the general *Aspergillus* and strain from two species namely *A. oryzae* and *A. niger* are used. Large amount of proteases are formed by these species when cultivated on solid substrate. The yield can be further increased by addition of inorganic nitrogen. Apart from proteases, relatively large amounts of α-amylase, glucoamylase, cellulases and pectinases are formed.

Aspergillus proteases are used for hydrolysis of soybean protein in the production of soya sauce, as a constituent of enzyme preparations for the treatment of digestive disturbances, and in the baking industry. The addition of proteases to flour partially hydrolyzes glutin and lowers the viscosity of dough and shortens the kneading time. Fungal proteases are deactivated at 50°C, so a rapid denaturation occurs in the initiation of baking process and prevents the complete hydrolysis of proteins.

Acid proteases are also obtained from *Mucor* strains *M. pusillus* and *M. michei*. In the fermentation of *Mucor* strains, esterases and lipases are also formed. They are mainly used in the manufacture of cheese.

2.13.5. Glucose isomerase (D-xylose isomerase)

Glucose isomerase is the first intracellular enzyme that has been used on large scale. It is used in the isomerization of glucose to fructose. The process is based on the hydrolysis of starch with α-amylase and glucoamylase and then isomerization to a mixture of glucose and fructose. The mixture contains 42% fructose, 50% glucose and 8% other mono and disaccharides used as liquid sugar in food industry. Fructose has a greater sweetening power than sucrose and glucose. Generally immobilized enzyme is used because use of soluble glucose isomerase is very expensive.

Glucose isomerase is produced by submerged cultivation of various organisms listed in table 2.19 in the pH range 6.5 to 8.5 at 30°C. The isolation of enzyme is usually omitted and whole or disintegrated cells are immobilized. For immobilization of glucose isomerase, adsorption or heat treatment together with cross linkage has been used.

Table 2.19 : Glucose isomerase sources and immobilization techniques

Name of organism	Immobilization technique	Final form
Actinoplanes missóuriensis	Mycelium encapsulated in gelatin cross linked with glutaraldehyde	Microspheres
Arthrobacter	Immobilized in the cells with a flocculating agent	Cylindrical particles
Streptomyces olivochromogenes	Aluminium oxide support	Powder
Streptomyces olivvaceus	Whole cell; cross-linked with glutaraldehyde	Granules

Various types of reactor have been tested and it has been found that continuous fixed-bed reactors are the most suitable. The isomerization is carried out in the pH range of 7.0 to 8.5 at 60 to 65°C. The substrate solution contains 40 to 50% glucose and oligosaccharide and has a viscosity of 0.8 to 3 mPaS. Magnesium salt (0.5 to 5 mM/lit) is added to activate and stabilize the enzyme.

Alkali catalyzed conversion of fructose into mannose and psicose is prevented by lowering the pH of the product solution. Purification of fructose syrup is carried out by treatment with activated charcoal and using ion exchangers. The fructose syrup is concentrated to 71% dry matter and supplied.

The flow diagram of production of fructose syrup is shown in figure 2.36.

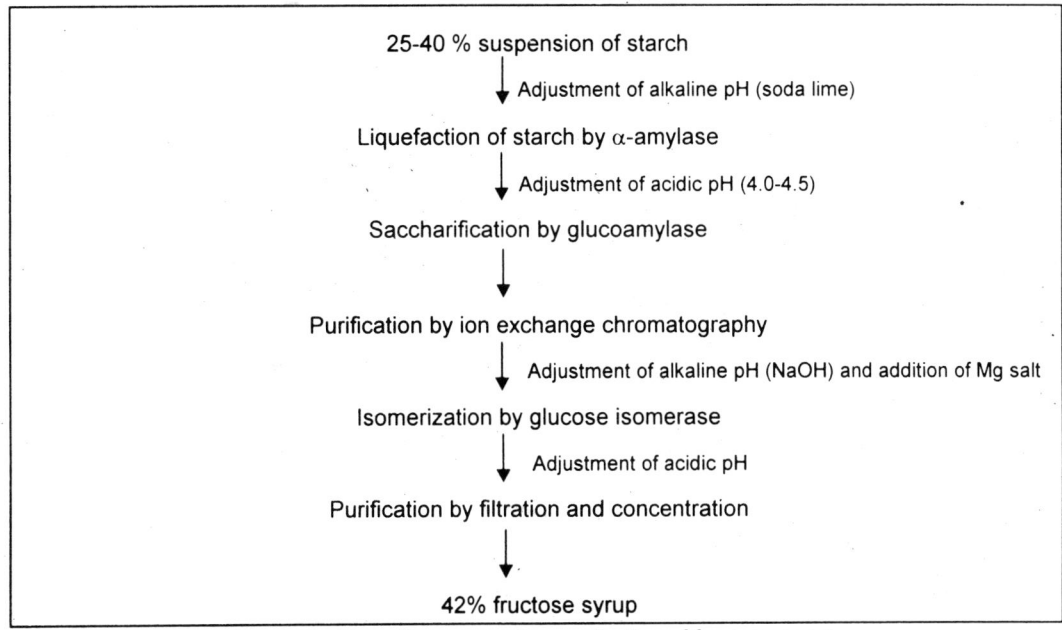

Fig. 2.36 : Flow diagram for the production of fructose syrup

2.13.6. Penicillinase

Penicillinase, a class of bacterial enzymes, which has gained wide publicity because of its inactivation property against the world's first antibiotic, the penicillin and certain cephalosporins. Penicillinase is not the only enzyme which can inactivate penicillin. There are several other hydrolytic enzymes which are also capable of inactivating penicillin. Penicillinase is produced by a number of pathogenic bacteria, notably of the *Staphylococcus* species and some gram negative bacteria of intestinal origin. This came into light when certain species showed resistance against penicillin. Especially, it was noted in patients infected by *Staphylococcus aureus*. The enzyme penicillin amidase is normally produced by many common genera of fungi, including *Penicillium*, *Aspergillus* and *Mucor*.

Penicillinase can be divided into two major classes based on their activity:

(a) Penicillin amidase or penicillin acylase, and

(b) β-lactamase or penicillinase

Penicillinase defeats the therapeutic potential of penicillins. The enzyme penicillin amidase is specific on attacking the acyl group attached to the basic nucleus, i.e., 6-aminopenicillanic acid (Fig. 2.37). Hence the name penicillin acylase. This enzyme is more specific with penicillin V and K. The other enzyme β-lactamase acts on the basic nucleus itself, i.e. by breaking the β-lactam bond and ultimately producing penicilloic acid. This enzyme is more specific with penicillin G, X and to a lesser extent against penicillin V.

As discussed above, some bacteria have the ability to produce penicillinase in constitutive, while in others it may be inducible. The latter can be demonstrated with the following example. When a patient is being treated with penicillin and if the concentration of the antibiotic is found to be non-lethal, then, it may induce the formation of penicillinase after which the bacteria becomes resistant to the antibiotic. A similar case is also observed when the penicillinase producing bacteria are more in number as compared to the concentration of antibiotic present at a particular time period. In this case, even though the bacteria when present in less number is susceptible to penicillin, becomes resistant to the same when they are more in number as the amount of penicillinase secreted by each bacteria mounts to a larger amount which as a result can sufficiently inactivate the antibiotic.

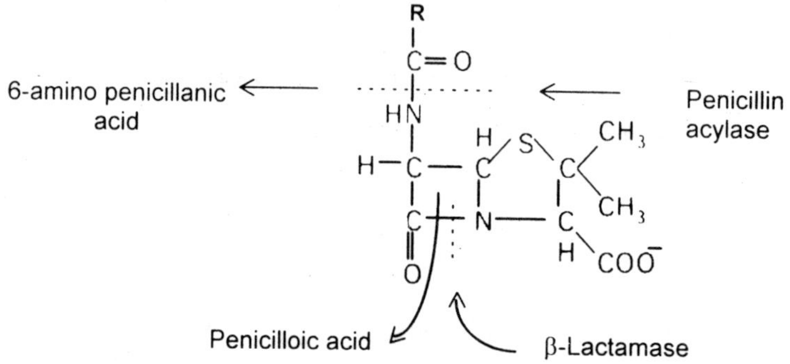

6-amino penicillanic acid ← ⋯ ← Penicillin acylase

Penicilloic acid ← β-Lactamase

Fig. 2.37 : Stucture of penicillin and its enzymatic conversion to 6-aminopenicillanic acid and penicilloic acid.

In many clinically resistant strains of bacteria, the production of β-lactamase is controlled by extra-chromosomal genetic elements. There exists a large number of striking differences between the enzyme produced by a gram positive and gram negative bacteria. The gram positive β-lactamases are of large molecular weight (28,000) while that of the gram negative are generally small (22,000). The amount of β-lactamase produced by gram positive bacteria are more in quantity and as the antibiotic is more specific against gram positive bacteria as compared to gram negative class so is the enzyme β-lactamase, more sensitive against penicillin when produced by gram positive bacteria. This is because the amount of enzyme produced by gram negative bacteria is far less and secondly they do not release the enzyme into the external environment. This can also be correlated in another way, i.e., as there is no β-lactamase released into the external environment, there is no dilution (loss) of β-lactamase takes place in gram negative bacteria and thus need for synthesis of β-lactamase by the cells is quenched.

2.13.7. Chloramphenicol acetyltransferase

Chloramphenicol a drug of choice in the treatment of typhoid fever and certain infections caused by organisms like *Haemophilus influenzae*. It was in Mexico when a major typhoid epidemic was encountered by chloramphenicol that certain strains of the gram negative bacteria *Salmonella typhi* came into light. It was further discovered that chloramphenicol resistance mediated by R-factors in gram negative bacteria and by transducible plasmids in *Staphylococcus aureus* is due to the presence of an enzyme chloramphenicol acetyl-transferase (CAT), which acetylates the **hydroxyl groups** of the side chain of the chloramphenicol (Fig.2.38).

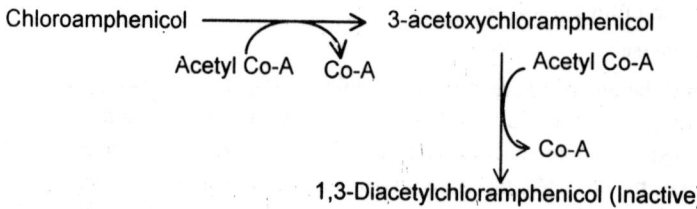

Fig. 2.38 : Two stage chloramphenicol inactivation reaction involving chloramphenicol acetyltransferase

The product obtained following the two stage inactivation process involving chloramphcnicol acetyl-transferase is 1,3-dicetoxychloramphenicol which is inactive. The synthesis of CAT in gram positive bacteria is induced by chloramphenicol. Chloramphenicol being an inhibitor of protein synthesis, shows an initial lag period wherein the antibiotic inhibits protein synthesis while simultaneous induction of CAT is called on. Hence, an initial low concentration of CAT does not affect the antibiotic however at a later phase, it brings down the inhibitory level i.e., when the concentration of CAT is sufficiently high enough to break down the drug moiety.

As discussed earlier under penicillinase, their exists a difference between enzymes which are secreted by a gram positive bacteria as compared to a gram negative bacteria. However, here, there is no such significant difference. The molecular weight of CAT synthesized by both gram positive and negative cells are nearly the same (80,000).

2.13.8. Aminoglycoside antibiotic inactivating enzymes

Aminoglycoside antibiotics are also susceptible to inactivation. Inspite of the variety of enzymes showing full or partial resistance to the antibiotic, there are only three types of inactivation reactions.

1. N-acetylation of susceptible amino groups
2. adenylation of hydroxyl groups
3. phosphorylation of hydroxyl groups

Table 2.20 shows various enzymes that are responsible for the inactivation of aminoglycoside antibiotics.

Table 2.20 : Various aminoglycoside antibiotic inactivating enzyme

Enzymes	Substrates (aminoglycoside antibiotics)
Gentamicin adenyltransferace	Kanamycins, gentamicins
Gentamicin acetyltransferases I and II	Gentamicin
Kanamycin acetyltransferase	Kanamycin A and B, neomycin, gentamicin
Kanamycin/neomycin phosphotransferases I and II	Kanamycins, neomycins, gentamicin A
Lividomycin phosphotransferase	Neomycin, paromomycin
Streptomycin/spectinomycin adenyltransferases	Streptomycin, spectinomycin
Streptomycin phosphotransferase	Streptomycin

Acetylation of the drug is carried out by acetyl-CoA which acts as the source of acetyl group. While the source of phosphoryl and adenyl groups is the adenosine triphosphate (ATP). Inactivation takes place in the periplasmic space (periplasm) or on the outer surface of the cytoplasmic membrane. Intracellular accumulation of active aminoglycosides appears to depend upon the induction of an energy-dependent process. Once the aminoglycosides are inactivated by the enzymes, the modified aminoglycoside is unable to induce intracellular accumulation. If at all they succeed in entering a cell, they are unable to interfere with the ribosomal function.

2.13.9. Fibrinolytic enzymes

The fibrinolytic system dissolves intravascular clots as a result of the action of plasmin, an enzyme that digests fibrin. Plasminogen, an inactive precursor, is converted to plasmin by cleavage of a single peptide bond. For this purpose, infusion of two types of enzymes can be considered, those with direct and general proteolytic activity such as plasmin or trypsin, and those such as the plasminogen activators which increase the level of native plasmin. In this respect, lyokinase plasminogen activator like streptokinase urokinase, and tissue plasminogen activator (t-PA) have received more attention.

2.13.9.1. Streptokinase

Streptokinase is a proteolytic enzyme (47-Kda protein) derived from the culture of β-hemolytic *Streptococci*. The protein molecule (mol. wt. 47,600 daltons) contains no cystein or cystine and has an isoelectric point of pH

4.7. The protein molecule possesses thrombolytic capability, catalyzing the transformation of human plasminogen to plasmin by hydrolytic cleavage of the arg-val bond. Its enzymatic action is based upon 1:1 noncovalent complex with the zymogen from which active plasmin is released. This complex has been dissociated into two components, one with plasmin activity along with other having plasminogen activity. Figure 2.39 schematically represents positive feedback mechanism, in which complexation first takes place between streptokinase and the plasmin contaminant of plasminogen. This complex, which is then free to transform a second plasminogen molecule.

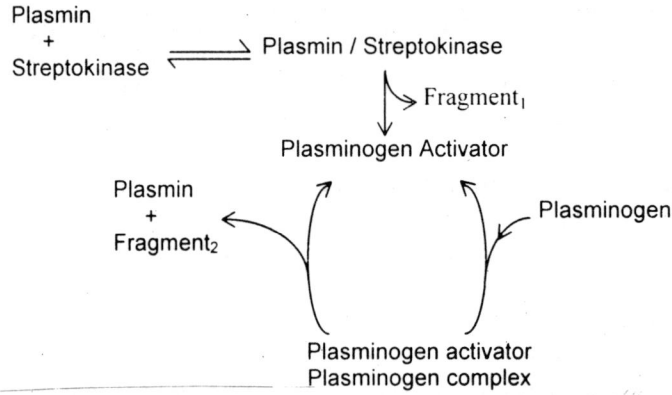

Fig. 2.39 : Proposed feedback mechanism attributed to streptokinase

Streptokinase have been found superior in the lysis of artificially induced coronary thrombi and pulmonary embolism. The superiority of streptokinase over heparin in reducing mortality in myocardial infection have also been established. A streptokinase-plasminogen complex (antistreplase) in which lys-plasminogen is acylated at its catalytic site, serine is also used for coronary thrombolysis. The acyl group is hydrolyzed *in vivo*, allowing the complex to bind to fibrin prior to activation, and this modification confers some specificity towards clots on the fibrinolytic process. Streptokinase is antigenic due to its bacterial origin and may bind to antibodies and nonspecific inhibitors. The immune response shown by streptokinase affects the alteration of urokinase.

2.13.9.2. Urokinase

Urokinase is a two chain serine protease containing 411 amino acid residues. Synthesized and isolated from cultured human kidney cells, the protein is a single polypeptide of molecular weight 54,500 daltons and is very stable to temperatures and extremes of pH.

It has been known for many years that urine can digest blood clots because of the presence of proteolytic enzyme, urokinase. Human urokinase can act as a plasminogen activator, its specificity is to cleave peptide bonds adjacent to lysine and arginine side chains, and being of human origin, it is non-immunogenic. Its enzyme action is similar to that of trypsin, catalyzing the activation of plasminogen in a first order reaction with cleavage of the arg-val bond.

2.13.9.3. Tissue plasminogen activator (t-PA)

t-PA is a proteolytic enzyme that has 527 amino acid residues. It binds to fibrin via lysine binding sites at its amino terminus and activates bound plasminogen several hundred fold more rapidly than it activates plasminogen in circulation. It is a poor plasminogen activator in the absence of fibrin. Under physiological conditions (5 to 10 ng/ml), the specificity of t-PA for fibrin limits systemic formation of plasmin and induction of a systemilytic state.

t-PA is effective in lysing thrombi during treatment of acute myocardial infarction. t-PA is produced by recombinant DNA technology It is currently recommended for coronary thrombolysis. The main side effect is severe hemorrhage. t-PA is expensive, costing several times more than streptokinase per therapeutic dose.

2.13.10. L-Asparaginase

In 1953 Kidd found that only adult guinea pig serum induced regression of lymphosarcoma and identified L-asparaginase as the source of activity. In *E. coli*, two isoenzymes with asparaginase activity EC-1 and EC-2 are present. Asparaginase I (EC-1) is constitutive and asparaginase II (EC-2) is included anaerobiosis and only latter has anti-leukaemic activity. Isoenzymes II from *E. coli* strain A1.3 have been purified to homogeneity and the amino acid sequence. Preliminary X-ray studies show a tetrameric quaternary structure with the four subunits related by 222 symmetry. The subunits are identical with molecular weight 34,080. *E. coli* asparaginase-II (EC-2) obeys Michaelis-Menten kinetics and has maximum activity between pH 6 and 8. Hydrolysis of asparagine and L-aspartyl-β-hydroxamate catalyzed by L-asparaginase is consistent with a "ping-pong" mechanism.

Normal tissues synthesize L-asparagine in amounts sufficient for protein synthesis. Acute lymphoblastic leukemic cells require an exogenous source of this amino acid. L-asparaginase, by catalyzing the hydrolysis of circulating asparagine to aspartic acid and ammonia deprives these cells of the asparagine necessary for protein synthesis, leading to cell death.

SUGGESTED READINGS

Barman, T.E., (1969) **Enzyme Handbook**, Spring-Verlag, Berlin, Heidelberg, New York.

Boyer, P.D. (Ed.), (1971)**The Enzymes**, Vol. 3, Acdemic Press, New York.

Colowick, S.P. and Kaplan, N.O. (Eds.), (1955) **Methods in Enzymology**, Academic Press, New York, Vol.I.

Enzyme Nomenclature : Recommendations (1978) of the Nomenclature of the International Union of Biochemistry on the Nomenclature and classification of Enzymes, Academic Press, New York, San Francisco, London.

Fersht, A., (1977) **Enzyme Structure and Mechanism**, Freeman, San Francisco.

Foster R.L., (1980) **The Nature of Enzymology**, Croom Helm, London.

Godfrey, T. and Reichelt, J. (eds), (1983) **Industrial Enzymology**, Macmillan Publishers.

Greenberg, D.M. and Harper, H.T. (Eds.), (1960) **Enzymes in Health and Disease**, Charles, C. Thomas, Spring-Field.

Hugo, W.B. (Ed.), (1971) **Inhibition and Destruction of Microbial Cells**, Academic Press, London, p 39-70.

Innerfield, I., (1960) **Enzymes in Clinical Medicine**, McGraw Hills, Blakiston Division, New York.

Kula, M.R., (1987) *Enzymes* In **Fundamentals of Biotechnology** P. Prave, U. Faust, W. Sittings, D.A. Sukatsch (Eds.), VCH Verlagsgesellschaft mbH, D-6940, Weinhein Germany, p 473

Lehninger A. L., (1990) **Principles of Biochemistry**, CBS Publishers and Distributors Pvt. Ltd., New Delhi, p 207-241.

Melling, J. and Phillips, B. W., (1975) *Practical aspect of large-scale enzyme purification* In **Handbook of Enzyme Biotechnology**, A. Wiseman (Ed.), Elis Harwood Ltd. Chichester, p 181-202

Moran, L.A. and Scringeous, K.G., (1994) **Biochemistry Resource Book**, Neil Patterson Publishers, Prentice Hall, NJ, USA, p 27-57.

Murry, P.K., Mayes, P.A., Granner, D.K., Rodwell, V.M. (Eds.), (1990) **Harper's Biochemistry**, 22nd edition, Prentice-Hall International Inc., p 58-89.

Neilands, J.B. and Stumpf, P.K., (1958) **Outline of Enzyme Chemistry**, 2nd edition, John Wiley & Sons, New York, p 132-169.

Ottaway and Apps, D.K., (1984) **Biochemistry**, Fourth edition, The English Language Book Society and Bailler Tindall, p 24-44.

Patel, P.R., (1985) *Enzyme Isolation and purificatio*, In **Biotechnology: Application and Research**, P.N. Cheremisinoff and R.P. Ouellette (Eds.), Technomic Publising Co. Inc., Lancaster, Basel, p 534-564.

Strove, E.A., (1989) **Biochemistry**, Mir Publications, Moscow, p 125-163.

Stryer, L., (1988) **Biochemistry**, Third edition, W.H. Freeman and Company, New York, p 177-257.

Weber, G. (Ed.), (1963-1977) **Advances in Enzyme Regulation**, Vol. 1-4, Pergamon Press.

West, E.S., Todd, W.R., Mason, H.S., VanBruygen, J.T., (1966) **Text book of Biochemistry**, fourth edition, The Macmillan Company Collier-Macmillan Ltd., London, p 419-490.

IMMOBILIZATION

3.1. INTRODUCTION

In modern therapeutics, physiologically active natural compounds, especially enzymes have gained considerable importance in practical medicine and in many of biotech events where they are being utilized, industrially. Moreover, in recent years quite a number of diseases, related to the lysosomal enzyme activities have been identified and discussed. These diseases theoretically can be cured by supplementation or replacement of defective or deficient enzyme. Furthermore, enzymes with very specific functionaries are generally involved in the catalysis of many reactions.

It should be realized with emphasis that a day to day use of enzymes in clinical therapeutics, as bioreactors, biosensor and in other enzyme based reactions is limited by a number of factors, i.e. high cost and low availability, quick inactivation under physiological condition followed by fast clearance, thus necessitating for higher requirement of enzyme in the course of treatment. Furthermore, possible antigenicity, inactivation by various endogenous natural inhibitors and lastly, difficult to build up a higher level for therapeutic activity are constraints which restrain the practical clinical use of enzymes. Despite of all constraints, enzymes have an enormous range of possible applications covering therapeutic, analytical and industrial. However, the enzymes per se demonstrated their application potentials unified by the unique enzyme characteristics of precise specificity for substrate and reaction catalyzed. In order to be practically acceptable, an enzyme should have superb catalytic behavior, with specificity, stability and reusability. It has been realized that most of the enzymes following their involvement in initiation of a particular reaction during latter phase due to the accumulation and detrimental effect of the reaction product become relatively less active. Enzymes being bioproteins are environmental sensitive in regard to pH, temperature and as a consequence their stability remains under constant challenges, thus entails for an effective cure of problems associated with enzyme and enzyme technology. The objective of immobilization is distinctively, economic application of enzyme systems. Other added advantages of the immobilized enzyme system are ease of control and uniformity of conversion. The key to qualify economic considerations is the determination of the cost of the components of the immobilized system versus the value of its performance.

3.1.1. Immobilization

Immobilization of enzymes may be defined as a process wherein an enzyme makes use of carrier phase for stealth, and safe homing. The immobilization matrix or support allows exchange with, but remains separated from the bulk phase in which substrate, effect or inhibitor molecules are present dispersed. It involves confining soluble protein catalysts, or individual buoyancy of cells in a reactor system which can repeatedly need fresh change of solution. The immobilized system is generally placed in a suitable column through which the charge is allowed to pass continuously. The definition may be expanded to cover intact cells and biocatalyst under the category of guest. The process of immobilization which in other words implies for restrictive localization of enzymes perhaps in the immediate future will have great potential in the development of biosensor, bioelectronic sensor in fermentation technology as well as in enzyme therapeutics. The carrier phase, also referred to as enzyme phase is typically a water insoluble but hydrophilic porous polymeric matrix, e.g. cellulose, agarose and acrylamide. In other words, particularly in biochemical control immobilization is a generic term that describes the retention of biologically active catalyst within a reactor or analytical system with the help of an appropriate carrier support. A special module is produced employing immobilization techniques through which fluid can pass easily, transforming substrate in to product under controlled enzymatic reaction and at the same time facilitating the easy removal of catalyst from the product as it leaves the reactor.

The immobilization or forced homing of enzymes is brought about via covalent coupling employing adsorption or physical entrapment of enzyme within the enzyme phase (polymeric matrix). The nature of immobilized enzyme is characteristically dependent upon the character of matrix and enzyme phase. The most common form of enzyme immobilization utilizes its anchoring on the surface of an insoluble polymeric matrix, i.e. cellulose or polyacrylamide through covalent bond formation. The enzyme phase however, may be in the form of fine particulate, membranous or monolithic spheres. The enzyme in turn may be bound to another enzyme via cross linking. Thus, rendering the overall composite to be an insoluble, but active polymeric enzyme system. When a support or carrier is used for the purpose of enzyme immobilization, the durability of that carrier during its use is equally important. The carrier, which may be a membrane or matrix, that is not stable at a particular pH, ionic strength and or under solvent conditions of the process, may be disrupted or dissolved releasing the enzyme component. This clearly suggests that it is not necessary for a carrier to be insoluble and durable at all pH, ionic strength or solvent conditions. Various methods most commonly used for enzymes immobilization using solid support can be classified into two main classes.

The major division of approaches is between those which are employed to restrain biocatalysts within the support and those which held biocatalyst on the surface of the support, each class has further division as covalent and non-covalent coupling methods for surface immobilization whereas cross linking entrapment and encapsulation techniques for immobilization in or within a support.

On surface immobilization

1. Covalent coupling with polymers employing their functional group for anchoring, moreover the groups must be non functional or non-essential for biological activity.
2. Adsorption on an inert support or ion-exchange resins.
3. Complexation and chelation

Within support immobilization

4. Cross-linking by multifunctional reagents, following entrapment within a structure of known/defined geometry.
5. Entrapment by
    a. occlusion within cross-linked gel.
    b. encapsulation in microcapsules, hollow fibers, liposomes, etc.

Immobilization often causes noticeable changes in apparent parameters of the enzyme related to the reaction it catalyses. The parameters include the reaction rate, effect of inhibitor which may be excluded altogether in the case of immobilized enzyme, Michaelis-Menten kinetics and optimum temperature and pH corresponding to maximum activity. The extent of variation in these parameters may not only be related to the method of immobilization selected but also to some extent to the enzyme reaction.

3.2. SURFACE IMMOBILIZATION BY COVALENT COUPLING

The covalent bond between biocatalyst and a support matrix forms a stable complex which is appreciably stable during functional use of enzyme. However, the process subjects the delicate three dimensional structure of the biopolymer to strong disruptive physical and chemical forces or stresses. Therefore, where superior form and stability of immobilized enzyme overweighs the irreversible loss of activity that inevitably associated with immobilization process, it is preferred over soluble form.

The functional groups present on enzyme proteins, through which a covalent bond with polymeric or other supports could be established should be non-essential for enzymatic activity. Moreover, the reactions which involve relatively mild condition and essentially utilize an aqueous media are preferred. This further necessitates the complete knowledge of amino acids and their active group involved in polymeric covalent bonding, possibility of chemical amelioration or specific chemical modification on activity, protection of active group(s) and three dimensional structure of enzyme under consideration. The protein functional groups which could be utilized in covalent coupling include:

1. NH_2 lysine, N-terminal of polypeptide
2.   COOH β and α of aspartic acid, glutamic acid respectively
3.   OH   Phenol ring on tyrosine
4.   SH   group on cysteine

5.   group on serine, tyrosine and threonine

6. indole group of tryptophan

7. imidazole group of histidine

On the other hand the polymeric supports which have been explored as support for covalent coupling based immobilization include:

1. Hydroxyl groups of polysaccharides, PVA, polymethyl methacrylate (PMMA) and inorganic glasses.
2. Amino and related groups of amino-ethyl coated polysaccharides and silica gel, poly(D-aminoglycine), etc.
3. Carboxylic acid and related groups of poly(glutamic acid), maleic anhydride co-polymers, poly(acrylamide) and carboxy methyl cellulose.
4. Aldehyde and acetal groups of polymers.
5. Amide group of polypeptides and polyamides (nylon).

The covalent coupling methods generally used for conjugation of enzymes with solid/matrix support are cyanobromide, cyclic trans 2,3-carbonates and acid anhydrides. Similarly, methods used for covalent anchoring via support activation are typically diazotization, Schiff's base formation, glutaraldehyde treatment, thiodisulfide and imido ester formation.

With the help of these coupling agents and selected method covalent bonds are formed between functional group on enzymes and respective counter groups on polymeric support with a net result of an immobilized enzyme system formation.

3.2.1. Polymers with hydroxyl groups

Polymers which contain free hydroxyl group have widely been used as supporting polymers for enzyme-localization or immobilization via covalent anchoring.

The most commonly used polymers are polysaccharides, polyvinyl alcohol (PVA), polyhydroxyethyl methacrylate (PHEMA), silica and porous glasses. The polymers may be engaged in direct coupling as well as could be modified and generated with other coupling functional groups. Polysaccharide supports are basically cellulose, starch, dextran and agar. The coupling and activation reactions are schematically presented in figure 3.1. The reactions most commonly used are discussed in this chapter. These chemical reactions are used to deal most delicate proteins and enzyme molecules for their immobilization as well as surface modification of carrier units using proteinaceous modules.

Commercially available dextran gel (sephadex) is a cross linked dextran where epichlorhydrin is used as a cross linking agent. Polysaccharide solid support immobilization is generally covalent anchoring of protein or peptide molecule. Various chemical covalent coupling method which could be exploited for surface anchoring or immobilization are discussed in this chapter.

3.2.2. Glutaraldehyde based protein coupling

Proteins and related components possessing free amino/amine groups could be immobilized utilizing these groups as anchoring points. Agents like glutaraldehyde with bifunctionality may be used. It could effectively hook up the amino group of two adjacent molecules of which one is essentially a protein whereas other obviously must be a support. The bifunctional agents however, could lead to cross linking as well as cross bridging amongst other proteins adjacent molecules.

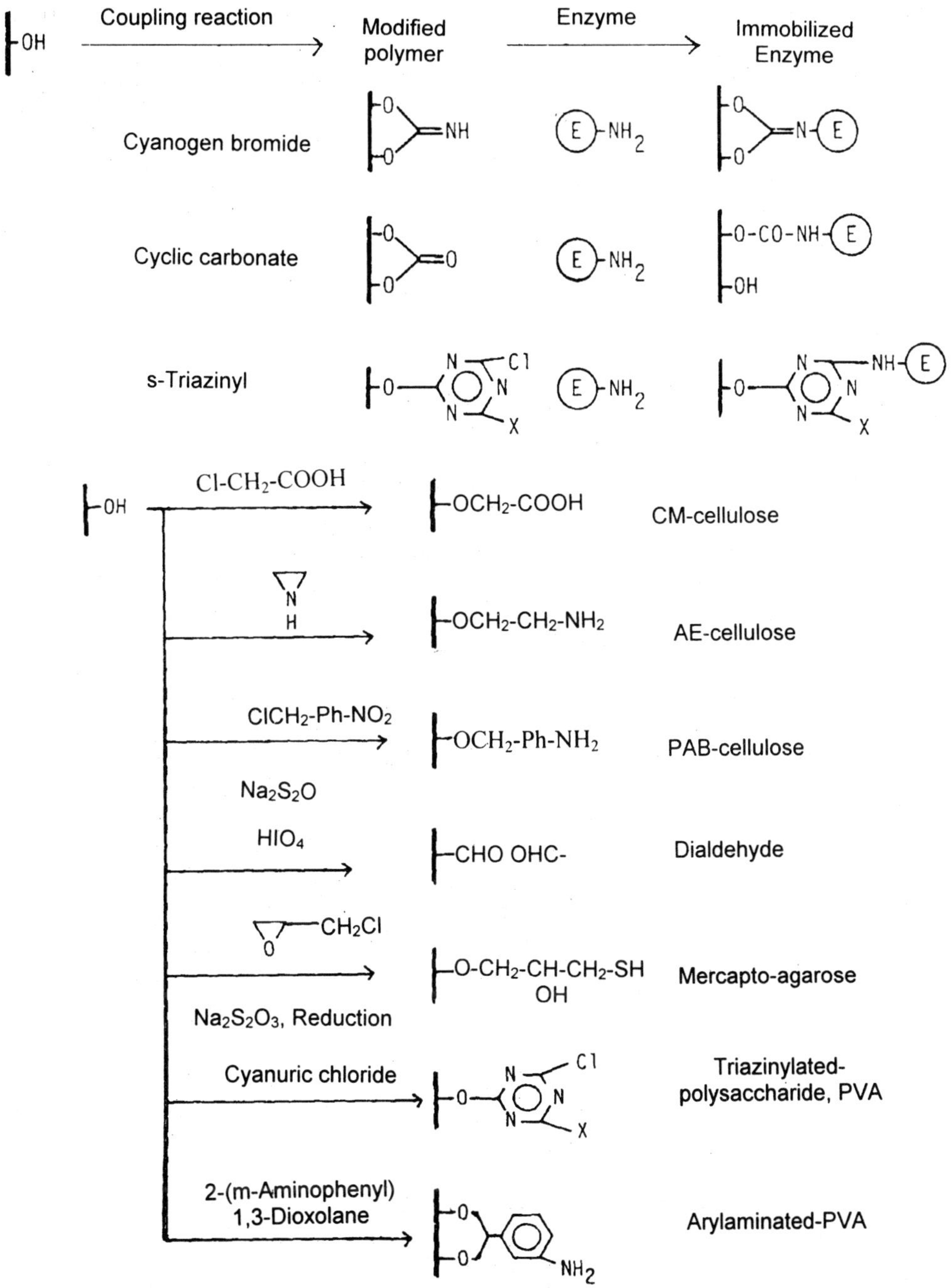

Fig. 3.1 : Schematic representation of hydroxyl group bearing polymer support modification

Thus, at large in contrast to desirable support-protein linking, protein-protein cross linking may also result, which in general is not a preferred state however, in other situations this cross linking phenomenon may be appreciated as **autoimmobilization**. The functional character of glutaraldehyde initiated covalent anchoring is schematically presented in figure 3.2.

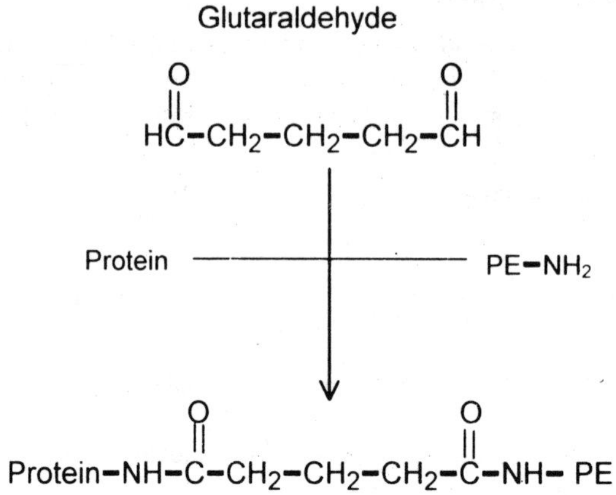

Glutaraldehyde

$$O \qquad\qquad O$$
$$\parallel \qquad\qquad\qquad \parallel$$
$$HC-CH_2-CH_2-CH_2-CH$$

Protein —————————————— PE—NH₂

$$O \qquad\qquad\qquad O$$
$$\parallel \qquad\qquad\qquad\qquad \parallel$$
$$Protein-NH-C-CH_2-CH_2-CH_2-C-NH- PE$$

Fig. 3.2 : Cross-linkage of protein and lipid with the homobifunctional agent glutaraldehyde

3.2.3. Covalent coupling employing N-succinimide activation

In another variation where surface fatty acylation is adapted as a strategy for protein or enzyme immobilization, the amino group of the protein could be covalently linked to the activated carboxyl group of a fatty acid. However, the latter needs preactivation which could be brought about by reacting fatty acids with N-hydroxy succinimide. The most widely used reaction is schematically presented in figure 3.3.

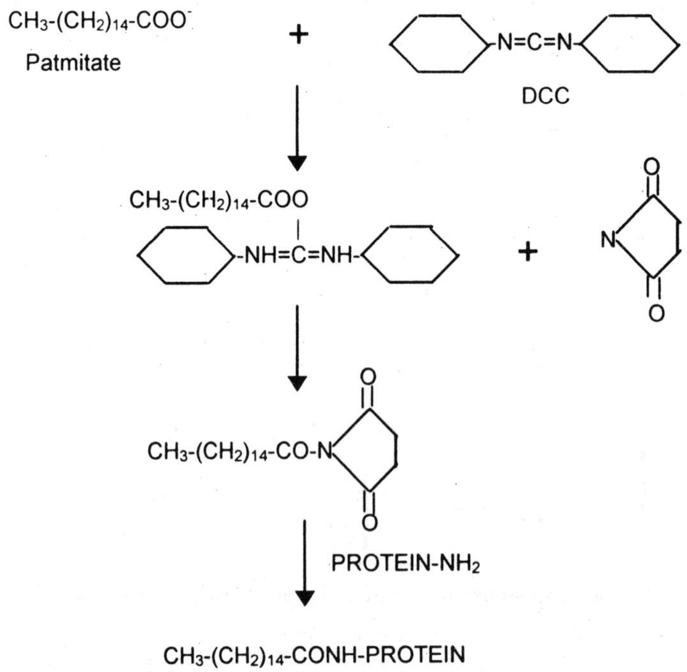

$$CH_3-(CH_2)_{14}-COO^-$$

Patmitate

$+$

⬡—N=C=N—⬡

DCC

$$CH_3-(CH_2)_{14}-COO$$

⬡—NH=C=NH—⬡

$+$

$$CH_3-(CH_2)_{14}-CO-N$$

PROTEIN-NH₂

$$CH_3-(CH_2)_{14}-CONH-PROTEIN$$

Fig. 3.3 : Coupling of the amine residue of protein to fatty acids via N-succinimide

3.2.4. Coupling through diacyl fatty anhydrides

The free amino groups of the enzymes and the protein could directly be reacted and conjugated with diacyl fatty anhydride(s). The covalent conjugation employing this method is shown in figure 3.4. Dodecanoic acid anhydride reacts with free amino group imparting fatty acylation to the protein molecule(s).

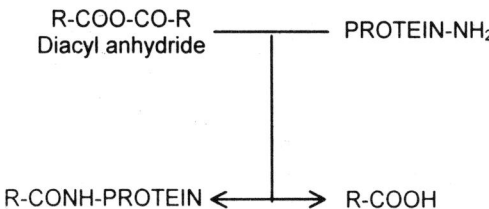

Fig. 3.4 : Reaction of diacyl acid anhydrides such as dodecanoic acid anhydride with the free amino group of the protein.

3.2.5. Schiff's base reaction and periodate activation

The free hydroxy group(s) of immobilization carrier is oxidized to produce active aldehyde group which reacts with free amino group of protein forming an amide/peptide bond. The bond is stabilized following the reduction with borohydride. The scheme is depicted in figure 3.5. In an alteration of this method the amino group of the protein or enzyme could be activated using periodate to form free aldehyde reactive group which in turn conjugates with free amino group of a hydrogenated polymeric support.

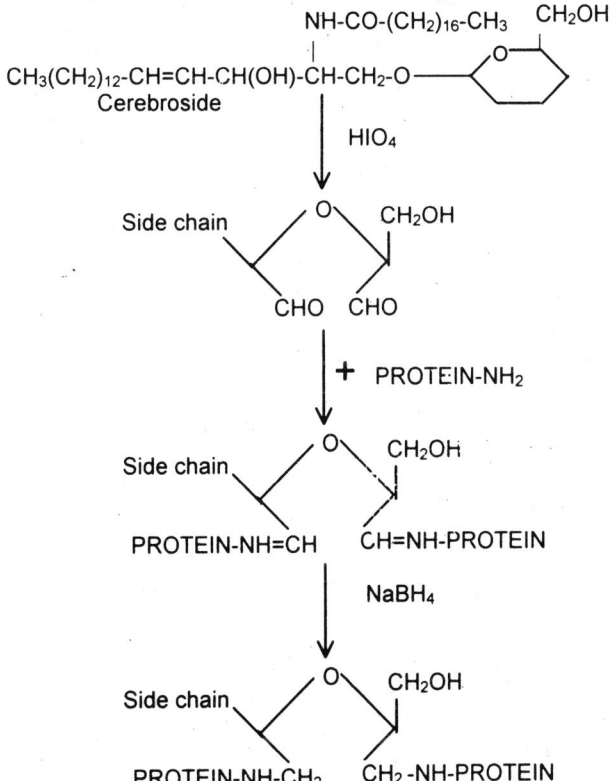

Fig. 3.5 : Schiff's base reaction between the periodate-activated carbohydrate function of a glycolipid and amine group of protein

3.2.6. Carbodiimide mediated coupling

Carbodiimide reagent has been extensively used in covalent coupling and thus in immobilization. This method essentially involves activated carboxyl group of amino acid/protein/enzyme using carbodiimide. So activated groups are then allowed to react with amine group of carrier support. Carbodiimide used for this purpose should be water soluble hence, 1-(3-dimethylaminopropyl)-3-ethyl carbodiimides are typically selected agents. Similar to glutaraldehyde the carbodiimide also causes cross linking of protein molecules through internal carboxyl and amine groups (fig.3.6). This could effectively eliminate the required citraconylation of the protein or enzyme molecules.

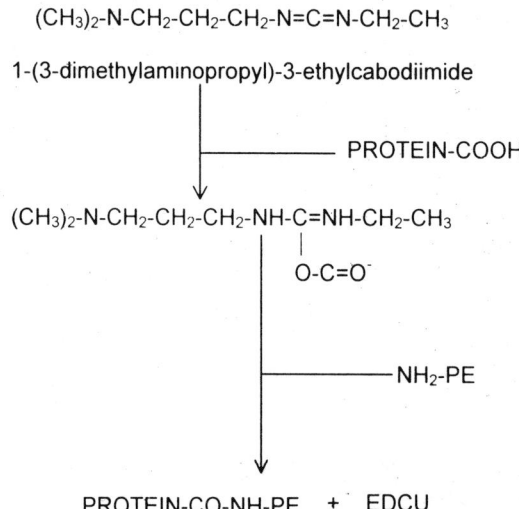

$$(CH_3)_2\text{-}N\text{-}CH_2\text{-}CH_2\text{-}CH_2\text{-}N=C=N\text{-}CH_2\text{-}CH_3$$

1-(3-dimethylaminopropyl)-3-ethylcabodiimide

PROTEIN-COOH

$$(CH_3)_2\text{-}N\text{-}CH_2\text{-}CH_2\text{-}CH_2\text{-}NH\text{-}C=NH\text{-}CH_2\text{-}CH_3$$

$$O\text{-}C=O^-$$

NH₂-PE

PROTEIN-CO-NH-PE + EDCU

Fig. 3.6 : Water-soluble carbodiimide coupling between the carboxyl function of the protein and the amine terminus of lipid.

3.2.7. Conjugation through phenolic group of protein or enzymes

The diazotization reaction typically involves coupling of proteins as an enzyme through tyrosine residues of proteins containing free phenolic group. The procedure is capable of avoiding homopolymerization reactions which are frequently encountered in the methods which employ bifunctional agents. Furthermore, it does not necessitate thiolation of proteins which is an essential step required with sulfhydryl reactive group.

3.2.8. Conjugation through sulfhydryl group

It is well established and known that the immunoglobulins interchange disulfide linkage, this later linkage offers useful strategies where sulfide reactive agents could be used for covalent conjugation without disrupting the immune reactivity. General, prerequisite is thiol modification prior to treatment of such proteins with disulfide reducing agent, i.e. dithiothreitol. However, the pretreatment step could be avoided by adapting the procedure which introduces new preactivated sulfhydryl group into the protein molecule.

The compound used for preactivation and incorporation of such groups into the protein molecules are exemplified by succinimidyl-acetyl thioacetate (SATA), exposure of free sulfhydryls conjugated to SATA can be a compressed by the addition of hydroxylamine, which need not to be removed thus obviates the need of subsequent conjugation procedure.

Similarly, a common sulfhydryl detecting agent, i.e. 5,5'-dithio bis-2-nitrobenzoic acid, which is referred to as Ellman reagent can be coupled to the carrier which has been activated at amine residue using 2-iminothiolane. The method is presented schematically in figure 3.7. Disulfide coupling with available sulfhydryl group of proteins occurs together with the production of thionitrobenzoate, which is water soluble hence could be removed through washings.

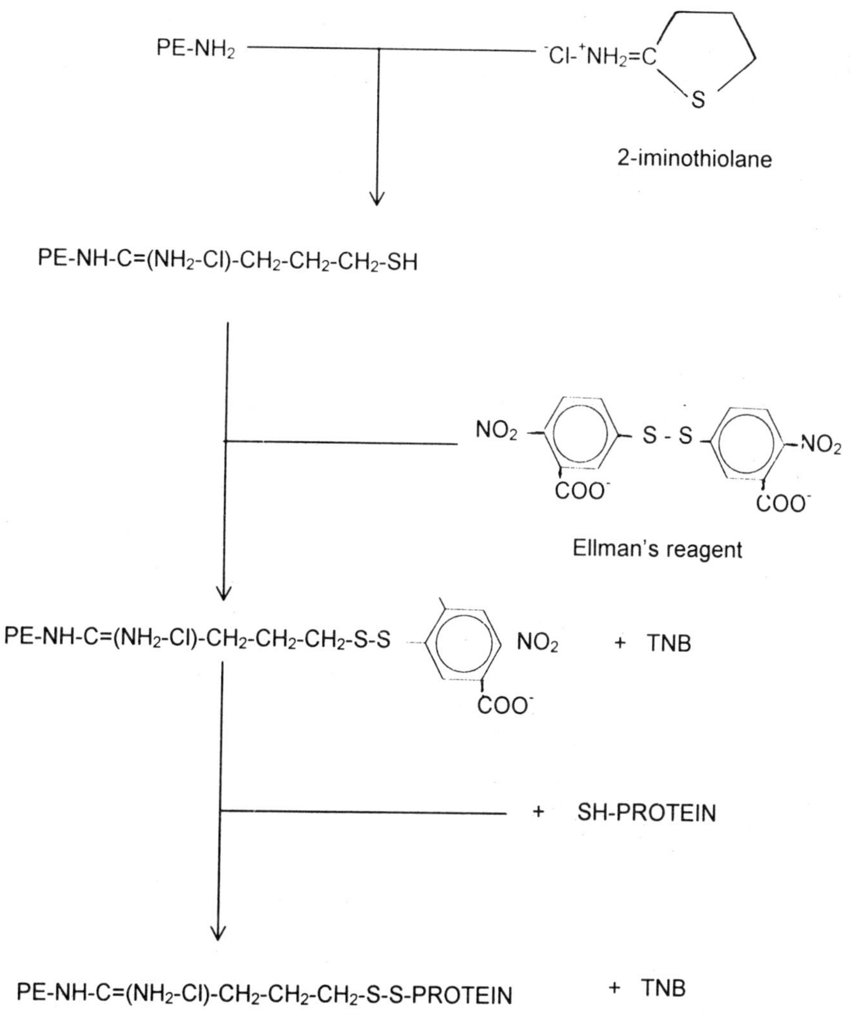

PE-NH₂ ——————————— Cl⁻·⁺NH₂=C⟨S⟩

2-iminothiolane

PE-NH-C=(NH₂-Cl)-CH₂-CH₂-CH₂-SH

NO₂ — S - S — NO₂
COO⁻   COO⁻

Ellman's reagent

PE-NH-C=(NH₂-Cl)-CH₂-CH₂-CH₂-S-S — NO₂   + TNB
                                      COO⁻

+   SH-PROTEIN

PE-NH-C=(NH₂-Cl)-CH₂-CH₂-CH₂-S-S-PROTEIN   + TNB

Fig. 3.7 : Thiolation of phospholipids and subsequent activation for reaction with the sulfhydryl functions of proteins

The group sulfhydryl has also been appreciated and used for covalent coupling using alkyl halides such as iodoacetate as an activator. The later, selectively blocks appropriate groups and allows possible linkage of protein sulfhydryl forming an iodoacetate modified carrier support. This alternative strategy is depicted in figure 3.8.

In essence the reaction can be concluded with the introduction of most widely used sulfhydryl linkers, which are typically heterobifunctional agents and succinylamine They offer an N-hydroxy succinimide function on one end of the molecules and either a pyridine or maleimide group on the other. The reaction is schematically presented in figure 3.9 and 3.10.

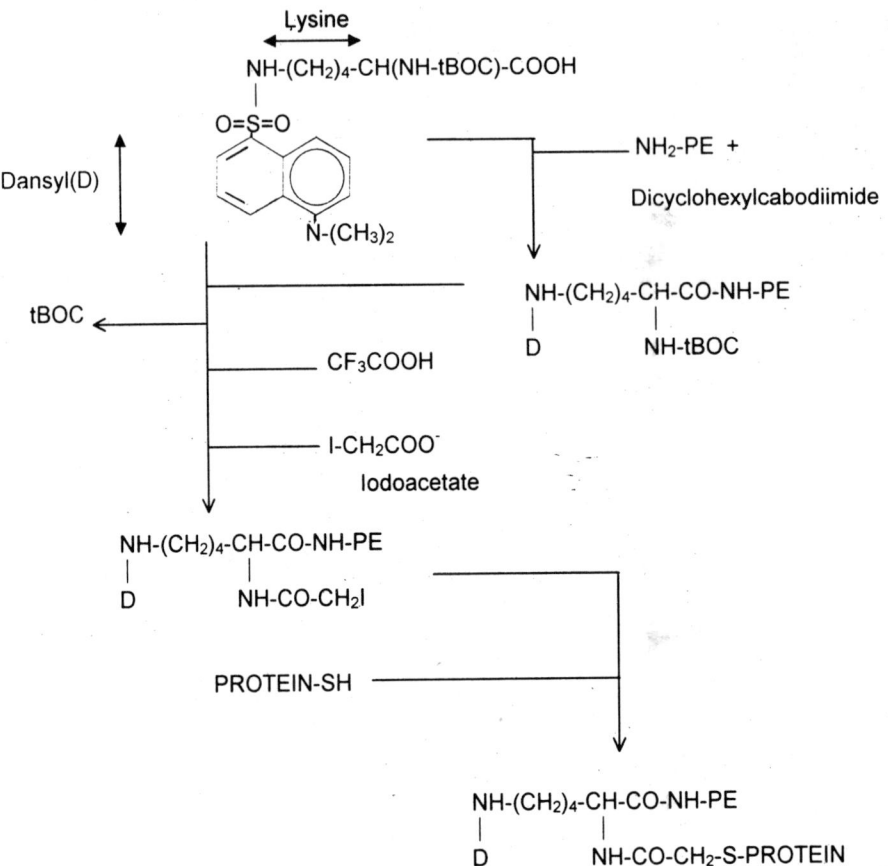

Fig. 3.8 : Reaction of protein sulfhydryl groups with iodoacetate-activated lipid-lysine conjugate

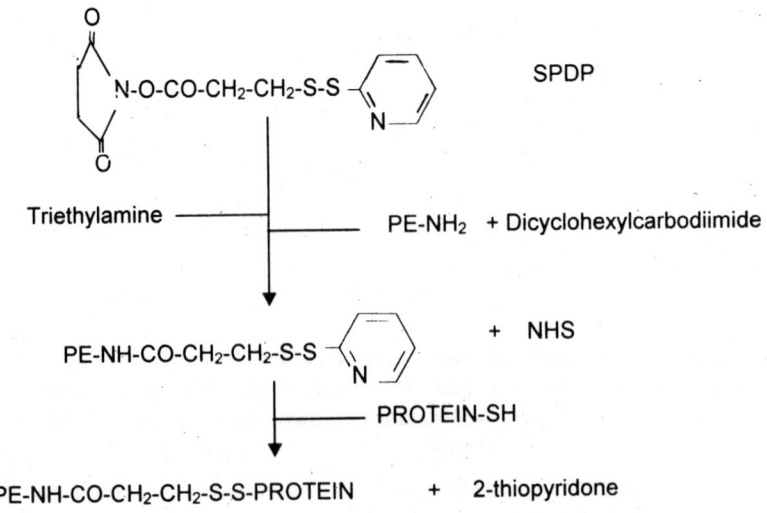

Fig 3.9 : Acitivation of phospholipids with the heterobifunctional agents SPDP
(N-succinimidyl proprionyl dithiopyridine) for reaction with sulfhydryl groups of protein

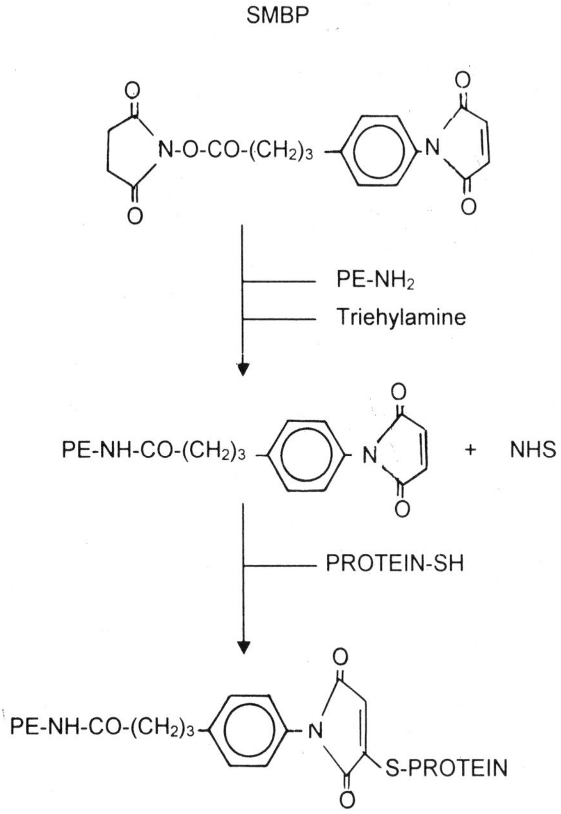

SMBP

Fig. 3.10 : Activation of phospholipids with heterofunctional agents SMPB
(N-succinimidyl 4-(p-maleidophyenyl) butyrate)

3.2.9. Application of covalent anchoring

3.2.9.1. Polysaccharide as solid support

Cellulose is essentially 1,4-linked β-D-glucose organized into fibers of high crystallinity and dextrans a linear water soluble polysaccharide that is a 1,6-linked α-D-glucose biosynthesized by a microorganism leuconostoc. Commercially available dextran gels (Sephadex) are epichlorhydrin-dextrin cross linked polymer. Agarose derived from agar, is a complex mixture of naturally occurring polysaccharide extracted from species of the Rhodophylaceae family of red sea water algae. The agarose molecule is composed of alternating 1,3 linked β-D-glucose, and 1,4-linked 3, anhydro-α-L galactose. These naturally occuring polysaccharides are activated and derivatized using different reagents and used as support for the immobilization of enzymes (Fig. 3.11). Some classical examples are polysaccharide containing alkylamino groups which have been derivatized as amino-ethyl cellulose(AE-cellulose), Diethylaminoethyl cellulose (DEAE-cellulose) and p-amino benzyl cellulose (PAB-cellulose). These polymers are firstly diazotized or subjected for isothiocynation before they are used for coupling.

One of the most extensively and successfully used procedure for enzyme immobilization involving polysaccharide support has been the cyano-bromide activation method. The method at low temperature has successfully been utilized to obtain high yield of conjugated protein. The method employs for activation of polysaccharide/cellulose involving cyclic trans-2,3 carbonate derivatives which are analogous to 2,3 trans-imido carbonate.

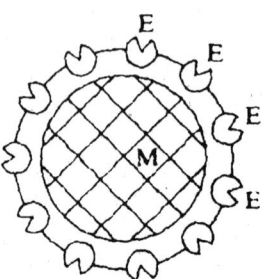

M = Water-insoluble matrix
E = Enzyme

Enzyme attachment to
matrix by covalent bonds

Cross-linked
enzyme matrix

Enzyme cross-linking by
multifunctional reagent

Fig. 3.11 : Diagrammatic representation of covalent and crosslinking technique

The later is assumed to be an active intermediate in cyanogen bromide activation. The method is schematically given in figure 3.12. Yet another interesting methods of cellulose modification are the formation of cellulose dialdehyde derivatives or dimethyl sulfoxides (DMSO) or an oxidation of vicinal hydroxyl groups. Partially oxidised cellulose binds enzymes presumably through Schiff's base formation and subsequent linkage with amino group of protein.

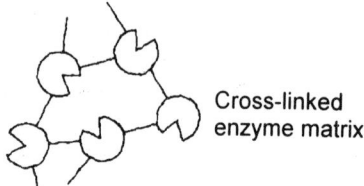

Fig. 3.12 : Schematic presentation of immobilization using cyanogen bromide method

Hydroxyl group containing vinyl polymers such as PVA (polyvinyl alcohol) and poly hydroxylethyl methacrylate are well accepted polymeric supports used for immobilization. Similarly, a co-polymer based on hydroxy-alkyl acrylate and/or hydroxy alkyl methacrylate monomers is a hydroxyl group containing polymeric support spherical in shape (as polymerized by suspension polymerization method) which has been proven to be suitable for enzyme immobilization.

The hydroxyethyl groups of spheron gel may chemically be modified by a set of chemical treatments including, diazotization, cyanobromination, trans 2,3-cyclo carbonation, and Schiff's base formation. As discussed in the case of polysaccharide(s), cellulose, chemical modification of spherons, can be conducted under relatively much more drastic conditions. Spheron gel may be activated using CNBr, diisocyanates, dithioisocyanate, anhydride and acid chloride, phosgene and number of other procedures.

The polymers containing functional amino groups have been used as polymeric supports. The activation of amine group could also be possible by phosgene or thio-phosgene to isocyanate or isothiocyanate. These activated group subsequently in turn could react with amine groups of enzymes.

The carboxylic group of amino acids however could directly be coupled with amino group of polymer(s) using carbodiimide to form an amide bond. Where as arylamino derivatives after diazotization can be used for coupling of protein mainly through tyrosyl or histidyl residues. Polymers containing alkylamino group have been prepared with polysaccharide, porous glass, polyacrylamide. Polysaccharide as DEAE, or AE cellulose. DEAE cellulose can be used in effective enzyme immobilization. These materials are commercially available. Polymers containing aryl amino group are poly (p-amino styrene), poly (acrylamido Co-p-amino acrylonitrile) enzyacryl), enzyacryl AA and poly(leucine Co-p-amino phenylalanine), p-amino benzyl ether of cellulose PAB-cellulose.

3.2.9.2. Polymers containing amide groups

Polymers that contain amide bonds, such as polyacrylamide and polyamides as nylon are useful electro-neutral hydrophilic supports. Preformed polyacrylamide beads as (bio-gel) can be chemically surface modified and activated for enzyme anchoring or coupling. Polymers containing amide in the main chain, i.e., polyamides, ω-amino carboxylic acids or dicarboxylic acids and ω-amines are called nylons. These supports are mechanically strong and non-biodegradable hence significantly useful in enzyme immobilization.

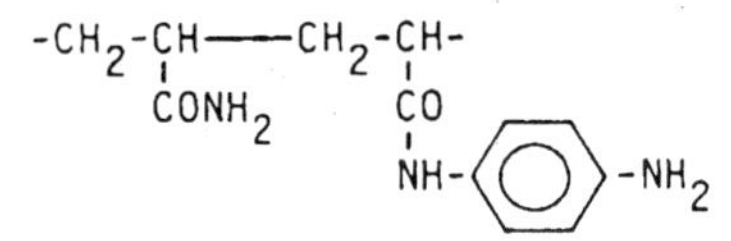

Poly(acrylamido-co-p-aminoacrylanilide) 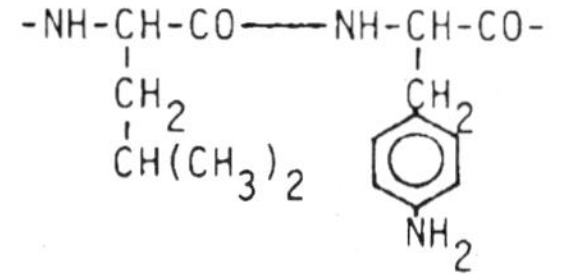   poly(leucine-co-p-aminophenylalanine)

Various coupling reactions including carboamylation, glutaraldehyde activation diazotization, etc., conventionally used for covalent anchoring of ligand molecules to polymeric supports with amino groups are schematically presented in fig 3.13.

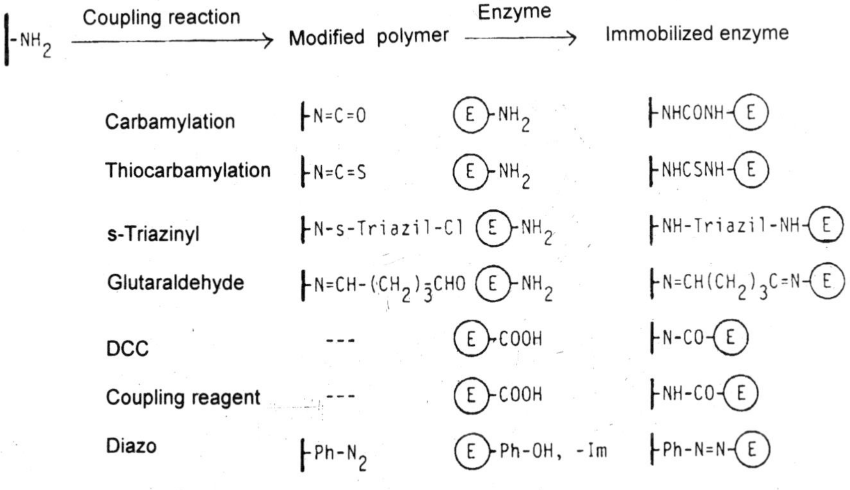

Fig. 3.13 : Schematic presentaion of immobilization on amine containing polymers using different coupling reactions.

3.2.9.3. Inorganic supports

Protocol for surface modifications by covalent enzyme immobilization begins with chemical modifications, activation, silanation, coating the surface with organic functional group bearing material using organo-functional silane reagent [$CH_3CH_2O)_3Si(EH_2)R$; where R is frequently [$(NH_2)'$] a widely used strategy in initial surface modification and subsequent utilization of inorganic materials as supports. In such coat native surface, amino groups are generally converted into aldehyde group- CHO using glutaraldehyde; Ar-NH_2 using p-amino benzoic acid or COOH using succinic anhydride.

Another procedure generally adapted for inorganic support(s) modification involves use of flexible spacer i.e., n-propylamine to which an enzyme is linked. Inorganic supports offer several distinctive advantages, such as they have high mechanical strength, resistivity to solvents and to bacterial attacks, regenerability and they remain unchanged over a wide range of pH variation. The materials which could be used as effective inorganic supports include alumina, bentonite gel, glass, nickel oxide, silica, titanium, zirconium and magnetic iron oxide powders. The inorganic supports and enzyme immobilization have most extensively been studied for ceramics, glass and Fe_2O_3 powder. Inorganic material surface is first treated with a trialkoxysilane derivative containing an organic functional group; i.e., γ-amino propyl triethoxy silane (PTES).

Polymerization most likely occurs between adjacent silanes product of reaction, thus alkyl amine glass can be converted to the aryl-amino derivative following the treatment with p-nitrobenzoyl chloride and its subsequent reduction.

3.2.9.3.1. Immobilization of enzymes on porous glass (alkylamine), as an inorganic support

Most of the inorganic materials are inherently strong and mechanically appropriate for use as an enzyme support. However, the methods which could effectively be used for covalent coupling of the enzyme(s) or proteins to inorganic supports are limited. The method that has been extensively employed for keying an organic or proteineous ligand to such support is essentially based on organo-silane, i.e. aminopropyl triethoxy silane. The reaction of organosilane with an oxide or hydroxide incorporates a relatively stable ligand processing a reactive amino (NH2) group which becomes incorporated rather integrated into the inorganic matrix through a silanaceous polymer.

An alternative to typical silanation method is coating of inorganic support using a polymeric solution where the organic ligands could subsequently be coupled to the polymer using conventional chemical covalent coupling methods as discussed in preceding part of this chapter. The concept has been discussed with the help of some interesting examples. Inorganic support immobilization process could be well appreciated by following representative examples:

Porous glass acrylamine support preparation: To a clean porous glass (nearly 1g), 18 ml distilled water is added with 2 ml of γ-amino propyl triethoxy silane. After addition of silane solution the pH of mixture is adjusted between 3 to 4 using 6N HCl. Following pH adjustment, the reaction is allowed to proceed in a water bath maintained at 72°C for 2 hours. Then the porous glass beads are filtered on a Buchner's funnel, washed well with approximately 20 ml of distilled water and dried by keeping them at 112°C in an oven for nearly 5 hours.

One gram of alkylamine glass is treated with 25ml of 2.5% v/v glutaraldehyde solution in 0.5M Na_2HPO_4 buffer solution of pH 7.0. The reaction is allowed to continue for at least 1 hour. The treated glass beads are filtered, washed well to ensure complete removal of glutaraldehyde.

Enzyme immobilization: To the glutaraldehyde treated alkylamine glass small volume 1% of enzyme in phosphate buffer pH 7.0 is added. The quantity of enzyme should be between 50-100 mg for 1 g of alkylamine glass support. Allow 2-4 hours for reaction. The unadsorbed excessive enzyme could be separated using urea. The immobilized enzyme so obtained should be recovered as damp mass, for storage at refrigeration temperature.

3.2.9.3.2. Succinyl chloride-activated succinamido-propyl glass :a releasable immobilized system

Covalent coupling: Molecules possessing primary amino or thiol groups (amino acid derivatives and proteins) react rapidly. The covalently coupled amino acids or proteins are not removed on washing with 8M urea or guanidinium chloride solutions.

Releasable protein immobilizing systems are achieved on incubation of activated beads with proteins at a pH between 5-8 and temperature between 10 - 40°C. A solution containing 6 mg of protein per ml of sodium phosphate at pH 7.0 can be recycled through a column of beads in a fluidized bed manner for 3 hours at room temperature. Immobilizable amount of protein normally equals the amount which could be immobilized on succinamido propyl-glass activated using water soluble carbodiimides. So immobilized protein can be exposed to denaturants which reductively cleave the disulfide bond without the loss of protein from the matrix. Thus, reductively denatured and refolded chymotrypsinogen from its random coil state could be obtained as immobilized protein. The immobilized protein or species can be released by its incubation in hydroxylamine solution at pH 7.0 at room temperature.

3.2.9.3.3. Tresyl chloride-Activated support for enzyme immobilization

Sulfonate esters are suitable affinity ligands for enzyme immobilization to hydroxyl group carrying supports, such as agarose, cellulose, glycophase glass, and glyceryl propyl-silica. The activation and coupling of the enzyme to the support is accomplished as follow:

Activation support-CH_2OH + R-SO_2Cl $\longrightarrow$ Support-CH_2-OSO_2R

Coupling support-CH_2OSO_2R + H_2N-Enzyme $\longrightarrow$ Support-CH_2H-Enzyme + $HOSO_2R$

Support-CH_2OSO_2R + HS-Enzyme $\longrightarrow$ Support-CH_2-S-Enzyme + $HOSO_2R$

(R= CH_2CF_3 OR $C_6H_4CH_3$), Tosylates (R=$C_6H_4CH_3$) and Tresylate (R=CH_2CF_3) are usual conventional reagents for enzyme immobilization.

Similarly, the activation can also be possible on hydroxyethyl methacrylate like polymer with tresyl chloride.

3.2.9.3.4. Metal ion activated alkylamine derivatives

A novel covalent process to immobilize enzyme was developed by Carbel et al The immobilized enzyme systems obtained using this procedure were of greater operational stability. The method involves activation of support with transition metal salts, usually titanium chloride (IV) followed by amination with a suitable diamine in an aprotic (hydrophobic) solvent in order to form an alkylamine derivative which on subsequent reaction with a bifunctional bridging agent, forms a bridge between alkylamine derivative of support and the enzyme. The influence of nature of amine on the activity profile of glucoamylase was studied. It was noted that when 1,6-diaminohexane was used as an anchoring agent, the resultant immobilized enzyme was most active. This has been interestingly found to be attributed to the spacing between two methylene group of the agent.

The alkylamine derivatives of transition metal solid support can also be activated by several procedures. In one of the method tannic acid as bridging agent has been used successfully. Another process which could be used for inorganic support based immobilization is **polymeric isocyanate** binding. According to the scheme a carbamate bond is formed between inorganic surface and isocyanate group. If enzyme is attached under alkaline conditions, a substitute urea bond is formed between amine of the protein surface (of enzyme) and the isocyanate whereas under moderate acidic conditions isocyanate reacts with hydroxyl group of the enzyme and a methane bond is formed.

A number of methods for immobilization of biological molecules are available however, they could not be considered to be perfect for all proteinaceous molecules. Covalent coupling moreover has been found to be an efficient method, which involves chemical modification or activation of support or matrix. The process nevertheless, may demand long reaction time or specialized conditions.

3.2.9.3.5. Thionyl chloride - activated succinamido propyl glass as reversible immobilization support

Covalent coupling of proteins or other biomolecules to an insoluble support in general relies on common organic reactions. The immobilization matrix does not allow for characterization of immobilized enzyme except kinetics or fluorescent spectroscopy. If selective release of loaded or immobilized moiety can be achieved, this would allow the application of different biochemical and physicochemical experimentation with the protein liberated in free form in solution. The methods of such immobilization are mainly based on bridging agents which when required could be cleaved selectively.

Succinimido propyl glass can be prepared from porous or non-porous conventional glass in the form of beads employing aqueous or non-aqueous derivatization processes. Aqueous derivatization produces more hydrous surface and contains more silane polymers as compared to that prepared using non-aqueous derivatization. The surfaces so obtained could then covalently be linked with protein or enzyme following activation with thionyl chloride. The immobilized enzyme can be released if required on subsequent treatment with hydroxylamine.

Glass beads are cleaned with acid, the surface impurities are removed by successive washings with acetone and toluene. Then the beads are treated with 4 volumes of 10% 3-amino propyl 3-methoxy silane and incubated for 3 hours at 80°C. The excess of reagents is decanted-off and the silanated beads are collected. Succinylation is subsequently performed by adding the beads to 4 volumes of 10% w/v solution of succinic anhydride in acetone containing 1% w/v triethylamine. The reaction is usually completed on 5 minutes incubation

3.2.9.3.6. Immobilization of glycoenzyme through carbohydrate chains

Glycoenzymes namely carboxypeptidase-Y (CPY), glucoamylase, peroxidase, glucose oxidase can be immobilized by forming enzyme EDTA/glycyltyrosine adducts. Generally, these enzymes are having residual amino acids (particularly lysine, tyrosine) on their surfaces.

The whole procedure involves the following steps:

1. Oxidation of glycoenzymes
2. Formation of EDTA/glycyltyrosine adducts
3. Enzyme immobilization

Oxidation of glycoenzymes

In order to make the glycoenzyme reactive, the carbohydrate chains of the enzyme are oxidized (Fig 3.14). Generally, sodium metaperiodate or other periodates or iodates are used as oxidizing agent. The pH of the medium is generally adjusted to be slightly acidic (pH 4.5-6.0) during oxidation reaction.

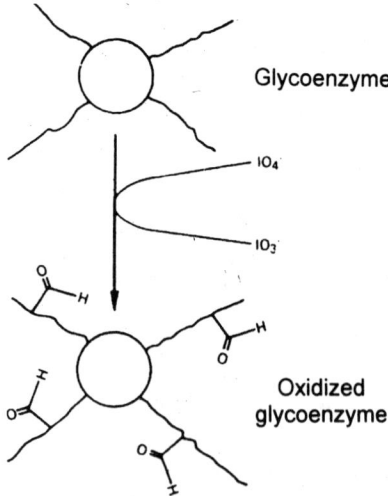

Fig. 3.14 : Oxidation of glycoenzyme

EDTA/glycyltyrosine adducts

The stable enzyme derivatives are formed by the attachment of EDTA or glycyltyrosine to the carbohydrate chain in the presence of sodium borohydride (Fig. 3.15). These derivatives are enymatically active and react well with solid support.

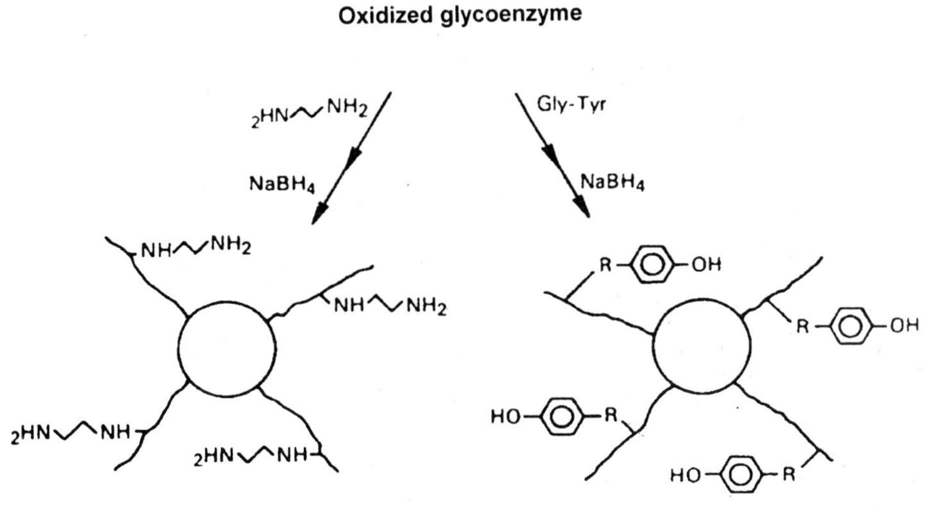

Oxidized glycoenzyme

Fig. 3.15 : Formation of stable enzyme derivatives

Enzyme immobilization

EDTA adducts are finally reacted and coupled with an active ester derivative of agarose by covalent binding (Fig. 3.16). The glycyltyrosine adducts are attached to diazotized arylamine supports via azo linkage (Fig. 3.17). The stability of aminoalkylamino derivatives of glycoenzymes is superior to the aldehydic enzyme that is formed by periodate oxidation alone. The immobilized system so obtained demonstrated well identified potentials.

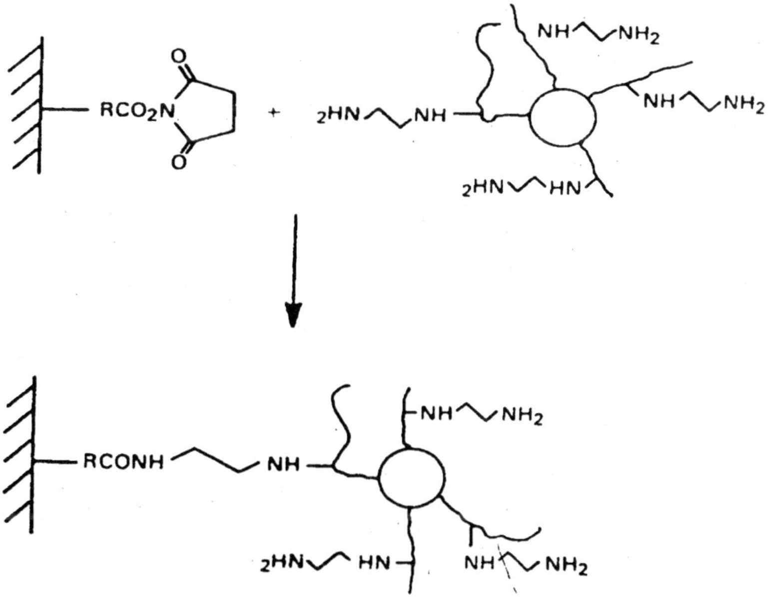

Fig 3.16 : Reaction of ethylendiamine adduct

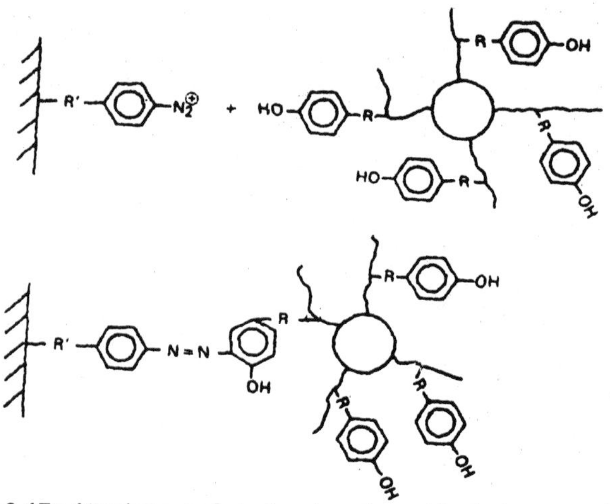

Fig 3.17 : Attachment of glycine, tyrosine adduct via an azo linkage

3.2.10. Avidin biotin affinity coupling

Avidin-biotin affinity coupling is a well known technique. Avidin is a tetrameric protein which has high affinity for co.-enzyme biotin. This strong however non-chemical, non-covalent binding has extensively been exploited for coupling of pilot ligand modules, i.e., monoclonal antibodies on the surface of a carrier system. One of the coupling component is covalently anchored on the surface of the carrier whereas other may be conjugated covalently to the other entity which has to be appended to a surface, i.e. biotinylation of antibodies. The coupling of this complex to the avidin is brought by its avidity to biotin. The biotin is the component of this system that is generally pre-anchored covalently to some carrier support (fig 3.18).

The methods which are frequently employed for covalent coupling of one of the affinity ligand to the carrier and support surface include; succinimide carbodiimide, or glutaraldehyde based activation and other coupling reactions.

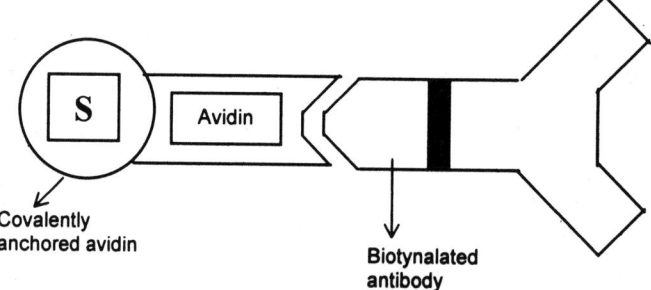

Fig. 3.18 : Schematic representation of avidin biotin affinity coupling

The reactions which are employed for incorporation or activation of reactive groups for biotinylation are summed up and given in table 3.1.

3.3. ADSORPTION

Although functionally at the level of operation, adsorption appears to be most economical and simple process, the forces involved are extremely complex. In fact almost no material is known which could be utilized for adsorptive immobilization with its own surface contribution. The bonds that exist between enzyme protein and carrier depend upon the nature of carrier and nature of enzyme protein surface. The bonds may be critically ionic, hydrogen, covalent, coordinated covalent or hydrophobic or even combination of any of these.

Table 3.1 : Reactive chemistry of biotinylation

Functional group	Reactive group	Linkage formed
Primary Amine	NHS-Ester/Sulfo-NHS Ester	Amide Bond

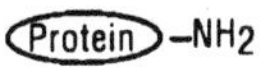

Primary Amine: (Protein)—NH₂

Reactive group: (Label)—C—O—N (NHS-Ester/Sulfo-NHS Ester)

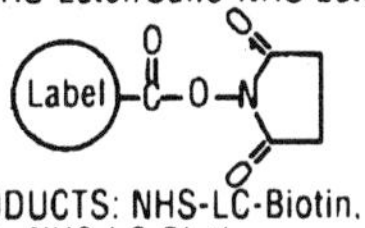

PRODUCTS: NHS-LC-Biotin, Sulfo-NHS-LC-Biotin, NHS-LC-LC-Biotin, Sulfo-NHS-LC-LC-Biotin, NHS-Biotin, Sulfo-NHS-Biotin, NHS-SS-Biotin

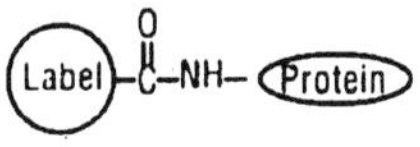

Linkage formed: (Label)—C—NH—(Protein) Amide Bond

Sulfhydryl: (Protein)—SH

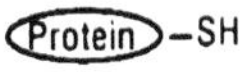

Maleimide: (Label)—N

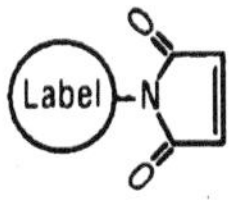

PRODUCTS: Biotin-BMCC, Maleimide Activated-HRP, Maleimide Activated Alk. Phos.

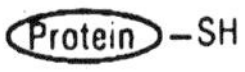

Thioether Bond: (Label)—N ... S—(Protein)

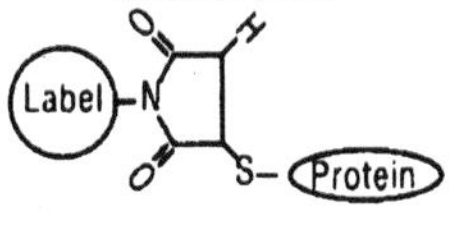

Sulfhydryl: (Protein)—SH

Iodoacetyl: (Label)—C—CH₂—I

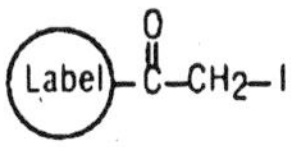

PRODUCTS: Iodoacetyl-LC-Biotin

Thioether Bond: (Label)—C—CH₂—S—(Protein)

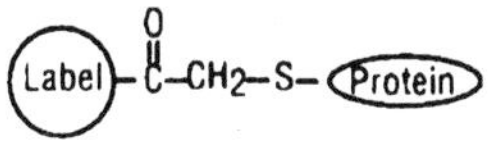

Oxidized Carbohydrate: (Protein)—C—H

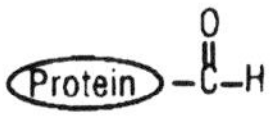

Hydrazide: (Label)—C—NH—NH₂

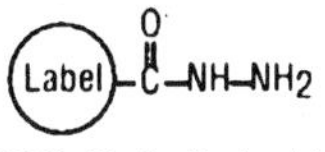

PRODUCTS: Biotin-Hydrazide, Biotin-LC-Hydrazide, Biocytin-Hydrazide

Hydrazone Bond: (Label)—C—N—N=C—(Protein)

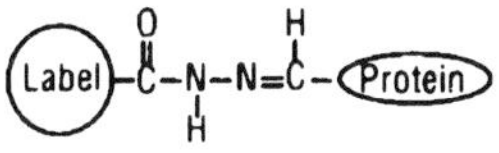

DNA/RNA Protein Carbohydrates

Azido (Photoactivatable): (Label)—N—⟨NO₂⟩—N₃

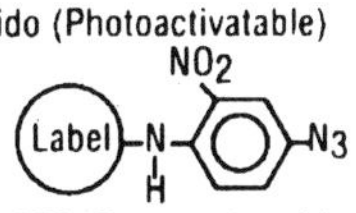

PRODUCTS: Photoactivatable Biotin

Nonspecific

Carboxyl: (Protein)—C—OH

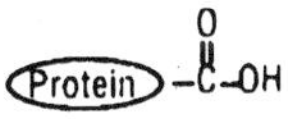

Other: (Label)—NH₂

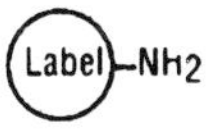

PRODUCTS: (Biotinamido)-pentylamine

Amide Bond: (Label)—NH—C—(Protein)

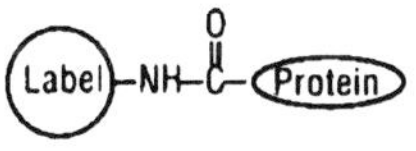

Reaction requires DC cross-linker

*Adapted from Pierce product catalogue, USA, 1997.

Immobilization can be brought about by coupling an enzyme either to external or internal surface of a carrier. In case enzyme is immobilized externally it is desirable that the particle size of carrier must be small enough to provide an appreciable surface for binding. These particles may have diameters ranging between 500Å to 1 mm. The external surface binding utilized in immobilization of enzyme is advantageous for it does not involve the conditions like pore diffusion. The disadvantages, however, include relatively low surface area for binding, exposure of enzymes to microbial attack, physical abrasion of enzyme or inhibitory effects, due to turbulence associated with the bulk solution. Lastly, smaller particles cause high pressure drop (gradient) in continuous packed bed reactors.

Although internal surface involvement of a porous carrier in enzyme immobilization has one of the marked disadvantage yet many advantages may be harvested from this approach. The major disadvantage of internal immobilization pertains to pore diffusion. Thus, it entails for proper optimization of pore diameter, surface area, surface charges, and other related parameters.

3.3.1. Forces involved in internal surface immobilization

The types of bonds formed between carriers and enzymes are dependent on the support materials selected for immobilization. The basic forces underlying the immobilization of enzymes on internal pore surfaces can be appreciated from the adsorption studies on porous glass. These studies suggested that there is a force involved to attract enzymes to the internal surface. In this case, the dissociated silanol negative charge on the glass attracts the positively charged amine groups associated with the surface of the protein. Finally, the coupling process involves multiple hydrogel bonds and ionic amine silanol bonds. It is apparent, that three forces involved in internal surface immobilization are attractive, diffusive, and multiple hydrogen bonds (Fig. 3.19).

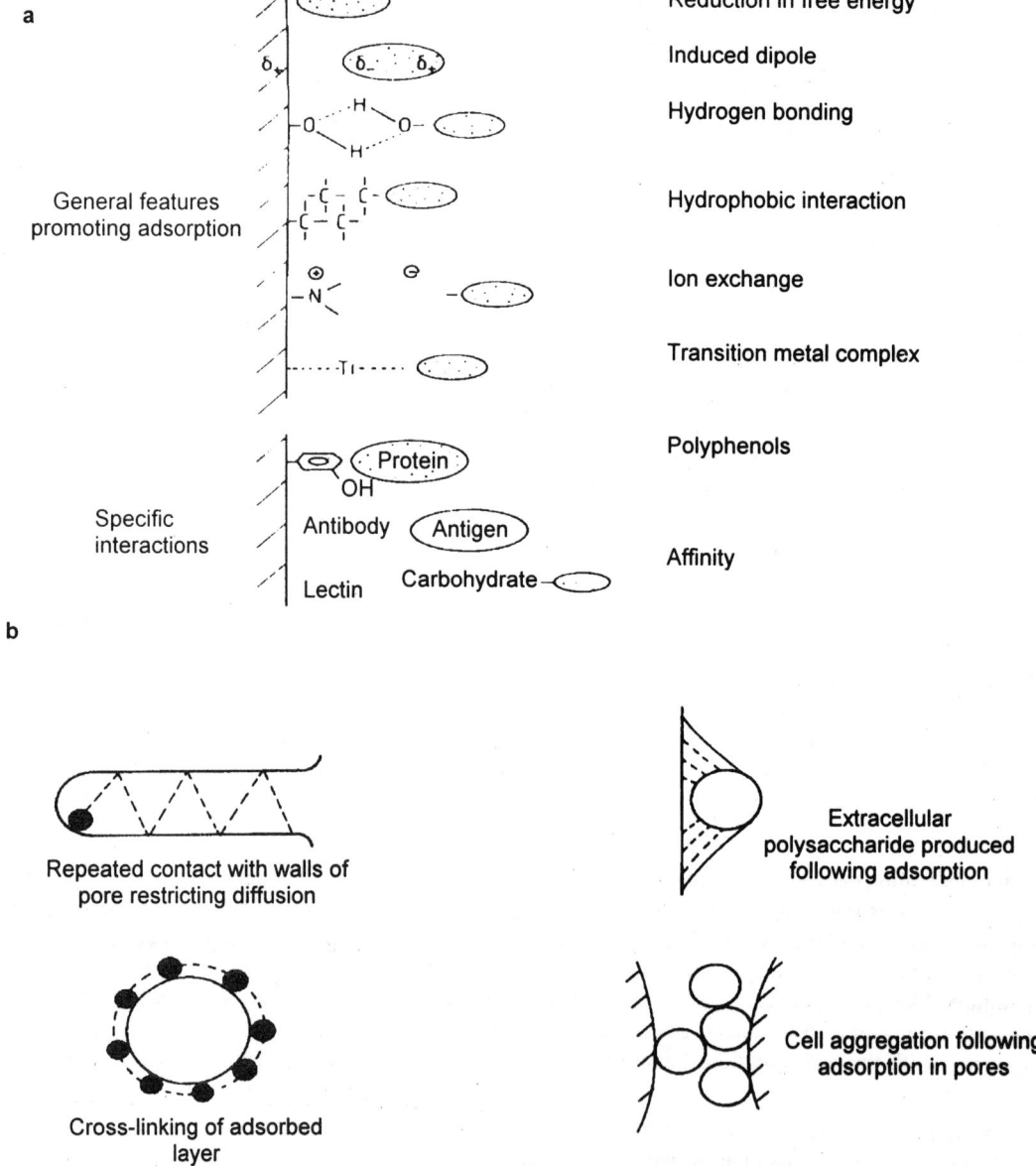

Fig 3.19 : (a) Forces involved in adsorption of biocatalyst on the support;
(b) Secondary features involved in improving the retention of adsorbed biocatalyst

In a given porous material having uniform distribution of pore diameters it could be realized that as the pore diameter decreases the resultant surface area increases. The effective bonding appears to be a function of pore diameter and molecular weight of the protein. Studies on glucose oxidation catalase related to pore diameter indicated that optimum diameter for immobilizing the highest quantity of active enzymes was related to major and main axis of units and dimensions of molecular structure rather than the molecular weight. Interestingly, it was noted that highest activity of an enzyme could be attained by internal surface immobilization when the pore diameter is chosen to be twice of the major axis of unit cell.

The carriers generally used for immobilization are characteristically very active materials. The major concern should be that these materials prior to use should be thoroughly cleaned and fully activated with respect to their surfaces before they are utilized for enzyme adsorption. Carrier materials may absorb volatile organic substances from the air as well as microbial contaminants. These contaminants may effectively mask the functional groups available on the surface and thus may prevent the immobilization of the enzyme. A very stable carrier may safely be cleaned using acidic solution, likewise, those which are stable in basic pH may be washed using alkaline solutions. Probably the most frequent and more costly process of immobilization is the preconditioning of the carrier surface. Each enzyme has its own stability status with respect to pH, ionic strength and against activators and cofactors. A frequent error encountered is the direct application of enzyme solution to the dry surface of the carrier without its prior exposure to the preferred pH or the salt conditions. A dramatic loss in total activity may thus result.

3.3.2. Methods for immobilization by adsorption

The adsorptive immobilization of enzymes (Fig. 3.20) may be affected by four methods namely static process, dynamic batch process, reactor loading process and electro deposition process.

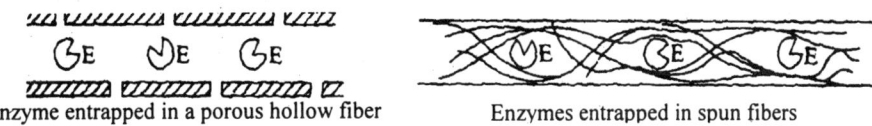

Enzyme entrapped in a porous hollow fiber   Enzymes entrapped in spun fibers

Fig 3.20 : Diagrammatic representation of adsorption methods

3.3.2.1. Static pores

The static process technique is considered to be the most efficient, however it requires maximum time. The enzyme is immobilized on the carrier by allowing the solution containing an enzyme to be in contact with the carrier without any agitation or stirring. Generally, loading of an enzyme on carrier surface is non uniform and rather low. The carrier must be exposed to an excessive concentration of an enzyme for a long period of time usually for days at low temperature in order to obtain modestly active immobilized enzyme system.

3.3.2.2. Dynamic pores

The dynamic batch process on the other hand, is a frequently employed procedure at laboratory levels. It typically involves the admixing of enzyme solution with the carrier under constant stirring or agitation using a mechanical shaker. The process convincingly effective and results into uniform and high loading provided an adequate concentration of enzymes is used. Precautions should be taken to ensure that agitation is not so vigorous that it may result into abrasion or disruption of the carrier. However it is required to be sufficiently effective to allow a low density carrier to come in intimate contact with the enzyme solution.

3.3.2.3. Reactor loading

The process most frequently referred to as a reactor loading process is employed for the commercial production of immobilized enzymes. The carrier is placed into the reactor and enzyme solution is transferred to the reactor loaded with carrier. Immobilization is normally accomplished through a dynamic environment by either circulating the enzyme or by the agitation of solution containing enzyme carrier mix.

3.3.2.4. Electro deposition

Lastly, the electro deposition process in which the carrier is placed just in proximal vicinity of one of the electrode in an enzyme bath and subsequently electric current is applied leading to the migration of enzymes towards the carrier thus resulting into its deposition on the carrier surface. However, it should be ascertained that the carrier system which is being employed for immobilization must be stable in an electric field.

3.3.3. Immobilization on self-assembling nanocrystalline ceramic core (Aquasomes)

Self assembling nanocrystalline solid ceramic core coated with a glass polyhydroxyoligomer can be used for immobilization of biochemically active molecules. The system namely 'aquasome' can carry different classes of biochemically active molecules which can be immobilized in a classical non-covalent manner. It has been reported that enzymes, antigens and drugs could be immobilized in these ceramic biomolecular delivery system. Delivery of biochemically important molecules have always presented problems as they are relatively labile. Many ways to prevent this have been proposed. One such effort is immobilization of bioactive proteins on nanocrystalline ceramic core. This system could effectively deliver viral antigens which pave way for newer generation vaccine adjuvants for therapeutic, industrial and diagnostic applications.

The study of the ceramic nanocrystals coated with glassy cellobiose for delivery of a wide range of biochemically active molecules include Epstein Barr Virus (EBV) and HIV to elicit immunity, muscle adhesive protein to elicit polyclonal antibodies for affinity chromatography and rpg 120 (HIV) to elicit polyclonal antibodies for ELISA-based immunoassays for HIV infection. Secondly, they can be effectively used for targeted drug delivery (See chapter 9).

Insulin has been immobilized on aquasomes prepared using degradable calcium phosphate nanocrystals coated with glassy pyridoxal-5-phosphate. The immobilized insulin demonstrated a significant fall in blood glucose level. Similarly, DNase a therapeutic enzyme used in the treatment of cystic fibrosis was successfully immobilized on aquasomes and targeted to the specific site and elicited significant therapeutic effect as desirable. The ceramic carbohydrate is essentially an aqueous colloid comprises of ceramic nanocrystals surface stabilized via carbohydrate epitoxial adsorption. The adsorbed carbohydrates provide a non-denaturing solid phase. The layer could retains its inherent water even under stern environmental challenges. The adsorptive immobilization of sugar on ceramic nanaocrystals is essentially epitaxial adsorption (Fig. 4.21). The sugars used include cellobiose, mallose, sucrose, trehalose, etc.

Surface immobilized antigens coated over ceramic cores were studied for their effective delivery potential of antigen and for appropriate antigenicity elicitation. In addition, they have been studied as artificial oxygen carriers wherein, hemoglobin was immobilized onto the coated brushite cores. From the oxygen affinity curves, it was concluded that the administration of this delivery system showed a remarkable effect.

3.4. COMPLEXATION AND CHELATION

3.4.1. Metal link chelation

This process offers an instantaneous coupling without chemical derivatization or activation of support or matrix. Method is essentially based on chelation properties of transition metals namely titanium and zirconium which appear particularly attractive for their nontoxic nature.

A system based on titanium chloride-cellulose illustrates the way of transition metal association-chelates formation. Titanium metal has property of octahedral coordination with ionic molecules which serve as ligands. In most of the cases these ligands are typical water molecules or chloride ions. In the case where chloride ion acts as a ligand, its excess electron density is utilized in the formation of partial-covalent bond with metal ion(Ti) as a result the overall positive charge of titanium is reduced by a unit (fig 3.22).

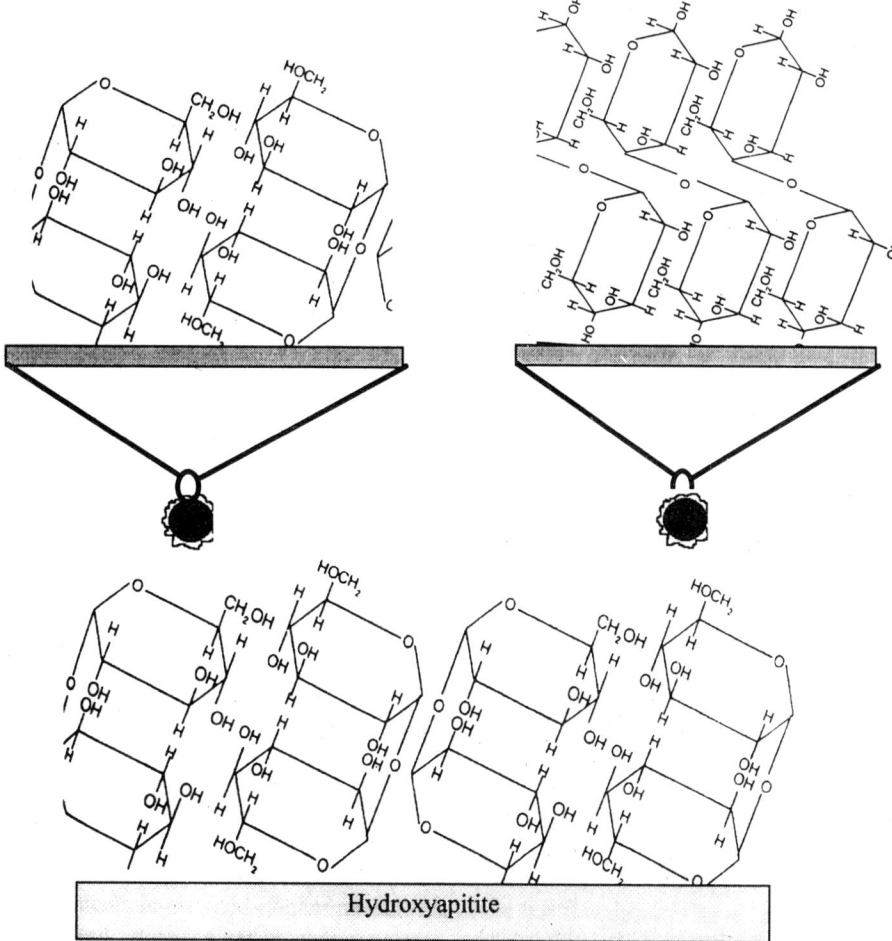

Fig. 4.21 : Epitaxial adsorptive coating of some sugars on ceramic nanocrystals

3.4.2. Chloroaquo complexes of titanium in HCl solution

These ligands may be replaced by other water based ligands or other electron donating groups. Critically the strength of association depends upon the chemical nature of the ligand. Hydroxyl ions are effective ligands for transition metals, therefore they may well be anticipated to complex with polysaccharide where new ligating hydroxyl ions may be replaced for preexisting if any. Some polysaccharides, i.e. cellulose contains **vicinal dio group** which are not involved in glycosidic linkage hence available for free chelation by transition metals. The chelate is a result of replacement of two ligands from titanium ion by polysaccharide hydroxyl groups. For steric reasons number of ligands which could be replaced by cellulose hydroxyl groups are restricted.

3.4.3. Hydrous transition metal oxides

The method uses hydrous metal oxides as support for enzyme or cell immobilization. The oxides could be produced by precipitation after the hydrolysis of the corresponding chloride. The mode of immobilization essentially remains to be chelation. Thus the precipitation affected in to an order to get respective hydrous oxide in the presence of enzyme results in effective and efficient immobilization. However, all precautions to understate the detrimental conditions should be taken. The metal chlorides which may be used for their conversion to hydrous oxides include cobalt(II), copper(II), iron(II), manganese(II), tin(II), zinc(II), chromium(II), vanadium(III), tin(IV) and zirconium(IV). The complexes retain significant activity profile of chelated immobilized enzyme. Owing to low operational stability of enzyme, immobilization on metal hydrous oxide, a cross linking step based on glutaraldehyde treatment has been suggested. The procedure so modified could prevent the protein loss into the solution during operation.

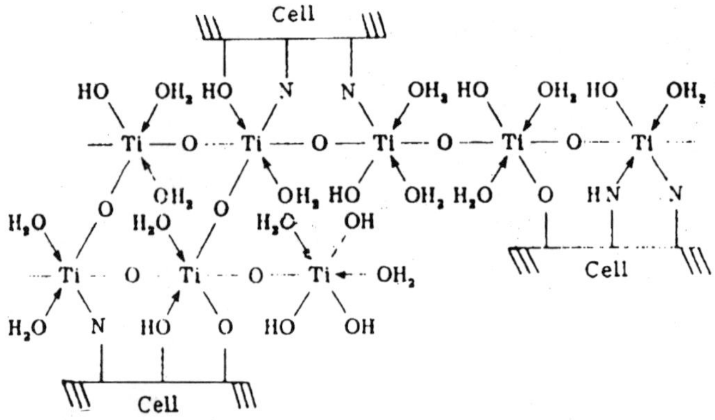

Fig. 3.22 : Representative structure of titanium (IV) oxide polysaccharide chelate

3.5. WITHIN SUPPORT IMMOBILIZATION

The entrapment or encapsulation of enzymes can be achieved via its inclusion in matrix that is based on highly crosslinked polymer, encapsulation in microcapsules or in distinct non-aqueous phases. The distinctive feature of these methods particularly matrix inclusion and encapsulation is that the enzymes is not attached to matrix therefore, any problem like steric blockade as associated with covalent or electrostatic binding is not encountered. The method provides scope for developing biocatalysts in various physical shapes and forms. Although beads are most common, fiber, sheets, emulsions, gels have been used in bioreactors. In summary immobilization using entrapment methods(Table 3.2) is an attractive option where difference in size of catalyst and substrate should be distinctively large. In practice membrane reactors are well adapted for enzyme which acts on low molecular weight substrate whereas three dimensional gel is preferred for immobilizing cellular/particular biocatalysts and thus apparently a method of choice for immobilization of live cells.

In general entrapment is performed by dissolving a enzyme in a solution that is required either for dissolution or for preparation of enzyme phase (carrier) and then treating this solution so that a distinctive and discrete biphasic system is created in the form of dispersion. Subsequently, the dispersed enzyme phase is stabilized via depletion of solvent or additional crosslinking of carrier mass(Fig. 3.23). Some of the representative examples of this class of immobilization are dealt in this chapter.

3.5.1. Entrapment

3.5.1.1. Three-dimensional gels

A large number of stable, three dimensional gels can be formed under mild condition in such a way that biocatalysts may get entrapped without loss of their activity. The most successful techniques use hydrogels since, in general, hydrogels provide maximum stabilization to the active structure and are easily wetted allowing the free access of the substrate (Fig.3.24). The main division in this group of techniques using hydrogels is between those which form a gel as a result of polymerization reaction in which new covalent bonds are formed and those methods which create a gel from existing pre-polymers with very little change in covalent bonds. The former yields very stable gels with well defined properties but can cause considerable deactivation of the catalyst, while the later, though formed under milder conditions, often have less satisfactory physical stability.

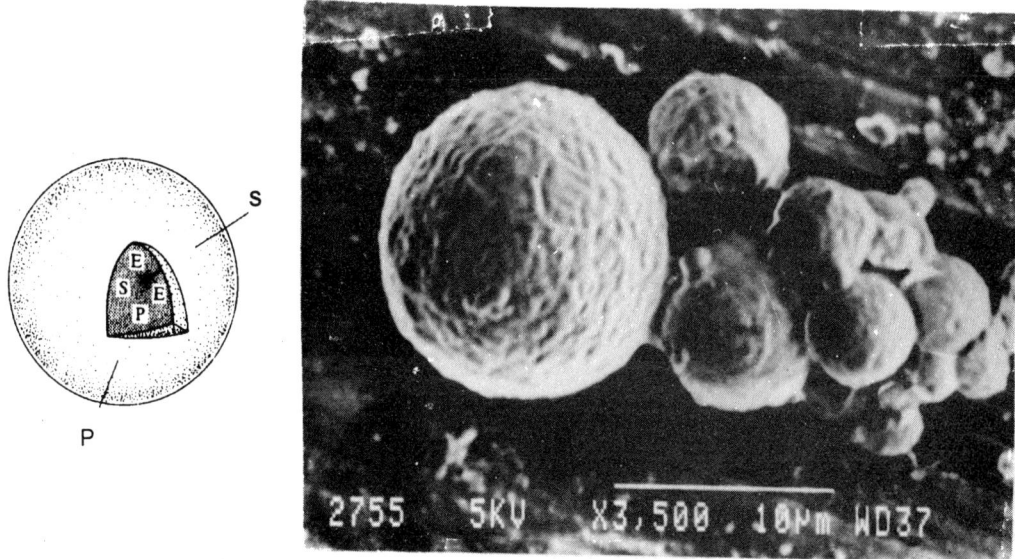

Fig. 3.23 : Diagrammatic presentation of enzyme entrapped in microcapsule

3.5.1.2. *In situ polymerization*

In the case of *in-situ* chemical reactions, chances of pre-polymeric weak-ionic or adsorptive interactions with the biocatalyst are likely. It is therefore, essential that biocatalysts entrapped by this technique are rapidly washed free of unreacted chemicals and other reagents. Crosslinked polymers of acrylamide have been used extensively in biochemistry as media for chromatography and electrophoresis. The hydrophilic nature of the gel, its high water regain, high porosity and low level of adsorptivity for biochemicals, lend it useful as a carrier for immobilizing biocatalyst, as well as in separation techniques.

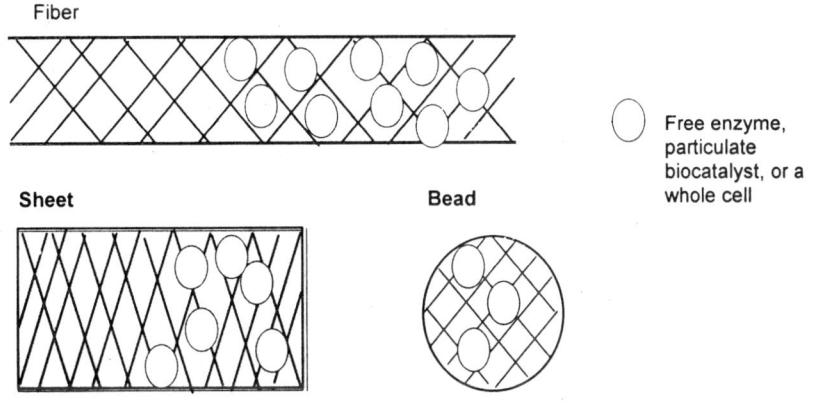

Fig.3.24 : Entrapment of biocatalysts in a three-dimensional porous matrix.

Table 3.2 :Selected examples of immobilization of enzymes by entrapment

Method	Matrix	Enzyme
Gel entrapment	Polyacrylamide	Glucose oxidase
		Urease
		Aminoacid oxidase
		Acetylcholinesterase
		Chymotrypsin
		Asperginase
		Glucose dehydrogenase
		Alcohol dehydrogenase
		Phenol-monooxygenase
		β-Galactosidase
		β-Fructosidase
		Asperginase
	κ-Carrageenan	Aminoacylase
		Aspartate ammonia-lyase
		Fumerate hydralase
	Acrylamide/glycidylmethacrylate/	AMP deaminase
	ethylene glycol 2-hydroxy-ethyl-	β-fructosidase
	methacrylate, 2-Hydroxyethyl-	Glucose isomerase
	methacrylate	Glucoamylase
		Cellulase
		Glucosidase
		Glucose oxidase
	Collagen	Amine oxidase
		Lactate dehydrogenase
		Alcohol dehydrogenase
		Glucose oxidase
		Sucrose
Microencapsulation	Phase separaton	Catalase
		Asperginase
		Urease
		β-Galactosidase
		Alcohol dehydrogenase

The basis of the method is to suspend or dissolve the biocatalyst in an aqueous buffer containing acrylamide and a bis-acrylate as a crosslinker. The vinyl polymerization of these two monomers is initiated by generating free radicals within the solution, either by incorporating a redox couple or by some form of energetic elecromagnetic radiation such as light or gamma rays. The mechanical strength of the gel is proportional to the square root of the acrylamide concentration but pore size falls to be smaller with increasing gel density so as to ensure free diffusion of solutes. The use of high-energy radiation to initiate the polymerization is restricted to the biocatalysts capable of withstanding the disruptive effect of such radiation, in such a condition the inclusion of glycoproteins being suitable. Other acrylates based on methacrylate monomers like hydroxy ethylmethacrylate (HEMA), bifunctional acrylates like PEG-dimethacrylates could also be used as gel forming polymeric matrices.

3.5.1.3. Polycondensations

The most common example of this group of reactions is the polymerization of bis-isocynates with polyalcohols or polyamines to give urethanes and the crosslinking of inactive proteins with the ubiquious bifunctional, glutaraldehyde. *Streptomyces rimoisus* cells are immobilized in urethane pre-polymers and used for the production of oxytetracycline. Similarly, bifunctional aldehyde like glutaraldehyde, reacts with the amine groups of proteins to give a crosslinked structure. For example, aqueous solution of gelatin containing urease can be entrapped by dipping the dried film into glutaraldehyde to fix up the matrix.

3.5.1.4. Immobilization of biocatalyst (enzymes) in gelatin

The protein nature of the gelatin, its high hydrophilicity and strong swelling power lend gelatin to be a suitable material for immobilizing cells and enzymes. The cells to be immobilized are dispersed in deionised water. The cellular aqueous dispersion is then added to 10%w/v gelatin aqueous solution at 30-40°C. The gelatin solution is added in volume so as to give a final cells to gelatin concentration ration 0.1%w/w. Immobilization of cells by suspending them in deionised water and dispersing into 10% w/v aqueous gelatin solution at 35-40^0 C to give a final cell to gelatin concentration ratio of 0.1% w/w. This cell-gelatin suspension is then poured into a cylindrical mold (0.3 cm;φ) immediately after mixing with hardening agents i.e., mixture of 20% w/v formaldehyde in 50% v/v alcohol. The molds are allowed to gel in deep freeze (about -25^{0}C). After 4 hours molds are brought to room temperature and cut into thin discs (0.2-0.4 cm). Then the gel discs can be stored under refrigerated conditions for months without any appreciable lose of enzyme (e.g. yeast cell invertase).

Immobilization of enzymes using gelatin is similar to cell immobilization except that it is preferable to mix gelatin and hardening agents first, immediately the defined volume of enzyme solution is then added to it. This has the advantage of reducing the exposure of enzyme to formaldehyde, so that active preparation can be obtained with retained enzyme activity.

3.5.2. Microencapsulation

Microencapsulation in classical sense can be defined as the process of spherical particles formation where a liquid or suspension is enclosed in a dense but semi-permeable polymeric membrane. The definition can further be expanded to lipoidal, non-ionic, or lipoprotein based membranes. Transport of nutrients as well as of substrate across the membrane could be a major limiting factor to the practical application of this technique. Particularly in the case of cell immobilization the effective use of technique has marked limitations. Three techniques can be employed in forming membranes for immobilization. The most defined membranes built in special reactors (sec.3.4.2.1). Alternatively stable emulsion of the biocatalyst in an aqueous phase can be formed (sec. 3.4.2.2) or the emulsion can be permanently stabilized by creating an interfacial polymeric membrane at the phase interface (sec.3.4.2.3).

3.5.2.1. Membrane reactors

A wide range of membranes with a variety of chemical composition are reported with their characteristics (Table 3.3). For establishing the reactors often required is a minor modification of standard equipment and techniques used for enzyme purification, merely involving the addition of substrate solution to the fluid held in the body of the reactor. Both reverse osmosis and ultrafiltration can be operated on immobilized enzyme or cell reactors, the only limitation being the size of substrate molecules which must pass through the membrane. The biocatalyst is normally retained behind the face of the membrane and the substrate is introduced directly into this enclosed compartment while the products of the reaction pass out as a permeate or filtrate (Fig. 3.25a, b). It is inevitable that concentration of solutes by membrane techniques results in a flux of solvent and small solutes through the membrane and a build-up of larger solutes on the inner face as a polarization layer. This can be understated during concentration-polarization by generating a tangential flow of fluid across the inner face of the membrane. The tangential flow however, can be achieved by stirring (magnetically) or by using thin channels near the face or alternatively by forming the membrane as thin hollow fibers. This means that the enzyme kinetics is similar to those of free enzymes and, in the case of cellular systems, the build-up of a biofilm layer does not operate to restrict the flux. Further it reduces the requirement of a large fluid volume and speeds up the reaction rate at the surface leading to an increased productivity (Fig.3.26).

Table 3.3 : Characteristics of common membrane materials

Material	Stable	Stability	Steam sterilizable
Polysulphone	pH 2-12	Most enzymes	Yes
Polyamide	pH 2-12	Most enzymes	No
Cellulose acetate	pH 4-9	Not cellulases or esterases	No

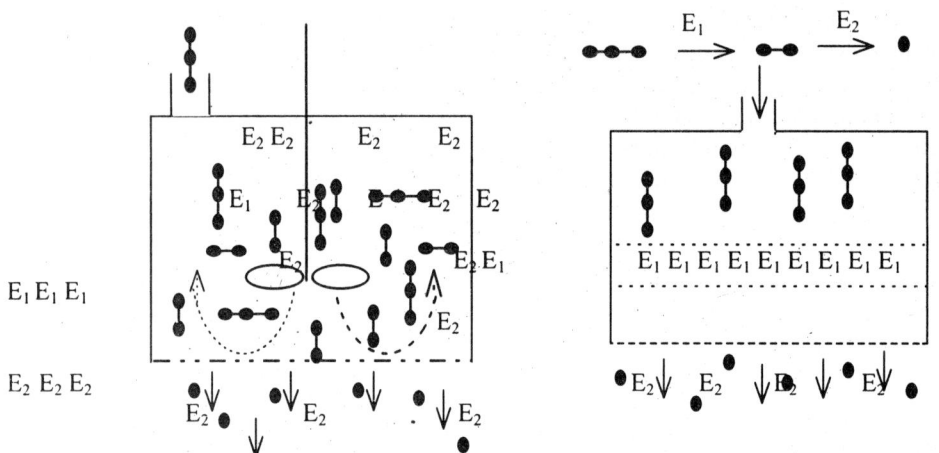

Fig 3.25a : Membrane reactors used in multienzyme processing. a) a well mixed system. b) Polarized cell.

Membrane reactors can be employed in a similar way to remove a product from a homogeneous cell reactor, and the use of such rigs to recycle or retain biomass in normal fermenters may be considered as an immobilization technique.

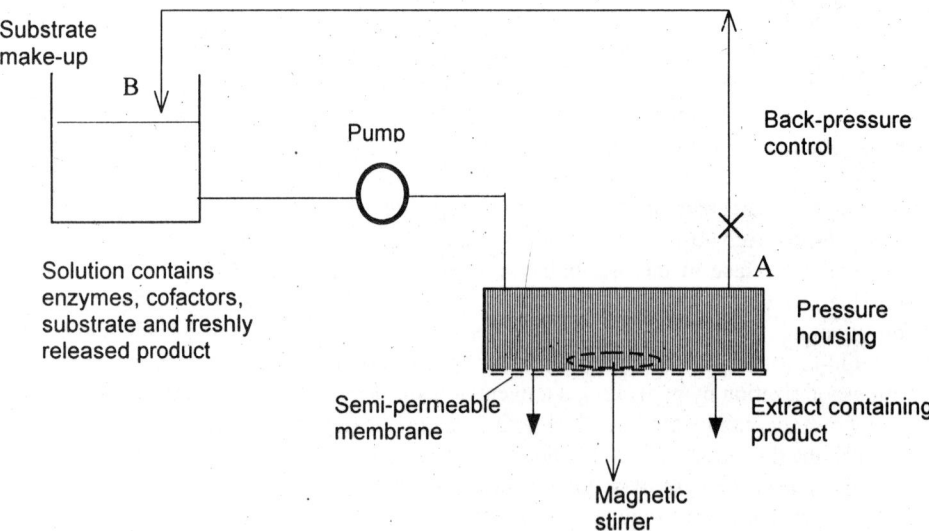

Fig. 3. 25b : Membrane reactor (recycle model). A single-pass system omits line A-B. The design of the pressure cell may provide high tangential flow without stirring.

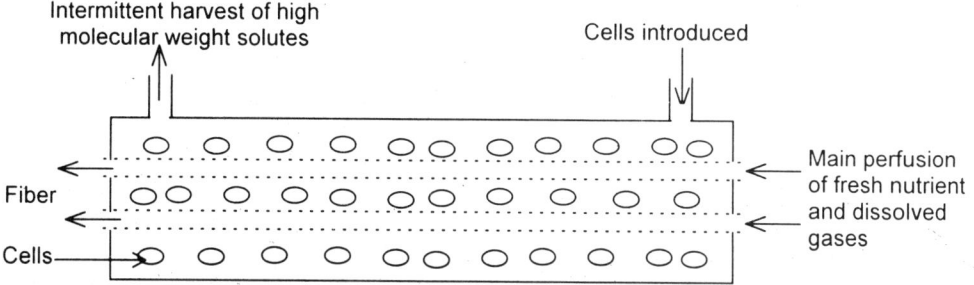

Intermittent harvest of high molecular weight solutes

Cells introduced

Fiber

Cells

←— Main perfusion of fresh nutrient and dissolved gases

Fig. 3.26 : Hollow fiber bundle used as immobilized cell reactor

3.5.2.2. Emulsions

This technique relies on a liquid phase boundary separating the enzyme from the bulk fluid. These emulsions are often stabilized by detergents to prevent coalescence and the loss of the surface area through which essential mass transfer of products must occur. However, emulsions can be used successfully with an aqueous bulk phase by generating a stable w/o/w emulsion to form a lipid membrane, rather similar to the bilayer around living cells, where, enzymes are confined effectively in hydrophilic phase (Fig.3.27).

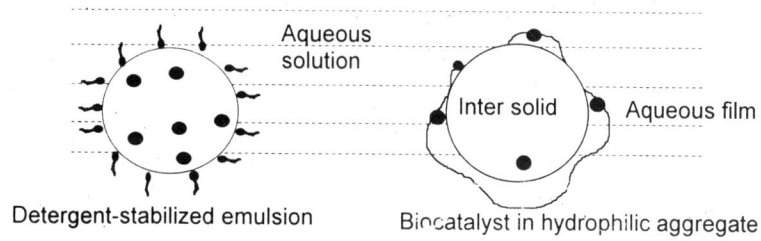

Aqueous solution

Inter solid   Aqueous film

Detergent-stabilized emulsion   Biocatalyst in hydrophilic aggregate

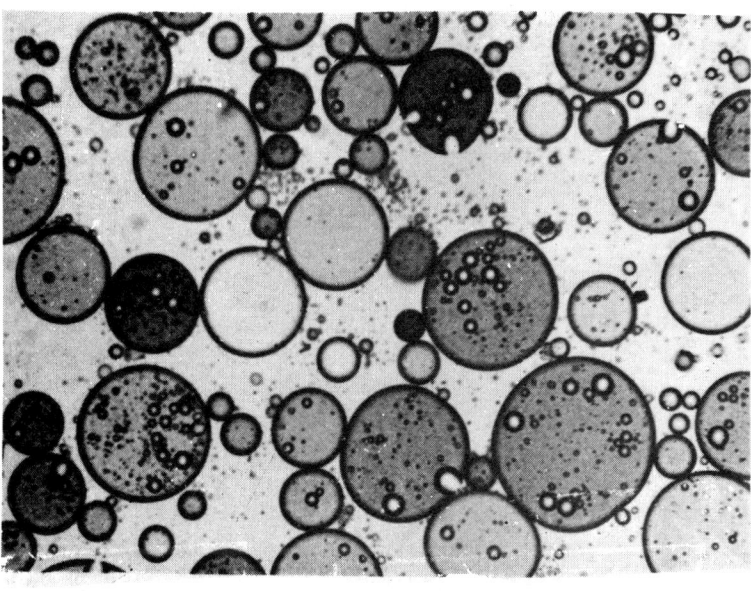

Fig. 3.27 : Emulsions used to immobilized biocatalysts

The enzymatic synthesis of peptides with chymotrypsin, in a etheylacetate-water system is a representative example. Thus, the enzymatic conversion of water insoluble, highly lipophilic substrates, such as steroids, can be carried out in a multiple emulsion (w/o/w) system. The enzyme is contained in a microdroplet 'water pool' whereas the organic phase contains the substrate solution.

3.5.2.3. Microcapsules

Liquid membrane systems is a biphasic system (Fig.3.28), where an organic intermediate phase imposes a barrier to the diffusion of enzyme molecules thus keeping them immobilized in the inner phase. A specific carrier system for substrate transportation can be utilized for an effective enzyme substrate interaction. On the other hand, microencapsulation recently has gained a special attention in connection with the immobilization of enzymes or mammalian cell lines. Emulsions can be permanently stabilized by hardening a polymer membrane at the interface to produce a microcapsule entrapping the droplet of biocatalyst and making it possible to subsequently transfer these membranous capsules to a fresh, non-emulsified solution. Stabilization can be achieved either by precipitating a water-insoluble polymer (coacervation) at the phase boundary or by promoting an interfacial polymerization between co-monomers present at the interface.

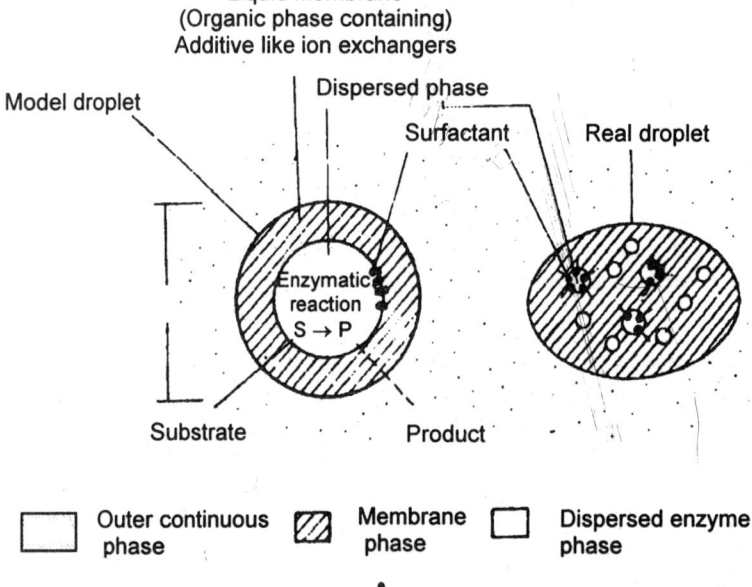

Fig. 3.28 : Diagrammatic presentation of liquid membrane systems

In a leading example, yeast cells have been encapsulated in microcapsules consisted of ethylcellulose, by coacervate phase-separation induced by solvent (hexane) addition. In brief, the organic solution of polymer (benzene/hexane 3:1) containing a surfactant, sorbitan monolaurate is maintained at 5°C and a saline (1%) slurry of cells is added under stirring to produce an o/w emulsion. This is then dropped into an aqueous PEG at 5°C while the stirring is continued to give a w/o/w emulsion around which the polymer gets precipitated by adding non-polar solvent (hexane). Further, hardening can be imparted by adding some cross linking\hardening agent, i.e. 1% chitosan to the cell slurry.

A classical example is the entrapment of enzymes or cells in an alginate beads followed by its treatment by polycationic solution like poly-lysine. This results into the formation of an insoluble polyelectrolyte complex possessing required membrane characteristics. The noncomplexed alginate can be redissolved from the microbeads leaving the cell in suspension as microcapsules. The method has been very successful in immobilization of pancreatic cells which were grown in a culture and were found to survive for six weeks as compared against their non encapsulated counter parts, (control cells) which could survive only for 24 days. Another attractive application of enzymes and cells microencapsulation is hybridoma cells. The successful application of technique demonstrates the special strength and potential of the method in the field of medicine and health care and most possibly in the development of artificial organ prostheses. The polymeric materials which have successfully been used for cellular/enzymic immobilization include cellulose acetate, ethyl cellulose, polyester cellulose diacetate, eudragits, liquid membranes (based on isoparaffin), alignate-poly-lysine complexes and nylons.

3.5.2.4. Dehydrated-Rehydrated vesicles (DRVs)

Encapsulated incorporation of proteins and enzymes in liposomal vesicles (dehydration-hydration vesicles) has been suggested by Gregoriadis et. al. The method effectively addresses osmosis, alliviate the constraints associated with other methods. The method essentially involves the formation of lipid vesicles wherein hydration fluid contains protein or enzyme to be incorporated in. The total content of the hydration stage are frozen followed by rehydration using plain phosphate saline buffer (PBS). The transformation stages involved in the form of rehydrated-dehydrated vesicles tend to produce uni- or oligo-lamellar liposomes capable of entrapping up to 70% of therapeutic protein as well as DNase. Further, the entrapment could be improvised by increasing the concentration of sodium or potassium chloride while incidental or intended incorporation of sugar or carbohydrates results into decreased entrapment of macromolecular bioproteins. It may presumably be due to the phenomenon referred to as cryoprotection offered by sugars which may prevent the membrane rupture, thus, the fusion process of the vesicle during dehydration phase. The fusion is an essential event for effective performance of this method particularly during freeze drying.

3.4.2.5. Reverse phase evaporation method (REVs)

Another method which could successfully be employed for incorporation of bioproteins including enzymes into liposomal construct is REV technique suggested by Szoka and Pappahajopolous. The method principally based on w/o emulsion formation which was considered to be the reverse of o/w emulsion involving removal of solvent from emulsion through evaporation. The water phase of the system contains bioproteins to be incorporated. The droplets resulted on removal of solvent or when subjected to sonication and the emulsion is dried to a semisolid stage in a rotary evaporation under reduced pressure. At this stage particularly the monolayers of phospholipids surrounding discrete water compartments are closely attached to each other. Whereas during second step where vigorous mechanical shaking is applied it affects collapse of water droplets. Thus, the resultant collapsed vesicles contribute their monolayers resulting into intact vesicles relatively larger in size. The aqueous content of aqueous droplets provide the medium that is required for the suspension of the newly formed liposomes. The other steps, i.e. harvesting of liposomes using dialysis or centrifugation remain to be the same as in the case of conventional liposomal preparations.

3.5.2.6. Immobilization of enzymes in reverse micelles

Enzymes are expected to work differently, if they are isolated from their natural environment (*in vivo*). They become unstable and are rapidly inactivated. Increase in stability of enzymes result from multipoint interaction with cell components, like lipids, polysaccharides and proteins into a supramolecular structure. This results in to natural immobilization. Similarly, reverse micelles possess a microenvironment in which multilayers of structured water exist. Reverse micelles are associated colloids of surfactant molecules in water immiscible organic solvents. The entrapped water resembles the water adjacent to biological membranes (Fig. 3.29). This makes the system as a tool to study enzymatic reactions. This system facilitates solubilization of materials of widely differing polarities in a single gel phase and is optically clear and thermodynamically stable.

Immobilization of the enzyme using reverse micelles has gained utmost importance because the conventional methods by which enzymes are dissolved using organic solvents, destroy the catalytic power of the enzymes due to their exposure towards the nonpolar groups. In addition, stability of an enzyme at a given temperature is highly desirable for their isolation, processing and storage at industrial scale. Experiments have been carried out in this direction and it has been proven to be successful with α-amylase, invertase, and arginase. The system based on reverse micelles could catalyze reaction in organic phases promoting synthetic chemistry to proceed under biocatalysis.

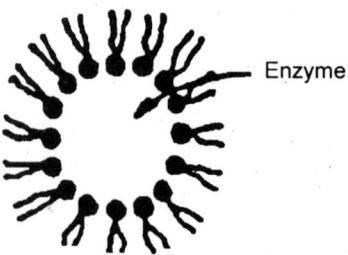

Fig 3.29 : Reverse micellar enzyme immobilization

3.6. CELL IMMOBILIZATION

Immobilization of enzymes has become a mature technology with number of immobilization methods developed. On the other hand, the innovative interest has moved onto development of immobilization of whole plant/animal cells which provides another route to highly specific enzyme processes aimed at multistage processing and biosynthesis of fine chemicals against first generation biocatalysts.

During the last decades, experiences and expertise in the immobilization of microbial cells has increased such that a range of mild techniques are now available to generate fine chemicals, cloths and membranes incorporating high number of viable cells. Drawing on experience from the fermentation industry immobilized microbial cells have been used over prolonged periods in continuous reactors to give extracellular products ranging from alcohol and pharmaceuticals to hydrolytic enzymes.

3.6.1. Unique features of plant and animal cells

In the field of cell immobilization research has been concentrated on using the prokaryotic bacterial cells as a subject. The differences between it and the eukaryotic cell are more distinguishable and involve size, form and function. As prokaryotes all of which are bacteria, lack of organelle, have a different cell wall composition and are typically one tenth the size or one thousandth the volume of the plant and animal cells. Eukaryotes, plant and animal cells have distinct subcellular, membrane bound organelles such as nuclei, mitochondria, lysosomes, vacuoles and various other plastids (Fig. 3.30). As a consequence of these differences the metabolic functions of eukaryotes proceed more slowly than those of bacteria.

Eukaryotic cells can express greater amount of genetic information in a number of ways, to produce distinct, differentiated (i.e., specific) cells which often function cooperatively to form tissues, organs or even whole organisms. Consequently, they evolve complex mechanism for both intracellular and intercellular control and informative transfer, involving hormones,. cell mediators and specific cell surface receptors. They are thus, capable of more sophisticated responses than the basic survival-related reactions of bacteria.

The overall complexity of their metabolism, affecting the gene expression in individual cells, presents problems in the maintenance and use of eukaryotes, even when successful immobilization has been achieved. However, these different levels of control could clearly provide valuable opportunities for manipulation of cellular activity. Unfortunately, these mechanisms are so incompletely comprehended at present that bacteria are likely to be preferred in an any applications where either cell types could be used.

3.6.2. Products from eukaryotes

The growing interest shown in large scale culture of plant and animal cells for the synthesis of high value pharmaceuticals, flavors, hormones and immunological products, despite the difficulties associated with them.

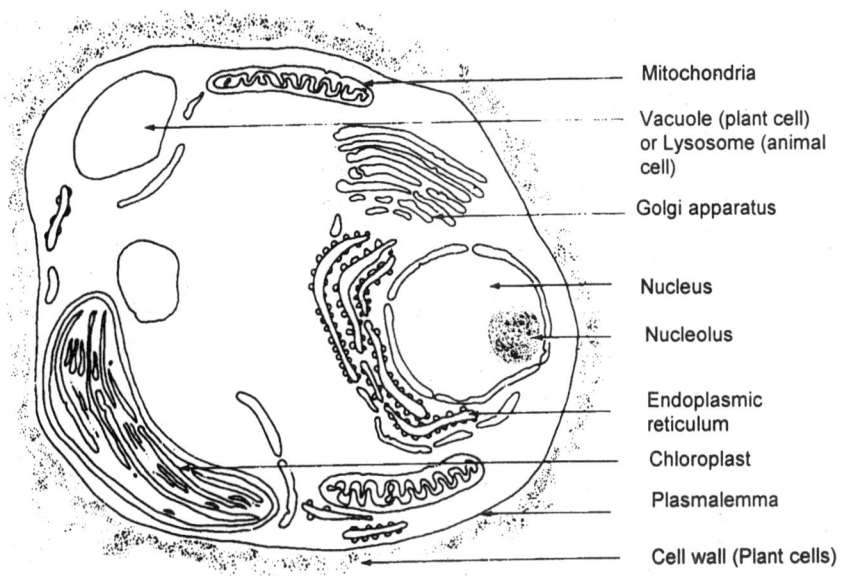

Fig 3.30 : Unique features of a eukaryotic cell

The complexity of organization and control of the biosynthetic pathways leading to secondary products in eukaryotes is likely to be beyond the practical or economic limits whereas to be beyond the practical or economic limits of genetic manipulation of bacteria it is still for sometime to arise. Furthermore, certain operational and post-translational modifications such as glycosylation, are unlikely to be achieved by inserting gene sequences into prokaryotes. It might also be argued that the most acceptable source of material for replacement therapy in the treatment of humans will be obtained from genetically engineered human cell lines, and that the best way of producing plant and animal cell products is by direct genetic manipulation of these cells and their use in an immobilized form.

3.6.3. Limitation of immobilization of eukaryotic cells

In comparison with enzymes, immobilized cells are less responsive to high substrate concentrations, surfactants, solvents and rapid changes in physical parameters. Thus process intensity and flexibility of response are likely to be lower. The substrate is often a major nutrient of the cell and in a single pass reactor, cells at the end of the process will either be subjected to nutrient starvation, or lower conversion must be accepted.

The sensitivity of higher cells to environmental factors e.g., osmotic shock, oxygen, shear, gas balance, pH, temperature and toxic chemicals is an obvious limitation to the methods which might be used for immobilization. However, these problems are to some extent offset by the capacity of cells to regenerate after immobilization, if maintained under appropriate conditions. The hormonal responses of eukaryotes allow addition at levels of control and flexibility compared to micro-organisms, which often only respond to nutrient levels or gross environmental changes.

To take maximum advantages of immobilization cells must be reused and thus must be kept in a healthy condition. The rich nutrient media, in which both plant and animal cells must be maintained are highly vulnerable to microbial contamination and so all operations must be performed under aseptic conditions. This further limits immobilization methods and adds to the cost and complexity of the techniques. In addition, stored medium can deteriorate and may become particularly apparent where continuous operation of a process is considered.

It can be seen that many of these limitations are actually associated with the cells rather than the immobilization process. If production by eukaryotic cells is selected, it has been discussed abcve that the benefit resulting from immobilization can, be very high, provided adequate process control is available. However, it is clear that the complexity involved in using cultured plant and animal cells will in general limit their application in production of high value compounds.

3.6.4. Immobilization of cells

In contrast to enzymes, the preferred methods of cell immobilization rely on entrapment of a cell suspension in a gel or within a membrane. Gels have the advantage that:

1. Any post-immobilization cell division can easily be accommodated in gel structures.
2. Cell itself need not be chemically modified during immobilization.
3. Cell is not subjected to strong asymmetrical forces such as those involved in adsorption on a surface, and
4. The whole gel volume can be used to hold cells. Hydrogels are particularly useful since their higher water content ensures open porosity and predominantly hydrophilic environment that is less likely to disrupt the cell membrane.

Knazek et al. first successfully immobilized the mouse fibroblasts and human choriocarcinoma cells cultured by using hollow fiber ultrafiltration units. However, unlike work on plant cells, the major drawbacks related to studies of animal cells have been the development of artificial organs from which hormones can be directly perfused into deficient animals. Thus, the biocompatibility of the immobilization systems has been a major consideration and the systems have been viewed as clinical aids rather than methods of producing fine chemicals.

The immobilization of animal cells may be of minor importance for the production of biochemicals since most important animal products are proteinaceous and thus amenable to synthesis by genetically engineered microbes. However, the large size of some proteins like immunoglobulin fractions and the post-translational modification which may be so important for full biological activity of the protein, (e.g. glycosylation) should ensure an important role of immobilized animal cells. It is to be hoped that cell metabolites such as interferon, plasminogen activators and some other potential drugs will make satisfactory progress in the therapy using substances which are homologous with respect to the natural acceptance of the body. The ideal method for the immobilization of animal cells should possess the following character.

1. the more complex nutrient requirement of animal cells, particularly for high molecular weight complexes such as growth hormones and transferrin.
2. the greater molecular size of potential products like protein and glycoproteins.
3. the absence of a rigid cell wall, making the cells more sensitive to osmotic changes.

The first two factors emphasis the need for a highly porous immobilization matrix, while the third imposses further restrictions on methods of forming the immobilizing gel. Polymerization, for instance, inevitably results in to a sharp fall in the osmolarity of the gel-forming liquids and could cause cells to swell and ultimately lyse.

3.6.5. Entrapment in porous polymeric carrier

It is basically a simple technique which in most of the cases possible by providing absolute cell retention with high degree porosity of substrate penetration and in turn for diffusive product transportation. It is obvious that polymeric network should essentially be formed in the presence of cells to be entrapped therefore, the reactions that lead to net work formation have to be adapted to the near physiological requirements desirable for the stability of enzymes or cells. The reaction conditions include the solvent (aqueous or non-aqueous), temperature, possible addition of catalysts and lastly the chemical composition, functionality and size of substrate molecules (monomers, oligomers, or polymers). The forces which may be involved in addition to physical trapping for effective association of cell and enzymes with the carrier are vander Waals, secondary valance bonding, ionic bonding and covalent anchoring particularly involved in crosslinking reactions.

Another method that could be employed for polymeric entrapment of enzymes or cell is by gelation. The method is a temperature controlled phase transition based phenomenon where a homogeneous polymeric solution is transformed in to a homogeneous gel without any change in composition. Usually it is brought about by lowering the temperature however, the systems are also known where the reverse phenomenon is observed to be responsible for gelation. Systems of latter type could be of interest for their application in immobilization of thermophilic organisms. The cells are mixed with polymer solution at an appropriate concentration get entirely immobilized via their entrapment in the solidified gel. The macromolecules other than gelatins used for immobilization are agar or agarose. Small particles discrete and regular in size have been prepare by application of temperature induced solidification of polymeric globules. The latter could be obtained in a biphasic system by the formation of suspension or emulsion. The much more practical procedure appears to be the use of water immiscible oil phase which could be a paraffin oil, soyabean oil or isoparaffin for the dispersion of solution and the conversion of this to an emulsion which is essentially water-in-oil type and its subsequent conversion into a solid-liquid dispersion by cooling or congealing of the whole system. Spherical particles of uniform size can be obtained. The size can further be modulated by the variation in degree of mixing. The system however, suffers mechanical strength and stability. Therefore, appears to be adaptive in situations where mild immobilization conditions are desirable rather than the mechanical properties. The reversibility of gelation renders the system to be reusable where the cellular or enzymatic components could be liberated free.

The entrapment could also be achieved in a polymeric carrier via precipitation of polymer where a polymer solution is used as a dispersion media for the moiety to be immobilized. In this case, the coacervation-phase separation followed by its coagulation is generally induced by changing the physicochemical parameters which involve temperature, solvent or pH. Since such precipitates are to be stable in aqueous media seemingly it is an imperative that the starting solution of polymers should be prepared with an organic solvent or water/organic solvent mixture. Water miscible solvents are dimethyl formamide, trihydro formamide, ethanol and acetone. The polymers which have been used successfully include cellulose triacetate, polystyrenes and Eudragits, whereas cells used for immobilization were *E. coli*, *Actnoplanes*, *Missourinsi* and *Candida tropicalis*. The only noticeable drawback of the procedure is an intensive exposure of cells or enzymes to the non-physiological solvent.

In a variation gelation of the polymeric systems is achieved by the addition of multivalent counter ions. The polymers typically used are hydrophilic polyelectrolyte in nature thus on addition of multivalent counter ions they form poly salt which gets precipitated as a solidified mass. Since this mass is distinctively a water swollen structure of controlled morphology hence termed as **ionotropic** gelation. The most popularly known example is calcium alginate gel which is obtained on gelation of a sodium alginate solution using calcium chloride bath. Some of the polymers and their respective counter ions which have been successfully applied for whole cell immobilization are presented in table 3.4.

Table 3.4 : Some polymers and their counter ions used in whole cell immobilization

Poly ions	Respective terminal ions	Counter ions
Alginate	CO_2	$Ca^{2+} Al^{3+}$, Zn^{2+}, Co^{2+}, Ba^{2+}, Fe^{3+}
Pectin		Ca^{2+}, Al^{3+}, Zn^{2+}, Co^{2+} and Mg^{2+}
Carboxy methyl cellulose		Ca^{2+}, Al^{3+}
Carboxy-guar-gum		Ca^{2+}, Al^{3+}
Copolystyrene-maleic acid		Al^{3+}
Phospho-guar-gum	PO_4^{2-}	Ca^{2+}, Al^{3+}
Carrageenan	SO_3^{3-}	K^+, Ca^{2+}
Furcellaran		K^+, Ca^{2+}
Cellulose acetate		K^+
Chitosan	NH_3^+	Polyphosphates $[Fe(CN)_6]^4$ $[Fe(CN)_6]$ polyaldehydocarbonic acid, poly-1-hydroxy-1-sulfonate-propene-2-ol

3.6.6. Entrapment of biocatalyst in chitosan

Chitosan is a partially deacylated chitin, formed by the reaction of chitin with concentrated alkali. Chemically, it is high molecular weight linear polymer having the composition of glucosamine 1→ 4 linkage (Fig 3.31). Chitosan crosslinked with high molecular weight counter ions results in capsules, while cross linking with low molecular weight counter ions (Table 3.5) results in globules in which biocatalyst gets entrapped. Using more hydrophobic counter ions (Table 3.6) it is possible to prepare hydrophobic carriers.

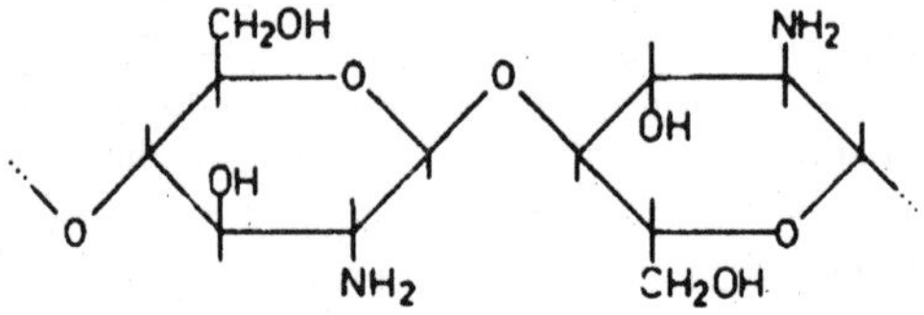

Fig. 3.31 : Chemical structure of chitosan

The method of beads formation are as follows : wet cells/enzymes suspended in 1% w/v chitosan acetate solution (which is prepared by mixing 1 gm of chitosan with 99 ml of water and 0.7 ml of glacial acetic acid under heat) using gentle mixing. This suspension is added dropwise (Fig. 3.32) under gentle stirring into 2% w/v counter ion. The pH of the medium should be maintained at 8.2 by adjusting with 5 mol alkali. After 4 hours the beads are collected by decantation of the supernatant or simply filtering the suspension.

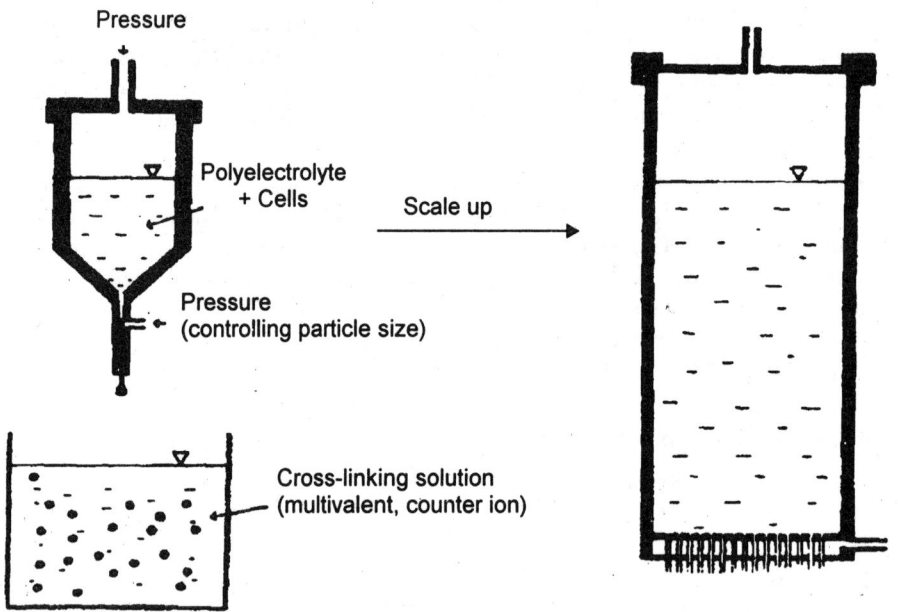

Fig. 3.32 : Schematic representation of bead formation technology

3.6.7. Entrapment of cells in beaded polymers

Various gel-forming polymers may be employed for the immobilization of the whole cells by entrapment. The biocatalyst is mixed with gel forming material. The resulting suspension is dispersed in an inert hydrophobic phase and gelation is induced. Subsequently, a washing medium compatible with the biocatalyst is added and the formed beads with biocatalyst entrapped are allowed to sediment under gravity or gentle centrifugation into an aqueous phase. The hydrophobic phase and most of the washing medium is aspirated and then the beads are washed with medium until they are free from hydrophobic phase. If necessary the formed beads are sieved on metal screens or nylon nets. Such sieving may be required to remove very small beads to avoid problems when operating a continuous reactor. It should be emphasized that the whole procedure may be carried out under the sterile conditions. The hydrophobic phase selected should be inexpensive, nontoxic, easily disposable and easy to separate from the aqueous phase. Vegetable oils, paraffin oil, silicon oil, tri-N-butyl phosphate and dibutyl phthalate are some examples of the hydrophobic phases that have been found to fulfill the above crite a. Paraffin oil is the only hydrophobic phase that has been successfully used for the entrapment of the animal cells. The above procedure is schematically outlined in figure 3.33.

Table 3.5 : Possible counter ions for ionotropic gelatination of chitosan

Polycation	Counterions
	Low molecular weight
Chitosan	Pyrophosphate
	Tetrapolyphosphate
	Octapolyphosphate
	Hexametaphosphate
	High Molecular weight
NH₃	Poly (1-hydroxy-1-sulfonate-2-propane)
	Poly (aldehydrocarbonic acid)
	Alginate

Table 3.6 : Hydrophobic counter ions for ionotropic gelatination of chitosan

Polycation	Counterions
Chitosan	Octyl sulfate
	Lauryl sulfate
	Hexadecyl sulfate
	Cetyl stearyl
NH₃	

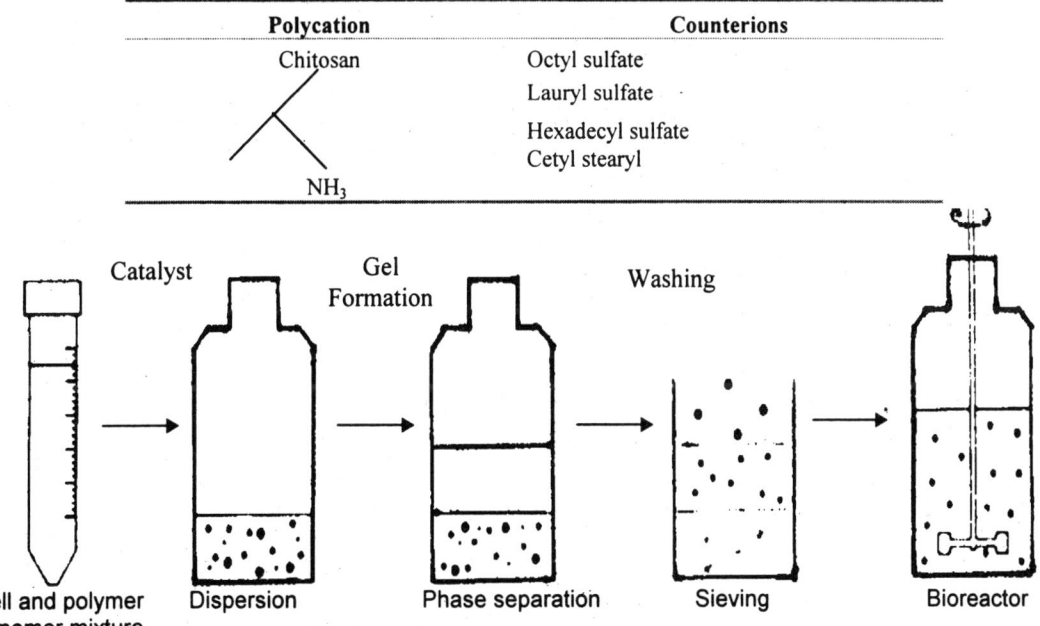

Fig. 3.33 : Two phase procedure for immobilization of intact cells in gel beads

3.6.8. Entrapment of biocatalyst in agarose

Agarose is a linear, neutral polysaccharide isolated from marine red algae. It is basically composed of repeating agarobiose units consisting of alternating 1,3-linked D-galactopyranose and 1,4-linked 3,6-anhydrous-L-galactopyranose. The polymer shows hysteresis which means it will dissolve in water at higher temperature above its gel-forming temperature. The gelling temperature may be influenced by chemical modification of the polymer (introduction of the hydroxyethyl group). The gel formed is non-charged, porous, resistant towards bacterial degradation and does not require counterions for stability. Different agarose qualities with gelling temperatures down (15°C) are commercially available. Normally agarose preparations with gelling temperature between 28 and 40°C are employed for the immobilization of viable cells.

An agarose solution 2.5% w/w equilibrated at 40°C is mixed with cells. The mixture is dispersed in vegetable oil and equilibrated at 40°C under magnetic stirring. The droplets size can be controlled by adjusting the rpm of the magnetic stirrer. When the droplets of appropriate size usually 0.5-1.0 mm are formed, the mixture is cooled on an ice bath under continuous stirring until the agarose beads are solidified (15°). Culture medium or buffer is added and the beads are allowed to sediment by gravity or gentle centrifugation into aqueous phase. The last step is repeated until the beads preparation is free from the organic phase.

3.6.9. Entrapment of biocatalyst in carrageenans

Carrageenans are naturally occurring hydrocolloids consisting of high molecular weight linear sulfated polysaccharide. They are prepared commercially by extraction from red algae, sea weeds and are widely used in the food and cosmetic industries as a gelling, thickening and stabilizing agent. They are mainly obtained from *Chondrus, Giger-tina, Eucheuma irideae* and *Hypnea*. There are three principle types of natural carrageenans i.e., kappa (κ), lota (ι) and lambda (λ). They are mainly composed of D-galactose, 3,6-anhydro-D-galactose and their ester sulfate derivatives. The molecular structure of three types of carrageenans is shown in figure 3.34.

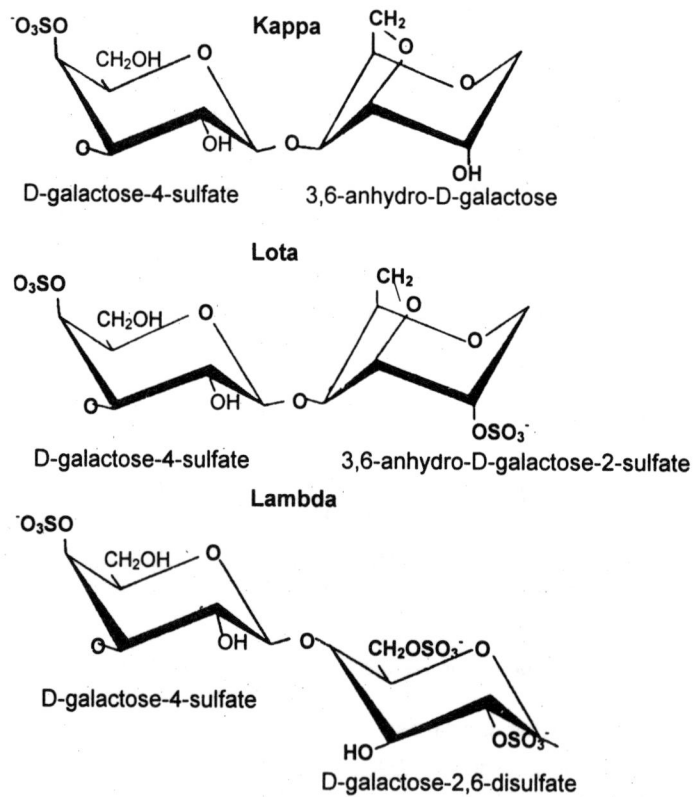

Fig. 3.34 : Chemical structure of carrageenans

κ-carrageenan in the potassium form that is insoluble in cold water and potassium salt of ι-carrageenan is also insoluble in cold water although it swells markedly. All salts of λ-carrageenan are soluble in cold water. κ- and ι-carrageenan form a thermoreversible gel when dissolved by heating followed by cooling below certain temperature whereas λ-carrageenan does not gel. The rigidity of λ-carrageenan gel in the presence of potassium ions increases with the increasing potassium concentration. κ-carrageenans have been used for the immobilization of biocatalysts. A one-step procedure which entraps a large amount of biocatalyst directly in carrageenan gel is discussed below.

In this procedure, large amounts of biocatalyst are homogeneously immobilized in carrageenans gel; the pore size of this gel matrix is small enough to prevent higher molecular weight compounds, such as enzyme proteins from leaking out from the gel lattice, although the lower molecular weight substrates and products may easily pass through the gel lattice. The immobilized biocatalysts are stable and a column packed with them can be used for continuous reaction for a long period. If the operational stability of the immobilized biocatalyst is unsatisfactory, preparation of higher stability can be obtained by further treatment with hardening reagents such as glutaraldehyde and hexamethylene diamine. Schematic procedures for immobilization of biocatalyst using κ-carrageenans is illustrated in figure 3.35.

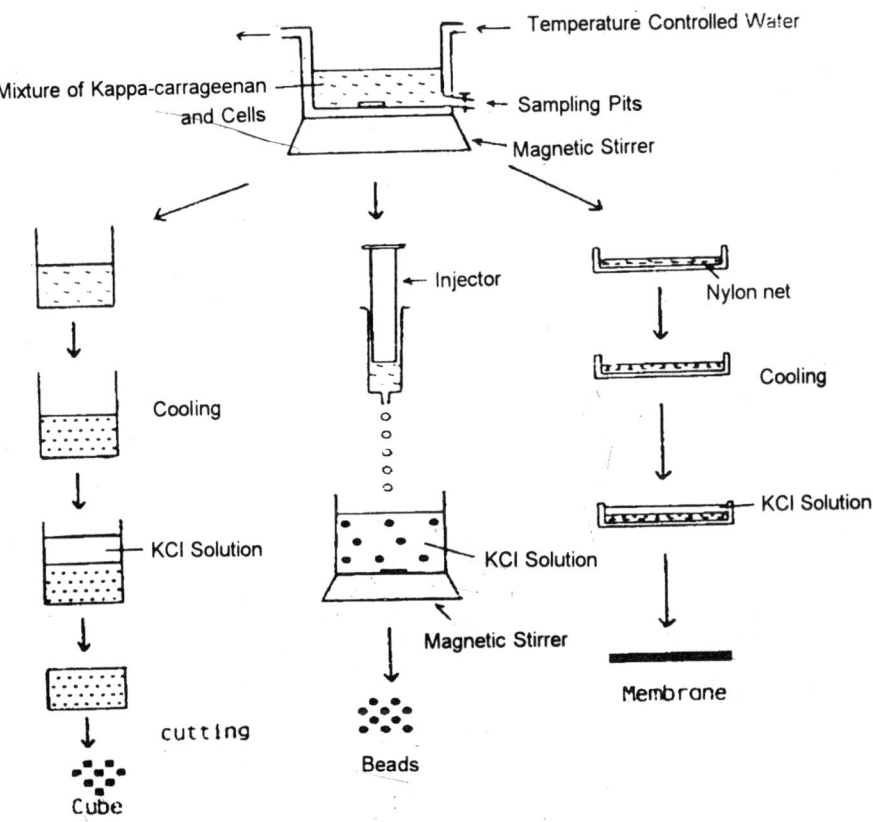

Fig 3.35 : Schematic procedure for immobilization of cells in κ-carageenan

The main advantage in this method is that the immobilization can be performed under very mild conditions without the use of chemicals which could destroy enzyme activity. Therefore, if a suitable gel-inducing reagent is selected for immobilization, a preparation of higher enzyme activity and operation stability can be obtained. In this method, various shapes of immobilized cells can be easily tailor-made for particular application purposes.

3.6.10. Entrapment of biocatalyst in polyacrylamide

In this case, the polymeric network is built up by polymerization of monomers. Acrylamide and N,N′-methylene bisacrylamide are the monomers which are usually used for immobilization. A stock solution of monomers is made from acrylamide and N,N′-methylene bisacrylamide in 50mM Tris-HCl buffer, pH 7.0. Monomer solution is mixed with biocatalyst and ammonium persulfate is then added. The biocatalyst suspension is dispersed in soya oil supplemented with 0.05% w/v Triton X-100. N,N,N′,N′-Tetra ethylenediamine is added to the dispersion when droplets of appropriate size are formed. On completion of polymerization the beads are collected and washed.

3.6.11. Inorganic support and microbial cell immobilization

Enzyme immobilization has received considerable attention and appreciation for quite some time and the possible applications of the system have been persuaded extensively. A logical extension of the approach towards multicomponent cellular system where more than one enzymes are responsible for a cascade of reaction, involving their joint action in the immobilization of cells.

Porous silica supports were activated by different procedures described for the enzymes such as alkylamine, the carbonyl and phenol derivatives of titanium activated support. To nearly 1 g of acid washed pumic stone approximately 3 ml of a 15% w/v titanium (IV) chloride solution in 15% w/w hydrochloric acid is added. The mixture is dried in an oven for 48 hours at 45°C (oxychloride derivative). So obtained oxychloride derivative is washed with distilled water yielding anhydrous oxide derivative. A 2% w/v suspension of *Saccharomyces ccrevisiae* (yeast) cells in 0.02 M sodium acetate buffer (pH 4.5) is added and kept aside for 2 h at 4°C. The excessive of suspension is then removed and separated, solid is washed with distilled water and 10ml of 0.01M sodium acetate buffer. The systems so obtained are considerably stable at 45°C. Long term batch operation stability at 45°C of yeast cells immobilized on different derivatives of titanium (IV) activated pumic stones has been reported. In another example the *S. uvaraum* cells are immobilized by suspending the cells in saline buffer pH 5.0 and percolating the suspension through a bed comprising of silica or brick in a glass column (fig. 3.36). The cell suspension is recirculated with the help of peristaltic pump at 25° C.

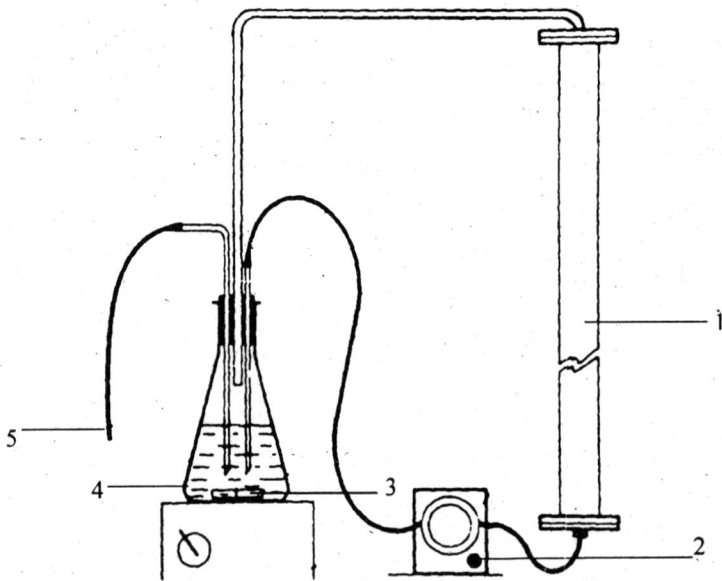

Fig. 3.36 : Reactor device used for microbial cell adsorption. 1. Reactor, 2. Peristaltic pump, 3. Magnetic stirrer, 4. Reservoir, and 5. Sampling duct.

·Number of recyclng of the cell suspension are dependent o the number of residual cells in the suspension which can be measured using the coulter counter device that allow approximation of the number of cells retained on the support.

Though, immobilization is dealt separately yet it is relevant to deal it with solid support particularly of inorganic types as to consolidate the precise application domain of the same. It could be drawn as a conclusion that methods classically leaded on the principles discussed in this chapter with modifications may be used for immobilization of bioproduct in order to assist them to function effectively as a stable system both in *in-vitro* and *in-vivo*. Additionally, judicious application of principle of immobilization may at large help developing dual systems with stability and function specificity.

SUGGESTED READINGS

Antonini and M.R. Rossi Faneli, (1987) *Immobilized Enzymes and Cells*, In : **Methods in Enzymology,** Vol.44, Klaus Mosback (Ed.) Academic Press Inc., Orlando, Florida.

Antonini, M.R. Rossi Fanelli, and E. Chiancone, (1975), In: **Protein-Ligand Interactions,** H.Sund, (Ed.), De Gruyter, Berlin.

Berezin and K. Martinek (Eds.) (1982) **Introduction to Applied Enzymology-Immobilized Enzymes,** MSU Press, Mosocow.

Buchholz, (1983), In: **Enzyme Technology,** R.M. Lafferty (Ed.) Springer-Verlag, Berlin and New York.

Byong-Kak Kim, E.B.Lee, C.Kim and Y. N. Han (Eds.) (1991) **Advances in New Drug Development,** The Pharmaceutical Society of Korea, Seoul, Korea.

Chibata and L.B. Wingard, Jr., (1983) **Applied Biochemistry and Bioengineering,** Vol.4, Academic Press, New York.

Chibata, (1978) **Immobilized Enzymes Research and Development,** Halstead Press, New York.

Chibata, and T. Tosa, (1978) **Immobilized Enzymes,** Wiley, New York.

Chibata, T. Tosa and T. Sato, (1983), In: **Advances in Biotechnological Process,** A. Mizrahi (Ed.), Alan R. Liss, Inc., New York.

Hermanson, G.T., Mallia, A.K., Smith, P.K., (1992) **Immobilized Affinity Ligand Techniques,** Academic Press, San Diego, CA.

Karl Schugerl and Wolfgang Sittig, (1987) *Bioreactors*, In: **Fundamentals of Biotechnology,** P. Prave, U. Faust, W. Sittig, D.A. Sukatsch (Eds.), VCH, Weinheim, Germany.

Klaus Mosbach, (1987) *Immobilized Enzymes and Cells*, In: **Methods in Enzymology,** Vol.135, Part-B, Klaus Mosbach (Ed.), Academic Press Inc., Orlando, Florida.

Martinek, V.V., Mozhaev and I.V. Berezin, (1980) In: **Enzyme Engineering: Future Directions,** L.D.Wingard, I.V. Berezin and A.A. Klyosov (Eds.), Plenum Press, New York.

Mattiason, (1983) **Immobilized Cells and Organells,** Chem. Rubber Publ. Co., Cleveland, Ohio.

Mattiason, (1983) In: **Immobilized Cells and Organelle,** Vol. 1&2, CRC Press, Boca Raton, Florida.

Rosevear and Lambe C.A., (1983) *Immobilized Plant and Animal cells*, In: **Topics in Enzymes and Fermentation Biotechnology,** Alan Wiseman (Ed.), Ellis Horwood Ltd., Chichester, West Sussex, UK.

Rosevear, Kennedy, J. F., and Cabrel, J.M.S., (1987) **Immobilized Enzymes and Cells,** Adam Hilger, Bristol, UK.

Sugiyama and Seki, J., (1991) *In Vivo Application of Lipoproteins as Drug Carriers*, In: **Lipoproteins as Carriers of Pharmacological Agents,** M.J. Shaw (Ed.), Marcel Dekker Inc., New York, 315-350.

Torchillin and Klibanov, A. L., (1993) *Coupling of ligands with liposome membrane,* In: **Liposomes in Drug Delivery,** G. Gregoriadis, A.T. Florence and H.M. Patel (Eds.,) Harwood Academic Publisher, Chichester, West Sussex, UK.

Torchinski, Yu. M., (1974) **Sulfhydryl and Disulfide Groups of Proteins**, Plenum, New York..

Ugi (Ed.), (1971) **Isonitrile Chemistry**, Academic Press, New York.

Vorlop, and Klein, J., (1983) In: **Enzyme Technology**, R.M Lafferty, (Ed.) Springer-verlag, Berlin and New York.

Zaborsky, O.R., (1973) **Immobilized Enzymes**, CRC Press, Boca Raton, Florida, USA.

APPLICATIONS OF IMMOBILIZATION

4.1. INTRODUCTION

Immobilized enzymes and cells are of use in industrial, clinical and analytical processes and in fundamental biochemistry and microbiology. The immobilization as such offers opportunities to improve existing processes, but more exciting is the prospects of totally new processes which are based on immobilized biocatalyst. In the forthcoming discussions the real and potential uses of immobilized biocatalysts are discussed with the help of special examples. The application domain of immobilization covers cell and animal cell, tissue(s), proteins and enzyme macromolecules immobilized in appropriate carrier system with distinctive advantages over their free or soluble counter parts. The applications include the use of technology in novel drug delivery system design, in extracorporeal hemoperfusion, in analytical technique(s), in secondary metabolite production, in designing of bioreactors and biosensors, in immunoadsorptive and affinity chromatographic separations, in apheresis, in drug targeting, in bioenvironment modification, in fabrication of surrogate organs and cellular systems, in blood detoxifiers designing etc.

The application potentials are mainly based on the concept that *in-vitro* simulation and culturing of biocomponents, cells and plants for biological activity under external manual control could be concluded for evaluations. The bioevents recorded *in*-vitro in immobilized system could be exploited judiciously for medicinal or clinical benefits. Similarly, sensitivity and selectivity could be utilized in qualitative and quantitative determination of bioeluate(s) also in extractive isolation events. The method ensures for longevity of cells and biologicals rendering them to be stable in *in vitro* as well as *in vivo*.

4.2. USES OF IMMOBILIZED BIOCATALYST

The most potential uses of immobilized biocatalysts have been appreciated and summarized as retention of catalyst, high catalyst concentration, microenvironmental control, fine process control and separating biocatalyst and process product. Some of the representative examples and process operations are discussed in this chapter.

4.2.1. Retention of catalyst

Retention of catalyst provided by immobilization process offers two types of distinctive benefits. Firstly, those where the catalyst is very expensive hence its use only can be contemplated by efficient reuse. Secondly, those where the presence of active or even inactivated catalyst in the product is undesirable due to continued changes in the product or toxicity effects.

Reuse for example, many traditional enzymes and cell processes have been evolved depending on low-cost catalyst which did not warrant recovery after a single use. However, recent advances in biotechnology have presented many processes for which a biocatalytic step might be integrated as one of the steps in a sequence of reactions needed to prepare a high-value product. Many of the enzymes required are significantly more costly than the crude hydrolases and require expensive purification if they are to provide with the specificity required for their use. The diversity of approach with immobilized catalysts is illustrated by variety of methods used to prepare α-keto acids (Fig. 4.1).

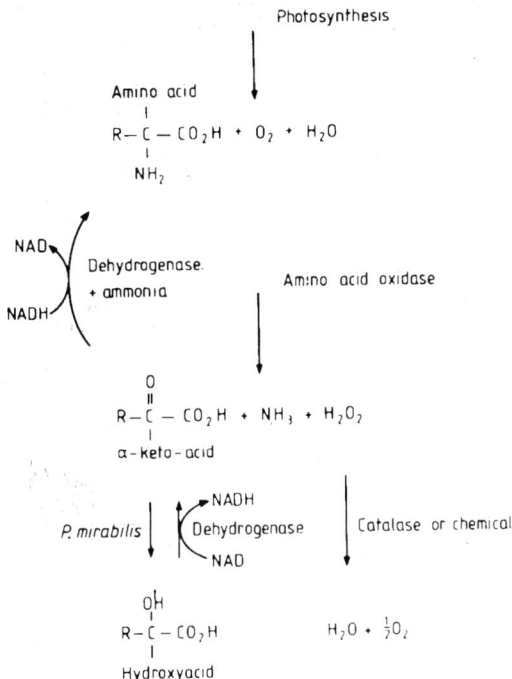

Fig. 4.1 : Interconversion of substituted organic acids by enzymatic reactions.

Trigonopsis variables whole cells were immobilized in calcium alginate beaded gel and used in bioconversion of amino acids to α-ketoacids. The trickle bed column was used for better oxygenation, where as manganese oxide was used for the decomposition of peroxide. Similarly, a coimmobilized system containing *Providencia* cells with oxidase activity and chlorella with photosynthetic character has been reported. The immobilization has been based on entrapment of these cells in alginate beads prepared by emulsion congealing method. In this system the co-immobilized chlorella cells supply oxygen to bacterial cells *in-situ*, thus facilitating ketoacid bioproduction.

In clinically applicable bioproducts it is sometimes desirable to remove biocatalyst totally for its antigenic nature, or systemic toxicity. To reduce the blood level of phenylalanine, an enzyme phenylalanine ammonia lyase is recommended and employed to reduce the level. However, this enzyme in free form can not be used. The higher levels of phenylalanine are particularly toxic to patients suffering from phenyl ketonuria. To circumvent this toxic situation Ambrus et. al., (1978) suggested immobilized enzyme based multitude reactor system using which 50% amino acid could effectively deleted. Similarly, sepharose bound heparinase in a blood purifying extracorporeal shunt has been used successfully where enzyme is not allowed to join systemic circulation thus immobilized enzyme system ensures an absolute safety.

The retention of enzymes in analytical devices such as enzymes non-invasive analysis is highly desirable, therefore immobilization is likely to be of increasing importance as new analytical enzymes are now available in large quantities. This is discussed later in brief under enzyme electrode (Fig. 4.2).

Immobilized enzymes have been proved to be useful in studies of cellular fundamental biochemistry. The immobilized cellular systems not only able to attack substrate selectively but also offer for their easy recovery hence the effect of a biochemical process on enzyme integrity could simultaneously be studied. The immobilization of neuraminidase on sepharose has made it possible to restrict the desialisation to the outer surface of cells. Otherwise, the enzyme penetrates in to the interior of cells, initiating a complex set of intracellular biochemical modifications. Similarly, immobilized trypsin could be used successfully in the study of neural cells dissociation without getting absorbed or bound to isolated cells.

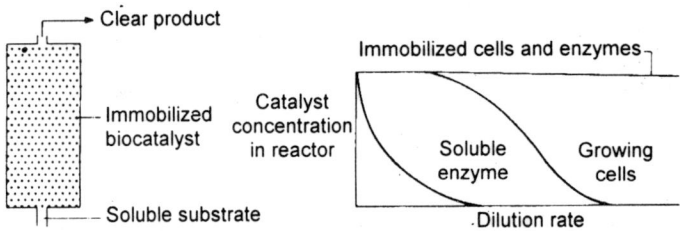

Fig. 4.2 : Potential of immobilization - retention of catalyst

4.2.2. High concentration of catalyst

The high catalytic density results in a more compact system, reducing capital cost but also reduces the volume of reactor which has to be specially treated or kept sterile. The high concentration of catalyst leads to two major benefits. One is the extreme rapidity of the enzyme reaction in the matrix and the other is the ability to generate specific compounds at high local concentrations. The speed of reaction in an immobilized enzyme reactor makes it feasible to process fluids which may not be sufficiently stable for treatment in the form of dilute enzyme solutions. Immobilized higher concentration peroxidases have been used to catalyze the bactericidal action of thiocynate and hydrogen peroxide and proved very useful for in-situ sterilization of reactors.

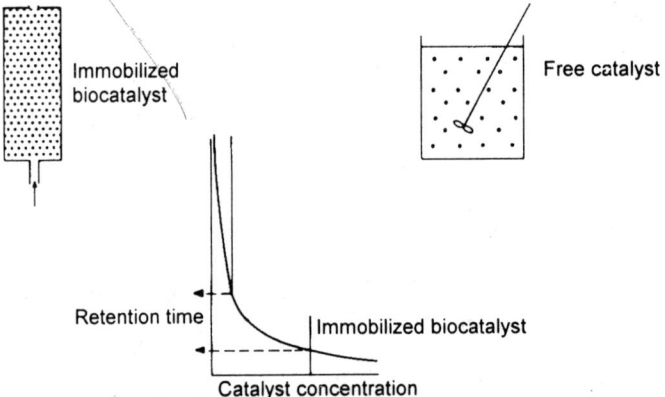

Fig. 4.3 : Potential of immobilization - high biocatalyst density

4.2.3. Microenvironmental control

The microenvironment in the vicinity of an immobilized catalyst distinctively differs from the homogeneous equivalent. Surface charge or hydrophobic regions on the matrix interact specifically with the catalyst, and even where this does not occur, effects on ionic balance, pH, water activity and osmolarity will directly contribute to and have an impact on the aqueous environment. These effects collectively can increase the thermostability of the enzymes by reducing the degree of freedom of the protein chain. The free movement of protease, which might cause autolysis as in soluble preparations, is restricted by immobilization. Thus, spectacularly reduces this mode of activity loss. Additionally, toxins and inhibitors can be excluded from the matrix (Fig. 4.4) while the biocatalyst is mechanically protected. This is particularly useful for very delicate cells such as those from plant and animal tissue culture. For example, calcium alginate gel can be used to stabilize human red blood cells against pressure changes and in addition cells with even very weak cell walls. The membranes of immobilized cells can be permeable without the risk of serious mechanical damage. This property has been used to remove intracellular products from *C. roseus* plant cells by treating them intermittently with medium containing 5% dimethyl sulfoxide to recover ajmalicine.

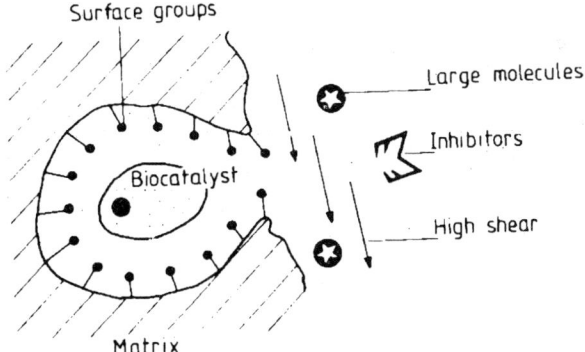

Fig. 4.4 : Microenvironmental control by immobilization.

Another microenvironmental effect which has not yet been fully exploited is the change in **cellular metabolism**, which could be successfully utilized particularly in secondary metabolite production. This offers more opportunities to manipulate cells than is the case in fermentation or tissue culture.

4.2.4. Quantitative and rapid removal of the catalyst (fine control)

This can be very useful, where the final product should be an intermediate or partially degraded product of an enzyme reaction. Since, once withdrawal of fluid from the enzyme reaction systems leads to the complete ceasing of the enzyme-induced changes. Immobilized enzymes have been used more generally as "off-the-shelf" reagents in organic synthesis where the need to stop a reaction at a specific point of time and prevention of carrying of catalyst is important to success. For example, caboxypeptidase-γ immobilized on CL-sepharose can be used for deprotection of growing peptide synthesis in aqueous medium. Similarly, immobilized lactoperoxidase can be employed as an easily removable reagent in the radio-iodine labeling of proteins.

4.2.5. Delinking growth and production

This property has most obvious application in the production of cell metabolites, by separating the growth and production phases. Conditions for each can be maximized so that in the former, suspension culture can be used to produce rapidly proliferating cells at low cell density while after immobilization the cell density can be increased leading to a greater diversion of energy into product formation. This is likely to find its most important use in complex slow-growing cells such as plant and animal cells, slow-growing fungi such as lichens are unusual organisms.

Immobilization creates conditions similar to those in whole tissue where blocks of non-growing cells exist in a vascular matrix. Consequently, cells bound to supports offer useful models to study the effects of compounds and conditions on the metabolism while avoiding the use of whole animals or the time-consuming task of raising whole plants.

4.3. USE OF IMMOBILIZED CELLS

The major use of immobilized cells is likely to be for the synthesis of secondary metabolites (Table 4.1). Most of these are small to medium molecular weight biochemical and can arise either by *de novo* synthesis from primary metabolites or by biotransformations of similar compounds from either from plant or animal kingdom (for details refer chapter 8).

4.3.1. Immobilized *E. coli* lysate for clean, easy removal of *E. coli*-reactive antibodies

Isolating a recombinant DNA clone that encodes a particular gene or mRNA sequence is accomplished by screening a recombinant DNA library. Once recombinant DNA is synthesized, it is necessary to introduce the hybrid molecule into bacterial cells, i.e., in *Escherichia coli* (*E. coli*) which is an usual bacterial host.

Table 4.1 : List of secondary metabolite from plant and animal cells

Cells	Immobilization Method	Product
Plant cell		
Biotransformation		
Digitalis lanata	Alginate bead	Methyl digitoxin → Methyl digoxin
Solanum aviculare	Polyphenylene oxide	Steroid glycosides
Daucus carota	Alginate bead	Digitoxigenin → Periplogenin
Biosynthesis		
Catharanthus roseus	Alginate bead	Tryptamine → Ajmalicine
Catharanthus roseus	Agar	
Catharanthus roseus	Gelatin	
Catharanthus roseus	Alginate	Sucrose → Ajmalicine
Catharanthus roseus	Alginate/Acrylamide	Sucrose → Ajmalicine
Catharanthus roseus	Xantham/Acrylamide	Serpentine
Nicotiana species	Xantham/Acrylamide	Sucrose → Alkaloids
Nicotiana species	Alginate beads	Sucrose → Nicotine
Capsicum		Capscicin
Animal cell		
Rat-Pancreatic β-cells	Hollow fibre units	Releasing insulin over the period of 40 days.
BHK cells	Hollow fibre units	Insulin
Hepatoma cells	Hollow fibre units	Bilirubin glucuronide
Rat-pancreatic β-cells	Very porous calcium alginate gels	Insulin
Hepatocyte	Calcium alginate beads	LDH
Adipocyte cells	Calcium alginate beads	free fatty acids after noradrenaline stimulation
Hybridoma cells	Microcapsules of porous carbohydrate	Monoclonal antibodies (MAbs)

The resulting library of clones is screened by immobilizing synthesized antigenic material onto a solid support and detecting with a sensitive procedure often using an enzyme-labeled secondary antibody. High background, or low signal-to-noise ratio, is often a problem during screening of libraries. There are many sources of high background localized and unexpected plaques appear to be positive, the primary antibody used may contain components that react with *E. coli* proteins. Crude antisera and ascites fluids often contain IgG components that bind to *E. coli* proteins. This could be especially problematic if the titer of binding affinity of the *E. coli* binding antibodies is higher than that of the antibody to the protein of interest, making the background of the false positive plaques. Optimizing the dilution of primary antibody for screening may eliminate some of the nonspecific background. By adsorbing the antisera or ascites fluid with an extract of the bacterial strain to inhibit or remove the anti-*E. coli* IgGs, the nonspecific binding may be further decreased. Another cause of localized background could be cross-reaction of the labeled secondary antibody with bacterial proteins. In this case, it may be beneficial to preadsorb the diluted secondary antibody conjugate with an *E. coli* extract immobilized on a support (Fig. 4.5).

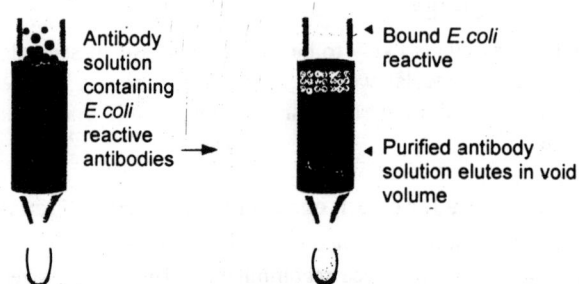

Fig. 4.5 : Principle of immobilized *E.coli* lysate

4.4. USE OF MONOCLONAL ANTIBODIES IN ACTIVE IMMOBILIZED ENZYME PREPARATION

Antibody based immobilization is a novel technique which produces highly active enzyme system. The method essentially involves binding of enzymes to a suitable carrier/support using monoclonal antibodies. The antibodies are selective and have higher affinity for enzyme bonding whereas inherent activity of enzyme is retained without any loss. Cell fusion (hybridoma) technique introduced by Kohler and Milstein makes it possible to clone up and harvest variety of monoclonal antibodies which specifically bind and directed towards respective antigenic site(s) of a protein. The studies suggest that an enzyme specific antibody with significant binding affinity $>10^8$ m^4 could be cloned up. The anchoring of such antibodies to a carrier support(s) thus results into the formation of a carrier monoclonal antibody conjugate which binds selectively with corresponding enzyme.

The desired MAbs (monoclonal antibodies) to carboxy peptidase A (CPA) were prepared and purified following standard method, the antibodies were covalently bound to Eupergit C3 via oxirane active group of the polymer. The Carboxy peptidase A was then incubated with antibody-carrier conjugate (Eupergit C-MAb or cellulose/sepherose protein A) to form MAb-Eupergit C-E system. Practically all of the bound enzyme moles retained their activity and could be stored in the cold for prolonged period.

4.5. IMMOBILIZED ENZYMES AND INDUSTRIAL PROCESSES

The use of immobilization technology has gained wide range of applications in the industrial field as well as in the medical and analytical field (Table 4.2). A brief discussion on the use of immobilized enzymes in the field of industrial processes is presented below. To start with, the use of immobilized enzyme in industrial processes includes their utilization in enzyme reactors.

Table 4.2 : Applications of immobilized enzymes

Industrial	Applications
Pharmaceuticals	Selective hydrolysis of penicillin G
	Steroid modification
	Production of monoclonal antibodies
	Animal vaccines
Food	Isomerisation of glucose to fructose
	Hydrolysis of sucrose
	Inversion of sucrose
	Transesterification of fats
	Amino acid synthesis
	Waste digesters
	Ethanol production
	Beer childproofing
Fine chemicals	Optical isomer resolution by hydrolysis of ester and amides
	$\propto$-keto acid production
	Redox reactions using dehydrogenases
	Cyanide detoxification
	Iodination of proteins
	Phenol degradation
	Radioactive chemicals
Analytical	Enzyme electrodes based on changes in pH, redox potential, oxygen tension
	Enzyme thermistors based on heat of reaction
	Bioprobes based on cellular metabolism
Medical	In vivo devices to treat failure of kidney, pancreas(Islets)
	Detoxification following drug overdose
	Body monitors for key electrolytes and glucose
Fundamental biochemistry	Study of enzyme interactions with other solutes
	Selective cleavage of biopolymers

4.5.1. Enzyme reactors

4.5.1.1. Batch reactors

These are enzyme reactors in which the immobilized enzymes and substrates are placed and the reaction is allowed to take place under constant stirring. Once the reaction is completed, the reactor is drained and the product is separated from the enzyme. Separation of enzymes is usually done by denaturing the enzymes. Again this is possible only with soluble enzymes. This type of separation when required at large scale, can be carried out only when the cost of enzyme used is less. If the availability of enzyme used is low, then such process would lead to a severe loss in production. To overcome such problems, the use of immobilization technique is highly appreciated. Using this technique the enzyme can be recovered intact without any significant loss in activity.

4.5.1.2. Continuous flow reactors

In a continuous flow enzyme reactor, the substrate is added continuously to reactor while simultaneous removal of product is taking place. Among the various types of continuous flow reactors, a few are discussed here :

4.5.1.2.1. Continuous flow stirred tank

These are reactors consisting of a continuously stirred tank with a separate inlet for the substrate while a product outlet is provided separately. The yield obtained can be increased by varying the input substrate quantity to minimum while the enzyme available to convert the same into a product will be at large, ultimately leading to a higher yield. Now the question arises how the immobilized enzyme used in the reactor could be retained while the product is recovered?. In fact, this is achieved by simply either filtering the product outlet or by using magnetically active particles for immobilization which can later be retained actively within a magnetic field whilst the product is still recovered.

4.5.1.2.2. Cell - free system and bioreactors

A typical cell free bioreactor(Fig. 4.6) for gene cloning principally works on the principle of immobilization of the required component(s) in chamber classically constructed using semipermeable membrane. Thus immobilization technique could effectively made it possible to synthesize and clone up the gene or other peptides which are amenable to the factoring and modifications. The principle of *in vitro* protein engineering may be referred in chapter 10.

4.5.1.2.3. Other reactors

The *packed bed reactor* is an enzyme reactor in which the immobilized enzyme particles are packed inside the column while the substrate is allowed to pass through the column.

The *hollow fiber reactor* is a variant of the packed bed reactor which uses walls made up of fibers permeable to the substrate and product while being impermeable to enzyme molecule. The substrate passes over the enzyme to react with it producing the required product. Further, the substrate diffuses out through the fibrous wall, reacts with the enzymes and the product diffuses through the fibrous wall. Another class of bed reactors is the fluidized bed reactors, the combination hybrids of packed bed reactors and constant flow stirred tanks. In this reactor, the immobilized enzyme is loosely packed into a column while the substrate stream is passed through the bottom of the column at a sufficiently high flow rate so as to lift and mix the packed immobilized enzyme thoroughly.

4.5.2. Industrial processes

Several large-scale industrial processes are already in operations employing immobilized-enzyme catalysts at some point. Two notable examples are the production of high-fructose syrups from corn starch and manufacturing of L-amino acid by resolution of racemic amino acid mixture (containing both D and L optical isomers). Also, immobilized penicillin acrylase has been used commercially in the manufacture of semisynthetic penicillins through deacrylation of penicillin G to 6-amino penicillanic acid (6APA) using macroreticular ion exchange resin as supports.

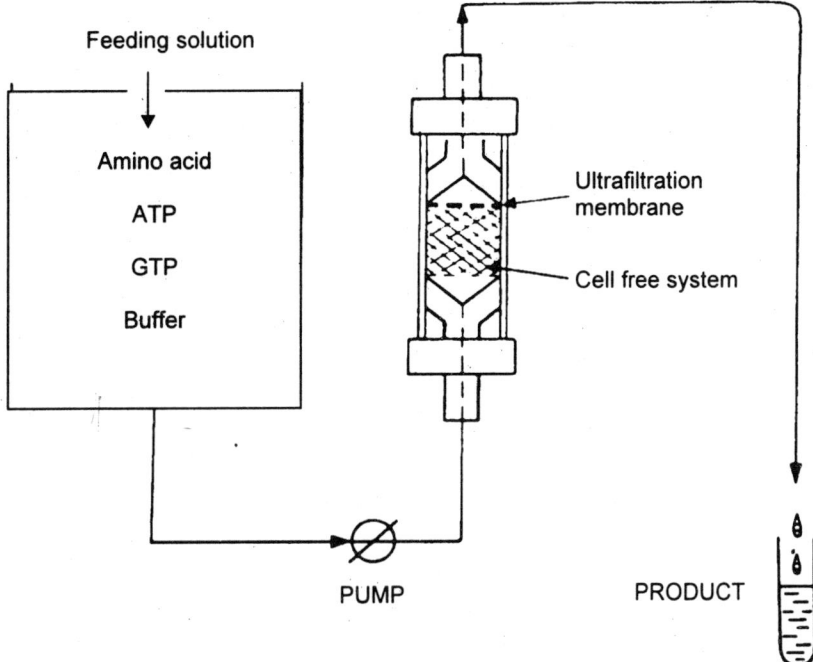

Fig. 4.6 : Sketch of bioreactor based on micro-column technique

4.5.2.1. Production of high-fructose syrups

D-glucose cannot be substituted directly for sugar (sucrose) because glucose is relatively less sweet also, glucose crystallization in concentrated solution can make subsequent handling and processing difficult. These problems are alleviated considerably by isomerizing some of the glucose to fructose, using the enzyme glucose isomerase.

The equilibrium constant of this reaction at 50°C is approximately unity. Consequently, the equilibrium product contains roughly a 1:1 ratio of glucose to fructose. Such a mixture has greater sweetness than glucose alone and is well suited as a substitute for sugar in many applications including soft drinks, processed foods and baking.

An intracellular enzyme, glucose isomerase, is produced by a number of microorganism, *Arthrobacter* and *Streptomyces* species being among the preferred sources. The need to disrupt cells without destroying the enzyme makes glucose isomerase substantially more costly than the extra-cellular hydralases. Also, glucose isomerase is very sensitive to several inhibitors. Therefore, the enzyme in immobilized form under well-controlled reaction conditions is desirable. Glucose isomerase can be immobilized in various carriers. In one of the method enzyme contained in whole cells, is held immobilized in matrix of collagen or other carrier systems.

4.5.2.2. Production of L-amino acid by resolution

The demand for L-amino acids in food and medical industries is increasing day by day. To meet the growing need, chemical synthesis is utilized in addition to the microbial process. The chemical method has the disadvantage that it produces a racemic mixture. The D-isomer in the mixture is of no nutritive value. To obtain a product containing only active L-isomer, Tanabe Seiyaku Co., Ltd., of Osaka, Japan designed a process based on immobilized enzymes. The optical resolution was catalyzed by the enzyme aminoacylase, the reaction scheme is as follows:

$$\text{D,L} \quad \underset{\underset{\text{NHCOR}'}{|}}{\text{R-CH-COO}^-} \quad \xrightarrow{\text{Aminoacylase}} \quad \text{L} \quad \underset{\underset{^+\text{NH}_3}{|}}{\text{R-CH-COO}^-} \quad + \quad \text{D} \quad \underset{\underset{^+\text{NHCOR}'}{|}}{\text{R-CH-COO}^-}$$

D,L-Acylamino acid ⟶ L-Amino acid + D-Acylamino acid

The next step is carried out in a column reactor containing immobilized aminoacylase, the desired L-amino acid is separated from the unhydrolyzed acyl D-amino acid based on solubility differences. The D-acylamino acid is then racemized to the DL-acylamino acid which is subsequently recycled through the aminoacylase column.

4.6. ANALYTICAL APPLICATIONS

4.6.1. Enzyme electrode

Enzyme electrodes are probes capable of generating an electrical potential as a result of a reaction catalyzed by an immobilized enzyme that is fixed onto or around the probe. The use of immobilized enzymes in automated analysis implies that the immobilized enzyme is used to replace the soluble enzyme in an existing automatic analyzer system. Ideally, analytical procedure should be :

- selective
- capable of determining a component in a complex mixture
- automated
- simple and rapid
- non-destructive
- requires use of small amount of material
- inexpensive and
- requires frequent standardization

Some of the above criteria are attributed to enzyme system used in the process. Major advancement was recorded when glucose oxidase was trapped within a polyacrylamide gel and layered with the film over the membrane of an oxygen electrodes. Where a redox enzyme confined close to the tip reduces the flux of oxygen reaching the detector by catalyzing a specific oxidation. This "enzyme electrode" was then combined with the selectivity of the enzyme for its substrate such as D-glucose and the sensitivity of potentiometric measurements.

The concept of generating physical changes in close vicinity of a detector by a biocatalytic process has been well appreciated and discussed elsewhere. **Thermistors,** which register the heat of the enzyme catalyzed exothermic reaction have proved effective detectors and similarly, no doubt that other physical factors could also be useful. **Bioprobes** consisting of living cells held close to oxygen or pH probes have also been suggested. Though they detect interesting metabolites directly they are far more susceptible to deactivation, interference and contaminative infections.

The first enzyme electrode to be reported was the glucose-sensitive electrode. In this electrode, the enzyme glucose oxidase was immobilized in a polyacrylamide gel and held in place around the electrode by a piece of cellulose acetate. The principle involved is the removal of oxygen from solution at a rate dependent upon the concentration of glucose present (Fig. 4.7A). One another example is the urea electrode. In this immobilized urease decomposes urea into ions which can be detected using standard electrochemical techniques (Fig 4.7B). Also, using immobilized-enzyme electrodes, standard biochemical tests can be automated. Examples, to determine glucose or lactate levels by employing immobilized glucose oxidase or lactate dehydrogenase, respectively substantiate practical application potentials of immobilized enzyme systems in the estimation of bioeluates (Table 4.3).

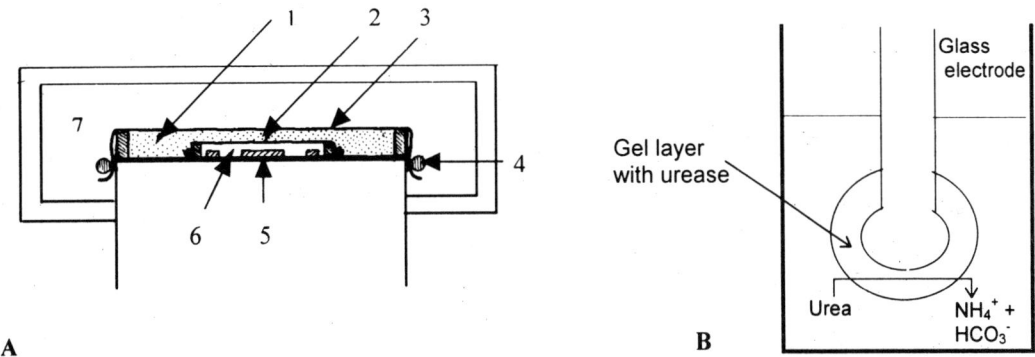

Fig. 4.7 : A model of substrate sensitive enzyme electrode; **A:**1. immobilized glucose oxidase; 2. Teflon membrane;3. Cellulose acetate membrane; 4. 'o'-ring seal; 5. Platinum-oxygen electrode; 6. Saturated KCl solution; 7. Sample solution; **B** : A model of urease electrode

4.6.2. Affinity chromatography and purification

Immobilized enzymes are also used in affinity chromatography. One species which has an extremely high affinity for the material to be removed from solution permits purification or analysis of enzyme inhibitors, cofactors, antigens, antibodies and other substances. For example, concanavalin A, a plant protein can be purified by passing the crude extract of the plant containing the protein through a column of beads containing covalently attached glucose residues. Concanavalin A has affinity to glucose and thus gets bound to the beads while the other proteins pass through the column.

Table 4.3 : Some examples of immobilized enzymes used in electrode constructs

Substance assayed	Enzyme immobilized	Electrode base
Adenosine monophosphate	AMP deaminase	NH_4^+
Alcohols	Alcohol oxidase	Pt/O_2
D-amino acid	D-amino acid oxidase	NH_4^+
L-amino acid	L-amino acid oxidase	NH_4^+
D-Glucose	Glucose oxidase	Pt/quinone
Glucose-6-phosphate	Alkaline phosphatase/glucose oxidase	Pt/O_2
Lactate	LDH	Pt/ferricyanide
Penicillin	Penicillinase	pH
Urea	Urease	pH or CO_2 or NH_4^+
Uric acid	Urease	Pt/O_2

The bound concanavalin A can then be released from the column by adding a concentrated solution of glucose. The glucose in solution displaces the glucose attached to the column from the binding sites on concanavalin A (Fig. 4.8).

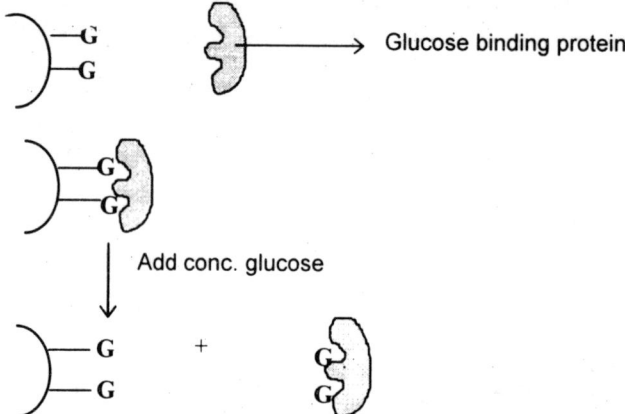

Fig. 4.8 : Affinity chromatography of concanavalin A

4.6.2.1. Immobilized receptor ligands for affinity cell sorting

The cell isolation affinity chromatography media principally based on immobilization of affinity ligands corresponding to the receptor which are specifically expressed by a particular cell line. The cells containing receptor or positive with regard to receptor are actively retained in the column producing that cell type negative elution. Thus with the combination of cell affinity media, cells can be isolated free of identified cellular contaminants some commercially available affinity media are Isocell™ for human T cell isolation, Isocell™ for CD8, Isocell™ for CD4, etc.

4.6.2.2. Immobilization in affinity purification

Based on avidin-biotin binding the immobilized systems have been developed where affinity binding has been taken advantage of, for the purpose of separation/purification. Avidin is covalently attached to a solid support, a biotinylated product or conjugate passing through is held strongly which can later be detached to let immobilized affinity support freely eluting LiM urea or 6M guanidine HCl. The biotinylated ligands include antigen, antibody, carbohydrates, cells, DNA, enzymes, haptens, lectins, peptides, proteins and receptors. The principle of affinity isolation based biotin-avidin interaction is represented in figure 4.9.

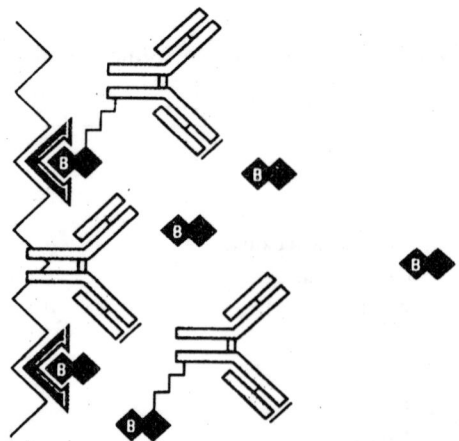

Fig. 4.9: Affinity purification: monomeric avidin-biotin binding

4.6.2.3. Immobilized avidin-biotin based systems

Immobilized avidin can be used in a variety of applications for the affinity purification of biotinylated macromolecules. Principally, an antibody that has an affinity for a particular antigen is labeled with biotin. Cells containing the antigen are lysed, then incubated with the biotinylated antibody to form a typical antigen/antibody complex. To isolate the antigen the crude mixture is passed through an immobilized avidin or streptavidin column, which will bind the complex. After appropriate washed, the antigen can then be eluted from the column with a pH 2.8 elution buffer. The biotinylated antibody is retained by the column.

Immobilized avidin are used for various purposes. They are:

• Purification of double-strand DNA.
• Binding biotinyl peptides and elution with a SDS/urea solution.
• Binding biotinylated antitransferrin for purifying transferrin from serum.
• Hybridization of biotinylated RNA to its complementary DNA and binding to immobilized avidin, with subsequent elution of the single-stranded DNA.

The interaction between biotin (a vitamin) and avidin (hen-egg white protein) has been extensively exploited to produce a variety of applications in the field of immunology. The figure 4.10 shows an example of avidin-biotin complex (ABC) systems for detecting antigen on solid support. A similar assay procedure can develop where, immunoassay reagent bounds to biotinylated enzymes or conjugates to enzymes. For example, DNA or RNA hybridization assays where a probe is biotinylated instead of an antibody and a few applications are exploiting the avidin-biotin interaction beyond assay developments. These are ELISA assays, immuno-histochemical staining, western blotting, DNA hybridization assays, immunoprecipitation, affinity chromatography, fluorescent activated cell sorting (FACS).

Similarly, purified streptavidin and lectin can be used in place of avidin in above system (ABC system). This modified system is broadly used in

• Enzyme immuno staining ,
• Cell and tissue staining (for light microscope),
• Blot immuno staining,
• Tissue staining, and
• Cell staining for fluorescent activated cell sorting.

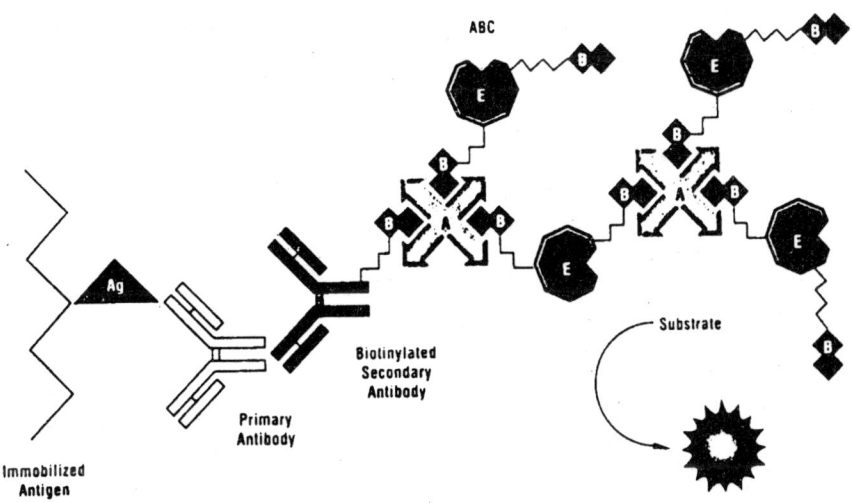

Fig. 4.10 : The ABC system.

4.6.3. Autoanalysis

Immobilized enzymes are mainly useful in two areas

1. repeated autoanalysis of small samples (e.g., blood samples)
2. continuous stream monitoring of large volume.

The conventional method has the disadvantage that an aliquot of enzyme is added to each sample which is subsequently lost. The alternative is to immobilize the enzyme and fix it in the sample stream. The enzyme may also be conveniently be attached to the inner wall of a narrow bore nylon tube, through which the sample stream is made to pass. Immobilized hexokinase and glucose-6-phosphate dehydrogenase have been used for the autoanalysis of glucose concentration. When large volumes are analyzed continuously the principle involved is the measurement of heat generated by an enzyme reaction. If a thermistor is held in the middle of a column of an immobilized enzyme as a substrate solution is passed through the column, the reaction catalyzed around the thermistor raises the temperature. The rise in temperature created by the reaction could be a measure of the substrate concentration. The advantage of using such a system is in checking contaminants in the production stream where the solvent stream is not required to be optically clear (used to monitor substances in blood).

4.6.4. Biosensors

A biosensor is a device, probe or electrode having immobilized biocatalyst which, upon making contact with an appropriate sample, converts the presence of the desired analyte into a physical, chemical, or electrical signals which can be measured. The concentration in the sample is measured as the electrical signal, or could be measured with the help of a suitable combination of a biological recognition system and an electrochemical transducer. Biosensors essentially respond in a reversible and specific manner to the concentration variation of biochemical event of great practical utility. The research drive has been propelled vigorously towards designing and development of precise biosensors as there is a continuous need of them. One common use of biosensor is quantitation of a drug substance in the finished drug product. Accurate measurements of drugs have been possible applying biosensing for all traditional dosage forms such as liquids, tablets, powders and ointments.

The biological recognition systems are typically some enzymes, organelles, microbial, plant or animal cell, tissue, slice, section, or immune binding or receptor protein. The system is responsible for the specific recognition of the analyte and subsequent response with a change in some measurable parameters. Various types of detection systems can be used in biosensing, They are namely, electrochemical detection system, thermal and mass detection, photometric detection, infra-red, fluorescence, surface plasmon systems and those based on signal processing and instrumentation (Fig. 4.11).

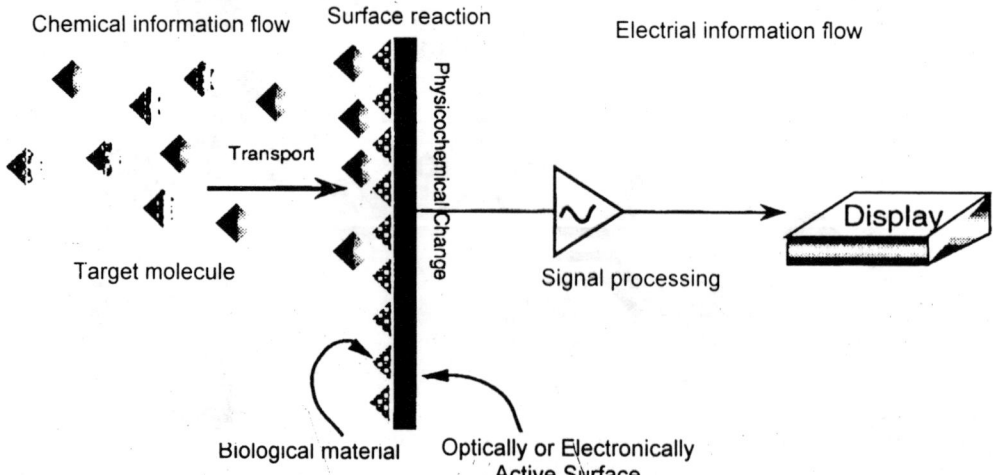

Fig. 4.11 : Schematic representation of a generic biosensor showing major components and the processes that contribute to signal generation.

A combination of immobilized antibody (or antigen) with an electronic device yields an **immunosensor**. In this system, the antigen acts as an analyte. Immunosensors are of two main types, namely, **labeled** and **non-labeled**. The frequently used labels are radioisotopes, enzymes, particles, and precipitins. Non-labeled immunosensors include potentiometric immunosensors with antigen (or antibody) coated membrane or potentiometric immunosensor with antibody-coated electrode. An interesting immunosensor has been developed for the diagnosis of syphilis. Principally, the antigen analyte due to affinity selectively binds to immobilized antibody and generates signals via labeled immunsorbent(s) which could be monitored electronically. This enables estimation to be rapid, precise, reproducible and continuous in nature.

4.6.4.1. Electrochemical sensors

Electrochemical sensors are subdivided into either amperometric, potentiometric or conductometric types. In the amperometric category, an enzyme is typically coupled to an amperometric electrode and as the enzyme reacts with the substrate, a current is produced that is correlated to the analyte concentration.

There are four common ways that an amperometric device could be constructed.

a) An oxygen consuming enzyme is immobilized on a platinum electrode where the reduction of oxygen produces a current that is inversely proportional to the analyte concentration.

b) An alternate approach is to provide for direct or mediated electron transfer from the electrode to the enzyme, thus eliminating the oxygen consumption at the electrode.

c) Utilizing an enzyme directly immobilized on to a polarized anode to produce hydrogen peroxide based sensors is generally better than oxygen sensing systems, but the selectivity is usually poorer.

d) Oxidizing the analyte with a dehydrogenase enzyme to produce a concomitant reduction of NAD^+ to NADH.

4.6.4.2. Potentiometric sensors

Potentiometric sensors utilize either an immobilized enzyme on the surface of a glass pH electrode or they are based on the production or consumption of protons by the enzyme which could be measured by the electrode. Measurements are usually done in the 'zero current' mode for both liquid and gaseous configurations. One of the major limitations of the potentiometric approach observed is activity of the enzyme sensitive to pH, ammonia, carbon dioxide, or other analytes endogenous to the sample volume.

Miniaturization of potentiometric biosensors is possible with ion-selective field effect transistors (ISFETs). Hundreds of sensors configurations have been proposed and developed for a wide variety of applications such as chiral amine salt detection, enzyme inhibitors of acetyl choline esterase, anionic surfactants like sodium dodecyl sulfate and dodecyltrimethyl ammonium bromide, concentrations in pharmaceutical preparations for cationic anesthetics such as procaine, tetracaine and lidocaine. Sensors for cardiovascular applications have also been developed. The intramyocardial pH is monitored by an ISFET biosensor during human open-heart surgery.

4.6.4.3. Thermal and mass calorimetric biosensor

The heat which is generated during enzyme/substrate reactions are used. Changes in solution temperature caused by the enzyme/substrate reactions are measured using a thermistor or transistor and compared to a sensor with no enzyme to determine the analyte concentration. Calorimetric microsensors have been manufactured for detection of cholesterol in blood serum based on the enzymatically produced heat of oxidation and decomposition. Industrial applications are possible for monitoring sugars and amino acids in biotechnology based processes and determination of water content in foods like jelly, chicken and fish. Femtogram levels of drug vapors have been detected with SAW resonators for forensic use and sub-nanograme amounts of particulates are detectable as a function of temperature and pressure. In liquid based systems, piezoelectric mass sensors based on AT-cut shear mode quartz crystals have been used as miniature viscometers. The system has successfully been used for the study of interfacial processes.

4.6.4.4. Optical biosensor

This is another version of biosensor which is a small device along with its measuring instrument, uses optical principles quantitatively to convert chemical or biochemical concentrations or activities into electrical signals. This type of sensor often incorporates biological molecules such as antibodies and enzymes as transducing elements.

The application of photometric assay techniques such as fluorescence, absorbance, chemiluminescence, internal reflection spectroscopy, etc. to biosensing has been adopted. Optical fibbers or light pipes are usually employed in photometric systems because of the added flexibility since the transducer element can be separated from the actual measuring instrument by relatively large distances with virtually no losses in sensitivity or selectivity. Optical based biosensors have many advantages over electrical based sensor. The biocatalyst or bioreceptor does not have to be in intimate contact with the optical fiber which allows for a wider range of non-invasive sensor configurations. Optical fibers permit the scientist to bring the spectrometer to the sample and apply many of the spectroscopic techniques on a sample volume of few microliters. The interference from electrical noise does not occur in optical based biosensors.

NIR (near I.R) spectroscopy has also been shown to be a valuable tool for real-time process control when combined with fiber optic probes or on-line flow-through cells. Diffuse reflected and **transmissive IR absorption measurements** have been simultaneously applied to blood serum analysis to measure blood analyte concentrations such as glucose. *In vivo* oxyhemoglobin measurements were first made using NIR reflection spectroscopy in conjunction with balloon catheters. ATR spectroscopy and IR spectroscopy were used in developing a biosensor based on the immobilization of enzymes on a chalcogenide optical fiber. NIR Raman spectroscopy proved to be effective as a medical diagnostic tool for identifying silicone gel materials in biopsy specimen taken from women who possess leaking breast implants. A personnel vapor detector badge has been developed for detecting the accumulated exposure to benzene vapor using small sections of optical fibers coated with a membrane that adsorbs ambient benzene vapor. After exposure, the badge is passed into a FT-IR spectrometer for quantitation thus enables estimation of degree of exposure.

An application of optical fiber sensing that has already become a commercial reality is in the area of blood gas monitoring. Combining three optical fibbers and a thermocouple with an appropriate gas sensing dyes produced a systems that accurately measures *in vivo* concentration of pH, pCO_2 and pO_2 for use in critical care and surgical monitoring. Respiratory gas measurements for the volatile anesthetic halothene were possible using the absorbance of UV radiation at 230 nm as measured by the change in fluorescence of a polymer film. Optical fibbers have also been applied to immunoassay systems.

One of the most incteresting application of optical biosensors is to combine bacterial magnitite with a chromophoric system to measure patient's blood glucose level through a colur develop(Fig. 4.12). Briefly, the glucose oxidase is immobilized on to bacterial magnetite which act as a reaction phase. The levels of glucose (in the range of 0.56 - 22 mM) are linearly proportional to the quantity of H_2O_2 produced, which moves through the inner membranes and alter the colour of chromphore, o-dianisidine. The intensity of colour is proportional to the quantity of glucose which is calculated ultimatly.

4.6.4.5. Acoustic biosensors

The piezoelectric devices have been formed to exhibit sensitivity towards frequency of interactions which pertain to surface mass. Principally, piezoelectric device based on acoustic principle that essentially relay on establishing vibrational wave in material i.e., under the influence of alternative current voltage apply through a electrode coated on its surface depending on the characteristics of acoustic waves which depend on the structure of device in terms they are known as quartz micro valence Saw(surface acoustic wave) lamb wave or acoustic plate based devices. When antibodies are coated on to the surfaces resulting constructs could selectively pick-up the load of complementary antigens. The resultant increment in the surface mass loading decrease the vibrational frequency which could be quantify as and has found to be proportional to the mass.

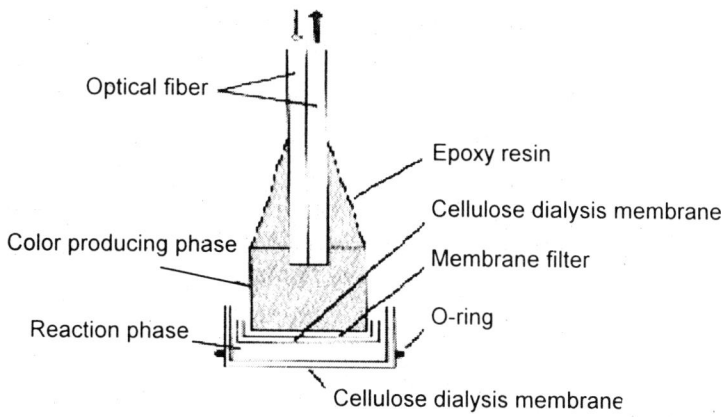

Fig. 4.12 : Optical fiber biosensor

4.6.4.6. Surface plasmon

Surface plasmon is a quasi-free electron cloud which is prepared by coating the core with a thin layer of silver approximately 600 A° thick. **Surface plasmon resonance** is used to measure concentration of sulfamethazine in bovine milk with standard digestion as low as 2.2%. It has also been used for kinetic analysis of low molecular weight compounds and (<5000Da.) by immobilizing receptors to the sensor surface. Kinetic measurements with an optical fiber sensor for the IgG anti-tetanus antibody gave approximately a 10 fold difference in the dissociation rate constant when compared with affinity constants determined by conventional solid phase enzyme immunoassays.

Biosensors are applied successfully in various fields. They replaced the existing inconvenient bioassays. It can be used for the monitoring of pollutants in water, monitoring of fermentation products and cell cultures, estimation of the concentration of various ions. NIR can be used as an in-process quality control tool for pharmaceuticals to measure particle size, moisture content, identity and quantitation of blends of polyacohols, celluloses and thickening agents. The polymer films and monolayers of metals can be analyzed by applying polarization modulation FTIR to the reflection spectra from the films. These instruments are used in the pharmaceutical manufacturing area where continuous monitoring of the gaseous environment is significant for ensuring good quality control and safety during production.

In manufacture of temperature-sensitive foods and pharmaceuticals for on-line process monitoring of the product sometimes biosensors are needed. A commercially available thermal profiler is able to make continuous on-line measurements of product temperatures in a non-conductive fashion based on IR sensor technology. Thin polymeric films and monolayers of metals can be analyzed by applying polarization modulation FTIR to the reflection spectra from the films.

Non-invasive sensors can be very powerful tools in pharmacokinetic and toxicokinetic studies. By using a NIR based finger region monitoring system in combination with an indocyanin green tracer, human clinical research has shown that the plasma disappearance rate and the blood retention ratio of a drug substance can be correlated with different liver diseases i.e., chronic liver disease, cirrhosis, chronic hepatitis, hepatocellular carcinoma. Cerebral hemodynamics were measured non-invasively in human adults during cerebral angiography using infrared tracer indocyanin green. Blood alcohol levels have been found to correlate well with the concentration of ethanol in vapour densified above the lacrimal fluid in the eye.

A paramagnetic oxygen sensor in combination with an infrared carbon dioxide sensor monitors oxygen consumption for patients with bacterial infections. Using pulse oximetry a non-invasive measurement can be made to get the informations regarding blood oxygen. This method is based on variations in the light transmission through the skin. An *in-vitro* testing procedure for assessing ocular irritancy is potentially based on a light addressable silicon potentiometric sensor that can be used during the evaluation of soaps, detergents and chemicals (the common irritants).

For investigating transdermal delivery of drugs and the impact of penetration enhancers on skin permeability, a non-invasive technique based on attenuated total reflection infrared spectroscopy can be used. The biosensors have some advantages which make them very useful in the field of biotechnology. With the help of biosensors, very low concentrations of biological substances (even about 10^{15} m) can be measured. It makes a wide range of sensitive and selective analysis to be possible. Continuous real-time assay can be performed with the help of biosensors. The major advantage of biosensor is its computer-compatibility, so that it can be used in adjunction with the computers.

Immobilization technology allows reuse of costly biological molecules as well as allows to bring about an analytical apparatus which is simple with precision. Enzymes are by far the most commonly used biological components in biosensor. Oxido-reductases and amperometric electrodes are the best combination, since an enzymatic reaction with substrates is easily and sensitively measured by electrochemical means.

Various methods have been described for enzyme or protein immobilization which can be used for biosensors. In general, biosensors using physical adsorption, chemical coupling and electropolymerization are evolved. Some of immobilized enzymes are used for the on-line determination in fermentation of cells, for example, determination of lactate and pyruvate concentrations in supernatants, using co-immobilized lactate dehydrogenase, glutamate dehydrogenase, and NAD and glutamate as a reagent. The evolved concentration of ammonium ions is measured, with the help of a biosensor. Following scheme represents the principle of the glutamate biosensor.

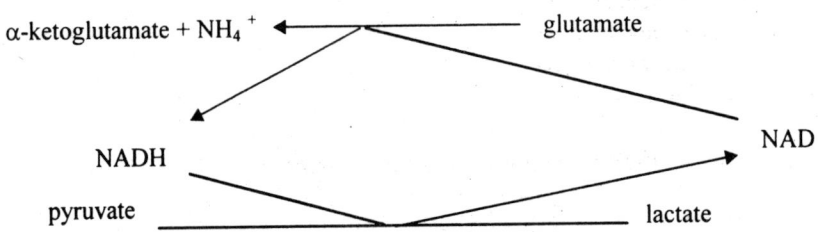

4.6.4.7. Glucose sensor

The determination of glucose is important for the process control pertaining to many nutrients metabolism. Assimilation of glucose by microorganisms can be determined by an oxygen electrode because respiration activity increases after assimilation of organic compounds. Therefore, it is possible to construct a microbial electrode sensor for glucose using immobilized whole cells which utilize mainly glucose and an oxygen electrode. A microbial electrode consisting of immobilized whole cells of *Pseudomonas fluorescens* and an oxygen electrode was developed for the determination of glucose. Furthermore, the microbial sensor was applied for continuous determination of glucose in molasses.

The typical membrane electrode is consisted of bacterial membranes and an oxygen electrode (Fig. 4.13). The bacterial membrane remains in direct contact with the oxygen electrode and is tightly secured with the help of rubber rings.

The microbial sensor is inserted into a sample solution and the sample solution is saturated with dissolved oxygen and stirred magnetically. The system has temperature control, maintained at $30.0 \pm 0.5°C$. The current is measured with the help of a milliammeter whereas signal is magnified and recorded.

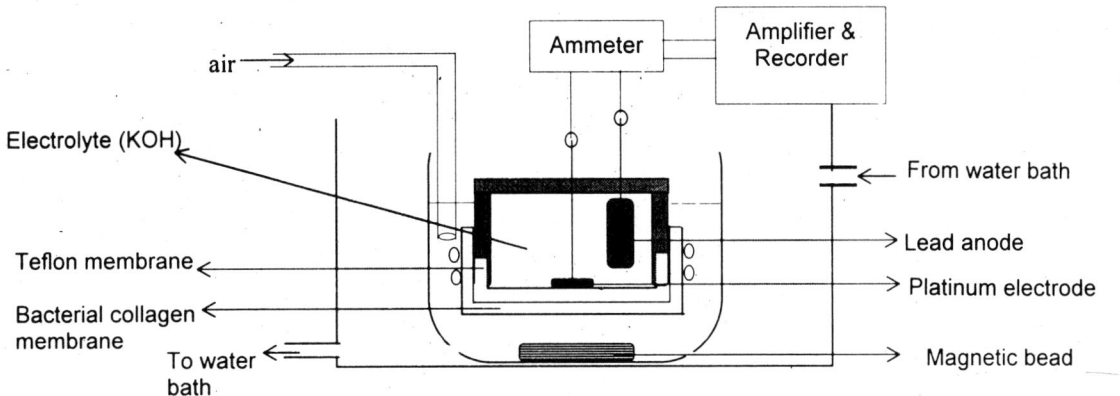

Fig. 4.13 : Membrane biosensor for glucose determination

4.7. APPLICATION OF IMMUNOADSORPTION TECHNIQUE

Immobilization with its enormous application has spread deep into medical research wherein it is of prime importance. Allergic diseases have caused certain concern, as a sizable population is suffering due to them. This made researchers to work on methods to diagnose and treat allergic diseases. Immunoglobulin E (IgE) has been found to play an important role in pathogenicity of type I hypersensitivity reactions. This can be cited with the example of production of both "allergen-specific" and "non-specific" IgE in atopic diseases such as asthma and dermatitis. Newer, biotechnological approaches have been devised for the diagnosis and treatment of IgE-mediated allergic diseases. These approaches are based on use of monoclonal antibodies (MBAs) to key components of IgE-system and recombinant analogs of components themselves (Fig. 4.14). An apheresis system principally houses monoclonal antibodies in its elution chamber could effectively sequester and remove IgE from blood when used as an extracorporeal immunoadsorptive system. The IgE serum load has been found to reduce significantly well below near normal (Fig. 4.15).

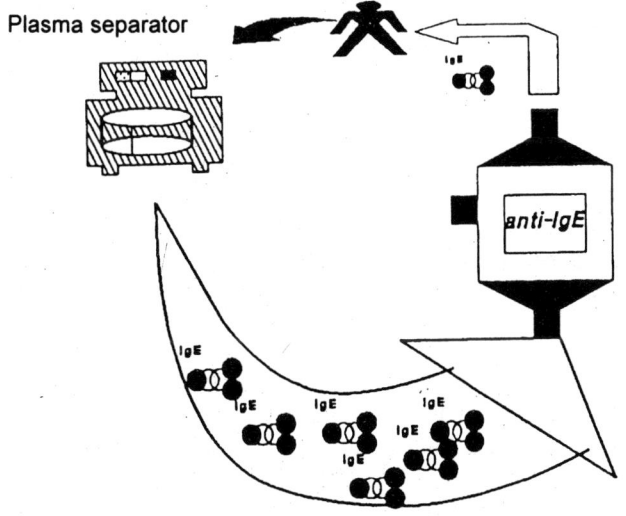

Fig. 4.14 : IgE apheresis by immunoadsorption

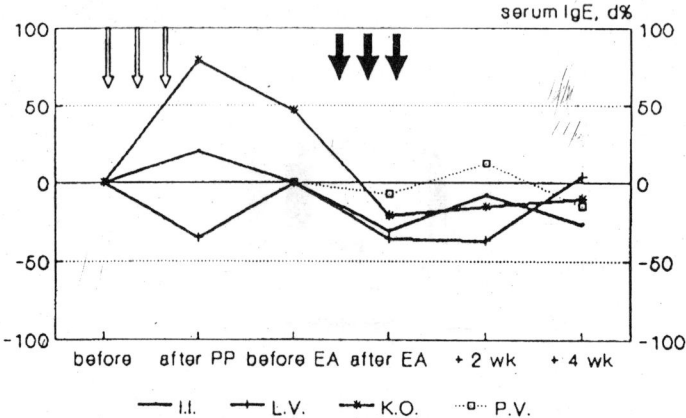

Fig. 4.15 : Clinical IgE apheresis; serum IgE levels.

Using immobilization technique measurements of IgE system as a component into clinical trials for **IgE apheresis** (EA) in atopic asthma, was possible due to the elaboration of **extracorporeal plasmaimmunoadsorption (EPIA) technique** using the principle of affinity chromatography. Clinical immunoadsorbent (IA) has been prepared from MBAs against IgE and their subsequent immobilization on a agarose gel activated by cyanogen bromide.

Monoclonal antibodies are produced against IgE using conventional hybridoma technique. However, to ensure epitope specificity immunochemical sorting is included as one of the step. The later is based on anti-IgE fragmentation, and chemical synthesis or cloning of domains. The specific antibodies effectively sequester and retain IgE and lend effluxed blood free of them suitable for perfusion.

DNA can be immobilized onto a polymer support and it can be potentially used as an immunoadsorbent for the therapy of systemic lupus erythematous for selective removal anti-DNA antibody by extracorporeal immunoadsorption. In the case of albumin coated artificial cells, the albumin on the surface of the acrylic acid (AAC) could also be used to remove antibodies to albumin from the circulating blood of animals. The synthetic immunosorbent is available for the removal of antibodies of blood groups. By incorporating the principle of artificial cells with an albumin collodion coating on the surface, the adverse effects on platelet elimination and particulate borne embolism are eliminated.

4.7.1. Immobilized enzyme based immunoassay

Immobilization technique has played a vital role in detection of microorganisms responsible for a particular disease. Enzyme immunoassay **(EIA)** a highly sensitive method developed for detection of microorganisms in food was first reported. The method involves a set of procedures which leads to quantitative estimation of the antigen present. The main step involved in the procedure is the antigen-antibody enzyme reaction and the detection of this complex. Initially, the method was cumbersome for the reason that the steps involved in the method were time consuming and involved difficulty in separation from one step to the other. To overcome such difficulties, a newer method which is the modification of EIA has been developed. The method, namely enzyme linked immunosorbent assay (ELISA) involves immobilization of antigen on a solid matrix (glass, membrane filter or polystyrene). **Enzyme-linked immunosorbent assay (ELISA)** is the latest technique available for detection of either antigen or antibody. The technique is widely acclaimed for its cheap cost and safety involved in it. The technique involves immobilization of antigen (indirect ELISA) or antibody (sandwich ELISA) onto a microliter well (plate). The excess antigen or antibody used for coating is washed off and counter antibody linked with an enzyme is added and allowed to react with the immobilized antigen or antibody, a substrate specific for the enzyme is then added and the color produced is used as a measure. For further details refer chapter 12.

Activated Horseradish peroxidase (HRP) conjugate can be used for ELISA, immunoblotting or histochemical applications. The principle, involved in this method is depicted in figure 4.16. Briefly amines residues are more abundant than sufhydryl residues on proteins (Ab) This means more available sites for attachment compared to maleimide chemical coupling. These amines are conjugated with activated sugar residues present on HRP.

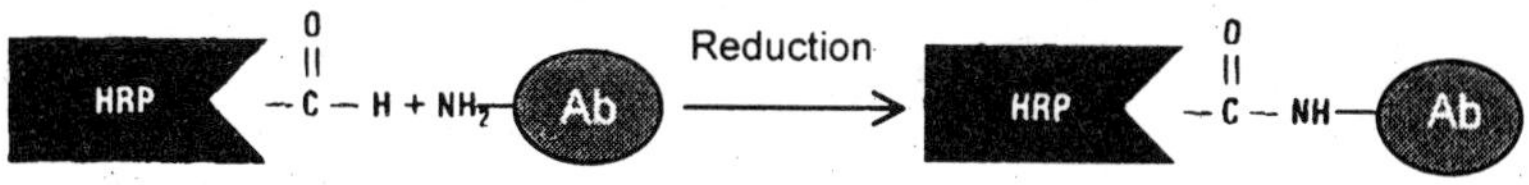

Fig. 4.16 : Active aldehyde reaction scheme.

EZ-link plus activated peroxidase kits are available commercially from pierce products, USA.

The cost of many analytical enzymes may lead to immobilization being appreciated as a sensible option for reducing the cost of analysis. However, the cost of equipment and manpower is the dominant factor and it is only where immobilized enzymes can be used is a fully automated system. A further limitation is the fact that, since they depend on biomolecules, these systems cannot be sterilized, therefore much of their present use is still awaited for rapid *in-vivo* analysis.

4.7.2. Immobilized haptens as immunopurifier

Affinity chromatography, which is used extensively for the purification of biological molecules, takes the advantage of the binding interactions that occur on the surface of a protein. There are number of different immobilization supports available, which could couple to a variety of different functional groups. These supports are useful for immobilization of the molecules like protein, antigen, antibody or nucleic acid. Among, two activated supports are particularly well suited for immobilizing antigens to affinity purifying antibodies. The solid phase matrices are reactive towards a functional group on the antigen such as a primary amine($-NH_2$) or a sulfhydryl (-SH) group (Fig. 4.17 & 4.18). The resulting covalent linkage immobilize the antigen permanently to the support. Antibodies recognizing the immobilized antigen or hapten can be purified from serum or ascetics.

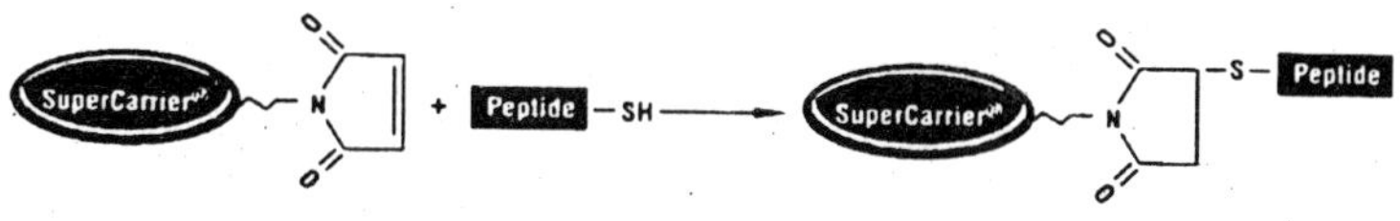

Fig. 4.17 : Hapten conjugation to melamine activated carrier.

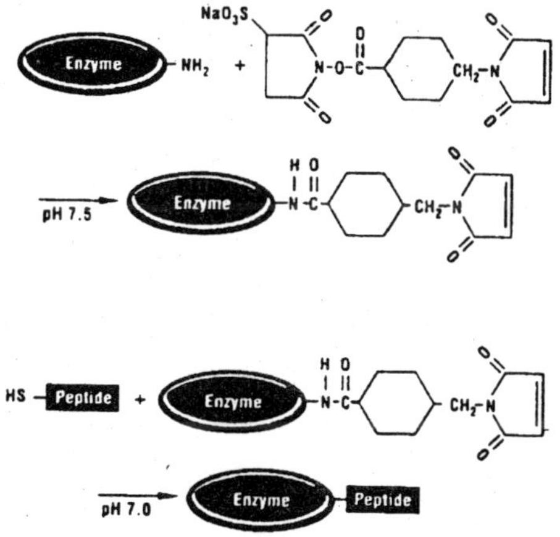

Fig. 4.18 : Hapten-carrier conjugation.

4.7.3. Immobilized protein A/G in IgM purification

Protein A and G are native and recombinant proteins of microbial origin. They have specific ability to bind to the Fc portion of mammalian immunoglobulin molecules. Immuno Pure® and Ultralink™ are commercially available forms for purification of specific antibody. The products are essentially based on immobilization principle where protein(s) are covalently coupled or entrapped in a gel or some biosupport. The protein and antibody interaction magnitude and degree of interaction varies. Table 4.4 enlists some affinity supports for different antibodies. Protein A and recombinant protein G are generally immobilized on agarose or sephadex via covalent linking and used as affinity chromatography medium a typical immobilized protein complex or conjugation is schematically depicted in figure 4.19.

Easy-to-use affinity matrix has been developed for purification of IgM fraction. The matrix based on an immobilized mannan binding protein (MSP) support, is most effective for purifying mouse IgM from ascites. Mannan binding protein is usually immobilized on agarose bead and used in affinity chromatography.

4.7.4. Radioallergosorbent test (Rast)

The Rast abbreviated test is based on absorption of IgE antibody by immobilized antigens and subsequently the degree of binding is quantified determined. For immobilization of antigen covalent coupling method(s) are employed where insoluble support i.e., cellulose or activated sepharose is used as solid support (Fig. 4.20).

Table 4.4 : Binding capacity of immunoglobulin proteins

Antibody	Protein A	Protein G	Protein A/G
Human IgG	s	s	s
Mouse IgG	s	s	s
Rabbit IgG	s	s	s
Goat IgG	w	s	s
Rat IgG	w	m	m
Sheep IgG	w	s	s
Cow IgG	w	s	s
Guinea Pig IgG	s	w	s
Hamster IgG	m	-	-
Pig IgG	s	w	s
Horse IgG	w	s	s
Donkey IgG	m	s	s
Dog IgG	s	w	s
Cat IgG	s	w	s
Monkey IgG (Rhesus)	s	s	s
Chicken IgG	nb	nb	nb
Human IgM	w	nb	w
Human IgE	m	nb	m
Human IgD	nb	nb	w
Human IgA	w	nb	m
Human IgG1	s	s	s
Human IgG2	s	s	s
Human IgG3	w	s	s
Human IgG4	s	s	s

w- weak binding, m - medium binding, s- strong binding, nb - no binding, - information not available.

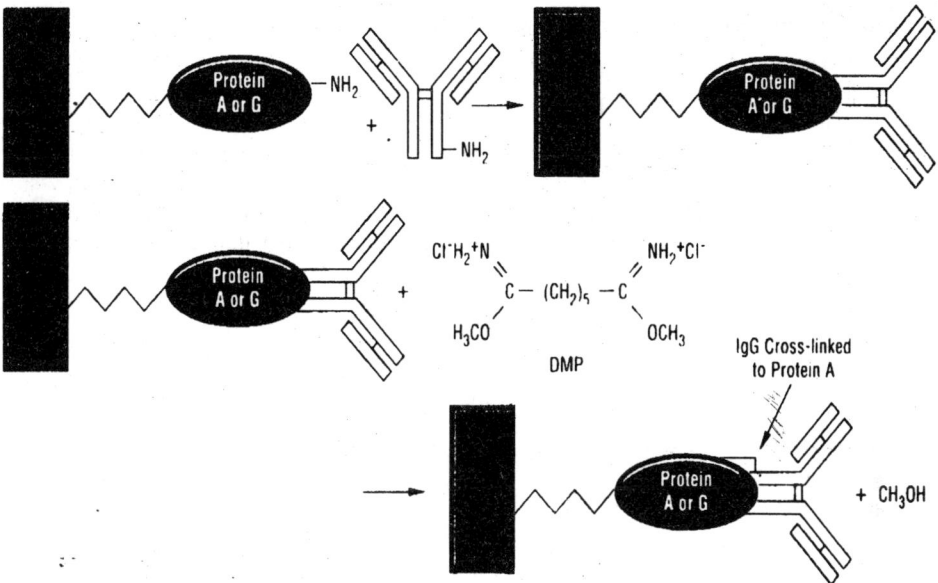

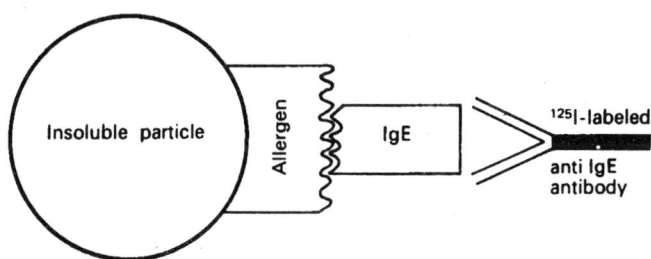

Fig. 4.20 : Radioallergosorbent test

4.8. THERAPEUTIC APPLICATIONS

The clinical uses of enzymes are still limited by a number of factors, which are:

a) availability of enzymes at site of interest is generally very poor unless, the high therapeutic dose is administered; which is often undesirable;

b) the sensitivity of enzymes to the action of various natural inhibitors;

c) the immunogenicity of many enzymes;

d) the destruction of the enzymes under the action of endogenous protease;

e) *in-vivo* inactivation and their fast clearance considerably increases the consumption of the enzyme in the course of treatment, and

f) the high cost and poor availability of pure enzymes.

In order to resolve the above listed problems, the immobilization of enzymes can be used to a great extent. Such a technique makes it possible to decrease the total dose of enzyme used, could prolong enzymatic activity at the site of interest, and at the same time could reduce undesirable side effects.

Preparation of immobilized enzymes for example fibrinolysis, streptokinase, urokinase in microgranules of sephadex can be effectively used for the treatment of thromboses, and thromboemboli of any vessels (for example atherosclerosis of coronary arteries, which is often the cause of myocardial infarction) that is accessible with the help of modern methods of catheterization.

An *in-vivo* experimental result demonstrated that enzymes bound to polysaccharides acquire many useful properties, stability against autolysis, thermostability and the action of protease. One of the most significant results of enzyme binding to natural polysaccharide is the considerable increase in the time of immobilized enzyme circulation in blood as compared to free enzyme. Thus, α-amylase and catalase bound to activated dextran demonstrated a very slow clearance from the circulation in an experiment conducted on rats. Similar, results have also been observed with immobilized trypsin, chymotrypsin, ribonuclease, catalase and α- and β-amylase.

Covalent bonding of carboxypeptidase G and arginase to soluble dextran noticeably increases the duration of enzyme circulation in the blood in healthy mice and mice with inoculated tumors. Similar results were noted with enzymes catalase, trypsin and urease which were covalently bound to PEG. Immobilized lysosomal hydrolase, β-D-N-acetyl hexosaminidase, are reported to be useful in the therapy of Tay-sachs disease.

In an other experiment conducted in animals, the immobilized kallikrein was reported to retain the ability to decrease the blood pressure. A most impressive study involved the use of glucocerebrosidase accumulated in the cells of the RES as a result of a deficiency of the corresponding lysosomal enzyme. Attentions have also been drawn as an attempt to treat a patient having type II glycogenesis caused by the deposition of glycogen due to a lysosomal aminoglucosidase deficiency.

1. A number of inborn human metabolic disorders, are related to the absence of a particular enzyme normally present in the body. For example, phenylketonuria, a disease leading to mental retardation, is thought to be caused by deficiency in the enzyme which leads conversion of phenylalanine into tyrosine. The latest therapy for this is encapsulative isolation of the enzyme within a microcapsule, fiber or gel. While membrane contained enzymes are not susceptible to antibody attack, protein build-up on bio-membrane surfaces adds mass-transfer resistance and causes decreasing efficiency of substrate utilization.

2. A variant of this strategy has led to the construction of a compact artificial kidney. In this device, urease and an adsorbent resin or charcoal are encapsulated together, so that ammonia produced by decomposition of urea is adsorbed within the microcapsule.

$$\text{Urea} \xrightarrow{\text{Diffusion into microcapsules}} \text{Urea} \xrightarrow{\text{Urease}} HCO_3^- + NH_4^+ \xrightarrow{\text{Adsorption on charcoal}}$$

3. Cortisol, a useful drug in arthritis treatment, can be made from a precursor 11-deoxycortisol using in a column of immobilized 11-β-hydroxylase, following which cotrisol can be converted into prednisolone by immobilized Δ^1 dehydrogenase (Scheme 1) in a subsequent packed-bed reactor.

4.8.1. Immobilization based novel drug delivery systems

4.8.1.1. Urea-urease modulated system

Urea-urease modulated system suggests the interesting possibility of using immobilized enzymes to alter local pH and consequently to change the pH sensitive polymer erosion rates. Urease converts urea to NH_4HCO_3 and NH_4OH and this causes an increase in pH. To utilize this reaction, a polymer whose erosion rate increases with pH is selected. A partially esterified copolymer of methylvinyl ether and maleic anhydride undergoes surface erosion at an erosion rate that is extraordinarily sensitive to small increase in external pH. The polymer dissolves by ionization of the carboxylic acid group as shown below and results in release of incorporated therapeutic agent.

Insoluble   Soluble

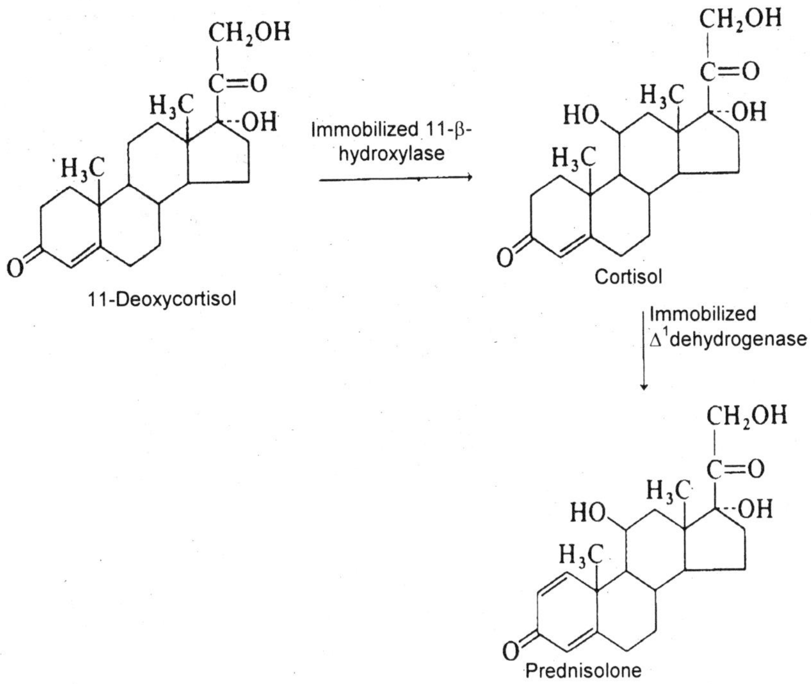

Scheme 1 : Enzymatic conversion of 11-deoxycortisol to prednisolone

The figure 4.21 shows the release of hydrocortisone from thin disks of the n-butyl half ester containing physically dispersed drug, as a function of pH and thus pH sensitivity of the polymer. Application of these systems as an enzyme-mediated self-regulated drug delivery system can be exemplified by the dispersion of hydrocortisone in a hexyl half ester copolymer and the dispersion surrounded by a hydrogel containing urease immobilized by glutaraldehyde cross linkinging. The device has no therapeutic relevance, as it depends strongly on presence and concentration of external urea for drug release, however it establishes the feasibility of this concept.

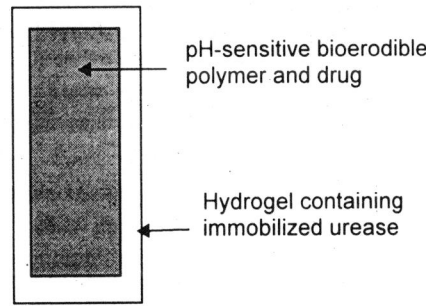

pH-sensitive bioerodible polymer and drug

Hydrogel containing immobilized urease

Fig. 4.21 : Pulsed and self regulatory drug delivery

4.8.1.2. Glucose oxidase-glucose modulated system

The search for a delivery system to replace parenteral administration of insulin by periodic injections has led to the development of an erodible polymeric system containing insulin which is modulated by glucose-glucose oxidase reaction (Fig. 4.22).

In this system a polymer is selected which shows increased erosion rates with decreasing pH. The pH is lowered by the production of gluconic acid from glucose. The conversion is catalyzed by the enzyme glucose oxidase. Poly (ortho esters), prepared by the reaction between polyols and the diketene acetal. 3,9 bis (ethyldiene 2,4,8,10-tetraoxaspiro [5,5] undecane) are ideal polymers for this system because of the pH sensitive linkage in the polymer back bone. Crosslinked poly (ortho esters) are produced by first preparing a ketene acetal-terminated prepolymer that is a viscous liquid at room temperature and then its cross linking with a triol. A therapeutic agent can be mixed into the prepolymer at room temperature and the mixture can be cross linked at temperatures that can be as low as 40°C; mild conditions being important for therapeutic agents (like insulin) which are protein.

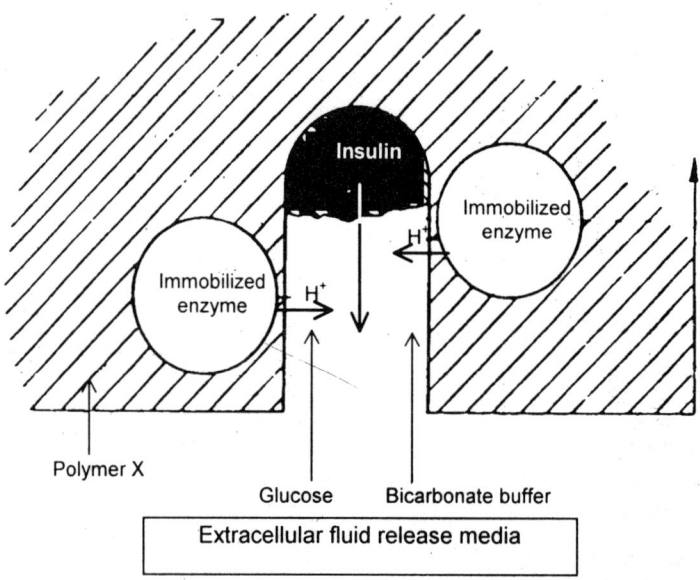

Fig. 4.22 : Schematic representation of the one dimentsional model for the release of insulin from the polymeric systems.

Acid sensitivity of these polymers can be studied by incorporating a marker molecule such as p-nitroacetanilide in the polymer and observing its release at different pH. Magnitude of change and response times in the process is not adequate. A self regulated insulin delivery system should respond within time not more than 15 minutes.

In order to increase the pH sensitivity of the system polymers prepared by using n-alkyl diethanolamines and triethanolamines were prepared. The acid sensitivities of polymers prepared from N-N-butyldiethanolamines and from N-methyldiethylanolamines can be observed. It has been observed that changing size of alkyl group on the amino portion of the diol has a significant effect on both degree of acid sensitivity and the pH range where maximum sensitivity occurs. The pH sensitivity of the polymer can be explained by swelling of the polymers induced by protonation of the tertiary amines in the polymer back bone. The observed effect of N-alkyl group size is consistent with decreased hydrophilicity as the size of N-alkyl group increases and to a lesser extent by changes in the pKa values. Polymers of varying degrees of cross-linking and consequently varying degrees of swelling have been prepared by varying the ratio of triol cross-linker and the bifunctional ketene acetal-terminated prepolymer.

4.8.1.3.. *Triggered drug delivery system*

Triggered drug delivery systems utilize a device containing the active agent placed subdermally or in other appropriate body sites where it remains passive until a specific molecule appears in tissues surrounding the device. This molecule triggers the programmed release of therapeutic agent from the device. Device utilizes highly selective sensing mechanisms to recognize the specific trigger molecule in a complex mixture of physiological fluid. Antibodies to the trigger molecule provide such high selectivity. Such triggered device may have many potential applications.

A device containing narcotic antagonist naltrexone can be implanted to opiate addicts undergoing rehabilitation, after the withdrawal therapy. The device is so designed that the release is triggered by morphine. Such device remains passive as long as the individual refrains from heroin and naltrexone is released upon heroin intake, morphine is produced as a result of metabolism and this triggers the release of naltrexone in amounts sufficient to replace morphine from its receptors and thus neutralizes the pleasurable heroin induced effect.

In designing such a device, a hapten (morphine in this case), is covalently attached to the enzyme, close to its active site, and the hapten is complexed with its antibody. Antibody being a very large molecule, sterically hinders access of enzyme substrate to the enzyme active site thus rendering the enzyme inactive. In the presence of free hapten, the complex dissociates to form separate antibody hapten complex and a substrate enzyme complex leading to enzyme action. This process has been illustrated in figure 4.23A. Figure 4.23B shows the design of a bioerodible polymeric device.

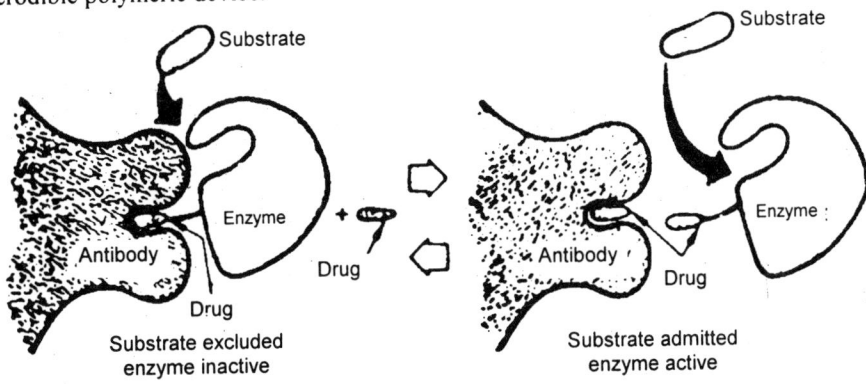

Fig. 4.23A : Reversible enzyme inactivation by hapten-antibody interactions

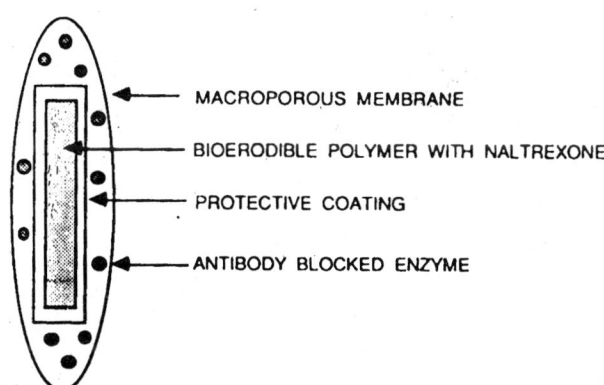

Fig. 4.23B : Schematic representation of triggered drug delivery device

This device contains a pH sensitive polymer capable of releasing naltrexone by an erosion controlled process at the physiological pH 7.4 but is stable at a lower pH. The polymer is surrounded by an enzyme degradable acidic hydrogel with an environment having a pH low enough so that no erosion and drug release takes place. This device also contains reversibly inactivated enzyme that in its activated state is capable of degrading the hydrogel. This enzyme is activated when morphine appears in the tissues surrounding the device and the enzyme then removes the protective hydrogel. Activated device releases an antigenic enzyme and antibody, so it is necessary that the components of the device are enclosed to permit passage of the opiate and naltrexone but which excludes the much larger molecules of enzyme and antibody.

4.8.2. Immobilization of artificial cell as artificial organs

An artificial cell is consisted of a spherical ultra-thin semipermeable membrane of cellular dimension, enveloping biologically active material. In this artificial cell system, the semipermeable membrane prevents external proteins, antibodies or cells from entering, but external permanent molecules can equilibrate rapidly to come in contact with enclosed materials. The artificial cellular units could be developed using various perm-selective membranes preferably based on biodegradable polymers. Some polymers of synthetic and of biological origins have been identified for their use and presented diagramatically in figure 4.24A. Artificial cells are being used as detoxifiers, artificial kidney, artificial liver, immunosorbents, blood substitutes and in other areas.

Almost any biologically active material such as enzymes, proteins can be enclosed within artificial cells. Magnetic materials have also been included within artificial cells to allow external magnetic fields to direct the movements of the artificial cells. Other materials which can be incorporated include radioisotope labeled enzymes, proteins, antigens, antibodies, vaccines, hormones, etc. The artificial cells can be used to immobilize enzymes and proteins. The enzymes immobilized in artificial cells remain in enzyme systems in red blood cells, especially as complex multienzyme systems. The advantage is that there is no limit to the number of different enzyme systems that can be enclosed immobilized together in a single artificial cell.

Enzymes, adsorbents or other material can be incorporated together with target enzyme into the artificial cells. Using artificial cells containing activated charcoal or ion exchange resin, toxic materials can be removed. Using the principle of artificial cells, extremely compact, efficient and simple artificial organs can be designed and constructed for example blood detoxifier, artificial liver, artificial kidney and immunosorbents.

Artificial cells containing multienzyme systems are used for the sequential conversion of substrates into products and at the same time to recycle the required cofactors.

Immobilized enzymes are generally recommended in replacement therapy needed in hereditary enzyme-deficiency conditions in the form of microencapsulated enzyme as cell immobilized catalase is used to effectively replace a hereditary catalase deficiency. Artificial cells containing tyrosinase have been used in extracorporeal hemoperfusion to lower tyrosine levels in rats. The therapeutic application of artificial cells for tumor suppression are well appreciated being distinctive and of therapeutic value. Artificial cells containing tyrosinase immobilized in a carrier system have been used for hemoperfusion in galactosamine-induced fulminate hepatic failure [FHF] in rats.

4.8.3. Artificial cells immobilized enzymes and multienzymes

In the body, enzymes and proteins are mostly located in the intracellular space. These proteins carry out their functions by acting sequentially on substrates, by oozing out through the cell wall by passive transportation or by special transport mechanism. In the deficiency of them, one cannot inject in solution of enzyme(s) into the body, since, the exogenously administered enzyme(s) are considered as foreign proteins in the free form, therefore, result into hypersensitivity reactions, production of antibodies is followed by rapid removal and inactivation. Free enzymes in solution cannot be kept at the sites where the action is desired. Enzymes in free solution are not stable, especially at a body temperature of 37°C. Furthermore, multienzyme systems require the enzymes and substrates to be in closer proximity and also for cofactor recycling preferably in an intracellular environment. In order to inculcate the whole benefits of treatment, the possible use of artificial cells as a system to immobilize enzymes and proteins could be considered. Unlike, enzymes immobilized by a conventional method, enzymes immobilized in artificial cells may remain in free solution as suspended cellular units. Therefore, systems function more like enzyme systems which operate in RBC, especially similar to a complex multienzyme system. There is no limit to the class of different enzyme systems that can be enclosed in one artificial cell.

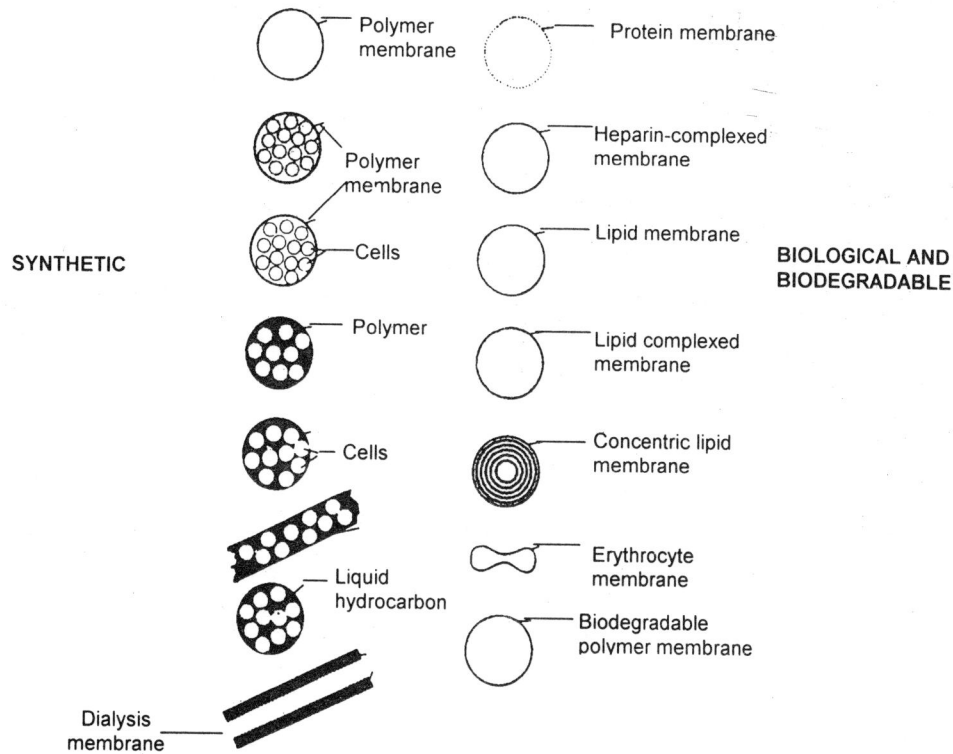

Fig. 4.24A : Artificial cells : Example of possible variations in membrane compositions and configurations.

Artificial cells containing simple enzyme systems may be obtained by selecting one of the many methods available (Fig. 4.24B), since all single enzymes tested so far can be successfully encapsulated within artificial cells.

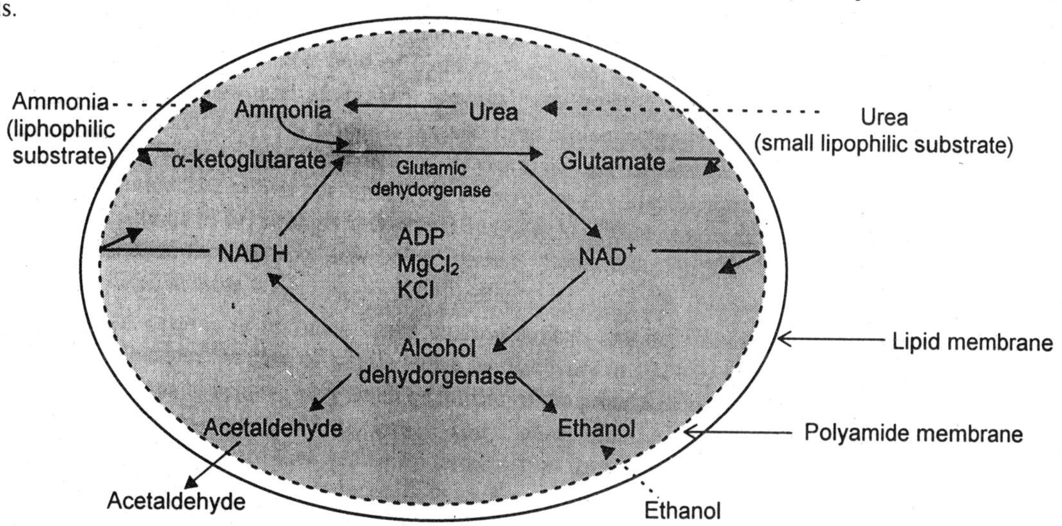

Fig. 4.24B : Representation of artificial cells containing multienzymes with cofactor recycling component

A 10 gdl^{-1} hemoglobin solution is usually present in the standard artificial cells. This simulates an intracellular environment, which is comparable to red blood cells. Thus, the enzymes enclosed in the artificial cells are cells are stabilized by the high concentration of protein(s). Similarly, multienzyme systems can also be generated. Since most metabolic functions are carried out in cells by complex multienzyme systems in coordination with cofactor. For example, artificial cells containing hexokinase and pyruvate kinase could recycle ATP for the continuous conversion of glucose into G-6-P and phosphoenol pyruvate into pyruvate; similarly, artificial cells containing alcohol dehydrogenase and maleic dehydrogenase can recycle NADH making use of NAD^+. A multienzyme system consisting of urease, glutamate dehydrogenase and glucose-6-phosphate dehydrogenase all within each artificial cell can convert urea into ammonia which then serves as substrate to $\propto$-keto glutarate which in the presence of NADPH forms an amino acid, glutamate with glucose-6-phosphate dehydrogenase to recycle the cofactor.

The above system suggests that it is feasible to prepare artificial cells containing multienzyme systems for the sequential conversion of substrate into products and at the same time to recycle the required cofactors. This principle is applicable in the conversion of waste metabolites in liver failure, renal failure or other metabolic disorders. Thus the concept opens up possibilities of management of disease related to organ failure via application of immobilized cellular unit(s).

4.8.4. Artificial Pancreas

Endocrine cells from heterogeneous sources could be enclosed within artificial cells and implanted. In this form the cells inside the artificial cells can respond to external substrate concentrations(e.g. blood glucose) and the required hormone (e.g. insulin) can be secreted into the systemic circulation. The microencapsulated rat-islet cells when implanted intraperitoneally into diabetic rats, could avoid rejection and functioned to maintain normal glucose levels in the diabetic animals.

4.8.5. Blood detoxifier

Artificial cells containing activated charcoal have been the basis for the construction of a novel detoxifier. A simple and inexpensive system uses $0.005\mu m$ thick collodion membrane coating on activated charcoal granules. An albumin coating can be applied to the collodion membrane to make the surface more blood compatible.

In coating activated charcoal with polymer membranes, the thickness, permeability are extremely important factors. One of the most effective blood detoxifiers consists of 80g of spherical petroleum-based charcoal (1mm diameter) coated by an ultra-thin collodion membrane. The principle of microencapsulation of ion exchange resin inside artificial cells can be also used, so that it prevents the ion exchange resin from adversely affecting blood cellular components. Circulating the blood from patients through these artificial cells detoxifying devices, purify it. This led us to apply detoxification based on artificial cellular detoxifier units in patients needing treatment for acute drug intoxication. The principle of working of a blood detoxifier is schematically shown in figure 4.25.

4.8.6. Artificial liver

The first partial success with an artificial liver support system was attained when a patient with grade IV hepatic coma was treated by hemoperfusion with an artificial cell detoxification device. Artificial cells containing multienzyme systems with cofactor recycling characteristics are being studied *in-vivo* for the sequential conversion of ammonia into different amino acids.

4.8.7. Artificial kidney

The blood detoxifier, consisting of artificial cells containing activated charcoal can maintain terminal renal failure as it eliminates uremic symptoms related to nausea, vomiting, fatigue, bleeding and others. But the above artificial cells containing activated charcoal fail to remove coated, electrolytes and urea. In patients who develop uremic symptoms despite standard hemodialysis treatment, the artificial cells approach can eliminate the complications of pericarditis, nausea, vomiting, peripheral neuropathy or others.

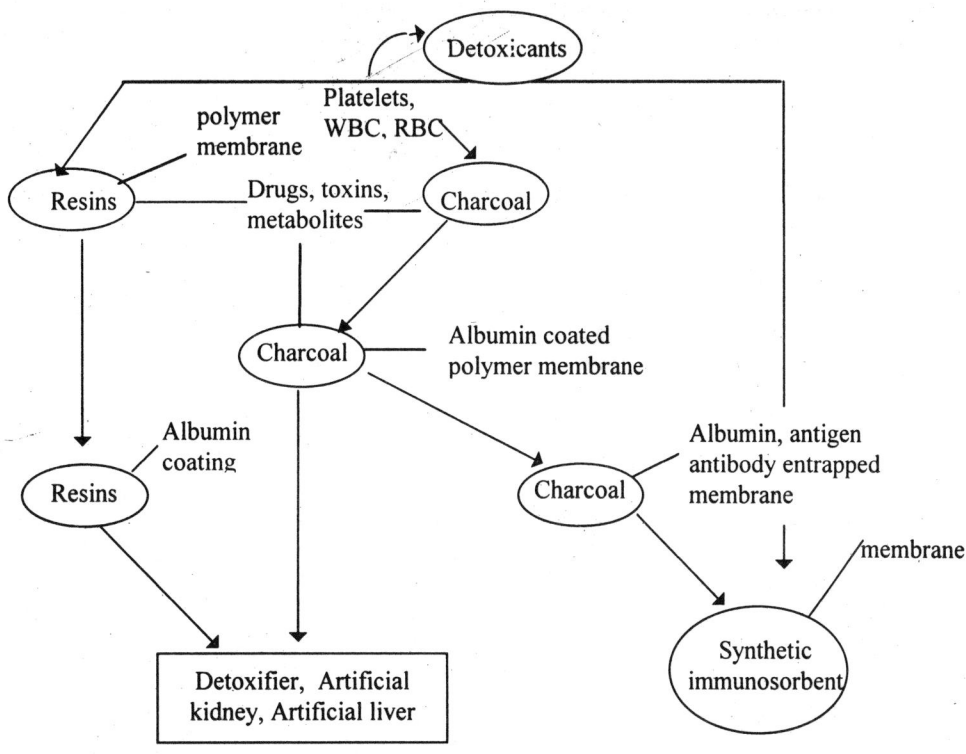

Fig. 4.25 : Development of artificial cells with adsorbents and immunosorbents.

However, the best combination is the artificial cell blood detoxifier combined in series with a small ultrafiltrator. In this way the artificial cells can remove the uremic water metabolites and toxins while the ultrafiltrator would effectively remove sodium chloride and water (Fig. 4.26). Still it may have the problem of removal of potassium, phosphate and urea. Potassium could be removed by the oral administration of potassium adsorbent, and the urea is removed by the use of artificial cells containing urease.

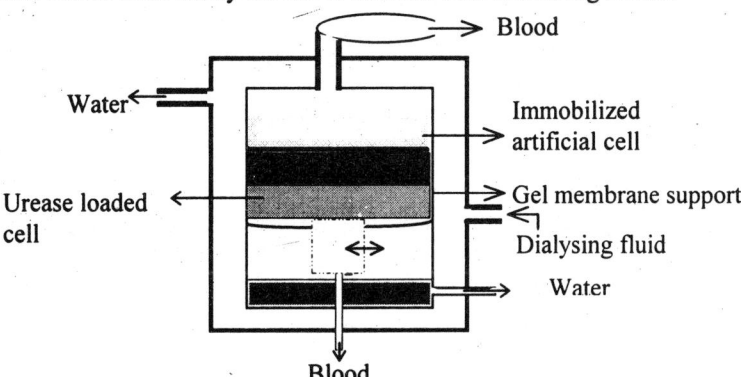

Fig. 4.26 : Schematic representation of artificial kidney.

4.8.2. Artificial Cells Used as blood substitutes (surrogates)

Artificial cells with hemoglobin and artificial cells with organic material are two systems being investigated as possible red blood cell substitutes. In the preparation of hemoglobin artificial cells, microdroplets of hemolysate solution with spherical ultra-thin membrane of cellular dimensions can be developed or by the use of cross-linking (Fig.4.27). There was no agglutination when the above two type of hemoglobin artificial cells were laced in contact with plasma even when the artificial cells were prepared using hemoglobin obtained from blood of a heterogenous sources with varied blood groups.

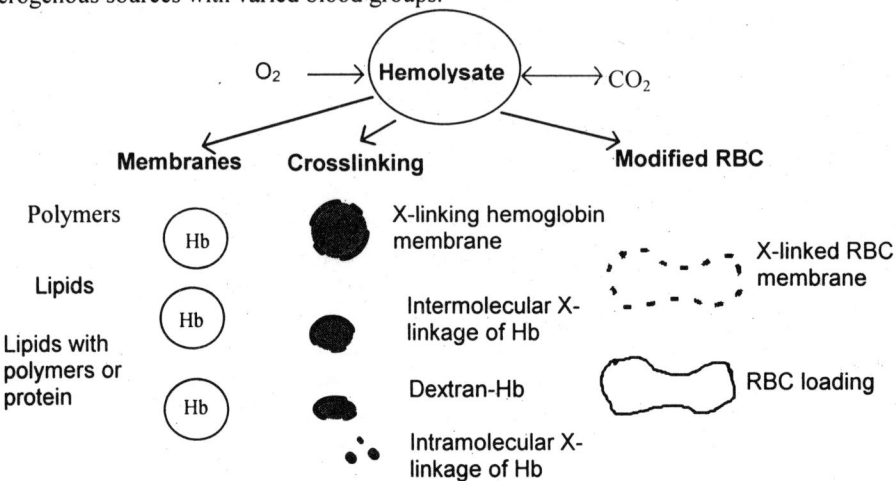

Fig. 4.27: Development of artificial red blood cells based on hemoglobin

The cross-linking hemoglobin artificial cells, each consisting of soluble poly-hemoglobin, survives significantly longer in the circulation when compared to free hemoglobin. A fine emulsion of fluororcarbon was used for the development of artificial cells based on organic material (Fig.4.28). These fine fluorocarbon emulsions were evaluated to be effective oxygen carriers. The fluorocarbon artificial cells are the first artificial cells ready for clinical trial ass a blood cell substitute. One of the advantages of hemoglobin artificial cell is the biodegradability of the hemoglobin content. Artificial cells can be prepared to fulfill a large number of potential function up to now, only comparatively simple artificial cells have been developed to a stage of actual application. Some of the classical examples of such systems are liposomes, nylon capsule, lipid nanocapsules, cross linked microsphere and aquasomes.

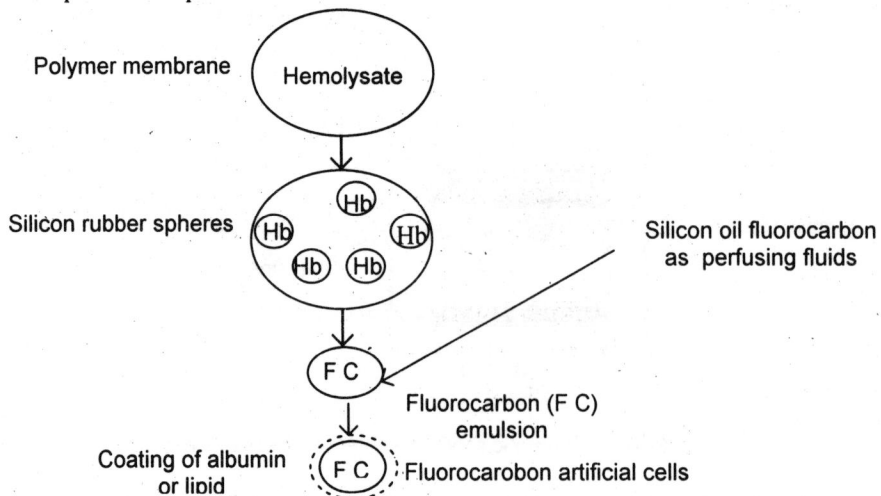

Fig. 4.28: Development of artificial blood surrogates based on microencapsulated hemolysate, in silicon rubber microsphere.

Immobilization has got a wide range of application which is well evidenced from the above discussion. To appraise the technique, another set of examples which plays an important role in gene analysis, namely gene probes and oligonucleotide probes, are discussed.

4.9. GENE PROBES

Gene probes are used to find genes of particular interest. This is done by using molecular hybridization technique, when two strands of DNA can be dissociated and reassociated *in-vitro*. Thus, one can identify the gene of interest by constructing a DNA with identical sequence which will anneal only to that particular gene but not to the rest of the DNA. Similarly, using the enzyme RNA-dependent-DNA-polymerase cDNA were synthesized from mRNA isolated from mammalian cells. Furthermore, if radioactive bases are added to the reaction, the synthesized cDNA could be used as a probe to look for complementary sequences. As the technique is versatile in gene identification and their production needing more precise technology, their long term utility was sort. At first, when the technology was introduced it was based on solution. Utilizing the latest technology, these DNA are now immobilized over nitrocellulose fibers which can act for a longer period of time.Human responses to foreign chemicals vary depending on their genetic make-up, predisposition and environmental exposures. This individual variation reflects differing degree of expression. The kind and amount of expression of these enzymes can determine whether a chemical is detoxified or activated to toxid metabolites. Using this, one can determine the gene or other biologically active system responsible for the metabolism or inactivation of the drug. One such example is the identification of specific cytochromes p-450 responsible for xenobiotic and endobiotic metabolism.

MAbs and cDNA have been used as bioprobes to identify the specific cytochrome p-450 responsible for xenobiotic and endobiotic metabolism. MBAs are specific to each epitope of p-450 and can phenotype, quantify levels of expression of individual p-450 and determine the contribution of individual p-450 forms to metabolism for reaction phenotyping. MAbs inhibitory to enzyme activity can determine the contribution of the MAb specific p-450 to the total reaction of an individual substrate in a tissue preparation such as microsomes. Inhibitory MAbs can also be added to the tissue preparation at saturating levels and inhibition can be observed. In addition to examining intertissue differences, interspecies comparisons can be made with activity inhibition experiments for different animal species.

While MAbs can be used as probes for the detection of p-450 proteins, p-450 cDNAs isolated from cDNA libraries and immobilized on a proper support can also be used as probes for the detection of mRNA transcripts of p-450 genes in different human organs and tissues and DNA fragments present in cells can be amplified by specific polymerase chain reactions (PCR).

4.10. IMMOBILIZATION AND DRUG TARGETING USING ARTIFICIAL CELLULAR SYSTEMS

Proteins, antigens and enzymes can be immobilized on the surface of artificial cellular systems, to confer specificity and cellular targetability, to make them to be long circulatory and to function as a cellular bioreactor. Immobilization can deter the contents from bio-environment vis-à-vis guide them to the proximity of target cell lines. Artificial cellular carriers investigated for immobilization and sequestration of contents as non viral vectors for drug and gene delivery include, bilayer vesicular systems including liposomes and niosomes, reconstituted viral vesicular system (virosomes), artificial viral envelopes (AVE), artificial red cells (ARC), erythrocytes (ghost and resealed), erythrosomes, endogenous carriers like lymphocytes and platelets. The traditional approach for immobilizing a biochemically active molecule in a delivery vehicle is through covalent anchoring. This is very much the case with various macromolecular vehicles, but also has been used to couple agents to the larger particulate carriers. The alternative approach, is the use of non covalent forces to promote "self assembly" of the biomolecule to the carrier. This has been exploited in liposomes, aquasomes and some complex polymeric carrier systems. For last few decades, delivery vehicles immobilized with site directing ligands have been studied for cellular targeting by presenting them to target cells, which express either cell surface antigens or cell surface receptors . In order to endow the same concept, several vector molecules have been evaluated as ligands for immobilization on the appropriate artificial cellular systems, for their drug and gene targeting potentials.

4.10.1. Bilayer vesicular systems as cellular carriers

Protein immobilization on the liposomal constructs have been studied with ligands like immunoglobulins (IgG) and their fragments Fab' or F(ab)₂, haptens, lectins, nonviral and viral spike glycoproteins, antigen presenting cells, and enzymes for their therapeutic possibilities and potentials. The targeted liposomes have been used for gene delivery, vaccine delivery, immunomodulator activity and for their potential as circulatory cellular bioreactor. Several strategies have been reported for the protein immobilization in the artificial cellular systems. Tetanus toxoid and IgG, model proteins for vaccine and targeting ligands respectively, were covalently coupled to preformed dehydration-rehydration vesicles (DRVs) to produce vesicles with surface immobilized proteins (DRV-Protein) or to preformed SUVs, which were used to generate DRVs with bound protein [(SUV-Protein)DRV]. Protein immobilization on the surface of liposome can also be achieved via carbodiimide activation in the presence of N-hydroxysulpho-succinimide. In this chapter, drug targeting potential of immobilized artificial cellular system, liposomal system in particular is presented.

4.10.1.1. Liposome appended with antibody (IgG) or their fragments and conjugates

As site directing ligands with selective receptor/antigenic site(s) on the target cell surface, is the well established approach of cellular targeting. Antitarget monoclonal antibody (MAb) immobilized via anchoring to liposomes (Immunoliposomes), specifically directed to carbohydrate containing antigens have been investigated to deliver the drugs like IUDR/ACV (Idoxyuridine/Acyclovir) in the treatment of herpes simplex virus (HSV) infections. The access of immobilized MAbs can be improved by employing immunologically active fragment Fab' or F(ab)₂, instead of complete IgG portion. It could be realized that bioprotein(s) of therapeutic values could safely administered if they are well immobilized on to an appropriate carrier equipped with site directing ligands. Furthermore, in a way ligand anchoring too, is achieved via the process of immobilization.

Recently, long circulatory high molecular weight soluble Fab aggregates of MAb have been immobilized on the surface of liposomal system and targeted to Fc/C3b receptor bearing necrotic tumor cell lines. Haptenated liposomes interact with Fc receptor bearing cells in the presence of antibody to the haptens and using this approach antitumor agents (mainly methotrexate) have been targeted to human/murine macrophages. Liposome immobilized immunotoxins have also been developed for the treatment of various tumors, the concept may be utilized for antiviral therapy. Liposomal system has also been introduced and demonstrated to function as a vector for diphtheria toxin to deter diphtheria toxin from immunoglobulins pool and destined them to the site of action. One of the future goals, as suggested by some of the authors would be the development of 'target-triggered release immunoliposomes'. These are novel derivatives of immunoliposomes evolving with a triggered release component to deliver their contents at the cellular level; and have been investigated as non viral vector for the succesful delivery of genes and antisense oligonucleotides. The constructs have been designed employing immobilization technique.

4.10.1.2. Immunoliposome : A total immobilization concept

Liposomes as an artificial cellular system can be appreciated as a vaccine carrier or as an adjuvant for vaccines, or otherwise as a carrier for vaccine adjuvants. Several strategies of vaccine delivery system relying upon immobilized cellular systems have been described, including incorporation of particulate (killed Bacillus subtilis and killed Bacillus calmette-Guerin) and soluble (tetanus toxoid) antigens in giant DRV vesicles prepared by double emulsion technique. The other strategy combines two technologies, the encapsulation of antigens within liposomes followed immobilization of liposomal constructs in hydrogels, to protect them from rapid degradation *in-vivo*. The technology has been adapted to increase the immunogenicity of poorly immunogenic peptides and protein vaccines.

Since, liposomes are known to act as immunological adjuvants and vaccine carrier, giant vesicles containing microbes (live or attenuated) and soluble antigens could be used as multiple vaccine to ensure simultaneous presentation of antigens to immunocompetent cells. Immunoadjuvant properties of liposomes have come to an age, with the first IRIV (Immunopotentiating reconstituted Influenza virosomes) liposome based vaccine (against hepatitis A) being licenced for use in humans. Vaccines based on novasomes (nonphopolipid, biodegradable, pausilamellar vesicle formed from single chain amphiphiles, with or without other lipids) have also been investigated. In the case of liposome, further improvement of adjuvanticity has been received by the use of immobilized co-adjuvants such as 'endogenous cytokines', namely, interleukines IL-2 and IL-6, interferons(IFN) and tissue necrosis factor(TNS) and "exogenous products"namely, muramyldipeptide(MDP), derivatives lipopolysaccharide(LPS) and o-polysaccharide(OPS) and positively charged lipids.

It has now become apparent that antigens, presented or constituted in liposomes, can promote humoral and cellular immune responses providing therapeutic and immunological status to many of the vaccines. Liposomes interact efficiently with macrophages, thus macrophages may serve as antigen presenting cells for liposomal antigens. Liposome immobilized vaccine against malaria have been found to be safe and fairly immunogenic, but exhibited inability to provide long term immune responses against the antigen, probably due to liposomal destabilization *in vivo*. This has switched interest to **microencapsulated liposomal systems (MLS)** to control the delivery of liposome associated macromolecules, *in vitro* and *in vivo*. The microencapsulated liposomes are engineered liposomes, encapsulated within polymeric microspheres made permeable to provide controlled release of antigens. The ability to control the presentation of liposomes associated macromolecules, from a long term depot such as MLS, makes these systems suitable as immunization vehicles. In one of the MLS system explored in literature, the liposomes were encapsulated within microspheres of calcium cross-linked alginate, with an additional membrane of alginate-poly-L-lysine (PLL). The system has been evaluated for *in vivo* performance demonstrating an appreciable presentation of model antigen ^{3}H-labelled BSA. At present the potential applicability of MLS is being explored in hepatitis B vaccination. Microencapsulated liposomal systems engineered with nylon walled, nylon-gelatin walled and nylon-gelatin-acacia walled microcapsules have been discussed for the controlled delivery of proteins and macromolecules.

4.10.1.3. Immobilized ligands as pilot module

Glycoconjugate ligands have been immobilized on liposomal surface to be targeted to specific carbohydrate recognition domains, mainly membrane sugar binding protein, lectins. The protein based glycoconjugates which have been investigated as an immobilized vector for the cellular targeting are glycoprotein and virus spike glycoproteins. Targeting potential of glycoprotein directed immobilized cellular system exploits the ability of sialic acid derivatives to interact with lectins receptors. Sialic acid residues immobilized on the liposomal surface have been reviewed for their biodistribution and cell targetability, e.g., sialoglycoprotein of human erythrocytes as glycophorin reconstituted liposomes, monosialo-ganglioside GM_1, sialoglycopeptide derived fetuin, sialic acid conjugated cholesterol substitued polysaccharide and sialoglycolipid, a novel synthetic sialic acid derivative.

The viral spike protein immobilized system named as virosomes (as viral vectors) may be target oriented and their fusogenic characteristics could be exploited in genome grafting and intracellular delivery of antisense oligonucleotides and plasmid DNA. Lectins (Con-A, WGA and RCA) upon immobilization on liposome retain saccharide specificity and ability to agglutinate red blood cells, and this immobilized system has been exploited as a means of targeting to a range of oral and skin associated bacteria. Surface immobilized lectins can promote binding to peyer's patches and the concept has proposed lectin modified polymerized liposome as a novel vehicle for oral vaccination.

4.10.1.4. Fusogenic liposomes or chimerasomes

Virosomes are the liposomes immobilized with virus spike glycoproteins, incorporated into the lipcsomal bilayers derived from reteroviruses. It has been used as a means of targeting to hamster hybridoma cells, murine lymph node T-cells, to elicit immune response in animals and in the mice and guinea pig. Commonly encountered problems with conventional liposomes is their internalization via endocytic compartment into lysosomal system. To directly introduce molecules into the cytoplasm, liposomes that merge with cell membranes have been developed. The principle mimics the way by which several viruses bind and merge with cell membranes at neutral pH, and therefore, release their genome into the cytoplasm. Reconstitution of number of spike glycoproteins including those of sendai virus, rabies virus, influenza virus, herpes virus, HIV- I and vesicular stomatis virus into liposomes has been described. Development of virosomes exploits the ability of spike glycoprotein to undergo a conformational change at the endosomal pH, resulting in exposure of their hydrophobic residues to initiate fusion with plasma membrane of the cell or in case of small liposomes, fusion with endocytic vacuoles.

An alternative strategy to the reconstitution of virus spike glycoprotein in liposomes, involves the reconstitution of the virus receptor of the target cell in the liposomes. Fusion between the receptor bearing liposomes and the target cell is then brought about by the virus particle. The virosomes may be target oriented and their fusogenic characterstics could be exploited in genome grafting and cellular microinjections. Proteoliposomes have been reported to deliver gene expression systems to cells. Liposomes prepared with fusion protein F of sendai virus, incorporated into lipid bilayers (reconstituted fusogenic viral membrane) have acquired the capacity to merge with cell membrane and some molecules with poor cellular membrane permeability (like the RNA duplex poly(rl), poly(rc)) have been very efficiently delivered to the cells.

4.10.2. Artificial cellular reactor

Artificial cellular carriers, engineered with encapsulated or immobilized macromolecular catalysts, as a homing device capable of providing them, the micro climate have been proposed (Immobilized bioreactors). Artificial cellular bioreactors, encapsulating enzymes have been proposed for lysosomal storage disorder and enzyme replacement therapy. The same model encapsulating plasminogen activators, like streptokinase and glu-plasminogen has been investigated for thrombolytic therapy in acute myocardial infarction. Artificial cellular bioreactor having a polymerase protein as a homing molecule, immobilized within phopholipid vesicles, has been employed for the production of RNA in the bioenvironment. It has been further described that immobilized RNA polymerase (template independent polynucleotide phophorylase) selectively interect with the externally provided substrate adenosine diphosphate (ADP) with the synthesis of long chain RNA polymers within the vesicles. A soluble-insoluble immobilized system has been engineered by immobilizing enzyme chymotrypsin on reversibly precipitable polymerized liposomes. This immobilized enzyme reactor was reusable and more stable at high temperature and long term incubation than native enzyme.

4.10.3. Artificial viral envelope (Ave) as cellular carriers

AVE have been investigated as pathophisiological approach to cellular drug targeting. The concept of molecular recognition of cell surface receptors by viral surface glycoproteins as a means for the selective intracellular delivery of macromolecules, has been exploited for cellular targeting. To accomplish this, artificial viral envelopes (AVE) resembling the HIV-1 were designed as a model system. Recombinant HIV-1 surface glycoprotein gp 160 (HIV-r-gp 160) inserted in the artificial envelope recognizes the CD4 cell surface receptor, selectively transfer ricin-A and FITC-dextran, encapsulated in HIV-1 r-gp 160 AVE into a CD4 positive cell line as against a CD4 negative cell line. The arrest of cell growth was reverted in the presence of excess anti-gp 120 monoclonal antibody. Viral mimicry using AVE may be a means for targeted intracellular delivery of immobilized bioproteins i.e., peptides, proteins, enzymes, toxins, oligonucleotides, gene constructs, and other nondestructive, labile or toxic macromolecules (readers may refer also chapter 16 for more details).

4.10.4. Erythrocytes and fused cells as potential cellular carrier

Erythrocytes (ghost and resealed), lymphocytes, fused erythrocytes, fused cells (erythrocytes/lymphocytes), erythrocyte fused lipid vesicles and other somatic cells have been porposed as novel cellular drug carriers for the delivery of enzymes, vaccines and drugs immobilized in them. The use of erythrocyte cells as carriers to modify the *in vivo* distribution of active principle was originally reported for entrapment of enzymes in the **ghost erythrocytes**.

Several reports exist in the literature which describe the entrapment of proteins and other macromolecules (DNA, RNA, antisense, etc.) into ghost cells by gradual hypotonic hemolysis and the subsequent fusion (induced by sendai virus) of these loaded cells with other culture cells. By this technique, the erythrocyte is used as a "syringe" to inject macromolecules or other agents in the bio-cells. This concept led to the development of **fused cell carrier systems**. Erythrocytes fused with unilamellar lipid vesicles containing inositol hexaphosphate(1HP) have been proposed for therapy of oxygen deficiencies. Immobilization of bioactive compounds into erythrocytes and lymphocytes by fusion with lipid vesicles displayed some decisive advantages that there is little or no loss of hemoglobin or other intracellular components.

On the same lines, a novel cellular drug carrier system has been evaluated that based on the cell to cell fusion of different cells (e.g. lymphocytes/erythrocytes tumor cells/lymphocytes, and tumor cell, erythrocytes) exploiting fusogenic potential of either PEG or sendai virus. Electric field method of fusing pairs of cells synchronously have also been reported as ideal vector for the delivery of immobilzed materials. The fact that lymphocytes can leave the blood vessels and may penetrate the BBB (Blood brain barrier) makes them particularly interesting candidate for target specific delivery of immobilized drugs to the brain tissue (Fig.4.29).

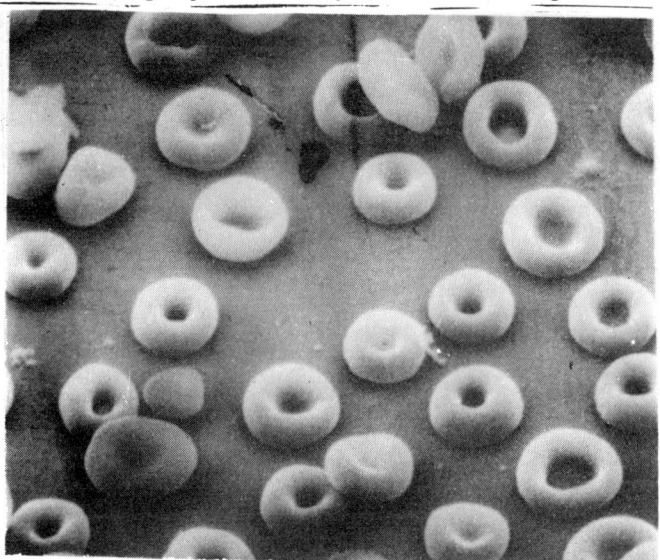

Fig. 4.29 : SEM of lyophilized, drug immobilized erythrocytes

In the last decade, it has been widely accepted that human and animal erythrocytes, (ghost or resealed) can be properly engineered to behave as passive carriers of immobilized bioactive molecules. These transport cell systems have been proposed for dissemination of incorporated active compounds through the organism. The major advantages of this strategy are the *in vivo* protection from premature degradation and immunological reactions, as well as widespread distribution via circulatory systems. Some reports of immobilized erythrocytes as delivery vehicle are as discussed below.

I. Enzymes immobilized in erythrocytes could be exploited for enzyme replacement therapy as well as for lysosomal storage disorders. The use of erythrocyte entrapment as a strategy to deliver and protect exogenously administered enzymes for replacement therapy in selected genetic diseases has been evaluated. The entrapment of β-galactosidase, invertase, urease, arginase, uricase, β-fructo-furanoside and asparaginase in erythrocytes has proved its potential as enzyme carrier. The results with enzyme loaded cell *in vivo* and *in vitro* demonstrate that it is possible in principle, to exploit such a system for the degradation of small molecules in the blood stream, provided that the cells are sufficiently permeable to the substrate and that they have a life span, long enough (circulating bioreactor). In addition to the therapeutic removal of small molecules in the blood stream, the treatment of lysosomal storage disorder, mainly Gaucher's disease can be performed in better way by use of erythrocytes immobilized with glucocerebrosidase compared to ghost resealed erythrocytes. This can also be achieved by glutaraldehyde cross linked enzyme loaded erythrocytes which are taken up by phagocytic cells of RES, and provide targeted delivery.

II. Erythrocytes as cellular carriers have been exploited in the targeted drug delivery to the liver and spleen. Asparaginase and methotrexate (antineoplastics) have been investigated for passive hepatic targeting potential of resealed erythrocytes. Modification of the loaded cells by such means as neuraminidase (sialic acid, specific glycocidase acting on glycolipids and glycoproteins) may result in long circulating half-life and other target site specifications. At present the most promising approaches to introduce target specificity into the cellular carrier systems are magnetic field techniques and local hyperthermia which could be used as physical tools for designing them for desired therapeutic benefits.

Erythrocytes have been reported as long acting operative system immobilizing recombinant human erythropoietin (Epo), a sialoglycoprotein hormone which is the principal physiological regulator of erythroid differentiation. Similarly, erythrocytes immobilized with inositol hexaphosphate (1HP, phytic acid) have been engineered and reported to be useful in oxygen deficiency therapy.

4.10.4.1. Erythrosomes

Erythrosomes are especially engineered liposomal system in which chemically crosslinked human eythrocytes cytoskeletons are used as a support upon which a lipid bilayer is coated. This can be achieved by the modified procedure normally adapted for reverse phase evaporation. This is proposed as a useful encapsulation system for drug delivery particularly for effective targeting of macromolecular drugs.

4.10.5. Artificial red cells (arc) as cellular carriers

The potential problem of HIV, hepatitis (virus) and infective micro-organisms in donor blood has led to the concept of artificial red blood cells. Artificial red blood cells (ARC) are red cells substitutes with encapsulated (immo ilized) hemoglobin. A number of approaches have been reported; synthetic polymer membranes ARC, bilayer lipid protein or bilayer lipid-polymer membrane ARC, biodegradable synthetic polymer membrane ARC, submicron lipid membrane ARC, biodegradable polylactide nanocapsules ARC, and most widely investigated bilayer vesicles, i.e., liposomes encapsulated hemoglobin as red cell surrogates.

Liposomes encapsulated hemoglobin (LEH) is extensively investigated strategy towards the development of red cell substitute as a high capacity artificial oxygen carrying systems. In LEH approach, modification through immobilization prevents the hemoglobin, a tetramer, from breaking down into dimers especially in the circulation. Also, the incorporation of the required cofactors improves the ability of hemoglobin to release the oxygen it carries. For example, fine tuning of the oxygen affinity of the Hb molecule is possible by co-encapsulating natural allosteric effectors, such as 2,3-diphosphoglycerate (DPG). Thus immobilized hemoglobin in synthetic membranes permits tailoring of its oxygen carrying properties. ARC prepared by immobilizing Hb with a polymerizable phospholipid was found to have almost the same oxygen transport capacity as those of RBCs. Liposome encapsulated hemoglobin, which inhibits tumor necrosis factor (TNF) release from rabbit alveolar macrophages has also been investigated (for further details readers may refer chapter 16).

Potential utility of ARC as an emergency blood replacement alternative and as an artificial oxygen carrier has been proved. There has been a significant demonstration that LEH delivers oxygen to peripheral tissues and improves the outcome of hypovolemic, hemorrhage shocks following total isovolemic exchange transfusion. Liposome encapsulate hemoglobin/hypertonic saline solution have been reported as a salutary resuscitative fluid. It has been recently observed that LEH has modulatory effect on MPS functions, by monitoring cytokine expression, phagocytosis and monocytes migration. Attempts should be made to permit the modification of the current LEH preparations devoid of potentially detrimental effects on MPS function.

4.10.6. Encapsulated cells

A number of encapsulation systems have been developed and refined in which immobilized living cells can be separated from the immune system of the body by a synthetic but selective permeable membrane. The membrane allows the free exchange of nutrients, oxygen and biotherapeutic agents between the blood/plasma and the encapsulated cells. ECT (encapsulation cell technology) may also modulate the bi-directional diffusion of antigens, cytokines and other immunological moieties based on the chemical characteristics of the membrane and matrix support. Cellular encapsulation may pave a way to establish prolonged survival of cell and tissue transplants in patients with diseases caused by the loss of specific differentiated cell functions. It has broad spectrum of applications in disorder originating from functional defects of native cell systems, viz., diabetes, Alzheimer's disease, Parkinson's disease, HIV and tumours.

A major focus of biotechnology during the past decade has been the development of genetically engineered cells that produce specific bioactive substances. The development of encapsulation system containing either bio-engineered or primary isolates of living mammalian cells offers enormous potential. Among the encapsulated devices investigated microparticles (microcapsules and microspheres) and micro-reactors have got much attention in recent years.

4.10.6.1. Bioartificial implants

Recently, encapsulated cells have been designed for sustained neurotransmitter delivery to central nervous system (bioartificial delivery system). Figure 4.30a illustrates an implantable bioartificial prosthesis composed of neurosecretory cell core surrounded by a semipermeable membrane. Immobilized cell devices of these types allow for site specific delivery for affected brain areas, but differs from other controlled release systems in that they incorporate living cells within the structure. The immobilized cells are kept alive by passive exchange of nutrients and waste products with surrounding extracellular fluid through semipermeable encapsulating device. Figure 4.30b illustrates the rationale behind the approach by presenting cells, which synthesize and spontaneously release appropriate neuroactive molecules, as a "biological sustained release system" for the treatment of Parkinson's disease. Bioartificial molecular delivery system releases molecules from prosthesis to diffuse into surrounding nervous tissues. A bioartificial system has both synthetic and release capabilities and may, therefore, deliver neurosecretory products longer than conventional controlled release devices.

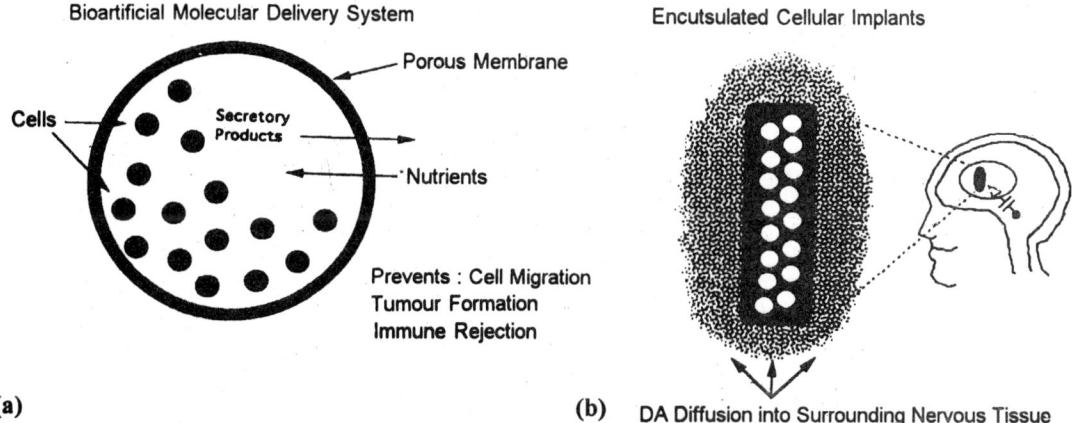

Fig. 4.30 : Schematic representation of a bioartificial molecular delivery system

4.10.6.2. Microparticles

Microparticles have been investigated as adjuvants in encapsulated cell technology for transportation of cells and tissues from either bioengineered sources or from primary animal isolates (or from cell culture grown using primary animal isolates). To date, most of the research in the area of cellular encapsulation has been carried out with pancreatic islets (for diabetes). Most of the procedures for fabricating microspheres involve extruding a mixture of cells and sodium alginate into a $CaCl_2$ solution. The negatively charged, gelled droplets can then be coated with positively charged poly-L-lysine (PLL). The islets within these biohybrid systems are generally immobilized in hydrogels, such as alginate or agar. One of the important functions of these gels is to provide more uniform islets distribution by preventing settling and subsequent aggregation of the islets into larger, necrotic masses. Alginate microspheres without the synthetic PLL membrane have also been evaluated for the prolongation of discordant xenograft survival in mice without immunosuppression. Successful long term implantation of microencapsulated allografts of PLL-coated microspheres have also been reported in higher animals.

4.10.6.3. Injectable microreactor

A new type of encapsulation technology with the potential for transplantation of islets across a wide species barrier without immunosuppression has been developed. These selective permeable "microreactors" (600-1200µ) are fabricated from biodegradable polymers that are slowly absorbed and excreted from the body. The rate of degradation of the micro-reactors can be adjusted to correspond to the functional longevity of the encapsulated islets. These microreactors have been tested in both small and large animal models for xenograft survival. Bovine and porcine islets were immobilized in the microreactors and implanted into the peritoneal cavity of diabetic rats without immunosuppression, and into dogs both with and without immunosuppression. When the xenografted islets were immobilized within the selectively permeable micro-reactors, viable tissue was observed both with and without immunosuppression. The result indicates that survival of discordant islet xenografts can be achieved in both rodents and dogs without immunosuppressive drug using microreactors fabricated from biodegradable materials.

SUGGESTED READINGS

Antonini, E. and Faneli, M.R.R., (1987) *Immobilized Enzymes and Cells*, In : **Methods in Enzymology,** Klaus Mosback (Ed.,) Vol.44, Academic Press Inc., Orlando, Florida.

Antonini, E. and Faneli, M.R.R., and Chiancone, E., (1975) In: **Protein-ligand Interactions,** H.Sund, (Ed.), de Gruyter, Berlin.

Berezin, I.V. and Martinek, K., (Eds.), (1982) **Introduction to Applied Enzymology-Immobilized Enzymes,** MSU Press, Mosocow.

Buchholz, K., (1983) In: **Enzyme Technology,** R.M. Lafferty, (Ed.), Springer-verlag, Berlin and New York.

Chang, T.M.S., (1977) *Encapsulation of Enzymes, cell contents, cells, vaccines, antigens, antiserum, cofactors, hormones and proteins.* In: **Biomedical application of Immobilized Enzymes and proteins,** T. M.S. Chang, (Ed.), Vol.1, Plenum, New York.

Chang, T.M.S., (1978) **Artificial Kidney, Artificial liver and Artificial cells,** Plenum, New York.

Chang, T.M.S., (1980) *New approaches using immobilized enzymes for the removal of urea and ammonia,* In: **Enzyme Engineering,** H.H. Weltall and G. P. Royer, (Eds.), Vol. 5, plenum, New York.

Chiancone, E., Gattoni, M. and Antonini, E., (1983) In: **Affinity chromatography and Biological Recognition,** I.M. Chaiken, M. Wilchek, and I. Parikh, (Eds.) Academic press, Orlando, Florida.

Chibata, I. and Tosa, T., (1978) **Immobilized Enzymes,** Wiley, New York.

Chibata, I., (1978) **Immobilized Enzymes Research and Development,** Halstead press, New York.

Chibata, I., Tosa, T. and Sato, T., (1983) In: **Advances in Biotechnological Process** A. Mizrahi, (Ed.), Alan R. Liss, Inc., New York.

Chibata. I. and Wingard, Jr. L.B., (1983) **Applied Biochemistry and Bioengineering**, Vol.4, Academic Press, New York.

Heller, J., (1990) *Use of Enzymes and Bioerodible polymers in self regulated and Triggered Drug delivery systems*, In: **Pulsed and Self-Regulated Drug Delivery**, Joseph Kost (Ed.,), CRC Press, Boca Raton, Florida, USA.

Hermanson, G.T., Mallia, A.K. and Smith, P.K., (1992) **Immobilized affinity ligand techniques**, Academic press, San Diego, CA.   •

Kim, B.K., Lee, E.B., Kim, C. and Han, Y. N., (Eds.) (1991) **Advances in New Drug Development**, The Pharmaceutical Society of Korea, Seoul, Korea.

Klein, J., Wagner, F., Kressdorf, B., Muller, R., Tjokrosoeharto, H. and Vorlop, K.D., (1985) In : **Application of Enzymes and Immobilized Cells to Biotechnology**, A.I. Laskin, (Ed.), Benjamin/cummings, Menlo park, California.

Martinek, K., Mozhaev, V.V. and Berezin, I.V., (1980) In: **Enzyme Engineering: Future directions**, L.D.Wingard, I.V. Berezin, and A.A. Klyosov, (Eds.), Plenum, New York.

Mattiason, B., (1983) **Immobilized cells and organells**, Chem. Rubber Publication Co., Cleveland, Ohio.

Mattiasson, B., (1983) In: **Immobilized cells and organelle**, (vol. 1&2), CRC Press, Boca Raton, Florida.

Mosbach, K. (Ed.), (1987) *Immobilized Enzymes and Cells*, In: **Methods in Enzymology**, Vol.135, part-B, Academic press Inc., Orlando, Florida.

Rosevear, A. and Lambe, C.A., (1983) *Immobilized Plant and Animal cells*, In: **Topics in Enzymes and Fermentation Biotechnology**, Alan Wiseman (Ed.,), Ellis Horwood ltd., Chichester, West Sussex, UK

Rosevear, A., Kennedy, J.F. and Cabrel, J.M.S., (1987) **Immobilized Enzymes and Cells**, Adam Hilger, Bristol, UK.

Schugerl, K. and Sittig, W., (1987) *Bioreactors*, In: **Fundamentals of Biotechnology**, P. Prave, U. Faust, W. Sittig, D.A. Sukatsch (Eds.), VCH Verlaysgesellschaft, Germany.

Shek, P.N., (1993) **Liposomes in Biomedical applications**, Harwood Academic Publisher, UK.

Sugiyama, M. and Seki, J., (1991) *In Vivo Application of Lipoproteins as Drug Carriers* In: **Lipoproteins as carriers of Pharmacological Agents**, J.M. Shaw, (Ed.), Marcel Dekker Inc., New York, 315-350.

Torchillin, V.P. and Klibanov, A.L., (1993) *Coupling of ligands with liposome membrane* In: ·**Liposomes in Drug Delivery**, G. Gregoriadis, A.T. Florence and H.M. Patel (Eds.), Harwood Academic Publisher, UK.

Torchinski, Y.M., (1974) **Sulfhydryl and Disulfide Groups of Proteins**, Plenum Press, New York.

Ugi (Ed.), (1971) **Isonitrile Chemistry**, Academic press, New York.

Vorlop, K.D. and Klein, J., (1983) In: **Enzyme Technology**, R.M Lafferty, (Ed.) Springer-verlag, Berlin and New York.

Zaborsky, O.R., (1973) **Immobilized Enzymes**, CRC press, Boca Raton, Florida, USA.

Malaria vaccine 'promising' . . . .

A clinical trial conducted by SmithKline Beecham showed that human volunteers were protected against malaria after vaccination with a experimental vaccine developed in collaboration with United States Army's Walter Reed Army Institute of Research. In tests on seven volunteers injected with the experimental vaccines, only one developed malaria. In contrast, all the non-vaccinated volunteers became infected. The researchers said the later versions of the vaccine would be tried on people living in malaria-infested parts of the world to make sure that it works. The first of these testes scheduled to begin in a few months in West Africa.

The new vaccine combines proteins from the parasite that causes malaria and from hepatitis B virus. If it succeeds, it will protect against both diseases. The study has been described by a few experts as "a considerable advance on the development of malaria vaccines". Detailed results have been published in the *New England Journal of Medicine.*

.... from Express Pharma Pulse Jan 16,1997.

5

FERMENTATION: GENERAL CONSIDERATION

5.1. INTRODUCTION AND HISTORICAL PERSPECTIVE

Fermentation may be defined as the process of growing a culture of microorganisms in a nutrient media and thereby converting feed into a desired end product. It is sometimes described as a biochemical reaction in which microorganisms serve (bacteria or fungi) as biocatalyst. The fermentation segment forms a major part of biotechnology industry. It has been for a long time, starting with the herbs, doctor, brewer, bakers, and cheese and wine-makers of ancient civilization who used empirical fermentation methods to achieve the desired products.

Going into the history of fermentation it takes back to two centuries behind. The first scientific report to the fermentation came with ethanol fermentation mechanism by Gay Lussac in 1700's. By the early 1800's the controversial works of Pasteur, Kutzing, Schwann and Cagniard-Latour indicated that the fermentation is caused by living organism. Biotechnology industry of today is a combination of pure research and its practical application and really began with the French genius, Louis Pasteur, who demonstrated that fermentation was caused by living cells, rather than by decomposition. Rudolf Virchow's work at the pathological institute in Berlin helped to establish a basis of cellular biotechnology. However, the work in the field gained an impetus in twentieth century. First world war was a major propeller for the growth of industrial fermentation and food storage which led to the large scale production of breweries yeast in Germany, and bulk chemical shortage led to large scale production of glycerol in Germany and acetone in Great Britain. Second world war led to the discovery of wonder drug *'Penicillin'* an antibiotic that revolutionized the field of pharmaceuticals.

The intensified research related to fundamental processes of life occurred during 1950 and 1960's and provided a newer dimension to fermentation as a discrete science. Microbes are now designed to produce bioactive proteins such as human type insulin, enzymes, vitamins, amino acids or specific antibiotics on a large industrial scale. A list of major industrial products prepared from fermentation is given in Table 5.1.

Table 5.1.: Major industrial fermentation products

S. No.	Fermentation product	S. No.	Fermentation product
1	Foods and beverages	7	Alcohol
2	Antibiotics	8	Carbohydrates
3	Vitamins	9	Enzymes
4	Amino acids	10	Single cell protein
5	Organic acids	11	Biological pesticides
6	Solvents	12	Miscellaneous products

The pharmaceutical industry uses fermentation for the manufacture of hormones, biologicals and biodrugs. Furthermore, the micro-organisms are used to convert waste products and raw material into energy or industrial chemicals. Especially microbes have an affinity for certain metals, they are used to mine low-grade ores of uranium, copper, etc. and also to remove or recover metals from industrial effluents and to enhance oil recovery.

5.2. THE FERMENTATION PROCESS AND OPTIMIZATION

As has been highlighted in the preceding paragraphs, process of fermentation is based upon utilization of metabolic and enzymatic activities of various micro-organisms so as to transform organic compounds. The aim of the present illustration is to make the reader well familiar with the latest techniques which have revolutionized the industrial process of fermentation. The study of kinetics of cell growth has put forth some of the applicability so as to obtain highest end product. Similarly with the technique of genetic engineering scientists are able to manipulate the genes controlling a micro-organisms protein expression system to produce desired biomolecular product. Fermentation generally encompasses processes and products, it is beyond the scope of this book to enlarge upon them. However where they appear to be relevant a brief accord is presented. The basic principles of fermentation remain nearly the same for all.

5.2.1. Kinetics of cell growth in fermentation optimization process

In order to design a maximal capacity fermenter, it is desired that there should be a proper understanding of the kinetics of microbial, animal or plant cell growth kinetics. Cell production kinetics revolves around the cell-growth rate and it is affected by various physicochemical conditions. It is appropriate to state that cell kinetics is the consequential interaction of numerous complicated biochemical reactions and transport phenomenon, involving multiple stages of multicomponent systems. The complete mathematical modeling of growth kinetics is not possible as a heterogeneous mixture of young and old cells continuously transforms and adopts to a changing environment during growth phase. Hence, in order to derive simpler models of fermenter operation and performance that can accommodate mathematical modeling, assumptions must be made regarding the involvement of various cellular components and cell population dynamics (Table 5.2)

Table 5.2 Kinetics growth and production of models

Population	Cell components Unstructured	Cell components Structured
Distributed	Cell represented by single component, which is uniformly distributed throughout the culture.	Multiple cell components uniformly distributed throughout the culture, interact with each other
Segregated	Cells are represented by single component, but form a heterogeneous mixture	Cells composed of multiple components and form a heterogeneous mixture

Among the models suggested, the simplest possible model is the unstructured distributed model. The model is classically based upon two basic assumptions:

(a) all the cells can be represented by single component such as cell mass; cell number etc.;

(b) cellular mass is distributed throughout the culture. In addition to the cells, the medium should be formulated such that *'one component may limit the reaction rate'*. All other components should present at sufficiently high concentrations so that the minor changes do not effect the growth significantly.

Growth rates based on the number of cells and on cells weight are not necessarily the same, as the average cell size may vary considerably from one stage to another. For example, when the mass of an individual cell increases without division, the growth rate based on cell weight increases while the growth rate based upon number of cells remains constant. However, during exponential growth phase, cell number based growth rate and growth rate based on cell weight are proportional. Furthermore, sometimes growth rate is confused with division rate (rate of cell division per unit time). Take the case of a vessel in which all the cells at time t = 0 ($Cn = Cn_0$) have divided, once after a certain period of time, the cell population will have increased to $Cn_0 \times 2$. All the cell are divided X times after time t, the total number of cells will be:

$$Cn = Cn_0 \times 2M \quad \text{---[5.1]}$$

Cn Vs t curve presents a relationship between growth and time where the growth rate is expressed as the slope of the curve (Fig 5.1). If fresh sterile medium is inoculated and the cell density is measured deriving subsequent growth as against time, the results could be distinguished as six stages in batch growth cycle.

(i)*Latent period*: The phase in which the cell number does not vary.

(ii)*Accelerated growth*: The cell number starts increasing and cell division rate accelerates.

(iii)*Exponential growth*: It is the phase of exponential increase in cell number.

(iv)*Decelerated growth*: The phase where growth rate is maximum and during this period growth and division rates start decreasing.

(v)*Static period*: Any further proliferation of cells is stopped and cell number reaches to a maxima point.

(vi)*Death period*: The period where limiting growth substances have depleted and cells begin to die.

The major applications of kinetic growth data and models are to predict the length of fermentation stage in order to estimate the necessary fermenter size before considering other more complex factors. Furthermore, the same models could be utilized in designing batch fermentation processes as well as to predict the fermenter size necessary for continuous culture fermentations.

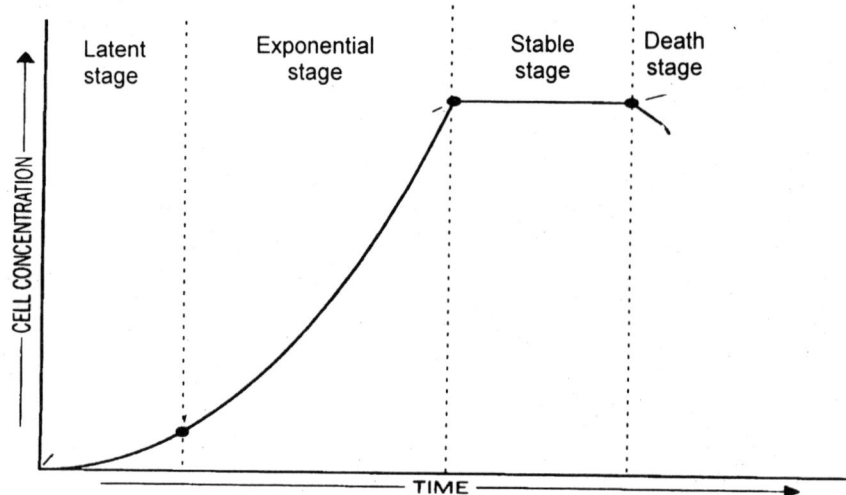

Fig. 5.1. : Batch fermentation stages

The foremost objective of fermentation is to support the growth of specific culture and to promote high end point yield. In certain conditions excess of essential nutrients concentration could extensively inhibit growth (or even kill off the culture), hence essential nutrients should not always be supplied in excess. It is precisely to correlate that the nutrient concentration in the broth should appropriately be optimized with respect to the requirement of the micro-organism involved in the fermentation process. For main application of the optimization process established on the requirements of nutrients by certain micro-organism is to study the kinetics of growth by limiting the concentration of one ingredient while keeping the others in excess. Hence, the growth increases exponentially until the essential (limiting) substance is depleted.

The prediction of kinetics for single cell growth is quite simple

$$\mu = \frac{1}{X} \frac{dX}{d\theta} \quad \text{--[5.2]}$$

where θ is time factor, μ is specific growth rate and X is the concentration of cells. However, for complex cell growth a Monod equation is utilized. It projects an empirical a... simplified model for complex cell-growth.

$$\mu = \mu_m \frac{[C_1]}{[C_1 + K_1]} \frac{[C_2]}{[C_2 + K_2]} \quad \text{--[5.3]}$$

The two limiting components C_1 and C_2 are the concentration.

$$\mu = \mu_m \frac{[C_i]}{[C_i + K_i]} \frac{[C_P]}{[C_P + K_P]} \quad \text{--[5.4]}$$

where K_P is the saturation constant for the products K_i and C_P is the product concentration.

The latent state as has been pointed out earlier is the stage where cell population growth rate is either null or negligible, although cells are still able to increase in size and it occurs while cells adjust to their newer environment. Some important factors such as cell type and age, inoculum size and culture conditions have to be carefully looked into. To highlight the importance of these factors consider the simplest case, when the cells from low nutrient concentration are inoculated into a high concentration media, the latent state size is considerably elongated. However, if the opposite set is followed, there is virtually no latent stage exists. Furthermore, the size of inoculum also effects the span of latent stage. Similarly, if a small number of cells are inoculated into a large volume, the latent phase elongates. In a large scale fermentation unit, the major objective is to shorten the latent stage and hence to inoculate a large fermenter, a series of progressively larger seed lots is created in order to minimize the latent phase.

When the case of batch culture is considered, it involves inoculating sterile medium with a seed culture of the cells to be grown. After inoculation apart from air addition to aerobic fermentation and removal of waste gases, usually nothing else is required to be added or removed from the batch. The rapid change in newer environment can affect four important variables which are discussed below:

1. inoculation into medium with high nutrient concentration can cause delayed cell growth until the culture adapts to new environment;
2. essential molecules synthesized by cell to promote growth (vitamins, activators) may be lost by diffusion out of the cells and may take time for replenishment;
3. the inoculum size and viable cell percentage greatly affect the duration of latent stage;
4. the maturity of the inoculum is important because newer cells are already in exponential growth.

For an optimum fermenter design it is the foremost requirement that the latent phase should be shortened. Hence, following three points are to be considered:

1. inoculum should be as active as possible;
2. inoculum medium should correspond as closely as possible to the fermenter;
3. reasonably large volume of inoculum should be used to minimize the loss of key metabolic intermediates by diffusion.

A proper consideration of all kinetics related factors and appropriate modeling of the fermentation unit should be considered for development and design of a fermenter.

5.3. IMPROVEMENT OF MICROBIAL STRAIN

In order to obtain the highest possible yield of the fermented product it is the major requirement that the micro-organism being utilized should have the highest productions capabilities. Recent advances have enabled the availability of various alternative methods of cell expression and production of recombinant proteins. The major key factors affecting the choice of an expression system are have been identified to be :

1. the required quantity of the designated protein; and
2. the proteins indigenous structural complexity.

Furthermore, products estimated market size, whether or not specific biological modifications are necessary for retaining biological activity and whether the product is chemically stable or not. The optimal expression system, then, would be the one that yields the maximum quantity of property folded, bioactive material. Although product yield could be improved by optimization of culture conditions, productivity is ultimately controlled by genome. Thus, to improve the potential productivity, the organisms genome must be modified.

A genome is defined as the set of nucleic acids (genes) which are responsible for the production of a particular component (primary or secondary metabolite). A detailed discussion of the concept has been dealt with at appropriate length in other chapters. This part of the chapter is focused upon, how this modification in the inherent genes could be brought so as to get the highest productivity of a fermented product. The gene modification could be brought about by two methods (a) mutation and (b) re-combination.

5.3.1. Mutations

When the natural cell division of a microbe takes place there are little probabilities of occurrence of inherited changes. However, still due to some environmental factors some strains exhibit a changed characteristics. These strains are termed as mutants, the factor due to which the change occurred is called as the mutagen and whole process is termed as mutation. The mutagenic agents could be *UV radiation, ionization radiation, chemicals like nitrous acid, nitrosoguanidin,* etc. The exposure to these agents leads to the death of most of the cells in a culture, however, some survivors may contain some of the mutants exhibiting changed characteristics. A small population of these cells could be the one which produces large amount of bioactive components of interest.

One major drawback of this mutation induced improvisation of cell strains is that, it is not always possible using standard mutation techniques, to predetermine the gene that will be affected by the mutagens because a mutagenesis is not site specific. Hence, it is the task of an industrial geneticist to differentiate a few superior producers found among the survivors of mutation treatment. This tedious task is further diluted, in the case of strains producing primary metabolites are selected for that it is for those producing secondary metabolites. For further consideration simple example of both the cases have been listed. The concept have been discussed in more details in chapter 10.

5.3.1.1. Selection of mutant producing improved level of primary metabolite

One of the most important commercially available primary metabolite is the amino acid. The most common organism for the production is *Corynebacterium glutamicum*. Originally *C. glutamicum* was isolated by Kinoshita and associates which was a biotin auxotroph, i.e. requires biotin for production of glutamic acid. Looking into the TCA cycle it could be inferred that glutamic acid is produced when the microbe lacks in the enzyme for conversion of α-ketoglutamic acid to succinic acid (Fig.5.2). *C. glutamicum* when grown in the culture media containing high concentration of biotin 25-35μg/mg/dry weight of cells, of glutamic acid was produced. However, when biotin concentration was limiting factor a higher yield could be obtained. Earlier low yield of glutamic acid could be accounted for the negative feed back inhibition due to glutamic acid. The explanation of excretion of glutamic in the biotin limiting condition is based upon the fact that it results into the cell membrane being deficient in phospholipids thus corrupts their selective permeability (Nakaao et al., 1973).

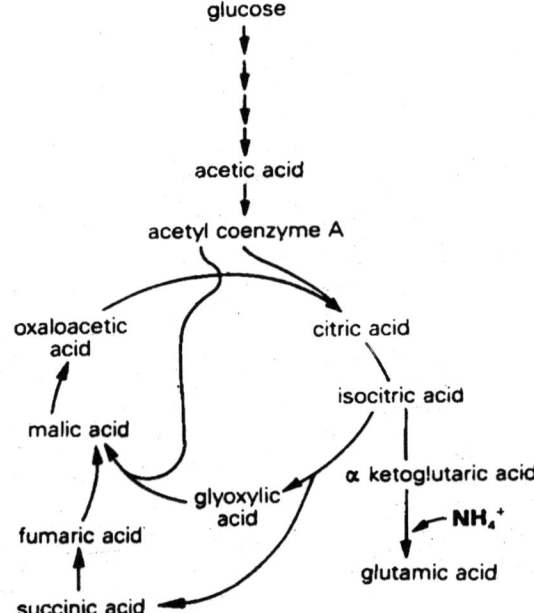

Fig 5.2: The TCA cycle and glyoxylate cycle in Corynebacterium glutamicum

Thus, the combination of a metabolic block in conversion of a TCA cycle intermediate results in a higher yield of glutamic acid. A major disadvantage of using biotin limitation as a controlling factor is that it precludes the use of biotin rich, crude carbohydrate carbon source. As an alternative some other growth factors such as penicillin and surfactant like fatty acid derivatives have been utilized so as to vary the permeability of the cell membrane.

Mutants of *C. glutamicum* have been extensively utilized for commercial production of a large number of amino acids. However, the wild type of strains produce the primary end product according to the requirement of the organism. The control over the production is typically a negative feed back control. Since the feed back control for *C. glutamicum* is quite easy for production of glutamic acid , hence the microbe has found a lot of application potentials for industrial usage. Furthermore, the use of mutant strains of *C. glutamicum* has been effectively utilized for the production of lysine.

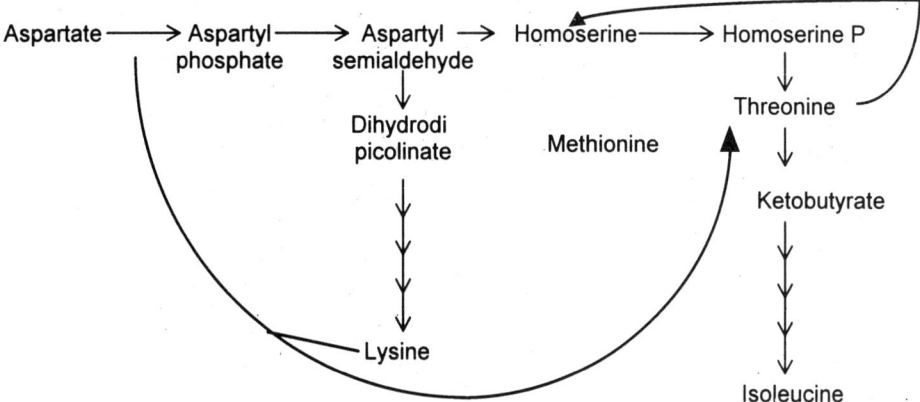

Fig. 5.3 : The control of lysine production in *Corynebacterium glutamicum* (feed back inhibition)

Figure 5.3 shows the control of lysine production in *C. glutamicum*. It could be inferred that aspartokinase, the first enzyme in the biosynthetic route, is inhibited only when lysine and threonine are present above threshold level. This type of control is termed as an absolute feedback inhibition. An important feature of the pathway is that lysine does not exert any control over the biosynthetic route from aspartic semialdehyde to lysine. A mutant which could not catalyze the conversion of aspartic semialdehyde to homoserine would be able to grow only in homoserine supplemented medium and the organism would be referred as a homoserine auxotroph. If such an organism were grown in the presence of very low concentration of homoserine the endogenous level of threonine would not reach the inhibitory concentration of aspartokinase control, then aspartate will be converted to lysine.

The knowledge of biosynthetic route allows the geneticist to develop a mutant of desirable characters. Using logical treatment Nakayama and associates isolated homoserine auxotroph of *C. glutamicum* using penicillin enrichment technique developed by Davis (1949). Under normal culture conditions an auxotroph is at a disadvantage compared with the parental (wild type) cells. However, penicillin selectively kills growing bacterial cells and therefore, if the survivors of a mutation treatment were cultured in a medium containing penicillin and lacking the growth requirement of the desired mutant only those cells unable to grow would survive, these are, the desired auxotrophs. If the cells were removed from the penicillin broth, washed and resuspended in a medium containing requirements of the desired auxotroph then the resulting culture should be rich in the required type. Nakayama's group succeeded in isolating a homoserine auxotroph of *C. glutamicum* which synthesized 44 g dm^{-3} lysine.

5.3.1.2. Selection of Secondary metabolite producing strains

Preceding discussion could highlight the knowledge of control systems which could assist in the designing of the procedures for isolation of mutants which could overproduce the primary metabolites. However, the procedures for isolation of mutants overproducing secondary metabolites are more difficult and complicated, due to the fact that far less information is available for control of production. The systems which could be evolved are based upon the direct empirical screening of the survivors mutation treatment for productivity rather than cultural systems which provided an advantage to potentially producing types. Hence, a typical screening for improved productivity mutants, would be to subject a population of cells to mutational treatment such that 1-5 % of the cells survived and to screen as many as survivors as possible for productivity. The procedure is surely very laborious and cumbersome. Several miniature cultures have to be developed and screened for mutant activity.

The empirical system for improvement of secondary metabolite production has met with selective success. However, some other systems such as isolation of auxotrophs, analogues resistant mutants and those resistant to auxotoxic effect of secondary metabolites have only been developed. In most of the cases there appears no correlation between compound and the secondary product synthesized. This could be due to the improved productivity. However, such systems may be exploited using nitrosoguanidine (NTG) as mutant. NTG causes cluster of mutations around the replicating fork of bacterial chromosome. Hence, if one mutation was selected (e.g. by auxotrophy) it may be possible to isolate a strain containing a selected mutation along with the non selected ones which also map close by. An efficient use of this approach would require an accurate knowledge of the position of the genes important in secondary metabolism so that neighboring appropriate mutation may be selected.

It has been successfully demonstrated that many secondary metabolites inhibit the producer strains if they are added during the growth phase of the organism. Furthermore, there appears to be a correlation between the auxotoxic resistance in growth phase and productivity in idophase. This ability of a survivor of a mutation treatment to grow in presence of high concentration of its secondary metabolites may be used as a selective characteristics for improved productivity. The technique has been combined with genetic manipulation techniques by Crameri and associates (1985) who cloned the gene coding for 6$^{/}$ N-acetyl-transferase into *Streptomyces kanamyceticus*, a kanamycin producer. The enzyme is involved in aminoglycoside resistance and the recombinants containing the cloned gene were more resistant to, and produced more of kanamycin. Thus, the application of the technique used in improvement of primary metabolite formation subsequently resulted in considerable progress in the secondary metabolite production.

5.3.2. Recombination

The first possibility of utilizing the genes in effective recombination so as to generate a new combination was proposed and investigated by Hopwood (1979). The utilization and practical applicability for strain improvement by utilizing this technique is quite less in context with improvement of industrial strains due to the basic reason of complexity of process and non availability of genetic literature of industrial strains. However, in the recent years considerable work is being undertaken in this direction. Relatively few industrially important organisms exhibit sexual reproduction as such, and the attainment of the recombinants of such types probably confines to commercial mushrooms and yeast strains used in baking brewing and distilling industries. However, recombination systems not associated with sexual reproduction are more common in industrially important strains. Recently developed experimental methodologies lend these systems easier to exploit. Some of these techniques applied for various fermentation products have been described in the following paragraphs.

5.3.2.1. Recombination systems utilized in earlier days

Earlier days of recombination systems development were based upon the concept of parasexual cycle. In this cycle the nuclear fusion and gene segregation could take place outside the sexual organs of fungus *Aspergillus nidulans*, *Pencillium chrysogenum*, etc. The nuclear fusion occurs in genetically indifferent nuclei when present in same the organism. Such an organism is termed as heterokaryon and is formed by migration of two cells when they come in contact with each other. The establishment of heterokaryon is a rare event and to aid its recognition, auxotrophic markers are used.

Nuclear fusion may occur between unlike nuclei in the heterokaryon and gives rise to a diploid clone. In rare cases the nucleus undergoes an abnormal mitosis resulting in production of a recombinant. The abnormal mitosis may involve mitotic crossing over, haplodization or a combination of both. The recombinants hence formed will be having the characteristics of both the nuclei.

Some agents like camphor vapors, UV light increase the frequency of nuclear fusion. Furthermore, utilization of X-rays, UV light and nitrogen mustards facilitates crossing over or haploidization. The technique has been utilized to study the genetics of *P. chrysogenum* and *A. niger*. However, the technique could not be successfully utilized due to one major difficulty in the establishment of a heterokaryon, that is fusion of cells from different strains, but the techniques of protoplast fusion have overcome the problem effectively and successfully effectively.

Another similar process of interest is conjugation. In this process in bacteria, the genetic information is transferred from one cell to another by cell to cell contact. The chromosomes of the 'donor' cell are mobilized by integration of a normal extrachromosomal DNA particle into chromosome. The transfer of genetic material is based on the time of contact. Further more, the DNA is transferred in a linear fashion; single strand of DNA is cut adjacent to the site of integration of the mobilizing factor and this strand passes into recipien cell, the mobilizing factor is the last element to be transferred. The transferred segment is incorporated into the recipient cells chromosomes by crossing-over procedure. Similar to the case of parasexual cycle different isolating procedures have to be applied so as to separate the most appropriate strain since the activity of conjugate is dependent upon the linkage of gene in the chromosome fragment. However, availability of genetic maps aids to the process, as the utilization of genetic markers could be used to screen certain recombinants. Moreover, the conjugation requires the complete genetic information about strain, which adds to the complexity of the process.

5.3.3. Protoplast fusion

A protoplast is defined as the cell which is devoid of the cell walls and could be prepared by subjecting cells to the action of wall-degrading enzymes in isotonic solutions. Cell fusion, followed by nuclear fusion, may occur between protoplasts of cells that not otherwise fuse, further following fusion protoplast regenerates the cell wall and grow as normal cells. It has successfully affected in filamentus fungi, yeasts, Bacillus sp., *Brevibacterium flavum* and *Streptomycetes*.

The process offers advantage over parasexual cycle in facilitating heterokaryon formation. Furthermore, the isolation procedures still required have offered a considerable success. Literature presents several citation regarding the strain improvement for industrially applicable strains: Hamlyn and Ball (1979) fused strains of *Cephalosporium acremonium*; Chang and associates (1982) utilized the technique for fusing the strains of *P. chrysogenum*. For more detailed consideration regarding techniques the reader may refer other chapters on Genetics in the same volume.

5.4. FERMENTERS

The heart of the fermentation process is the fermenter. A working definition of a fermenter is a container in which, is maintained an environment favorable to the operation of a desired biological process. Fermentation is typically either batch operated or continuous in operation mode. In the case of batch operated, fermentation proceeds for defined period and terminated when the product concentration reaches a preselected level. The fermenter contents are then harvested, separated, recovered and purified. In the case of continuous culture fermentation, there is a requirement for sterile medium for continuous feeding and medium containing desired end product should continuously exit the vessel at the same rate. The major advantage with continuous culture fermentation is the productivity rate. However, factors like maintenance of aseptic medium and steady state environment are to be carefully considered and monitored.

A fermenter is frequently confused with a bioreactor. However, the major difference between the two is the type of cells being grown. A fermenter grows a prokaryotic cells such as bacteria, fungi etc. while a bioreactor grows eukaryotic cells such as insects, mammalian cells etc. In practice, many manufactures and bioprocess scientists still refer them as fermenters. Furthermore the bioreactors differ from fermenters in their parts such as agitators and mixers.

The word 'fermenter' tends to conjure up the vision of large, shiny, stainless steal vessels bristling with sophisticated instrumentation. While most of the industrial ferementers are indeed like that, several large-scale biological processes are carried in equipments which are considerably less sophisticated and considerably cheaper. In fermentation engineering the statement of 14th century philosopher should be borne in mind '*entia non sunt multi pli canda praeter necessinatron*' which means the system should not be more complicated than really necessary.

An optimum design of a fermenter is to maintain an environment suitable for the controlled growth of microorganisms, so regulating the environment and maintaining aseptic conditions are their prime functions regardless of size. Growth medium must be regulated with respect to agitation, temperature, aeration, pH concentration dissolved oxygen, foam control and other parameters. To overcome the difficulty of purifying the product, the fermenter must be made up of non-corrosive and non-toxic material that could be readily sterilized. Small fermenters are usually made from borosilicate glass while the pilot size systems are made up of stainless steel. Furthermore, each fermenter should be so assembled that most of the parts could be separated for cleaning purpose.

5.4.1. Structure of a fermenter (with appropriate configuration)

A typical fermenter consists of three major parts :

1. the culture vessel
2. associated supply and environmental systems
3. its measurement and control systems.

Various important factors responsible for optimized fermenter design are enlisted in table 5.3.

Table 5.3 : Various important fermenter design considerations

S No.	Factor	Importance
1.	Maintenance of sterility	So as to allow only desirable micro-organism to grow
2.	Oxygen transfer rate	For optimum growth of the micro-organism in aerobic conditions
3.	Heat transfer	For maintaining optimum temperature which changes due to growth of cells
4.	Instrumentation and control protocols	For continuous fermentation process monitoring
5.	Biological kinetics	So as to decrease latent phase
6.	Mass transfer of the substrate to micro-organism	For attaining higher yield
7.	Mass transfer of product out of micro-organism	For attaining higher yield
8.	Safety (fail-safe control; pressure build up; micro-organism escape)	Production hazards

After a careful consideration of all these factors in designing of a typical fermenter some more operational characteristics have to be looked into which are listed in table 5.4. Basically from a bench type fermenter to a production scale fermenter, they are essentially similar and are simply closed, temperature controlled culture vessels. Further the maximum instrumentation, controls and accessory equipments differ from requirement to requirement. Fig 5.4 shows a typical fermenter design.

Table 5.4 : Characteristics of typical fermenter

S.No.	Characteristics	S.No.	Characteristics
1	Alarm and fail safe system	9.	Integrated piping system
2.	Batch or continuous operation	10.	Interchangeable peripherals
3.	Computer controlled operation	11.	Multiple entry and exit ports
4.	convenient aeration	12.	Physical integrity
5.	Ease of installation	13.	Programmable inputs
6.	Foam control	14.	Reliability
7.	Heating and cooling	15.	Sterilizable peripherals
8.	In situ sterilization	16.	Suitable contact surface

5.4.2. Size and scale of process

As the complexity of a fermenter increases there originates the need for increasing peripheral equipment and instrumentation, particularly measurement and control systems. Essential features which have to be considered in selecting fermenters are the product reliability, multipurpose flexibility, interchange ability, level of sophistication, compatibility and range of monitoring instrumentation available for the system.

Most frequent classification of fermenters is based upon their size and accordingly they are grouped as given below:

(a) Laboratory and research (bench scale) fermenters, that are generally ranging from 1-50 liter.
(b) Pilot plant fermenters that typically ranging from 50-1000 liter.
(c) Production scale fermenters, usually larger than 1000 liter.

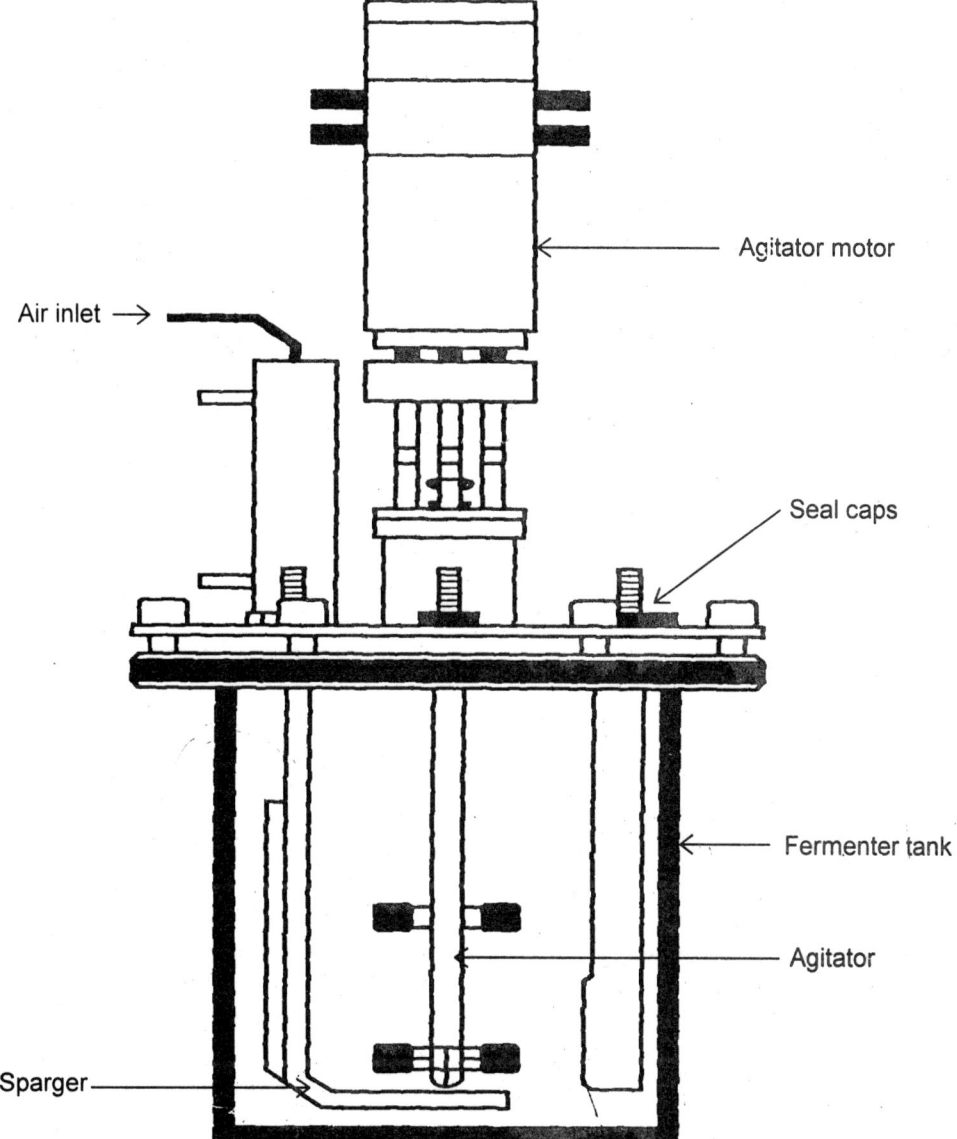

Fig. 5.4 : Three liter bench top stirred tank fermenter

However, the division appears to be arbitrary, it has generally been adopted at industrial level. The large number of fermenters currently available cover a wide spectrum that blurs distinction between one class and another, especially when dealing with smaller production quantities of high-value added substances such as cytokines or interferons. A comparative account of all the three classes of fermenters is presented in table 5.5 and figure 5.5.

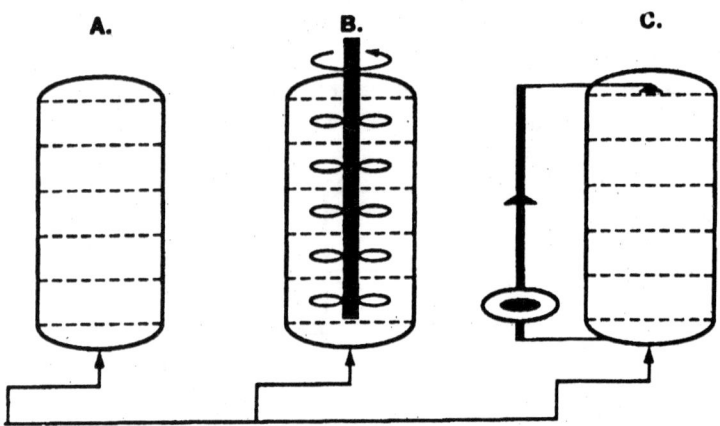

Fig. 5.5 : A schematic view of a Column Fermenter

Table 5.5 : Stirred tank fermenter (STF) : a comparison

Feature	Small Bench	Large bench	Pilot scale
Size:	1-10 L	10-100 L	100-1000 L
Sterilization:	Autoclave	*in situ*	*in situ*
Mixing:	Air lift	Bladed turbine	Impellers
Drive:	←	Direct drive or magnetically coupled	→
Fittings:	Autoclavable	← sterilized *in situ*	→
Seals:	←	Autoclavable O-ring seals	→
Jacketing:	←	Yes, with internal baffles	→
Ports:	4-10	4-10	10-20
Surface:	←	Electropolished stainless steels, Pyrex	→
Parts:	←	interchangeable impellers and fittings	→
Others:	bottom aeration by sparging; maximized oxygen transfer; remote valve process control; view window; sterile compressed air between agitator seals; distinctive safety features.		

5.4.3. Culture vessels

As has been discussed in the preceding discussion that culture vessel forms the major part of a fermenter is common and to all types regardless of their size or utility. Most bench-scale fermenters are made up of borosilicate glass and/or stainless steel. The selection of both the materials is based upon the conceptual understanding of process as both of them are nontoxic, non corrosive, easily cleanable and could be steam sterilized. As an example a cheap and simple to maintain fermenter culture vessel could be made up of glass cylinder with stainless steel head and bottom plates, lending an opportunity for viewing of fermentation. The head plates provide ports for nutrient media and gas input as well as waste product removal. For linking vessel and head plate, silicon rubber O-rings are utilized so as to provide seal and autoclaving is utilized for sterilization.

Stainless steel vessels on the other hand provide strength as well as a double jacketed steam sterilization equipments could be utilized. However, the hindrance in visualization is considered as a major drawback. To overcome the problem many sealed glass windows could be utilized. Interestingly contamination problems have been attributed to glass vessels rather than to stainless steel vessels, further self sterilizable stainless steel vessels typically offer greater protection against contamination than glass vessels, silicon rubber seals, etc.

5.4.4. Agitation systems

Agitation systems form the major requirement for all fermenters. On small scale units agitation is generally accomplished by direct-drive mechanical stirring through seal in the head plate. Some models offer either magnetically coupled agitators or air-lift systems to eliminate mechanical seals (Fig. 5.6). For large scale fermenters, use of baffles and paddles on the mechanical agitator offer advantages. At the lower end LSL **BioLafitte** for example offer a fermenter with an overlay of pressurized sterile air between the two impeller shaft seals and an automatic monitor of seal wear.

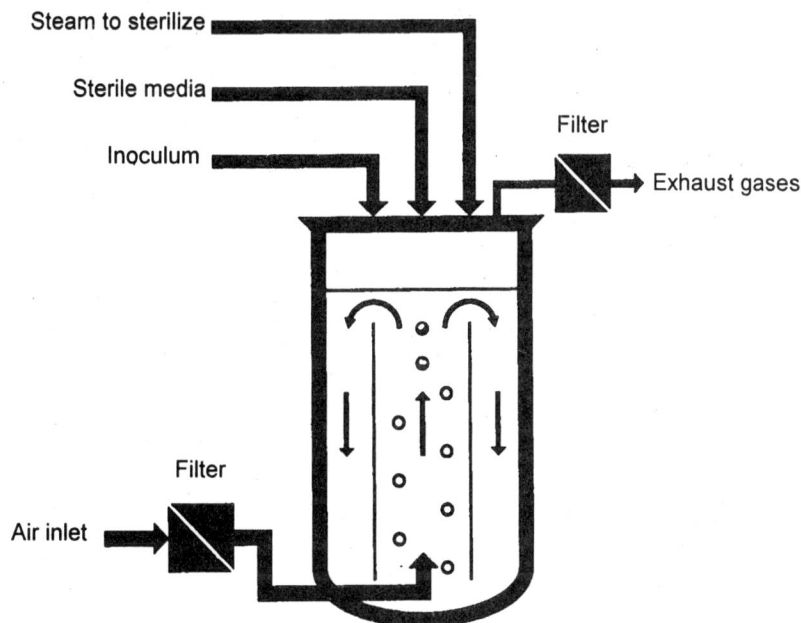

Fig. 5.6 : A typical agitator commonly used in fermenters

5.4.5. Size and capacity

Regardless of size, the basic fermenter design remains the same. However, as fermenter size increases, special and more complex features tend to multiply. Large fermenters usually vary in the additional devices incorporated into the large units such as additional entry and exit ports frequently used to accommodate more monitoring probes that are required by the large vessels, although sometimes extra ports are utilized so as to separate various components before adding them to culture vessel.

Although large scale fermenter adds to the complexity of operation, but also allows greater control, for example, increased thermal mass of a larger vessel permits better temperature control and its large volume facilitates closer pH regulations and buffering precision of the medium. Large scale also allows the employment of process equipment unavailable for small vessels. A Chemp's Chemical system that enables efficient bubble free medium aeration and cell separation and thereby avoids growth limitation for metabolic waste products build up. The major consideration in large scale equipment is proper agitation and *in-situ* control monitoring.

5.4.6. Process monitoring and control

Process monitoring and control are issues at leading edge of fermenter development. With the recent advents in bioanalytical techniques and vast array of probes have been developed and are being utilized. The controls applicable in the fermentation process are enlisted in table 5.6. Furthermore, the process monitoring parameters are listed in table 5.7.

Table 5.6 : Typical fermenter control ranges

S No.	Control	Range
1.	Temperature	8°C above coolant to 60°C $\pm$ 1°C
2.	Agitator Speed	0-1000 rpm
3.	Stability	>98%
4.	pH range	2-12 $\pm$ 0.1
5.	Pressure	2000mbar
6.	DO_2 range	0-100 %
7.	Air flow	0-6 liters/minute

5.4.7. Cleaning and sterilization

A bioprocessing facility that is an ability to be cleaned is a crucial element in designing and construction. Piping, inlet and outlet ports, valves, sensors, regulators, and other components must be designed to eliminate dead spaces, ridges and cervices where material can accumulate and must be constructed to resist the wear and corrosion that could produce areas of surface deterioration (preferential sites for micro-organism growth and substance contamination).

Cleaning process begins when a fermenter is empty following completion of a culture run. Clean-in-place (CIP) and sterilize-in-place (SIP) systems minimize disassembly and down time. CIP and SIP systems, sanitary design verification and sterile operation are critical components of fermenter system validation. Fermenter cleaning and sterilization systems should be designed as integral components with validation maintained from the start. Most industrial fermentations are carried out in pure culture. If foreign organisms proliferate in the medium or on any of the equipment that may lead to a situation where producing organisms are forced to compete with the contaminating organisms for the nutrients.

Table 5.7 : Fermentation process control monitoring parameters and methodology

S No.	Process control	Monitoring device
1.	Air flow	Flowmeter
2.	Coolant water flow	Flowmeter
3.	Power input	V.O.M.; torque
4.	Temperature	Resistance thermocouples thermistors diodes
5.	Rheology	Tube viscometer Cone and plate viscometer, concentric cylinder viscometer Infinite sea viscometer Foam control
6.	Redox potential	pH Dissolved oxygen (DO_2), Polarographic probes, Galvanic probes, Permeable tube/oxygen analyzer, Dissolved carbon dioxide(DCO_2)
7.	State of culture	Enzyme probes metabolic heat substrate analysis
8.	Cell concentration	Gravimeteric dry weight turbidity
9.	Immunocytometry	Cell number, Impedance, Carbon dioxide production, Oxygen production, DNA content, Cell particle size distribution
10.	Gas analysis	Oxygen analyzers, Carbon dioxide analyzers, Mass spectrometry, Gas chromatography

Foreign organisms also produce metabolic byproducts that limit the producing cultures growth. Therefore, before starting a fermentation, the medium, additives, and all equipments must be completely sterile and aseptic conditions should be maintained. Steam sterilization is desirable because it destroys contaminants as well as effects cleansing of the system as the steam reaches all systems contact sites, process liquids and gases. Continuous steam flow during processing provides a sterile barrier with process liquid on one side and steam on the other. Media and equipment is generally performed by destroying all contaminating organism with:

1. Dry or moist heat
2. Ultra violet radiation
3. Chemical agents
4. Ultra filtration
5. Ultra sound (Mechanically disrupting contaminating organisms)

Heat is most widely used as a means of sterilization and is employed for both medium and heatable fermenter parts. It can be applied either dry or moist (steam). Moist heat is more effective for sterilization because vegetative bacterial heat resistance is greater in dry state resulting in death kinetics that are much lower for dry cells than for moist ones. Laboratory autoclaves are usually operated at pressure of about 30 psia, corresponding to 121°C where bacterial spores are rapidly destroyed.

UV light is absorbed by the cells causing DNA damage leading to cell death. The best bactericidal efficiency is at wave length around 265 nm. Its use has been limited to microbial population in areas such as clean rooms and sterile chambers due to its limited ability to penetrate non-biotic matter.

Oxidizing and alkaylating chemicals kill micro-organisms but they are not used for medium or fermenter sterilization because residual antiseptics inhibit fermentation. Some of the major antimicrobial chemical agents are phenol and phenolic compounds, ethanol, halogens, detergents, dyes, quaternary ammonium compounds, acids, alkalis and gaseous sterilizing chemicals (ethylene oxide, propiolactone, formaldehyde, etc.).

Ultrafiltration can be effectively used for removing micro-organisms from the air or from other gases; and with liquids. Ultrafiltration is used for thermolabile products such as sera and enzymes. Ultrasound of sufficient intensity can disrupt microorganisms. This technique is usually employed for extracting cellular components rather than for sterilization.

5.5. TYPES OF FERMENTERS (BIOREACTORS)

In the large scale biological processes various different types of vessels are utilized. The degree of sophistication vary from sensitivity of the process to the environment to be maintained within the vessel. In some previously established processes like brewing and production of penicillin, the fermenter design has evolved from that of a simple container into a more complex modification as understanding of biological process mechanisms has been extended. In the simplest case, the fermenter is a vessel in which reagents, substrates and organism are brought into contact with provisions of their addition and removal. Broadly the fermenters could be grouped under two classes

(a) Submerged fermenters (suspended-growth systems)

(b) Surface fermenters (supported-growth systems)

However, most of the industrial fermenters/bioreactors contain the elements of both. In suspended growth systems, the organisms are immersed in and dispersed throughout, their nutrient medium and their movement follows that of the nutrient liquid. In the case of supported growth systems the organisms grow as a layer or a film on a surface in contact with a nutrient medium. Practically, the suspended growth systems have a film of the organisms on the surface of the container, and supported growth systems usually have organisms dispersed in the nutrient media.

5.5.1. Submerged fermenters (Suspended growth systems)

It is one of the simplest fermenter in the form of an open tank in which the organisms are dispersed into nutrient liquid. These types of fermenter tanks were successfully utilized by brewing industry for generations, and in the anaerobic fermentation, a foam cover of carbon dioxide and yeast develops which effectively prevents access of air to the process. Cooling coils can be fitted for control of temperature during fermentation. Open concrete pools can be used, frequently in the preliminary stage of production of synthetic hormones, where chopped yams are fermented to release a steroid from its glycoside by enzymatic hydrolysis. Open pools or 'lagoons' are widely used for low rate biological waste water treatment, where the liquid surface allows the dissolution of oxygen from the air and escape of carbon dioxide Agitation which will bring this effect, can be carried out with a mechanical stirrer or by the rise of gas bubbles through the liquid. With aerobic processes, the sparging of air into the liquid provides oxygen for the process as well as agitation. In anaerobic process, gases released by the fermentation can provide agitation, using a pump to recirculate the gas through a sparger, or by arranging for the gas bubbles to be evolved during fermentation. The latter effect is utilized in the 'conical fermenter' used in brewing, which is a tall cylinder with a conical base section. For aseptic conditions, closed tanks must be used The conventional fermenters used for aerobic processes are closed vessels, sparged with air, having additional mechanical stirrers.

The submerged reactors could be grouped into three major types:
1. Reactors with mechanically moved internal members.
2. Reactors with forced convection of liquids (by pump).
3. Fermenter with pneumatic operation (by compression of air).

5.5.1.1. Mechanically stirred fermenters

Stirred tank fermenter is one of the most highly applicable fermenter in the modern fermentation industry. The basic advantage of this type of fermenter is the flexibility of its design. A schematic view of the typical fermenter is presented in figure 5.7.

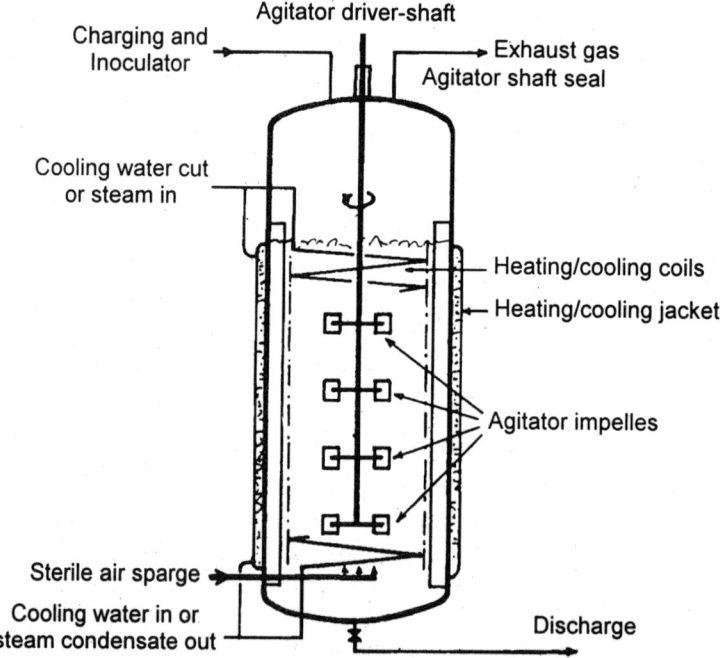

Fig. 5.7 : Stirred tank fermenter in a schematic view

They are equipped with a mechanical agitator so as to maintain homogeneity, to attain rapid dispersion and mixing of injected materials and to enhance heat transfer in temperature control and mass transfer in dissolving sparingly soluble gases such as oxygen. These stirred tank fermenters are the most versatile fermenter and are used in a range of sizes from one liter laboratory unit to production scale vessels of typically 100 ton capacity. The configuration of the fermenter vessel itself is derived from that of conventional pressure vessels which are widely used in industrial processes and for which detailed and comprehensive design procedures have been developed. The fermenter is usually constructed as an upright cylinder with dished ends to facilitate liquid drainage during medium discharge and of splashes and disrupted foam during operation. The volume of vessel is about 30 to 50 % larger than the required culture volume leaving a head space allowing disengagement of the liquid droplets from the exhaust gas and room for foaming.

The agitators consist of one or more impellers, mounted on a shaft, usually suspended on a thrust bearing above the vessel and entering the vessel through a gland or a mechanical seal. The shaft is driven by a motor via a flexible coupling clutch or on smaller units a belt drive or universal joints. With very long shafts one or more steadying bearing are used to reduce vibration and bear on shaft seal. Such bearings must be of very simple types, lubricated by the nutrient medium and capable of repetitive sterilization. The gland or seal through which the shaft enters the vessel is a major contamination risk point, and must provide a tight closure between the vessel and the atmosphere, while allowing the shaft to rotate reasonably freely. The elements of mechanical seals, illustrated in figure 5.7, are two seal rings with accurately flat faces rotating against each other and forming the boundary between the fermenter and the outside atmosphere. A soft seal ring of carbon rotates with the shaft and is held in contact with a hard seal ring of ceramic or hard faced stainless steel by spring made of metal, rubber or plastic. The seal is cooled and lubricated by a flow of sterile liquid usually a steam condensate. Additional security against contamination is obtained by mounting two such seals 'back to back' to form a double mechanical seal.

In conventional stirred tank fermenters, the turbulence required for satisfactory mixing, heat and mass-transfer is obtained with the add of four baffles attached or close to vessel wall. The width of vessels is usually 10-12% of the vessel diameter as the mixing effect is increased only by a little wide baffles, but decreases sharply with narrower baffles. The agitator power dissipation is in production-scale fermenter is about 1-2 kW/m^3.

Some of the other types of mechanically stirred fermenters are given below. They are:

1. Draught tube reactor;

2. High power stirred tank reactor;

3. Stirred multistage fermenter;

4. Paddle wheel reactor; and

5. Mechanically stirred loop reactor.

5.5.1.2. Forced convection fermenters

In some of the newly designed fermenters the agitation is affected by using a pump instead of a mechanical stirrer so as to circulate liquid medium from the fermenter vessel through a gas entertainer and then back into the fermenter. This separates the liquid movement and gas dissolution functions in separate specialized units, and the two designed have evolved using this principle. The 'loop fermenter' and the 'deep jet fermenter'. In the loop fermenter the gas dissolution device is a subsidiary vessel into which the gas is injected and the gas saturated liquid is circulated into the main growth stage. In the deep-jet systems, gas is entertained into a high power jet of liquid injected into the liquid in the fermenter, reentering the gas from the vessel head-space. Exhaust gas is purged partly from the vessel head space and partly form the specially designed separating pump, form which the degassed liquid passes through a supplementary cooler before passing through a gas entrained. This system gives high gas dissolution rates but has a correspondingly high power consumption compared to conventional systems. The liquid and entrained gas can also be introduced into the fermenter through a 'bell' which holds the gas bubbles in contact with the circulating liquid to enhance the gas utilization. Both this and the plunging jet techniques are successfully used in biological water treatment.

5.5.1.2.1. Gas-lift and sparged tank fermenters

The fermenter has no mechanical stirrers and the power dissipation for mixing and gas dissolution is imparted by the movement of gases through the liquid medium. The gas from the compression systems is used as the source of power transmission. The design has been sorted to have some basic advantages over the conventional stirred tank fermenter like:

1. The absence of any rotating agitator shaft removes the major contamination risk at its entry point of the vessel.

2. The very large vessels require a high power input for the agitators and hence multiple agitators are required for proper stirring of the medium as a result the entry points are increased leading to higher risk levels for contamination.

3. The evaporation of water vapors as stream makes a small contribution to cooling of the fermentation.

The fermenter interior does, however need for a careful design so as to ensure that the movement pattern of the gas through the system produces sufficient agitation. It cannot be increased just by increasing the gas flow as there is the upper limit beyond which the quantity of liquid may be carried out of the vessel in the gas stream. This is expressed in terms of *superficial gas velocity* which is the velocity of gas attained if it passes through the empty vessel at a uniform rate; mathematically it is the volume gas flow-rate (m^3/s) divided by the cross sectional area of the vessel (m^2). At a high superficial gas velocities, the gas bubbles coalesce to form 'slugs' which not only carry liquid out of the system but also reduce the efficiency of the gas dissolution by reducing the gas-liquid interfacial area. Fitting horizontally helps in the breaking of the slugs and redisperse them as bubbles and liquid carry-over can be reduced by installing a disentertainment device before the gas outlet.

The point to be considered is that the superficial gas velocity is a scale-dependent parameter. In the case of the vessels with the same volume gas flow-rate per unit volume, increases proportionately to the vessel volume where as the superficial gas velocity increases proportionately with the cube root of the vessel volume, i.e. the large vessels operate closer to the limiting superficial gas velocity than smaller ones.

Two different designs are available or the air agitator systems, gas-lift (including air-lift) fermenters and the sparged tank (or bubble column) fermenter. In the latter the gas is introduced at the bottom through a single nozzle or a perforated or porous distributor plates. The gas bubble rises through the liquid in the vessel and may be redispersed by a succession of horizontal perforated baffle plates sited at the intervals up the column. Temperature controls are maintained by the temperature jacket or the internal coils. In the anaerobic digestion, the gas evolved can be recirculated through spargers to maintain homogeneity and enhance temperature control, but since gas dissolution is irrelevant, baffle plates are not used

In the gas-lift fermenters internal liquid circulation in the vessel is achieved by sparging only part of the vessel with gas. The sparged volume has a lower effective density than the bubble-free volume and the difference in the hydrostatic pressure between the two sections drive the liquid circulation upward in the sparged section and after gas disentertainment, it moves downwards in the bubble free section. The two sections may be separated by a vertical draught tube. Overall, the vessel acts more or less as a completely mixed system but within the circulation loop has the properties of a typical plug flow system as well.

5.5.2. Supported growth (surface culture systems)

This is a standard laboratory technique in which growing micro-organisms are cultured on the surface layer of the nutrient medium held in a dish or a tray, usually called as surface culture. Penicillin was originally produced by surface culture before being superseded by deep tank culture. Surface culture is still used for the industrial production of citric acid by the mould *Aspegillus niger* and for nicotanic acid by *Aspergillus terrus*. The mould is grown on the surface of a suitable medium such as molasses in shallow trays, kept in stacks in a constant temperature room with air blown over the trays to provide oxygen. This method is useful in utilizing low grade molasses.

Microbial films can be developed on the surfaces of a suitable packing medium. This can be in the form of a fixed bed, of stones, plastic pieces or ribbed plastic sheets, through which the nutrient liquid is trickled to contact the microbial film on the packing surfaces. This system is widely used in biological waste water treatment, and for aerobic processes, the liquid flowing rate is normally kept low enough to leave room in the packing for circulation of air to supply oxygen. For anaerobic or anoxic processes, the packing is flooded and held in a closed container. Such closed systems can be used for aerobic processes, with air sparged directly into the flooded packing or by predissolving the high purity oxygen into the nutrient liquid field. Vinegar can be made by trickling dilute ethanol solution, beer or wine, through a bed of beach wood shavings on which a culture of acetobector develops. As an alternative to trickling the nutrient liquid through the packing, the packing can be moved through the liquid. This moving bed approach can be effected in two ways;

(a) as a fluidized bed

(b) as a coherent moving bed

In **fluidized beds,** the biological film is developed on particles which are suspended in an upward flow of liquid in which they are then free to circulate. Thus a fluidized bed has features of both, suspended and supported growth systems. The support particles can be solids such as sand or glass beads or porous such as plastic or stainless steel mesh. Porous particles allow growth within the particle as well as on the surface and they have been used successfully in the pilot scale production of citric acid by *A. foetidus*. Among the advantages of fluidized bed include avoidance of blocking of the packing by luxuriant biological growth which happens with fixed packed beds, and the loss of biomass by 'washout' which can happen in continuos suspended growth systems. Oxygen supply of fluidized beds can pose problems, and they are most readily used in anaerobic processes such as brewing, or in anoxic processes, such as denitrification, or where the oxygen demand is very low, as in drinking water treatment. For aerobic systems, oxygen can be supplied by the predissolution of high purity oxygen in the feed stream to the process. Fixed and fluidized bed systems are also used in immobilized enzymes and immobilized cell reactors.

The **Coherent moving bed systems** have the packing with its associated microbial film mounted on a shaft and rotating in the bath of nutrient media. The packing may be affixed bed type held in a cage or in the form of the disc. Closed versions of this have been developed for aseptic aerobic operation and for anoxic denitrification of washed water.

Tray reactors: The growth rate of the microorganisms is having a direct correlation with the rate of nutrient substrate when grown on solid nutrient substrate. This obstacle has been overcame by introduction of 'fermenter tray process' in which a liquid is used in place of jelly-like nutrient medium. The process is applicable only to the culture which can float on the surface. It is intended that once the closed culture is prepared the liquid could be replaced by a fresh one so as to make the process continuous. Figure 5.8 shows the reactor.

Film reactor: These reactor/fermenter are based on the solid packing support/bodies of regular (or even irregular) structures vertically arranged in bundles of tubes or channels upon which the nutrient solution is distributed from above. The air of incubation as a rule fed in at the bottom so that counter current flow condition are generated.

Immobilized cells : All 'surface fermenters' which supply cells settled on the solid surface with feeds of nutrient solution and gas works basically with immobilized cells. This method has been utilized due to the reason that it prevented the washing out of cells in continuous fermentation even at high dilution rates. The method offers the advantage of lowering the ratio of necessary production of cell mass to amount of substrate converted. The method has been further expanded by introducing particles upon which the mycelium can grow into submerged reactors. The particles could be restrained within the reactor by means of sieves or continuous centrifugation.

The fermenters or bioreactors belonging to various categories could be compared based on the mechanism of working, agitation speed as well as the product to be obtained (Fig. 5.9).

5.6. FERMENTER DESIGNS

Environment sensitive processes require a closed and a controlled environment to be maintained within the fermenter however, maintaining an aseptic entry and outlet for the nutrient media, air and control fluids and provision for heating , cooling and agitation. However, these fermenters are highly maintainable as compared to the chemical reactors in terms of corrosion and contamination. The fermenter design is quite simple and a lot of efforts have been devoted for an efficient fermenter design so as to increase the versatility of the process and hence to evolve a generalized design for a fermenter to be applicable to all the biological processes. The current intensive development in biotechnology will undoubtedly affect the design and will lead to the development of the novel processes whose technology will be used to modify the conservative design.

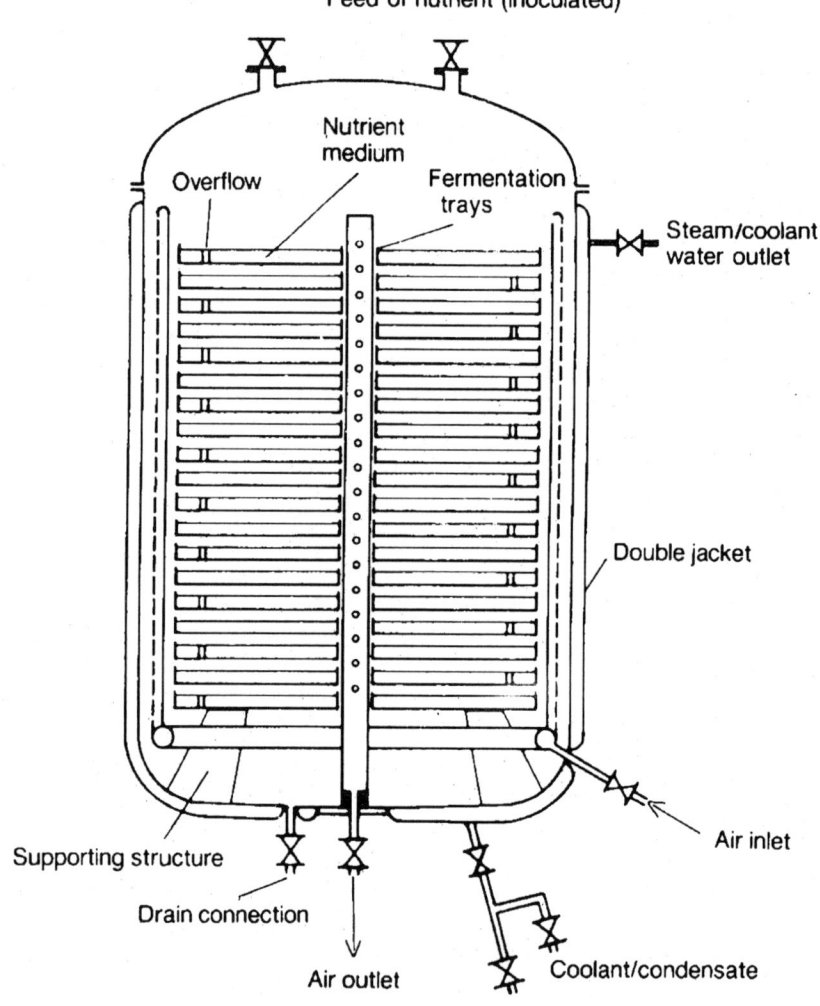

Fig 5.8: Tray fermenter as a continuous process

5.6.1. Fundamental rules in designing of a fermenter

The fundamental grounds for the design and construction of aseptically operated plant are based on the precept that micro-organism are extremely small with dimensions much less than normal engineering tolerance that is a satisfactory tight closed container in a non-biological process could afford ample space for the passage of micro-organisms. This leads to a conclusion that strictly aseptic conditions have to be maintained however, the maintenance of such conditions leads to high expenses and inconvenience in construction, operation and maintenance of plant.

In order to maintain aseptic operation the mechanical integrity of the plant should be maintained. Entry points to the aseptic region of the plant such as mechanical seals for agitators and pump shafts, valve closures, probe insertions, sample ports and joints are loci of contamination risks and should be as few in number as possible. The structure as far as possible should not be all welded with mechanical closures, however flanged, O screw joints etc. can be replaced by welded joints.

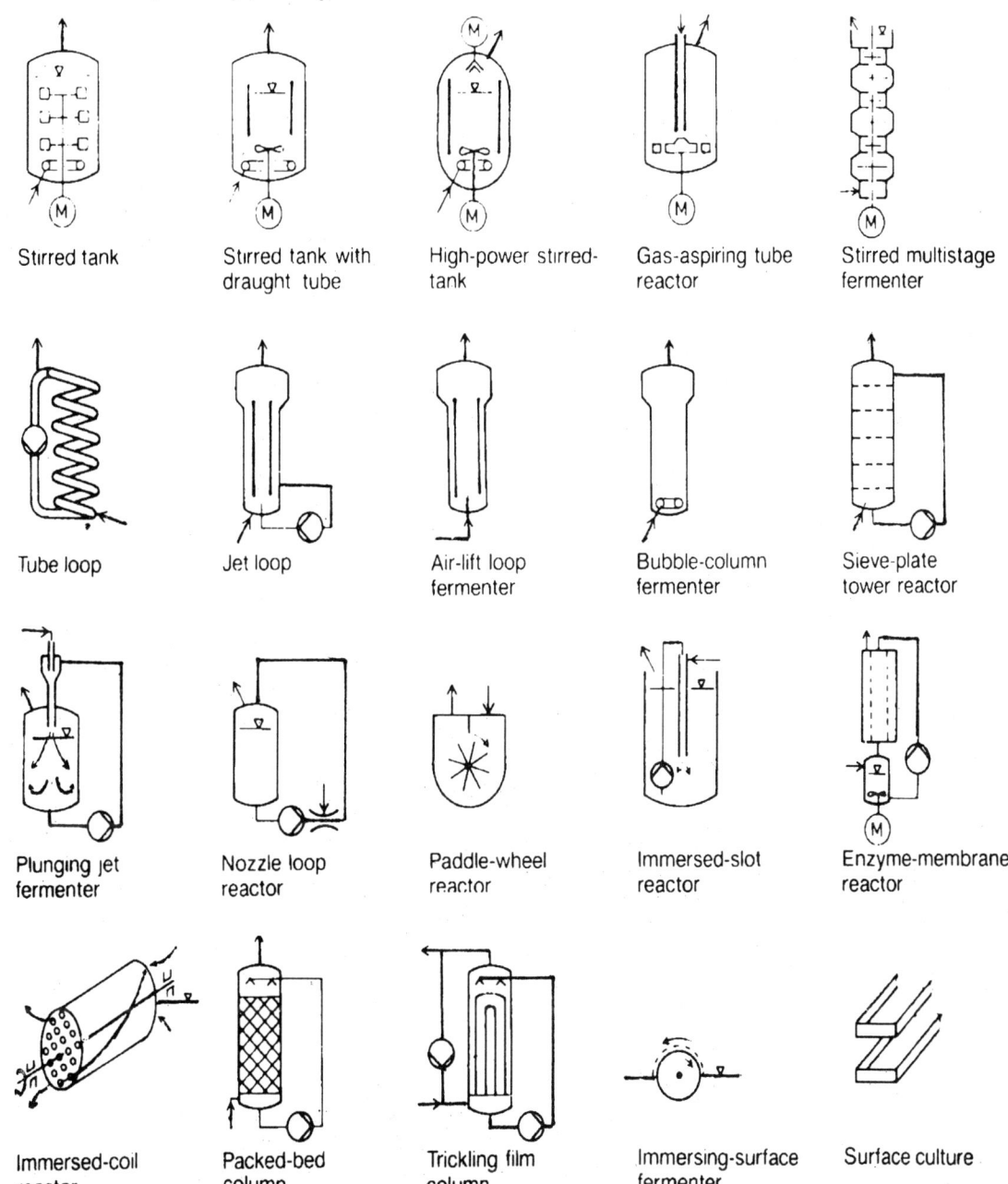

Fig. 5.9 : Comparative presentation of various fermenters / bioreactors

The resulting maintenance problem where removal and replacement of a component involves cutting and re-welding is justified by avoidance of contamination. Where ever such closures are not possible there should be a steam box surrounding the joint. All other connections to the aseptic region of the plant should be steam sealed, including the glands of the valves used to control liquid flow in the pipe and steam flow in the pipe and steam flow to the steam lock and there should be no connection between the sterile and non sterile section of the plant. Figure 5.10 shows the simple steam locks.

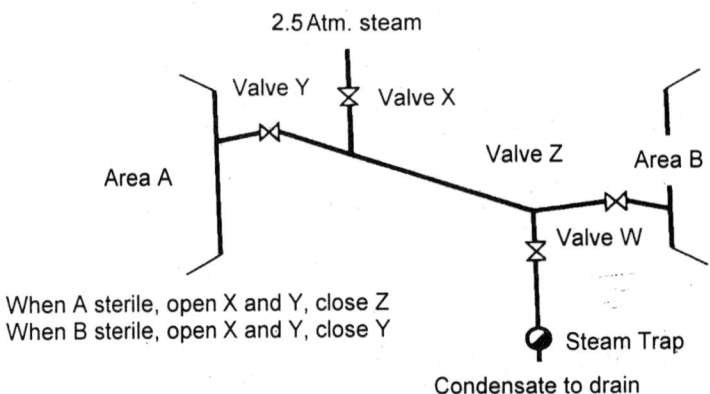

When A sterile, open X and Y, close Z
When B sterile, open X and Y, close Y

Fig 5.10: Simple example of steam lock

Pipeline should be kept under steam when not in use and should be constructed to slope to a definite drain point so that stagnant liquid cannot accumulate at any point. The steam is fed at top of the slope and the condensate is allowed to drain through a steam trap at the drain point. The general design should also avoid stagnant regions, dead spaces, pockets, pipe branches and cervices which cannot only collect stagnant liquid and micro-organisms but also difficult to sterilize effectively. Such areas are also more liable to corrosion.

5.6.2. Materials and components

Suitable grade of stainless steel is one of the most common type of construction material used in the production scale fermenters. Different formulations of steal with differing mechanical strength, corrosion resistance, ease of fabrication, availability and cost effectively are available and could be selected according to the requirement of the operation. Stainless steal is the most reliable than the ordinary mild steal due to its high mechanical strength as well as corrosion resistance due to the chromium oxide layer and its resistance to the oxidizing conditions. Some of its drawbacks are the ease of damage by the reducing agents, chlorides and high cost as well as difficulty to weld. The alloy containing 18% chromium, 8% nickel and 3% molybdenum is refereed as the best one.

Valves are needed to regulate fluid flow and should be capable of handling hot and cold liquids possibly containing suspended solids and steam. They represent for an infection risk point since they inevitably involve a joint or mechanical closure. Diaphragm valves are widely used in fermentation, or for strictly aseptic conditions, a piston valve with a steam sealed gland is used.

Pumps should be avoided wherever possible hence as an alternative the gravitational movement for the flow of fluids should be utilized as there are moving components which could serve for contamination risk points. However wherever necessary they could be supplemented with an intermediate sterilization stage. Centrifugal pumps are commonly used in the biological industry with a seal on the rotating drive shaft and for strictly aseptic operation steam sealed piston pumps are commonly utilized.

Furthermore, in order to impart flexibility to the operation the main plant section should be capable of independent sterilization but must be connected through a steam lock to prevent unsterilized plant to be connected to sterile plant. As shown in the figure 5.10 the valves are protected by circulating steam through their glands. A full scale plant should have a large number of such locks so that sterilization of units and transfer of material round the plant involves hundreds of sequential operations of valves, instruments and pumps. in such cases a computerized controls could serve effectively to ensure the precise sequence .

In the case of aerobic biological process the major requirement is of a perfectly sterile air supply. A typical fermentation batch has to be supplied with hundreds of tons of perfectly microbe free air. The most effective method to achieve this is the utilization of deep fibrous filters for rendering air free of contaminating micro-organisms. The effect of the depth of the pad on the particle removal is logarithmic, i.e. each unit depth of the pad removes the same proportion of the passing particles from the air in an exponential fashion. The pads are routinely cleaned and sterilized by passing steam through it. The simplest example of these filters are the HEPA (high efficiency particulate air filters) made of the membranous fibrous supports. These filters have got the pores so as to retain the bacterial particulate form the air i.e. a pore size of 0.22μm and hence resulting in an absolute sterilization of the air. These filter media are made up of high tensile cellulosic fibers, unglazed ceramics, and porous plastics.

5.6.3. Selection of the fermenter

The selection of the type, size, mode of operation and the pattern of the fermenter to be used in the particular biological process is based on the following characteristic of the biological process which are predetermined ones:

5.6.3.1. Characteristics of the microorganisms to be used

The mode of operation depends substantially on the type and the stability of the microbe stain. The operation conditions are decisively selected by the factor that the stain is aerobic or anaerobic. In the breeding of the aerobic strains adequate amounts of the oxygen is required. Since the solubility of the oxygen in the medium is low and hence it should be available at a continuos rate. The size and the shape of the cells also have considerable effect on the design of the fermenter. Spherical cells are usually smaller and less sensitive to shear than the filamentous organisms. The former needs a higher degree of dispersion of the air than the filamentous mycelia. Small dimensions ensure a high surface to volume ratio and a high rate off uptake of substrate and therefore a rapid growth. Aerobic cells with high rates of growth exhibit high rates of oxygen consumption.

Many organisms tend to grow on the surfaces. In the case of metabolite-producing organisms or of sewage treatment, these properties may be desirable if continuos operation is required. If this property is pronounced than the surface reactors must be used. In general the film formation is not desirable. If cells show a tendency to grow on the surface, the formation of the stagnant region at the surface must be avoided by a suitable fermenter design.

5.6.3.2. Characteristics predetermined by the properties of the Medium

The choice of the strain generally determines not only the culture medium but also exerts a pronounced influenced on the choice of reactor The characteristics of the medium such as physical properties, biokinetics , difficulty in sterilization, rheological behaviour are the most important properties to be considered for the selection of the reactor. The physical properties of the substrate used generally differ like gaseous (e.g., methane), liquid and water-soluble (e.g., methanol, ethanol), solid and water-soluble (e.g., glucose, lactose), liquid and water-insoluble (e.g., gas-oil and paraffin) and solid and sparingly soluble or insoluble in water (e.g. starch, cellulose). On the other hand the biokinetic effects of the substrate or the products also affect the choice of reactor. In the case of substrates showing inhibition or repression of growth, the process is carried out either in semicontinuous operation with sustained feed of the substrate ("extended culture" or "fed batch culture") or in a continuous culture. In the case of the thermolabile components of the medium requires special measures and, frequently, separate sterilization of these materials.

The rheological behavior of the medium has very great influence. An increasing in viscosity may influence in the rheological properties of the medium, which may arise together:

- The secretion of highly viscous products, e.g., pullulan and xanthan particularly in batch operation at the end of the formation of product;

- High concentration of substrate; and

- The morphology of the organisms.

When substrate or product is responsible for the high viscosity, the medium frequently has a new-toning behavior. A high apparent viscosity due to the morphology of the organisms is almost always associated with a non-Newtonian behavior.

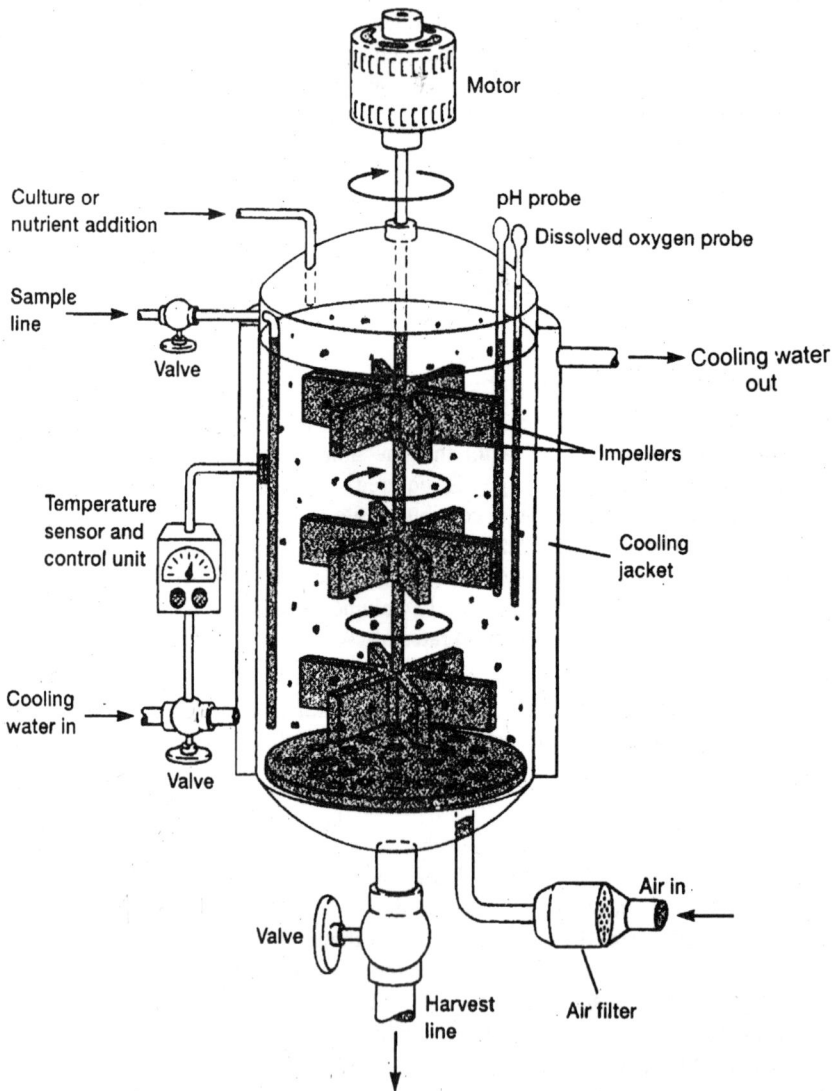

Fig. 5.11 : An industrial fermenter and its accessories

5.6.3.3. Characteristics predetermined by the parameters of the biomedical process

A fundamental factor influencing the choice of the fermenter in the cultivation of aerobic organisms is the specific oxygen transfer rate in the medium. In the case of the continuos fermentation the processes are never carried out in the regime of unlimited growth, since here the fermenter is unstable. The rate of growth and of the product formation are temperature dependent. Consequently the cultivation and the formation of the product are usually carried out at controlled temperatures. To facilitate the removal of the process heat from the fermenter to the cooling water, the highest possible temperature and hence the use of thermophilic organisms is favorable. As the volume of the fermenter is increased a limit is reached at which the heat produced cannot be removed solely via the cooling jacket.

The pH of the cell cultivation is determined by the optimum pH desired for reaction. The lowest possible pH f꞉vorable in order to suppress any infection by the organisms.

Table 5.8 : Fermentation based commercial products

Product	Microorganism
Industrial chemicals	
Ethanol (from glucose)	*Saccharomyces cerevisiae*
Ethanol (from lactose)	*Kluyveromyces fragilis*
Citric acid	*Aspergillus niger*
Gluconic acid	*Aspergillus niger*
Acetic acid	*Acetobacter spp.*
Lactic acid	*Lactobacillus delbrueckii*
Amino acids	
L-lysine	*Corynebacterium glutamicum*
MSG	*C. glutamicum*
Glutamic acid	*C. glutamicum*
Vitamins	
Riboflavin	*Ashbya gossypi*
Vitamin B_{12}	*Pseudomonas denitrificans*
Ascorbic acid (L-sorbose)	*Gluconobecter oxidans*
Enzymes	
Amylase	*Aspergillus oryzae*
Cellulase	*Trichoderma reesii*
Invertase	*Saccharomyces cerevisiae*
Lipase	*Saccharomyces lipolytica*
Protease	*Bacillus*
Polysaccarides	
Dextran	*Leuconostoc mesenteroids*
Xanthan gum	*Xanthomones compestris*
Pharmaceuticals	
Penicillin	*Penicillium chrysogenum*
Cephalosporin	*Cephalosporium acemonium*
Amphotericin B	*Streptomyces nodosus*
Kanamycin	*Streptomyces kanamyceticus*
Neomycin	*Streptomyces fradiae*
Streptomycin	*Streptomyces griseus*
Gramicidin S	*Bacillus brevis*
Polymyxin	*B. polymxa*
Chroamphenicol	*Streptomyces venezuelae or chemical synthesis*
Erythromycin	*Streptomyces erythreus*
Steriodal transformations	*Rizopus nigricans*
Steriodal transformations	*Arthrobacter simplex*
Viva A (adenine arabinoside)	*Streptomyces antibiotioticus*

5.6.3.4. Characteristics predetermined by the site

The choice of the fermenter depends on the production site. A number of factors which are repressible for its determination are:

1. Trading facilities for the product as well as the raw material.
2. Market features (stable sales-single product works or when a variable sales a flexible plant is required).
3. Availability of the raw material and their supply.
4. The cost of the raw material and the labor (skilled or unskilled).
5. Cost of the energy and cooling water.
6. The economical use of the by products.
7. Working and safety regulations.

All these aspects have to be carefully scanned and then the choice of the fermenter is to made.

In general depending on the size of the production to be planned, the number of fermenter units should not fall bellow a minimum. However the plant should be capable of producing more than one product so that an economical utilization the same could be assured. Experience proves that although the plant is utilized for a single product however a flexible design comprising of considerable reserves for the flows of materials and drives must be utilized.

The correct manipulation of the parameters as well as the choice of the producing strain and media composition is the major consideration so as to achieve a high yield in the fermentation production.

SUGGESTED READINGS

Aharonowitz, Y. and Cohen, G. (1981), **Sci. Am.**, 245, 140-152.

Atkinson, B. and Mavitana, F. (1991) **Biochemical Engineering and Biotechnology Hand Book**, Stockton Press, New York.

Chang, L.T., Terasaka, D.T. and Elander, R.P., (1992) **Development in Industrial Microbiology**, Vol-23.

Davis, B.D., (1949) Proceedings National Academey of Science, USA, ,35, 1-10

Demain, A.L. (1981) **Science**, 214, 987-995.

Fiechter, A. (1978) **Dechema Monogr.**, 82, 17.

Hochfeld, W. L. (1994) **Growth and Synthesis Fermanters, Bioreactors, and Biomolecular Synthesisers**, Interpharm Press Inc., Buffalo Grove, IL.

Hodgkin, D.C., Pickworth, J., Robertson, J.H., Tru blood, K.N., Prosen, R,J., White, R., Bonnette, R., Cannon, J.R., Johnson, A.W., Suther Land, I., Todd, A.R. and Smith, E.L. (1955) **Nature**, 176, 325-330.

Hollaender, A (Ed.) (1982) **Genetic Engineering of Micro-organisms for chemicals**, Plenum Pres, London.

Hopwood, D.A., (1979) **Genetics of Industrial Microorganisms**, Sebek, O.K. and Laskin, A., I (Eds), American Society for Microbiology, Washington.

Nakayama, K., Kituda, S. and Kinoshita, S., (1961) **Journal of General and Applied Microbiology**, 7, 41-51.

Prave, P., Faust, V., Sitting, W., Sukatsch, D.A. (1987) **Fundamentals of Biotechnology**, VCH, Germany

Prekop, A., Erckson, L.E., Frenandez, J. and Humphery, A.E., (1969) **Biotechnol. Bioeng.**, 11, 945.

Prescott, S.C. and Dunn, C.G. (1959) **Industrial Microbiology**, III Ed., McGraw-Hill Book Co. Inc., New York.

Riviere, J., (1986) **Industrial Applications of Microbiology**, Halstead Press, New York.

Stanier, Roger, Y.,Ingraham, J.L., Wheelis, M.L and Painter. P. R., (1987), **General Microbiology**, 5 Ed, Macmillan Education Ltd., London.

Taguchi, H. (1971) **Adv. Biochem. Eng.**, 1.

Trehan, K. (1994) **Biotechnology**, Wiley Eastern Ltd., New Delhi, 17-102.

Vandamme, E.J.(Ed.) (1984) **Biotechnology of Industrial Antibiotics**, I Ed., Marcel Dekker Inc., New York.

BIOTECH IN NEWS . . . .

New Vaccine to counter Typhoid...

With typhoid now seriously resistant to common antibiotics, doctors advice a new-generation vaccine as the best way to counter the pestilence. Thanks to indiscriminate use of antibiotics in India, Multi-Drug Resistant Typhoid (MDRST) has reached epidemic proportions and some strains are now resistant to Chloromphenicol, Ampicillin and Co-trimoxazole, says a Heart Care Foundation of India (HCFI) paper.

Although the WHO classifies typhoid as a diarrhoeal disease it is a serious blood disease and victims are likely to have constipation as diarrhoea. In such a scenario, the importance of vaccination rather than antibiotic treatment, has grown and mercifully there is now available in India a single-shot vaccination, "Typhim-vi" which directly addresses typhoid as a blood-disease. The blood poisoning or septicaemia caused by typhoid is linked to the vi-antigen, and germs isolated from the blood of patients with typhoid fever invariably possess the vi-antigen. This means that vi is essential for the survival of salmonella typhi in the blood, according to the HCFI paper, which also said the antigen gives the germ resistance to phagocytes and to the natural bactericidal effects of serum. It is the vi-antigen which allows the bacteria to penetrate into the blood where through the joint action of endotoxins and speticemic diffusion, the typhoid germ produces typhoid fever.

For effective protection against typhoid, anti-vi antibodies are essential according to WHO trials, and only the new vaccine, Typhim-vi, confers this, the HCFI paper said. There are several advantages of Typhim-vi in Indian conditions, foremost among them being that the temporary increase of storage temperature as a result of breakage in the transport and storage "cold chain" does not affect its efficacy. Because of its purity, Typhim-vi is well-tolerated and it produces fewer local and systematic reactions than the earlier injectable whole cell vaccines and this makes it deal for public health programmes. Large-scale vaccinations during epidemics using Typhim-vi can be effective while groups like travellers can be vaccinated a short while before departure. Also Typhim-vi is well-tolerated by children.

. . . . . . *The Hindustan Time, New Delhi, dated 05/05/'97.*

6

FERMENTATION: INDUSTRIAL PRODUCTS

6.1. ANTIBIOTICS

The research efforts made in the field of antibiotics research has been undulating, where following the discovery of penicillin, amazingly no other antibiotic was introduced into the market for quite some time. Thus with the introduction of second generation lactam type antibodies, the research in particularly revitalized. Thus conferring thence time as if golden era in antibiotic research. Since the discovery of penicillin in 1942, more than 5,500 natural microbial compounds which display antibiotic activity have been discovered. Only a relatively small number of these products has found to be practically applicable; about 150 antibiotic compounds are currently being produced exclusively by the fermentation process. These antibiotics have distinct and find applications in medical, veterinary and agriculture practices.

    The term antibiotic appeared as early as 1928 in the French microbiological literature related to antibiotics. The word antibiotic in its present retrospective meaning- 'a biosynthetic product of microbial origin which has the capacity of inhibiting growth, and even distorting other micro-organisms in dilute solutions'. Although most of the antibiotics are produced by fermentation, however, to discuss all in detail is beyond the scope of the book. Some of the important antibiotics with their production strategy are discussed here.

6.1.1. Tetracycline

It is now 30 years since tetracycline has been discovered as an antibiotic. Biological research till date has been focused on its production organism (morphological and physiological studies, improvement procedures, genetic analysis, etc.), on biosynthetic and its metabolic and genetic controls, on the mechanism of antibiotic action and origin of resistance as well as on various pharmacological aspects of tetracycline application. Table 6.1 shows the chemistry of tetracyclines.

Table 6.1: Chemistry of tetracyclines

NAME	R^2	R^5	R^6	$R^{6'}$	R^7
Chlortetracycline	H	H	OH	CH_3	Cl
Oxytetracycline	H	OH	OH	CH_3	H
Tetracycline	H	H	OH	CH_3	H
Demeclocycline	H	H	OH	CH_3	H
Methacycline	H	OH		$=CH_2$	H
Doxycycline	H	OH	H	CH_3	H
Minocycline	H	H	H	H	$N(CH_3)_2$

6.1.1.1. Strain improvement and genetics of tetracycline producers

Tetracyclines are produced mainly by *S. aureofaciens* and *S. rimosus*. With the recent advents of newer technologies, it is now possible that the production of tetracycline could be increased many folds by utilizing various breeding techniques. As discussed in the previous chapter on Fermentation : A general consideration, the strain improvement technique, i.e. mutation could be utilized. In the case of tetracycline the technique, could increase the antibiotic titer by 30-500%, depending on the strain, the mutagen and a number of selection steps. The best results were obtained with the mutagens like UV light, ethyleneimine, X-rays, Υ-radiation and nitrogen mustards, alone or in combinations. Further, by utilizing an appropriate selection systems like, isolation of prototrophin revertants from auxotrophs, producing revertants of non producing mutants, etc., some good strains for better selection were developed, however, the hybridoma techniques could not contribute much in the strain improvement as compared to the mutational selection. All the above results were obtained in basic research using strains with antibiotic titer value of 3000µg/ml. No data till date is available regarding improving high antibiotic producing industrial strains of *S. aureofaciens* and *S. rimosus*.

As far as the genetics of the organism is concerned, the circular linkage map of *S. rimosus* for nutritional marker has been constructed. The oxytetracycline production in biosynthesis of tetracycline takes place due to some loci present in lower arc of the map but further conversion takes place due to some genes located on small chromosomal segments located between markers i.e., ProA and adeA. Results of experiments with plasmid-curing agent indicate that extrachromosomal DNA participates in biosynthesis of oxytetracycline. Still further study is required regarding genetic manipulations of the tetracycline producing strains.

6.1.1.2. Fermentation processes

As compared to the abundant literature available on medical and technological applications of tetracyclines, references on process technology are rather scant. This is surprising as the tetracyclines are in the hundred million dollar fraternity. The fermentation technology of five of the principle tetracycline antibiotics was protected by 33 US patents. Most of the patents reported tetracycline yields up to hundred or thousands of µg/ml of fermenter broth, the existing industrial yield are above 20,000 µg/ml following about 200 hours of fermentation.

6.1.1.2.1. Equipment

The fermentation tanks described previously can be utilized for an appropriate production of tetracyclines. However, for proper growth, a fermenter should provide facility for oxygen supply (0.4-0.8 µ mol/liter per min.) in a fermenter of 100-150 m³ working volume. It should have three open turbines 1460-2100 mm in diameter and maximum speed of 80 rpm, and a power input of 300 kW at the axle which corresponds to 3 kW/m³ of fermented broth. Variable revolution stirrers are often advantageous, so as to solve the inverse relationship between oxygen transfer into the liquid by the stirrer and the shear stress of the biomass, and they can better cope with foam formation particularly when the stirrer cannot be switched off. The supply of oxygen should be carefully monitored for proper yield of tetracycline.

6.1.1.2.2. Preparation of inoculum

For prolonged preservation, the strains for industrial fermenters are maintained either by freeze drying or at liquid nitrogen temperature as spore stock. A step wise flow sheet (Fig. 6.1) shows the preparation of *S. aureofaciens* inoculum.

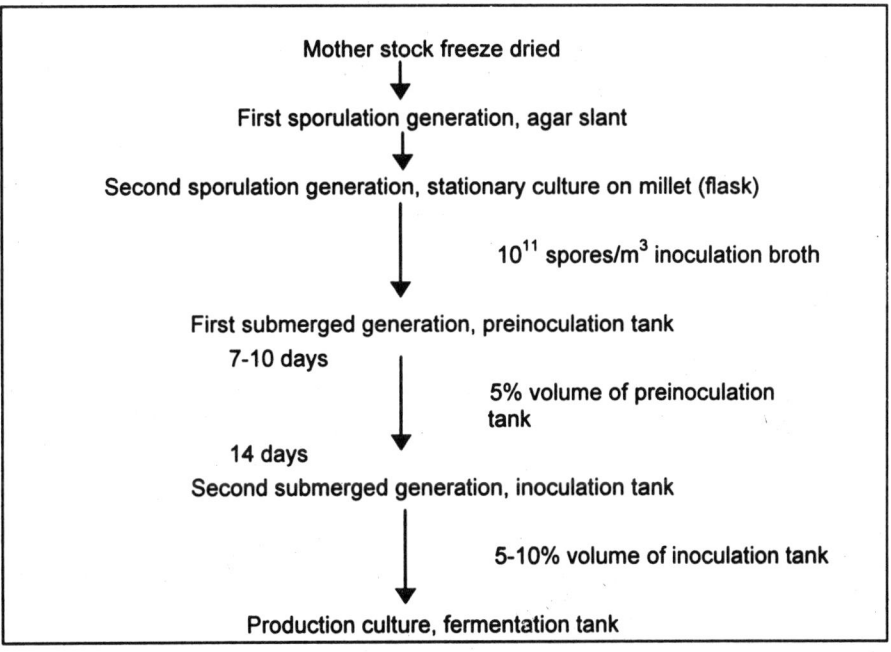

Fig. 6.1: Preparation of inoculum

A temperature of 29°C is suitable for fermentation. The composition of inoculum medium is similar to that in the production tank. The nutrient media is composed of :

Carbohydrate sucrose and maltose	2.5% w/v
Organic nitrogen source soyabean meal or corn steep liquor	1.7% w/v
Buffer; calcium carbonate and inorganic salts (NaCl & KH₂PO₄)	0.2-0.3% w/v
Vegetable oil	0.2% w/v

The culture is monitored for pH, residual sugar, respiration (CO_2) and increase of biomass both in volume and morphology.

6.1.1.2.3. Nutrients

Commercially produced strains utilize sucrose (molasses), starch or technical glucose as cheap carbon sources. Starch being a polysaccharide is particularly suitable for prolonged fermentation of about 200 hours. The organic nitrogen sources include corn-steep, Soya bean meal, peanut meal. Calcium carbonate not only helps in maintaining pH, but also binds the formed antibiotic from the heterogeneous phase of complexes insoluble above 1500 μg/ml and thus decreases the inhibitory effect of their own products on the product ions. Animal or vegetable lipids are used as antifoaming agents and even as carbon sources. Chloride ions serve as processors of chlortetracycline biosynthesis, while benzyl thiocyanate is used as an inhibitor of undesirable metabolic pathway particularly during lack of oxygen.

6.1.1.2.4. Process parameters in production

The sterilization of liquid nutrient broth is undertaken either at 120°C for 40 minutes or at 140°C in 1 min interval (carbon and nitrogen separately). Stirring uses 2.5-5 kW/ m³ medium, revolutions can be varied up to a peripheral velocity of the propeller equal to 500m/min., aeration ranges up to 0.8 medium vol./min., and oxygen over pressure up to 0.1M psi. The temperature (29±1°C), pH, oxygen content of medium (at least 20% saturation), and CO_2 in outcoming air are monitored continuously.

6.1.1.2. 5. Product recovery and purification

The major aspect of isolation process focuses around the amphotropic nature of the substance and the possibility of their polymerization and rearrangement. A dozens of cases have been reported with different methods of isolation and purification of various tetracyclines as reported in various patents. Some of them are compiled herewith and presented below:

   i. Adsorption on diatomaceous earth or active charcoal.

   ii. Chromatography or selective extraction.

   iii. Extraction from acid or alkaline medium. The most frequently used extraction agent is 1-butanol, owing to its suitable partition coefficient and economic availability.

   iv. Direct mesh extraction based on solubilization of the antibiotic by acidification, precipitation of Ca^{2+} with ammonium compounds as carriers, and extraction of metabolites with an organic solvent usually one of methyl alkyl ketone type.

   v. Precipitation (dry salt) process based on precipitating the antibiotic from dilute aqueous solution of aryl azosulfonic acid dyes. Tetracyclines are precipitated as complexes with alkaline earth metal compounds or with primary and secondary alkyl amine.

   vi. Solvent extraction of antibiotic with salt, based on salting out (NaCl) of the antibiotic from the aqueous to the organic phase (1-butanol). This method is also suited for refining of a crude product.

The preparations are purified by crystallization as salts (e.g., hydrochlorides) or bases. Particularly efficient is crystallization from boiling solvent, such as lower alcohols, ketones or aliphatic ethers of ethylene glycol, which yield non-hygroscopic preparations. The specific crystal surface depends upon temperature, stirring and pH value.

6.1.2. Streptomycin

Aminoglycoside antibiotics form a major group of products utilized in the treatment of mycobacterium infections. Streptomycin is the most important product of this group. The aminoglycoside antibiotics (or aminosides) possess an aminocyclitol, linked to one or several sugars which are in most cases ammoniated. The first aminoglycoside antibiotic discovered, was streptomycin, isolated from culture broth of an *Actinomyces*, *Streptomyces griseus*, by Waksman and associates. The therapeutic importance of these antibiotics is due to their highly potent nature as compared to other antibiotics reported so far. They are having a very broad spectrum of antimicrobial activity, i.e. they are active against both gram negative as well as gram positive bacteria. Furthermore, their main use is due to their bactericidal activity against *Mycobacterium*. Hence, they are in wide clinical use despite of their severe side effects, viz. nephrotoxicity, ototoxicity, etc. The other antibiotics except streptomycin of this group are kanamycin, novamycin, spectinomycin, gentamycin, lividomycin, neomycin, etc.

The first structural elucidation of streptomycin was done by Kuehl et al.. He showed that the molecule looks like a trisaccharide and is formed from three subunits an aminocyclitol, the streptidine linked to a disaccharide streptobiosamine, composed of α-streptose and N-methyl-α-glucosamine. Table 6.2 shows the structure of streptomycin and some semisynthetic derivatives of commercial utilization. Table 6.3 presents the list of most of the main micro-organisms utilized in producing streptomycin and its two important derivatives. All of them are *Streptomyces*. Within them the most famous is the *Streptomyces griseus*.

6.1.2.1. Production Technology

The industrial streptomycin is prepared by fermentation tanks of 100 to 200 m^3; it is then isolated and purified through various methods.

Table 6.2: Chemistry of streptomycin

Name of antibiotic	R$_1$	R$_2$	R$_3$	R$_4$	R$_5$
Streptomycin	CHO	OH	H	CH$_3$	H
Dihydrostreptomycin	CH$_2$OH	OH	H	CH$_3$	H
Hydroxystreptomycin	CHO	OH	OH	CH$_3$	H
N-Demethylstreptomycin	CHO	OH	H	H	H
Deoxydihydrostreptomycin	CH$_2$OH	H	H	CH$_3$	H
Mannosidostreptomycin	CHO	OH	H	CH$_3$	M*
Mannosidohydrostreptomycin	CH$_2$OH	OH	H	CH$_3$	M*

6.1.2.1.1. Strains

Since Waksman's discovery and thereafter up to the present date, the industrial productivity of streptomycin using *S. griseus* strain has increased over 100 folds by using classical programs of mutation involving physicochemical agents.

Table 6.3 : Different producers of streptomycin and their derivatives

Antibiotic	Producer strain
Streptomycin	*S. griseus*
Streptomycin	*S. bikiniensis*
Streptomycin	*S. clivaceus*
Streptomycin	*S. rameus*
Streptomycin	*S. galbus*
Streptomycin	*S. erythrochromogenus var. narutoensis*
Dihydrostreptomycin	*S. humidus*
Hydroxystreptomycin	*S. grisecarneus*
Hydroxystreptomycin	*S. subrutilus*

Another attempt to increase the productivity was made by varying the culture conditions so as to achieve better yield. An overview of culture media manipulations for selected mutants so as to increase yields are presented in table 6.4.

Table 6.4 : Improvement of streptomycin production by *S. griseus*

Culture media	Yield (gm/lit)
Glucose-peptone-meat extract	0.1
Glucose-proline	1
Glucose-yeast-ammonium sulfate	1
Glucose-soyabean-distiller's soluble	1
Glucose-soyabean-yeast	2
Glucose-soyabean	3.4
Glucose-soyabean-ammonium sulfate	5-10
Glucose-ammonium sulfate	1.3

6.1.2.1.2. Culture media

Similar to the other fermentation producers a nutrient media should contain carbon source, nitrogen source and some essential minerals. Among carbohydrates the starting point in streptomycin fermentation; glucose has always been the product of choice for its production. However, other simple or complex sugars, i.e. fructose, maltose, lactose, dextrin, starch, etc. can be used.

Most of the industrial strains require complex nitrogen source for optimum production. In beginning Waksman used peptone and meat extract, but Rake and Donovik showed that the soyabean flour could be much more favorable, besides, it is more economical. No nitrogen source has been exploited for use since then. The stimulating effect of ammonium ions on the production has been known for long times and it is recently been utilized. Other rich nitrogen sources such as corn steep liquor, distiller's soluble, are sometimes added to complement soyabean flour. Some of the commercially available culture media are listed with their components in table 6.5.

Table 6.5: Composition of some culture media used in streptomycin production

Nutrient	Schartz media	Rake and Donovik's media	Merck's media	Singh's media
Glucose	10	10	10	60 (+10)*
Peptone	5	--	--	--
Meat extract	3	--	--	--
Soyabean extract	--	10	20	--
Distiller's soluble	--	--	--	30
Corn- steep (100% solid)	--	--	--	
Ammonium sulfate	--	--	--	4
Sodium chloride	5	5	10	9(+ 1.5)*
Potassium dihydrogen phosphate	--	--	--	2.5
				0.025
Calcium carbonate	--	--	--	0.5
Soyabean oil	--	--	--	7

* complementary addition during the fermentation

Various other substances are present which stimulate the production but their beneficial effect is particularly noticeable when low production strains and synthetic media are used. These are:

(i) Barbital: It delays mycelium lysis in the end of fermentation and hence prolongs antibiotic secretion.

(ii) Factor A: a component secreted by streptomycin producing strains, that stimulates both production of streptomycin and formation of spores.

(iii) Sclerine: favorable effects on the production.

(iv)Myoinositol: the precursor of streptidine subunit of the streptomycin molecule.

6.1.2.1.3. *Process parameters*

The precise fermentation conditions vary with the strains and nutrients used, in the scale up considerations and to provide 'know-how' proper to each manufacturer. However, the general outline is based on small scale production method described by Singh et al.

The laboratory operation starts with; spores which are kept lyophilized and usually mixed with soil are spread on soyabean flour admixed with agar medium, in petri dish or Roxus bottles. After 2-3 weeks of incubation at 27°C, the culture obtained is well sporulated. The spores are harvested and used to prepare the inoculum intended to seed the fermenter. The laboratory scale fermentation has been represented schematically in figure 6.2.

The inoculum is usually processed in two stages, the first one in the laboratory, in 0.5-2 litre flasks and agitated on a shaker and the second one in a fermenter. In both the cases, the composition of the medium is relatively close to that of the medium of production; temperature is maintained at about 26°C, the duration of culture varying from 2 to 4 days. The production fermenter is then inoculated at a rate of 5-10% (v/v) per minute. The pH, which is around 7.0 at the start, is mostly maintained in the range of 6.5-7.5 during the course of the fermentation, which can last up to 8 days. Vigorous agitation and much aeration are necessary to obtain good streptomycin production yields. In case of restricted aeration, glucose is rapidly consumed, with the formation of lactate and pyruvate, and as a result streptomycin production is lower. Excess of phosphate in the medium leads to a similar situation.

The fermentation has a biphasic characteristics, as is the case with production of numerous antibiotics. During the first stage (trophophase), the growth of *Streptomyces* takes place. At the end of this phase and at the beginning of the second stage (idiophase), the enzymes involved in streptomycin biosynthesis are suddenly depressed, initiating the production, which is exocellular although part of the streptomycin usually remains bound to the mycelium.

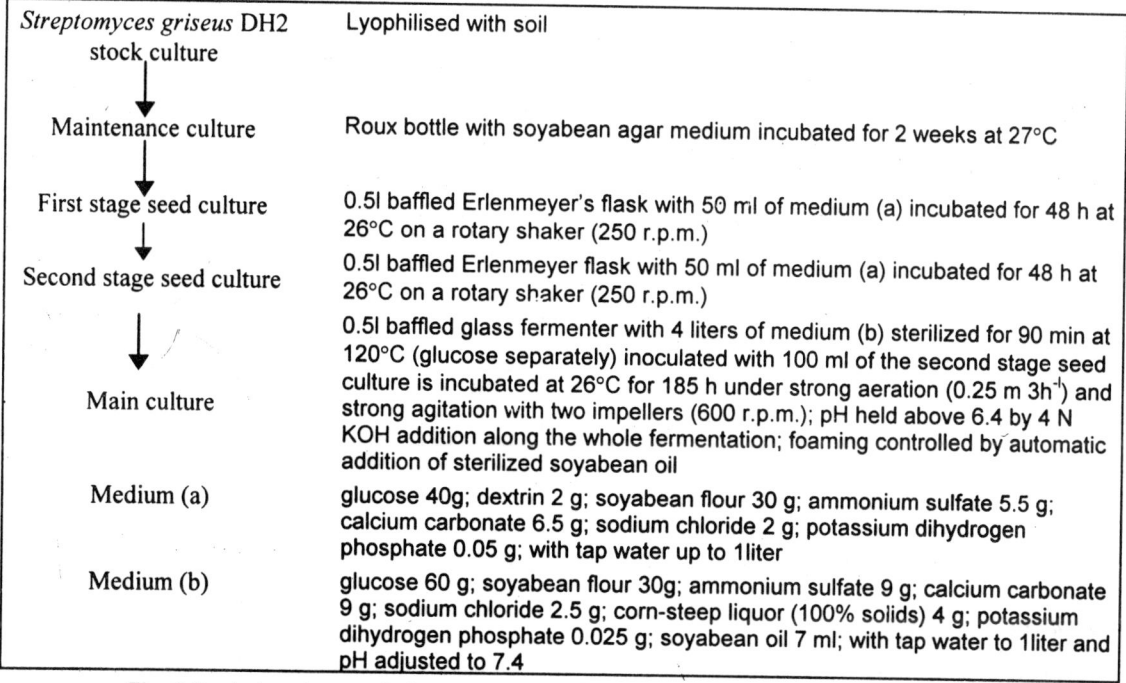

Streptomyces griseus DH2 stock culture	Lyophilised with soil
Maintenance culture	Roux bottle with soyabean agar medium incubated for 2 weeks at 27°C
First stage seed culture	0.5l baffled Erlenmeyer's flask with 50 ml of medium (a) incubated for 48 h at 26°C on a rotary shaker (250 r.p.m.)
Second stage seed culture	0.5l baffled Erlenmeyer flask with 50 ml of medium (a) incubated for 48 h at 26°C on a rotary shaker (250 r.p.m.)
Main culture	0.5l baffled glass fermenter with 4 liters of medium (b) sterilized for 90 min at 120°C (glucose separately) inoculated with 100 ml of the second stage seed culture is incubated at 26°C for 185 h under strong aeration (0.25 m 3h^{-1}) and strong agitation with two impellers (600 r.p.m.); pH held above 6.4 by 4 N KOH addition along the whole fermentation; foaming controlled by automatic addition of sterilized soyabean oil
Medium (a)	glucose 40g; dextrin 2 g; soyabean flour 30 g; ammonium sulfate 5.5 g; calcium carbonate 6.5 g; sodium chloride 2 g; potassium dihydrogen phosphate 0.05 g; with tap water up to 1liter
Medium (b)	glucose 60 g; soyabean flour 30g; ammonium sulfate 9 g; calcium carbonate 9 g; sodium chloride 2.5 g; corn-steep liquor (100% solids) 4 g; potassium dihydrogen phosphate 0.025 g; soyabean oil 7 ml; with tap water to 1liter and pH adjusted to 7.4

Fig. 6.2 : Laboratory scale fermentation process utilized for considering parameters to industrial scale (adapted and modified from Singh et al. 1976)

Mannosidostreptomycin, an undesirable product which is not an obligatory intermediate in streptomycin biosynthesis, but which is produced concurrently, is hydrolyzed with a release of streptomycin only at the end of the fermentation. The main reason for the late appearance of mannosidostreptomycinase is the catabolite repression by glucose. The regulation of biosynthesis of this enzyme and its properties have been thoroughly examined by Demain and Inamine. Mannosidostreptomycin can account for up to 40% of the total amount of streptomycins produced in a fermentation, but this percentage probably has been brought down to a much lower level with the mutant strains used at present in industry.

Streptomycin production comes to an end when the culture autolysis finally takes place. The improvement of the production capacities of the strains, the adjustment for optimized media and the addition of supplementary nutrients during the fermentation have allowed the increasing delay of the autolysis phenomenon and prolonging the streptomycin production phase. The evolution of such an operation is shown in figure 6.3.

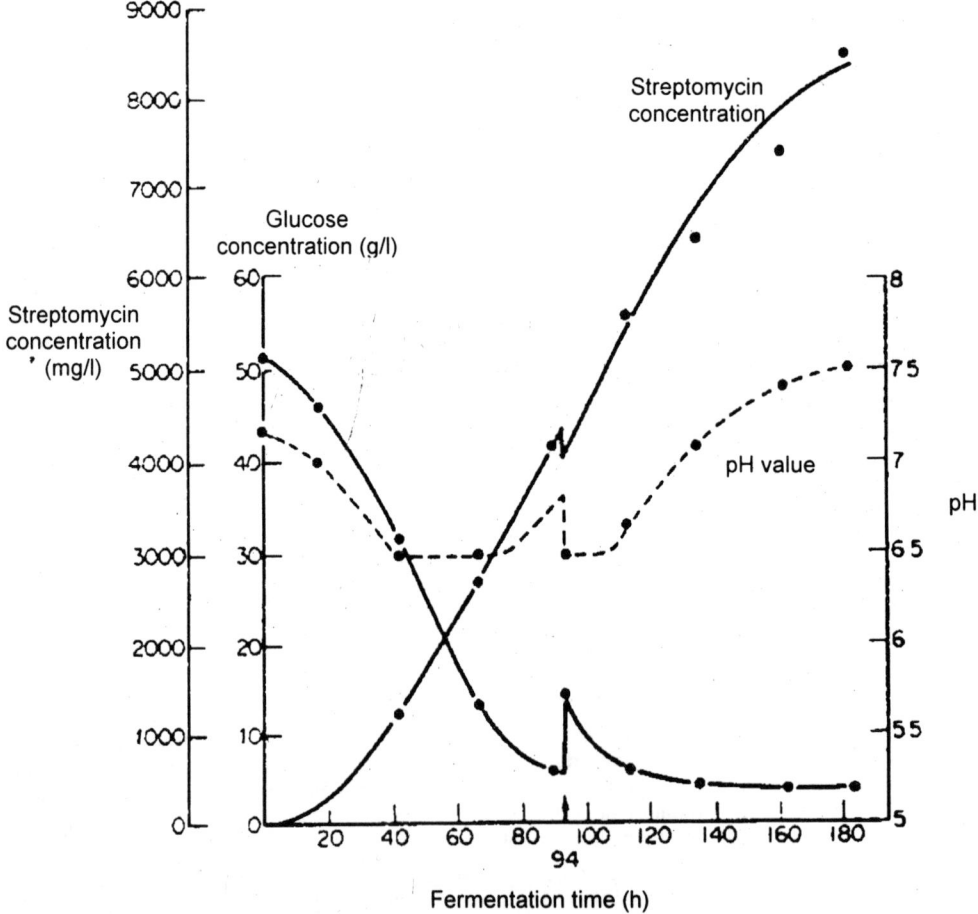

Fig. 6.3 : Time course of streptomycin production in a 5 liter fermenter

6.1.2.1.4. Product recovery

Numerous processes, often rather complex, have been used to recover the streptomycin present in fermentation broth, and to purify it in the form of various salts (sulfate, chlorohydrate, calcium complex, etc.). They always involve several steps requiring some of the following techniques:

(i) Adsorption on a support, followed by elution: the support can be activated carbon (Norite), with elution with a lower alcohol in aqueous acid solution (such as methanol-water-formic acid, for instance) or non-ionic resin (such as Amberlite XAD 1 or XAD 2) with elution with methanol or methyl ethyl ketone;

(ii) Fixation by ion exchange on a carboxylic type of a weak cationic resin (Amberlite IRC 50, XE 89, XE 222, Wofatit CP 300), with elution with a diluted mineral acid, HCl or H_2SO_4;

(iii) Chromatography on alumina, followed by elution with methanol;

(iv) Extraction with a water-immiscible solvent in the presence of a carrier (for instance a 5% mono-2-ethylhexyl phthalate solution in chloroform; Novo, 1967) followed by a re-isolation with water having acidic pH;

(v) Selective precipitation as helianthate, picrate, silicotungustate, reineckates, various sulfonates, etc., which are then converted into chlorohydrate or sulfate;

(vi) formation of Schiff's base by reaction with an amine (benzylamine, phenyethylamine, dibenzylmethyl-amine, etc.); the crystallized product obtained is recovered and later subjected to the action of an acid, sulfuric acid, for instance, which leads to the formation of streptomycin sulfate (Olin-Mathieson, 1963).

In addition to these operations, in which streptomycin is primarily involved, there are certain number of other processing steps which are used to eliminate impurities without directly interfering with the antibiotic.

The steps for industrial utilization have to combine at best, the simplicity, economy, yield and quality of the final product, according to the broth treatment (composition of the medium, streptomycin concentration). Most of the time, in production plants, after preliminary treatment of the broth (acidification, filtration, neutralization), the antibiotic is successively fixed and eluted through one or several ion-exchange columns; it goes as a solution through different ion-exchange columns (demineralization, neutralization columns, etc.) to get rid of various impurities; the operation ends with decolorization with carbon, followed by concentration under vacuum and drying or lyophilization. A patent was taken out by Squibb (1969) (Fig. 6.4) for a process based on this principle, which is much simplified and therefore very attractive.

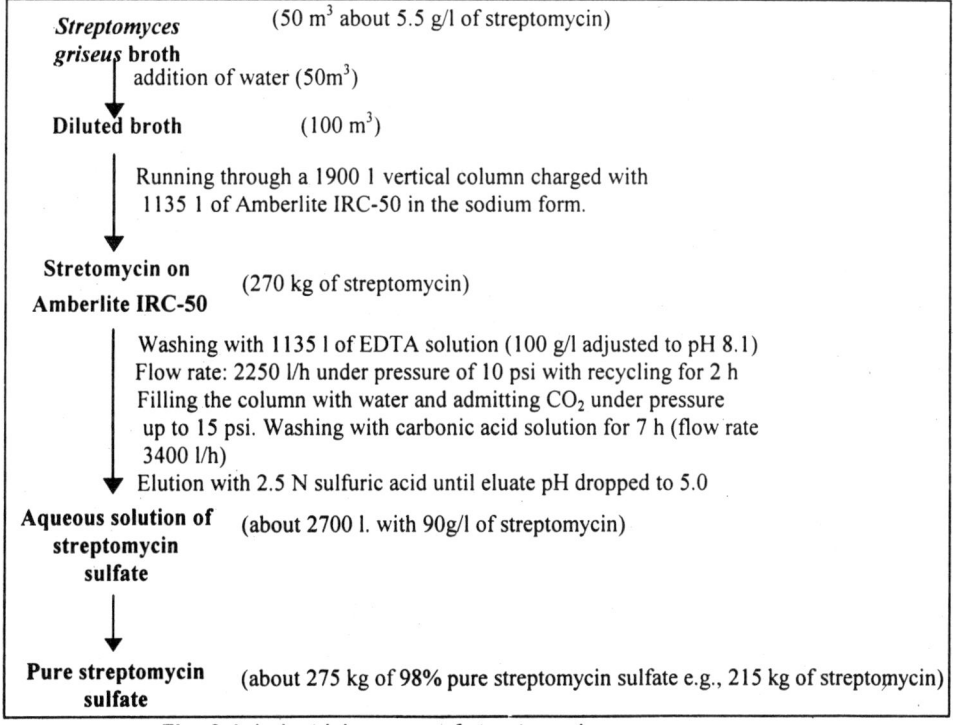

Fig. 6.4: Industrial process of streptomycin recovery

Streptomycin is usually obtained, industrially, as a sulfate salt with approximately 90% purity (790 mg of streptomycin base per gram of sulfate). The global yield of the preparation, as streptomycin base in the final product in comparison with the broth, is between 75 and 85%.

6.1.3. Penicillin

In 1928 Alexander Fleming's curiosity was aroused by zones of inhibition surrounding mould colonies contaminating a used petri dish. On further investigations he concluded that the mould had secreted a compound which has activity against several pathogenic bacteria. He named the lytic filtrate of the mould *Penicillium notatum* as penicillin. Further development of this compound has revolutionized the treatment of bacterial infection and has led to the discovery and served as a model for the development of numerous pharmacologically active compounds produced by fermentation. In 1941, when penicillin manufacturing began in United States, the process was to grow the *P. notatum* on the surface of a simple medium for 5-10 days and to use the liquid underlying the culture which contained the penicillin in concentration of 10-20 Oxford units per ml (an activity equivalent to 0.006-0.012 mg pure benzyl penicillin sodium salt). A solvent extraction procedure was used to isolate the material for clinical, pharmacological and chemical characterization.

6.1.3.1. Process overview

The technology of the manufacturing process is still regarded as highly proprietary in nature by the major commercial firms even though excellent fermentation technology and organisms have been publicly available for purchase. Similarly, purification of these compounds is thoroughly described in the literature. The distinguishing aspects of commercially acceptable process are based on operational simplicity and cost effectiveness. This explicitly entails for process optimization and development of better alternative options.

The process, involving culture maintenance fermentation and isolation, is presented in figure 6.5 and 6.6. Nutrient utilization and accumulation of the microbial mass and penicillin are presented in figure 6.7. In analyzing data of the type presented in figure 6.7 a quantitative approach, which clearly presents rates of utilization and production, is essential for understanding process behavior. In fact it is difficult to maintain a competitive position without making some efforts in each area of the process developments related to strain, fermentation and separation.

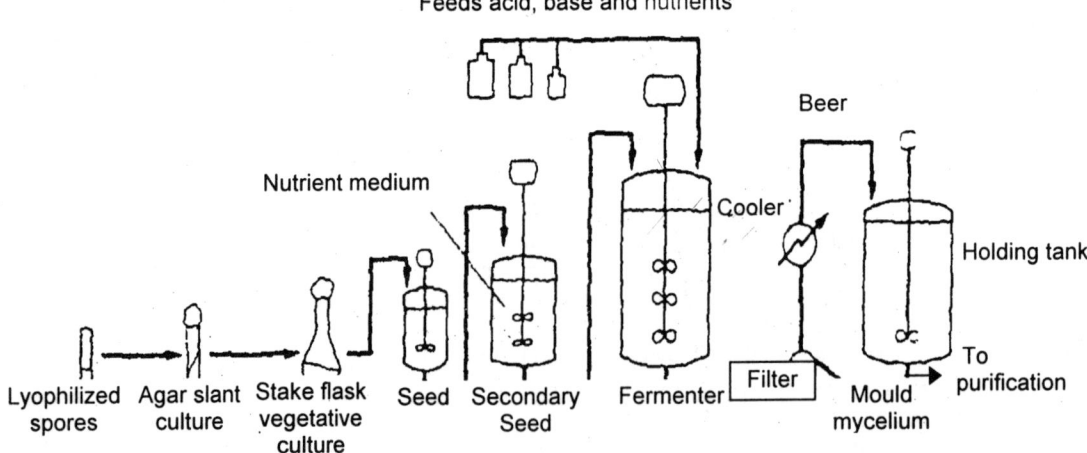

Fig. 6.5 : Penicillin production

Various penicillins viz., penicillin G and penicillin V, are produced by *P. chrysogenum* provided the appropriate carboxylic side chain is added to the medium in sufficient quantities. Basically the process involves the

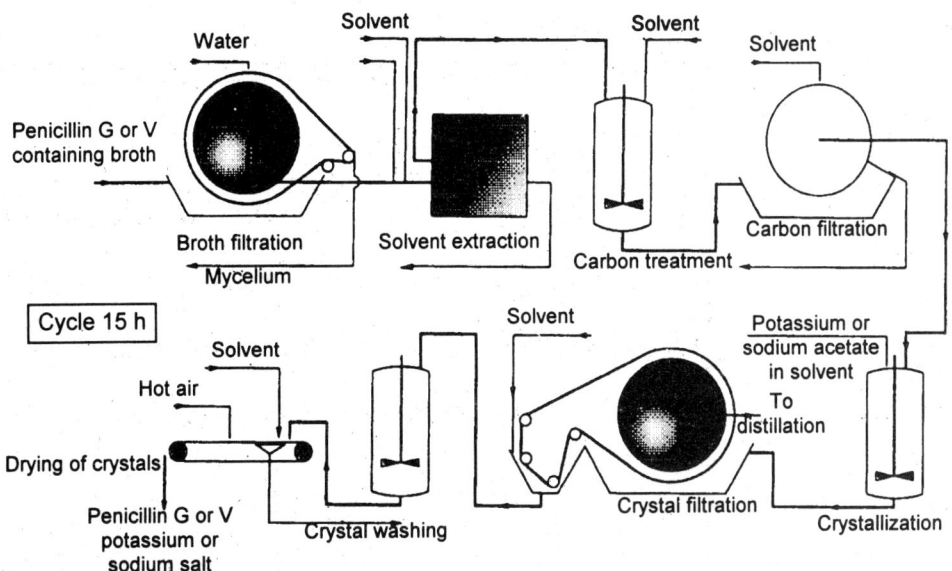

Fig. 6.6 : Purification of penicillin by Gist-Brocades process

cultivation of *P. chrysogenum* in vessels of increasing size up to 200,000 litters beginning with a slant or a vial of frozen vegetative mycelium. As harvest, the batch is filtered to remove the mycelium and the filtrate is extracted and crystallized or precipitated by acidification.

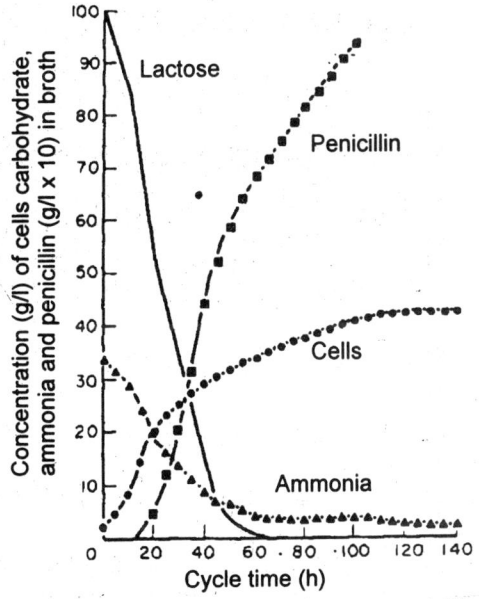

Fig. 6.7 : The time course of carbohydrate, nitrogen, penicillin and biomass concentration during a penicillin formation

6.1.3.2. Strain development

6.1.3.2.1. Strain maintenance and initial seed

The process begins with lyophilized spores of selected production strain. Alternatives are to store the master or secondary cell bank in the form of spore suspension in liquid nitrogen or as frozen vegetative material with glycerol and/or lactose as suspending agents at either -70°C or in liquid nitrogen. Frozen spores are inoculated on slants and allowed to sporulate, then transferred to a vegetative culture in Erlenmeyer flask containing a vegetative medium generally of similar composition as of the production medium.

6.1.3.2.2. Mutation

Lein diagramatically represented the pathway to secondary metabolites as:

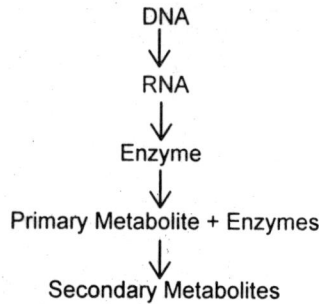

This has drawn attention to the complex multigene pathway which is strongly influenced by genetic and physiologic factors. Until the middle 1960's, UV irradiation and nitrogen mustards were the preferred mutagens used in penicillin strain improvement. Table 6.6 lists various mutagens which have been used. In recent years, NTG, a mutagen providing extremely high mutation rate over to killing effect has become the preferred compound for this reason and simply because its mechanism that differs from the techniques previously emphasized, NTG has the potential thereby of inducing different groups mutational events.

Screening (i.e. examining all members of the population which has been mutagenized) has been the most significant technique adapted for increasing the penicillin yields to date. One approach to improve the efficiency of the procedure is the potency index agar plate technique used by Ball *et al.* for the improvement of high yielding cultures. In this case the zone size was reduced by incorporating penicillinase in agar to reduce the sensitivity to a useful range.

Table 6.6: List of various mutagens used in the improvement of penicillin yields by *P. chrysogenum*

Methylbis(2-chloroethyl)amine	Ethyl methanesulfonate
Ultraviolet light irradiation (275 and 253 nm)	X-rays
N-methyl-N'-nitro-N-nitrosoguanidine	γ -rays
Nitrous acid	Ethyl amine
Diepoxybutane	

6.3.1.2.3. Selection

The proven success of the empirical approach had been appreciated widely (mutation and screening for increasing potency) nevertheless it was a tedious procedure. A specific selection procedure designed to identify those organism producing and possessing a desired phenotype (generally by allowing only that group to survive) can greatly increase the effectiveness of the program provided that the trait is selected from the whole population so as to improve the final yield. Several different and quite successful selective techniques are described in literature. The improved yield has been achieved largely through the sequential application of the selective procedure involving high concentration of the amino acids, biosynthetic intermediates and amino group analogues. These selective techniques presumably lead to the organisms with the higher levels of amino acids and intermediates. Specific selection procedures leading to the improvement in the strain selection were presented by Lein and associates. Changes recorded in the colony morphology during the program are presented in figure 6.8. An important contaminant of the high potency broth turned out to be oxidized parahydroxy form of phenylacetic acid, which when incorporated interferes with the semisynthetic chemistry of the analogs. An interesting selection technique used by Pan Labs involved selection and further evaluation of small colonies from plates with phenylacetic acid as sole carbon source, except for just enough glucose to produce a small colony.

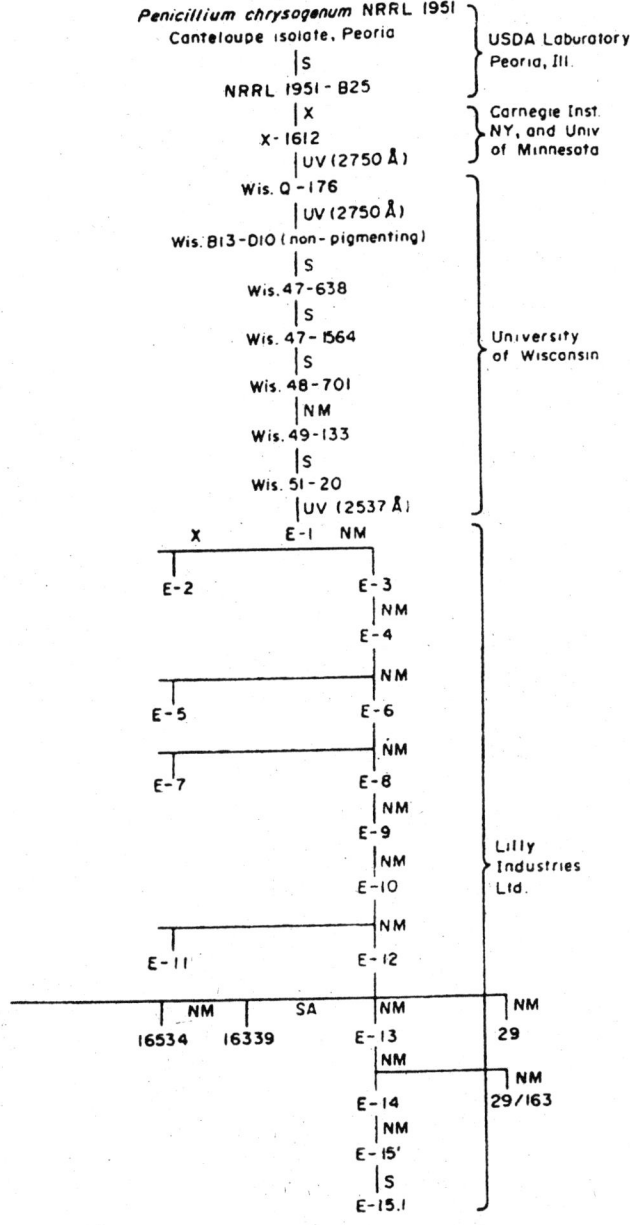

Fig. 6.8 : Strain linkage in the *Penicillium chrysogenum*

Thus the small colonies selected were those impaired in the ability to oxidize the side chain precursor. The technique was successful and as a result several commercial users of P14B-4 and its progeny are concerned about interference by *p*-hydroxy penicillin G. Also this loss of precursor is eliminated. The literature is mainly useful as source of information on approaches which may prove useful in the development of other strains such as those producing cephalosporin C and helping the physiologist to understand the organism for which the nutritional environment must be optimized. The strain improvement and selection procedures have yielded the development of the linkage between the whole process as outlined in figure 6.8.

6.3.1.2.4. Genetics

Genetics of penicillin producing organism has been reviewed by Ball , O'Sullivan and Ball and MacDonald . The biology of Penicillium has been reviewed by Peberdy. The biosynthetic pathways to the penicillins have been intensively worked out. Genetic studies were utilized in two ways to improve penicillin production. First, studies with blocked mutants have led to an understanding of the pathways and suggested appropriate selective techniques described previously. Second, two techniques have allowed the merging of potentially desirable traits. These are parasexual breeding and protoplast fusion. The parasexual breeding techniques basically involve the construction of complementary auxotrophs block or different resistance mutations in two strains having traits deemed desirable to incorporate in a single strains. The parents are grown together on complete medium, then selected for the presence of both markers, allowed to sporulate, and stable diploid spores are then isolated. After various treatments to allow recombination, haploid colonies are derived and evaluated for production and other characteristics. Recombinants with superior yields over the parents have been effectively utilized for the industrial strain improvement.

6.1.3.2. Fermentation process

6.1.3.2.1. Facilities

Production of penicillin G or V by fermentation is carried out in liquid culture. In modern practice the culture volume is typically 40,000-200,000 litters although one or two plants may successfully be operating with somewhat larger vessels equipped with air lift. The process is aerobic, having a volumetric oxygen uptake rate in the range of 0.4-1.0 mMol/l/min. and an RQ of approximately 0.95. Oxygen is supplied by passing air through the culture at a rate of 0.5-1.0 volumes of air (volume of fluid)$^{-1}$ min^{-1} and the air is vigorously contacted with the fluid using turbine agitators of various designs.

Power introduced to the culture is generally of the order of 1-4 Wl^{-1} including that introduced by the air stream. Other fermenter designs, including Waldhof fermenters and air-blown columns, are used, some of which are more energy efficient than the conventional designs, or offer other advantages in terms of capital costs or higher oxygen-transport capacity. The time-course of penicillin production is depicted in table 6.7 and presented graphically in figure 6.7.

6.1.3.2.1. Inoculum development

The main purposes of vegetative cultures and subsequent inoculum development steps are to increase the biomass to give a population which can be added to the next stage, such that each step will be reasonably short and large-scale equipment could be used efficiently.

Inoculum development stages are typically conducted at 25^0 C in shake cultures and agitated vessels. A typical vegetative or seed-stage medium contains an organic nitrogen source, such as corn-steep liquor, and sufficient concentration of a fermentable carbohydrate, such as 2% (w/v) sucrose or glucose. Calcium carbonate is often included as a buffer at 0.5-1.0% (w/v) concentration level. Other inorganic salts required for proper growth are also incorporated. Lag-phase growth is usually desirable in these stages, and a mass-doubling of time of about six hours (minimum for typical production strains) is achieved. Problems with growth rate or inoculum quality are usually associated with raw materials variability and mishandling of earlier inoculum steps of culture steps. Criteria for monitoring the inoculum stages, include cycle time, change in pH value, residual carbon source concentration, packed cell volume and respiration rate.

6.1.3.3. Culture medium

6.1.3.3.1. Carbon source

Penicillium chrysogenum can utilize a variety of carbon and energy sources. Various carbon sources used for penicillin production are sucrose, dextrins, and starches. Crude carbohydrates of low purity such as molasses have also been used. Animal and vegetable oils and ethanol inclusion has also been reported. Stoichiometric ratio number of moles of oxygen consumed by kilogram of sugar is constant at 33, regardless of growth rate and that the concentration of glucose after the rapid growth phase remains constant within a range of glucose feed rate to the fermenter. This indicates that under certain conditions the carbon in the fat, glucose is completely combusted for energy production and is not incorporated into cell mass.

Table 6.7: Changes from fed batch or semicontinuous penicillin fermentation

Time	0-40 h	40-?	?-harvest
Penicillin production	Slight	High, the rate peaks then declines over the most of the period	Some production occurs but at a low and a declined rate
Specific growth rate	8-20h; 0.07/h 20-40h; 0.01-0.02/h	40-75h; 0.009/h	115-209 h; ~ 0/h
Carbon and energy source, used	Organic nitrogen (e.g., corn steep liquor and/or carbohydrates, oils)	Carbohydrates, triglyceride oils, ethanol fed or hydrolyzed slowly and the generally thought to regulate growth	Various energy sources, as available sometimes insufficient for maintenance. Growth limitation may shift to other nutrients
Nitrogen source used	Mainly organic nitrogen	Organic nitrogen and/or ammonium and/or nitrate salts depending on the process. Used for cell growth and product formation	Nitrogen source may become growth-rate limiting. Cell lysis may occur
Sulfur source used	In crude organic nitrogen and inorganic salts e.g., ammonium sulfate. Used rapidly for cell growth	Often fed as an inorganic salt. Used for penicillin synthesis and slow cell growth.	
Phosphorous source used	In crude organic nitrogen and as inorganic salts	very little if any is fed as quantitative needs are very low. Growth-rate limitation may be harmful.	
Other nutrients	Required for cell growth	some like Iron may be regulatory.	

6.1.3.3.1. Nutrients other than carbon-energy sources

In general the media used in the earlier years of penicillin production and what being used now are quite similar. Table 6.8 presents typical formula of the media commonly used.

Table 6.8: Typical fermentation media for production of penicillin G or V in 1945 and 1967

1947	Concentration	1967	Concentration
Lactose	3-4%	Glucose or molasses (by continuous feed)	10% total
Corn steep liquor solids	3.5%	Corn steep liquor solids	4-5%
Calcium carbonate	1%	Phenylacetic acid (by continuous feed)	0.5-0.8% total
KH_2PO_4	0.4%	Lard oil (or vegetable oil) antifoam (by continuous feed)	0.5%
Lard oil antifoam	0.25%		

6.1.3.3.3. Nitrogen source

Until 1975 most industrial processes included corn steep liquor as an organic nitrogen source in the media. This was included due to a marked increase in the yield of penicillin after its addition because it is a component precursor of side chain. Later reports suggested that cotton seed meals can also be a satisfactory substitute for corn steep liquor.

6.1.3.3.4. Side chain Processor

Recent studies have demonstrated that the side chain attachment is relatively non specific and that relatively high concentrations of phenylacetic acid and phenoxyacetic acid (sodium salts) have to be included in the medium or in feeds to the fermenter, if the desired single component penicillin is to be obtained. In order to avoid toxicity of sodium phenyl acetate as well as its deterioration due to hydroxylation by the microorganism, it is fed at a well defined rate continuously throughout the process.

More than 90% conversion of phenyl acetic acid into penicillin G side chain has been obtained through continuous feeding of one of its salts to maintain a low residual concentration. The penicillin V precursor phenoxy acetic acid may be fed in a few large doses. More than 80% of the material can be incorporated into the penicillin V side chain.

6.1.3.3.5. Sulfur source

Ammonium sulfate is a common ingredient used in the production media for providing nitrogen and sulfur in the proportions necessary for penicillin synthesis. Sulfur is also provided in significant quantities by the organic nitrogen sources used in media.

6.1.3.3.6. Phosphorous source

Phytic acid in corn steep liquor is an important source of phosphorous. Phosphorous may also be added in the form of inorganic salts and can be maintained by feeding inorganic phosphorous salts. A level of phosphate phosphorous of 250 to 500 µg/ml is optimum for penicillin production.

6.1.3.3.7. Other nutrients

Inorganic salts of potassium and magnesium as well as additional nitrogen, phosphorous and sulfur are necessary for growth and product formation. Chemically defined media include, requirements for phosphorous, sulfur, potassium, magnesium, manganese, zinc, cobalt and copper.

6.1.3.4. Recovery of penicillin

6.1.3.4.1. Carbon process (obsolete)

The original commercial process of penicillin recovery from the fermentation broth was based upon the adsorption of the product on the activated charcoal. The carbon was collected, washed with water and the carbon adsorbate was eluted with 80% acetone. The penicillin was concentrated by distillation or evaporation under vacuum at 15-32°C. The remaining aqueous solution was cooled to 2°C, acidified to pH 2.0-3.0 and the penicillin extracted into amyl acetate from which it was crystallized with excess mineral salts of buffer near neutral pH under vacuum. As higher quantities of penicillin were produced, this approach became impractical because of increased carbon requirements.

6.1.3.4.2. Solvent extraction process (industrial standards)

An outline of the current standard process is presented in table 6.9 and figure 6.9. Solvent extraction forms the basis of isolation and purification.

Table 6.9 : Outline of the penicillin purification process

Steps	Purpose	Equipment	Bases
Filtration	Separate mycelia from penicillin	Rotary drum vacuum filter	Size of particles
Extraction	Remove soluble contaminants	Counter current extractors	Differential extraction based on pH chain
Carbon treatment	Remove soluble contaminants	Mixer and drum filter	Adsorption of impurities
Crystallization	Further purification and stabilization	Tank and drum filter, settlers, or basket centrifuge	Via addition of Na or K salts
Drying	Stabilization	Horizontal belt filters/warm dry air	Dry solvent vacuum or air

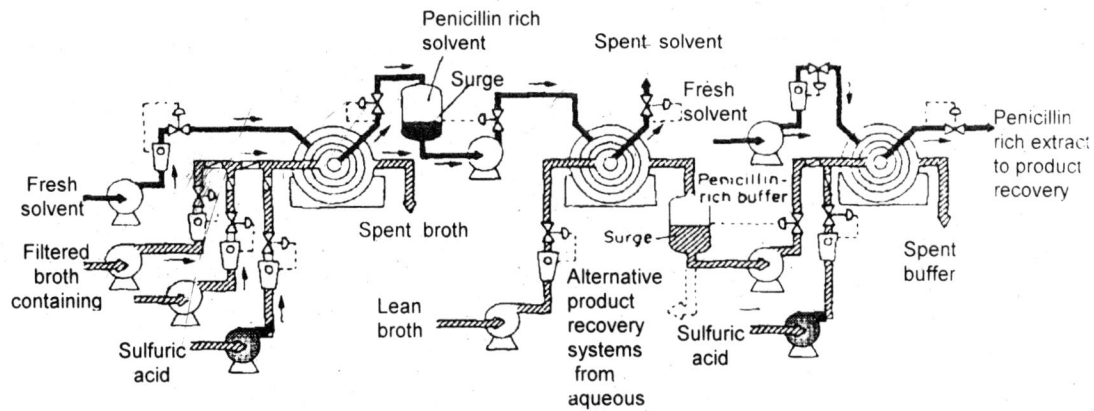

Step 1: Acidification and extraction of penicillin from filtered broth to solvent   Step 2: Extraction of penicillin from solvent to fresh buffer   Step 3: Acidification and reextraction of penicillin from buffer to fresh solvent

Fig. 6.9: Diagram of a three stage extraction/purification process used in penicillin production.

The basic process has changed very little since late 1940s except for the addition of automatic controls and simplifications permitted by broth of higher potency and purity, by increased scale of operation and by improved design of specific equipment. Typical steps and related yields for the solvent extraction process are presented in table 6.10.

Table 6.10: Typical yields in penicillin purification

Step	Yield
Holding	95% but losses can even be large if broth is not rapidly chilled or if microbial contamination occurs
Filtration	90-95% based on filtrate assay. 5% of the loss is accounted for insoluble solids in the broth Other losses are due to degradation and leakage to drain.
Solid extraction	
Single stage	80-90%
Lead-Trail	92-96%
Aqueous (back) extraction	95-97%
Crystallization	95%
Drying	95%
Overall	~ 78%

6.1.4. Clavulanic acid

Clavulanic acid, a lactamase inhibiting agent was discovered independently by Brown and co-workers in 1976 and Napier and co-workers. It was found to inhibit the activity of β-lactamase enzymes which are produced by many penicillin and cephalosporin resistant clinical pathogens. Clavulanic acid is a fused bicyclic β-lactam structurally different from the penicillins and cephalosporins in having an oxygen atom in place of sulfur.

Clavulanic acid

Besides being a potent β lactamase inhibitor, it also possesses weak broad spectrum antibacterial activity.

6.1.4.1. Clavulanic acid producing micro-organisms

Clavulanic acid an was antibiotics obtained initially by *Streptomyces clavuligerus*. Later on like *Streptomyces jumonjinensis* and species designated as *Streptomyces* sp.6621. Studies aimed at finding biosynthetic pathways of clavulanic acid have revealed that labelled [^{13}C] acetate enters the clavulanic acid molecule via the tricarboxylic acid cycle and 2-oxoglutarate, which provides, probably via glutamate, a five-carbon skeleton to be a part of clavulanic acid molecules (carbons 9,8,2,3 and 10). This conclusion was supported by evidence suggesting direct incorporation of 3,4 [^{13}C] glutamate.

It was postulated that if reduction of γ-carboxyl group of glutamic acid was to take place before closure of oxazolidine ring, then α amino-δ-hydroxy valerate (AHV) might be a clavulanic acid precursor, and indeed the labelling pattern resulting from feeding 3,4 (^{13}C$_2$) AHV was consistent and concordant with this view.

6.1.4.2. Fermentation process.

6.1.4.2.1. Inoculum preparation:

Highest yielding isolate is selected from a number of single colonies obtained by plating out the culture collection organisms from single colony isolates. Isolates are tested for clavulanic acid yield in shake flask fermentations using 100ml of production medium in 500ml conical flasks which are incubated for 3-5 days at 26°C on a rotary shaker. The concentration of clavulanic acid in the fermentation may be estimated using a microbiological assay method or the automated enzyme inhibition assay or by employing high performance liquid chromatography.

The selected isolate is preserved as a master stock either in lyophilized form in ampoules or as soil stocks in tubes of desiccated soil. Working slant cultures of agar are prepared from the master stock, as secondary culture to produce spores inoculum for fermenters. Examples of solid media which are suitable for slant culture are as follows:

Medium A : 10% glucose, 0.1% yeast extract 0.1% beef extract, 0.2% N-Z amine A, 1.5% agar, pH 7.3 (Benett's agar)

Medium B : 1% soluble starch, 0.1% potassium dihydrogen phosphate. 0.1% MgSO4. 7H2O, 0.1% sodium chloride, 0.2% (NH$_4$)2SO$_4$, 0.2% calcium carbonate, 1 ml trace salts solution (trace salts solution = 0.1% FeSO$_4$. 7H$_2$O, 0.1% MnCl$_2$. 4H$_2$O, 0.1% ZnSO$_4$.7H$_2$O) pH 7.0 - 7.4.

The inoculum preparation for a large scale fermentation the medium (A or B) is set in a Roux bottle to give approximately 200 cm^2 of agar surface. This is then uniformly inoculated with a suspension of spores in sterile water and incubated for 10 days at 26°C. The sporulating aerial mycelium from a Roux bottle is used to inoculate a stirred tank seed stage which provides vegetative growth for inoculum for the final fermentation. The medium used for the seed stage contains 1.0% soyabean flour, 2.0% dextrin, and 0.03%v/v antifoam consisting of 10% Pluronic L81, a block polymer of ethylene oxide and propylene oxide dispersed in soyabean oil; 75 liters of medium is prepared and steam sterilized in a 100 liter stainless steel fermenter. Agitation is provided by means of a flat-bladed turbine impeller, the overall impeller diameter being 19 cm.

Seed stage medium is inoculated with the suspension obtained from scrapings of spores and aerial mycelium from agar surface of Roux bottle and sterile water. The seed stage is then incubated for 72 hours at 28°C with stirring at 140 rpm and airflow of 1000 liters per minute.

6.1.4.2.2. Fermentation Nutrients

Soyabean protein has been found to be the most important nutrient for clavulanic acid biosynthesis. A suitable production fermentation medium described consists of 1.5% soyabean flour, 1.0% glycerol, 0.1% KH$_2$PO$_4$ and 0.2%v/v of 10% Pluronic L81 antifoam in soyabean oil. Another medium obtained by substituting a lipid for glycerol at the same concentration (1.0%) and omission of the antifoam showed improved results. Natural oils such as lard oil, maize oil, peanut oil and soyabean oils all give better results than glycerol, but the best clavulanic acid yield resulted from the use of Prichem P224, which is a triglyceride of a fatty acid mixture containing 65% oleic acid.

An alternative medium for *S. clavuligerus* fermentation is described, containing 3.0% soyabean meal, 4.7% soluble starch, 0.01% $FeSO_4.7H_2O$, 0.01% K_2HPO_4 and 0.05%v/v silicone antifoam emulsion. This gives results comparable with to the above media.

6.1.4.2.3. Production stage procedure.

Production is carried out in a 200 liter fermenter containing 1500 liter of medium. The medium is steam sterilized in the fermenter at 121°C for 30 minutes. The contents of a 75 liter seed stage is kept for 72 h are transferred as an inoculum to the production medium. The production fermenter is a conventional stainless steel reactor fitted with baffles and a mechanical agitation device. The agitator is fitted with two flat bladed turbine impellers, each with six blades and of overall diameter 48 cm., the impeller diameter tank diameter ratio being 0.43. After incubation with constant agitation (106 rpm) at 26°C and with an airflow of 0.75 v/v per minute, the production medium containing lipid as carbon source (soyabean flour, Prichem P224, and inorganic phosphate; pH adjusted to 7.0 before sterilization), the clavulanic acid concentration in the brew usually reached the maximum after approximately 90 h of incubation. Typically the maximum titer was about 500 µl/ml. Evidence has been presented to suggest that in stirred *S. clavuligerus* fermentation, with a medium containing 0.52% distillers soluble, 0.52% casein hydrolysate, 2.1% soyabean meal, 4.7% soluble starch, 0.78% glucose, 0.01% $FeSO_4.7H_2O$ and antifoam, an improvement in the amount of clavulanic acid product has been obtained if pH of the fermentation is controlled at about 6.5 and within the range 6.3 - 6.7 through out the fermentation. The procedure has been summarized in fig 6.10.

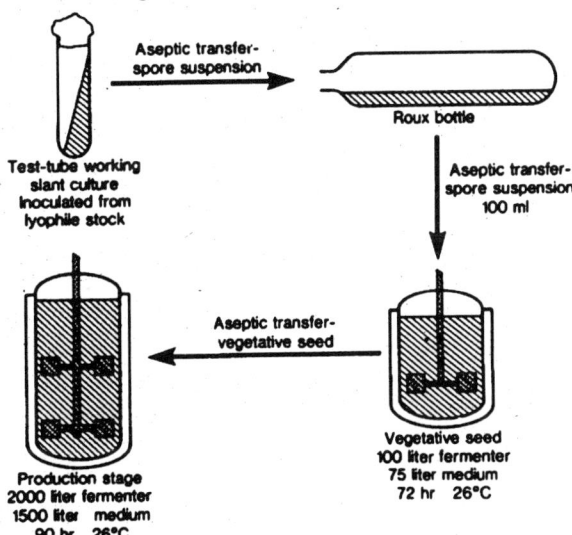

Fig 6.10: Fermentation process of clavulanic acid

6.1.4.3. Product recovery and purification

After fermentation the broth is first clarified by filtration or centrifugation of *S. clavuligerus*, mycelium is discarded. Variety of fractionation methods may be adapted for primary extraction from clarified broth. Larger scale processing may be done by (1) extraction from acidified fermentation broth into a water immiscible organic solvent and (2) adsorption onto an aqueous salt solution. Purification of the primary extract is achieved by further chromatographic procedure, particularly the use of ion exchange chromatography. The final high purity product is obtained by freeze drying or crystallization from aqueous solution.

In one procedure, for primary butanol extraction and subsequent purification of the sodium salt by column chromatography, the culture filtrate at 2-5°C is acidified to pH 2.0 and extracted with n-butanol by means of a continuous flow multistage counter current extractor; at the ratio of solvent to aqueous phase being 0.75. An aqueous back extract is then obtained by efficiently mixing the extract with 1/20 volume of water while maintaining the pH at 7.0 using 20% sodium hydroxide solution. The aqueous extract-butanol mixture is then separated in a liquid-liquid separator. Recovery of clavulanic acid from clarified broth to aqueous back extract is approximately 40% during which the temperature of aqueous back extract is maintained at 5°C. The back extract is percolated through a column of Permutit Zerolit FFIP (SRA62) anion exchange resin in chloride form. The active fractions are combined and concentrated before desalting on a column of Bio-Rad Bio-Gel P2. Alternatively, desalting may be achieved by using a polystyrene-divinylbenzene copolymer such as Amberlite XAD-4, which adsorbs clavulanate but not inorganic salts; this operation also results in additional purification of the clavulanate. After elution with 1.0% n-butanol solution (or demineralized water in case of XAD-4), combined salt free fraction containing clavulanate are vacuum concentrated to a suitable volume before freeze drying to give the solidified sodium salt.

A strong basic anion exchange resin column (Zerolit FFIPS RA61 resin) can be employed for primary extraction of clarified broth. After percolation the broth is adjusted to pH 6.2, the column is washed with chilled water and then eluted with chilled 1.0M aqueous sodium chloride. Combined fractions containing clavulanate adjusted to pH 6.2 before desalting on a column of Amberlite XAD4 resin. The combined active fractions are then concentrated by reverse osmosis prior to purification, for example, by the method employing SRA 62 resin described above for aqueous back-extract from primary n-butanol extraction.

Secondary purification can also be achieved by conversion of the partially purified clavulanate to the benzyl ester, which is then dissolved in ethylacetate and subjected to two chromatographic steps using Sephadex LH 20 and silica gel; the purified benzyl ester is then hydrogenated over 10% Pd/C in the presence of sodium bicarbonate to yield sodium clavulanate tetrahydrate.

6.2. AMINO ACIDS

6.2.1. L-Lysine

A considerable amount of attention has been concentrated in various parts of world in regard to the production of amino acids by fermentation process. L-lysine is being manufactured now a days by a process protected by United States patents.

A large number of microorganisms have been identified which produce free extracellular lysine in small quantities. Richard and Haskins screened some 600 fungi in order to determine their ability to form free, extracellular lysine in submerged culture conditions. However, further investigations put forth some other microorganisms producing a considerable yield of lysine. Dulaney obtained yield of about 400 µg/ml of extracellular lysine in shaken flasks using strains of *Gliocladium* species and a strain of *Ustilago maydis*.

6.2.1.1. Fermentation process for production of lysine

The commercial production of lysine based on a two step process is generally followed at industrial scale. Diaminopimelic acid is first produced by microorganism (*Corynebacterium diphtheriae* and *Mycobacterium tuberculosum*). It is then converted into L-lysine as described by Casida (1968) as shown in the following reaction.

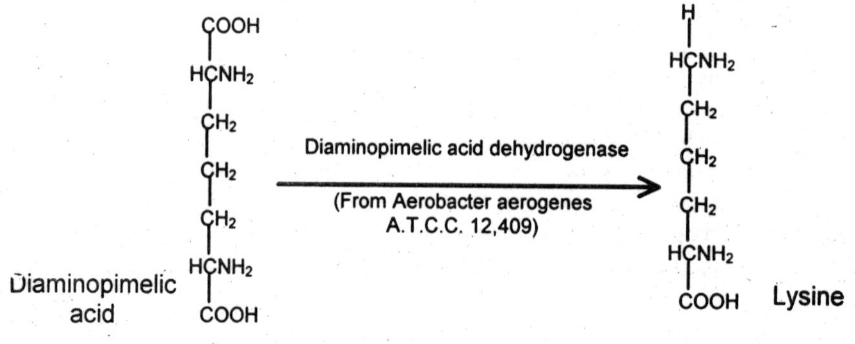

6.2.1.2. New strain development and improvement

Although the industrial production of L-lysine is generally undertaken by the above process. Nevertheless, some work on mutation and selection principles has suggested some newer strains which could alternatively be utilized. Furthermore, the use of mutant strains of *C, glutamicum* has been effectively utilized for production of lysine.

Figure 5.3 shows the control of lysine production in *C. glutamicum*. It could be inferred that aspartokinase, the first enzyme in the biosynthetic route, is inhibited only when lysine and threonine are present above their respective threshold levels. An important feature of the pathway is that lysine does not exert any control over the biosynthetic route from aspartic semialdehyde to lysine. A mutant which could not catalyze the conversion of aspartic semialdehyde to homoserine would be capable of growth only in homoserine supplemented medium and the organism would be described as a homoserine auxotroph. If such an organism were grown in the presence of very low concentration of homoserine the endogenous level of threonine would not reach the inhibitory concentration of aspartokinase control, then aspartate will be converted to lysine. The knowledge of biosynthetic route allows the geneticist to construct a mutant of desirable characters. Using the logical treatment Nakayama and associates isolated homoserine auxotroph of *C. glutamicum* using the penicillin enrichment technique developed by Davis. Under normal culture conditions as auxotroph is at a disadvantage compared with the parental (wild type) cells.

Sano and Shiio attempted to isolate mutants of *Brevibacterium flavum*, the control of lysine production in *B. flavum* is the same as shown for *C. glutamicum*. They demonstrated that the lysine analogues (2-aminoethyl)-cysteine (AEC) could inhibit growth completely in the presence of threonine which indicates that AEC combined with threonine, caused concerted feed back inhibition of aspartokinase and deprived the organism of lysine and methionine. Mutants capable of growing in the presence of AEC and threonine were isolated by plating the survivors of mutation treatments onto agar containing the two factors. A relatively high proportion of resulting colonies were lysine over producers, the best of which was found to produced more than 30g/dm.

6.2.1.3. Commercial production process

A two stage process is used for the commercial production of lysine. First step involves the production of diaminopimelic acid and the second step involves its conversion to L-lysine.

6.2.1.3.1. Step 1: Diaminopimelic acid production

A large number of organisms have been found capable of producing the acids. Work (1951) reported its production utilizing *Corynebacterium diphtheriae* and *Mycobacterium tuberculosum*. Davis (1952) reported high yield by some lysine requiring auxotrophs of *E. coli* (A.T.C.C. 12,408), which is a lysine auxotroph and also unable to decarboxylate diaminopimelic acid to lysine. For industrial production A.T.C.C. 12,408 strain of *E. coli* is utilized.

Inoculum preparation

The inoculum for production medium could be prepared by growing *E .coli* A.T.C.C., 12,408 for 20 h at 28°C with proper agitation and aeration in a medium of following composition:

Glycerol	0.5%
Corn-steep liquor	0.5%
$(NH_4)_2HPO_4$	0.5%

pH of the medium is adjusted to 7.5 with KOH. The medium is sterilized at a pressure of 20 psi for 30 min.

Instrumental requirement

The fermenter design is quite similar to those mentioned earlier. The fermenter tank should be equipped with an agitator and an appropriate air supply should be maintained. The temperature should be controlled at 28°C.

Growth media

One production media, cited as an example in the patent issued to Casida, contained:

$(NH_4)_2 HPO_4$	4%
$CaCO_3$	0.5%
Glycerol	6%
Corn-steep liquor	4%

The pH of the medium is adjusted to 7.5 with KOH and medium is sterilized. The medium may be seeded with 1 to 5 % of inoculum and incubated at 28°C with agitation and aeration (1% v/v of medium per minute). Traces of soyabean oil or DC antifoam-A may be added.

Process control

During the fermentation, it is important to maintain the pH in the range of 7 to 7.5. After about 24 h it is necessary to add an alkali, ammonium hydroxide being preferred (but KOH and NaOH are satisfactory), after about 64 hours, it may be necessary to add H_2SO_4. Aeration of broth is an important factor and should be controlled. The temperature should be maintained up to 29°C. Optimum yields (about 9 mg/ml) are obtained in about 3 days.

6.2.1.3.2. Step 2: Decarboxylation of diaminopimelic acid to L-lysine

The enzyme diaminopimelic acid decarboxylase that converts diaminopimelic acid into lysine, is produced by a number of bacteria, for example by strains of *Aerobacter aerogenes* and of *E. coli* which do not require lysine for growth. Casida reported that a strain of *A. aerogenes* (now designated as A.T.C.C.,12409), has been found particularly for converting diaminopimelic acid into lysine. This organism lacks the enzyme lysine decarboxylase. *A. aerogenes*, A.T.C.C., 12409, may be grown in the same medium and under similar conditions which are favorable for the propagation of inoculum for the mutant strain of *E. coli*. In general, the conversion of diaminopimelic acid to lysine may be carried out at about 28°C which is completed in approximately 24 h. Furthermore, the addition of 0.004 to about 0.032 molar citric acid and EDTA sodium salt favors the conversion.

6.2.1.3.3. Recovery of lysine

After conversion of diaminopimelic acid to lysine, the reaction mixture is filtered and the lysine is absorbed on a cation-exchange resin, such as Amberlite IR-120, and eluted with dilute alkali by passing it through a weak cation-exchange resin such as Amberlite IRC-50. The eluates are pooled and dried to crystallize lysine which may be recrystallized for purification.

6.2.2. L-Glutamic acid

It is an essential amino acid and could be produced by a number of ways: by the hydrolysis of wheat glutin, soyabean cake or by other protein rich food materials; by cleavage of pyrrolidone carboxylic acid found in stiffens molasses; or by one step fermentation process using single microorganism; or by a two step process involving α-ketoglutaric acid by fermentation and its conversion by another microbe or by an enzyme process. The discussion is limited to the production of glutamic acid by fermentation process, by single stage and two stage process.

6.2.2.1. Single stage fermentation process for production of glutamic acid

The commercial process is mainly used in Japan that employs sweet potatoes as chief raw material and is based on a Commonwealth of Australia patent application (1956). The process utilizes the strain of *Micrococcus*, No. 541 for production of glutamic acid. The strain is biotin auxotroph and requires 0.5-5 µg per liter of biotin for good yields. The carbon source may be glucose, fructose, sucrose, maltose, xylose or hydrolyzed starch. Nitrogen source contains at least one of the following components: urea, ammonia, ammonium salts, peptones, corn steep liquor, hydrolyzed caseine, meat extract or digested soyabean meals or fish meal. The pH of the media should be maintained within a range of 6-9, however, the optimum range found to be 7.0 - 8.5. Ammonium ion is essential for growth. The temperature of the fermenter should be maintained within the range of 27-30°C. Proper aeration of culture is essential for good production.

For better understanding of strain improvement and biosynthetic pathway the reader should refer earlier chapter on introduction to fermentation where mutation and selection based techniques have been discussed.

6.2.2.2. Production by Cephalosporium species

L-glutamic acid is directly produced by means of a strain of *Cephalosporium*, such as *C. salmosynnematum* NRRL 2271, *C. diospyri* ATCC 9066 or *C. acremorium* ATCC 10141. The mould is cultivated in nutrient media containing a carbohydrate source and urea at pH 4-9 under aerobic conditions. The fermentation is continued until appreciable amounts of L-glutamic acid accumulated.

6.2.2.2.1. Two- stage process for production of glutamic acid

The two step process of L-glutamic acid production involves:

(i) Formation of α-ketoglutaric acid.

(ii)Conversion of α-ketoglutaric acid in to L-glutamic acid via enzymatic conversion or by microorganism.

$$
\underset{\text{Ketoglutaric acid}}{
\begin{array}{c}
\text{COOH} \\
|\\
\text{C=O} \\
|\\
\text{CH}_2 \\
|\\
\text{CH}_2 \\
|\\
\text{COOH}
\end{array}
}
\quad\xrightarrow{\text{Microbial enzymes}}\quad
\underset{\text{L-glutamic acid}}{
\begin{array}{c}
\text{COOH} \\
|\\
\text{CHNH}_2 \\
|\\
\text{CH}_2 \\
|\\
\text{CH}_2 \\
|\\
\text{COOH}
\end{array}
}
$$

The process of production of α-ketoglutaric acid by fermentation has been described by many authors (Lockwood and Stodala; Katagiri et al.) utilizing different microorganisms and shown improved productivity.

Microorganisms being utilized

Although considerable work has been carried out regarding the utilization of an appropriate microorganism involved in the production of α-ketoglutaric acid yet there is a need of work to establish, identify an appropriate mutant strain which should be utilized for production. The discussion on the general mutation based improvement of microorganism may be referred by the reader for further clarification. Table 6.11 indicates various types of microorganisms which are utilized for improved production of α-ketoglutaric acid.

Table 6.11 :   Various strains producing L-glutamic acid with their respective yields

Strain No.	Name	Approximate yield
--	*Bacterium α-ketoglutaricum*	50-60 %
--	*Bact. Succinicum*	13.6 %
1	*Bacillus megatherium*	20.6 %
1	*B. natto (var.B. subtilis)*	14.6 %
3	*Escherichia coli*	40-60 %
7	*Escherichia coli*	40-60 %
5	*E. freundii*	40-60 %
9	*E. freundii*	40-60 %
12	*E. freundii*	40-60 %
8	*Aerobacter cloacae*	40-60 %
84 C	*Kluyvera citrophila* var. α	40-60 %
11	*K. citrophila* var. α	40-60 %
NRRLB-6	*Pseudomonas fluorescens (reptilivora)*	47.9 %
18	*Serratia marcescens*	49.3 %

Nutrient requirements

The production medium contains a carbon source, a nitrogen source, minerals, and occasionally some vitamins. The most widely used source of carbon is glucose, however, the other sources of carbon like fructose, sucrose or some organic acids such as acetic acid or succinic acid could also be utilized. Nitrogen source contains at least one of the following components: urea, ammonia, ammonium salts, peptones, corn steep liquor, hydrolyzed casein, meat extract or digested soyabean meals or fish meal or some other compounds. The minerals like magnesium sulfate or potassium acid phosphate may be added to the synthetic or semisynthetic media. Addition of traces of iron enhances the yield. Yeast extract has been utilized in some of the media as the source of some vitamins.

6.2.2.2.2 Process Parameters

Two organisms have been utilized for production of α-ketoglutaric acid, namely *K. citrophila* var.α and *Pseudomonas fluorescens*.

Production from Pseudomonas fluorescens

The media for production consists of glucose, ammonium sulfate, potassium acid phosphate, magnesium sulfate, calcium carbonate(sterilized separately) and ferrous ammonium sulfate using *Ps. fluorescens* B-6 strain. It was dispersed in a 200 ml portion in a 1 liter Erlenmeyer flask, sterilized, cooled, inoculated and incubated at 28^0C on a reciprocating shaker. There was a marked effect of nitrogen supply on the yield of α-ketoglutaric acid. It was found that at 25 µM/ml nitrogen level an incomplete fermentation resulted; whereas at above 50 µM/ml yield of α-ketoglutaric acid was low or absent but the rate of fermentation was considerably rapid. Therefore, 25 µM/ml nitrogen level was used for the production of α-ketoglutaric acid.

Production from Kluyvera citrophila var. α

The media used for production consisted of fructose, $NH_4H_2PO_4$, $(NH_4)_2SO_4$, KH_2PO_4, $MgSO_4.7 H_2O$, NaCl, $CaCO_3$ (sterilized separately), $Fe_2(SO_4)_3.7 H_2O$. By this method yields of up to 56% of α-ketoglutaric acid was obtained from a 10.4 % of glucose solution after 72 h with *Bacterium* strain No. 84C (*Kluyvera citrophila* var. α). 50 ml portions of the medium were dispensed in 500 ml flask sterilized, inoculated and incubated at 30^0C on a reciprocating shaker. For maximum yield nitrogen concentration of 0.05% was found to be optimum in the case of *Kluyvera citrophila* var. α.

6.2.2.3. Transformaing α-ketoglutaric acid to L-glutamic acid

Two methods for conversion of α-ketoglutaric acid to L-glutamic acid have been reported: by microorganism and by enzymatic conversion.

6.2.2.3.1. Microorganism based conversion

Microorganisms belonging to following enlisted genera are able to accumulate glutamic acid : *Pseudomonas, Xanthomonas, Erwinia, Serratia, Bacillus, Micrococcus, Escherichia, Aerobacter, Hansenula, Debaxyomyces, Mycotorula* etc. Three different media are frequently used for these microorganisms for growth and hence conversion to L-glutamic acid. These are designated as A_1, A_2 and A_3. Their compositions are as follows:

Medium A$_1$

Sodium-α-ketoglutarate	1% (as free acid)
Glucose	0.1%
NH_4Cl	0.5%
$K_2 HPO_4$	0.1%
$MgSO_4 .7H_2O$	0.05%

Medium A$_2$

Medium A$_1$ plus 0.01% caseine-tryptic-hydrolysate

Medium A₃

Medium A₁ plus 0.008% caseine-tryptic-hydrolysate plus 0.007% yeast extract.

A 1:1 mixture of distilled water and tap water was used in the preparation media. The pH of each medium was adjusted to 7.

6.2.2.3.2. Conversion by enzymes

Enzymatic methods for converting α-ketoglutaric acid have been developed. Two procedures have been developed for undertaking the conversion of α-ketoglutaric acid and ammonium ions to glutamic acid using:

1. A biological catalytic system, containing a reversibly oxidizable and reducible nicotinic acid containing co-enzyme.
2. A water soluble hydrogen donating reactant.
3. A dehydrogenase system specific for this reactant.

The hydrogen donor oxidizes the coenzyme of dehydrogenase and as a result glutamic acid is formed. The reaction is undertaken at a pH of 6.0-8.5 and the temperature 20-45°C. The hydrogen donating reactant may be citric acid, maleic acid, or glucose-6-phosphate.

6.3. VITAMINS

Vitamins are the essential components of the human diet which are required for a normal physiological behavior of the body. These products are now a days being produced by the micro-organisms using the fermentation principles. Various vitamins have been identified till date and their production strategies designed, however, our discussion will be limited only to two of these category, i.e. riboflavin (vitamin B₂) and ascorbic acid (vitamin C).

6.3.1. Riboflavin

Riboflavin also known as vitamin B₂ was first isolated from milk and synthesized in 1935. It occurs as intense yellow color due to the presence of complete isoalloxazine ring system. Chemical structure of riboflavin is shown as follows. Riboflavin is hygroscopic and sensitive to alkalies and is decomposed by ultraviolet and visible light. It is essential for growth and reproduction in mammalians.

Riboflavin may be produced by a number of microorganisms including yeast-like microbes, and bacteria. The most important of these are *Eremothecium ashbyii*, *Ashbya gossypii*, and certain *Clostridium* species (Table 6.12).

6.3.1.1. Production by A. gossypii

A. gossypii is the causative organism of a disease of cotton bolls (especially in South Africa), which produces rooting and staining. It may also cause infection to beans, citrus fruits, coffee, okra and tomatoes. Since the organism is highly pathogenic, it is essential to sterilize all fermentation residues and cultures before they are discarded.

Table 6.12 : Various sources of riboflavin

Bacteria	Yeast	Yeast like
Clostridium butyricum	Anascosporogenous:	Ashbya gossypii
Cl. acetobutylicum	Candida arborea	Eremothecium ashbyii
Cl. felsineum	C. flareri	
Cl. roseum	C. utilis	
Aerobacter aerogenes	Ascosporogenous:	
A. cloacae	Hansenula suaveolens	
Azotobacter chroococcum	Saccharomyces sp.	

6.3.1.1.1. Nutrient requirement

In order to achieve maximum yield of riboflavin commercial glucose and sometimes sucrose and maltose are used as the source of carbon. Peptone and animal stick liquor are used as nitrogen source and corn-steep liquor as plant protein source. Biotin, thiamin, and *meso*-inositol are also required for the optimum growth of micro-organism.

6.3.1.1.2. Stock culture

A. gossypii may be transferred at weekly intervals on a medium containing:

Peptone	0.5%
Yeast extract	0.3%
Malt extract	0.3%
Commercial glucose	1.0%
Agar	2.0%

Incubation temperature 27-30°C

6.3.1.1.3. Inoculum development

Pfeifer et al., (1950) described a method for preparing an inoculum for pilot-plant fermentation. A loopful of a 24 h old culture of *A. gossypii* NRRL Y-1056 placed in 100 ml of the following medium in a 500 ml flask and incubated for 24 h on a reciprocating shaker at 26 to 30°C.

Glucose	2.0%
Peptone	0.5%
Corn-steep liquor	1.0%
Water	to 100 ml.

The pH of this medium before sterilization for 30 min. at 121°C was 6.5. The contents of the flask were used to seed 6 liter of sterilized medium of the following composition contained in a 9 liter glass bottle:

Glucose	2.0%
Corn-steep liquor	1.0%
Animal-stick liquor	0.5%
Water	to 6 liter

The pH of the medium before sterilization for 45 minutes at 121°C was 6.5. The organism was grown for 24 h with aeration provided by passing sterile air through a perforated tube located at the bottom of the bottle. This culture can be used to inoculate 200 or 300 gallons of sterilized medium in a fermenter.

6.3.1.1.4. Production

For maximum yield of riboflavin the following composition of media is recommended and used:

Glucose	2.0%
Corn-steep liquor	1.8-2.1%
Animal-stick liquor	1.0%
An antifoam agent	Small amount

The medium has been sterilized at pH 4.5 and at a temperature 135°C for 5 minutes. An inoculum of 0.5 to 1.0% has been used for seeding fermenters. Sufficient aeration for adequate mixing of the medium but not hampering growth should be provided. An aeration rate being maintained at about 0.25 vol. of air per vol. of medium per min. is satisfactory. Fermentation is carried out at a temperature of 28 to 30°C for 96 to 120 h. The yields have been 500 to 600 μg/ml. of riboflavin. The fermentation liquor thus produced may be evaporated to a syrup and then dried on drum dryers to yield a concentrate containing 2.5% of riboflavin.

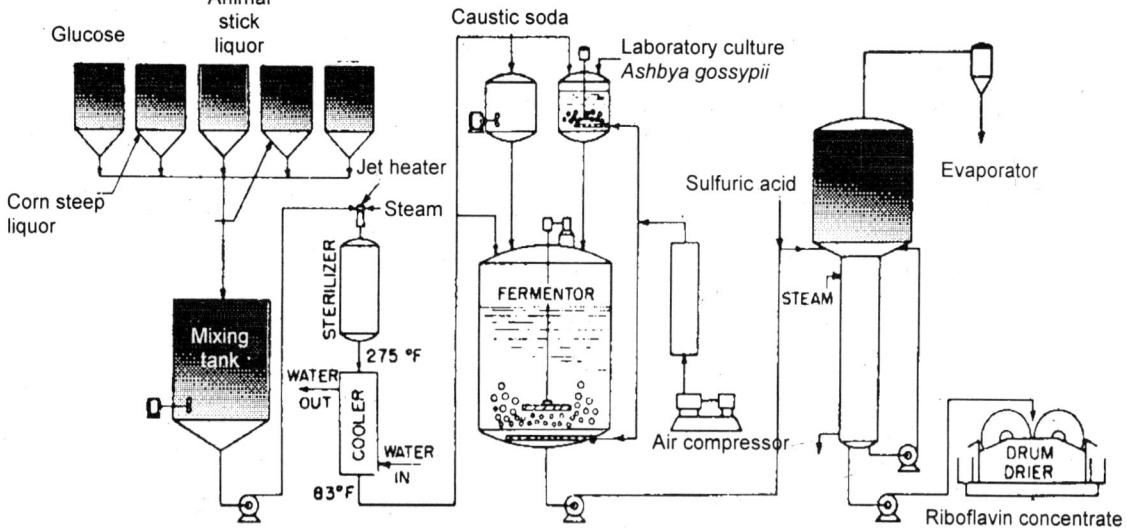

Fig. 6.11 : Flow diagram for the fermentation based production of riboflavin

6.2.1.2. Production by E. ashbyii

Riboflavin is produced industrially from *E. ashbyii,* a yeast like organism belonging to the *Ascomycetes.* Various patents describe the methodologies for riboflavin production. The methods described by Rudert (1945) for its production from *E. ashbyii* from subsequently carbohydrate-free media is based on the total weight of nutrients, the medium contains 10-90 % of proteinaceous materials, a metabolizable lipid and nutrient such as peptone or a combination of salts (0.05%, KH_2PO_4,0.07% $MgSO_4.7H_2O$),0.107 NaCl and 0.01% $FeSO_4.7H_2O$). In carrying out production, the following procedure is illustrative of Rudert's invention:

The media are adjusted to an initial pH of 5.5 to 7.5 and dispensed in containers to give a depth of 0.5 inch, sterilized at 20 psi for 45 minutes, cooled to 30°C, and inoculated with 0.7% of an active culture of *E. ashbyii.* During production, the temperature is maintained between 20 and 34°C and the medium is aerated with 1.5 to 2 Cu ft of sterile air/ min/sq. ft of mesh surface. At the end of 50 to 90 h, the conversion is completed. The dried residue contains 200 to 6000 μg/g of riboflavin.

Gaden, Petosiava and Winokar (1954) reported on the production of riboflavin from citrus molasses, using *E. ashbyii* NRRL 1363. The citrus molasses were clarified by settling followed by decantation. The inoculum was prepared by growing the microorganism for 24 h in a sterilized medium containing:

Clarified citrus molasses 1.5%
Yeast extract 0.3%
Peptone 1.0%
pH adjusted to 6.6 to 6.8

The use of an initial concentration of citrus molasses equivalent to approximate 6.0% reducing sugar, fortified by the addition of a commercial enzymatic yeast hydrolysate at a concentration of 0.3% has been recommended for the production of highest yields of riboflavin. The pH of the production medium was adjusted between 6.5

to 8 before sterilization, which generally resulted in a pH of about 6.4 to 6.8 after sterilization. This production medium was inoculated with 4% by volume of inoculum. Yields of as much as 729 μg/ml of riboflavin were obtained on 7-9 days of incubation at 27°C to 30°C in shaker flasks.

6.3.1.3. Production by Candida species

Burkholder (1943) found that *Candida guilliermondia* grew and produced riboflavin satisfactorily in media containing dextrose, mannose, levulose, or sucrose. Aspargine and glycine were found to be suitable and relatively inexpensive sources of nitrogen for riboflavin production by *C. guilliermondia* (A.T.C.C. 9058).

Medium

	g/l		PPM
KH_2PO_4	0.5	Boron	0.01
$MgSO_4.7H_2O$	0.5	Manganese	0.01
$CaCl_2. 2H_2O$	0.3	Zinc	0.07
$(NH_4)_2SO_4$	2.0	Copper	0.01
KI	0.1	Molybdenum	0.01
Aspargine	2.0	Iron	0.01
Dextrose	20.0	Biotin	1 μg

Most satisfactory results were obtained when the pH was adjusted to 5 to 6 and temperature was maintained at 30°C. An increased yields of riboflavin were obtained by adding small amount of sterile potassium cyanide to the medium under vigorous fermentation.

The fermentation time was 6-7 days. Tanner and Van Lanen (1947) have patented a method for producing riboflavin from *C. flareri*. The method briefly consists of fermentation under aerobic conditions at 30°C for about 7 days using other suitable *Candida* species, in a medium containing a fermentable sugar, an assimilable source of nitrogen, non iron salts, biotin and less than 10.3μg of iron/100 ml. The preferred species of candida are *C. flareri* and *C. guilliermondia*.

6.3.1.4. Recovery of riboflavin

Riboflavin may be recovered from production substrates by a variety of procedures, many of them are patented. Keresztesy (1944) patented a procedure for extracting riboflavin with butanol, followed by the use of other solvents, such as petroleum ether and acetone. McMillan (1945) patented a chemical precipitation method in which a soluble reducing agent and a finely divided diatomaceous earth were used. Hines (1945a) described a method wherein riboflavin was absorbed on fuller's earth, silica gel, or other adsorbent and eluted with an aldehyde, ketone or alcoholic solution of an organic base. Another procedure by Hiner (1945b) related to the conversion of riboflavin to a less soluble form by the action of reducing bacteria, such as *Streptococcus faecalis*. Dale (1947) has patented a method for securing crystalline riboflavin from the precipitate produced by the reduction of this vitamin to a less soluble form by either reducing bacteria or using some chemical reducing agent.

6.3.2. Ascorbic acid (vitamin C)

Vitamin C, (L-ascorbic acid) was isolated from lemons, capsicum fruit, adrenals etc., prior to 1930s. In 1933 Reichstein and associates as well as Haworth et al., independently published first synthesis of vitamin C. Industrial production of Vitamin C is based chiefly on Reichstein procedure. Some other procedures have also been developed afterwards.

6.3.2.1. Reichstein synthesis

In this method D-glucose is hydrogenated chemically to produce D-sorbitol. A deionized enzymatic hydrolysate of starch obtained following the action of mould glucoamylase, is directly hydrogenated in a contemporary method, instead of using crystalline glucose.

Non isolated sorbitol thus produced in the form of 20% or more concentrated solution, is then subjected to biochemical dehydrogenation, by *Acetobacter suboxydans*, to yield L-sorbose. L-sorbose is then isolated and condensed with acetone to form 2,3,4,6-diisopropylidene-L-sorbose (so called diacetonesorbose). This offers protection to L-sorbose from an advanced oxidation. In the above mentioned step: 2,3,4,6-diissopropylidene-L-sorbose is oxidized to diacetone-2-keto-L-gulonic acid, which after hydrolysis, enolization, and lactonization yields L-ascorbic acid. By this method, production of 1kg of vitamin C requires 2-4 kg of glucose. Thus, the process is highly economical.

6.4.1.1. Sorbose fermentation

Initially employed *Acetobacter xylinum* (previously named 'sorbose bacterium' by Bertrand), when used in surface fermentation process yields 40-60% sorbose after about 6 weeks. Other species of Acetobacter were also studied. *Acetobacter suboxydans* was discovered later, yields after 7 days of surface fermentation, 80-90% sorbose. For the preparation of inoculum, a medium containing 10% sorbitol, 0.5% yeast extract, 1% glucose, and 3.1% calcium carbonate were used by Wells et al (1939).

Culture media for *Acetobacter suboxydans* for the growth of microorganism required an inclusion of (apart from assimilable sources of carbon, organic nitrogen and mineral salts), pantothenic acid. It does not require riboflavin and biotin. Sorbitol serves as the source of carbon whereas other nutrients are supplied by dried yeast extract (0.1-1.0.%), yeast autolysate, or corn steep liquor. Industrial production of sorbose requires cheap materials as corn steep liquor, a decoction of waste brewers yeast, acidic yeast hydorlysate, and alfalfa extract. Generally 0.3% of corn steep liquor is used but its concentration can be lowered to as low as 0.1% according to later experiments. Studies have shown that organic sources of nitrogen may be partly replaced by ammonium sulfate, phosphate or nitrate. Cells grown in media with a high content of organic nutrients show higher growth rate and lower dehydrogenation activity than those grown in less nutrient media. Amounts of phosphate, i.e., 10-50 mg/ml were found to be optimal. It was found earlier that the sorbitol concentration in the medium may be as high as 35%, in such cases the sorbose content attainable per 100ml of the medium is 28g after complete fermentation. On the production scale sorbitol concentration 20g/100ml; as a rule was used. In such concentration inoculum can be cultivated in the same whenever possible, inoculum used should be collected from the preceding batch at time when the culture achieves the highest activity. Fresh inoculum is prepared only in the cases of contamination or where decreased activity of the culture is observed. The amount of inoculum added varies between 5 and 20%. Use of small amount of inoculum extend, the duration of fermentation. If media with higher sorbitol concentration are to be used, it is of advantages to begin with the fermentation in a less concentrated medium (e.g., 10-20 g/100ml), and subsequently to enrich it by gradually adding concentrated solution of sorbitol (if necessary with respective nutrients added) until the total amount of sorbitol added corresponds to an initial concentration of 28 g/100ml of the medium. Intense aeration is required during the preparation of inoculum as well as fermentation. Fermentation may be accelerated by increasing the air pressure in the fermenter. Substitution of air by oxygen under increased pressure substantially shortens the duration of fermentation where *Acetobacter xylinum* and *Acetobacter suboxydans* were used. Some investigators have reported that oxygen content elevated over its usual percentage in the air inhibited the activity of some species, i.e., *Acetobacter melanogenum*.

Right time to interrupt the sorbose fermentation is when concentration of reducing sugars, calculated as sorbose, reaches about 96-99% of refractometrically estimated drug sugars in the solution, the latter is filtered or centrifuged and the clear liquid is then thickened under reduced pressure (at a temperature not exceeding 50°C) for crystallization. Deionization prior to thickening leads to increased yield. It has been observed that crystallization at pH 3.0 gives an increased yield and better quality of sorbose. Yields have been reported in the range of 70-80% and with previous deionization as high as 87% of sorbitol used. On the laboratory scale, production of other reducing sugars as D-fructose, 5-keto-D-fructose (2,5-D-threodi-ketohexose) has been also recorded in small amounts as a result of side metabolism.

Initially sorbose fermentation was carried out in rotating drum with an air under pressure of 30 psi over periods of 33-45 h and yields obtained were approximately 98%. A defoamer 0.08%, octadecanol was sometimes added to the rotating drum. Later an conventional type vat fermenters were developed which were equipped with means like perforated papers for dispersion of air. Because of high toxicity of nickel for *Acetobacter suboxydans*, equipment was constructed in high purity aluminum or nickel free stainless steel. Defoamers employed in these were 0.1% octadecanol, soyabean oil and liquid portions of cord. Activated charcoal was also recommended for this purpose. Later on cylindrical fermenters equipped with mechanical stirrers and aeration devices, similar to those commonly used in production of antibiotics were developed.

The problem of sensitivity of commonly used Acetobacter to nickel has been studied in detail. Nickel may be present in sorbitol because of use of Raney nickel present in sorbitol, was removed by using disodium hydrogen phosphate. Presently if necessary, it is removed with the use of catexes (cationic exchange resins). Removal of nickel by precipitation with raw protein contained in the nourishing additive e.g. corn steep liquor is advantageous. Precipitate formed by boiling is removed by filtration or centrifugation, thereby subsequently reducing the nickel content. Besides these approaches, in laboratory conditions *Acetobacter suboxydans* has been adapted to tolerate concentrations of nickel as high as 600 mg/l of fermentation medium. Normal upper limit for the organism is 10mg/l.

Efforts to simplify Reichsteins synthesis has been directed mainly towards finding a process which would allow direct oxidation of sorbose to 3 keto- L- gluconic acid. Initially direct chemical oxidation of sorbose to 2 - keto-L-gluconic acid gave yields of 15 - 20 % because of concomitant side reactions. Newer processes use slow air oxidation, catalyzed by platinum, with stated yields of 60 - 65%. A Pfizer patent uses 0.5 - 2% solutions of sorbose that are oxidized by selected strains of genus *Pseudomonas* in a weakly alkaline medium. The process lasts for 50-70 hours. One another process utilizes *Pseudomonas* species mutant, for fermentation of 2% solution of sorbose. About 16% conversion of 2 keto-L-idonic acid takes place, 0.8% sorbose remaining in the solution. Japanese patents use selected species of genera *Acetobacter* or *Pseudomonas* for oxidation up to 5% sorbitol solutions directly to 2 keto-L-idonic acid, this acid may be, if separated from the solution with the help of an annex (anionic exchange resin) or esterified without previous isolation, and converted to L-ascorbic acid. Yields of isolated 2-keto-L-idonic acid reaches about 8% of the sorbitol used; the fermentation lasts for 150 hours.

6.3.2.2. Newer processes for vitamin C preparation

Bernhaner's team produced calcium 5-keto-D-gluconate (5 keto L-idonate) and calcium 2, keto-D-gluconate for the first time by fermentation. In this process glucose is converted by biochemical dehydrogenation in the presence of calcium carbonate to calcium 5,keto-D-gluconate. D-gluconic acid is an intermediate product. According to the original procedures calcium 5,keto-D-gluconate was catalytically dehydrogenated to a mixture of calcium-D-gluconate with calcium-L-idonate in a 1:1 ratio. Only L-idonate component of the mixture can be used for further preparation stages of L-ascorbic acid. The D-gluconate processed analog yields isoascorbic acid (a-D-arboascorbic acid)that possesses only about 1/20 of the biological activity of L-ascorbic acid (VI). Therefore, the reduction mixture was to be processed further in order to separate out either hexonate or at least to isolate L-idonate component from the mixture.

Several separation processes have been used; some of which are as under

1. Chemical separation by formation of slightly soluble dibenzyl L-idonic acid and likewise slightly soluble binary salt which consists of cadmium (II) L-idonate and cadmium (II) chloride or bromide.

2. Calcium-D-gluconate present in reduction mixture is dehydrogenated, using a suitable strain of *Acetobacter suboxydans* back to slightly soluble calcium 5,keto-D-gluconate; this salt is returned into the process while calcium L-idonate remains in the solution. The yields obtained from this relatively simple procedure are not satisfactory.

3. The reduction mixture is directly hydrogenated by bacterial strains capable of selective dehydrogenation of hexanoic acid in position 2. It was found that, in this case, D-gluconate is first dehydrogenated to 2-keto-D-gluconate (2-keto-D-mannolate (VIII) which is totally degraded during further course of the process, while 2-keto-L-idonate (2, keto-L-gulonate)(V) remains in the solution. This simple process of separation directly

yielding the intermediate product has the disadvantage of loosing one half of the material at the third stage of synthesis.

6.4. ALCOHOL FERMENTATION

Alcohol fermentation is known since ages. Ayurveda also deals with alcoholic preparations made by fermentation of crude drugs. Asavas and aristas are the alcoholic ayurvedic preparations prepared by fermentation of crude drugs. Louis Pasture, almost a century ago, first reported the yeast mediated fermentation of sugars for the production of alcohol.

The chemical name of alcohol is ethyl alcohol or ethanol and its chemical structure is CH_3CH_2OH. The term alcohol is named to indicate the source of raw material from which it is manufactured, or to indicate the general purpose for which it is used. For example grain alcohol are alcohol made from grains such as whey, rice or corn. Industrial alcohol is ethyl alcohol which is used in various industrial purposes. Alcohol finds a large number of application in the pharmaceutical industry. It is used in the preparation of various formulations, extraction of active constituents from crude drugs as well as in disinfection.

6.4.1. Raw material

Ethyl alcohol may be produced from frementable sugar by yeast under suitable conditions. Starches and certain carbohydrates, may be hydrolyzed to fermentable sugars by biological or chemical means.

Raw materials for alcohol fermentation may be classified into three categories:

1. Sucrose containing or the saccharine materials - for example, corn, sugar beets, molasses and fruit juices.
2. Starch containing materials such as wheat, rice, corn, malt, barley, rye, oats, sorghum, potatoes, etc.
3. Cellulose containing materials such as wood, and waste sulfite liquor.

Various types of raw materials used in alcohol production are listed below:

1.Cellulose pulp; crude ethanol mixtures	1.Ethyl sulfate
2.Cerelose	2.Ethylene gas
3.Corn syrup	3.Grain and grain products
4.Corn sugar by- products	4.Molasses
5.Citrus waste concentrate	5.Potato and potato products
6.Fermented liquor	6.Sulfite liquor
7.Fruit juices	7.Whey

Molasses and grains are the principal carbohydrate materials used in the production of ethanol by fermentation.

6.4.2. Ethanol from molasses

Molasses is the main source of industrial alcohol. It is the by-product of sugar industry. It is mainly a syrupy substance that is left after the recovery of crystalline sugar from the concentrated juice of sugar cane. It usually contains 48-55 % of sugars of which major proportion is represented mainly by sucrose. There are seven steps involved in production of ethanol from molasses. They are as follows:

1. Selection of yeast
2. Preparation of starter
3. The molasses and its preparation for fermentation
4. Optimization of process parameters
5. Distillation and recovery
6. Yield
7. Purification
8. Storage.

6.4.2.1. Selection of yeast

Various strains of *Saccharomyces cerevisiae* are commonly used, but other yeasts such as *S. anamensis* and *Schizosaccharomyces pombe* are also employed under certain conditions in the fermentation production of alcohol.

6.4.2.2. Preparation of starter

After selection of the yeast for the fermentation and its isolation in pure culture, a starter is prepared and the large quantities of starters are used to 'pitch' or inoculate the main mesh. About 10 ml of sterile wort is inoculated from a pure culture of yeast using aseptic technique. After incubation for suitable time period at a temperature 25-30°C, the culture is used to inoculate a flask containing 200 ml of sterile mesh. After incubation, the contents of flask may be used to seed a sterile mesh of about 4 liter capacity. Aeration is used to increase the production of yeast cells. The automatic systems are used for preparing the starter instead of the above method. In these types of system a stock of the pure culture is maintained in the upper drum of the apparatus (Fig. 6.12). Meshes are inoculated using this pure culture.

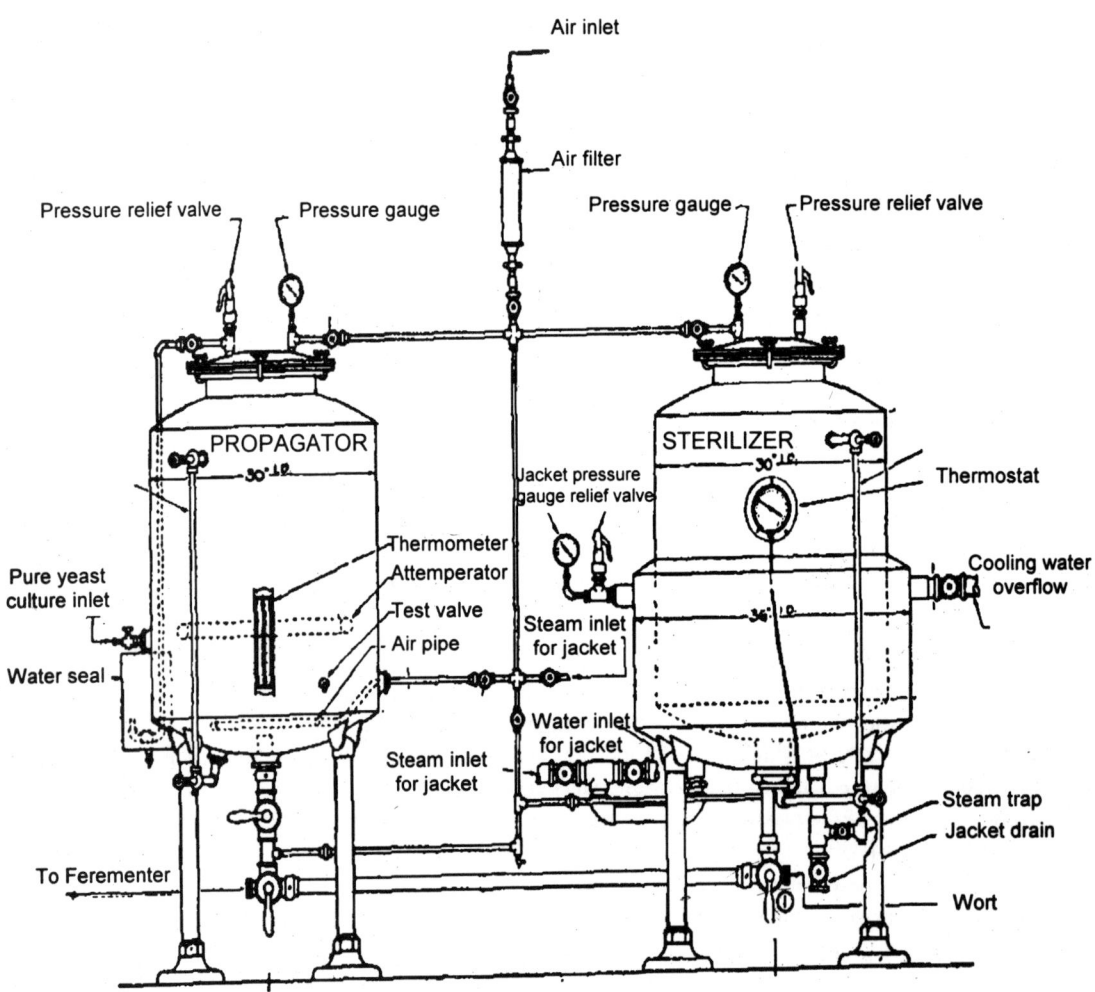

Fig. 6.12 : Pure yeast propagator

6.4.2.3. The molasses and its preparation for fermentation

Molasses is the main source of industrial alcohol, which is a byproduct of sugar industry. It is the syrup that is left after the recovery of crystalline sugar. It usually contains 48-55% of sugar mainly sucrose.

6.4.2.3.1. Adjustment of concentration of sugar

Higher concentration of sugar inhibits the action of yeast. As a consequence of this, the fermentation time is prolonged leaving some sugar unutilized. The use of very low sugar concentration on the other hand is uneconomic. A sugar concentration of 10-15% is found to be optimum for alcohol production. In practice 12% sugar concentration is used. Molasses is diluted to desired sugar concentration with water. The sugar concentration in wort is determined by means of Balling hydrometer.

6.4.2.3.2. Nutrient Substances

Generally molasses contains most of the nutrient substances required for fermentation, however ammonium salts such as ammonium sulfate or phosphate are added to the mesh to provide nitrogen and phosphorous supply.

6.4.2.3.3. pH of the mesh

The optimum pH for the fermentation is 4.0-4.5. This pH favors the growth of yeast but at the same time inhibits the growth of many types of bacteria. Sulfuric acid is commonly used to adjust the pH of mesh. Sometimes lactic acid may be used. Lactic acid favors the growth of yeast but inhibits the growth of butyric acid bacteria which has the detrimental effect on the development of yeast.

6.4.2.3.4. Oxygen tension

Large amount of oxygen is required in the early stages to facilitate the maximum reproduction of yeast cells, however, it is not required for the bioproduction of alcohol. During fermentation carbon dioxide is evolved which creates anaerobic condition

6.4.2.3.5. Temperature

The mesh is inoculated at a temperature between 18 to 28°C. Heat is evolved during fermentation resulting in to an increased temperature of mesh. To maintain suitable temperature of mesh, cooling with sprays on the outside of the tank are utilized. At the temperature above 28°C, alcohol evaporates very rapidly favoring bacterial growth, which effectively modulates the temperature.

6.4.2.3.6. Time required for fermentation

A fermentation is usually completed in 50 h or less, depending on the temperature, sugar concentration and other factors.

6.4.2.4. Distillation

The fermented mesh 'beer' is distilled to separate the ethyl alcohol and fused oil from other constituents of the mesh. Fractions containing different concentration of alcohol and slops are separated. The fraction containing 60 to 90% of ethanol is known as 'high wines'. These fractions are concentrated to 95% ethanol concentration level by further distillation fractionation.

6.4.2.5. Yield

Approximately 90% of the theoretical yield is achieved on the basis of the amount of fermentable sugar. However, the yield of the product could be specifically increased by variation of the process parameters as per the available plant facilities.

6.4.2.6. Purification

The 95% alcohol is further purified, dehydrated or denatured. The flow chart is presented in figure 6.13 representing various steps involved in the purification and the recovery of the alcohol. The facilities and the processes vary in regard to the starter and the nutrient used for the initiation of the process.

6.4.3. Ethyl alcohol from whey

The main constituent of whey is lactose 5%. Lactose fermenting yeast are used in production of alcohol from whey. Some of the yeast most often used in alcohol fermentation are enlisted below.

Torula cremoris	*Saccharomyces fragilis*	*S. lactis*
Torula sphaerica	*Z. lactis*	*T. kefir*
Torula lactosa	*S. anamensis*	*M. lactis*

Torula cremoris (renamed as *Canadian pseudotropicalis*) is generally used because the rate of lactose fermentation is high as compared to other micro-organism. 2 % w/w yeast is required for seeding as compared to lactose present in the whey before fermentation 33-34°C as an optimum temperature maintained for fermentation. However, at 37°C the fermentation is more rapid, nevertheless, the evaporation of alcohol is also more.

6.4.3.1. Production methodology

The whey is heated to boiling, and pH is adjusted to 5.0 by adding acid, followed by filtration of the proteins. The pH of the clarified whey should be between 4.8 to 5.2. The pH of the whey mesh is adjusted to a range of 4.7 to 5.0. The fermentation profile and apparatus are schematically presented in figure 6.14.

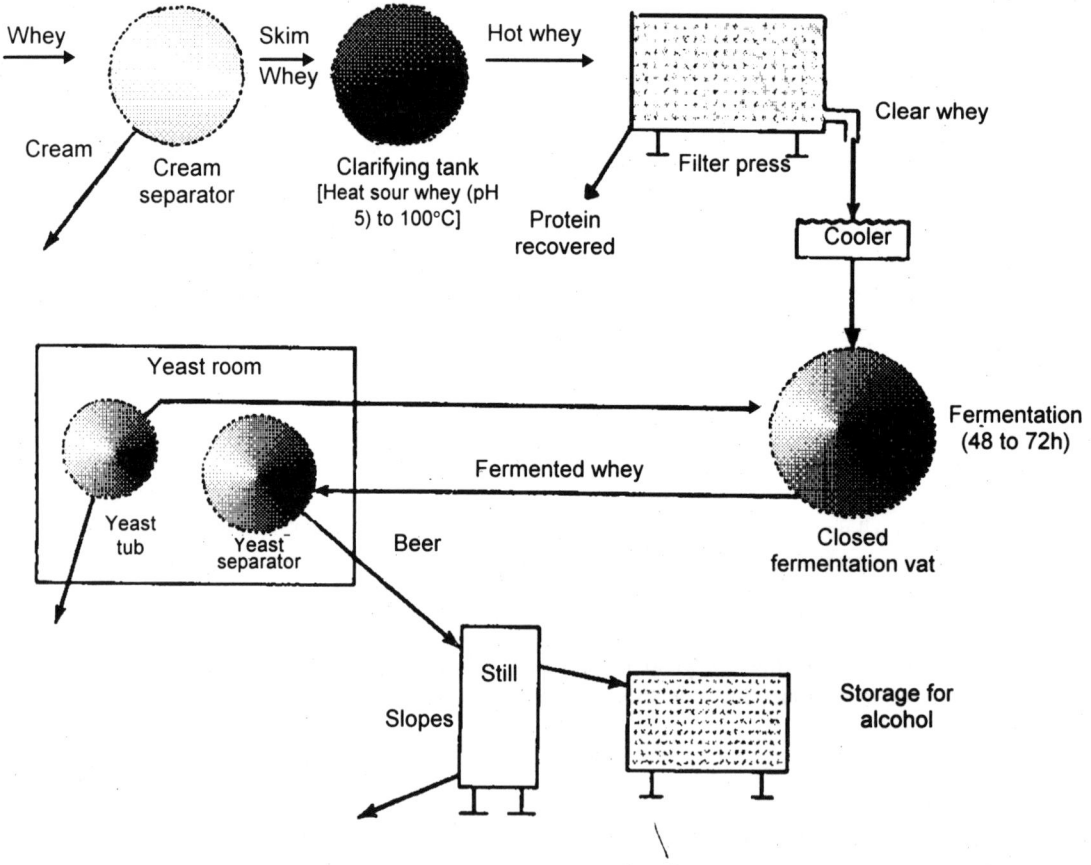

Fig. 6.14: Production of alcohol from whey

The clear whey is cooled to 34°C and 500 g of *C. pseudotropicalis* added per 1000 liter of whey. Fermentation is carried out at 33-34°C for 48-72h. The yeast is separated out and alcohol is distilled off. A 90% yield of alcohol is obtained on a laboratory scale and 84% under semiplant conditions.

SUGGESTED READINGS

Asai, T., Aida, k. and Oisho, K., (1957) *L-Glutamic Acid Fermentation*, **Bull. Arg. Chem. Soc., Japan**, 21, 134-135.

Barnhauer, K., (1950) **Erged. Enzym. Forsch.**, 11,151.

Brown, A.G., Butterworth, D., Cols, M., Hanscomb, G., Hood, J.D., Readings, C. and Rolinson, G. N., (1976) **J. Antibiot.**, 29, 668.

Campbell, A.M. (1954) **Research**, 6, 42-50.

Casida Jr., L.E., (1956) **Preparation of Diaminopimelic Acid and Lysine**, US. Patent No. 2,771,396.

Casida Jr., L.E., (1968) **Industrial Microbiology**, New Age International (P) Ltd. Publ., New Delhi.

Chang, L.T., Terasaka, D.T. and Elander, R.P., (1992) **Development in Industrial Microbiology**, Vol-23.

Davis, B.D., (1949) **Proceedings National Academey of Science**, USA, ,35, 1-10

Demain, A.L. (1981) **Science**, 214, 987-995.

Fiechter, A. (1978) **Dechema Monogr.**, 82, 17.

Growich Jr., J. A. and Deduck, N., (1963) **Tetracycline Fermentation**, U.S. patent No. 3,092,556.

Gupta, P.K. (1997) **Elements of Biotechnology**, Rastogi Publication, Meerut.

Hockenhull, D.J.D., (1960), *The biochemistry of Streptomycin Production*; In: **Progress in Industrial Microbiology**, D.J.D. Hockenhull (Ed.), Vol. II, Interscience Publishers, Inc., New York, 131-165.

Hodgkin, D.C., Pickworth, J., Robertson, J.H., Trublood, K.N., Prosen, R,J., White, R., Bonnette, R., Cannon, J.R., Johnson, A.W., Suther Land, I., Todd, A.R. and Smith, E.L. (1955) **Nature**, 176, 325-330.

Hodgkin, D.C., Pickworth, J., Robertson, J.H., Tru blood, K.N., Prosen, R,J., White, R., Bonnette, R., Cannon, Johnson, J.R., Suther Land, A.W., Todd, I. and Smith, E.L. (1955) **Nature**, 176, 325-330.

Hopwood, D.A., (1979) **Genetics of Industrial Microorganisms**, Sebek, O.K. and Laskin, A., I (Eds), American Society for Microbiology, Washington.

Katagiri, H.I., Imai, K., Tochikura, T., (1957) **Process for Producing α-Ketoglutamic Acid by Bacteria of Coli-Aerogens Group**, U.S. Patent No. 2786, 799.

Lockwood, L.B. and Stodala, (1946) **J. Biol. Chem.**, 164, 81-88.

Nakayama, K., Kituda, S. and Kinoshita, S., (1961) **Journal of General and Applied Microbiology**, 7, 41-51.

Pfeifer, V.F., Vojnovick, C. and Heger, E.N. (1954) **Eng. Chem.**, 46, 84?.

Prave, P., Faust, V., Sitting, W., Sukatsch, D.A. (1987) **Fundamentals of Biotechnology**, VCH, Germany

Prekop, A., Erckson, L.E., Frenandez, J. and Humphery, A.E., (1969) **Biotechnol. Bioeng.**, 11, 945.

Prescott, S.C. and Dunn, C.G. (1959) **Industrial Microbiology**, III Ed., McGraw-Hill Book Co. Inc., New York.

Reichstein, T., Grussner, A. and Opperauer, R. (1933), **Nature**, 132, 280.

Richards, M. and Haskins, R.H., (1957) *Extracellular Lysine production by various fungi*, **Can. J. Microbiol.**, 3, 543.

Riviere, J., (1986) **Industrial Applications of Microbiology**, Halstead Press, New York.

Stanier, Roger, Y., Ingraham, J.L., Wheelis, M.L and Painter. P. R., (1987), **General Microbiology**, 5 Ed, Macmillan Education Ltd., London.

Sylvester, J.C. and Coghill, R.D., (1954) *The Penicillin Fermentation;* In: **Industrial Fermentations,** L.A. Underkofler and R.J. Hickey (Eds.), Vol. II, Chemical Publishing Company Inc., New York., pp 219-263.

Taguchi, H. (1971) **Adv. Biochem. Eng.,** 1.

Trehan, K. (1994) **Biotechnology**, Wiley Eastern Ltd., New Delhi, 17-102.

Underkofler, L.A. and Hickey, R.J. (Ed.), (1954), **Industrial Fermentation,** Chemical Publishing Company Inc ., New York.

Vandamme, E.J.(Ed.) (1984) **Biotechnology of Industrial Antibiotics**, I Ed., Marcel Dekker Inc., New York.

PLANT CELL AND TISSUE CULTURE

7.1. INTRODUCTION

Tissue culture is an experimental technique through which a mass of cells (callus) is produced from an explant tissue. The callus produced through this process can be utilized directly to regenerate plantlets or to extract or manipulate some primary and secondary metabolites. Plant tissue culture is used as a gross term for protoplast, cell, tissue and organ cultures grown under aseptic conditions. The term 'cell culture' covers the growth of any cell, be it a microbe or a plant or animal cell. On the other hand 'tissue culture' refers to the cultivation of a plant or mammalian cell which normally forms a multicellular tissue. In these cultivation processes, the cells used for culture may be isolated from nature or the strains improved by selection, mutation or genetic manipulation.

When grown on agar medium, the tissue forms a callus or a mass of undifferentiated cells. The technique of cell culture is convenient for starting and maintaining cell lines, as well as, for studies pertaining to organogenesis and meristem culture. The liquid suspension cultures are comprised of mixtures of cell aggregates, cell clusters and single cells. Generally, the growth rate of such cultures is much higher than on solidified medium and a better control over the growth of biomass is offered as the cells are surrounded by the nutrient medium, and for the same reason, the cell material could be probably more uniform physiologically. Both callus and suspension cultures can be derived from tissues of most of the species, but the ease of starting the cultures varies with the type of plant and the origin of tissue. A callus and a suspension culture can be induced from any part of the plant. These necessary tissues can be obtained from roots, stem, seedlings, poller and leaf portions and they usually grow as a mass of undifferentiated cells on enriched solidified medium. Some of the salient features of tissue culture are :

1. The culture of the cells/tissues is carried out in a sterile medium under controlled conditions.

2. Clones generated through tissue culture are identical in terms of size, developmental stage and rate of metabolic activities.
3. The rate of tissue multiplication is rapid within a small area.
4. The clones are capable of performing the transformative activity which involves biotransformation to produce primary and secondary metabolites in the tissue culture medium.

7.2. HISTORICAL BACKGROUND

Over the years there has been an outstanding and spectacular progress in the area of tissue and cell culture. In the last six decades, this technique has reached a stage that is nothing short of phenomenal. Deliberate, however, well aimed *in vitro* culture of the plant and animal cell, tissue and organ has always fascinated the biotechnologists. A brief review of the work done in the direction of tissue culture is presented in table 7.1.

Table 7.1 : Work carried out in the direction of tissue culture

Researcher(s)	Work carried out
Haberblandt (1902)	First visualized the science of tissue culture. However, his attempts to obtain continuous culture of cells failed. His methods had a couple of blind spots viz., the nutritional and growth factors involved in cell growth were overlooked and plant materials used were unsuitable to culture
Robbins and Kotte(1922)	First to develop a technique for culture of isolated roots using maize roots. Efficiency of vitamins as growth promoters was established. But cultures had short survival time due to the faulty selection of materials
White (1939)	Successful culture of organized structures such as storage roots of carrot was achieved
Gautheret et al (1939-1957)	Studied histophysiological changes in explanted tissues brought about by addition of B-vitamins, cysteine HCl, glucose and indole acetic acid in basic media. Also examined the effect of growth hormones in cyto-differentiation and morphogenesis
Van Overback (1941)	Culture of plant embryo
Street (1950)	Role of vitamins in plant growth and shoot-root relationship established
Muir (1953 & 1958)	Developed single cell culture by the paper-raft 'nurse technique'
Welmore and Sorokin (1955); Wetmor and Rier (1963)	Established the role of auxins and vitamins as growth controlling factors
Skoog and Miller (1957)	Demonstrated that organogenesis had hormonal control over it
West and Kika (1957)	Callus production achieved
Torrey (1957); Jones (1960)	Single cell culture was developed by the micro-chamber method (hanging drop culture)
Reinert (1958); Steward (1959)	Demonstrated the development of embryoids from carrot cells in suspension
Tulecke (1959)	Developed submerged suspensions
Bergmann (1960)	Developed clones from a large number of cells
Kohienbach (1966)	Demonstrated the development of embryoids of leaf mesophyll cells of McCleayer cordata
Cocking (1970)	Protoplast fusion
Carlson et al (1972)	Production of first somatic hybrid
Nitsch (1974)	Discovered the chromosomal doubling in haploid tissues in the medium
Melchers et al. (1978)	Performed successful parasexual hybridization between potato and tomato
Bajaj et al. (1976)	Regenerated plants from cryopreserved plant tissues
Murashige (1977)	Proposed artificial seed production
Melcher (1978)	Production of somatic embryos by using the protoplast fusion technique
Barton et al. (1983)	Demonstrated gene transfer into the protoplast by using plasmid vectors
Lazar et al. (1983)	Production of cybrids by protoplast fusion technique

7.3. BASIC REQUIREMENTS FOR A TISSUE CULTURE LABORATORY

Tissue culture technique requires a controlled, aseptic environment to proceed with the establishment of callus in the nutrient media. In addition to this, some quanta of light is required by the plant cell during their growth and proliferation phases. The important requirements of a tissue culture laboratory are presented below:

7.3.1. Area for medium preparation

It should be separate and away from the working laboratory. This area is to be utilized for preparation of culture media and should be equipped with glassware, laminar air flow bench, weighing balance, a pH meter, a deep freezer and an autoclave.

7.3.2. A sterile room for inoculation

A sterile area is imperative for the tissue culture practice, viz., for distribution of medium into plates/flasks, for transfer of explants to the medium and for subculturing. Sterile room or a sterile air cabinet or laminar flow bench can serve the purpose.

7.3.3. Various glassware, apparatus and instruments

These include:

1. A large flask for preparation of nutrient media.
2. A pH meter for adjusting the pH of the medium.
3. Conical flask for the distribution of culture and culture medium.
4. Test tubes, pipettes, measuring cylinder, petri dishes for the preparation and transfer of culture media and culture.
5. Scissors, scalpels and forceps for explant preparation from excised plant parts and for their transfer.
6. Spirit lamp for carrying out the aseptic transfer.
7. A balance with appropriate weights to weigh various nutrients for the preparation of the medium.
8. An autoclave to sterilize the glassware, scissors, forceps and scalpels prior to use.
9. An incubator for maintaining constant temperature to facilitate the culture of callus and its subsequent maintenance.
10. A fluorescent tube light to ensure proper light required for normal growth and development.
11. A shaker to maintain cell suspension culture. This helps in growth of plant cells as individual cells and also provides adequate aeration.

7.4. CULTURE CONDITIONS AND PREPARATION OF CULTURE MEDIA

7.4.1. Culture conditions

For the successful culture of isolated plant cells and tissues on artificial media, many formulae have been developed. These have been based on the nutritional and hormonal requirements of the whole plants and these serve to suit the nutrition of particular tissues, be they free cells in suspension, somatic embryos or protoplasts. The components of the media are modified and adapted according to the objective of experimental studies of regeneration, micropropagation, cytodifferentiation, experimental androgenesis, biosynthesis of secondary metabolites or biotransformation of cells. Furthermore, in addition to an appropriate medium, maintenance of temperature, agitation, aeration, an optimum pH is essential for promoting growth or differentiation of cultured cells or tissues.

7.4.2. Culture media

The plant cells and tissues require a proper medium for their growth and development. The nutrient media for plant cell is a well defined mixture of inorganic salts and typical carbon sources like sucrose and glucose. In majority of cells, supplementary constituents are required which are essentially growth regulators, i.e. indole acetic acid (IAA), kinetin and NAA, vitamins like thiamin and nicotinic acid, amino acids, inositol and sugar alcohols. The various components of tissue culture media essentially involve the following ingredients.

7.4.2.1. Ingredients

Basically a complete media has the following ingredients:

I. Inorganic elements
a) Macro-elements (in mmol/l), e.g., N, P, K, Ca, Mg, S.
b) Micro-elements (in μmol/l), e.g., B, Mn, Zn, Cu, MO, Cl, Ni, Al, etc.

II. Organic components
a) Sugar (mmol/l)
b) Vitamins (μmol/l), e.g., thiamin, riboflavine, ascorbic acid, etc.
c) Phytohormones, eg., auxins, cytokinins, abscisic acid, etc.

III. Complex extract(s): This includes natural plant extracts and other undefined components. (e.g., coconut milk, yeast extract, malt extract, potato extract, tomato juice, casein hydrolysate, etc.).

IV. Water : Demineralized and double distilled water.

V. Agar: As a gelling agent when solid surface is required for growth.

The composition of Murashige and Skoog medium, the most widely used medium, is outlined in table 7.2.

Table 7.2 : Composition of Murashige and Skoog Medium

Compound	Conc. in medium mg/L	Amount in stock solution	Stock vol. ml
NH_4NO_3	1650	8.25g	
KNO_3	1900	9.50 g	
$MgSO_4.7H_2O$	370	1.85g	
KH_2PO_4	170	0.85 g	
KI	0.83	4.18mg	400
$MnSO_4.4H_2O$	22.30	111.50mg	
$ZnSO_4.7H_2O$	8.6	43.00mg	
Myo-inositol	100	0.50g	
$CaCl_2.2H_2O$	440	2.20g	
$FeSO_4.7H_2O$	27.8	139.25mg	100
$Na_2EDTA.2H_2O$	37.3	186.25mg	
$CuSO_4.5H_2O$	0.025	12.5mg	100
$Na_2MoO_4.2H_2O$	0.25	12.5mg	10
$CoCl_2.6H_2O$	0.025	12.5mg	100
Nicotinic acid	0.50	25.0mg	10
Pyridoxine-HCl	0.50	25.0mg	10
Thiamin-HCl	0.10	5.0mg	10
Glycine	2.0	100mg	10
Sucrose	30g/L		

7.4.2.2. Stock solutions

The word 'medium' refers to the basic culture medium devoid of any organic solution or growth hormones. In the preparation of media, usually a series of stock solutions is employed. Solutions of micro-elements and vitamins are made in 1000x final concentration and stored in the freezer. Stock solutions of KI can also be prepared. Calcium and magnesium sulfates and phosphates however should not be combined keeping in view their insolubility and consequent precipitation. Hormones should be dissolved in a little of ethanol and their volume should be made up with water to yield a concentration of 2-3 mM. Alternatively, they can be dissolved in dimethyl sulfoxide. Care should be taken to quantify media components in molar units rather than by weight. This enables to make possible the valid comparison and interpretation of concentration effects of equimolar concentration of various constituents.

7.4.2.3. Preparation of the media

The various steps involved in the preparation of media can be outlined as :

1. Macronutrients are dissolved in 200 ml of distilled water.
2. Micronutrients are dissolved in 200 ml of distilled water in another flask.

3. Vitamins are dissolved in 100 ml of distilled water in a separate flask and stored at refrigerated conditions.

4. Growth hormones are also dissolved separately in 100 ml of distilled water and stored in a cool place.

5. To prepare 1 liter of the media the above solutions are mixed together.

6. Sucrose and amino acids (if any) are added to the medium.

7. The volume of the media is made up to 950 ml by the addition of distilled water.

8. The pH of this solution is adjusted to 5.6 with 0.1M sodium hydroxide solution or 0.1M hydrochloric acid solution.

9. Finally the volume of this media is made up to 1 liter with distilled water.

10. The prepared media is transferred to conical flasks and the mouth of these flasks are plugged with non-adsorbent cotton. If a solid medium is desired, agar amounting to 2% w/v is added to each flask.

11. The above conical flasks are autoclaved and used for tissue culture.

7.4.2.4. pH of the media

pH of the media greatly affects the uptake of ingredients, solubility of salts and gelling efficiency of agar. An initial pH of the media prior to autoclaving is measured although it undergoes changes during culture. The pH is adjusted by a pH meter using 0.1M NaOH or HCl. Optimum pH depends upon the particular strain of tissue but a pH of 5.6-5.8 is often suitable for maintaining all the salts in a near buffered form. In spite of the initial adjustments, the pH of the medium usually changes after autoclaving and the media composition also gets affected. Normally, plant tissue culture media are poorly buffered, still pH remains stabilized to some extent as the media contains both nitrate and ammonium ions. Further it is highly desirable to maintain the pH at optimum value as agar may fail to gel at a low pH.

7.4.2.5. Sterilization of media

Sterilization of media can be carried by autoclaving at 15 psi for 20 minutes. Thermolabile components like certain carbohydrates, vitamins, growth regulators and plant extracts can be conveniently sterilized by micro-filtration and then added aseptically to the sterile medium (after it has been autoclaved but before it has reached the solidification temperature of agar).

7.4.3. Isolation of organs, tissues and cells

As discussed earlier all the manipulations involved in isolating and establishing plant tissue *in vitro* are conducted under aseptic conditions in a transfer chamber or transfer room. The basic necessary tools for plant tissue culture work include transfer loops, microspatulas, scalpels and forceps. These tools may be placed upright in alcohol and flamed and cooled prior to use.

7.4.3.1. Explant preparation

An explant is a detached portion of the plant body which is used in tissue culture to produce callus tissues. The age of explant (i.e., the age of meristematic tissue) plays a vital role in the production of callus. The desired portion is excised from the parent plant and utilized for callus induction. Seeds and grains are also considered to be good sources for preparation of explants. Seeds and grains after surface-sterilization are germinated aseptically in nutrient media by placing them on double layers of pre-sterilized filter paper in petri dishes moistened sufficiently with sterile distilled water or on moist cotton plugs in petri dishes or culture tubes. After few days, they germinate into seedlings, which are removed and surface-sterilized. These can then be used as a source of explants.

7.4.3.2. Surface sterilization of explants

In general, to carry out fresh isolation of tissues or organs, the surface sterilization of the plant materials should be kept at minimum. Commonly used surface sterilizing agents are sodium hypochlorite (1-2%), bromine water (1-2%), hydrogen peroxide (10-12%), mercuric chloride (0.1-1.0%) and silver nitrate (1%). The aerial portion of plants such as bud, leaf and stem sections are sterilized by submerging for 2-3 min in 70% ethanol, followed by 2-3 rinses with sterilized distilled water.

7.4.4. Establishment of cultures

7.4.4.1. Agar gel culture

The surface sterilized plant material is aseptically transferred onto solidified nutrient medium in flasks, glass jars or culture tubes and then incubated at 26-28°C in dark. After 3-4 weeks, the callus should be about 5 times the size of the explant. Many tissue explants possess some degree of polarity with the result that callus is formed most easily at one surface. In stem segments, callus is formed particularly from the surface which *in vivo* is directed towards the root. The callus often develops more readily from the tissue not in contact with and particularly not immersed in the solidified culture medium. The maintenance of growth in callus tissue by subculture requires the transfer of a piece of healthy tissue every 4 weeks into the flasks containing fresh solidified nutrient medium. Many cultures shall, however, remain healthy and continue a slow rate of growth for much longer periods without subculturing, if the standard incubation temperature of 26°C is lowered to 5-10°C. It has been observed that the growth of many cultures and particularly of those which form chlorophyll is stimulated by low-intensity illumination. Light either on a 12 h cycle or continuously, therefore, usually provided in the incubation chambers by fluorescent tubes.

The well-developed callus is cut into small pieces with a sterile knife. The pieces of callus are then transferred to another media, the **proliferation media**, to induce proliferation of callus. In this media the callus tissue multiplies more rapidly. 2,4-D is avoided in the proliferation medium as it induces callus product in most tissues. Instead the callus segments are cultured in the media containing growth hormone like IAA, NAA, 6-benzyl amino purine, kinetin. IAA induces callus production in the dicots but high concentration reduces callus production in monocots.

Sub culture of callus after the proper growth of callus tissues is usually developed as it is transferred to a fresh medium at regular intervals. This transfer of callus tissues facilitates the maintenance of the cells in a viable condition. The previously cultured tissues serve as an explant for establishing the secondary culture. This process of culture is also referred to as **sub-culture**. Generally, this process of sub-culture is practiced at regular intervals of four weeks. All steps involved are represented in a scheme in figure 7.1.

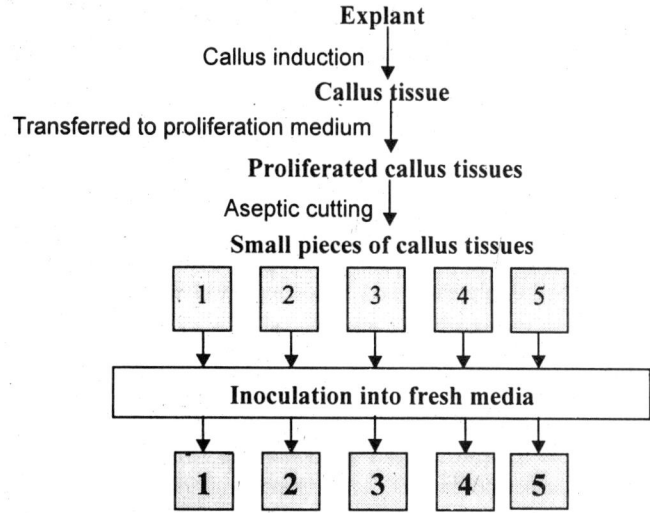

Fig. 7.1 : Various stages involved in callus induction, proliferation and sub-culture

7.4.4.2. Suspension culture

This culture essentially contains homogeneous individual plant cells in its liquid medium. The suspension cultures are generally initiated by transferring an established callus tissue to an agitated liquid nutrient medium in Erlenmeyer culture vessels (30-60 ml medium per 250 ml flasks). The composition of the medium for the establishment of suspension cultures could be the same as defined for callus cultures except for the addition of agar. The soft callus generally forms in a suspension culture without much difficulty. The release of cells and tissue fragments from less friable callus masses and the maintenance of a good degree of cell separation may often be promoted by the presence of a high auxin concentration and with an appropriate balance between yeast extract and auxin or between auxin and kinetin. The suspension cultures are usually incubated at 25°C in darkness or in low intensity fluorescent light. Continuous agitation of flask cultures is most commonly achieved by using horizontal rotary shaker which rotates at between 100 and 200 revolutions per minute. The culture flasks are sealed with double aluminum foil or parafilms to reduce evaporation during the process of culture growth. A cell suspension is generally formed within 4 to 6 weeks. The cells grown in cultures are **meristematic** and usually undifferentiated and there is no evidence that cells of shoot or root origin are metabolically different. The suspension cultures are **subcultured** by the transfer at regular intervals of untreated or fractionated aliquots of the suspension to fresh medium.

7.5. GROWTH PROFILE OF THE PLANT CULTURE AND ITS MEASUREMENT

7.5.1. Growth Profile

7.5.1.1. Cell culture

The various stages of the growth exhibited by the plant cell culture are to a great extent similar to those of the microorganisms. The various stages of growth are displayed in figure 7.2 and can be enumerated as:

1. **Lag Phase:** Here following subculture into the fresh medium, the cell regains the ability of division and the tissue shows slow growth.
2. **Exponential phase:** This stage involves rapid cell division. The duration of this stage varies according to the cell and its nutrient regime. In majority of the cases it is a short one and lasts for only 3-4 generations.
3. **Linear phase:** The growth in this phase follows a linear pattern with respect to time.
4. **Progressive deceleration phase:** In this stage the rate of cell division declines with the aging of the culture.
5. **Stationary phase:** During this phase the rate of production of cells is equal to the rate of their death.
6. **Senescent phase:** During this phase the cells are dying.

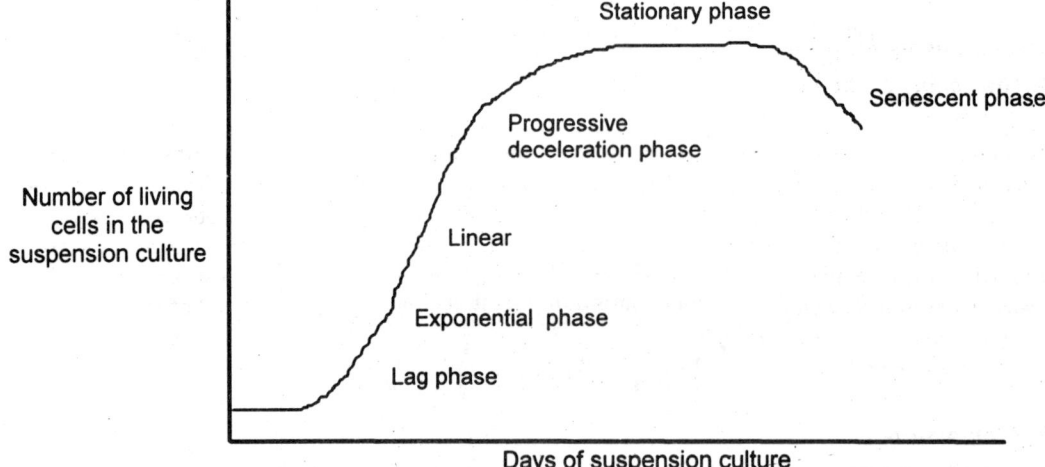

Fig. 7.2 : Model growth curve of single cell culture

7.5.1.2. Callus culture

The growth profile for the callus to a great extent is similar to that of cells suspension culture and presented in figure 7.3. The various stages of growth are:

1. **Lag phase:** Following inoculation of an explant, there is a lag time before the cells undergo cell division. Then a few cells start to divide and the tissue resumes its growth, albeit a slower one.
2. **Exponential phase:** This stage involves vigorous growth owing to the rapid cell division. During this phase, the tissues consume nutrients from the medium leading to their depletion.
3. **Decline phase:** The depletion of elements from the medium leads to starvation of some cells. This leads to a decline in the growth of callus tissue.
4. **Stationary phase:** From this stage onwards no growth is evident. For further growth and development subculture is an imperative.

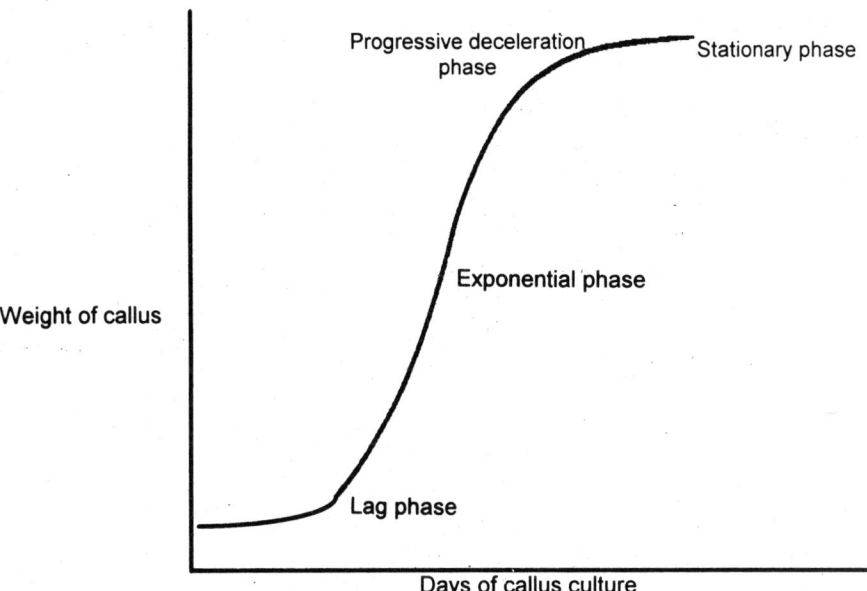

Fig. 7.3 : Model growth curve of callus culture

7.5.2. Requirements for growth of callus cultures

7.5.2.1. The acidity of the medium

The acidity of the medium is often adjusted to an initial value of pH 5.5-6.0. However, the optimum acidity depends upon the particular strain of tissue employed, usually the acidity of the medium drifts toward neutrality from more acid or alkaline conditions during the growth period. Studies have also indicated that the tissues could change the pH of the medium in the areas of the medium they occupy and grow. Tobacco tissues from the hybrid (*Nicotiana glauca* x *Nicotiana langsdorfii*) for example grow best on media with initial acidity averaging pH 5.0 to 5.4 and final acidity from pH 5.5 to 5.9. Similarly, corn endosperm grows best between pH 6.0 and 7.0. It was observed that regardless of the initial pH, the acidity of the medium at the end of the growth period drifted towards pH 6.0. Thus, when graphs indicated growth of cultures on originally more acid or alkaline media, it was observed that growth actually occurred when the final pH values were close to 6.0.

7.5.2.2. Temperature

The optimum temperature for growth of callus cultures varies with the strain of tissue. However, the temperature of the growth room is generally maintained at 26°±1°C. The temperature requirement variability is best exemplified by tobacco hybrid (*N. glauca* x *N .langsdorffii*) that grows best between 28°C and 32°C and sunflower crown gall tissue that grows best between 24°C and 28°C.

7.5.2.3. Light

Routinely, the tissue cultures are maintained in the light or dark environment. When the chlorophyll production by the callus in the light is undesired, the tissues are best grown in darkness. Quality of light and length of darkness have also been identified to have some effect on the growth as well.

7.5.2.4. Inorganic nutrition

The nutritional requirement of callus tissues has been discussed earlier. After much precise work other media for specific tissues have also been developed. The proper balance of mineral and the concentrations of both minor and major elements in the media are usually critical for optimum growth of specific tissues. However, the isolated cell masses are generally tolerant to a wide range of concentration of the various ingredients in media.

7.5.2.5. Carbohydrate nutrition

In order to achieve *in vitro* growth of isolated callus tissues an outside source of carbon is desired. Freshly isolated tissues, in some cases, may remain alive for months but eventually they die if an organic carbon source is not provided. Commonly utilized sources of carbon are dextrose, levulose, mannose, sucrose, maltose, cellobiose, dextrin, pectin, starch, etc. Tissues from sunflower and tobacco grow more on dextrose, levulose, sucrose, maltose, cellobiose, pectin or dextrin. The concentration of sugars and polysaccharides are found to be important for growth. Often a concentration range of 0.5-2% has been found to be optimum for growth. Alcohol and organic acids alone are generally not good sources of carbon. However, in the presence of 2% sucrose all species grow more or less on media with methanol, ethanol, glycerol, erythritol or mannitol, but the growth is very poor.

7.5.2.6. Nitrogen nutrition

To ascertain the growth of the tissues the types and concentrations of nitrogen present in the media are important. Many organic and inorganic compounds have been tested as nitrogen sources for tissues of many species. Nitrate nitrogen often supported excellent growth of the tissues. Urea as the sole source of nitrogen promoted good growth of sunflower crown gall tissue. Amino acids have been tested in concentrations from 0.256 to 0.00006 M as source of nitrogen but they failed to turn out as a good source. However, with ammonia, alanine, glycine, arginine, asparagine and aspartic acid good to poor growth resulted. Good growth has also been observed with casein hydrolysate, peptone and yeast extract. Once the amount of nitrate present was sufficient to promote excellent growth, the growth was inhibited by progressively increasing amounts of arginine and ammonium salts. Growth was also inhibited by nitrite, asparagine and all amino acids at 0.001M and higher concentrations. Aspartic acid, alanine and glutamic acid permitted growth favorably at 0.064M concentration. Transamination studies carried out to study the effect of the amino acids suggested that the amino acids are converted to the keto acids during transamination. Some studies have indicated that the optimal concentration of inorganic nitrogen is 8mM. The pH also influences the utilization of nitrate and ammonia. Among the nitrogen compounds tested as sources of nitrogen, only aspartic acid and urea have been found to be effective. Arginine, aspartic acid, glycine, proline and threonine are utilized little at a concentration of 0.002M. But in the presence of 0.004M nitrate, the same amino acids at the same concentration were rarely utilized.

7.5.2.7. Vitamins and growth substances

Many callus tissues synthesize vitamins and growth substances to meet their requirements. Thus, additional requirements are limited to few vitamins either alone or in combination with other metabolites. Vitamin B_{12} was found to be most beneficial for callus from white spruce, pantothenic acid for *Crataegus*, p-amino benzoic acid for *Jerusalem antichoke* and ascorbic acid for *Juniperus*.

The requirements for growth substances vary with the isolate and the species. The growth hormones employed include auxins, cytokinins and gibberellins and are listed in table 7.3.

Table 7.3: The commonly used auxins and cytokinins

Auxins	Cytokinins
Indole-3-butyric acid (IBA)	Benzyl amino purine (BAP)
Napthaleneacetic acid (NAA)	Isopentenyl adenine (2 IP)
p-Chlorophenoxyacetic acid (p-CPA)	Furfurylaminopurine (FAP)
Naphthoxyacetic acid (NOA)	N-Methylaminopurine (MAP)
Trichlorophenoxyacetic acid (2 4 5-T)	
Dichlorophenoxy acetic acid (2 4 -D)	
Indole acetic acid (IAA)	

Gautheret *et al.*, have demonstrated that requirements for IAA of callus may be of three types:

1. some species grow indefinitely on media without added IAA;
2. certain species or strains of tissues require IAA in varying concentrations as a supplement;
3. the habituated strains of tissue require added IAA during the first few weeks or months in culture and following transfer, synthesize their own requirements.

The effect of antibiotics on growth of callus tissue has also been studied. The growth of sunflower tissue was found to be stimulated by penicillin. Penicillin, streptomycin, terramycin and bacitracin stimulated growth of Rumex tissue. The polymyxin and chloramphenicol inhibited the tissue growth while terramycin has been found to be toxic to marigold tissue of crown gall origin.

7.5.2.8. Nucleic acids, purines and pyrimidines

Depending on the species and concentration of the nucleic acids, certain purines and pyrimidines may inhibit or stimulate the growth of the callus tissue. The growth of *Rumex virus* tumor tissue was improved by ribonucleic acid (RNA) at concentrations from 0.2 to 0.8 mg and impaired by deoxyribonucleic acid (DNA). Adenine, adenosine and adenylic acid inhibited the callus growth. Guanine, uracil, xanthine and hypoxanthine showed some beneficial effect. However, uric acid has been found to be toxic. The RNA has been found to be a good nitrogen source for tobacco tissue but not for marigold tissue however DNA could not serve as a good nitrogen source for either of the tissues.

7.5.2.9. Complex extracts

To induce continued growth in certain tissues various plant and animal extracts have been employed in addition to supplements like basic mineral salts and sucrose. These include yeast extract, malt extract, tomato, and other vegetable juices, casein hydrolysate and various liquid endosperm including those from horse chest nuts, coconuts, and corn. Malt extract has been beneficial for pure tissue culture whereas casein hydrolysate has been shown to stimulate growth of many species e.g., normal sunflower stem callus and carrot callus.

7.5.3. Growth determination

There are several techniques that are available for measuring culture growth. They are discussed in the following paragraphs.

7.5.3.1. Cell number

This method furnishes the most accurate information about cell growth as it involves direct counting of cells. This method, however, demands a high percentage of countable single cells. But plant cell suspension mostly comprises of cell clumps of varying sizes. Thus, for determination of cell numbers an additional step for disruption of cell clumps into single cell is required. This disadvantage can be circumvented by the treatment of cells with pectinase, a macerating enzyme or chromic trioxide before counting. Nevertheless, the entire process becomes lengthy.

7.5.3.2. Packed cell volume

This method gives very quick results however, they are more or less rough approximations only. This method involves the centrifugation of a known volume of suspension culture for favoring the deposition of the cell at the bottom of the tube. Following settlement, the total volume of packed cells is measured. The concentration of cells in the culture can be calculated in terms of percentage with reference to the total volume of suspension.

7.5.3.3. Fresh and dry weights

This is the most widely used method for the growth determination. During the linear phase, plant cells synthesize cell wall material and starch from available carbohydrates. As the cell enters the progressive deceleration and stationary phases, all the available carbohydrates are metabolized by the cells. Accumulation of starch is thereby stopped. Therefore, there is a decline in the dry weight corresponding to the metabolism of accumulated starch. But at this stage a progressive increase in fresh weight is observed as the cells are larger and they trap culture medium on the filter bed.

7.5.3.4. Nutrient uptake studies

Analysis of growth medium for certain nutrients like sucrose, glucose, fructose, nitrate, inorganic phosphates, etc. indicates if a particular component is limiting at any stage in the culture cycle. Carbon conversion efficiency of cell suspension culture can be calculated from the data of carbohydrate analysis and biomass measurements.

7.5.4. Cell viability measurements

The term viability can be defined as the capacity of a cell or an organism to live and grow. When it comes to measuring viability, measuring some parameters of metabolic activity is more reliable and informative than the growth measurements. Based on these metabolic functions, the viability tests can be categorized as follows:

7.5.4.1. Cytoplasmic streaming

This is a nondestructive assay method. A serious limitation of the method is that, it could only be applied to cell suspensions, protoplasts and single clumps of cells through which light can pass. Even in single cells and protoplasts, the observation of cytoplasmic streaming is hampered by large vacuoles.

7.5.4.2. Measuring membrane integrity

This can be applied to virtually all types of cultured plant material. However, an erroneous interpretation may be drawn if there is a lack in homogeneity in tissue composition. There is always a possibility that different cell types in the tissue would leak electrolytes at different rates. Also, typically the conductance of distilled water containing a tissue sample, that is employed for assessing electrolyte leakage may give some clumping and misleading results. Thus, electrolyte loss is measured only from cells having a contact with the water.

Another approach of stain exclusion assays is limited to cell suspensions and protoplasts or small clumps of cells through which light can pass. Also, a possibility of misinterpretation exists in the presence of dead cells which have lost their cytoplasm. These cells are not stained and they may be considered as if alive. Some dyes (like phenosafranine) are bound to cell walls of *Zea mays* and thereby any exclusion or cytoplasmic binding could be hindered.

7.5.4.3. Measuring biochemical activity

This is performed by the reduction of 2,3,5-triphenyl tetrazolium chloride (TTC) and fluorescein diacetate (FDA) stains. TTC is water soluble and gives a colorless solution. Within a live cell it is reduced to water insoluble red formazan by dehydrogenase activity or mitochondrial electron transport chain. In a dead cell, mitochondrial activity would be absent and TTC would remain unreduced. Thus, in a TTC solution a live tissue will turn red whereas dead tissue will not change color. This assay can be quantified by extraction of red precipitate from the tissue with ethanol and measuring its absorbance spectrophotometrically.

FDA is a nonpolar, nonfluorescent molecule. It enters plant cells where esterases remove the acetate moiety. The resulting fluorescence is retained in the cell owing to its polar nature and is unable to cross plasmalemma. Dead cells have limited esterase activity and have leaky membranes as well. As a result they would produce less fluorescein in comparison to live cells and the fluorescence produced would not be retained. Thus, after exposure to FDA, live cells will fluoresce whereas dead cells will not. In comparison to TTC reduction, FDA is faster and can be visualized within cells microscopically. Therefore, in addition to general viability assay it can be utilized to determine the number of live cells in a population.

7.6. TYPES OF CULTURE

7.6.1. Callus culture

Callus culture is a mass of cells or tissue resulted subsequent to initiation and continued proliferation of the undifferentiated parenchyma cells from parent tissue on a clearly defined semi-solid media (Fig.7.4). This is observed when an explant from a differentiated tissue is cultured on a medium. The quiescent (non-dividing) cells undergo changes to achieve meristematic state. This phenomenon of mature cells reversion back to the meristematic state leading to the formation of callus growth is called **dedifferentiation**. Moreover, the cells from callus are capable of generating into whole plant, a phenomenon referred to as **redifferentiation**. These two typical characters are components of **cellular totipotency**. These cultures present a convenient mode for the long term maintenance of cell lines, as such culture can be maintained for extended periods via subculturing at 2-4 weekly intervals. Cell suspension is usually derived from the callus culture and the plant regeneration is often initiated from them as well.

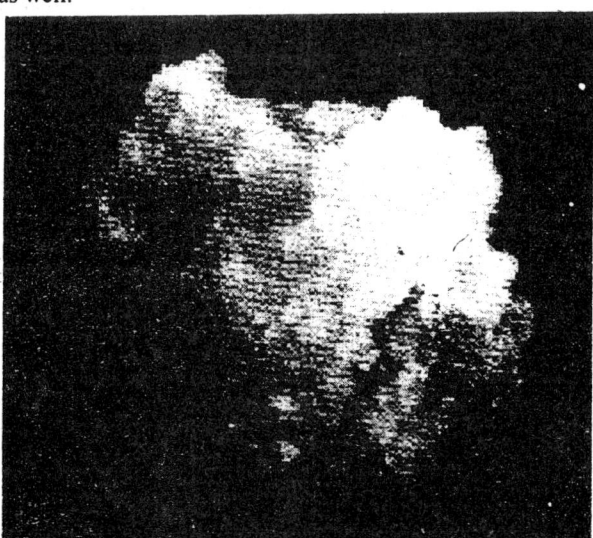

Fig.7.4 : Callus culture of *P. tomentosum*

Callus is frequently formed *in vivo* as a result of wounding at the cut edge of a stem or a root, that follows invasion by the microorganisms or damage by the insect feeding. The callus formation is controlled by the endogenous auxin and cytokinin. *In vitro* callus formation on the explant of the parent tissue can be induced by incorporating the above mentioned plant growth regulators into the growth medium. Organogenesis can be initiated and regulated in the callus culture by the manipulation of the ratio of auxin and cytokinins. With a few exceptions, a high ratio of cytokinin to auxin results into the shoot formation whereas a high ratio of auxin to cytokinin gives rise to the root formation. There are a number of plant tissue culture media documented in the literature that facilitate callus formation. One such media is that of Murashige and Skoog. Other techniques involved in the induction of organogenesis proceed via selection of a suitable inoculum and control of the physical environment

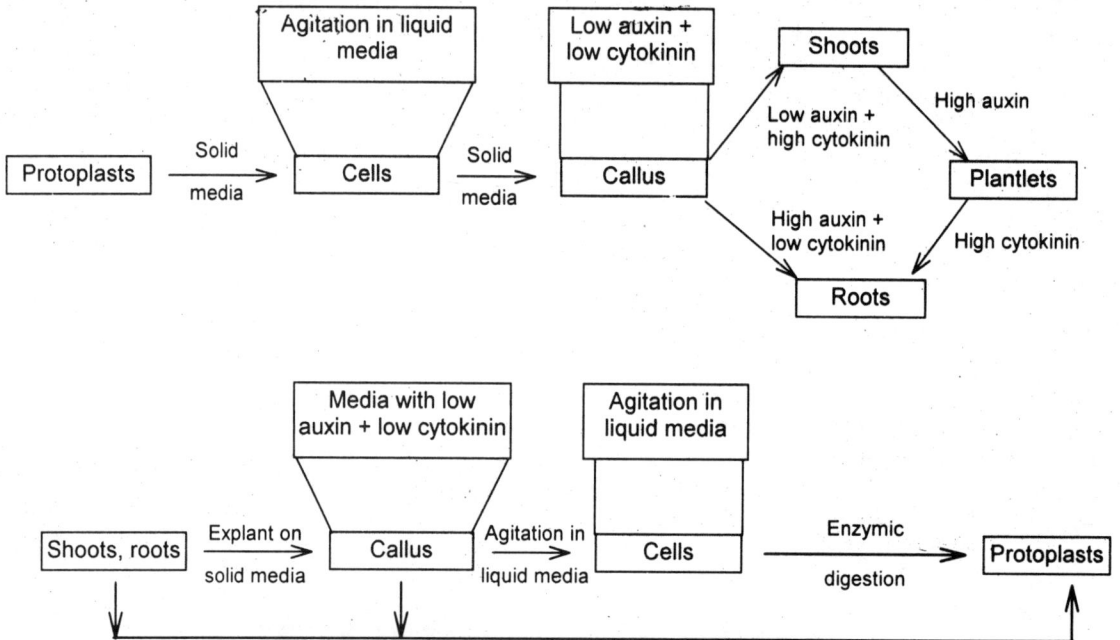

Fig. 7.5 : Schematic representation of different manipulations possible with plant cell, tissue and organ culture

7.6.2. Meristem-tip culture

Meristem is the mass of undifferentiated parenchyma cells found at the extreme tip of the shoot and root systems. They have the totipotency to regenerate into plantlets. In meristem-tip culture the organized apex of the shoot from a selected donor plant is excised for subsequent *in vitro* culture. The culture conditions are manipulated to permit only for organized outgrowth of the apex directly into a shoot, without the intervention of any adventitious organs. The meristem-tip is excised by sterile dissection under the microscope and is often kept less than 1mm in length. The excised portion excludes any differentiated provascular or vascular tissues and contains the otical dome and a limited number of youngest leaf primordia (Fig. 7.6).

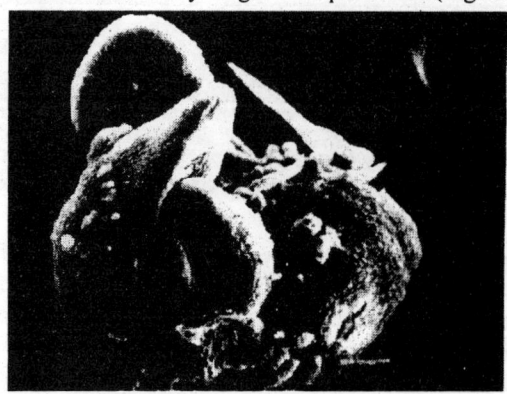

Fig. 7.6 : Meristem-tip culture of potato

Some of the advantages of the meristem culture are given below:

1. Viral, bacterial and fungal pathogen free stock for the propagation can be effectively prepared even from the infected donor plants. This is possible because the terminal region of the shoot meristem that is used for the culture is unlikely to contain pathogenic particles.
2. *In vitro* clonal propagation with maximal genetic stability is possible since plantlets production through adventitious organogenesis or any callus tissue formation can always be avoided.
3. The meristem tip is sufficiently small and the tissue is homogeneous. Thus, it provides a practical propagule for cryopreservation and other techniques for the culture storage.
4. This technique preserves the precise arrangements of the cell layers necessary for micropropagation of chimeral material. In a typical chimera, the surface layers of the developing meristem are from different genetic background. It is only their contribution in a particular arrangement that elicits desired characteristics to the plant organ.
5. These cultures are usually acceptable for international transport as they comply with quarantine requirements and regulations.

7.6.3. Shoot-tip culture

The shoot apex or shoot-tip consists of the apical meristem and one to three adjacent leaf primordia, whereas the apical meristem refers only to the portion of the shoot apex lying distal to the youngest leaf primordium. Although true meristem culture has been widely employed to eliminate virus infestation, the small size of this explant (80-100μm) limits its utility. Thus, usually virus eradication is achieved using the shoot apex, which includes the meristem and 2-3 primordial leaves. This method is widely used with both monocot and dicot species.

Some of the crop species that have been freed of viruses by this technique, they include horseraddish, soyabean, sweet potato, cauliflower, sugar cane and rhubarb. There are no reports of variant plant types resulting from this explant in culture. As the plants are derived from a preexisting shoot meristem, the true genetic type and agronomic and phenotypic characters are maintained.

Asexual reproduction using shoot tip or axillary bud explant, generates plants that are genetically identical to the stock plant. On the other hand, in plants arising from callus culture or suspension cultured cells, the somatic embryo or shoot meristem develops adventitiously. These plants thereby exhibit a variety of culture-induced changes termed as **somaclonal variations**. Somaclonal variation is the genetic variability observed in plants derived from a callus intermediate.

The adaptation of this procedure to transformation studies can eliminate many of the present restrictions relating to species and variety that arise due to the lack of an appropriate *in vitro* regeneration method. Transformed plants can be obtained using shoot apex explant in co-cultivation with *Agrobacterium tumefaciens*.

7.6.4. Flower organ culture

Flower formation in tissue culture has been observed in several plant species and is reported to arise from a variety of explant sources. There are variety of factors that contribute to flower induction in nature. It is assumed that various factors are mainly responsible for *in vitro* flowering. Reasons for studying flower formation in tissue culture include:

1. It provides a model system for studying whole flower development from an excised part of the flower (e.g., ovary culture).
2. It provides an opportunity for conducting microbreeding.
3. It provides a source of biochemicals and pharmaceuticals.

Thus, by using appropriate plants like *Amaranthus* there is a possibility of completing an entire life cycle of a plant. This leads to a model system useful in studying microclimates or nutritional effects on the vegetative and reproductive processes of the plant (Fig. 7.7). Explants in either the vegetative or the reproductive state can induce flowering in culture. Flower induction may be stimulated by both chemical and physical means.

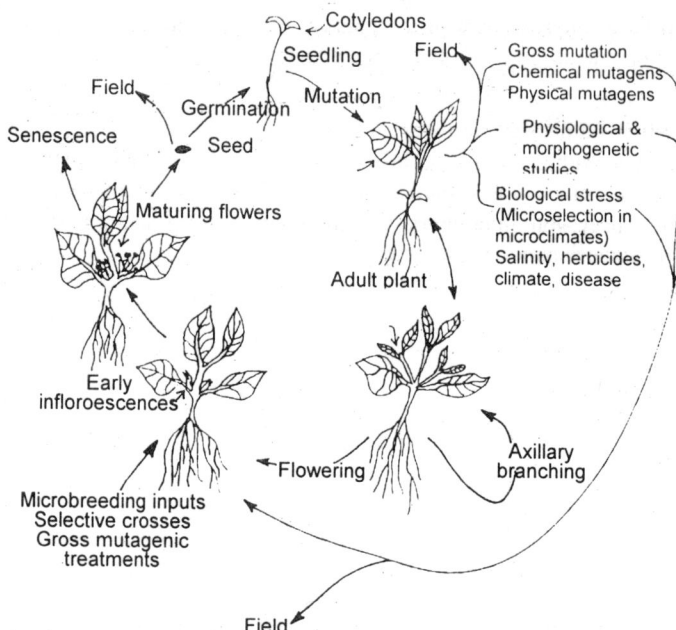

Fig. 7.7 : *Amaranthus* culture system and its potential study applications

7.6.5. Fruit organ culture

The culture of fruit tissues as whole organ or isolated tissue sections has been experimented and carried out with various species (Fig. 7.8). Whole, isolated ovaries have been successfully cultured to give rise to mature fruits (e.g., strawberry). Usually when an isolated portion of the fruit tissue is introduced into a sterile environment, it immediately loses structural integrity and degenerates into a rapidly dividing callus mass. Loss of structural integrity is associated correspondingly with an alteration of physiology that is subsequently reflected in the production of an altered metabolism. Thus at times, it is not possible to make a meaningful study of fruits development using callus derived from fruit tissues.

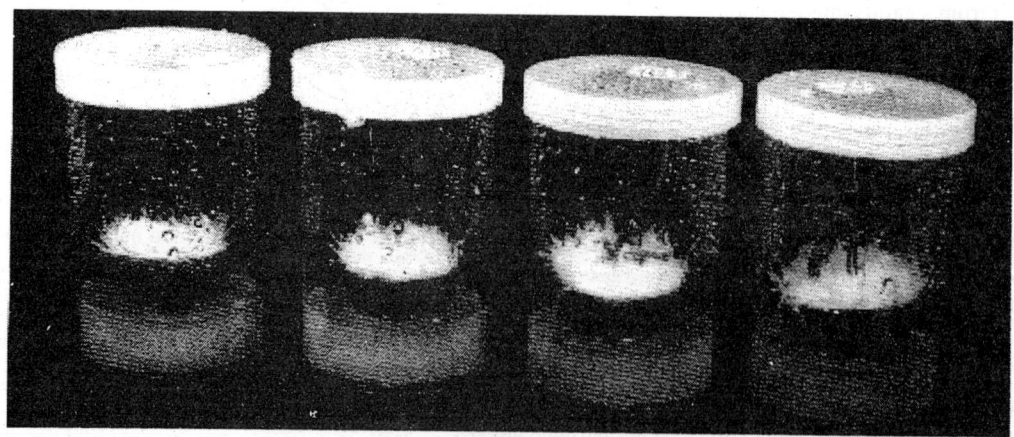

Fig. 7.8 : Whole fruit culture of lemon

At present, the use of fruit culture is to serve as a bioassay system to study fruits maturation events within a controlled environment. The reports of these studies can then be extrapolated for the improvement of field grown crops. A large quantity of extractable plant biochemicals and pharmaceuticals are derived from flowers and fruits. Seemingly, with an improvement in the present status of fruit culture technology, edible products from cultured fruits would be one of the possible future perspectives.

7.6.6. Microspore and anther culture

Microspore culture offers a powerful alternative to the protoplast culture as a single cell culture method. In microspore culture a true **haploid cell** system is utilized. Haploids are sporophytes with gametophytic chromosome number. For successful microspore culture the following factors have been appreciated and identified which play an important role:

1. Growth profile of donor plant;
2. Genotype of donor plant;
3. The pretreatment;
4. The developmental stage of microspore;
5. The culture medium and the conditions during culture growth.

The various steps involved in anther and microspore culture are outlined in figures 7.9 and 7.10 respectively.

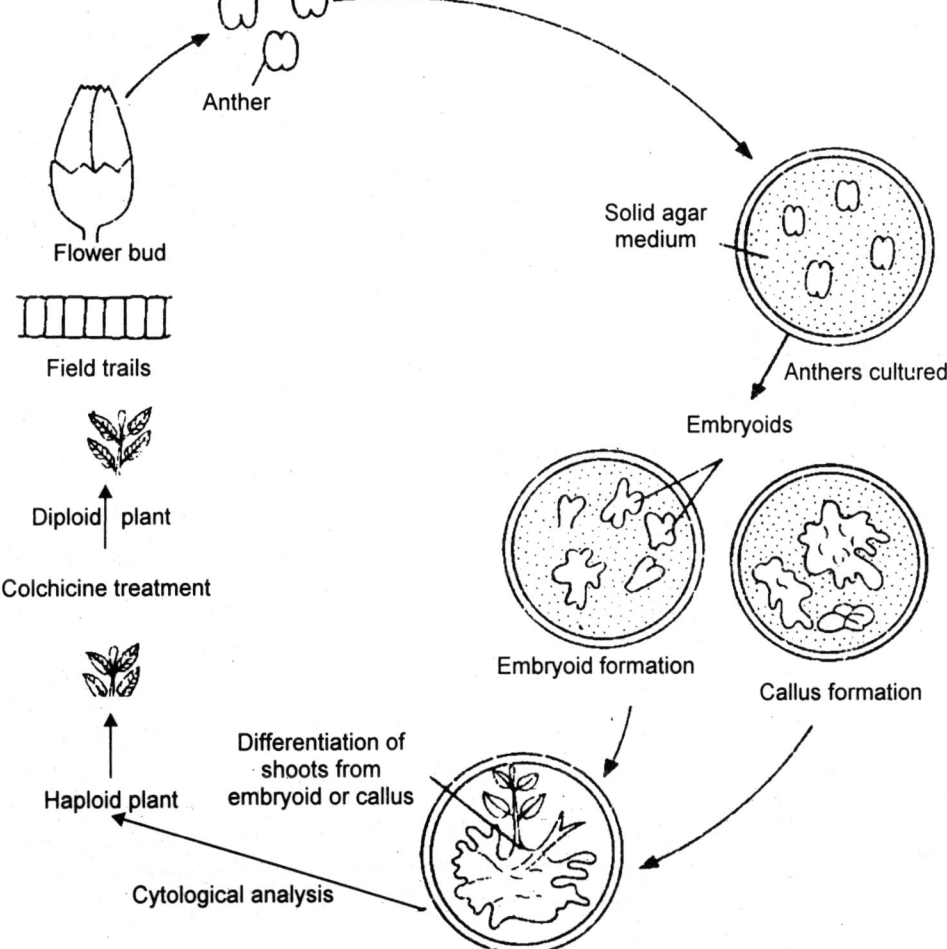

Fig. 7.9 : Various steps involved in the production of haploid plants from anther culture

Microspore culture is usually preferred over the anther culture even though the former has been successful in some species only.

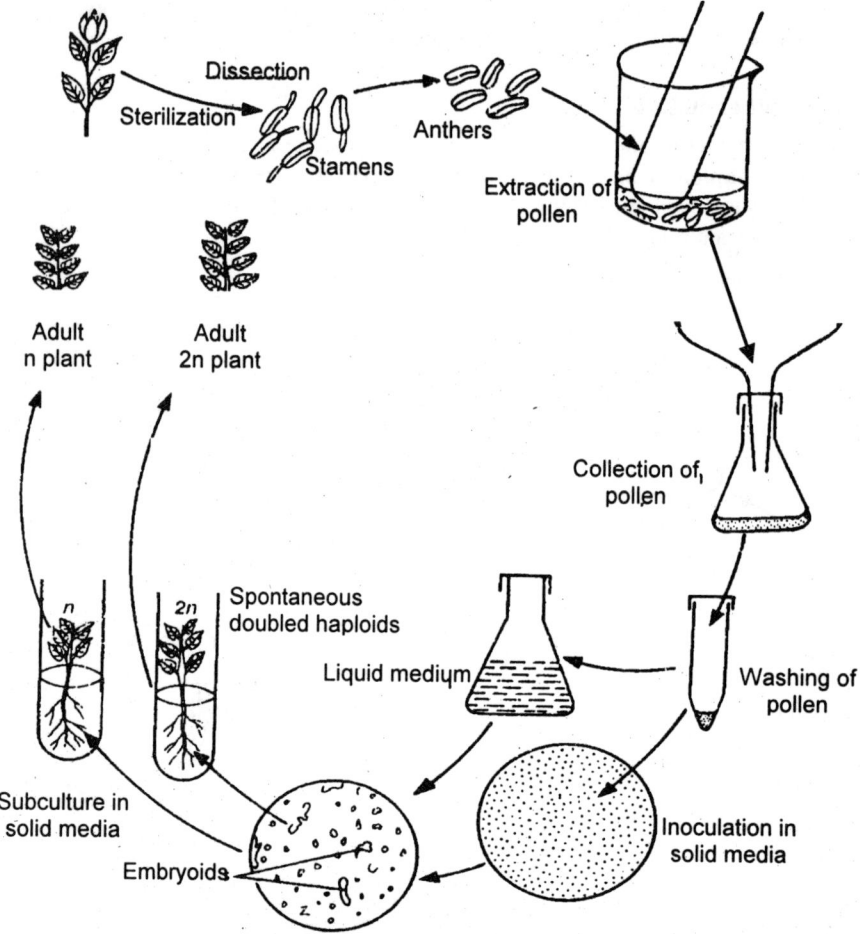

Fig. 7.10 : Various steps involved in the production of haploid plants using isolated pollen grains

The haploid production using isolated pollen grains involves following steps:

1. Dissected pollen grains are taken in a beaker containing liquid medium, they are skewed with the help of a glass rod or syringed piston;
2. The suspension is then filtered through a millipore nylon filter and the filtrate is collected. It contains only microspores;
3. Microspores containing filtrate is centrifuged at 1000 rpm for 5 minutes;
4. The pellet is resuspended in a fresh medium;
5. Microspore suspension is used as an inoculum and transferred on a solid/liquid medium maintained at 25°C for 10-15 h.

Microspores may develop directly into embryos within 15 days. In anther as well as microspore culture spontaneously doubled haploids are also generated hence requiring no colchicine treatment.

Similarly, haploids can be produced from female gametophytes. Haploid production with gymnosperms has been successful, Zamia, Ephedra and Cycads are some representative examples of this class. Nevertheless, the results were found to be promising and now haploids could be obtained from cultured ovaries in a few crop species like tobacco, barley and wheat. The haploid production technology seems to be possible with a number of plant species and thereby holds great potential to be an effective tool in plant species modifications.

Some of the inherent advantages of the microspore culture are:

1. The large somaclonal variations associated with protoplast selection in protoplast culture are largely eliminated.
2. A more synchronized embryo development facilitates accurate mutation and selection methods.
3. A high plant regeneration frequency (more than 80%) can be readily obtained.
4. The entire sequence from microspore isolation to plantlet development takes place in as little as 4 weeks time.

7.6.7. Dual fungal and plant cell culture

Success with combined fungal-plant cultures has been variable, especially in terms of establishing cultures that may be maintained in a balanced state for prolonged periods. But, undoubtedly such cultures are of immense utility for studying cell-cell interactions. Callus culture provides the host tissue that can be maintained in an undifferentiated state with the help of supplements and nutrients in a controlled environment. The tissue is axenic and cell population is nearly homogeneous. By judicious manipulation of growth conditions tissue differentiation can be affected and from sterile tissue, a plant similar to that of the intact plant can be obtained.

The interaction between pathogen and its host plant involves complex recognition and response mechanisms. Studies have indicated that some resistance genes can operate in callus tissue and thus tissue culture can be exploited for programs that could be utilized for screening of disease resistance. Investigation of the physiological and biochemical aspects of host-pathogen interaction and operation of resistance mechanisms at the cellular level can be carried out with dual cultures. The protocol for the dual fungal and plant cell culture is schematically presented in figure 7.11.

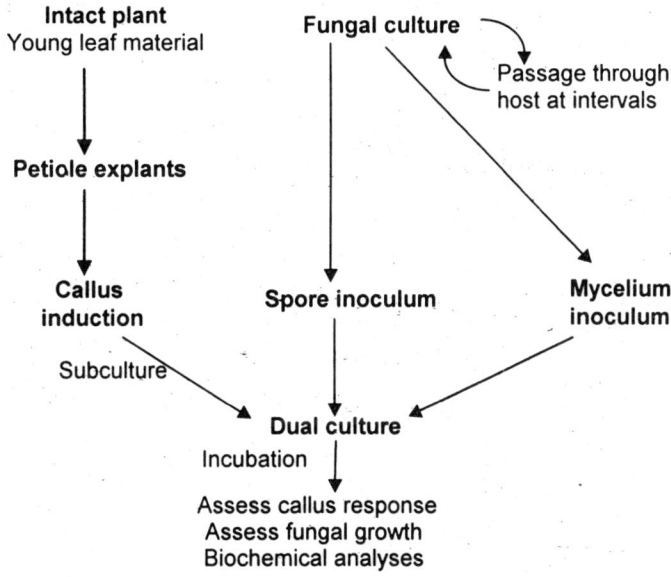

Fig. 7.11 : Summary protocol for dual fungal and plant cell cultures

7.6.8. Protoplast culture

A protoplast is a cell without a cell wall. They contain all the normal cell organelles plus the nucleus. The nucleus expresses totipotency through conversion of the protoplast to the regenerated plant. The cell wall of a plant cell can be decomposed and removed by the treatment of the lytic enzymes like cellulase and pectinase. Studies conducted with the regenerating plantlets from the protoplast culture indicated that all the clones regenerated from the protoplasts are not identical but exhibit some variation in their characters. This type of variation is referred to as somaclonal variation or **somatic variation**.

The salient features of protoplast culture are:

1. The somatic protoplasts are prone to fuse with one another, thereby leading to the formation of somatic hybrids. These somatic hybrids can be used for regeneration of plantlet having new characters, the ones that are not found in their parents.
2. The isolated protoplasts have the tendency to take up the foreign gene from culture. Following this uptake, the protoplast undergoes genetic modification. This feature can be exploited for crop improvement in agriculture.
3. The protoplasts are also capable of engulfing larger particles such as the isolated cell organelles present in the culture. For genetic manipulation of crops isolated chloroplasts, mitochondria, nucleus and chromosomes can be added to the protoplast culture (Fig. 7.12)
4. Protoplasts are also utilized in the establishment of cybrids through the fusion of protoplasts.
5. The plants regenerated from protoplasts, the somatic variants, show some variations in their character as discussed earlier. These somatic variants are used in crop improvement.

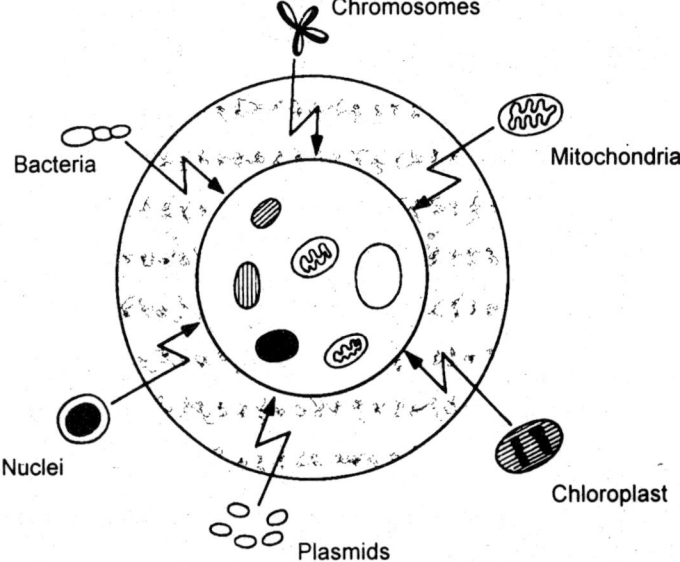

Fig. 7.12 : Various biological components that can be taken up by isolated protoplasts

The above mentioned applications are only possible if the isolated protoplasts have the element of **totipotency**. With the passage of time protoplasts synthesize new cell walls around themselves. These cells are cultured in a medium for the plantlet regeneration. This property of the plant cells is referred to as totipotency. If the isolated protoplasts lack their totipotency, the protoplast technology fails to give its beneficial results.

7.6.8.1. Methods of isolation of protoplasts

The two methods commonly used in the preparation of plant protoplasts from the cultured plant tissues are mechanical method and enzymatic method. In the mechanical method, removal of cell wall is facilitated by the aid of needles, forceps and scissors. In the enzymatic method the protoplasts are prepared by treating the cells with an enzyme like cellulase and pectinase which selectively digest the cell wall. Figure 7.13 and 7.14 explains the various stages of single step enzymatic isolation method used in protoplast isolation.

7.6.8.2. Applications of protoplast culture

The protoplast can be utilized for a variety of studies including the following:
1. Uptake of exogenously supplied materials like bacteria, algae, virus and macromolecules like DNA.
2. For physiological investigations.

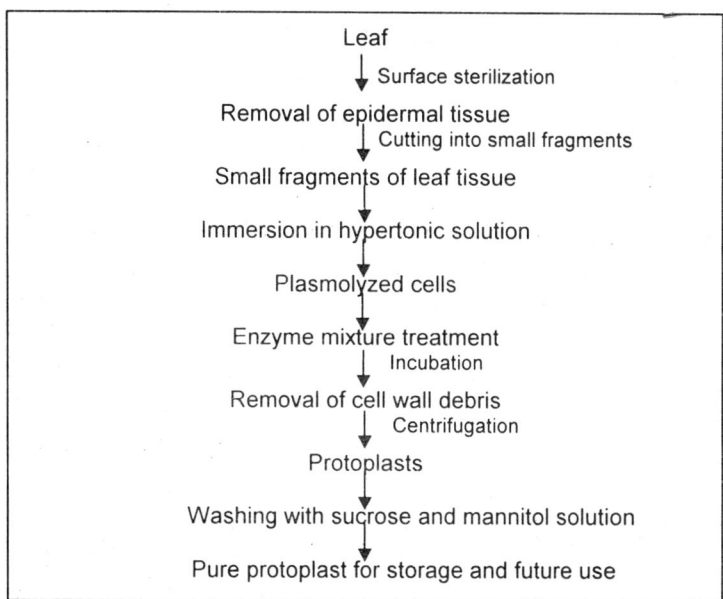

Leaf
↓ Surface sterilization
Removal of epidermal tissue
↓ Cutting into small fragments
Small fragments of leaf tissue
↓
Immersion in hypertonic solution
↓
Plasmolyzed cells
↓
Enzyme mixture treatment
↓ Incubation
Removal of cell wall debris
↓ Centrifugation
Protoplasts
↓
Washing with sucrose and mannitol solution
↓
Pure protoplast for storage and future use

Fig. 7.13 : Stages of single step enzymatic isolation method of protoplast isolation from leaf tissues.

3. In the ultrastructural studies.

4. For transformation assessments

5. For the isolation of subcellular components like nuclei, vacuoles and chromosomes.

In its simplest form the protoplast is used as the starting point in the manipulation for genetic (somaclonal) variation following the mass generation of the plants. The source of the protoplasts can be of whole plant or tissue culture. Leaves, *in vitro* grown shoots or callus/cell suspension culture give high yields of the protoplasts.

Electromanipulation i.e., electroporation has been utilized to introduce foreign DNA into plant protoplast. In this method, protoplasts are exposed to high voltage electric pulse of short duration (micro or milli seconds). The pores are induced in the plasma membrane. Through these pores exogeneous molecules and macromolecules including dyes, nucleotides, RNA, DNA and even small proteins can be taken up. Such electric fields stimulate protoplast division and increase the throughput of protoplast derived cell colonies.

The outstanding aspects of electroporation are its simplicity and its general effectiveness with a wide range of cell types. Due to its general efficacy this technique is becoming a valuable method for introduction of DNA into cell types that resist transformation by other procedures. Increased shoot regeneration capability through the influence of low voltage electric impulse on auxin metabolism has been reported in such colonies.

Another important and effective technique for transforming animal cells is through microinjection. This technique of introducing DNA to plants is sufficiently well developed and can be more generally adapted. One of the methods developed for protoplast microinjection involves the use of low melting point agarose, both for holding protoplasts during microinjection and for their subsequent culture.

Protoplasts are useful for micro-injection only on the day of their preparation, and possibly on the following day. This is due to the fact that after this period of time cell wall reformation starts and this makes the penetration with the needle difficult. Alternatively, time available for microinjection can be extended by delaying cell wall reformation by holding them at a lower temperature.

7.6.8.3. Protoplast fusion

Protoplast fusion is of great significance for hybridization between species and genera which are not amenable to crossing by conventional method of sexual hybridization.

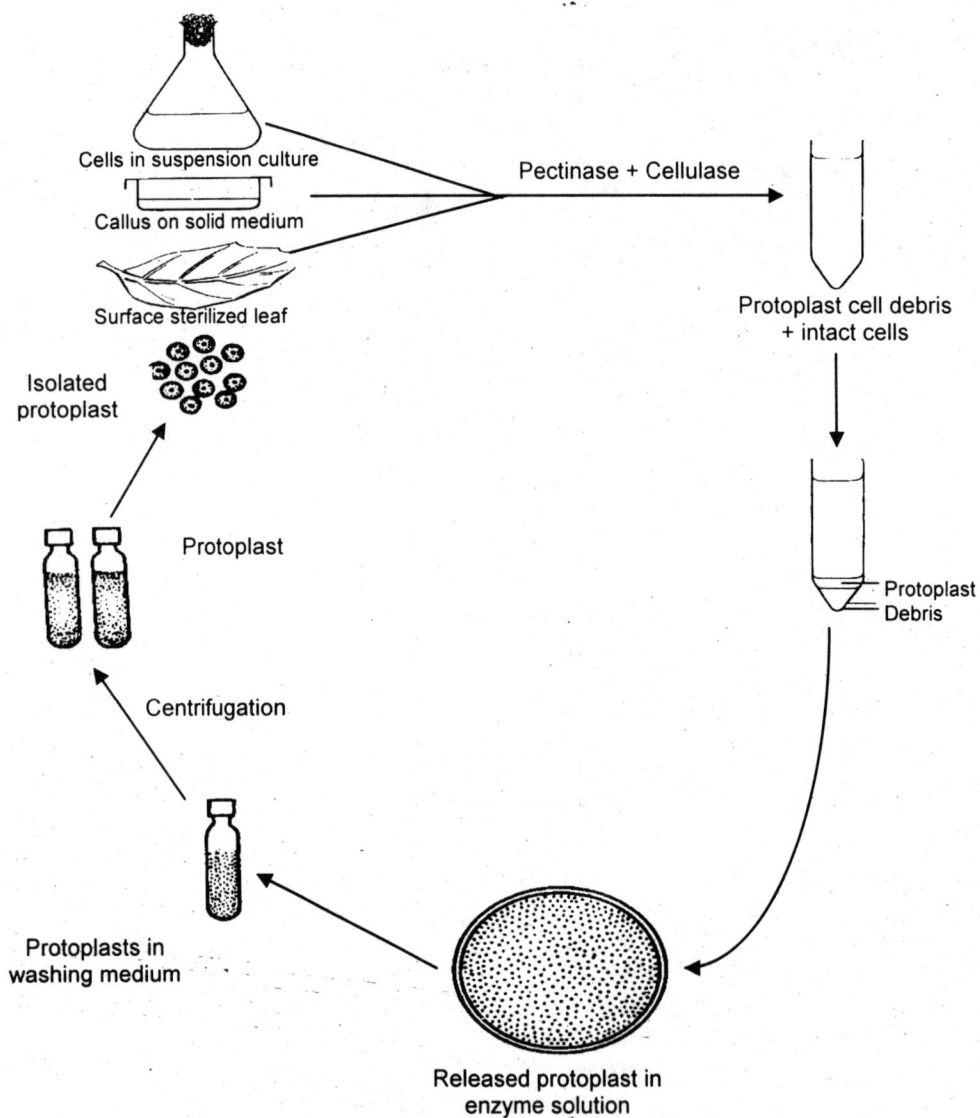

Fig. 7.14 : Schematic presentation of enzymatic isolation of plant protoplast

7.6.8.3.1. Techniques of protoplast fusion

1. Spontaneous fusion: Enzymatic degradation of cell walls is performed during isolation of protoplasts. During this process some of the protoplasts lying in close proximity may undergo fusion to produce homokaryons or homokaryocytes which contain 2-40 nuclei. If protoplasts are prepared from actively dividing cells, the frequency of multinucleate fusion bodies are more. But this spontaneous fusion is intraspecific. Another approach of inducing spontaneous fusion is by bringing protoplasts into intimate contact using micropipettes and micromanipulators. It has been observed that protoplasts isolated from young leaves are more prone to spontaneous fusion.

2. Induced fusion: Induced fusion is of great utility when fusion of protoplasts from two different species(intersepcific fusion) or from two different sources of same species has to be achieved. In this technique a fusogen is employed for inducing fusion. Inactivated sendai virus is often used in animals for fusion induction, whereas in plants the inducing agent brings the protoplasts together and this is followed by adherence to one another and finally that have been exploited for fusion of plant protoplasts. The fusion strategies are illustrated in figure 7.15.

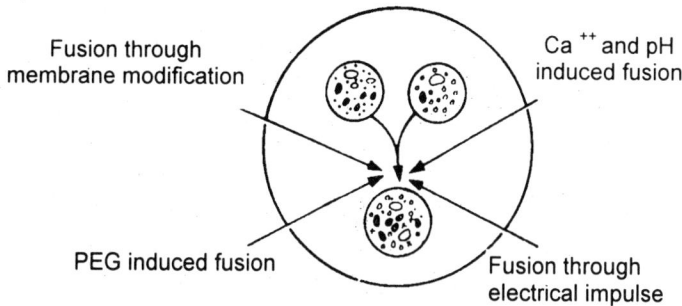

Fig. 7.15 : Experimental methods employed for induction of protoplast fusion.

1.Sodium nitrate treatment: In this method the isolated protoplasts are suspended in an aggregation mixture comprising of 5.5.% sodium nitrate in 10% sucrose solution and incubated at 35°C to induce fusion. To improve the frequency of fused protoplasts, centrifugation of the mixture followed by resuspension of the pellet and incubation for additional cycles can be opted. As the final step liquid medium is used to replace the mixture and protoplasts in this mixture are incubated once again and then protoplasts are plated on a solid medium. The various steps are outlined in figure 7.16.

2. Treatment with calcium ions at high pH: In this method protoplasts in a fusion inducing solution ($0.05M$ $CaCl_2.2H_2O$ in $0.4M$ mannitol at pH 10.5) are subjected to centrifugation for 30 min. at 50g. The fusion of 20-50% protoplasts is completed after it is incubated at 37°C for 40-50 min. In some cases the high pH may be toxic and a constraint in its application.

3. Polyethylene glycol (PEG) treatment: This approach has several advantages including low cytotoxicity, high fusion frequency and reproducibility. Moreover, this technique can be employed for fusion of soybean-barley, soybean-tobacco, etc.,). During PEG treatment, agglutination of protoplasts is performed by any of the following methods:

a) when the quantity of protoplast is sufficient, protoplasts suspended in 1ml. of culture medium is added to 1ml. of PEG solution (56%). The tube is shaken for 5 sec and protoplasts allowed to sediment for 10 min. Protoplasts are then washed with growth medium and observed for successful agglutination and fusion.

b) when the amount of available protoplasts is small i.e., in microquantities, drop cultures are preferred. The two types of protoplasts are taken and mixed in equal quantities. 4-6 microdrops or 100µl. of each are transferred to petri plates and allowed to settle for 5-10 min. at room temperature. From the periphery in each plate 2-3 microdrops of 50 µl of PEG added and incubated at room temperature (24°C) for 30 min. Once the agglutination of protoplasts is complete, the protoplasts are gradually washed and then the PEG is replaced by culture medium to facilitate the growth of fused protoplasts.

4. Electric fusion: In this approach protoplasts are placed in culture cell containing electrodes and a potential difference applied. This induces the protoplasts to line up between the electrodes. Fusion of protoplasts is subsequently achieved by application of a short square wave electric shock.

7.6.8.3.2. Selection of fused protoplasts

The protoplasts population after fusion treatment comprises of a mixture of parental types, heterokaryons and homokaryons. Heterokaryons are potential source of future hybrids and are only 0.5-10% in composition. Selection of heterokaryons or calli derived from the same has been attempted by employing these methods:

1) Growing hybrids on a medium on which the parent protoplasts fail to grow e.g., the hybrids *Nicotiana glauca* x *N. longsdorfi*.

2) Selection of hybrids in the form of green callus which represents only hybrid cells, e.g., hybrids of *Petunia parodii* x *P.inflorata, Datura innoxia* x *Atropa belladonna*.

3) Labeling of protoplasts of two parents by different fluorescent agents, e.g., hybrids of genus Nicotiana.

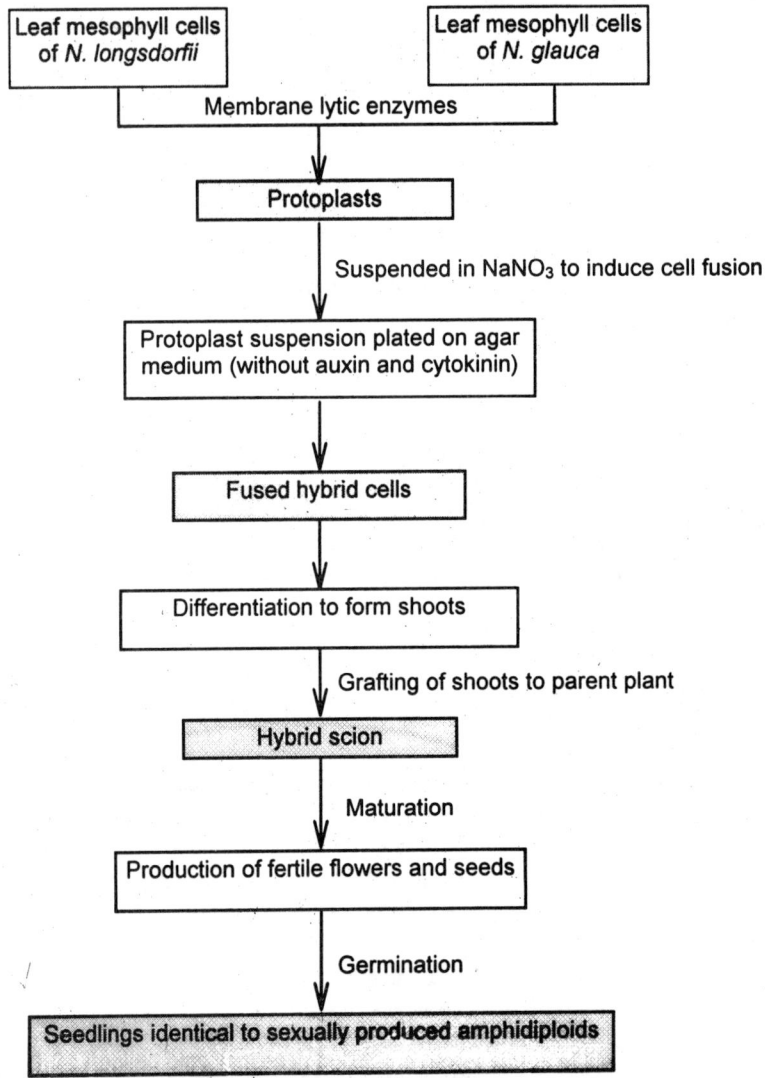

Fig. 7.16 : Various steps for production of interspecific somatic hybrids in the genus *Nicotiana* by sodium nitrate treatment.

In theory, the protoplast fusion technique promises to open up the potential 'gene pool' of a plant to every other living cells. However, in practice a few technical problems are confronted. One of the major problems encountered is due to the diminishing capacity of a cell culture to regenerate plants over a time period. This causes difficulties in cell selection techniques, because by the time the selection and testing stages are completed, the selected cells may fail to regenerate. These problems are to be sorted out so that the protoplast and somatic cell fusion techniques can be exploited for obtaining improved and desirable chemical products and biochemicals from plants.

7.7. MODIFICATION THROUGH TRANSFORMATIVE CELL CULTURE

Gene transfer can be achieved in higher plants by cell or protoplast culture and genetically modified cells could be regenerated into whole plants. Alternatively other meristematic cells, zygotes or pollens can be utilized for gene transfer. Totipotent characteristics of the plant cells lends them amenable to *in vitro* regeneration into whole plants via **embryogenesis** or **organogenesis**. A major constraint of *in vitro* plant regeneration, through a callus phase in particular is the occurrence of genome stress that may lead to somaclonal variation. However, genetically transformed gametes obtained by gene transfer into pollen/egg cells can be used for *in vivo* fertilization to generate transformed whole plants. Another approach is the insertion of DNA into zygote and subsequent to this by embryo rescue, individual cells in meristem/embryo can also be used for production of transformed plants. Table 7.4 enlists various target cells and the methods that are used for regeneration of whole lants from them.

Table 7.4 Methods used for regeneration of whole plants from various target cells

Type of target cell	Regeneration method employed
Cultured cells or protoplasts	Organogenesis or embryogenesis via callus phase
Meristematic cells from immature embryo or organ	In vitro plant regeneration from transformed cells
Cells from immature embryos, shoot and flower meristems	In vivo development by use of transformed pollen from chimeric plant to produce transformed seed
Pollen	Pollen treated with DNA and used for pollination leading to the production of transgenic plants
Zygote	In vivo development of transgenic plants

The DNA mediated transformation established in prokaryotes has been postulated to be a useful gene transfer process for higher plants. There are ample evidences which establish the uptake and integration of bacterial DNA into plants following the application of donor DNA to seeds. Generally, most of the foreign DNAs are broken down and reutilized and in some cases may escape destruction that persists in the plant tissues. The foreign DNA either stays free or it binds to the DNA of the recipient cells. DNA mediated transformation has been reported both in plant and animal cells, e.g. *Petunia* and *Arabidopsis*.

The general requirements for DNA mediated transformations include the following:

1. easy uptake of DNA
2. replication of DNA in the recipient cells
3. expression of newly introduced foreign DNA

Exogenous DNA has been introduced into very young isolated pollen grains and using these pollen grains haploid cells, a changed genetic constitution can be raised. An example, being the pollens from *Nicotiana glauca* using Rhizobium DNA. In some dicotyledonous plants direct gene transfer has been simplified and facilitated by the use of *Agrobacterium* species, the Ti plasmid of *A. tumefaciens* in particular, the latter is a natural plant-host vector system. *A. tumefaciens* is the bacterium responsible for crown gall disease. However, this species fails to infect the monocots (e.g. cereals), *A. tumefaciens* brings about transformation in plant cells by transfer of the T-DNA of the Ti plasmid to the host genome and here the genes contained in the T-DNA are expressed.

To bring about a successful transformation of a host the following criteria should be fulfilled:

1. *Agrobacterium* should recognize a suitable host.
2. Attraction and invasion of the host cells.
3. Excision of the T-DNA via the formation of a circular subgenomic molecule.
4. Integration of the T-DNA into host nuclear chromosome.

The tumorous properties of crown of all tissue include its ability to cause an overgrowth when grafted onto a healthy plant, the capacity for unlimited growth as a culture in tissue culture media devoid of the plant hormones (which are necessary for *in vitro* growth of normal plant cells), and the synthesis of opines (which are unusual amino acid derivatives not found in normal tissue). The type of opine produced is determined by the bacterial strain and not by the host plant. In general, the bacterium induces the synthesis of an opine which it can catabolize and use as its sole energy source, be it carbon and/or nitrogen. Thus bacteria that utilize octopine induce tumors synthesizing octopine, and those that utilize nopaline, induce tumors which synthesize nopaline.

7.7.1. The tumor-inducing principle and the Ti-plasmid

There are four well identified regions commonly found in most of the Ti plasmids.

i. Region A is responsible for tumor induction therefore mutation in this region obviously leads to the genesis of tumors with altered morphology as the gall could be shooty or rooty mutant. The sequence of this region are transferred to plant nuclear genome hence this region is most popularly referred to as T-DNA or transferred DNA.
2. Region B is mainly a region responsible for replication.
3. Region C brings about infectivity and conjugation.
4. Region D is virulent in nature, obviously mutations in this region reflect directly on virulence hence the region is also known as virulence (*vir*) region.

T-DNA consists of (I) One region with three genes represented as tms1 and tms2 for shooty locus and tmr for rooty locus. The genes of this regions have been appreciated to be responsible for the biosynthesis of phytohormones indole acetic acid (IAA) and isopentyl adenosine 5'-monophosphate as they express phytohormone synthesizing respective enzymes. Thus incorporation of this region along with its genus into plant cells endow them with biosynthesis property for these phytohormones. These phytohormones at large are attributed for initiating and propagating the growth of crown gall.

7.7.1.1. OS region

This region is accounted to be responsible for the synthesis of amino acid polymorphs or sugar derivatives these bioproducts are referred to as **opines.** The substance may be derived from various sources or compounds of cellular origin. The most frequently occurring opines are octopine and nopaline (Fig. 7.17). The enzymes octopine synthase and nopaline synthase are expressed by genes coded by T-DNA. Accordingly octopine synthase and nopaline synthase expressing T-DNA are referred to as octopine type Ti plasmid and nopaline type Ti plasmid respectively. Outside but adjacent to T-DNA region, the Ti plasmid contains genes that express enzymes and other bioproteins capable of catabolizing opines in order to utilize them as source of carbon and nitrogen.

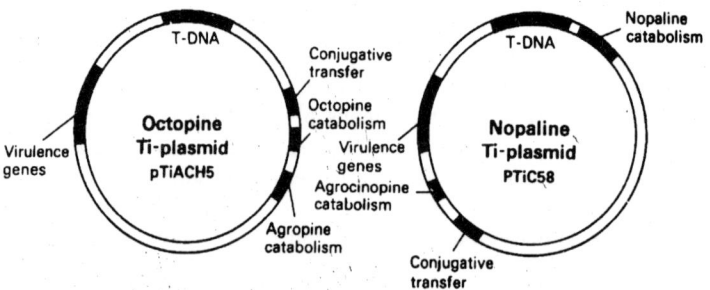

Fig. 7.17.: Ti-plasmid gene maps

The T-DNA regions of Ti and Ri plasmids are flanked by nearly 25bp repeat sequences with *cis* configuration and known to be essential for T-DNA transfer. It is this 25bp repeat sequence which imparts transfectivity to any DNA. In addition to the 25bp flanking border sequence, *Vir* region also contribute significantly in T-DNA transfer. Unlike 25bp border sequence, the *vir* region is capable of active functioning even in *trans* orientation.

Therefore, separation of T-DNA and *vir* region on two different plasmids has been found not to affect T-DNA transfer provided either of the plasmids are contained in the same *Agrobacterium* cell. The *vir* region which is approximately 35kbp is consisted of 6 operons which are named as *vir A, vir B vir D, vir E and vir G*. Out of these four operons are polycystronic. It was elucidated that operon A, B, D and G are absolutely essential for virulence activity whereas genes namely C and E have been found responsible for tumor formation. *Vir A* and *vir G* genes express the products which in turn regulate the expression of other *vir* loci. Generally *vir A* product is located on the inner membrane of *Agrobacterium* cells and functions as a chemoreceptor which senses the presence of phenolic compounds such as aceto and β-hydroxy aceto syringones. Furthermore, signal transduction has been recorded to proceed via activation of *vir G*, which is a product of *vir G* gene. This product may induce the expression of other virulent genes (Fig.7.18).

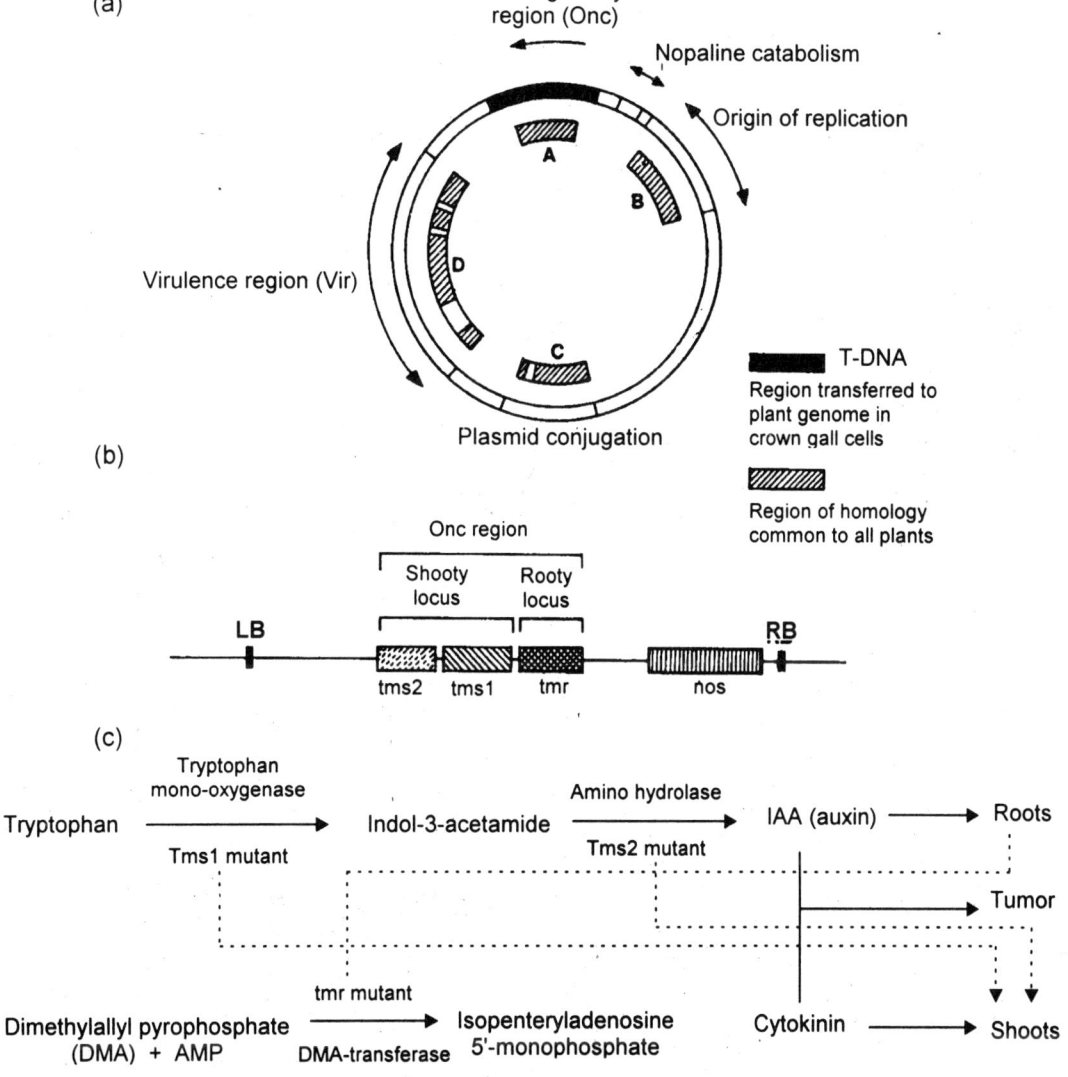

Fig. 7.18 : (a) General features of Ti-plasmid (b) General structure of T-DNA, (c) Biosynthesis of phytohormone in crown gall tissue (**Adapted from Gupta, P.K., (1997) Elements of Biotechnology*)

7.7.2. Incorporation of T-DNA into the nuclear DNA

The transfer of T-DNA proceeds with the formation of nick at the Ti plasmid DNA at two specific sites each between third and fourth base of the bottom strand of 25bp repeat. At the loci of nick DNA synthesis initiates in the right hand 25bp repeat sequence in 5'-3' direction. As a result a single T-DNA strand is displaced. This T-DNA single-strand then forms a complex with *vir E* protein and consequently transported to plant nucleus. The *vir D* operon that encodes for endonuclease expresses the enzyme that produces the nicks in the border sequences. Several other *vir B* operons may guide and direct T-DNA transfer extracellularly.

Additionally the genes which are located on *Agrobacterium* chromosomes also help in virulent activities. These genes characteristically synthesize and secrete glucons, cellulose, fibrils and cell-surface proteins. There are some active loci which play a more general role in the virulence of *Agrobacterium* and as a result *Agrobacterium* mediated gene transfer.

7.7.3. Disarmed Ti-plasmid derivative as plant vectors

In genetically engineered plant cell Ti-plasmid is a natural vector as it can transfer its DNA from the bacterium to the plant genome. But wild type Ti-plasmids are not suitable as general gene vectors because due to the effects of oncogenes in the T-DNA they cause disorganized growth of the recipient plant cells.

The tumor cells resulting from integration of normal T-DNA have proven to be recalcitrant to attempts to induce regeneration, either into normal plantlets or into normal tissue which can be grafted onto healthy plants. However, it was also observed that tobacco callus transferred with wild-type Ti-plasmid could rarely regenerate into shoots. On grafting these shoots onto healthy plants, some of the grafted shoots were found to be fertile and produced seed that developed into apparently normal plants. But these plants lacked opine and almost all the T-DNA had been deleted from them.

The observations made above indicate that for efficient regeneration of plants, the vectors used should be the ones in which the T-DNA has been disarmed by making it non-oncogenic, and this can be achieved by simply deleting all of its oncogenes (Fig.7.19).

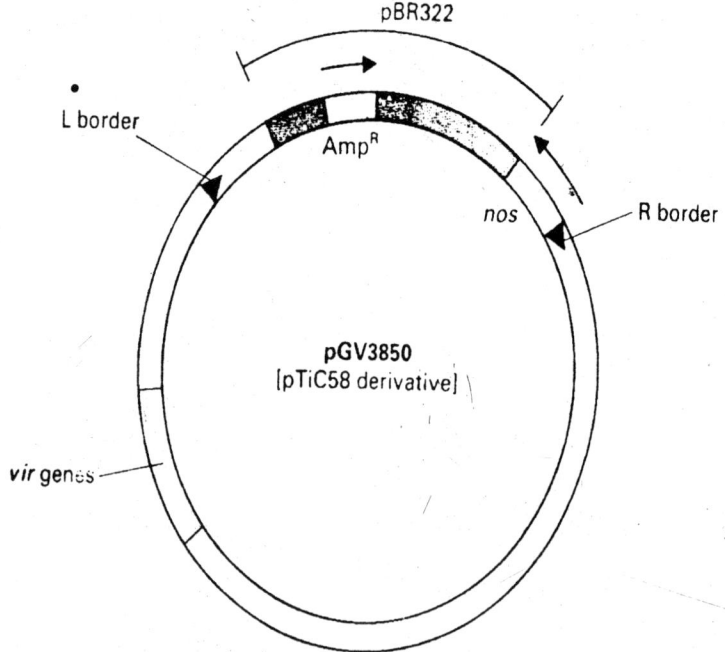

Fig. 7.19 : Structure of the Ti- plasmid pGV3850, in which the T-DNA has been disarmed.

7.7.4. Transfer of foreign DNA into T-DNA

Large size of wild-type Ti plasmids render them unsuitable as experimental gene vectors. Large size means that it is impossible to find adequate unique restriction sites in the T-region, and other procedures are also cumbersome. In an attempt to alleviate this problem intermediate vectors (IV) have been developed. In IV (a vector) the T-DNA has been subcloned into conventional small plasmid vectors of *E. coli*, standard procedures can then be employed to insert the desired DNA into the T-region of such vector. The IV, vector containing foreign DNA in the T-region, can be transferred to *A. tumefaciens* by conjugation. Since IVs are conjugation-deficient, conjugation ought to be brought about by a helper vector (a conjugation-proficient plasmid which can mobilize the IV).

The whole process of transfer proceeds with a typical 'triparental' mating. In these matings three bacterial strains are mixed together. They are:

1. The *E. coli* carrying the conjugation-proficient helper plasmid,

2. The *E. coli* strain carrying the recombinant IV,

3. The recipient *Agrobacterium*.

During the course of the incubation the helper plasmid transfers recombinant IV to the *E. coli* strain which is subsequently mobilized and transferred to *Agrobacterium*. The *Agrobacterium* recepient frequently receives both the IV and the helper plasmid. Following the introduction of vector IV into *Agrobacterium*, *in vivo* it is homologous recombination event that inserts vector IV into a resident nonrecombinant Ti plasmid.

The process essentially involves genetic engineering strategy as discussed below:

1. Identification and isolation of target gene from appropriate source.
2. Construction of intermediate plasmid vector e.g., pBR 322 from coli E1 plasmids.
3. Isolation of Ti plasmid from *A. tumefaciens* with the help of enzymes and separation of T-DNA.
4. Insertion of T-DNA in PBR 322 plasmid through gene cloning technique thus formation of a shuttle vector capable of replicating in either of hosts, i.e., *E. coli* and *A. tumefaciens*.
5. Cutting of cloned T-DNA with the help of restriction enzymes and insertion of foreign DNA.
6. Insertion of so formed chimeric DNA into *E. coli*. The uptake by *E. coli* is affected in the presence of calcium chloride solution.
7. Transformed *E. coli* cells are then added to a culture of *A. tumefaciens* and incubated for a few hours. This results into the transfer of chimeric DNA to *A. tumefaciens* cells through cytoplasmic factors of *E. coli*. The transformed *A. tumefaciens* cells are endowed with terramycin resistance acquired through *E. coli* pBR 322 plasmid.
8. Selection of transformed *A. tumefaciens* by culturing in a kanamycin containing medium.
9. The selected transformed cells are then used to infect the culture plant cells whose genome is to be manipulated for improvement.
10. Regeneration of plantlets from modified plant tissue using standard tissue culture techniques.

7.7.5. *A. rhizogenes* and Ri-plasmids

A. rhizogenes, incites a disease which is known as hairy root disease, in dicotyledonous plants. A large plasmid, the Ri (root inducing) plasmid, is responsible for pathogenicity and induction of opine synthesis. The Ri plasmids are thus analogous to Ti plasmids. They have been of interest for vector development as opine-producing root tissue. Ri T-DNA is transmitted sexually by these plants and affects a variety of morphological and physiological traits but generally does not appear to be deleterious. Therefore, Ri plasmids are apparently equivalent to disarmed Ti-plasmid. Thus, many principles of the disarmed Ti-plasmids and Ri-plasmids are similar. An intermediate vector co-integrating system has been developed and applied to the study of modulation in transgenic legumes, *Lotus corniculation*.

Agrobacterium containing both a Ri plasmid and a disarmed Ti plasmid can frequently co-transfer both plasmids, and this fact has been exploited. The Ri plasmid induced hairy root disease in recipient *Arabidopsis* and carrot cells, served as a transformation marker for the co-transferred recombinant T-DNA, and also allows regeneration of intact plants. With this plasmid. combination there was no need of incorporation of drug resistance marker on the T-DNA.

7.7.5.1. Hairy root cultures

Ri-plasmid has been utilized for genetic engineering as :

1. A gene coding for glyphosate resistance.
2. A chimeric leghemoglobin gene.
3. Various other genes have been inserted into plant cells employing Ri-vectors.

Although plants regenerated from hairy roots usually possess an abnormal phenotype, a semi-disarmed vector can be constructed to eliminate undesirable characteristics of these hairy root phenotypes. The various applications of *in-vitro* hairy root cultures can be enlisted as follows:

1. For studies of obligate root parasites or symbionts that cannot be grown in isolation and for carrying out investigations of root microbe relationships.
2. In contrast to the untransformed root in axenic culture which normally requires growth regulators as a constituent in culture medium for continual growth, transformed roots are capable of exhibiting high growth rate even on simple media lacking growth regulators.
3. *In-vitro* production of secondary plant products from hairy roots has been observed for the same spectrum of compounds as with nontransformed roots, at similar or increased concentrations. However, increased production of secondary plant metabolites has been reported by selecting high-yielding cell lines or enhancing product synthesis and release through treatment with elicitors. For example, treatment of hairy root of *Nicotiana tabacum* with elicitors derived from *Botrytis fabae* led to an increased nicotine synthesis and release (Fig. 7.20).

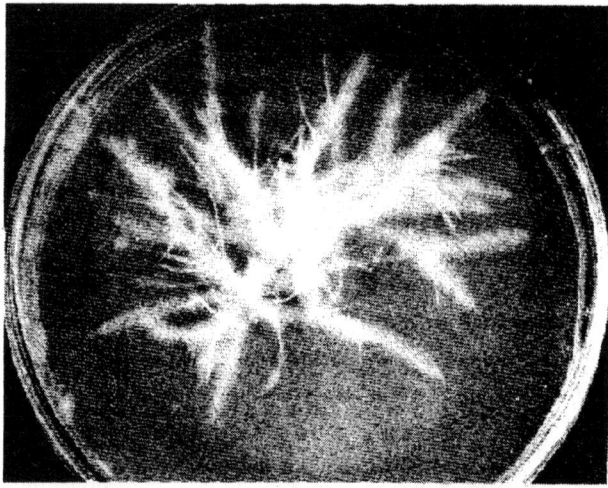

Fig. 7.20 : Tobacco hairy root culture on MS media and ampicillin.

Some hairy root cultures have been found to release a large fraction of the secondary products into the culture media which could certainly be considered as a bonus for the harvest of cell products. It is reported that this secondary metabolite production by transformed roots is stable during many generations.

7.7.6. Raising mutants in plant cell culture

With the advent of tissue culture, the techniques those were limited to microbial genetics are now being applied in higher plant cells as well. By exposure of plant cells to chemical and/or physical mutagens, genetic variability may be induced. Each plant cell has an equally good potential as any other microbial entity and may be used for induction and isolation of mutants and variants.

Isolation of variant cell strains with characteristics different from those of cells in the original cultures is possible by techniques which are utilized in microbial studies. One such method discusses the application of mutagens to plant cells. This technique increases the frequency of variant strains in population of cells so that their identification and selection become easier. However, in several cases the chemicals known to be potent mutagens in microbial cells were found to be marginally or in some cases not at all effective when used on cultured plant cells.

The mutagenic nature of a compound depends on the expression of an easily recordable characteristic in remarkably different form of the variants derived from plant cells after treatment with the agent. Parent cells growing in culture are highly resistant to 6-azauracil (a nucleic acid precursor analog), but the variants resistant to it can be easily identified and the difference can easily be assayed. This difference in sensitivity is attributed to the deficiency of an enzyme, uracil phosphoribosyl transferase (that actually kills the cell) in the variant cells. Strains of cells from diploid *Haplopappus gracilis* and haploid *Datura innoxia* lacking the enzyme and resistant to the analog have been isolated. Auxotrophic mutants requiring amino acids and vitamins have been raised in *Todea barbara*. On the same line mutants that require amino acids, vitamins and purines have been isolated in *Nicotiana tabacum*. Mutants that are resistant to antibiotics (streptomycin for instance) and base analogs (e.g., 5-bromodeoxyuridine and 80-azaguanine) have also been isolated. Resistant and auxotrophic mutants serve as markers in analysis of genetic linkage, complementation and recombination. Metabolic inhibitors are also important tools in understanding different metabolic processes. Inhibitors are substances that restrain the natural activity of a particular function or metabolic activity of an organism. They thereby interfere with the biological processes and lend to understand different metabolic processes. Cellular metabolism can be blocked at a specific site by a particular metabolic inhibitor. By examining the consequences of such blockages, the nature of the pathway and the factors controlling the process can be elucidated. A particular step in DNA, RNA or protein synthesis can be controlled by inhibitors and thereby the metabolic processes of an organism can suitably be manipulated. In addition, the mutants can be used in selecting products of fusion between cells of different genetic backgrounds. Further, the mutants recovered from cultured plant cells can be an aid in solving problems related to nutrition, agriculture and industry.

7.7.7. Phage mediated gene transfer

7.7.7.1. Gene transgenesis

Bacteriophages have been employed as vectors to facilitate the transport of genes into higher plant cells. They protect the donor DNA from nucleases and its entry into plant cells is also effected. Specially constructed transduction phages may also serve to carry bacterial genes. The phenomenon of gene and subsequent phenotypic expression is referred to as *gene transgenesis*. DNA viruses are now successfully employed as vectors in bacterial and animal systems.

For the study of DNA multiplication and gene expression in plants a simple genetic tool is offered by DNA plant viruses. The 6 genes in these viruses are believed to be regulated in the same manner as other plant genes. The DNA replicates in nuclei and may be associated with histones, the nuclear proteins.

The cauliflower mosaic virus (CMV) has been intensively studied during the past years. DNA from two strains of this virus has been completely sequenced. In its circular chromosome, an isolate was found to have 8,031 pairs of nucleotides. With the help of sequence of nucleotides and other information, a physical map of the virus chromosome has been constructed. Out of the 6 genes of this virus, one gene, gene II is not essential for reproduction, enclothement or expression of protein, or cell-to-cell movement. It has been postulated that this gene II may be involved in infective transmission of the virus in nature. Foreign DNA can be inserted in these dispensable regions of the virus chromosome, which is subsequently carried into the plant and replicated along with the DNA of the infecting virus.

In the CMV chromosome another region, gene VI, responsible for the severity of disease has been identified. Even a single change in this gene was found to have a profound effect on disease expression or presentation. This was exemplified by insertion of 12 base pairs at a particular location in gene VI and this change almost abolished the disease. Plants that are infected with this mutant of the virus exhibit only mild symptoms of the disease and have a growth rate similar to that of healthy plants. Thus, control of disease expression can be achieved if portions of the viral chromosome are eventually used as a recombinant DNA vector for plants. CMV has been used as a vehicle to reproduce foreign DNA in plant cells and to carry this particular DNA to each cell of the plant. However, a serious limitation of this process is the inability of inserting enough foreign DNA into the viral chromosome to bring about useful transformations of plant. This has been attributed to the low accommodating capacity of the viral particle for additional DNA. The assembly of DNA and coat protein to form viral particles seems to be a prime necessity prior to the movement of DNA from cell to cell in the plant. Therefore, it appears that the virus in its present form will be of limited use as a recombinant DNA vector. But, undoubtedly, this virus has an important role in defining the biological activity of the sequences involved in replication and expression of DNA in plants.

7.7.8. Cell culture, gene transfer and seed banks

For the transfer of genes into plants, methods which have been used extensively include the use of recombinant vectors based on Ti plasmid of *Agrobacterium tumefaciens* and delivery of foreign DNA directly into the protoplast. But there are certain drawbacks and limitations associated with these techniques. For instance, delivery of a recombinant Ti plasmid infection by *Agrobacterium* is desired and under normal conditions, monocotyledons are not susceptible to the *Agrobacterium* with some rare exceptions. Although monocot cells can be transformed by DNA delivered directly to protoplasts but it has been neigh impossible to regenerate transformed whole plants from the transformed cells.

A different approach to transfer foreign genes in *Secale cereale* L. (rye), a cereal species was attempted by the Pena, Lorz and Schell in 1987. They observed that during the development of the male germ of rye plant, the archesporial cells were particularly receptive to foreign chemicals such as **caffeine** and **colchicine** on their injection into developing floral tillers about 14 days before the first meiotic metaphase. Construction of a recombinant plasmid was carried out so that amino glycoside, phosphotransferase expressions, which confers resistance to kanamycin under the control of nopaline synthase promoter, derived from Ti plasmid of *Agrobacterium* could be achieved. This plasmid was injected into floral tillers. Once the pollen formation completed, the seeds were obtained by crossing injected plants. The seeds were tested for the presence of the plasmid DNA by germination and growth in the presence of kanamycin. The proposed alternative for the mode of inheritance can be any of the following:

1. The exogenous genome is integrated into the eukaryotic genome where replication is controlled by the host.
2. In another possibility, the donor genome is maintained as a cytoplasmic plasmid, resulting into an apparent failure of integration.

The entering exogenous DNA may retain its activity for a short period however, the autonomous state is lost owing to the lack of integration. Lately an electrochemical method for transfection of genes in microbial cells has been devised by Japanese workers. This method is based on the principle that electric impulses of high field strength increase the permeability of protoplast membrane and thus facilitate entry or uptake of DNA molecules by the cells provided that DNA is in immediate proximity of membrane.

7.8. REGENERATION OF PLANTS

The callus tissue growing on the tissue culture medium undergoes redifferentiation into tissue systems and organs, this is followed by its development into new young plant, the plantlet, or an embryo. This process is referred to as plant **regeneration**. The tissue culture technology is dependent on this concept of regeneration of plantlets. Without the plantlet regeneration callus induction, subculture, protoplast culture, etc. would achieve no end. Almost all the applications of tissue culture technology depend entirely upon this reproductive and regenerative capacity of plant cells. The term '**totipotency**' was coined by Steward in 1965 to describe this capacity.

7.8.1. Physiology of plant regeneration

The callus tissue comprises of a mass of parenchymatous cells, differentiates into different kinds of cells and tissues in the culture medium. This process proceeds through redifferentiation and dedifferentiation giving rise to new plantlets as discussed earlier in this chapter.

7.8.2. Types of plant regeneration

Depending on the nature of plant tissue undergoing differentiation the plant regeneration can be categorized as:

7.8.2.1. Embryo culture

The isolated immature embryo undergoes differentiation and develops into a plantlet. In some plants although fertilization takes place but the fertilized egg fails to develop into an embryo. In such cases, the immature embryo or proembryo is separated from the ovary and cultured in a chemically defined medium to facilitate the generation of a new plant. This process is referred to as **embryo rescue.**

7.8.2.2. Regeneration of embryos from cultured tissues

The tissue or cultured callus tissue undergoes differentiation and develops into embryos. Depending upon the origin of embryos the plantlet formation can be further categorized as somatic embryogenesis and organogenetic embryogenesis.

A. The **somatic embryogenesis** refers to the technique of production of embryo-like structures on the cultured callus tissue. The embryo is produced from a single cell or a tissue or an organ during the tissue culture. This embryo-like structure is known as **embryoid.** Under *in vitro* conditions, several species like *Coffea arabica, Citrus sinensis, Saccharum officinarum, Brassia oleraceae* are reported to produce somatic embryo. A schematic diagram of the procedure used for induction of direct somatic embryogenesis and regeneration is presented below (Fig. 7.21).

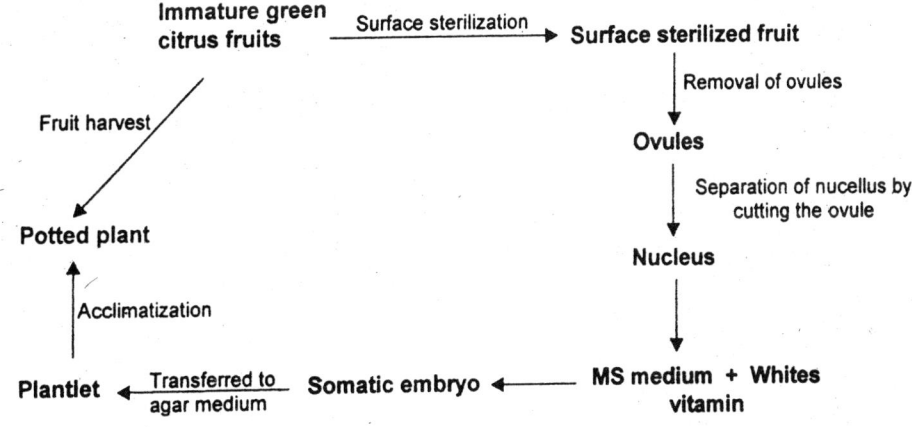

Fig. 7.21 : .Procedure for induction of direct somatic embryogenesis and plant regeneration in *Citrus*

Studies have indicated that not only egg cell but any cell of the embryo sac or any other part of the sporophyte is capable of generating an embryo. Generally, embryos fail to develop outside the ovules. However, there are certain exceptions to this, for instance in *Citrus* and *Mangifera* species adventive embryos (embryos developing from sporophytic tissue) are known to develop from nucellar cells or integuments of the ovule, outside the embryo sac. But, these embryos undergo maturation only when pushed into the embryo sac. So for the formation of somatic (bipolar) embryos in culture a special environ is to be provided. Somatic embryogenesis in culture has been carried out successfully in many species. Physiological status of calli, plant extracts and growth regulators is reported to affect somatic embryogenesis.

B. The **organogenetic embryogenesis** refers to the formation of plantlets through the formation of adventive shoots or roots from the callus tissue. These shoots or roots arise directly from the callus tissue. The plantlets produced are thus unipolar in nature, i.e. only shoot or root arise directly from the callus, but the other portion (i.e. root or shoot respectively) arise just away from the site of the origin of the shoot or root. So there is no direct physical contact between the root and shoot of the plantlet. The various types of organogenetic embryo development are:

(a) The production of plantlets from the callus tissue through the formation of adventitious organs.

(b) The production of adventitious organs directly from the explant tissue.

The highlight of this method is the absence of callus phase. Differences between organogenetic plant regeneration and somatic plant regeneration are given in table 7.5.

Table 7.5 : Differences between organogenetic plant regeneration and somatogenetic plant regeneration

Organogenetic plant regeneration	Somatogenetic plant regeneration
Embryos are unipolar in nature	Embryos are bipolar in nature
Organs arise only from the callus or an explant	Callus or explant directly develops into embryo in the culture medium
Different organs are attached with the tissue of their origin. All the shoots and roots are connected by the callus	Embryos are physically attached with the tissue of their origin
Organs produced only by a portion of callus	A few cells may also develop into an embryo

It has been demonstrated that regeneration from leaf explants, callus or plant protoplasts leads to the generation of considerable variation, described as 'somaclonal variation'. This variation includes sterile plants, aneuploids and morphological variants. In addition to phenotypic variation involving nuclear and organellar DNA, variation in chromosome number is also observed in plants regenerated from long time callus cultures.

The variation may either be genetic or epigenetic. Out of these only the former is transmitted to the next generation and is of importance in crop improvement. The genetic basis of somaclonal variation is supposed to be due to variation in number and structure of chromosomes. Aneuploidy, polyploidy, inversions, deletions, translocations, meiotic cross-over are reported to be responsible for these variations. The various steps involved in generation and utilization of somatic variation in plant breeding are presented in figure 7.22.

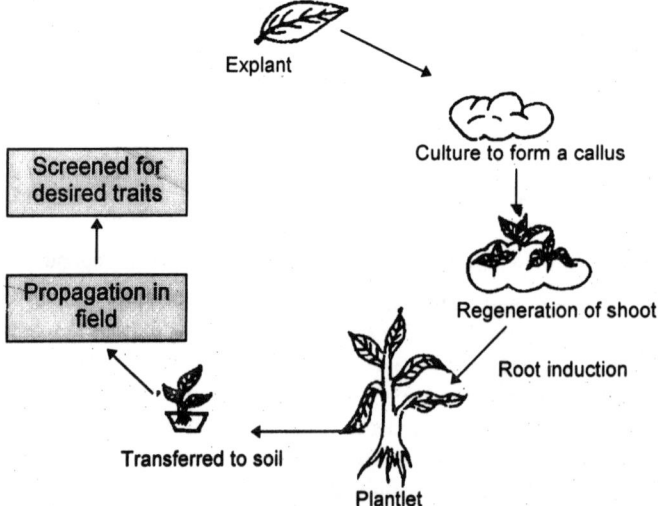

Explant

Culture to form a callus

Screened for desired traits

Propagation in field

Regeneration of shoot

Root induction

Transferred to soil

Plantlet

Fig. 7.22 : Various steps involved in the generation and utilization of somatic variation

Useful genetic somaclonal variations are selected at:
1. The cellular level by screening for the well defined derived traits like resistance to a particular herbicide, fungal toxin, extreme temperatures, etc. in the cultured cells. At the cellular level millions of cells can be screened with relative ease and minimum resources. Nevertheless for traits like flower characters, this method is unsuitable. Also, there is the possibility that the characters expressed by the selected cells may not be displayed by the regenerated plants. Thus, the phenotypes for which selection has been made at cellular level have to be cross-checked in the regenerated plants to confirm its presence.
2. The phenotypic level in the regenerated plants.

7.9. TISSUE CULTURE AND BIOSYNTHESIS OF SECONDARY PRODUCTS

Attention have been diverted towards exploration of possibilities of tissue culture as a tool for the purpose of micropropagation particularly in horticulture and agriculture. The potential for synthesis of chemicals by plants is enormous. It covers a wide range of compounds of pharmaceutical value as well as complex food materials. Growing research in practical tissue culture technology provides with the opportunity of the biosynthesis of a variety of natural products using tissue culture. The various compounds which have been modulated, synthesized and modified include alkaloids, anthraquinones, plant phenolics and volatile oil, etc. The production of chemicals using plant tissue cultures has attained a remarkable status.

Table 7.6 : Natural product yields from cell cultures and whole plants

Natural product	Species	Cell culture yield	Whole plant yield
Anthraquinones	Morinda citrifolia	900 nmol/g dry wt.	Root 110 nmol/g dry wt.
Anthraquinones	Cassia tora	0.34% fresh wt.	0.209% seed dry wt.
Ajmalicine & serpentine	Catharanthus roseus	1.3% dry wt.	0.26% dry wt.
Diosgenin	Dioscorea deltoidea	25 mg/g dry wt.	20 mg/g dry wt. tuber
Ginseng saponins	Panax ginseng	0.38% fresh wt.	0.3-3.3% fresh wt.
Nicotine	Nicotiana tabacum	3.4% dry wt.	2-5% dry wt.
Thebaine	Papaver bracteatum	130 mg/g dry wt.	1400 mg/g dry wt. leaf and 3000 mg/g
Ubiquinone	Nicotiana tabacum	0.5 mg/g dry wt.	16 mg/g dry wt. leaf

Tissue cultures of a number of plant species have been proposed and the cell extracts have been analyzed for biosynthesis of different classes of secondary products. Plant cell suspension culture is especially regarded as a suitable system particularly for the production of phytochemicals. Plant secondary metabolites are the compounds which are not required for normal plant growth and development by metabolic pathways common to all plants. Out of various products, medicinals are of great value for their effective use in health care. Narcotics from *Cannabis*, opium and heroin from *Papaver*, stimulants, i.e. caffeine from *Coffea arabica*, *Camellia synensis* (tea) and anthraquinone from *Cassia podocarpa*, are some of the compounds which can be considered as a group of the natural products. Similarly analgesics, antifertility agents, antimicrobial, cardiovascular and antimalarial drugs are other compounds which could be derived from natural sources. A comparative account of yields from cell culture and whole plants of different natural products is presented in table 7.6. Different substances as hitherto reported from plant cell cultures are tabulated in table 7.7.

Product biosynthesis has been related to three basic levels of cellular organization, i.e. cell suspension, callus and organ explants. A careful survey of literature reveals that cell culture is the best technique wherein modification in biosynthetic compounds can be affected. It has been noticed that secondary product from intact plants are produced at generally higher level as compared to their production from tissue cultures. Explanted materials of an alkaloid producing plants cultured *in vitro* have been found to attain capacity to synthesize alkaloid identical to that alkaloid in the intact plant. In some of the cases altered biosynthesis or metabolism have been noticed particularly in the case of cell suspension culture or callus culture. *Atropa* callus produces tropane alkaloids, when the roots are differentiated whereas no such compounds are synthesized in non differentiated callus tissue. Thus, it was suggested that during culture process the production of metabolites is mainly dependent on organ differentiation. Therefore, potential for production of secondary metabolites is not lost, however, due to some unknown reasons they are not expressed or produced. There are reports regarding organogenesis in the form of roots in *Dioscorea deltoidea* and *Bulbils* and *Agar wighii* capable of producing metabolites particularly sapogenins. High yields of indole alkaloids are reported in tissue culture of *Rauwolfia serpentina*. Plant natural products and cells cultured *in vitro* could be produced through different metabolic pathways or synthesis generally referred to as biotransformation which could be used as a route to the synthesis of the novel products not found in the parent plants. Compounds like diosgenin, saponin, etc., were produced in culture in quantities comparable or even higher than in the intact plant. With the advancement in the knowledge of biochemistry and biology of cell culture there have been reports on cell culture(s) claiming for reasonably higher yields of the compounds such as anthraquinone, diosgenin, nicotine, thebaine. Some of the cultures have been reported to yield higher amounts of the compounds as compared to their production in intact plant. The cell suspensions are ideal as they can be grown in simple bioreactors and could provide opportunities for scale up.

Table 7.7 : Substances reported from plant cell cultures

Alkaloids	Allergens	Anthraquinones	Antileukaemic agents
Antitumor agents	Antiviral agents	Aromas	Benzoquinones
Cardiac glycosides	Carbohydrates (including polysaccharides)	Chalcones	Dianthrones
Lipids	Latex	Naphthoquinones	Nucleic acids
Nucleotide	Oils	Opiates	Organic acids
Peptides	Perfumes	Phenols	Pigments
•Enzymes	Plant growth regulators	Enzyme inhibitors	Proteins
Flavonoids	Flavones	Steroids and its derivatives	Flavors (including sweeteners)
Furanocoumarins	Tannins	Hormones	Sugars
Terpenes terpenoids	Insecticides	Vitamins	

7.9.1. Factors affecting biosynthesis

Various factors which could affect the biosynthetic process, its rate and as a consequence the yield may typically include origin of tissue, media formulations, carbon sources, incorporation of plant growth regulators and precursor feed. Amino acids particularly tryptophan, phenylalanine and ornithine can be used as precursors. Feeding of phenylalanine to the culture of *Capsicum frutiscence* and 4-hydroxy-2-quinoline to the culture of *Butea graveolance* for obtaining better yield of alkaloids are the classical examples of precursor feed based amelioration and biotransformations. The effect of addition of precursors during the course of alkaloid synthesis by suspension culture technique particularly in the case of *Solanaceous* plants and of *Catharanthus roseus* and *Cinchona ledgeriana* has been investigated. The concentration level at which the precursor is added to the media is critical as at one concentration, it may respond as an initiator and promoter of biosynthesis while turns to be inhibitor at another (higher) concentration.

The presence of amino acids was found to be toxic when added to the culture media in concentration more than 2 mM causing cell death. However, accumulation of number of indole and quinoline derivatives has been reported. Cell culture techniques offer exciting opportunities in the production of various novel compounds. Cells in culture can be channeled into particular biochemical pathways as exemplified by the production of rutacultin by tissue cultures of *Ruta graveolens*. However, the process was found to be prohibitive and nonadaptive on the basis of cost factor. Production of medicinal alkaloids such as opiates and indole using cell cultures of *C. roseus* has been of prime interest in the research of modern times. Some of the alkaloids such as ajmalicine, reserpine, vinblastine, vincristine and vincanine are derived from the precursor tryptophan. The commercial production is however, not appreciable due to poor yield.

Furthermore, the poor yields of secondary metabolites appear to be due to:

1. differences between young, dispersed and rapidly dividing cells, akin to meristem tissue,
2. nature of slow-growing cells in organized mass,
3. variation in product formation as a function of time in culture repressing or dormancy of desired biosynthetic pathway and
4. non-excretion of products from cultured cells.

To overcome these problems, development of hairy root cultures, immobilized cell systems and techniques to encourage excretion of desired products into medium are being attempted. However, examples do exist that show that callus and suspension culture can synthesize secondary metabolite with yields that are comparable to the intact plant. In some cell lines the rate of production of secondary metabolites was found to be exceedingly higher to that found in the intact plant, e.g., jatrorrhizini from berberis, shikonin from *Lithospermum,* berberine from *Coptis* and rosamarinic acid from *Coleus.*

From a biotechnological point of view, suspension cultures are the most appropriate systems for the production of secondary metabolites on an economical scale. The productivity of metabolites synthesized by cell culture is a function of the amounts of metabolite in the cells and of growth rate of cells. A majority of the secondary metabolism activities are repressed in cultured cells and thus it becomes difficult to produce useful secondary products using them.

Some of the pharmaceuticals that have been successfully isolated from plant tissue cultures are listed in table 7.8.

Table 7.8 : Some pharmaceutically significant metabolites produced by plant tissue culture

Compound	Plant species	Culture type
Ajmalicine	*Catharanthus roseus*	Suspension
Anthraquinones	*Cassia angustifolia*	Cell
Atropine	*Atropa belladonna*	Hairy root
Berberine	*Coptis japonica*	Cell & suspension
Caffeine	*Coffea arabica*	Cell
Cardenolides	*Digitalis purpurea*	Cell & suspension
Codeine	*Papaver somniferum*	Suspension
Digoxin	*Digitalis lanata*	Suspension
Diosgenin	*Dioscorea compositae*	Cell
Hyoscyamine	*Hyoscyamus niger*	Suspension
Indole alkaloids	*Ipomoea violacea*	Cell & suspension
Morphine	*Papaver somniferum*	Suspension
Nicotine	*Nicotiana tabacum*	Suspension
Papain	*Carica papaya*	Cell
Quinine and Quinidine	*Cinchona ledgericna*	Root culture
Reserpine	*Rauwolfia serpentina*	Suspension
Rosamarinic acid	*Coleus blumei*	Cell & Suspension
Tropane alkaloids	*Datura innoxia*	Suspension
Vinblastine	*Catharanthus roseus*	Cell
Xanthotoxin	*Ruta graveolens*	Suspension

Sometimes, cell cultures have been reported to produce compounds which are not found as normal constituents of that species. For example, unusual ether lipids, 1(3),2 diacylglycero 3(1)-O-4'-(N,N,N-trimethyl) homoserines have been isolated from algae cultures of *Chlorella fusca.* Some other promising commercial products include a new CNS-active indole alkaloid percine and a new anti-inflammatory lignin.

Large scale production of bio-mass containing useful secondary metabolites has been achieved, however due to economical constraints the tissue culture technique is limited only to a few constituents only. To date more than 30 classes of compounds have been identified to be produced by plant cell cultures in appreciably high quantities some of the classic examples are digitalis glycosides, diosgenin-derived steroid hormone precursors, shikonin, rosamarinic acid, opium alkaloids (codeine and morphine), ginsenosides, ajmalicine and other indole alkaloids, including vinblastine and vincristine and possible complex mixtures such as rose and jasmine oil.

Mitsui petrochemical industries of Japan has been producing shikonin (a red colored phenolic naphthoquinone compound used as a dye and astringent) from cell cultures of *Lithospermum erythrorhizon*. A German pharmaceutical company is producing digitalis glycosides by biotransformation in cell cultures.

7.9.2. Indole alkaloids

Several important drugs, such as ajmalicine, phytostigmine, reserpine, vincristine and vinblastine belong to the class of molecules referred to as indole alkaloids (Fig. 7.23). These alkaloids are found in plant family Apocynaceae, Loganiaceae, Rubiaceae, and Fabaceae. Out of these vincristine and vinblastine are complex dimeric mono terpene indole alkaloids. They are used as antineoplastic agents. Although extensive work has been undertaken to produce these compounds using classical plant tissue culture techniques but the efforts have so far failed. Only by the induction of differentiated surface cultures via the addition of phytohormone benzyladenine into the growth media vindoline production has been demonstrated. The media alteration however, to some extent has been reported to be instrumental in modulation of the yield. The alteration of the media typically included the addition of sucrose as a carbon source and some phytohormones. Bioregulators like dimethylaminoethyl-1-2,4-dichlorophenyl ether on incorporation have been reported to increase the ajmalicine content by 270-570% and the production of catharanthine by 82-146%.

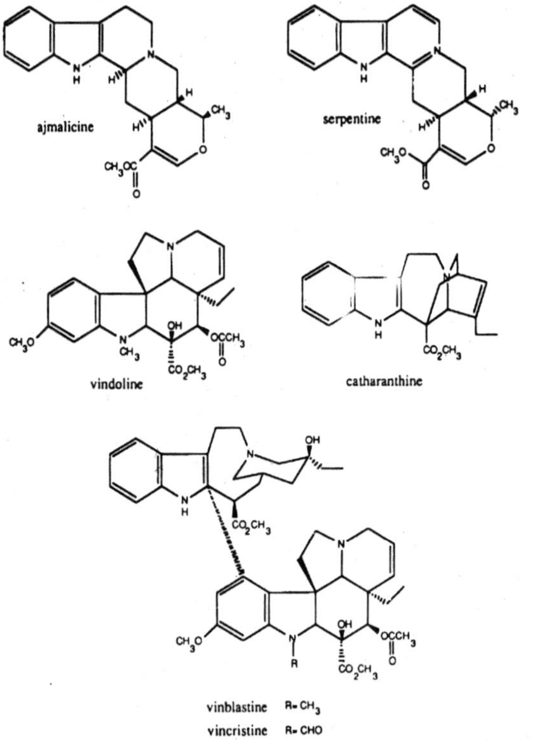

Fig. 7.23 : Representative examples of indole alkaloids

In another approach Eilert et al., transformed *C. roseus* cells with *Agrobacterium tumefaciens* to produce tumorous cell lines which was thought to be able to produce ajmalicine 0.060 mg/g fresh weight. Such modifications are referred as crown gall culture and reported to produce monomeric units. Catharanthine however failed to synthesize vindoline. Another interesting report relating to the transformation of *C. roseus* cell with a mild *A. rhizogenes* which resulted in production of hairy root culture showed a 20 fold increase in cell mass over a 28 day growth period. The cultures have been reported to synthesize high yields of wide variety of monomeric indole alkaloids including catharanthine, ajmalicine and vindolinine.

7.9.3. Tropane alkaloids

Tropane alkaloids which occur in plants of Solanaceae, Convolvulaceae, include several important pharmaceuticals most notably scopolamine, hyoscyamine (Fig.7.24), atropine and cocaine. The plants from Solanaceae family are highly responsive to cell culture techniques and plants producing these alkaloids have been studied extensively. Plants from these species synthesize biologically active compounds mainly in their roots. Therefore, attempts have been made to produce crown gall culture. *A. rhizogenes* to form hairy root culture exhibited a 20 fold increase in cell with an alkaloid content of 0.68% of the dry weight, wherein hyoscyamine and scopolamine were present in a comparable ratio of whole intact plant. Another solanaceous species, *A. belladonna* on transformation is with *A. rhizogenes* produced a hairy root culture with around 60 fold increase in cell mass over a 28 day growth period and synthesized scopolamine at 0.02% of the dry weight, whereas the content of hyoscyamine was estimated to be 0.371% as dry weight. The results with crown gall culture of *H.muticus*, *S. japonica* also exhibited increased production of tropane alkaloids in hairy root culture as compared with normal culture or suspension culture.

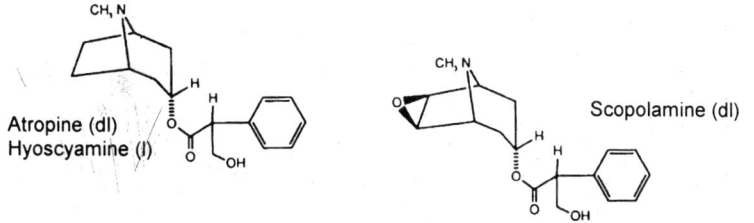

Fig. 7.24 : Representative examples of tropane alkaloids.

7.9.4. Quinoline alkaloids

The alkaloids mainly quinidine and quinine (Fig.7.25) are of particular importance in treatment of malaria and in restoring normal heart rhythms. These are the contents belonging to the family Rutaceae, where commercial source of quinine and quinidine is *Cinchona*. The cell culture and production of these alkaloids was experimented and revealed that cell suspension and callus culture failed to produce significant quantity of the either alkaloids. Whereas differentiated shoot systems demonstrated bio-synthesizing capacity. The transformation of this species using *A. tumefaciens* to form hormone independent undifferentiated cell-suspension culture (i.e., crown gall culture) exhibited promising results. The average quinoline alkaloid content of these cells was 5-6 times greater than previously studied untransformed form. The most recent reports on hairy root culture *C. ledgeriana* transformed with *A. rhizogenes* indicated 2-3 times alkaloid content of the most of the products of dark grown crown gall cells, with the methoxylated quinoline, in quinine and quinidine yielding up to 50-70% of total alkaloids.

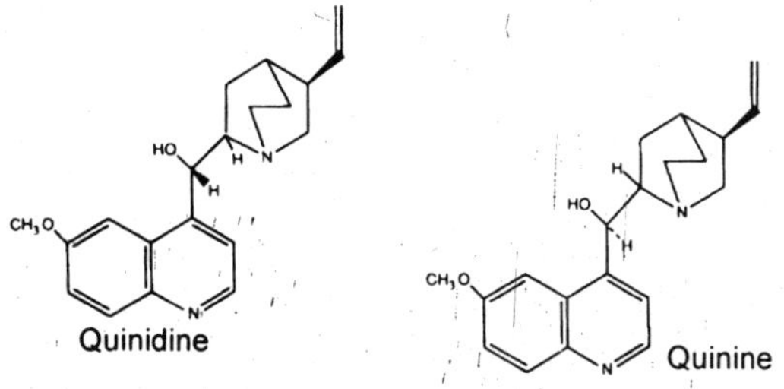

Fig. 7.25 : Representative examples of quinoline alkaloids.

7.10. APPLICATIONS

There are immense possibilities for basic studies using plant tissue culture methods. This technology can be exploited for the procurement of commercial products as well. Details of the specific applications are discussed below:

7.10.1. To study respiration and metabolism

Studies of respiration of whole pieces of callus tissue, homogenates and cellular fraction provide means of separating normal and diseased growth. For example, enzymatic differences in tissue of crown gall and normal origins exist even after growth in culture for extended periods. A reduction in respiratory levels in crown gall tissue culture has also been noted. There was an apparent increase maintained in endogenous auxins synthesis by crown gall tissue culture. C^{14} labelled fructose, sucrose and glutamine absorption and their incorporation into the alcohol insoluble fraction by crown gall tissues of *Parthenocissus* were lower than in normal tissue culture.

An increment in oxygen uptake by Rumex tissue has been demonstrated when 2-4-D, IAA and 2,3,5-triiodobenzoic acid and colchicine were used at concentrations from 0.001 to 1 mg/liter, and decreased on their incorporation at higher concentrations. The secretion of an α-amylase enzyme by this tissue accounted for the utilization of starch. The metabolism involved in cell enlargement of cultured tobacco pith parenchyma and transformations of carbohydrates by carrot tissue have also being studied and described. Tissue on IAA media in comparison to those on media lacking auxin displayed a rise in respiratory rate, an increment in ascorbic acid oxidase activity, a rise in intact cells to oxidize SH groups of cysteine and glutathione within 72 hours, increase in invertase and pectin methylesterase activity and a decrease in peroxidase activity. Changes in the media composition were followed by an increase or decrease in respiration and ascorbic acid oxidase activity. Phenylthiourea at critical concentrations inhibited ascorbic acid oxidase activity and the growth, whereas a large respiratory increase of auxin was permitted. Changes in the composition of the medium altered different phases of metabolism that control cell enlargement, or growth.

The oxidative and phosphorylative activities of cytoplasmic particles from crown gall and normal tissue cultures of tomato were studied and found to be qualitatively similar but quantitatively different. Both tissues had relatively constant respiratory activity during the active period of growth of tissues, but this activity period of growth of tissues decreased as growth leveled off. Crown gall tissue gave a lower activity profile than normal tissue on a dry weight basis however the values were comparable on nitrogen basis.

7.10.2. To study polarity and organ function

Isolated tissues are useful for conducting studies related to polarity and organ function. Gautheret has described three major types of proliferations developing in isolated tissues, viz. of unorganized parenchyma, of specialized cambial layer or that of organized growing points. These may develop in fresh explants or in established cultures. Variations in these types of proliferation may be observed in a variety of tissues from many species. For instance, proliferation from a fresh stem or carrot section commonly occurs as a layer of new growth over the cut surface. Proliferation may also occur from preexisting cambia or from diffused cambia scattered in the tissue. Isolated tissue often produces root or bud meristems. Various types of proliferation have been observed in established strains of tissue as well. Cultures originally parenchymatous may develop vascular bundles, with phloem and xylem, after several transfers, and eventually root and stem primordia may be developed.

Outstanding efforts have been made to clarify cell growth, cell division, callus differentiation and organ formation in terms of growth substances and balances of common metabolites. Interactions between IAA and adenines were found to be related to bud formation in tobacco callus. IAA prevented and adenine promoted the process of bud formation. Concentrations were found to be critical and the adenine-IAA ratio determined quantitatively the degree of bud formation. The tobacco callus cells enlarged enormously without dividing when supplied with auxin alone. In the presence of auxin, cell division resulted by contact with vascular stem tissue, or by adding coconut milk or malt extract. Kinetin was isolated from DNA and was noted to be highly active in promoting cell division in the tobacco callus.

The callus tissue masses may or may not change morphologically and/or physiologically with change in time. Tissue changes, if recorded, have been correlated with auxin requirements (habituation), with pigment formation and with varied sucrose concentration or light conditions. Similarly, for growth substances such as coconut milk or 2,4-D, modifications in rate of growth and firmness of tissue mass were observed. Nutritional requirements differ depending on the length of time in culture as in insect gall tissue and normal tissue, whereas crown gall tissues are remarkably constant in nutritional and growth substance requirements.

7.10.3. Studies of plant diseases and their elimination

A comparison of normal and diseased tissues of various plants can be made by tissue culture. White and Brawn demonstrated the possibility of growing crown gall tissue *in vitro*. The gall tissue was found to be more growth substance active than normal tissue. Detailed study has been performed to clarify the pathological nature and physiological differences between normal and gall tissue.

Tissues of gall of genetic origin were among the first grown *in vitro*. Galls of virus origin established in tissue cultures have been examined for nutritional requirements and metabolism. Callus tissues infected with TMV and other viruses have been examined to clarify virus infection and multiplication. The amount of virus in the tobacco callus cultures varied depending on the strain of host tissue and the nutritional and physical environments. The amount of virus in tobacco tissue cultures was influenced by the growth substances. The number of tobacco tissue pieces artificially infected with TMV exhibited dependence on the type and number of injuries caused and induced at inoculation time. Depending on the concentration, nucleic acids, purines, pyrimidines and analogs influenced the growth of the TMV infected tobacco tissue and the infectivity of the TMV. The plants free from pathogens can be raised from the existing infective plants. Since the pathogens infect almost all the portions of plants except the growing buds, disease-free plants can be raised through the meristem and callus culture method. Alternatively meristems can be treated with heat shocks to inactivate the virus. Virus infection can also be eliminated through repeated subculturing.

7.10.4. Single cell cultures of higher plant cells

Over the years tissue culture methods have expanded from organ culture to cell culture. It is now even possible to isolate and grow single cells of higher plants. But the critical question remains whether all the cells in a callus tissue mass are similar or not. If variation of cells exist, what are their types that make up the mass. Single cell clones are a valuable means to study similarities and differences between normal cells and various kinds of diseased cells. Single cell clones of tissue from marigold crown gall tissue have shown constant differences in growth rate, texture and color. Some clones with varied media developed shoots or roots in culture. Single cell clones of tissue derived from isolated single cells of tobacco crown gall teratomas were developed into masses of tissue of morphologically abnormal structures. These structures were typical of the teratoma cultures from which they were derived. Single cell clones of tobacco (*N. tabacum* x *N.glutinosa*) callus tissue demonstrated considerable variation in growth rate, morphology, color, texture and nutrient requirements. The amount of TMV in respective clones also varied greatly after 4 successive monthly passages of inoculated clones in virus-free liquid, shake cultures. Furthermore, it was observed that young largely meristematic single cell clones of the hybrid tobacco tissue were more resistant to TMV infection and subsequent multiplication of TMV than were older cultures (containing largely enlarging or senescent cells). When a single cell clone of *N. tabacum* was infected with a mixture of TMV strains, a single mild strain of TMV was selected. This mild strain multiplied in the tissue culture whereas the other strains in the mixture were lost. Single cell clones of tissue reisolated from two parent single cell clones of the hybrid tobacco tissue, maintained differences in growth rates which were observed between the two parent clones. The clone reisolates from a single parent displayed differences in color and consistency.

Phylloxera gall and normal grape stem tissues have also been used to establish their respective single cell clones. The clones varied in color, growth rate, texture and the ability to grow on media with various combinations of casein hydrolysate, growth substances and other nitrogen and carbon compounds as substitutes for coconut milk. The growth of the single cell clones coming from the gall and normal grape stem tissues was influenced by the type and concentration of sugar.

The single cell methods have enabled to carry out many new studies that were previously impossible. Single cell clones may be further evaluated for additional chemical, morphological, genetical and pathological similarities and differences. Clarification of the mechanism of virus infection and multiplication and location of the virus in the host cell may be carried out. In a similar fashion, mutation of cells, the process of habituation, the action of chemical growth regulators and of pathogenic agents (other than virus) may be further delineated. The possibility of developing an entire plant from a single cell (as from cells in mixed cultures) is also high. All the more, the somatic cells growing in microculture provide a simple experimental method for carrying out detailed cytological studies of both normal and diseased cells. This material is free of artifacts that are common with killed and stained preparations. The physical and chemical microenvironments can be controlled to observe the effects over a prolonged time period, e.g., for metabolites, growth substances, toxic materials and disease incitants.

7.10.5. Procurement of commercial products

Commercial products like cardiac glycosides, morphinone alkaloids, essential oil and original rubber can be procured by exploiting tissue culture which otherwise are to be obtained from plants. But in spite of the fact that plant cell cultures can accumulate sufficiently high concentration of secondary metabolites to render its production viable to commercial use, the compounds at these levels are not of great commercial importance. Commercially significant plant products are either not found in cell cultures or even if present they are only in very small concentrations. Interestingly, cardiac glycosides are found only in morphologically differentiated cell cultures with concentration of only 1mg/l suspension. Even morphine and codeine are found in about 1.5 mg/gm dry weight in the cell cultures of Papaver species.

The technical problems encountered in quantitative recovery of useful products in cell culture are:

1. Several metabolites are released in cell vacuoles and not in the medium, thus they are in a way locked and not available.

2. To release the product continuously, the viability of the cells must remain unaltered.

Since time immemorial, the plants have been utilized as an inexhaustible source of medicinal extracts, with the latest techniques the active constituents of these extracts have been isolated and characterized, their phyto-therapeutic activities verified and the dose-response relationships have been specified. Conventionally, the plants from which important pharmaceuticals are obtained are grown on large scale plantations. Nevertheless, if a factory-type production of biomedicinals could be possible, it would undoubtedly be of interest and shall attract the pharmaceutical industry. An interesting alternative for controlled production of plant constituents, like secondary metabolites is the tissue culture technique. The technique of plant tissue cultures can offer possible solution to some of the problems surfacing due to current rate of extinction and decimation of floras and ecosystems.

7.10.6. Germplasm storage

Generally most of the plants are stored in the form of seed or as growing plants. But some seeds fail to develop into plants while others fail to retain their originality. This limitation can be successfully eliminated to raise identical clones by employing tissue culture technique. The plant materials can be collected and stored in a minimal medium with low light intensity and low temperature without any appreciable loss in its viability. This helps in reducing the growth rate of plant tissue meanwhile the totipotency of tissue is retained. Thus, a large number of individual tissue can be stored in a limited area. This type of storage is referred to as **germplasm storage**. The sub-culturing of these tissues can be performed at regular intervals of one year. Germplasm can be stored in the form of seeds, buds, protoplasts, shoot tips, etc. The germplasm in the growing stage is used for storage of tissues. Their growth is suspended by any of these techniques:

1. Addition of hormones or other chemical retardant;
2. Lowering temperature;
3. Reduction in oxygen concentration.

Out of these storage at low temperature using liquid nitrogen i.e. cryopreservation is the most effective method. Whenever required, germplasm can be used following rapid thawing.

7.10.7. Embryo rescue

In some plants, normal fertilization occurs but the ovule fails to develop into a mature seed. In such instances, the fertilized egg on immature embryo is removed from the immature fruits and cultured in the tissue culture medium. The individuals so generated are hybrids which show a few new characters. This process of embryo culture is also referred to as embryo rescue and can be used for embryo culture, ovule culture and ovary culture. In the cases where it is not feasible to excise embryos due to small size whole ovules can be cultured. Even if ovules cannot be excised whole ovaries may be cultured.

7.10.8. Somaclonal variation or modification

Generally, the clones released through tissue culture bear uniformity in their characters but at times few clones show variations. These variant clones express new characters which were absent in their parent cells. The formation of variant clones from the cultured callus tissues is called **somaclonal variation**. The somaclonal variants can be desirable or undesirable. Desirable variants are useful in crop improvements whereas the undesirable ones are not. A variety of somaclonal variants have been raised from plants like sugarcane, maize, rice and other cereals. The regenerated variant clones are tested for their resistance to herbicide, temperature and heavy metals. The resistant clones are further tested for their productivity.

7.10.9. The production of haploids

The haploid plants are characterized by having only a single set of chromosomes in their cells. Production of haploids is relatively easy when anther, ovule or pollen grain culture is established in the medium. These haploid plants are employed in improving the field and agricultural crops. The detection and selection of recessive mutants for a few characters can be performed with haploid plants. Pollen incompatibility can be removed by mentor pollen technology.

7.10.10. Production of artificial seeds

An artificial seed is a synthetic seed which is made up of a somatic embryo surrounded by the nutrient medium and this as a whole protected by a thin synthetic membrane. In comparison to natural seeds, these artificial seeds are smaller in size. They are identical and contain only the somatic embryos of a known strain. They can be stored even for a period of one year without any appreciable loss in viability. The seeds are encapsulated in a synthetic membrane made up of polyoxyethylene, sodium alginate or polyacrylamide gel. The pattern of germination in artificial seeds is similar to that of natural seeds and can be directly sown in the soil but unlike natural seeds do not need hardening in green house. High cost of production seems to be the only limitation.

7.10.11. Clonal propagation and micropropagation

Clonal propagation involves the propagation through the techniques of cell, tissue or organ culture. The advantages of this method are rapid multiplication of superior clones, maintenance of genetic uniformity and multiplication of sexually derived sterile hybrids. In this technique shoot tips or axillary buds are utilized for propagation on culture media without the intervention of callus phase.

Micropropagation is the most common used technique being used both at the research level and commercial level. It can be employed for the mass production of plants including nursery stock species, ornamental vegetables and field crops. The method as such enables large production of selected genotypes. It provides a process which could effectively eliminate pathogens from viral and bacterial origin. It is desirable that a microproagation system developed should produce a large number of uniform plants which are genotypically and phenotypically the same as plant from which they are produced. Most suitable technique is the multiplication using axillary buds. This method could produce genetically stable plants under sterile conditions where a minimum possible stress is generated on the growing plants. The method allows for easy manipulation and strict control over environmental and nutritional levels. However, the main disadvantage of this method is meager possibilities for physiological experimentation because the plants produced are generally juvenile in nature, which tend to suffer epicuticular wax(s) removal/reduction. Palisade cell layer is smaller with larger mesophyll air sacs and disrupted stomatal physiology. Microproagation is conducted in four main stages as shown in figure 7.26.

1. Selection and sterilization of elite plants;
2. Establishment of axillary buds and culture;
3. Multiplication in culture; and
4. Rooting of *in vitro* plants and transfer to compost.

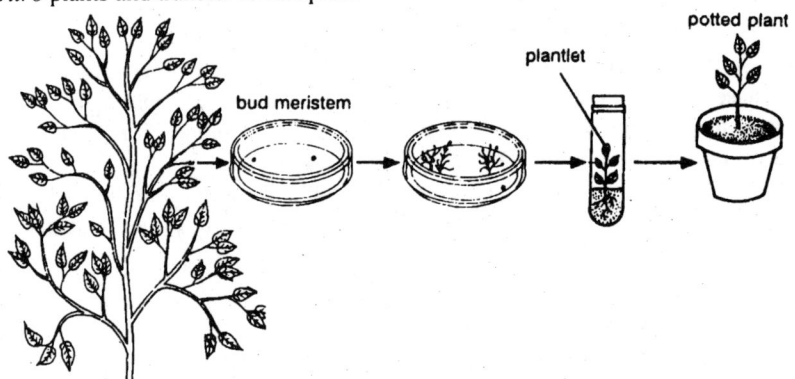

Fig. 7.26 : Steps involved in microproagation of plant material.

1. **Selection of elite plants:** Plants are selected which are apparently free from any disease, stress or surfacial blemishes. This material is preferably grown in an environmentally controlled growth cabinet or clean glass houses and should have been tested for the presence of any specific virus using sophisticated diagnostic tests like ELISA. The selected elites are washed with 70% ethanol containing 4-5 drops of surface active agents in 100 ml solution, followed by 2% chloros and 4 drops of surfactant per 100 ml of solution at room temperature. Using a clean sharp blade axillary buds of the desired variety were excised and stored in distilled water until enough buds have been collected. In a laminar flow bench a maximum 20 buds are kept in a sterile test tube and filled up to the brim with ethanol solution and left impregnated for 1-1.5 minutes. The ethanol is decanted off and the tube refilled with chloros solution. Agitation is provided out at 120 strokes/min for 12 min using an arbitrary hand wrist action shaker. The chloros rinse decanted off with sterile water 3 times and stored in sterile and distilled water.

2. **Establishment of axillary buds and culture:** Axillary buds are taken out in an empty sterile petri dish. Up to 4 buds are placed in a 50 ml petri dish containing medium 1 (M&S) and all essential medium components and nutrients. The base of bud is stuck firmly in the media. But buds should not be buried into the media. The petri dish is sealed in such a way that adequate gaseous exchange is ensured. This is transferred to the room temperature in an incubator for 1-2 week/months.

3. **Multiplication in culture:** When shoot appears extending, the apical part is cut and the cuttings and internodal cuttings are transferred to a sterile jar containing appropriate media in such a way that basal portion of stem is inserted into the media without burying the explant.

4. **Rooting of *in vitro* plants and transfer to compost :** The *in vitro* plant is pieced into 5 mm fragments and transferred into a fresh appropriate medium, left for 5 days until some sturdy roots are visible. Each plant is

removed carefully from the jar and then transferred into a damp compost in 50 mm pots. The high humidity is maintained for 12-24 hours. Then the pots are placed in a glass house under shed protected from light until plants are approximately 70 mm high and have begun to lose their juvenile nature or character. They can be transferred to the larger pots or to the fields.

7.10.12. Mutant selection

Mutant selection is an important tool effectively utilized in crop improvement. Cells are subjected to mutagenic treatments and subsequently mutants are selected. The selection of mutant cells is usually performed by addition of toxic substances to cells followed by isolation of resistant cells. In this manner cell lines resistant to these toxic substances can be efficiently selected. By exploiting this approach, cell lines resistant to antibiotics, amino acid analogs and fungal toxins have been isolated. Alternatively indirect selection can also be performed. For example, nitrate reductase deficient cell lines can be selected as chlorate resistant cells. On similar lines cell cultures of Nicotiana were selected, for resistance against herbicides like sodium chlorate, sulfometuron and amitrol. Cell lines of potato resistant to 5-methyltryptophan were selected and these cultures permitted the accumulation of free phenylalanine, tryptophan and tyrosine.

In haploids only one set of chromosomes is present and thereby even the recessive mutations are expressed immediately. Thus, the desirable mutants can be isolated among haploids derived in culture. Pollens can be grown as single cells on solid medium and a larger population can be screened in the laboratory and thereby precluding the phase of initial growth of plants in the field.

7.10.13. Endosperm culture

Tissue culture techniques are utilized for endosperm culture. Endosperm is triploid in its chromosome constitution. It supplies nutrition to the developing embryo. Triploid plants are useful for production of seedless fruits of banana, watermelon, etc. Production of trisomics for cytogenetic studies has also been reported. Triploids are generally obtained by crossing colchicine induced tetraploids with diploids and this is followed by rescue of triploid embryos. Strong crossability barriers at times preclude production of triploids from 4x X 2x crosses and in such cases endosperm culture may be used as an alternative strategy for triploid production.

The various steps involved in the endosperm culture are:

1. Aseptic dissection of immature/mature seeds;
2. Excision of endosperms along with embryos;
3. Culturing of excised endosperms on a suitable medium;
4. Removal of embryos after initial callus growth;
5. Embryogenesis or shoot bud differentiation of the callus;
6. Development of shoots and roots;
7. Establishment of complete triploid plants.

7.10.14. Nucellus culture

In some plant like Citrus, adventative embryos develop from nucellar cells. In such cases nucellus from pollinated flowers can also be utilized for micropropagation. It can be grown on White's medium supplemented with casein hydrolysate to obtain callus. This callus may give rise to pseudobulbils differentiating into embryoids. These embryoids eventually develop into seedlings. Nucellus obtained from unfertilized ovules are also capable of developing embryoids. The seedlings obtained from the nucellar tissue are of parental type. Thereby they are important for maintaining purity of horticultural stocks.

7.11. CONCLUSION

It is obvious that since last two decades there have been considerable efforts in the use of plant cell cultures in bioproduction, bioconversion or biotransformation and biosynthetic studies. The potential commercial production of pharmaceuticals by cell culture techniques depends upon detailed investigations into the biosynthetic sequences. Recent advances in sensitive analytical techniques, particularly of enzyme assay and radio-immunoassay have enabled biogenetic investigations within plant cell cultures to proceed at a faster rate than before. The potential use of cell cultures in the production of valuable secondary products is being viewed with a great sense of optimism and enthusiasm by biotechnologists. The key to commercially promising production of biomedicinals is clearly the induction and selection of high-yielding cell lines. The recent advances in plant biotechnology offer several mechanisms for unlocking the diverse and potentially profitable synthetic capabilities of cultured plant cells.

Some of the major advantages expected from tissue culture systems over the conventional cultivation techniques are presented below:

1. Availability of uniform plant material at all times and manageable under regulated and reproducible conditions.
2. Synthesis of those chemical compounds which are impossible or too difficult to synthesize chemically. Further, the compounds from tissue cultures may be more easily purified because of simpler extracts and absence of significant amount of pigments.
3. Production of natural compounds under controlled environmental conditions, independent of soil conditions and changes in climate.
4. Biogenesis of the secondary metabolites can be studied. Labelled precursors can be fed to the cell cultures and interpretations pertaining to the metabolic pathways of the desired compound can be made.
5. They offer an opportunity to attempt envisaged biotransformation or bioconversion reactions. It is expected that specific modification of chemical structures of certain compounds may be achieved more easily in cultured plant cells in comparison to micro-organisms or chemical synthesis.
6. The technique provides completely controlled conditions to elucidate growth and physiology of cells and to study host-parasite interaction at cellular level.
7. The cells of any plants, tropical or temperate, could be multiplied to yield specific metabolites produced by them.
8. Cellular totipotency, the unique potency of plant cells can be revealed. All living cells, irrespective of their potency level can potentially give rise to whole plants. It offers an efficient, safe and economical methods of plant propagation.
9. The cultured cells could be maintained free from any microbial contamination and insect attack.
10. Immobilization of cells can be carried out which could be used for various biotransformation and biochemical reactions.

At times, it is possible to store plant germplasm in tissue cultures at refrigerated temperature more economically and safely than by conventional methods. The feasibility of growing single cells and protoplast fusion of completely unrelated species has opened up new avenues for plant improvement.

SUGGESTED READINGS

Anderson, P.G., (Ed.) (1986) **Plant Tissue Culture and its Agricultural Applications**, Butterworths, Stoneham, Massachussets.

Barz, W., Reinhard, E. and Zenk, M.H., (Eds.) (1977) **Plant Tissue Culture and its Biotechnological Applications,** Springer-Verlag, Berlin and New York.

Bengochen, T. and Dodds, J.H., (1986) **Plant Protoplasts: A Biotechnological Tool for Plant Improvement**, Chapman and Hall, London, New York.

Bhojwani, S.S. and Razdan, M.K., (1983) **Plant Tissue Culture: Theory and Practice,** Elsevier, Amsterdam.

Dixon, R.A., (Ed.) (1985) **Plant Cell Culture: A Practical Approach**, IRL, Oxford and Washington DC.

Evans, D.A., Sharp, W.R., Ammirato, P.V., and Yamada, Y., (Eds.) (1984) **Handbook of Plant Cell Cultures**, New York.

George, E.F. and Sherrington, P.D., (1984) **Plant Propagation by Tissue Culture**, Exegetics Ltd., Reading U.K.

Green C.E., Somers, D.A., Hackett, W.P. and Biesboer, D.D., (Eds.) (1987) **Plant Tissue and Cell Culture**, Liss, New York.

Gupta, P.K., (1997) **Elements of Biotechnology**, Rastogi Publications, Meerut.

Hartman, H.T. and Kester, D.E., (1983) **Principles of Tissue Culture for Micropropagation**, Prentice Hall, New Jersey.

Ingram, D.S. and Hegelson, J.P., (Eds.) (1980) **Tissue Culture Methods for Plant Pathologists**, Blackwell Scientific, U.K.

Murashige, T., (1974) *Plant Propagation Through Tissue Culture,* **Ann. Rev. Plant Physiol.**, 25, 135-166.

Pollard, J.W. and Walker, J.M., (Eds.)(1990) **Methods in Molecular Biology ,Volume 6, Plant Cell and Tissue Culture**, Humara Press, Clifton, New Jersey

Sharp, W.R., Larsen, O.P., Paddock, E.F. and Raghavan, V., (Eds.) (1979) **Plant Cell and Tissue Culture**, Ohio State University Press, Ohio.

Thorpe, T.A., (Ed.) (1978) **Frontiers of Plant Tissue Culture**, IAPTC, Calgray.

Thorpe, T.A., (Ed.) (1981) **Plant Tissue Culture: Methods and Applications in Agriculture**, Academic, London and New York.

White, P.R., (1963) **A Handbook of Plant Tissue Culture,** Jacques Cottel Pennsylvania.

Withers, L.A. and Alderson, P.G., (Eds.) (1986) **Plant Cell Culture and its Agricultural Applications**, Butterworths, UK.

Yeoman, M.M., (Ed.) (1986) **Plant Cell Culture Technology** Blackwell Scientific, Oxford.

Engineered microbes may hold key to powerful vaccines...

Researchers decoding the genes of disease-causing microbes are finding new targets for vaccines against such age-old scourges as malaria, tuberculosis and syphilis, says a noted infectious disease expert in a recent issue of *The Lancet*. Over the past three decades, molecular biologists could successfully decode the genomes of more and more pathogens. Researchers in this field have already determined the complete DNA sequences of the all the genes of eight major disease-causing bacteria, including the bacteria that cause stomach ulcers, lyme disease and syphilis and they will soon decode the genomes of dozens of more pathogens, including the genomes of the bacteria that cause gonorrhea, tuberculosis, malaria, cholera and meningitis.

One area which knowledge of microbial genomes will certainly prove useful is vaccine development. Genetically attenuated vaccines could prove to be ideal for they would so closely resemble the disease-causing organism that they would elicit a strong immune response to the disease-causing versions of the microbe, but because they lack their virulence factors would be unable to cause disease and, thus, would be safer than many current vaccines. Research is now underway to identify the genes. One way to do this is simply to identify a suspect gene in a microbe, perhaps one that resembles a known virulence gene in another organism, and then make a strain of the microbe that lacks that gene. If that "gene knock-out" strain of the microbe cannot cause diseases, then it is likely the missing gene plays an important role in the production of a crucial virulence factor. Researchers can then take copies of that gene and, using genetic engineering techniques, produce large quantities of the virulence factor. It is then possible to analyze the factor to determine what it does and how a vaccine might be made to attack it.

. . . . *The Hindu, 13/11/'97*

CELL, TISSUE AND ORGAN CULTURE

8.1. INTRODUCTION

The term animal cell culture implies for the maintenance and propagation of animal cells in a suitable nutrient media. Currently, various laboratories are interested in the commercial production of a variety of pharmaceutically important macromolecules such as hormones, enzymes, antibodies, interferons, cytokines etc., Besides these categories of products, the animal cell culture technique has been successfully established in a number of scientific fields, particularly in the diagnostic virology, in the analysis of oncogenics, aging research, in the determination of cytostatic substances, in amniocentesis, gene mapping and in cell-cycle related events. The developments have been possible because of the feasibility of *in vitro* cultivation of animal cells their bio-products.

Before going into the details of the biotechnological aspects, it is necessary to know a few terms commonly used herein. The culture produced by the cell or tissue taken from an organism is termed as **primary culture**, and the term '**cell line**' implies to the sequence of culture obtained from the first subcultivation of the primary culture. This differs from cell strain derived from a clone of cells with specific stable properties like having marker chromosomes, marker enzymes, antigens, etc. By culture alteration one can produce **continuous (permanent) cell lines**. This has the potential for an unlimited subcultivation *in vitro*.

In the present state of our knowledge, it is impossible to determine the moment when the transition to continuous cell line has taken place. However, generally it takes at least 70-fold subcultivation (passage) at the intervals of about 3 days. The result of culture alteration is formerly called **transformation**; however, this term should now be used only in those cases in which the alteration can be ascribed unambiguously to foreign genetic materials.

8.2. MEDIA FOR THE CULTURE

All media for animal cell cultures contain at least the following components: a hexose (glucose or galactose), 13 essential amino acids, 7 to 8 vitamins of B-series, choline, inositol and inorganic salts. Such an isotonic nutrient solution can be used for the maintenance of many types of cells however, it cannot will not promote cell proliferation. The minimal media are proposed for use in combination with blood serum i.e., with an addition of 5-20% of a homologous or heterologous serum. Although great efforts are being made to replace these components since they are most variable and expensive additives.

Certain properties of sera (promotion of cell attachment and proliferation, inhibition of proteases) can be imparted by the use of substitutes. In addition to the nutritional requirements, the optimum pH (6.9 to 7.8) should be established and known for each cell line. The use of antibiotics in media is disputed for controlling the accidental contamination of micro-organism. A routine test for mycoplasma must definitely be advised, particularly since convenient methods of detection based on fluorescent dyes, are available.

8.3. CULTIVATION

The fundamental requirement for a successful cultivation is equipment and environment under which animal cell culture proceeds. In general, the working area and the equipment should be sterile. The same method and procedure can be used here also as described in tissue culture technique (chapter 7).

8.3.1. Sources of explant tissue

An explant could be an excised portion of the body of an animal which is generally used for the culture of animal cells in a suitable, chemically defined nutrient medium. The major explant tissues are collected from laboratory animals like rabbit, mice, guinea pig and hamsters. Usually from human endothelial cells hepatocytes, smooth muscle cells, alveolar cells, macrophages, amniotic cells, leukocytes, myocardial cells, etc., the explants are taken and cultured in simulated media.

8.3.2. Collection of explants

Excised tissues/cells from the explant source are immediately transferred to an adequate volume of sterile nutrient medium or a well balanced salt solution. Antibiotics are usually added to the medium to avoid accidental contamination.

The collected explant tissues or cells are cultured in an artificial medium for callus production. The explant culture is best suited for culturing animal cells when explants are available in small number. Each explant is cut into small pieces generally the size of 1-2mm^3 is preferred for the culture, and then the pieces of tissue are transferred to a culture vessel for inducing growth. Generally, three methods namely sandwich, etched 'Xs' and dissociation methods are employed for the culture of explants.

8.3.2.1. Sandwich method

Each piece of explant is aseptically placed in a sterile culture dish. Then a small, fine, thin sterile cover-slip is placed over the explant. The cover-slip prevents the floating of explant segments in the medium during the pouring of the medium into the culture dish. After the addition of sufficient nutrient medium, the culture dish is incubated at 37°C for favoring the growth of the explant segment.

8.3.2.2. Explant culture using Etched 'Xs'

In this method 'X'-shaped etches are made in a sterile culture dish with the help of a sterile scalpel. Then each piece of explant is placed on the 'X' mark and gently pressed. The small raised lines created by etching prevent the floating of explants during the pouring of the media. After the addition of medium the culture dish is incubated at 37°C.

8.3.2.3. Dissociation method

The prepared explant tissue is cut into small pieces. The pieces of explant are then transferred to a trypsinization flask. Fresh media is added into the flask. An enzyme solution containing trypsin, pronase or collagenase is added into the trypsinization flask and continuously agitated using a metabolic shaker, so that the cells dissociate from the explant. The dissociated cells are again filtered through the fine muslin cloth to remove the cell clumps. The suspension of isolated free cells is centrifuged for removing the liquid medium. The concentrated cell suspension thus obtained is inoculated in a fresh medium and incubated at 37°C,

Using above stated methods, viable young daughter cells can be produced within 1-2 days. In general the culture requires 2-3 days for producing new daughter cells. But some cultures require even a week for inducing the callus production. Some important consideration which should be appreciated are as follows:

1. Diploid cells require for their growth a solid substrate with a defined surface charge. For that, commercial 'tissue-culture grade' flasks and dishes are available with a coating of poly-D-lysine. The coating with poly-D-lysine helps cultivating cells at reduced levels of serum proteins.
2. Cultivation temperature should be maintained at 37°C. Since, most of the cell lines are processed from warm-blooded animals. This can be performed by using incubators with an adjustable supply of carbon dioxide and oxygen which are necessary for a controlled progression of cell metabolism.
3. Nutrient media which are used for this purpose should be sterile. Autoclaving in general should be avoided, since most of the components are thermolabile. High pressure membrane filtration(0.2μ; φ) is advisable for the same.
4. Cryopreservation of animal tissues and cells can usually be attained satisfactorily by controlling the critical temperature interval between +20 and -70°C. For long-term preservation, temperatures below -70°C are

required, and for this purpose Dewar vessels with liquid nitrogen or more sophisticated 'liquid nitrogen refrigerators' are required. The cryoprotective reagent, 10% glycerol is the preferred additive except for cells which are permeated too slowly and may require a cytotoxic agent like 7.5% dimethyl sulfoxide. An alternative for the cryoprotection of critical lymphoid cells can be an addition of 10% polyethylene glycol (PEG 20,000).

8.3.2.4. Plasma clot method

The method in principle remains to be the same as discussed earlier in the chapter. 15 drops of plasma and 5 drops of embryo extract are mixed in a watch glass. The watch glass is placed over a pad of cotton wool contained in a petri dish. The cotton wool is kept moist to prevent evaporation in the dish. A carefully dissected piece of tissue on the top of plasma clot is placed. In an alternative a raft of lens paper or rayon net is used to place the tissue. The movability of the raft allows for easy transfer of tissue, feeding of culture and replacement of media (Fig. 8.1).

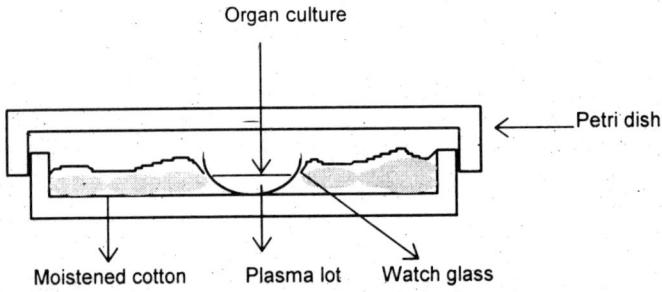

Fig. 8.1 : The classical organ culture technique

8.4. THE SETTING UP OF A CELL CULTURE

For establishing a primary culture, the source of the cell lines is required with markers, the number of passages, the feeding conditions, the survival rate, the growth rate, the plating efficiency, morphology, density of a monolayer, and sterility. The methods, which are used for setting up a culture generally based on a combination of the following:

- mechanical comminution of a tissue;
- chemical breakdown by chelating agents such as EDTA; and
- treatment with enzymes.

The most common enzyme used for this purpose is a crude trypsin preparation with chymotrypsin trace activities elastase, DNase, etc. Enzymes such as collagenase, pronase, and hyaluronidase have not found the same broad use still they are important in combination with trypsin.

After such pretreatments, the cover-slip method can be used for fibroblasts in order to supply a fragment of tissue between microscope slides with plasma or medium. On incubation, an exuberant growth of cells takes place. The grown cells can be removed from the glass support and transferred into a monolayer culture.

Organs with small proportions of connective tissue (liver, kidneys) can be perfused with an enzyme-EDTA mixture and subsequently be broken down immediately after they have been dissected out or even *in situ*. After mechanical dissection, pieces of tissues or individual cells can then be transferred to culture bottles. Even embryonic and cancer-like tissues are susceptible to mild processes, since they contain a weak matrix. For other differentiated tissues, more intensive methods are necessary in order to degrade intercellular materials (fiber proteins, mucopolysaccharides).

Treatments with oncogenic chemicals, transformation by viruses, or the fusion of the primary cells with cancer cells are suitable process options for the deliberate conversion of diploid primary cells into continuous cells.

8.4.1. Cultured cells and cell lines

The cultured cells are classified mainly as:

1. Precursor or stem cells or master cells are capable of proliferation, however they need stimulant or inducing conditions till then they remain undifferentiated. On stimulation under appropriate conditions some or all of the cells mature up to differentiate. These cells are referred to as **totipotent** or **pluripotent**. The stem cells exhibit varied levels of stemness, e.g., totipotent stem cells can generate cells capable of entire blood cellular components production including immune system. They can be differentiated from pluripotent cells which are less general, however can be differentiated into several types;

2. The second category referred to as committed precursor cells; and

3. Differentiated matured cells.

The cell culture therefore may be perceived as a mass of culturing cells under the state of equilibrium between the multipotent stem cells, undifferentiated but committed precursors and mature differentiated cells. The equilibrium as such could shift depending upon the environmental conditions as under high serum concentration in medium and growth factors, a low density cell mass will promote proliferation of the cells while under low serum concentration in the presence of appropriate hormone a high density cell mass may promote differentiation. Further, the cell types in a particular culture is determined by the source of culture. The concept can be clarified with the help of following example;

1. Cell lines of embryo origin, may contain relatively more stem cells (precursor cells) capable of cell renewal.

2. Similarly, the cultures from tissues undergoing continuous renewal *in-vivo* i.e., intestinal epithelial, epidermis, haemopoietic, vaginal endometrium possess stem cells despite they are derived from adults.

3. Some of the tissues renew under stress conditions include fibroblasts, muscles and glia. These cells contain basically committed precursors which have very short (limited) culture life span. Using any one of these cells derived from primary explant it is possible to develop respective cell lines after first subculture, the primary culture becomes cell line in itself which can be propagated and sequentially subcultured several times. It is interesting to note that every successive cell culture process provides proliferating population component predominantly and at the same time it may be observed that non-proliferating slowly growing cells get diluted out.

The cell lines may be propagated for a limited number of generation beyond which they may die off or give rise to a continuous cell lines. The latter are aneuploids with larger amount of variation in chromosome number while the finite cell lines are often euploid with a little variation particularly in the number of chromosomes. The process by which a culture transforms and gives rise to a continuous cell line is termed as *in vitro* transformation. This transformation may at large be induced by viruses or some chemical reactions. Furthermore, this term (transformation) is implied for continuous cell line due to the reason that the culture undergoes not only morphological and kinetic alterations but the cell lines are more frequently accompanied with an increased tumorogenicity. They exhibit malignant transforming properties reflected in their characteristics as asking for a reduced serum requirements, reduced density with limitation of growth or aneuploid.

8.4.2. Maintanance of culture cell lines

During the process of culturing owing to differentiation and proliferation the medium is largely consumed and the substrate is occupied by growing cells and entails for subculturing. Obviously, the heterogeneous primary cultures containing various types of cells, generate homogenous cell lines on subculturing. This culture is referred to as cell lines which can be propagated, characterized, preserved and stored. The term cell line defines the presence of several cell lineages which may be similar or distinct. A particular cell lineage may have specific properties which are well identified and distinctive in bulk of the cells. This cell lineage is referred to as **cell strain**. The cell strain or line may be finite or continuous depending upon whether the life span is limited or immortal in culture. Finite cell lines may extinct following 20-80 population propagation.

8.4.2.1. Maintenanace of adherent cell lines

Most of the primary cultures are continuous cell lines grow in the form of monolayers requiring continual however periodic change of medium irrespective of the situation whether cells are proliferating or not. The adherent cell line subculturing involves:

1. removal of medium;
2. dissociation and segregation of cells in the monolayer using tyrosine or other enzymes.

Highly proliferative cell lines HeLa are subcultured once per week likewise media is replaced four days later. In the case of slowly growing cells, they are subcultured every 2,3, or 4 weeks while medium is changed weekly between subcultures. The factors and steps involved in the maintenance of cell lines are presented in figure 8.2.

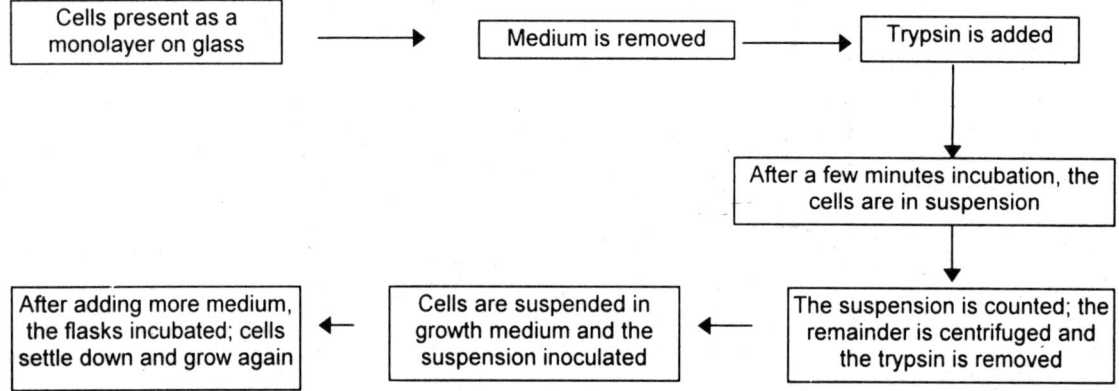

Fig. 8.2 : Maintenance of a cell line

8.4.3. Cloning of cell lines

From a heterogeneous culture pure cell lines can be produced employing cloning technique. However, cloning seems to be successful in the isolation of variants in continuous cell lines because most of the cultures have a finite life span. The mutants or variants may typically be biochemical mutants and strains with marker chromosomes. A method based on dilution cloning has been proposed by Sanford followed Puck and Marcus (1955). In this method trypsinized individual cells are seeded at low density concentration level in multi-well dishes or in petri dishes or plastic bottles. The seeded cells are incubated until colonies are formed. The colonies are isolated and propagated independently as a well identified clone of cells.

8.4.4. Cell-culture system

A variety of cells can be cultured by using any one of the above methods. For example, bone marrow cells and leukocytes cells are directly collected from patient or animal, and could directly be inoculated to a culture medium. Variety of cell cultures and cell lines are used in immunological research include primary lymphoid cells, cloned lymphoid cell lines, and hybrid cells.

8.4.4.1. Primary lymphoid cell cultures

Many *in vitro* culture techniques are available for the culturing of lymphocytes. Primary culture of lymphoid cells can be obtained by isolating the lymphocytes directly from lymph or blood or from various lymphoid organs by tissue dispersion. The isolated cells are grown in a chemically defined nutrient medium consisting of sodium chloride, carbohydrates, proteins, vitamins, trace elements and other nutrients to which various serum supplements are also added. In some cultures, serum-free media are employed. This is because, the *in-vitro* culture techniques require 10-100 folds specific cells than *in vivo*, so that, the immunologists can assess the functional properties of minor subpopulations of lymphocytes. For example, functional differences between CD4$^+$ T helper cells and CD4$^+$ T cytotoxic cells could be studied precisely with the help of cell culture techniques. These techniques have also been used as diagnostic tool for identifying various cytokines involved in the activation, growth and differentiation of various cells of the immune system.

8.4.4.2. Cloned lymphoid cell lines

Tumor cells or normal cells mutated with chemical carcinogens or viruses, are multiplied indefinitely in the suitable nutrient cultures. Because of growing nature, the multiplication of the specific defined cells is very fast unlike normal mammalian cell growth, these highly proliferating cells are referred to as **cell lines**.

The first cell line-the mouse fibroblast L cells was cultured in the 1940s for mouse connective tissue, mutated chemically by exposing to methylcholanthrene over a period of 120 days. Similarly, cell-lines can be obtained directly from culturing infected cells like HeLa cells derived by cultured human cervical cancer cells.

Various techniques are available for ensuring whether a cell line is derived from a single parent cell or not. Such a cloned cell line possesses a population of genetically identical cells that can be grown indefinitely in suitable culture (Table 8.1). In other cases the cell line can be obtained by transformation of normal lymphoid cells by viruses such as Abelson's murine leukemia virus (A-MLV), Simian virus-40 (SV-40), Epstein-Barr virus (EBV) and human T-cell leukemia virus (HTLV-1).

Table 8.1 : Cell line commonly used in immunological research

Cell line	Description
L-929	Mouse fibroblast cell line; often used in DNA transfection studies and to assay tumor necrosis factor (TNF)
SP2/0	Non-secreting mouse myeloma; often used as a fusion partner for hybridoma secretion
P3X63-Ag8.653	Non-secreting mouse myeloma; often used as a fusion partner for hybridoma secretion
MPC 11	Mouse IgG2a-secreting myeloma
P3X63Ag8	Mouse IgG1-secreting myeloma
MOPC 315	Mouse IgA-secreting myeloma
J558	Mouse IgA-secreting myeloma
ABE-8.1/2	Mouse pre-B cell lymphoma
7OZ/3	Mouse pre-B lymphoma; used to study early events in B-cell differentiation
BCL 1	Mouse B-cell lymphoma that expresses membrane IgM and IgD and can be activated with mitogen to secrete IgM
LBRM-33	Mouse T-cell lymphoma that secretes high levels of IL-2 after mitogen activation
CTLL-2	Mouse T-cell lymphoma that secretes high levels of IL-2 after mitogen activation
C6VL	Mouse thymoma expressing CD3 and CD4
Pu 5-1.8	Mouse monocyte-macrophage line
P338 D1	Mouse monocyte-macrophage line that secretes high levels of IL-1
WEHI 265.1	Mouse monocyte line
P815	Mouse mastocytoma cells; often used as target to assess killing by cytotoxic T lymphocytes (CTLs)
YAC-1	Mouse lymphoma cells; often used as target for NK cells
COS-1	African green monkey kidney cells transformed by SV 40; often used in DNA transfection studies

8.4.4.3. Hybrid lymphoid cell lines

Hybridoma cells are obtained by somatic-cell hybridization. For more details reader may refer chapter 13. In brief, during the hybridization, due to fusion of normal B or T lymphocytes with tumor cells in presence of polyethylene glycol after random loss of some chromosomes a hybridoma is formed, consisting of single nucleus with mixed chromosomes from each of the fused parent cells (Fig. 8.3).

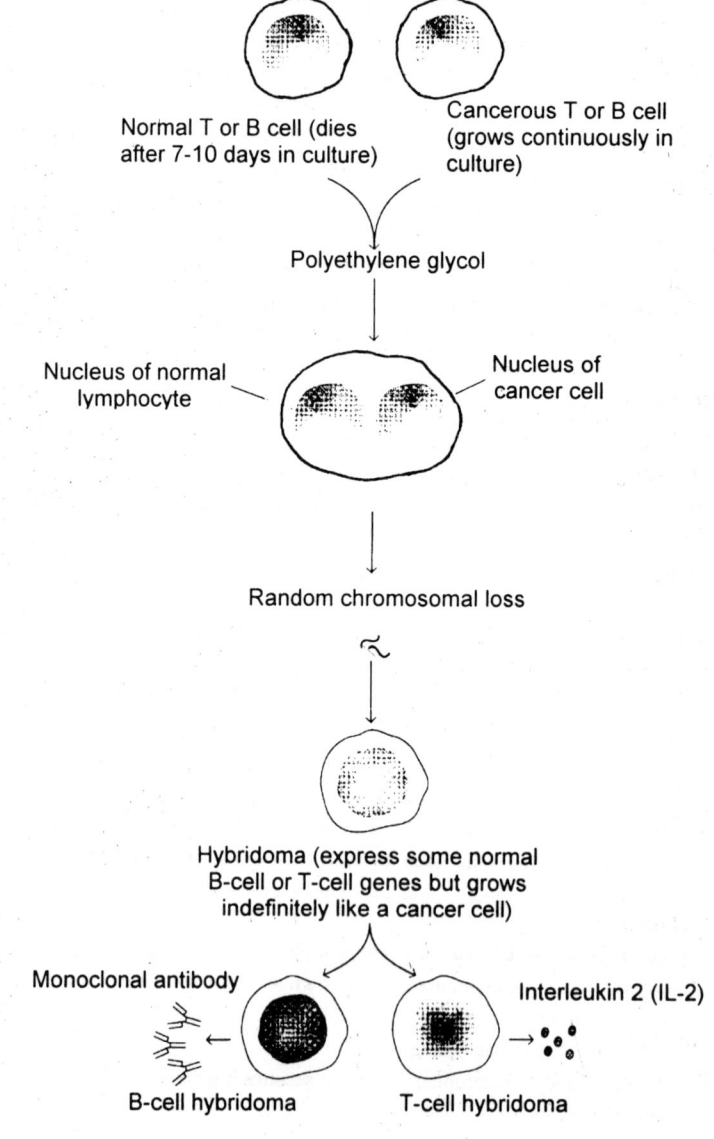

Fig 8.3 : Somatic cell hybridization

The formed hybridoma cells are competent to express the antibody genes of the normal B or T lymphocytes with rapid growth characteristics. These hybridoma cells are cultured in defined nutrient media to propagate the antibody secretion with a single antigenic specificity called monoclonal antibody as it is derived from a single clone.

8.4.5. Whole embryo culture

The whole embryo culture technique is well exemplified and represented by the work on embryonic development by Spratt (1956,57). A 40 hours old embryo was used. The technique involved preparation of well defined suitable medium. One ml aliquots of medium were added to sterile watch glasses placed on moist cotton wool pads in pertidishes, incubated hence at 38°C for 40-45 hours to provide a dozen embryos. Alcohol wiped egg cells were broken in a sterile evaporating dish containing chick saline nearly 50 ml. A circular cut was made with the help of scissors into the allantoin membrane around the blastoderm. The blastoderm was transferred to a petri dish containing BSS. The adherent allontoin with the help of a forcep and embryo was microscopically observed for any damage. The blastoderm was then transferred over the top of the medium in the watch glass after spreading on agar gels. Excess of BSS was removed and culture was incubated at 37.5°C.

8.4.5.1. Culture of mammalian embryo or ova

Two to eight celled fertilized ova have been cultured. The embryos were observed to develop up to blastocytes. So developed blastocytes or embryo can be re-implanted to give rise to healthy animals. The media used for mammalian embryo culturing varied from 100% serum to simple Kreb's ringer solution supplemented with 1% of white egg yolk or bovine albumin. The embryo can be cultured in pre-implantation state or at the post implant stage, however, in the post implantation stage a special care is needed in the removal of embryo in an undamaged form.

8.4.5.2. Flask culture methods

The flask culture technique is mainly used to establish and maintain a strain of fresh explant tissue. The flasks possess excellent optical properties or microscopic examination. In place of glass based flasks, polystyrene based flasks can equally be suited provided they have a wide neck for convenient handling of explants. The method is critically endowed with following advantages:

1. Tissue can be maintained for months or even for years in the same flask.
2. A scale up or handling of large amount of culture and tissue is possible.

The culture flask techniques are mainly of two types: thick clot cultures and thin clot cultures. The technique essentially involves 3 steps, i.e. preparation of flask cultures, renewal of medium and transfer of culture.

8.4.5.2.1. Preparation of flask cultures

Up to 6 carrel flasks (d-3.5) are placed in a rack after flaming their necks and pointing to the right, a drop of the plasma is placed on the floor of the flask and carefully spread in the form of a circle, with the help of a spatula desired number of explants are transferred to the flask to the plasma and clotting is allowed, after plasma clots and explants get fixed up in position, extra medium is added for thick clots measuring up to 1.2 ml of diluted plasma and for thin clots 1.2 ml of diluted serum in place of plasma. The flasks are gassed.

8.4.5.2.2. Renewal of medium

The renewal of medium may be undertaken periodically where old fluid is drawn off with the help of a pipette while 1.2 ml of fluid medium is added as a replacement, followed by supply of gas.

8.4.5.2.3. Transfer of culture

The culture grown in a flask needs to be removed, cut into pieces when it is to be transferred where the pieces serve for re-plantation as usual.

8.4.5.3. Test-tube culture

Test tubes can conveniently be used for the purpose of tissue culture where large number of cultures could be prepared. The tubes can be placed on a stationary rack or roller drums. The tissue culture technique suffers from poor optical properties for microscopy, high risk of contamination. The method however, remains to be the same as discussed for flasks. But tissues may be grown on the test tube without growing over plasma clots. The feeding, patching renewal of medium, transfer of culture and other steps are followed as they are used in case of other primary explanation techniques.

8.4.6. Organ cultures

Organ culture technique employed culturing of organ piece in vitro with an objective of viability. It is essential that tissue chosen should be undamaged. This necessitates careful handling hence method is much more sensitive and sophisticated than tissue culture. The basic media used are more or less the same as they are used for tissue culture.

8.4.6.1. Organ culture on agar

Solidified agar is used for organ culture. The agar media typically consist of 7 parts of 1% agar solution, 3 parts of chick embryo extract and 3 parts of horse serum. Media with or without serum may also be used. This method has advantage that support does liquefy thus requiring for no additional support. The embryonic organs are found to grow well on these media.

8.4.6.2. Culture of embryonic organs

The culture of embryonic organs is easier as compared to the culture from adult. Embryo organs can be cultured using plasma clots, agar substrates or fluid media methods.

8.5. REQUIREMENTS OF LARGE SCALE CULTURE AND PRODUCTION

8.5.1. Basic techniques for deep culture

The preferred technique of treating mammalian cells *in-vitro* is the deep culture, in which the cells are kept in surroundings of liquid nutrient medium. Other techniques such as cultivation on soft agar, etc., play a minor role in systems which are used for large scale production. A critical evaluation shows that only a few basic functions are realized in all of these constructions. The sequential operation is schematically presented in figure 8.4.

For a continuous spectrum of cell types, which are at their extremes either strictly anchorage dependent or prefer developing in free suspension, a broad assortment of matrices is available, whereby the matrix itself may serve several functions such as a growth supporting anchor, as well as an immobilizing vehicle, a protective macromolecule or as a multifunctional accessory. In the static culture, i.e. the Roux bottle type, the material communication between cells and throughout the liquid bulk is limited to diffusional driving forces. A homogeneous supply of nutrients to the cells is limited and will only be possible in small bioreactors with low cell densities. Both, either gently moving the cell supporting matrix (e.g. roller bottle type film reactor) or the liquid bulk respectively (e.g. perfused cell bed reactor) lead to improved mass transfer between the immobilized cells and the liquid bulk surrounding the cells. The diffusional transfer of masses between the different phases (cell phase, liquid phase, gas phase) is thereby dependent on more or less short distances across stagnant film at interfaces. According to mass transfer models, an increase of the velocity gradients between the different phases will reduce the thickness of stagnant liquid interface films and as a result decreases the distance for the diffusion of masses.

The highest interfacial mass transport can be achieved in systems in which both the cells, (or the cell carriers) and the liquid bulk are moved (or mixed). Fluidized beds and purely submerged cell cultures maximize the interfacial mass transfer due to the highest possible interfacial area created and high velocity gradients between the phases. The velocity gradients between the phases can only be intensified to a certain maximum beyond which the resulting shear forces become particularly evident under submerged culture conditions; hence the protective cloud of macromolecular substances coming from serum or other macromolecular additives seems to be an essential requisite for maintaining the activity relating to their functions.

8.5.2. Biological requirements

8.5.2.1. Cell specific productivity

The term implies, for the number of cells which are required to produce a unit amount of crude cell culture product in a batch. The typical illustration is shown in figure 8.5 for the efficiency of mammalian cells in product formation.

CELL TYPE	MATRIX FOR GROWTH IMMOBILIZATION OR PROTECTION	DEEP CULTURE TECHNIQUE
ANCHORAGE DEPENDENT	SOLID SURFACE TRAYS DISCS PLATES TUBES ETC.	STATIC — MATRIX (FILM REACTOR)
	SOFT MATRIALS LAYERS BEADS MEMBRANES FIBRES GELS	MOVED — LIQUID (PERFUSED PACKED BEDS)
	POLYMER BEADS MICROCARRIER MICROCAPSULES	MATRIX & LIQUID (FLUIDIZED BEDS)
FREE SUSPENSION	MACROMOLES	SUBMERGED

Fig. 8.4 : Techniques used for deep culture of animal cell

8.5.2.2. Surface area for growth and immobilization of cells

Most animal cells even hybridomas, which are often considered to belong to the suspension cell type and which can be propagated for large scale cultivation units such as the airlift reactor and in stirred tank reactors, tend to give increased specific production titers when they are treated like anchorage dependent cells. Most of the anchorage dependent cell types require much higher specific growth supporting surface areas, however they are less sensitive to a change in velocity gradients.

8.5.2.3. Cultivation method and physiological patterns

In general, cell culture behaviour is often different with the cultivation method, as it could be a closed (batch) culture or an open cultivation system such as the chemostat or perfusion culture system. A generalized scheme of physiological patterns of cell cultures in response to the method of cultivation is presented in figure 8.6.

The batch culture yields the lowest cell density(C) in a given growth medium and the cell specific productivity of product formation(Qp) tends to be variable during the course of the batch culture. Both, cell densities and productivity, are affected by varying concentrations of nutrients, depletion of essential substances due to consumption, inactivation, accumulation of metabolites, etc.

By simply changing the cultivation method from closed to open and in a chemostat the cell densities achieved with a medium increase up to several folds and the cell specific product formation rates become more stable. With respect to those physiological patterns the chemostat is therefore most often used for the mass propagation of cells whereas the continuous perfusion of immobilized cells has become the preferred and an acceptable method for product formation.

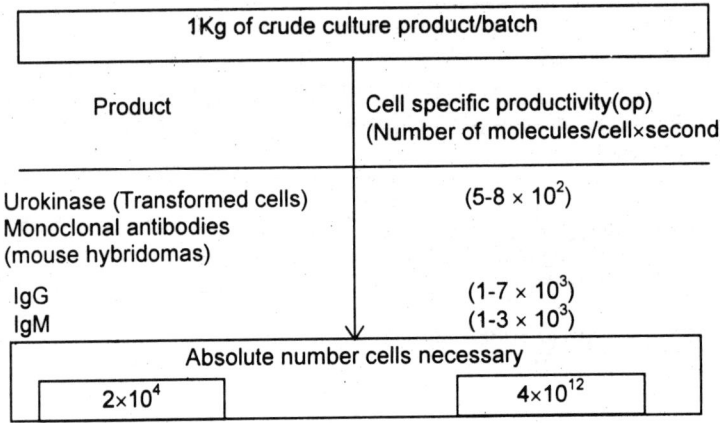

Fig.8.5 : Schematic representation of mammalian cells efficiency

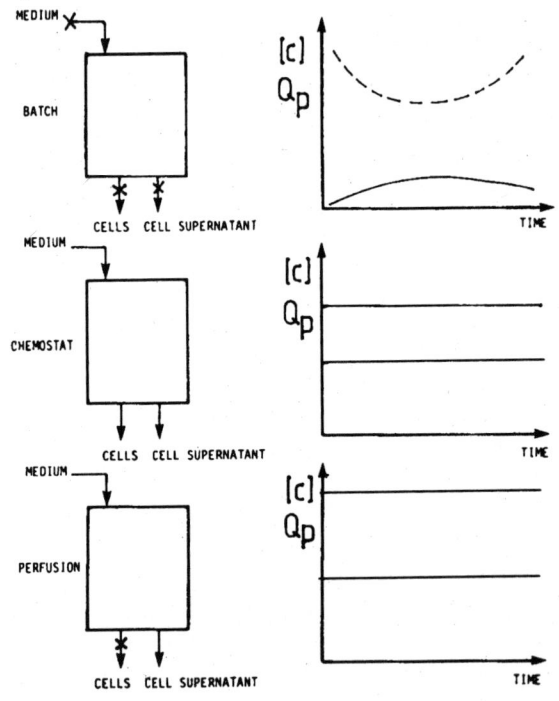

Fig. 8.6 : Cultivation methods and physiological patterns

8.5.2.4. Specific oxygen demand

Another point of interest is the oxygen demand of cells *in vitro*. Superficially a consideration of this factor seems negligible as shown in figure 8.7, animal cells generally exhibit low oxygen demand rates between 0, 15 µM per 106 stationary phase cells in 1 hour for propagating cells and around 0.03 micro Moles per 106 cells in stationary phase in 1 hour. Figure shows the oxygen requirements as calculated for a high cell density immobilized cell reactor for propagating cells and stationary phase cells respectively.

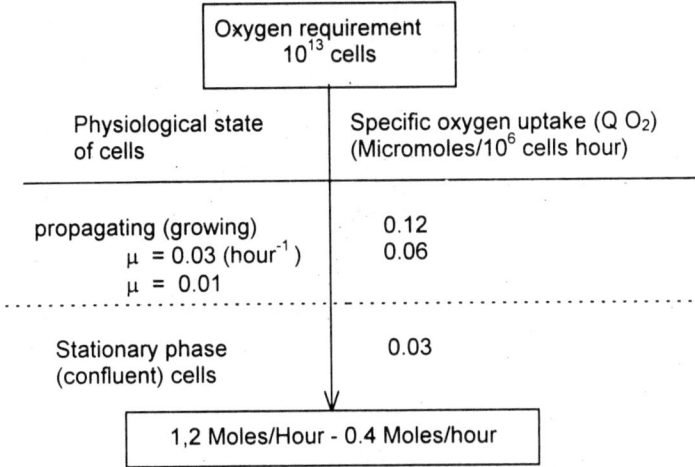

Fig. 8.7 : Oxygen requirement for propagating and stationary phase cells

8.5.3. Animal cell reactor : (Bioreactor / Fermenter)

Generally, bioreactors are large sized vessels that provide a controlled environment for the mass culture of process organisms. Most of the fermentation reactions are carried out in bioreactors.(*see chapter 5*). Designing consideration of the ideal reactor for the animal cell culture should be based on the basic requirements of large scale culture and production, for details about reactors designing readers may refer chapter 5.

For animal cell culture, the bioreactors should have good gas/liquid mass transfer provision, which is essential for oxygen supply and also for the control of pH. Three alternative methods for mass transfer have been suggested are:

1. Diffusional transfer across gas/ liquid interface;

2. Permeation through gas permeable membrane; and

3. Sparging of gas as bubbles.

8.5.3.1. Design

In one approach the reactor functions have been divided into a cell growth and cell immobilization unit, in which the supply of cells with all nutrients is achieved by diffusional transport whereas the physically supported mass transfer of the cell is performed in a distinct and separate device (Fig. 8.8).

Precautions

• More frequent recycling of media is required to alleviate problems due to higher growth capacity of the cell containment.

• Spatial concentration gradients build up in cell containment, results into certain degree of non-homogeneity in oxygen tension and pH. The degree of non-homogeneity depends on parameters such as the metabolic activity (e.g., cell density), the flow rate through the reactor and the distance between the inlet and the outlet in growth containment.

Conventional unit processes (Fig. 8.9) are coupling biological demand and physical supply of masses in close vicinity (Rushton type bioreactors). This results, into a high degree of homogeneity particularly in systems in which direct sparging of gas is possible or where gas permeation through membranes is applied. The air lift reactor is more simple and transparent in scaling up. The larger the scale the better its performance. Moreover compact geometric configurations are preferred.

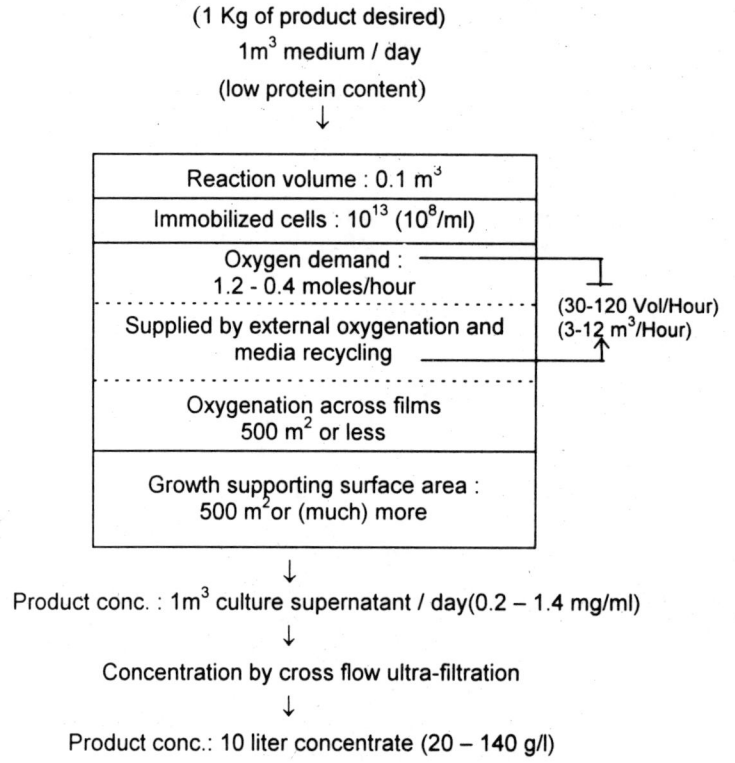

(1 Kg of product desired)
$1m^3$ medium / day
(low protein content)
↓

Reaction volume : $0.1 \ m^3$
Immobilized cells : 10^{13} (10^8/ml)
Oxygen demand : 1.2 - 0.4 moles/hour
Supplied by external oxygenation and media recycling
Oxygenation across films 500 m^2 or less
Growth supporting surface area : 500 m^2 or (much) more

(30-120 Vol/Hour)
($3-12 \ m^3$/Hour)

↓
Product conc. : $1m^3$ culture supernatant / day(0.2 – 1.4 mg/ml)
↓
Concentration by cross flow ultra-filtration
↓
Product conc.: 10 liter concentrate (20 – 140 g/l)

Fig. 8.8 : Idealized and optimized production unit for animal cell products

8.5.4. Biological film reactor (mammalian reactor)

The design of the fermenter is like roller bottle with slight modification which are fabricated according to fulfill the following principles.

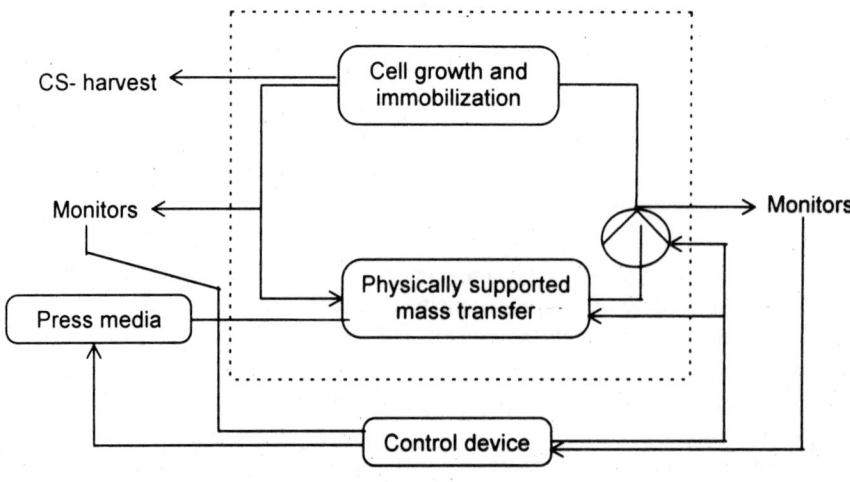

Fig. 8.9 : Unit process

- Peristaltic transportation of bulk masses,
- Diffusional mass transfer,

- Lamellar folded membranes creating distinct compartments,
- Having modified surface etc.

8.6.4.1. Cultivation

A cylindrical vessel is filled with a pack of lamellar disc shaped matrix. Roughly 20% of the reactor is filled with the liquid in films. The head space is gassed with the desired mixture of gases. During rolling a continuously renewed and aerated liquid film is built up. Several inlet and outlet sites for feeding and withdrawal of the liquid medium make any method of continuous cultivation possible. The ratio of liquid film surface area to liquid bulk volume is generally kept in a constant proportion and this enables a perfect control over film based mass transfer.

For the cultivation of anchorage dependent cells the packed lamella matrix surfaces serve as both the cell carriers and liquid film carriers (Fig. 8.10). Chemical modification of the matrix surfaces opens up unlimited uses of the reactor for any desired cell type.

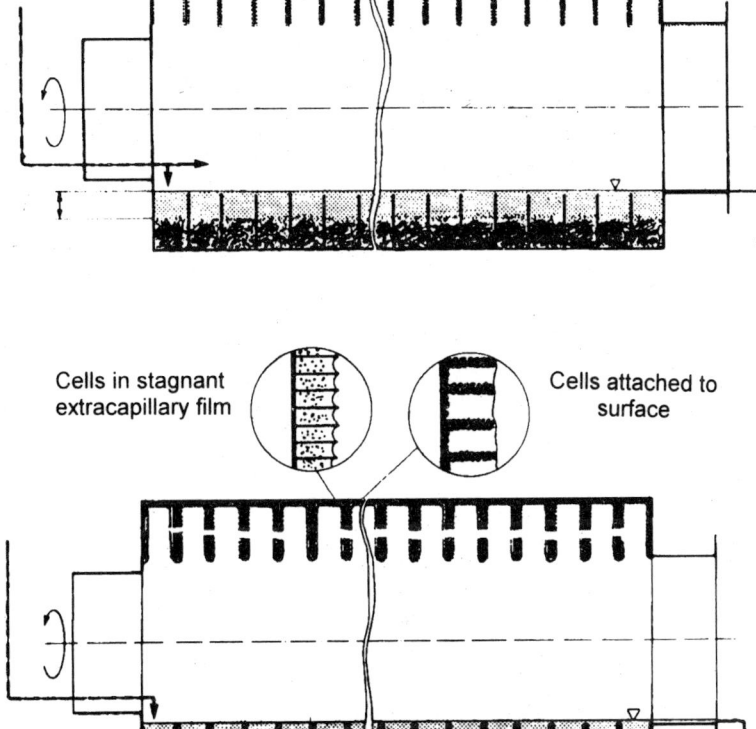

Fig. 8.10 : Above -- Principle of tubular liquid film reactor (cells retained by sedimentation)

Below – Principle of tubular biological film reactor (cells anchored)

The beard like physical surface modification shown in figure 8.11 may demonstrate that x-fold increase of the cells carrying surfaces can be achieved. Similar effects are possible when fleece like surface modification are considered. By means of these modifications it is possible to shift the proportion of gas/liquid film interface area necessary for oxygenation across the films on the one hand, and the cell carrier surface area on the other.

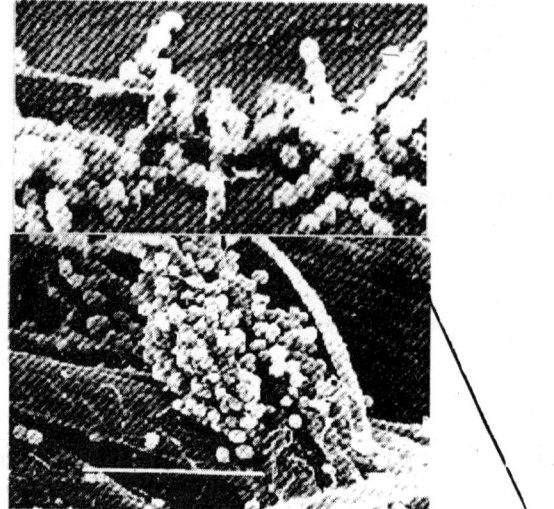

Fig. 8.11 : A live murine hybridoma adhering to fibrous polyester surface

8.6. SINGLE-CELL PROTEIN

The mass production of bioprotein from the single-cell organism like bacteria or fungi termed as microbial biomass or single cell protein (SCP). In technical fermentation process, in addition to the final desired product of natural substances e.g., penicillin, vitamins, the multiplication and growth of culture of microbes itself also takes place. These microbial cell masses or microbial biomasses, form a class of useful products (Fig.8.12). So that biomass production with the substantial exclusion of accompanying processes has been the subject of new development, the production of single-cell protein or microbial biomass.

Germans are the pioneer in the production of single-cell proteins. During the first world war Germans faced the problems related to food demand at the time, the group of scientists led by Delbruck first established the culture of *Saccharomyces cerevisiae* for the production of SCP. The biomasses were utilized in the forms of soups and sausages. The group of same Germans could develop the culture of *Candida aroborea* and *C. utilis* during the second world war as an alternative to foods.

In 1982, scientist of Kuwait Institute of Scientific Research, developed the cultures of fungi, Torulospsi and bacteria *Methylomonas clara, Methylophilu methylotrophus* and Alcaligenes for the production of SCP by using carbohydrate source as methanol. A Belgium Botanist J. Leonard harvested the biomass from *Spirulina platensis* in alkaline lakes as a feed stock. In 1982, Tochaix et al. developed the series of culture of green algae such as *Chlorella pyrenoidosa, Scenedemus acutus, Chlamydomonas reinhardii* for the consumption of human beings. In India, research work is in progress at CFTRI (Central Food Technology Research Institute) Mysore, on spirulina and others to develop some single cell proteins as a supplement to food.

The production of microbial biomass is a manufacturing process of the cell mass of microbes from suitable organic raw materials in a fermentation process. Here, selected strains of micro-organisms are multiplied on suitable raw materials in a technical cultivation process directed to the growth of the culture, and the cell mass so obtained is isolated by separation processes. Process development begins with microbial screening, in which suitable production strains are obtained from samples of soil, water, and air or from swabs of inorganic or biological materials (mineral ores, fruit peel) and are subsequently optimized by selection, mutation or other genetic methods. Then the technical conditions of cultivation for the optimized strains are worked out and special metabolic pathways and cell structures are determined (biochemistry, molecular biology). In parallel to these biological investigations, process engineering and apparatus technology contribute to the technical performance of the process and the apparatus in which the production of bioprotein is to be carried out in order to make them ready for use on large technical scale. The need of research to adapt novel technological aspects on the large-scale production of SCP is very much to fulfill the demand of conventional food production.

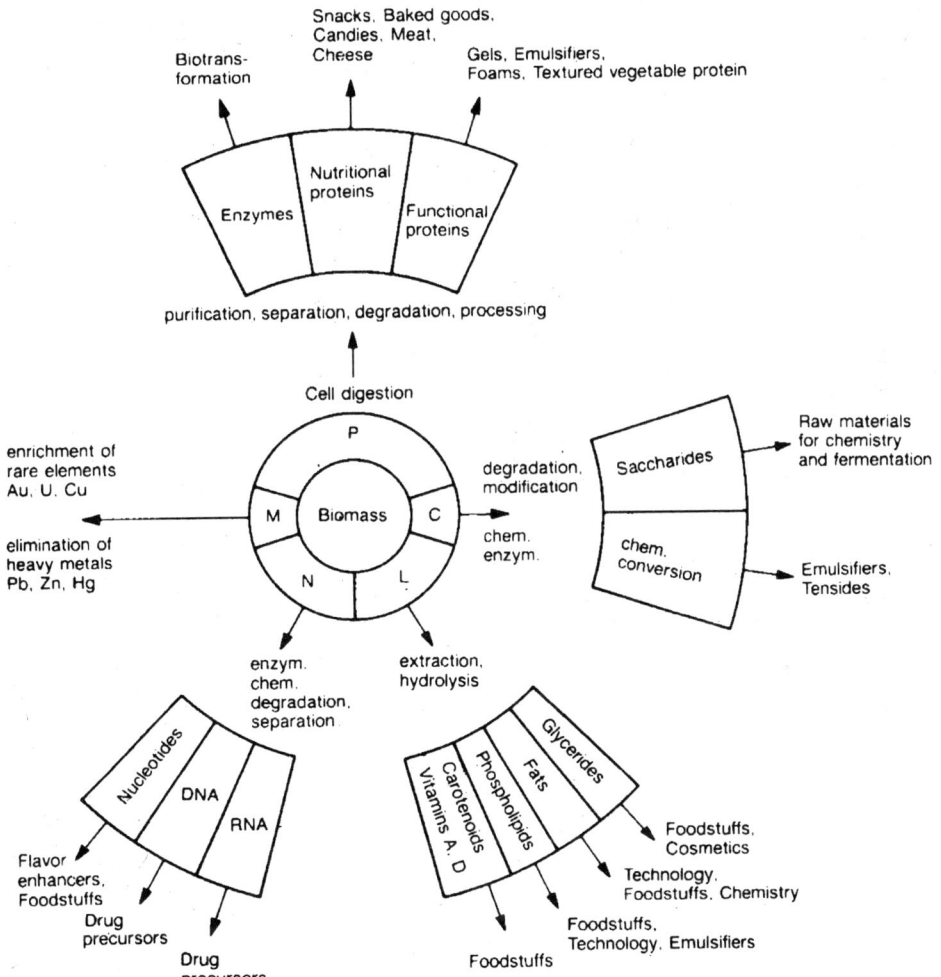

Fig. 8.12 : Various potential uses for components of SCP ;
-P = protein; C = carbohydrates; L = lipids; N = nucleic acids: M = minerals

8.6.1. Strain selection

Best strains of micro-organism are selected on the basis of following requirements .

• It should be genetically stable.
• should be usable in continuous cultivation.
• Provide high substrate yield.
• Less nutrient demand.
• Flexibility in substrate specificity.
• Submerged process in large bioreactor.
• Easy separation of the biomass from the culture.
• High quality and good composition of SCP.

8.6.2. Source of single-cell proteins

Certain microbes which have high protein content (Table.8.2) are considered to be very much beneficial for the production of SCP. Such prepared biomasses can be utilized for the human consumption as protein rich food. Generally, these microbes can grow in an industrial bioreactor with the utilization of common wastes such as sewage, animal excreta, agricultural wastes, petroleum wastes, crude oil waste, paper, textile industry wastes, saw mill wastes, starchy waste from potato industry, beverage industrial wastes and distilleries waste.

Table 8.2 : Source of single-cell protein

Active assimilator	Bacteria / Yeast /Fungi	Feed stock
Carbohydrate	*Endomyces vernalis* *Saccharomyces cerevisiae* *Candida utilis* *Kluyveromyces fragitis* *Aspergillus niger* *Cellulomonas alcaligenes* Thermoactinomyces *Trichoderma harzianum*, viride Gliocladium sp. *Endomycopsis fibuligera* *Debaromyces kloeckeri* *Sperotrichum pulverulentum* Brevibacterium sp. *Candida lipolytica*	Pentose containing raw materials like, waste from wood and processing industry, agricultural waste, n-paraffin.
Ethanol and Acetic acid	*Candida utilis*	Ethanol, microbial waste.
Methanol	**Substrate:** Methane, methanol, acetone **Bacteria** Methylobacter, Methylococcus, Methylomonas, Methylocystis, Methylosinus, Facultative methylotrophs **Substrate:** Methanol, carbohydrates, organic acid. Arthobacter, Bacillus, Pseudomonas, Streptomyces, Vibrio, Hyphomicrobium, Rhodopseudomonas, **Yeast and Fungi** Candida, Pichia, Hansenula, Kloeckera, Trichoderma, Torulopsis.	Waste of fruit products, dead marine animals. Methanol, n-alkane, fuel oil, diesel crude oil.
Methane	*Methylomonas methanoxidans* *Methylococcus capsulatus* Pseudomonas sp.	Agricultural wastes, wood wastes from saw mill, paper industry, alkaline lakes.
Carbon-dioxide	Scenedesmus sp., Chlorella, *Spirulina maxima*, *Rhodopseudomonas gelatinosa*, *Botyococcus braunii*	Alkaline lakes, domestic sewage.

8.6.3. Production of SCP

The production process of SCP usually consists of following operational steps namely,

- Preparation of nutrient media,
- Fermentation,

- Separation and mechanical concentration of SCP
- Drying of the SCP
- Final processing of the SCP

8.6.3.1. Preparation of nutrient media

The process is further divided on the basis of components of media as these based on;
- solid component of the media;
- liquid component of the media;
- gaseous component of the media;

The components of solid media include mineral salts, cellulose, starch and sugars which are comminuted and dissolved or suspended in water at definite concentration levels. Depending on the raw material and the production strain a substantial digestion of cellulose and starch can be brought by the addition of cellulases or amylases and glucoamylases.

Liquid components include, methanol, glucose, ethanol, acetic acid, molasses, syrup, whey, cane sugar juice, normal paraffin, and phosphoric acid, sulfuric acid (if desired). The above desired components are mixed, purified/sterilized (if necessary can be achieved by filtration) and transferred in to a suitable bioreactor.

Finally, gaseous components, like, air, pure oxygen, methane, ammonia, hydrogen, and carbon dioxide are passed through the sterile-filter under pressure. The sterile gas is usually passed through a metered valve into the reactors. In order to provide uniform distribution to the nutrient medium the gaseous media may also be predispersed through blast nozzles.

8.6.3.2. Fermentation

The biotechnologist should play an important role in the selection of fermenter. He should made certain demands on fermenter, so that, the yield of biomass should be maximized with better quality. The demands could be for:

- continuous operation
- sterile operation (in required case)
- rapid and uniform distribution of all the reactants over the whole reaction volume
- consistency in temperature and pH control
- energy saving operation
- high oxygen transfer
- high substrate yield
- realization on the large technical scale.

Technical and construction features of fermenter are discussed in chapter on fermentation and general considerations. The production of SCP on the large technical scale is usually, followed using submerged fermentation technique. All substrates and water as nutrients to the medium are fed continuously in accurately metered volume under high homogenization of the mixture. The temperature and pH of the medium are constantly monitored and controlled. Similarly, other physical parameters and supplies like, oxygen, free substrate concentration, ionic concentration of the medium, pressure at the head of the reactor, state of media filling, are monitored with the help of suitable probes (Fig. 8.13).

The inoculation of culture is an important event of the fermentation process. Considering the large fermenter, the production strains are stock cultured in an small pre-sterilized fermenter filled with required nutrient media with proper aeration. After a short initial growth phase, continuous flow is switched on. Thus, produced biomass (Fig. 8.14) is contained in dilute suspension after the completion of this process step.

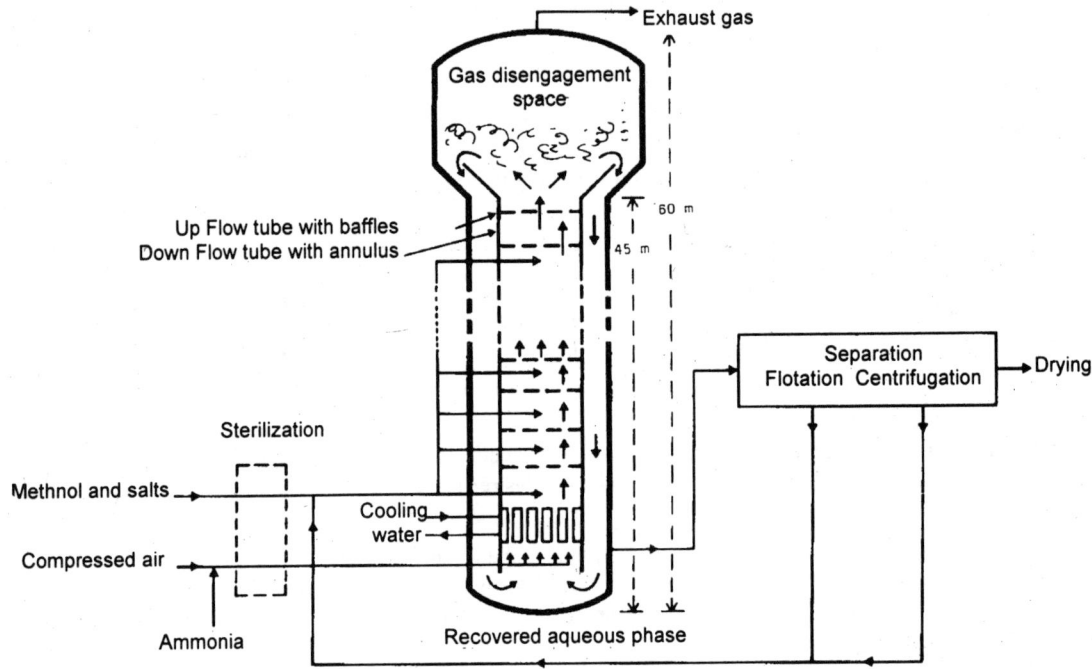

Fig. 8.13 : Pressure cycle airlift fermenter for bacterial SCP from methanol

8.6.3.2. *Processing*

This step includes of separation and concentration of produced SCP, drying operation and final processing of the SCP. Usually, separation of SCP can be performed by either centrifugation or decantation. This is only possible if the product of interest (SCP) is of high solid content e.g., fungal mycelium can be filtered off from yeast cultures. But as in the case of bacterial biomass, separation is carried out by adding ionic or non-ionic flocculant or by changing pH, or by simply heating or by application of an electric field.

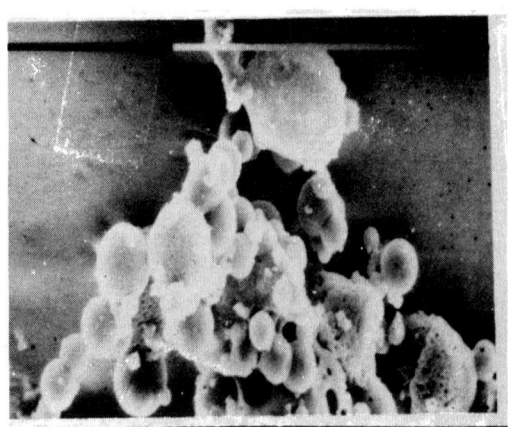

Fig 8.14 : Lyophilized cell mass cultured for SCP

After the flocculation of SCP the medium is concentrated and SCP is separated by decantation followed by centrifugation. The concentrated biomass is sterilized using moist heat sterilization or other suitable sterilization method in order to block the intact pathogenic microbes/ enzymes (thermolysis). The sterilization is only required if the SCP should not have any pathogenic characteristics. Otherwise, crude biomass may be processed and subjected to direct drying step.

8.6.4. Nutritive value of single-cell protein

In general, SCP has more nutritive value than the normal living cells. The composition of an ideal biomass is based on components (Table 8.3) which are carbohydrates, proteins, vitamins, lipids and trace amount of mineral and salts. Besides, these nutritive components SCPs also contain nucleic acid, basically purine bases. Unfortunately, human body systems do not have any excretion pathway for the metabolic product of purine bases, namely uric acid. This may restrict the utility of SCP which contain higher content of purine base nucleic acid (Adenosine and Guanosine). Generally, the bacterial biomass contains relatively higher proportion of purine base nucleic acid as compared to other sources of SCPs.

Table 8.3: Composition of an ideal biomass

Biomass products	Bacteria/ methanol	Yeast/ paraffin	Yeast/ carbohydrates	Fungi/ Carbohydrates	Algae/ carbon dioxide
Crude protein (%)	80	55-60	45 -50	35-45	40-60
Fat (%)	8	9	8	2-5	5-9
Mineral substances (%)	7-8	8	7	5-10	10-15
Nucleic acids (%)	10-15	5-8	5	10	6
Amino acids (g/16 g of nitrogen)					
Alanine	7	6	6	6.5	
Arginine	4.5	3.5	4.5	5	9-10
Aspartic acid	9	8	8	9	
Glutamic acid	10	9	10	2	
Glycine	5.5	3	5	5	
Histidine	2.5	2	3	2	1.8
Isoleucine	4.5	3	4.5	5	5-6
Leucine	7	5.5	6.5	7	8-9
Lysine	6	6.5	6.5	6.5	4-5
Methionine	2.5	2.	1.5	2	2-3
Phenylalanine	3.5	2.5	3.5	4.	4-5
Proline	3.5	2.5	`3.5	4	
Serine	3.5	3	2.5	4	-
Threonine	4.5	3.5	5.5	4	5
Tryptophan	1	0.5	1	1	1
Tyrosine	3	3	3.5	3.5	5
Valine	5	3.5	5	5	6-7

8.6.5. Consumption of SCP

Although, some other SCPs (few species of bacterial biomass) can not be directly consumed by the human beings as food, because of high content of purine base nucleic acid. But, it can be consumed through birds and animals as its eggs and fleshes. Birds and animals have excretion capacity for the uric acid which is the metabolic product of purine based nucleic acid in SCPs (Fig. 8.15).

8.6.6. Advantages of SCP

- The amount of biomass produced by bacterial and algae is enormous. This is because of their short lift-cycle.
- Large amount of proteins are present in these cells of micro-organisms.
- These micro-organism can be easily grown. Their feed stocks include waste products also.

- Large scale culture of these micro-organism also produces some valuable secondary metabolites.
- The quantity and quality of protein produced by these organism can be improved by changing their genetic composition employing genetic engineering methods.

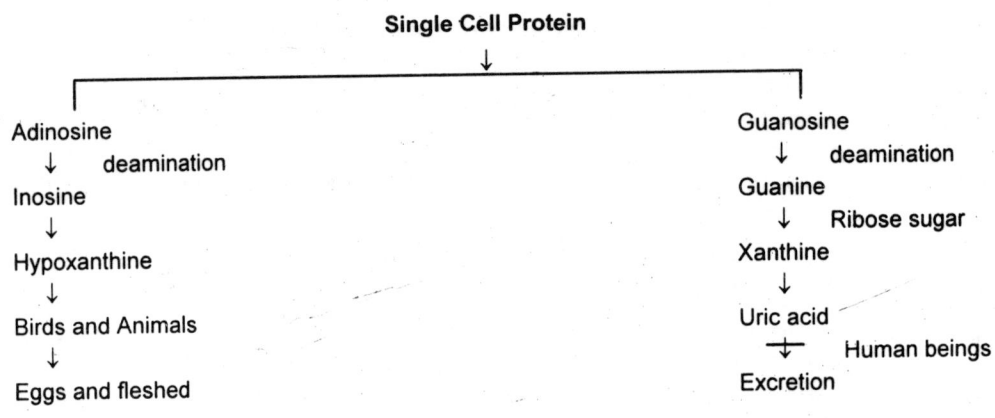

Fig. 8.15 : Utilization of SCPs in human diet.

8.7. PHARMACEUTICAL APPLICATIONS OF ANIMAL CELL CULTURES

The most important commercial utilization of animal cell cultures at the present time is still the multiplication of viruses for the manufacturing of vaccines, which offers considerable technological advantages over conventional production, e.g., in incubated eggs. In addition to this, there is a series of substances which are on the verge of being manufactured on the larger scale using cell culture technique.

Viruses require a living substrate for their multiplication. Previously, duck embryos or organ cultures from animal nerve and kidney tissues were used for the manufacture of virus vaccines. Such explants consist of different types of cells with different demands on the medium and have the identified disadvantage that comprehensive sterility tests must be carried out before they could be used. Furthermore, tissues from the kidneys of wild apes frequently contain simian viruses (SV-5, SV-40) or their constituents. Side reactions are also not infrequent after the administration of such vaccines. The setting up of characterized cell cultures under sterile conditions therefore provides a decisive advantage.

The production of polio vaccines by the replication of the virus on simian kidney cells has been carried out by Meigneir et. al., 1979. After becoming attached to the support, the primary cells are grown for 7 to 8 days with no change of medium, which leads to a ten fold increase in their number. In this phase, sterility tests and chromosome analysis can be carried out on aliquots. Three days after infection by polio virus, the culture becomes ready for the preparation of vaccine by concentration, chromatography method (Sepharose-6B & DEAE-Sephadex) and inactivation (Formaldehyde). Similar processes have been used for the production of rabies vaccine via dog kidney cells. Human diploid fibroblasts have also been successfully grown with cellulose fiber micro carriers using suspension culture techniques. The polio titer yield from this technique has been more than polio titers from cultures of veso or monkey kidney cells.

The production of cell surface antigens at a large scale is performed for several purposes. They are used to raise antibodies against themselves, which may then be used for therapeutic and diagnostic purposes. However, the efforts put into the production of antigens by cell culture techniques have been discouraged by the dramatic advances in recombinant DNA technology, which makes it possible to synthesize them at a large scale. Antilymphocyte serum (ALS) is an immune serum that is used as an alternative for proliferation inhibiting medicaments after organ transplantation in order to suppress the immune defense. Surface antigens from cultivated continuous human lymphoma or leukemia cell lines leading to the synthesis of far more specific antibodies can be used as an alternative to ALS.

Carcinoembryonic antigen (CEA) is a tumor associated glycoprotein used for diagnosis and monitoring of cancer patients. CEA is expressed in significant amounts during embryonic life, especially by the fetal colon. In healthy adults the antigen is expressed in small amounts (< 2.5 ng/ml) in normal colonic mucosa and in serum saliva, feces and colon lavages. CEA can be detected in relatively high concentrations (> 20ng/ml) in the sera of patients with metastatic colonic cancer and in moderate to low levels in the sera of patients with primary lesions of various cancers. Low levels of CEA were also found with various non-malignant inflammatory diseases, particularly those of the liver, lung, pancreas and bowl. In current clinical practice, CEA serum levels are used for monitoring cancer patients for their response to therapy and for an early detection of recurrences.

Many cell types are involved in an immune response. Besides B-cells, the antibody producing cells, and T-cells which are responsible for the cell-mediated immunity, macrophages, T-helper cells and many others are parts of a complex network where they communicate via several dozens of soluble factors (cytokines), particularly lymphokines (lymphocyte-derived) and monokines (macrophage-derived). There are three techniques by which lymphokines can be produced with the help of T-helper cells : Stimulation of lymphocytes from buffy coat or spleen cells by non-specific stimulators such as plant lectin, using certain continuous tumor cell lines, and synthesis by immortalized lymphocytes that have been obtained by hybridoma techniques. An alternative method of producing lymphokines is the construction of monoclonal **T-T hybridoma** which secretes distinct lymphokines. By adapting the hybridoma technology for T cells, one can select T hybridomas which may serve as a constant sources for the production of uniform and well defined lymphokines. Similarly, B cells growth factor is (lymphokines) primarily produced and secreted by activated T-cells. The growth factor stimulates and regulates the proliferation of B cells in culture and can maintain continuous growth of human B-cells. One of the putative uses of this factor might be the establishment of monoclonal B-cell lines which secrete specific antibodies. These antibodies could be used for passive immunization or *in-vivo* immuno-diagnostics. A factor interleukin 2 (formerly 'T-cells growth factor') is attracting great current interest. Its synthesis triggers antigen-specifically *in vivo* but once synthesized it has an antigen-nonspecific proliferative and differentiating action upon cytotoxic T cells (CTL) which, in turn communicate with natural killer (NK) cells via interferon-γ. Since CTL and NK cells are the most important in cellular immunity, interleukin 2 shows great promise as an agent through which the immune response can be regulated by direct application in certain immune deficiency diseases or indirectly by growing antibodies and using them for the intermediate suppression of unwanted responses.

Animal cell cultures are of growing importance for the mass-production of certain proteins. These fall into two classes: monoclonal antibodies obtained from hybridoma cells, which are mainly used for analytical and separation purposes and require only a modest degree of purification, secondly, proteins for therapeutic use., e.g. growth factors, immuno-modulators or hormones produced in recombinant cell-lines. These proteins often have to undergo post-translational modification e.g. correct glycosylation, which cannot be performed in recombinant micro-organisms.

Today, the antiviral action of interferons is well understood and interferon therapy is about to become routine in viral diseases like herpes zoaster and virus encephalitis. The bulk of α-interferon is being obtained by a process from buffy coats (leukocyte pellets) which are available as a waste product from blood banks. The leukocytes can be brought into suspension (107 cells/ml) and induced to secrete interferon with newcastle-disease or sendai virus. Human β-interferon is usually produced by cultivation and induction of human primary fibroblast cells, e.g. FS4 cells but alternatively it can be done with recombinant mammalian cell lines (e.g. mouse L-cells).

The species specificity of many polypeptidal hormones makes it necessary to develop highly productive strains of human origin, of which however, only a few have so far been described. Thus calcitonin secreting cell lines from thyroid tumors ceased their growth after a few months. A cell line 'Be Wo' (ATCC No. CCL 98) from a placental tumor is available which efficiently secretes human chorionic gonadotropin (HCG). It represents the only bulk producing source for a human hormone that has been established *in vitro*. A cell line from kidney carcinoma secreting erythropoietin has not acquired the same importance since the optimum conditions for cultivation are yet to worked out. However, the availability of both human insulin and human growth hormone from recombinant technology has discouraged the corresponding attempts to establish human cell lines for *in vitro* production purposes.

The production of enzymes by using cell culture is not a familiar strategy as compared to other fields. Although, few homologous enzymes can be produced by cell culture techniques. The plasminogen activator namely urokinase from a continuous line of porcine kidney cells (LLC_PK1; ATCC, No. CL 101) has been patented by the Lilly Research Laboratories. An another example for the source is the Bowes melanoma cell line. The enzyme is mainly expressed during cell growth phase rather than from stationary culture cells. The production of enzymes has to be a 2-step operation with initial growth to about 70% confluency in the presence of serum followed by a change in serum-free conditions for the final period of growth after which the enzyme is harvested. To increase the enzyme yield, means of amplifying enzyme expressions, using a serum-free medium so that the enzyme can be continuously harvested have been suggested. The stimulation of stationary phase cells can be improved by the inclusion of number of mitogenic lectins (15-20 fold increase of enzyme yield).

8.7.1. Cell culture models for examining intestinal absorption of peptides

The absorption of peptide across cellular barrier to mainly brought about by two general pathways namely paracellular and transcellular. In most of the cases it is molecular size of peptide that screens up their intestinal, brain or liver absorption through paracellular route. Obviously, the main route for peptide absorption remains to be transcellular which could be of passive or non-passive nature. Cell culture techniques provide for estimation of intestinal absorption of peptides. The passive diffusion has been observed to be low, because major fraction of peptide degrades by enzymatic reactions. These finding were substantiated using caco-2 culture model. A few number of peptides have been observed to undergo low level of non-saturable, bidirection diffusion across the monolayers. Thus, using this particular character, cell culture model could be utilized for examining the physicochemical properties. The significance of hydrogen bonding in passive diffusion across caco-2 cell monolayer has been established. The result indicated that hydrogen bonding has inverse relation to the corresponding permeability across caco-2 monolayers.

Similarly, intestinal absorption of di- and tri-peptides including cephalosporin antibiotics has been found to be facilitated by di-peptide transport/carrier system. The presence of the later has been confirmed by using the enzymatically stable cephalosporin. The absorption of cephalosporin is typically pH-dependent, with a maximum up-take at pH.6. In another set of study, it has been established that uptake of cephalexin in caco-2 monolayers is inhibited, competitively by various types of peptides and similar were the findings in in-vivo. Likewise, using caco-2 cell monolayer carrier system for cepharidin has been discovered, to be γ-GTP, located on the artificial plasma membrane. Active intestinal absorption of peptides by fluid phase or receptor mediated endocytosis is another route for transporting peptides across GI barrier. The use of in-vitro caco-2 cell to assess endocytic transport of drugs is a potential application for which in-vitro culture model suited to be the best. Horseradish peroxide in combination with caco-2 cell culture has been used to elucidate absorption mechanism of proteins following fluid phase endocytosis. The receptor mediated endocytosis of transferrin has been examined using caco-2 cell line and receptor binding in transferrin was found to be polarized to the basal side of the caco-2 cell membrane. These examples, suggest that a near approximation of qualitative and quantitative in nature could be arrived in regard to absorption of protein drugs following oral administration using *in vitro* cell lines techniques.

8.7.2. Cell culture model for examining peptide absorption in the BBB

DSIP peptides are known to cross BBB via passive diffusion pathway and vasopressin, via apical to basolateral route. The cell culture technique allows to study the effect of conformation of structure of proteins on their invasive BBB permeability. In general, it is the hydrophilic nature of peptide that presents major obstacle to passive diffusion across BBB. In an attempt to increase diffusion of peptides through the BBB the functional groups of peptide have been modified to be more lipophilic. The substitution of D-alanine at position 4 of DSIP (Delta sleep inducing peptide) by a glycine residue increases the lipophilicity of the analogue which has higher permeability profile across primary culture bovine BMC. Studies evaluating carrier-mediated transport across cultured BMC are somewhat limited. Moreover, cell culture study, could establish selective carrier system for AVP which is saturable in nature. However, carrier mediated transport of AVP (Arginine, vasopressin) was found to be in the basolateral to apical direction suggesting that it cannot be utilized for successful delivery of peptide to the brain. Similarly, carrier systems for the apical to basolateral transport of both glucose and biotin have been identified using cell culture technique. Such carrier holds promise in peptides transport promotion across the BBB. However, the confirmation of contribution remains to be established. Using cell culture technique it was found that epiratide, a cationic adrenocorticotropic hormone (ACTH) is transported across primary culture bovine BMC through endocytosis pathway. This has led to the development in designing of chimeric peptides consisting of β-endorphin and cationized albumin. The resulting system, shown significantly higher permeability across the BBB suggesting that cationization may be the viable method for the enhancement of peptides and proteins transport across the BBB. Thus, using cell culture strategies towards improvisation of BBB permeability profile of proteins could be studied in-vitro.

8.7.3. Cell culture models for examining hepatic absorption of peptides

Similar to the epithelial intestinal barrier and endothelial BBB, the tight junctions on the sinusoidal and cannicular membrane of hepatocytes limit the passive cellular clearance of peptides. Therefore, passive diffusion of peptides must occur through interactions with the plasma membranes of the hepatocytes. Cell culture study, can be used in determination of cellular engineering employing the technique if a drug molecule accumulated in hepatocytes otherwise, not permeable across the cellular barrier. Peptides smaller in size and lipophilic in nature, undergo passive clearance by hepatocytes, majority of peptides are absorbed through receptor mediated endocytosis. This has been successfully studied and confirmed using cell culture technique. Various cell culture techniques studied, for receptor mediated uptake are presented in table.8.4.

8.7.4. Strategies of foreign gene expression

E.coli has been utilized to harbor for several eukaryotic gene and for the expression of respective proteins. The production is significantly high however, there stands to be an accumulation of proteins in the cell as insoluble inclusion bodies, which have to be dissolved by the application of chaotropic agent such as urea or guanidine-HCl. This inducts for refolding the proteins as per its required structural configuration which is a far difficult task. Most of the proteins which of pharmaceutical interest fortunately soluble and secretory proteins, e.g. growth factors, hormone, serum proteins. Therefore, it is realized that an alternative host *Saccharomyces cerevisiae* could be an appropriate system for the expression of secretory proteins. This system unfortunately was noticed to be plagued by low expression levels and altered pattern glycosylation.

Meanwhile, animal cell culture techniques have occupied center position in the field of biotechnology, allowing the production of biological reactive proteins and cloned gene including genes for expression of interferon hepatitis-B (sAg), tissue type plasminogen activator, herpes simplex glycoprotein (gD). In many cases, tumor cell lines are available which over produce protein of therapeutic values. However, in some other cases gene engineering is of great significance for improvisation of production via introduction of cloned gene into animal cell. The processes of gene expression and animal cells culture essentially involve gene engineering then cloning and transfection of cloned gene in to the cultured cell line with the help of appropriate means followed by its harboring under optimized culture condition for optimum expression of protein of interest. It also involves removal and purification processes in most of the situations as they are used in culture technology that operates at batch level. It is also note worthy that choice of cell line is critical. Let us consider a case of cloned immunoglobulin-G(IgG) for regulation of expression in tissues specific manner. It is the first example of an expression system based on an enhancer sequence. The promoter could be substituted by viral promoter and enhancer, yet other sequence that had an intragenic restricted expression to lymphoid cells may also be used.

So the restriction sequence limits the choice of cell line as in stated case it can only feasibly be conducted in lymphoid cells. Here, availability of such a cellular culture may not be a problem, but other cell line specific problems could crop up a set of problems mainly regarding to their availability, as well as *in-vitro* culture feasibility.

Table 8.4 : Representative receptor and transport systems expressed in the various cell culture models.

Receptor and Transporter	Caco-2	BMEC	Hepatocytes
Amino acid	+	+	+
Angiotensin II		+	+
Asialoglycoprotein			+
Atrial natruiretic factor		+	
Bile acid (taurocholate)	+		+
Biotin	+, -	+	-
Cobalamine (Vit. B12)	+		
Choline		+	
Dipeptide	+		+
Epidermal growth factor	+		+
Ferritin			+
Folate	+		
Glucose (Na-dependent)	+	+	+
Immunoglobulin A			+
Insulin		+	+
Insulin-like growth factor I		+	
Low density lipoprotein	+	+	+
Methyldopa	+		
Monocarboxylic acid		+	
Nucleotide		+	
P-glycoprotein	+	+	+
Peptide YY	-		
Phosphate	+		
Spermidin	-		
Transferrin	+	+	+
Tissue plasminogen activator			+
Vasoactive intestinal peptide (VIP)	+		+
Vasopressin		+	+

Note: BMEC is brain microvessel endothelia cells, either functional or biochemical, of the various receptor and transport system listed. (+) indicates studies showing expression and (-) indicate studies that were unable to show expression.

8.7.5. Eukaryotic and prokaryotic cultures and secondary metabolites

Biotransformations can be defined as chemical transformations which are catalyzed by microorganisms or their enzymes. Enzymatically catalyzed biotransformations are superior to chemically catalyzed reaction because of:

Reaction specificity: Only one type of reaction takes place and hence no side reactions occur;

Regiospecificity: Biotransformations are specific in relation to the position of the reaction in substrate molecule;

Stereospecificity: Only one enantiomer can be selectivley or at least preferentially transformed out of a racemic mixture;

Mild reaction conditions: Biotransformation can be carried out under mild conditions of temperature (less than 40 C); pH (in vicinity of 7); and in aqueous solutions;

Lowering of activation energy: This permits accessibility to relatively non activated positions in the substrate molecule for selective transformation under mild conditions. Biotransformation can be carried out by growing cells, stationary cells, spores or immobilized cells or enzymes. Cell culture can successfully be applied in biotransformation in two ways e.g., growing cells and stationary cells;

Growing cells: In this technique substrate to be transformed is added during growth phase of cells at most favorable moment determined experimentally. This method is simple and used for screening of desired enzymatic activity in cells. But good conversions are often achieved in the stationary phase;

Stationary cells: Cells of biomass are harvested by centrifugation or filtration after cultivation in growth media. These are resuspended in transformation medium and substrate is added. Buffers are used to maintain optimum pH. Certain nutrients are also added to maintain viability for long period, growth and biotransformation can take place independently while growth inhibiting effects of substrate or products are eliminated. Biotransformation of certain important classes of compounds is discussed here.

8.7.5.1. Steroids

Steroids in the form of hormones as androgen, progesterone, estrogen, glucocorticoid and mineralocorticoid, perform central functions in human metabolisms. Their natural structures and derivatives also exhibit important pharmacological activities as anti-inflammatory, anabolic, sedative, cytostatic and contraceptive effects. Hormone antagonists have been also obtained from hormones by chemical modifications.

Diosgenin (from root of Mexican yam *Dioscorea composita*); stigmasterol (from soyabean), deoxycholic acid (from animal bile) serve as starting material for chemical synthesis of steroidal structures. But chemical synthesis requires many steps and the process is very lengthy. For example, anti-inflammatory compound, cortisone when synthesized from deoxycholic acid requires 31 steps for completion (Fig. 8.16). Similarly, nine steps are required for displacing 12-α,hydroxy group to form a keto function in position 11.

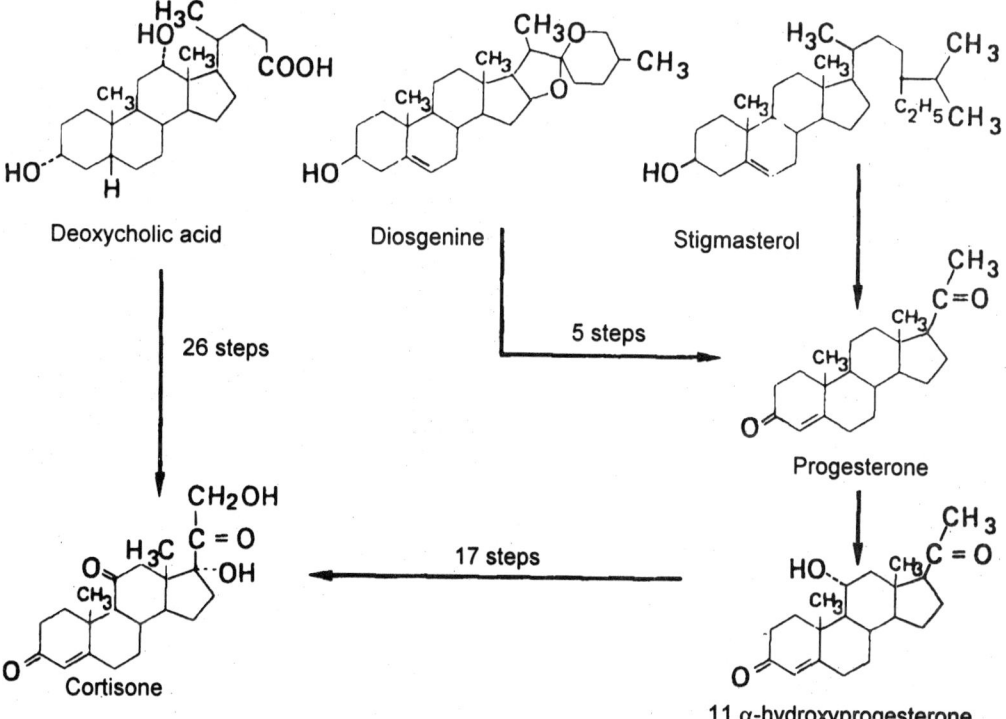

Fig. 8.16 : P_duction of cortisone from natural sterols

But efforts of investigators in Upjohn company resulted into decisive simplification of the synthesis of these hormones. Hydroxy group into the 11α position of progesterone was introduced with *Rhizopus arrhigus* or *Rhizopus nigricans* in yields more than 85%. This made available the important corticosteroid hormones with characteristics oxygen function in position 11 from the cheap natural products stigmasterol or diosgenin.

Introduction of a hydroxy group on 11β position was also achieved with *Cunnighamella blakesleeana* by which hydrocortisone was obtained directly from Reichstein's compounds These results paved the way for biotransformation to become an important technical method.

Chemical modifications in steroids which can be attempted applying biotransformation are:

1. 11α-Hydroxylation

The cultures of fungus *Aspergillus ochraceus* can be used for 11α hydroxylation of progesterone with substrate concentration of 50g/l of culture broth. Other suitable strains of fungi also affect biotransformation. But with *Aspergillus ochraceus* very small amount of the by product 6 β, 11α-dihydroxyprogesterone is formed. A number of other steroid structures can be hydroxylated at 11α position with high regio and stereo- specificity.

2. 11 β hydroxylation

Reichstein's substance S and its analogues can be hydroxylated at 11 β position with *Cunninghamella blakesleena* but paralleled 6 β hydroxylation and its subsequent oxidation to 11 ketones also occur, which can be partially suppressed by special enzyme inhibition, thus reaction rate could be modulated.

Fungus *Curvularia lunata* also carries out 11 β hydroxylation and is more frequently used nevertheless it performs unwanted hydroxylation at 7α, 9α and 14α positions. Use of 17-acetate of Reichstein's substance S excludes these side reactions as sporry-filling ester residue exerts protective effect on the rear(α) side of substrate against undesirable attack without affecting the 11 hydroxylation of the front (β) side. Similar screening effects are possible by substituting the 16 α position. In the β hydroxylation of the D-homo analog of Reichstein's substance S to D-homohydrocortisone with an anti-inflammatory action, the altered linkage blocks position 14 (Fig. 8.17).

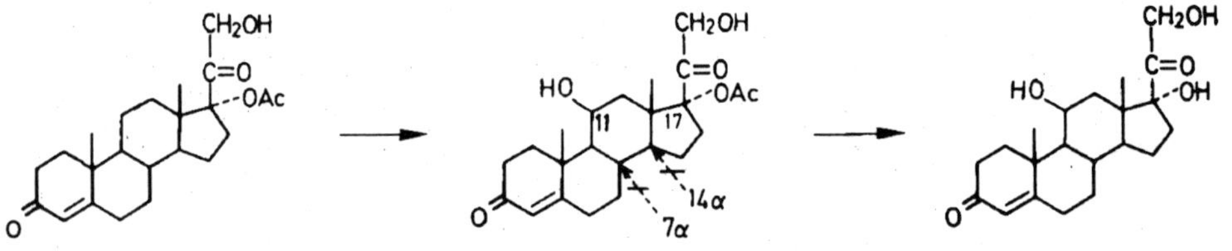

17-Acetate of Reichstein's substances Hydrocortisone 17-acetate Hydrocortisone

Fig. 8.17 : 11β-Hydroxylation of the 17-acetate of Reichstein's substance S by *Curvularia lunata*

3. 16α hydroxation

Strains of *streptomyces* have been utilized for the 16α hydroxation for the synthesis of Triamcinolone (an inflammation inhibiting agent) (Fig. 8.18).

4. Hydroxylation of other positions

Hydroxylation at other positions has been found useful in the production of new steroid structures with varied or new pharmacological activities. Hydroxylation at any position of steroid can be carried out using very diverse strains of fungi or more rarely with species of bacteria.

Broad systemic investigations have made possible the development of an enzyme-substrate model which permits approximate predictions of the type of attack in mono and dihydroxylations according to the position of a polar group of the substrate for enzymatic action process. Non-polar substrates often undergo introduction of two hydroxyl groups which can likewise be used for preparative purposes.

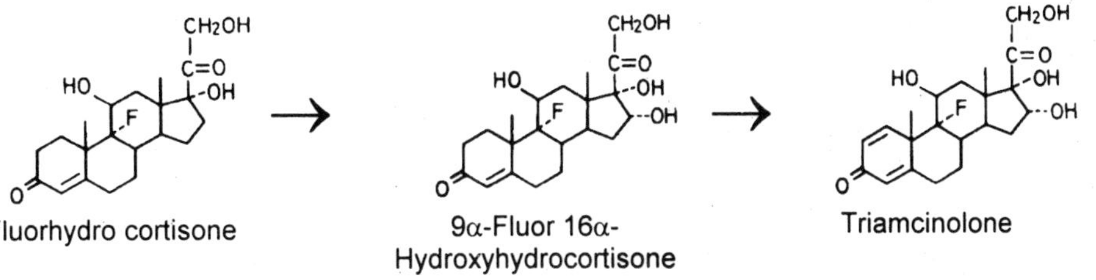

| 9α-Fluorhydro cortisone | 9α-Fluor 16α-Hydroxyhydrocortisone | Triamcinolone |

Fig. 8.18 : 16α-Hydroxylation of 9α-fluorohydrocortisone by *Streptomyces sp.*

5. 1,2-dehydrogenation

Prednisone, prednisolone, triamcinalone, 6-methylprednisolone, dexamethasone formed by the dehydro-genation of the corresponding 1,2 saturated structures possess significantly enhanced anti-inflammatory activity. This has led to the development of method of 1,2 dehydrogenation using *Bacillus sphaericus*, *Bacterium cyclooxydans* and *Arthrobacter (Corynebacterium) simplex* at technical scale.

Using *Arthrobacter (Corynebacterium) simplex* in a special process substrate concentrations up to 500 g of hydrocortisone per liter of culture broth can be converted to prednisolone in yields of over 90% in five days. The substrate is added in micronized form without a solvent and hence process has been termed as **pseudo-crystallofermentation.**

6. Ester saponification and oxidation of hydroxy groups

The wide distribution of hydrolyzing enzymes in microorganisms often couples ester saponification with other microbiological reaction in one step fermentation which can be used in practice when flavobacterium dehydrogenase is used to transform triolone diacetate into Reichstein's compound S, the acetate groups in positions 3 and 21 are hydrolyzed off before the oxidation of 3β-hydroxy-5-ene system to 3-keto-4-ene structure takes place (Fig. 8.19). If the pH is kept constant carefully at 6.6 in the corresponding 3 β,17α,21 tri-acetate, the 17α ester group is retained which leads to the 17-acetate of Reichstein's substance S, an advantageous starting material for the commercial preparation of hydrocortisone.

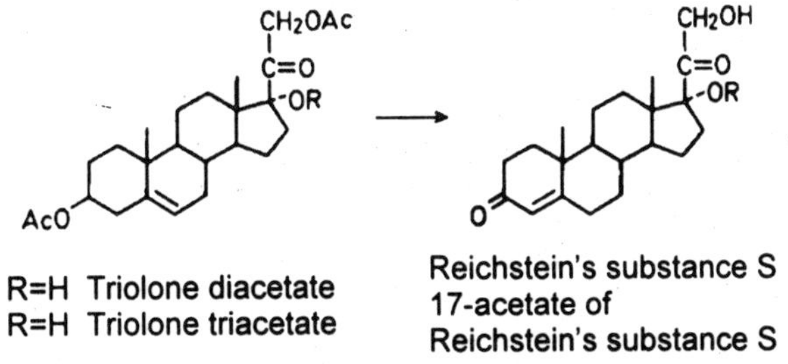

R=H Triolone diacetate
R=H Triolone triacetate

Reichstein's substance S
17-acetate of
Reichstein's substance S

Fig. 8.19 : Coupled saponification and oxidation of triolone acetates by *Flavobacterium dehydrogenans*

7. Reduction of keto group

Reduction of 17-keto group is utilized in the production of testosterone from androst-4-ene,3,17 dione (Fig. 8.20).

The process utilizing yeast was the first steroid transformation for which a patent was granted. Additionally, if a chiral or prechiral diketones are taken as substrates, then microbial reduction can selectively form four possible enantiomers. The introduction of first center of asymmetry by enzymatic reaction made it possible to synthesize steroids economically for the first time.

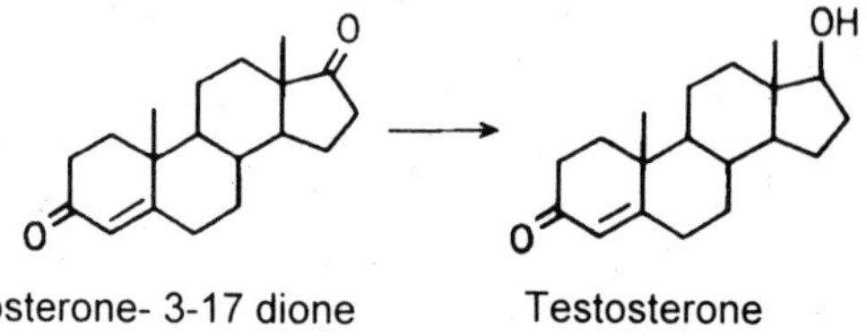

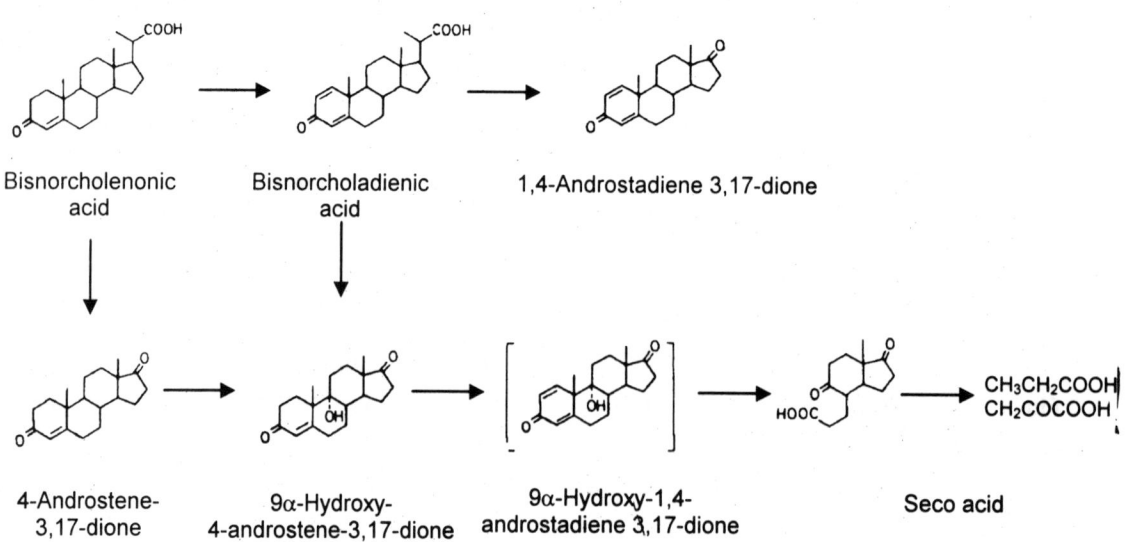

4-Androsterone- 3-17 dione   Testosterone

Fig. 8.20 : Stereoselective reduction of 4-androstene-3,17-dione to testosterone

One of the two equivalent keto groups of secodione can be steriospecifically and regiospecifically reduced to secolone which doubles the yield by eliminating the formation of racemate. An excellent application of the procedure lies in the manufacture of D-norgesterol, an important contraceptive. The bioconversion is schematically depicted in figure 8.21.

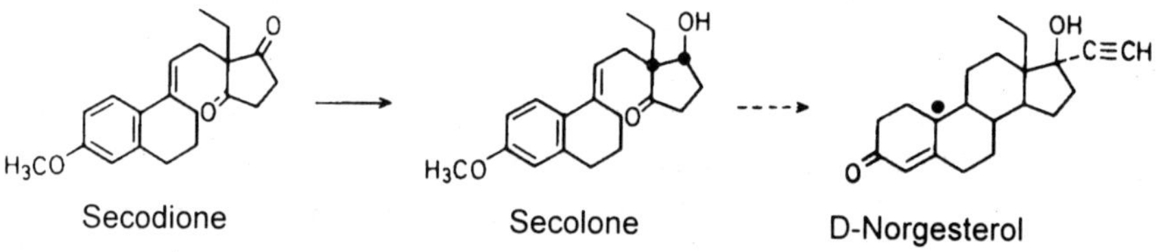

Secodione   Secolone   D-Norgesterol

Fig. 8.21 : The stereospecific reduction of a seco-dione yields secolone,
a constructional unit for the total synthesis of steriods (e.g., D-Norgestrel)

8. Sterol side-chain degradation

The several possibilities exist for suppressing the undesirable degradation of steroid skeleton and side chain can be degraded alone by microbial degradation. These possibilities can be unraveled from elucidation of enzymatic reaction mechanism. Various strategies which could possibly be employed for the purpose are schematically shown in figure 8.22.

Bisnorcholenonic acid   Bisnorcholadienic acid   1,4-Androstadiene 3,17-dione

4-Androstene- 3,17-dione   9α-Hydroxy- 4-androstene-3,17-dione   9α-Hydroxy-1,4- androstadiene 3,17-dione   Seco acid

CH_3CH_2COOH
$CH_2COCOOH$

Fig. 8.22 : Pathway of enzymatic degradation in steroids

One of the possibility is the inhibition of formation of 9α-hydroxy adrossa-1,4, diene 3,17 dione which is unstable and initiates total degradation. Sterol side chain degradation permits the use of cholesterol as a starting material for steroids. Besides cholesterol stigmasterol, sitosterol and mixture of sterols containing compesterol, stigmasterol, siboester can be used with equivalent possible potentials. These products are obtained on large scale cheaply from soyabean and til oil. Optimized procedures have been developed for the large scale production and technical manufacture of androst-4-ene-3,17 dione and androsta-1,4-diene 3,17 dione. These require special media additives and substrate. Yields of more than 80% of 17-ketosteroids are obtained with suitable mycobacteria in fermentation times of 3-4 days when susbtrate concentration is kept at several grams per liter.

9.Miscellaneous biotransformations

Various other types of reactions in microbiological biotransformation of steroids include:

1. Oxidation: It involving aromatization of ring A during dehydrogenation of 19 norsteriods ; oxidation of pregnan-20-ones to testolactone structure and epoxidation of double bonds.

2. Reduction: It includes hydrogenation of double bond and dehydrogenation.

3. Hydrolytic reactions (possibly oxidative): Cleavage of phenolic 3-methylethers as well as cleavage of glycosides.

4. Glycosidation of the glycosides at phenolic 3-OH group and 16-OH group is included in this class of biotransformation.

8.7.5.2. Prostaglandins

Prostaglandins are lipoidal and pharmaceutically important compounds which occur in low concentration in nature and require expensive purification methods for isolation. Initial total synthesizes were generally limited because of production of racemic mixtures as even simplest prostaglandins possess 3 to 5 centers of chirality (Fig. 8.23).

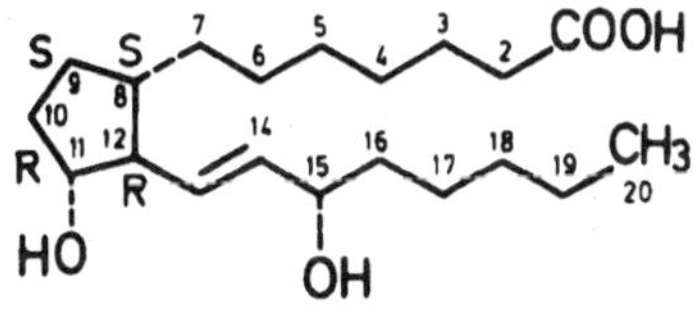

Fig. 8.23 : Structure of prostaglandins

Pure chiral structures can be obtained by following ways:

1. By initiating biogenesis with incorporation of native constructional units;

2. By chemical synthesis using an enzymatic-generally microbial reaction step to introduce the first chirality which directs the subsequent pathway of chemical synthesis to the desired enantiomers;

3. Microbial transformation of native or synthetic prostaglandins to obtain new types of structures with changed action profiles.

Prostaglandins are biologically synthesized from essential fatty acid by enzymatic cyclization resulting in to the formation of a cyclopentane ring with α and ω-side chains. Microorganism can produce prostaglandins from unsaturated fatty acids with a 1,4-diene system oxidation. Strains of species subphylum have been utilized with polyunsaturated fatty acids substrates. Mixture of PGE and PGE_2 is formed from substrate arachidonic acid (Fig. 8.24). Microorganism driven biotransformations are schematically presented in figure 8.25.

Hydroxylation at position 18 or 19 in arachidonic acid is carried out with *Ophibolus graminis* and can be chemically oxidized to corresponding keto compounds. These keto compounds can be cyclized with animal enzymes to yield corresponding hydroxy or oxo-PGE structures. For example, stereospecific reduction of a 2-

(6-methoxycarbonyl hexyl) cyclopentane-1,3,4 trione [1] with D*iplodascus uninucleatus* gives a 4 (R)-alcohol [2] in 75% yield which can be converted in two subsequent chemical steps into the desired cyclopentylsynthon [3]. *Aspergillus niger* ATCC 9142 can also be used for production of cyclopentyl synthon[3] by microbiological hydroxylation of a 2-(6 carboxyhexyl) cyclopent-2-en-1 one [4].

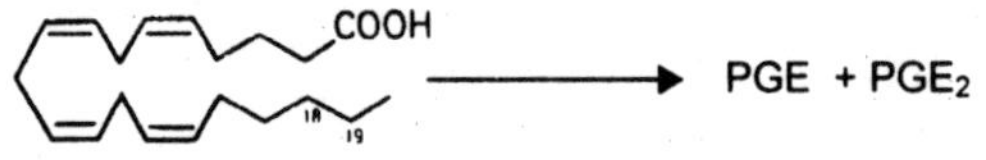

Fig. 8.24 : Arachidonic acid as prostaglandin precursor

Yield is 67% but optical purity of the product is poor. Lithium cuparate of a (+)-3(s)-indooct-1-en-3-ol [6] is used as octenyl synthon for introduction of ω-side chain. This chiral alcohol can also be obtained from the corresponding 3-ketone [7] similarly 2-(6 methoxycarboxylhex-cis-2 enyl) cyclopentane-1,3,4-trione can be used as cyclopentyl synthol to start preparation of PGE$_2$.

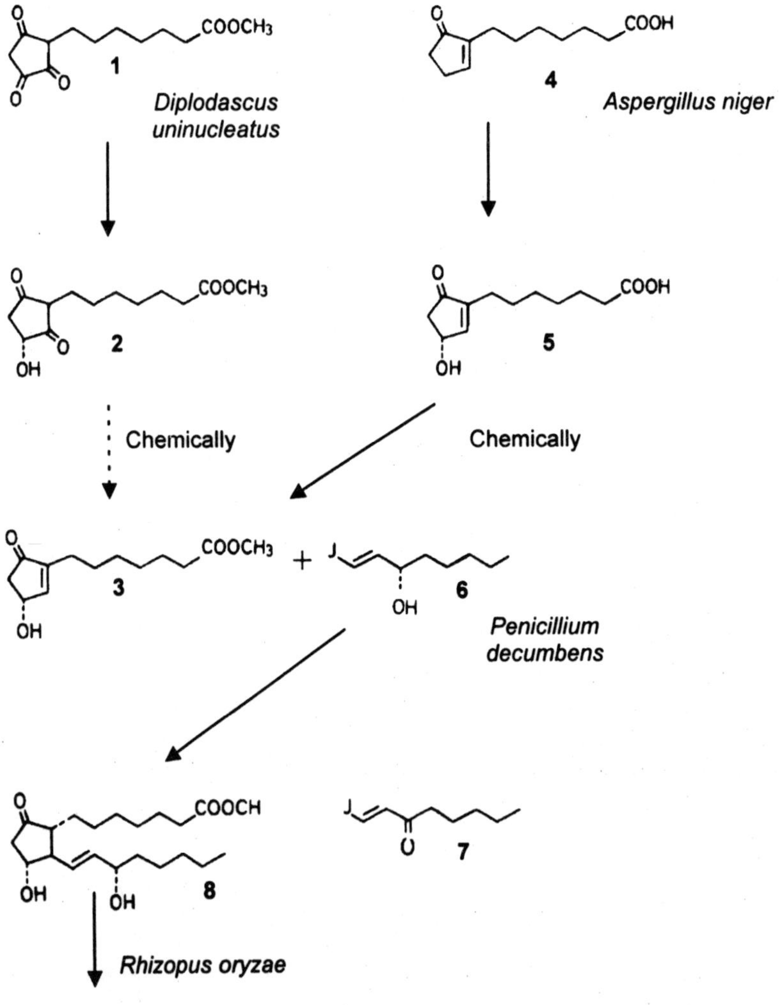

Fig. 8.25 : Synthesis of PGE$_1$ with the aid of microbiological reaction steps .

In an another synthetic pathway, the reduction of 15 keto group leads to a $\Delta^{8(12)}$-15-keto structures with racemic 11 hydroxy group [9] via the undermentioned pathways:

a. *Flarobacterium sp.* NRRLB-3874 gives the transdiol [10] in 30% yield;
b. *Pseudomonas sp.* NRRLB-3875 gives the transdiol [11] in 24% yield;
c. *Rhodotorula glutinis* gives only a d,l-transdiol;
d. *Flarobacterium sp.* NRRLB-5641 gives a mixture of cis-diols.

The bioconversions are presented in schematically in figure 8.25 and 8.26.

An active compound sulprostane [12] has been synthesized with the avoidance of racemate by specific reduction of an analogous conjugated keto group with *Kloeckera jensenii sp* (Fig. 8.26)

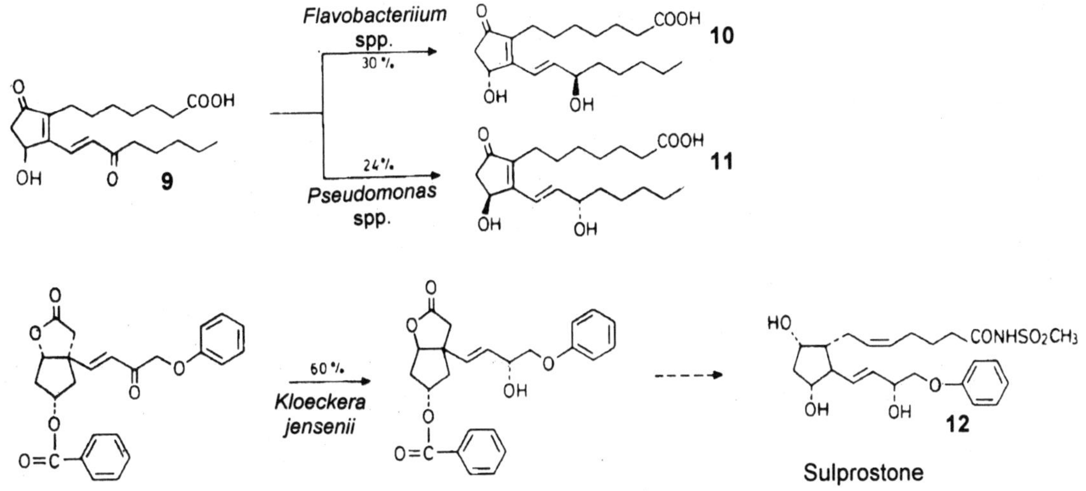

Fig. 8.26 : Enantioselective reductions of ketones

Biotransformation can also be initiated and employed in selective resolution of racemates by the saponification of esters of the 11-hydroxy group, an intermediate stage of this synthesis Saccharomyces sp.1375-143 hydrolyzes the acetate, propionate or isobutyrate of the R form steriospecifically giving 52% yields of R-alcohol.

The 3(R)-acetoxy-5(R)-hydroxycyclopent-1-ene [14] can be obtained to a maximum yield of 11.5% by careful control of saponification which is also a desirable prostaglandin synthon. The corresponding pure cis-diacetate [15] gives with *Bacillus subtilis* a 56% yield of the 3(s)-acetoxy-5(s)-hydroxy product [16], which is converted chemically into a lactone [17] with the desired absolute configuration. Although optical purity of up to only 35% is obtained, still the lactose is considered to be an important intermediate in various prostaglandin synthesis.

One of the most interesting application of biotransformations is that they could be used in the synthesis of artificial biotransformation also. For example, *Saccharomyces cerevisiae* ATCC 4125 has been used in 15 keto reduction of 9,15-diketo-11-deoxyprostanic acid. Another example is of *Trechispora brinkmanii* CMI 80439 which being used in reduction of 15 dehydroprostaglandins.

Besides synthesis, interconversions like reduction of nat PGE_1 to $PGF_{1\alpha}$ and nat PGE_2 to nat $PGF_{2\alpha}$ by baker's yeast have also been carried out. Here 9-keto group was reduced to a 9(S)-OH group without the formation of the 9(R) byproduct. When methyl ester is used in this process, saponification takes place prior to keto reduction. When racemic mixture of PGE_1 and PGE_2 is taken both enantiomers are reduced to nat $PGF_{1\alpha}$, nat $PGF_{2\alpha}$, nat $PGF_{1\beta}$ and nat $PGF_{2\beta}$, but side reactions limit maximum yield to 10%.

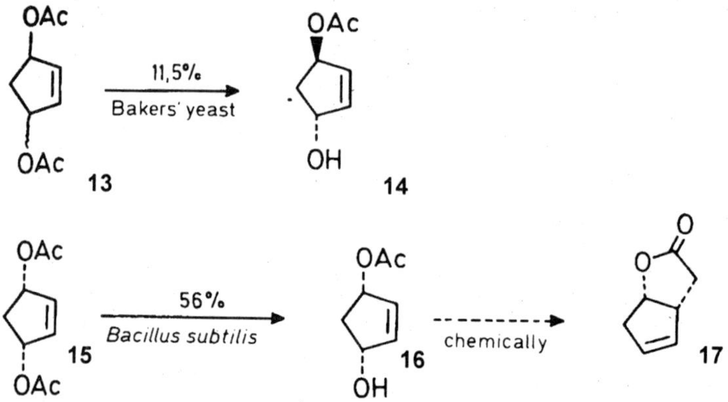

Fig. 8.27 : Regio- and stereoselective hydrolysis of 3,5-diacetoxycyclopentenes.

The PGA$_2$[18] can be transformed into 15 hydroxy-9 oxo prosta-5,13 dienoic acid [19] by the hydrogenation of 10,11-double bond with *Cephalosporinum sp.* NRRL 5499. *Dactylium dendroides* NRRL 2572 gives as a by-product 9,15-dioxaprost-5-enoic acid [20] and 9,15-dioxoprosta-5,8 (12)-dienoic acid [21]. An analogous 18-hydroxylated product [22] is formed in addition to 10,11-dihydrocompound by *Cunnighamella blakesleena*. 10,11-double bond can be reduced while hydrolyzing ester group by *Corynespora cassiicola* IM1 560007. Pseudomonas and streptomyces species can also perform this in case of 15-epiprostaglandin A$_2$.

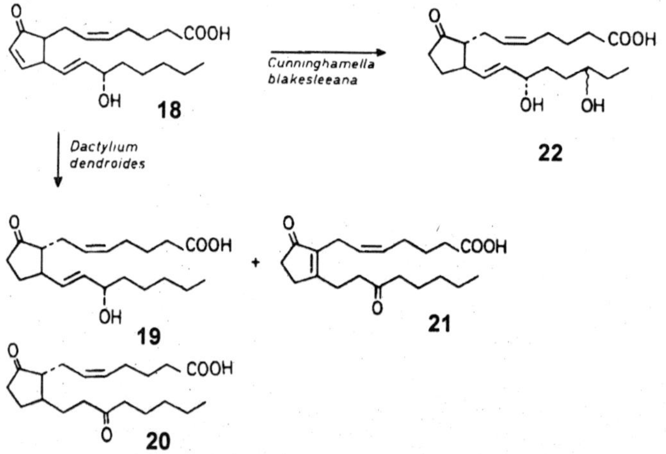

Fig. 8.28 : Biotransformation of PGA$_2$.

Interestingly, structures of new types have been obtained by microbial β oxidation of natural and synthetic prostaglandins. Pencillium sp. M8904 converts prostaglandins B$_2$ and A$_2$ into tetranor structures and attacks only α side chain forming various by-products. *Mycobacterium rhodochrons* UC6176 can also perform oxidative degradation to tetranor or dinor structures.

A summary of these biotransformation is presented in table 8.5.

Table 8.5: Hydroxylation in prostaglandins.

PGF$_{2\alpha}$	Streptomyces UC 5761	18-OH ; 19-OH
PGE$_2$	Streptomyces UC 5761	18-OH ; 19-OH
PGEA$_2$	Streptomyces sp.	17-OH : 18-OH ; 19-OH
Various prostaglandins	Streptomyces sp.	17-OH : 18-OH ; 19-OH ; 20-OH
d,l-Prost-13-enoic acid	Microascus trigonosporus	18-OH ; 19-OH

8.7.6. Miscellaneous products

8.7.6.1. Dihydroxyacetone

Dihydroxyacetone is an important agent in cosmetic preparations for promoting suntan. Acetobacter species, particularly *Acetobacter suboxydans* oxidize glycerol regioselectively to give dihydroxyacetone. Optimum concentration of glycerol is 110g/l and yield is 82% after 72 hours. *Gluconobacter melanogenus* also performs the same reaction and the rate of conversion can be increased at least three fold by enriching the aeration flow with pure oxygen.

8.7.6.2. L-Maleic acid and L-tartatic acid

L-Maleic acid, is used in the treatment of liver diseases and as an additive to infusion solution. It is an important intermediate in tricarboxylic acid cycle. *Brevibacterium* ammonia genes cells immobilized in polyacrylamide gel or *Brevibacterium flavum* cells immobilized in carrageenan have been used for the production of L maleic acid by asymmetric addition of water to fumaric acid. Immobilized cells are treated with bile extract for suppressing the undesirable by-product synthesis of succinic acid. Enzyme responsible is fumarase of which highest activity and the longest half life (160 days at 37°C) were observed with *B.flavum* immobilized in carrageenan.

L-tartaric acid production involves initial oxidation of maleic acid to cis-epoxysuccinic acid by hydrogen peroxide (H_2O_2) and then asymmetric hydrolysis of epoxide by using microorganisms *Nocardia tartaricus* or *Achromobacter tartarogenes* cells immobilized in polyacrylamide gel as biocatalysts.

8.7.6.3. Sugar transformations

Although many sugar transformations have been studied; three processes which are, particularly important from technical application point of view are being discussed.

a. Isomerization of glucose to fructose to enhance sweetening effect has been carried out by using *Bacillus coagulans* immobilized with glutaraldehyde; *Streptomyces phaeochromogenes* immobilized in polyacrylamide and *Achromobacter missouriensis* immobilized on cellulose fibers. Use of *Bacillus coagulans* make possible conversion of 1000 Kg glucose to a mixture of 45% fructose and 55% glucose per Kg of biocatalyst. Transforming enzyme present in the microbes is glucose isomerase.

b. Hydrolysis of raffinose to sucrose and galactose by α galactosidase to increase yields of sucrose from beet sugar molasses. Mycelial pellets formed naturally by *Mertierella vinacea* var raffinoseutilizer are rich in α galactosidase and have been used for continuous hydrolysis of raffinose.

c. Lactose in skimmed milk has been hydrolyzed by cells with high β-galactosidase activity *Lactobacillus bulgaricus, Escherichia coli, Kluyveromyces lactis* immobilized in polyacrylamide gel to produce lactose free milk products. Products formed are glucose and galactose. This process is also useful in utilization of whey.

8.7.5.4. Hycanthone and oxamniquine

Drug hycanthone is active against *Schistosoma mansoni*. The activity is enhanced by selective hydroxylation of an aromatic methyl group with *Aspergillus sclerotiorum*. The more potent drug formed is Hycanthone.

Oxamniqnine, a schistosomacidal drug produced from corresponding methyl compound by *Aspergillus sclerotiorum* (Fig. 8.29).

8.7.6.5. Biotransformations of antitumor drugs

Biotransformations have also been employed to many antitumor drugs. Reductive cleavage of glycosides, reduction of ketone groups in anthracyclines hydrolysis of amine moiety of bleomycin, regioselective hydroxylation in **withaferrin A** and in aromatic rings of acromycin (acronin) and vinblastine, N-demethylation in D-tetrandrine and vindoline, the formation of ether derivatives and the dimerization of vindoline and the opening of quinone ring in lapachol are some of the representative examples. Unfortunately these and other biotransformations have not led to development of products with significantly enhanced activity or reduced toxicity.

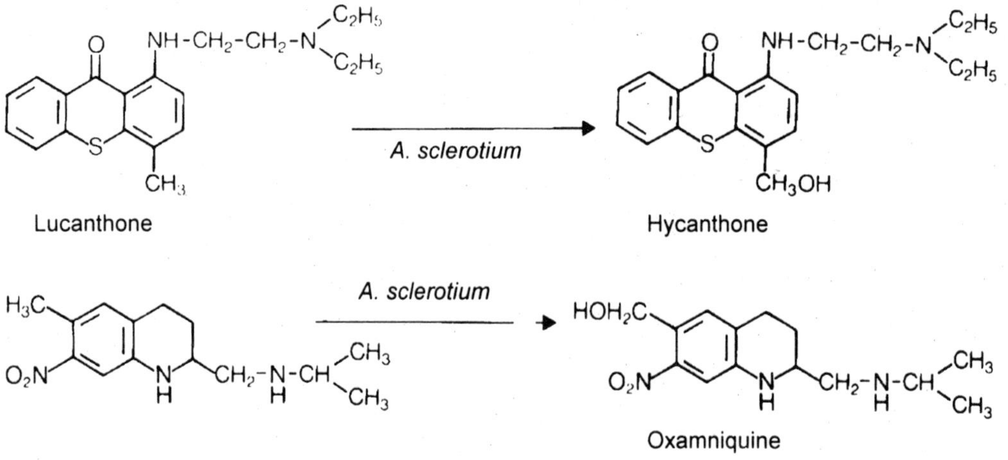

Fig. 8.29 : Production of hycanthone and oxamniquine by the selective hydroxylation of an aromatic methyl group.

8.7.6.6. Oxidation of naphthalene

Pseudomonas putida degrades naphthalene by reductive dihydroxylation to give cis 1,2-dihydroxy-1,2-dihydronaphthalene. Cis isomer formed is an important precursor for pesticides. Trans 1,2-dihydroxy-1,2-dihydronaphathalene is formed by *Nocardia sp.* NRRL 3385. Subsequent oxidation proceeds through several steps to salicylic acid, however its production by this method is insignificant even with the most suitable strain, *Corynebacterium renale* ATCC 15070.

SUGGESTED READINGS

Capek, K.A., Hanc, O. and Tadra, M., (1966) **Microbial Transformation of Steroids**, Akademia Press, Prague.

Cass, E.A., (1990) **Biosensors,** IRL Press, Oxford.

Fonken, G.S and Johnson, R.A., (1972) **Chemical Oxidation with Microorganisms**, Marcel Dekker, New York.

Hall, E.A., (1990) **Biosensors,** Open University Press, Milten Keynes.

Hopkinson, J., (1985) **Biotechnology, 3,** 225-230.

Jizuka, H., Naito, A., (1967) **Microbial Transformation of Steroids and Alkaloids,** University of Tokyo Press, Tokyo.

Kieslich, K., (1980) *Steroid Conversions*; In: **Economic Microbiology-Microbial Enzymes and Transformation**, Vol. V, 369-465.

Meyers, R.A., (1995) **Molecular Biology and Biotechnology**, VCH Publishers, Inc., New York, 110-113.

North, J.R., (1985) **Trends in Biotechnology, 3,** 180-186.

P. Prave, U. Faust, W. Sittig, D.A. Sukatsch, (Eds.), (1987) **Fundamentals of Biotechnology,** VCH, Verlagsgesellschaff mbH, D-6940, Weinheim, Germany.

Prescott, L.M., Harkey, J.P. and Klien, D.A., (1993) **Microbiology,** Wm. C. Brown Publishers, Dubuque, 905-906.

R. Spier, W. Hennessen (Eds.) (1985) **Developments in Biological Standardization,** Vol. 66., Academic Press, San Diego, CA.

Schaller, F. and Schubert, F., (1992) **Biosensors,** Elsevier, Amsterdam.

BIOTECH IN NEWS . . . .

Indigenous Hepatitis B vaccines...

Indigenously developed vaccines against Hepatitis B are holding out the promise that people can be protected against this fast spreading disease at much lower cost, making a nationwide mass immunization program feasible.

The first vaccine against Hepatitis was derived from the plasma of carriers. his vaccine went into general use in 1981 and by 1987 there were 12 commercial concerns manufacturing it worldwide. With modern recombinant DNA technology, however, a gene from the Hepatitis B virus could be introduced in cells so that they produced a viral protein. Using these techniques, genetically engineered yeast were developed which could synthesize one of the proteins found in the outer coat of the Hepatitis B virus. The modified yeast would be grown in fermenters and then chemically broken open so that the viral protein they produced would be released. After purification, the protein could be given as a vaccine. In 1986, this type of Hepatitis B vaccine entered general used in the US

SmithKline Beecham was one of the first to develop the technology for the recombinant Hepatitis B vaccine. Its vaccine, manufactured in Belgium, is used widely in India. Now two Hyderabad (India) based companies have indigenously developed the technology to manufacture the Hepatitis B vaccine, using genetically engineered yeast. They believe they can supply the vaccine at far lower prices.

The vaccine developed by **Shanta Biotech** was released in Hyderabad in the last week of August. The vaccine, which will be marketed under the brand name 'Shanvac-B', was made not with the conventional strain of yeast, *Saccharomyces cerevisiae*, but another strain, *Pichia pastoris*.

The *Pichia* strain has the advantage that it can grow to greater cell densities. As a result, *Pichia* is reported to give five times more yield than *Sacchraromyces*. The project was partially supported by Central Government's Technology Development Board for commercializing its technology.

Another Hyderabad based company, **Bharat Biotech's** first vaccine, which is expected to complete clinical trials and enter use early next year, uses the conventional *Saccharomyces strain*.

Use of *Pichia* for producing human vaccines had so far been cleared only in Cuba and India.

. . . .*The Hindu, 04/09/'97*

INTRODUCTION TO GENETICS

9.1. INTRODUCTION

The last few decades of twentieth century has brought about a revolution in the field of life sciences research with the advent of a modern science known as genetics. Virtually every aspect of the biological science as well as medicine has been profoundly affected by the discoveries which explored molecular basis of the gene. The research has thrown light on various structural and functional aspects of the cell leading to the development of the newer conclusions being arrived, both in the case of the biological science and the disease physiology. The aspect of genetics which has affected the development to the most is the molecular biochemistry combined with molecular physics leading to molecular biotechnology. The collaboration of these sciences has opened up newer vistas in the modern era. The first breakthrough in the field was in 1953 by James Watson and Francis Crick when they postulated the double helical structure of deoxyribonucleic acid (DNA). Their hypothesis was further verified by different experiments, representing the confluence of genetic theory, which contributed the concept of coding of the gene. Physics, helped in the determination of the molecular structure with the help of X-ray analysis vis-à-vis biochemical research could be accounted for its contribution in determination of the chemical structure of DNA and these sciences jointly contributed in building the basis of modern genetics.

In the modern era of computers and super computers in their most compact form; we are all aware of their abilities of labor-saving, data compilation, data interpretation, processing, and retrieval of information. All these systems work as a digital system in which the units for storage of information is in the form of *bits* (abbreviated from a binary digit) which means the amount of the information required for making a decision when two possibilities are present. The number of bits increase with the increase in the number of possibilities in a geometric progression. A similar system exists in the biological cell. However, the amount of the information coded and supplied within one cell is much more larger than that of the world's largest computer. As in the computer the information is stored in the form of bits, cell contains the information in the form of genes which are the set of various nucleosides with varying purine and pyrimidine sequences. This all has been revealed by the modern genetics. Recently one group of workers in Canada has prepared a computer microprocessor with a drop of DNA solution. The computer hence prepared was found to have the capability of working at much higher speeds than its normal counterparts as well as could store much more data, however, the tasks performed were much different from those performed by the normal computer.

The genetic materials and components particularly nucleic acid was first isolated in 1868 by F. Miescher. He established the material isolated containing phosphorus what today known as nucleoprotein. Cells possessing large nucleus have proved to be the best source of nucleic acid hence thymus gland was widely used as a source for nucleic acid isolation. Hydrolysis of nucleic acid from thymus yielded purine and pyrimidine bases (adenine, guanine, cytosine and thymine), 2 deoxyribose and phosphoric acid. The acid has been named as **Deoxyribonucleic acid (DNA)**. From bacteria, yeast, another nucleic acid was isolated that contained uracil instead of thymine and ribose in place of deoxyribose. This has been called as ribonucleic acid (RNA). The concentrations of RNA and DNA in cells have been recorded to be dependent on the functional state of the cell in Spermatozoa, the amount of DNA reaches approximately 60% of the dry cell weight, in other cells it remains to be 1-10% where as in muscles 0.2%. The amount of RNA by and large comes to be 5-10 times as much as that of DNA. Thus, the ratio of RNA/DNA in liver, pancreas, embryonic tissue varies from 4 to 10. The bacterial cells which are devoid of **true nucleus** (prokaryotes) the DNA molecules exist in nucleosides. DNA bound to cellular membrane of a bacterium in an invaginated region referred to as **mesosome**. A small portion of DNA may localize outside the chromosomal region. Such extreme chromosomal DNA is called as **plasmids**. The plasmids which irreversibly integrate in the host DNA are called **episomes**. In cells having distinctive nucleus (Eukaryotics) DNA is distributed between nucleus and mitochondria.

9.2. DNA IS THE MOLECULE OF HEREDITY

This has been proven experimentally that DNA is the molecule of heredity. The importance of nucleus which contains DNA was identified by the observation, that nuclei of male and female germicells (reproductive cells) fuse during the process of fertilization. It had been observed that there existed thread like objective inside the nucleus that was visible under light microscope. This structure was referred to as chromosomes. The chromosomes demonstrated typical splitting behavior during cell division, in which each daughter cell formed as a result of cell division received identical complement chromosomes. The number of chromosomes was observed to be constant within each species. The chromosomes which had been studied extensively by about 1900 found to be the carrier of genes. There had been number of indirect evidences suggesting close relationship between DNA and genetic material. However, the indirect evidence seemed to be unconvincing, as crude chemical analysis has suggested that the DNA lacks chemical diversity which is needed for a genetic substance. On the contrary, proteins were known to be highly diversified assemblages of molecules. Subsequently, it became widely accepted that proteins were the genetic material and the DNA nearly provides the structural framework of chromosomes. Hence, experiment purporting to demonstrate that DNA is the genetic material also had to prove that proteins were not responsible for genetic inheritance, and as a result could not be considered genetic material as such.

Streptococcus pneumoniae is known to cause pneumonia and measles and is able to synthesize a complex carbohydrate capsule around the bacterium, the later is accounted for the capability of bacteria to escape from host defense mechanism. Thus, allows it to cause the diseases. The culture of the bacteria on a solid support results into a colony, that was a visible clumps of cells. The enveloping capsule imparts the colony gellesting or smooth(s) appearance. However, some strains of *S. pneumoniae* are not able to synthesize the capsular polysaccharide and as a result their colonies appear to have a rough surface and these are referred to as R-cells. It had been established through experiments that R-strain is non-virulent for it cannot escape immune system of the host. When mice are injected either with a heat killed (attenuated) S-cells, they remain healthy. Subsequently in 1928 it was observed that inoculum based on R- and heat killed S-cell mixture could cause mortality into a large number of mice. The bacteria isolated from blood samples of the dead mice produced only S-culture with a capsule typical of the injected S-cell but the injected S-cells were dead. It appears reasonable to assume that injection material containing dead S-cells must have incorporated into the living R-bacterial cells rendering them to resist the immunological system of the mouse as a consequence could multiply to cause pneumonia. Furthermore, it could be inferred that there had been a total transformation of R-bacteria cells into S-bacteria without inheriting new characteristics different from the parents.

In 1944, the experiment that is considered as a milestone had been reported by Ostwald Avery, Colin MacLeod, and Maclyn McCarty. They suggested that substance causing the transformation of R-cell into a S-cell was DNA. In a well designed experiment, the extracted DNA from a cell was added to the growing culture of R-cell, it was observed that few of S-cell types were produced. DNA was analyzed for protein content, however the treatment of protein for destruction could not be eliminated. The experiment concluded that the substance responsible for genetic transfer or transformation is DNA the genetic material. It has also been proven through set of experiments that the transmission of DNA is a link between generations. The base pair can be arranged in any sequence, the sequence can vary from one part of molecule to another and from species to species. Thus DNA has virtually unlimited potential to code for a variety of protein molecules. DNA, in fact is a very dynamic molecule that remains constantly in motion. Obviously, in some reforms the strands may be separated transiently and then may come together again in the same conformation or in some events it may be different. Although typical right handed double helix is considered to be the standard form, DNA can form more than 20 identified variants of right handed helices. And in some of the regions even strands with left handed twist can be seen. In some of the DNA strands the complementing structures are likely to exist in the same strain, hence can fold upon itself to form hair-pin like structure. Each original strand in the doublex serves as a template for the formation of new complement strands. The primary function of replication is to copy the base pair, from the parent molecule. Nucleotide monomers are added sequentially one by one to the growing end of strand. The addition of nucleotide is brought about by an enzyme called **DNA polymerase**. The sequence of bases in newly replicated strands is obviously complementary to the base sequence of the original strands (parent strands) being replicated; wherever, adenine nucleotide is present a thymine nucleotide is added to the growing strand (or daughter cells). Obviously it is inferred that the nature of DNA for its replication is typically semi-conservative. This was demonstrated and proved with the help of experiment by Matthews Meselson and Franklin, Stahl in 1958. RNA is distinct from DNA and is found distributed throughout the cell indicative of dynamic and active functioning of RNA. In eukaryotes nearly 11% of total RNA could be accounted for nucleus where as 15% and 50% for mitochondria and ribosomes respectively. In cells, most of RNAs are bound to various proteins and exist as ribonucleic protein (RNP).

9.3. STRUCTURAL CONSIDERATIONS OF DNA AND RNA

9.3.1. Nucleosides the bases of RNA and DNA

Compounds which are based on pentose sugar linked with nitrogen bases are referred to as nucleosides and phosphoric acid esters of nucleoside(s) with deoxyribose/ribose a pentose sugar are termed as nucleotides. Nucleotides are building blocks of most important genetic material, i.e. DNA and RNA. The phosphate group can add to the 3' or 5' position of deoxyribose nucleotides. Free nucleotides which are involved in biological synthesis carry a PO_4^{2-} group in 5' position (Fig. 9.1).

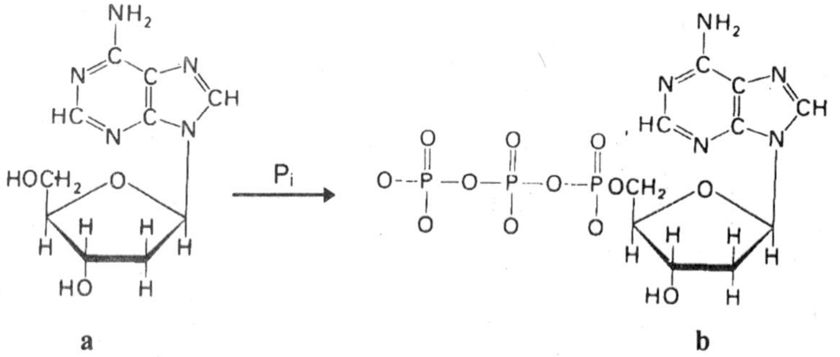

**Fig. 9.1 : Structure; a. Deoxyadenosine (a nucleoside) ;
b. Deoxyadenosine 5' triphosphate (dATP) (a nucleotide)**

9.3.2. Secondary and tertiary structures of DNA

9.3.2.1. Secondary structure of DNA

Chargaff in the year 1949, established a number of important relationships concerning the contents of individual bases in DNA. These relationships helped in clarifying the secondary structure of DNA. They are known as **Chargaff's rules**:

1. the total number of purine nucleotides (A+G) is equal to the total number of pyrimidine nucleotides (C+T), i.e. (A+G)/(C+T)=1;
2. the amount of adenine (A) is always equal to the amount of thymine (T): A=T, or A/T=1;
3. the amount of guanine (G) is always equal to the amount of cytosine (C): G=C, or G/C=1;
4. in the bases constitutive of DNA, the number of 6-amino groups is equal to the number of 6-keto groups; G+T = A+C;
5. the numbers (A+T) and (G+C) are the only variables. If (A+T) > (G+C), the DNA is said to belong to the AT-type; if (G+C) > (A+T), the DNA is of GC-type.

The above rules indicate that the buildup of DNA is effected in a strict conformity with the pairwise interactions thymine-adenine and cytosine-guanine rather than with a indiscriminate pairing of purine and pyrimidine bases.

9.3.2.2. Tertiary structure of DNA

The tertiary structure of DNA looks like a supercoil or like a bent double helix. It emerges as the double-helical DNA molecule is twisted in space.

9.3.2.2.1. Structural organization of DNA in chromosomes

In higher organisms, the DNA is located in chromosomes. They are characterized by a complicated structural organization. The shape of the chromosomes varies depending upon the location of the centromere or constricted portion of the chromosome. Each chromosome contains a single giant DNA molecule of molecular mass about 10^{11} and a few centimeters long which constitutes the basis for chromatin. Chromatin is a supramolecular structure made up of a double-stranded DNA which forms a complex primarily with protein and to a lesser extent with RNA and inorganic compounds. The composition of chromatin in percentage is: DNA,

30-45% ; histones, 30-50%; nonhistone proteins, 4-33%; and RNA, 1.5-10%. Only 2-11% portion of chromatin is active, depending upon the cell. The highest content of chromatin is found in the brain cells (10-11%), followed by liver cells (3-4%), followed by kidney cells (2-3%).

The electron microscopic structure of chromatin resembles a string of beads (globular bulges) with a diameter of 10nm spaced apart by thread-like linkers. These globular bulges are called *nucleosomes*. Each nucleosome contains a length of double-stranded DNA equal in extension to 140 base pairs, and eight molecules (an octet) of histones (Fig. 9.2). The histone octet is composed of four pairs of histones of H_{2a}, H_{2b}, H_3 and H_4. The thread-like linkers of double-stranded DNA that is composed of 30-60 base pairs having histone H_1 each, the linker lengths being different in various cells.

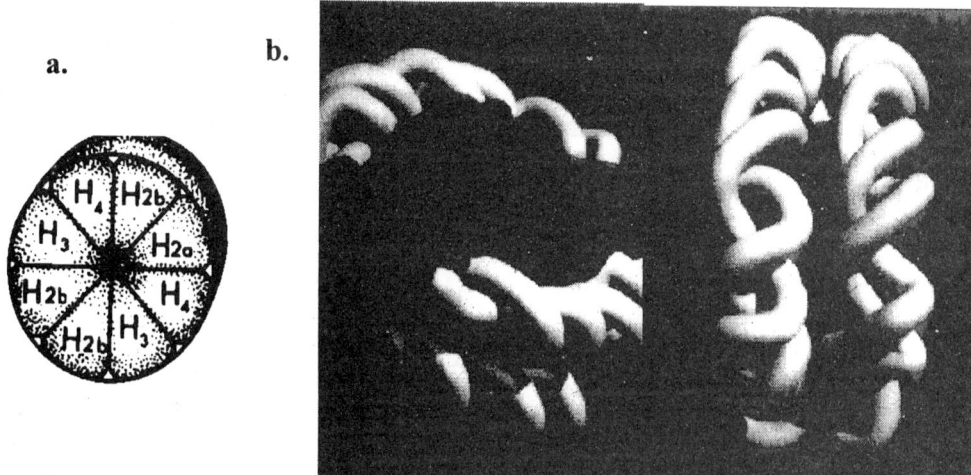

Fig. 9.2 : a. Octet structure of a histone; b. X ray crystal structure of nucleosome core particle at 7Å resolution [adapted from Richmond et.al., (1984) Nature, 311, 532]

The DNA double helix entwines round the protein core of the nucleosome on the outside hence forming a tertiary structure. At the binding sites the classical DNA structure is broken down and negatively charged DNA phosphate groups adhere to the positively charged protein beads made up of histones. Recent reports suggest that nucleosomes are the fragments of genetically inactive chromatin (heterochromatin), while the linkers represent the genetically active chromatin (euchromatin). However, the nucleosomes can unfold to adopt a linear form. In the unfolded nucleosomes, chromatin regains its full activity, which is a spectacular demonstration of structural relationship. The whole nucleosome chain containing nonhistone protein and RNA is multiple coiled and is packed in a chromosome as a solenoid.

9.3.3. The bases are genetic information carrier

In 1953 Watson and Crick proposed a model for DNA on the basis of X-ray diffraction data. It is composed of two right handed helices around a central axis. The two strands are anti parallel meaning there 5' and 3' phosphodiester link seen in opposite direction. The bases are stacked inside the helix. The bases of DNA carry genetic information, whereas their sugar and phosphate groups perform a structural role. The strands are typically complementary to each other thus serve as template during replication to each other.

9.3.3.1. The bases are of four kinds

The bases contained on either of helix are complementary to each other and pairs form the stacks (Fig. 9.3 a). The pairing is specific. The base are AGCT; adenine, guanine, cytosine, and thymine. Base pairing is typically pyridine, purine hydrogen bonds based interaction. It was deduced that adenine should pair with thymine where as guanine with cytosine for steric reason and on the basis of hydrogen bond formation as well (Fig. 9.3b).

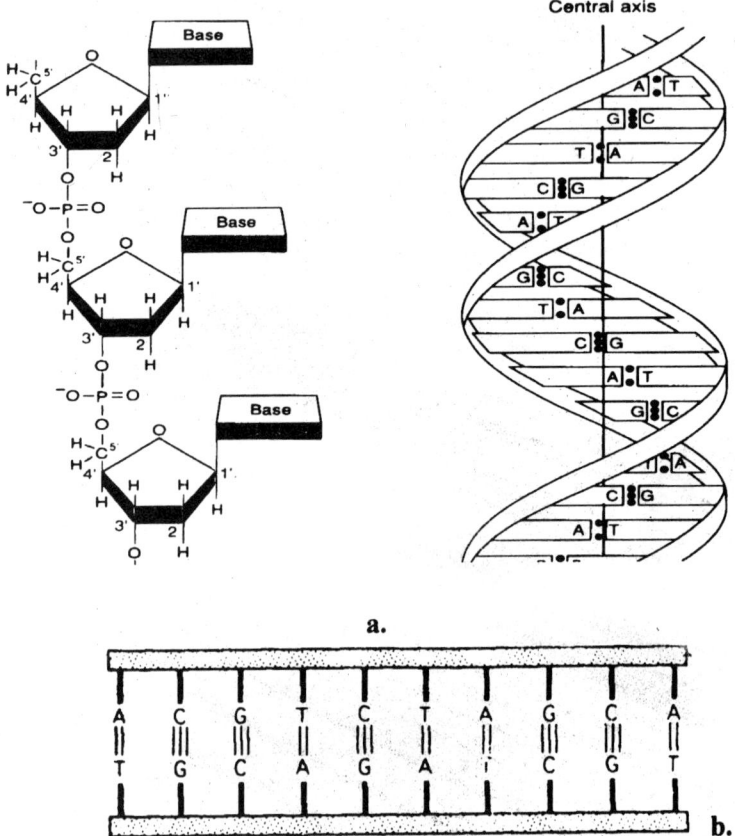

Fig. 9.3 : a.; Structure of DNA b.; Base pairing sequence

It is important to note that two hydrogen bonds are formed between A and T and three between G and C hence G≡C pair is relatively more stable than the A=T pair. The axial sequence along one chain may vary significantly however, it must be complementary on the other chain. During replication the two chains dissociate and each one serves as a template for the synthesis of new complementary strand (chain). This also suggests that the replication of DNA is semiconservative. As one of the strand of each daughter molecule is newly synthesised while other (template) is passed on unchanged from parent DNA molecules. This distribution of parent atom is referred as **semiconservative** (Fig. 9.4).

An interesting character of DNA molecules which occurs naturally is their length. It must be long to encode for all required cellular functional proteins. *E. coli* chromosome is consisted of single DNA molecule has 4 million base pairs. The mass equal to 2.6×10^6 kd length of DNA mole is 14×10^6 Å and diameter 20Å. The largest chromosomes discovered by Brunozimm was of *Drosophila melanogaster* containing single stranded DNA molecules with 6.27×10^7 base pairs, length 2.1 cm.

9.3.3.2. Supercoiled DNA

From many sources the DNA molecules have been observed to be circular. The gene linkage map constructed for *E. coli* gene was circular which suggested its chromosomes shape to be circular which was eventually confirmed. DNA molecules are highly condensed material. All DNA are not necessarily circular. The bacteriophage DNA adapts linear and circular shapes. The linear is traced inside cell where as outside the cell it turns to be circular. Sometimes the axis of circular molecule may be twisted over itself thus forms a **superhelix**. A circular DNA with superhelical configuration is known as **relaxed molecule**.

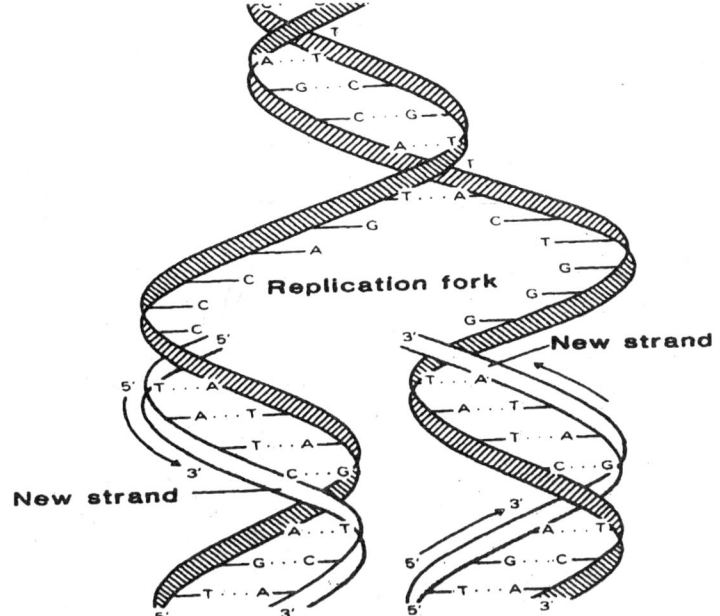

Fig. 9.4 : The semiconservative mode of DNA replication

9.4. REPLICATION OF DNA

DNA replication is continuous on 5'-3' strands while it is discontinuous on 3'-5' strands. DNA polymerase was first isolated in 1958 from *E. coli* by Arthur Kormberg and colleagues. The enzyme catalyses DNA synthesis. It was named polymerase I. There involves interdependent, independent and coordinated events of nearly 20 proteins. DNA-polymerase I is a 103 kD single polypeptide chain capable of step-by-step addition of deoxyribo-nucleotide units to a DNA chain.

$$(DNA)_n + dNTP \longleftrightarrow (DNA)_{n+1} + APP_1$$
dioxyribonucleoside triphosphate

9.4.1. Unwinding is must for replication

It has been indicated as a conclusion of experiment that the bacterial chromosome is circular in appearance. Replication circle appears as Greek letter θ therefore, mode of replication is generally called θ-replication. An important geometric feature of semi-conservative replication could be understood from circularity of replicating molecule. There are nearly 4,70,000 turns in an *E. coli* double helix. Since, two chains of replicating molecules must undergo full rotation to unwinding each of these gyres, some kind of swivel, must be created in order to prevent the tangling of entire structure (Fig. 9.5). The axis of rotation for the process of unwinding is provided by nicks made in the back bone of one of the strands of the double helix during the course of replication. After unwinding each cut is repaired rapidly.

An enzyme that could generate cuts and nicks and repairs them quickly is called **topoisomerase**. The position just adjacent to the cuts or nicks is called **replication origin** and the region where parent strands tend to separate allowing the synthesis of new one (daughter cell) is referred to as **replication fork**. The process responsible for generating new fork is termed as initiation. At one extreme end, initiation does take place at random position; at the other end, the origin is a unique site. This is not always true as in most bacteria, bactriophages and viruses, DNA replication is initiated at a unique origin rather than at random position.

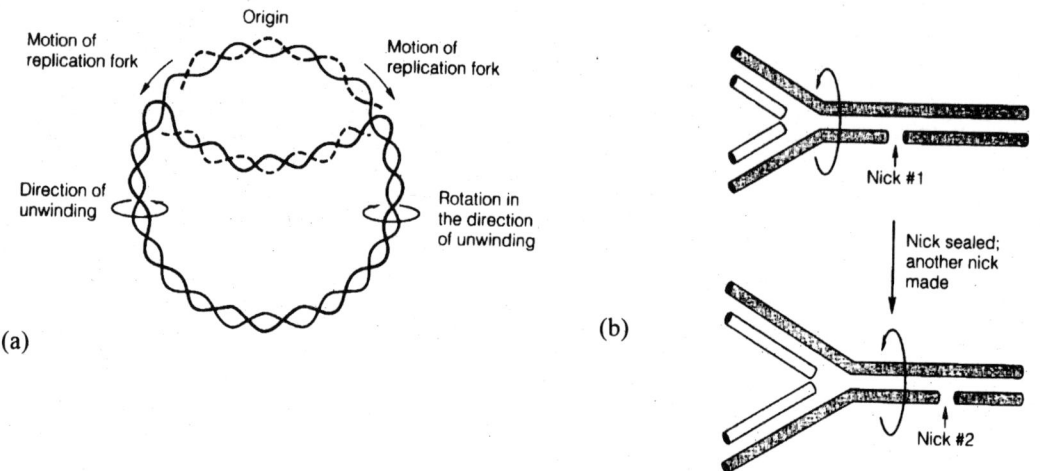

Fig. 9.5 : Replication of a circular DNA molecule: (a) unwinding motion of the branches of a replicating circle; (b) mechanism for breaking (nicked) of a single strand ahead of the replication fork allowing rotation.

9.4.2. DNA contains multiple origin of replication

The eukaryotic DNA is linear molecule that replicates bidirectionally. The replication could be initiated at a time at many sites in DNA. This results into appearance of multiple loops along a DNA molecule. The multi loops replication process reduces the replication time significantly. The replication of an *E. coli* DNA molecule containing about 4.7×10^6 nucleotide pairs takes nearly 40 min. The finding allows as to compute that two replication forks generated at the single origin move at a rate of about 60,000 nucleotide per min. Similarly it has been observed in case of replication of DNA molecules of phages. The moment of replication is found to proceed relatively much slower in DNA molecule in *D. melanogaster* (Fig. 9.6).

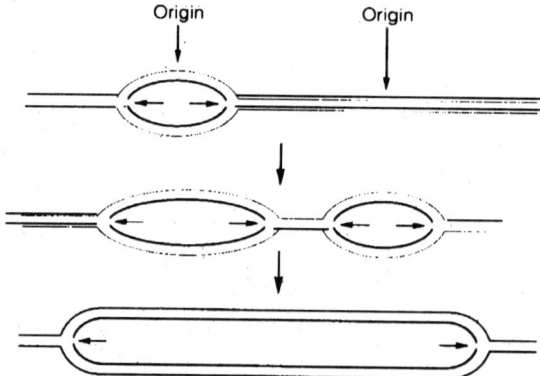

Fig. 9.6 : Schematic representation of loop merging

9.4.3. DNA Polymerase responsible for new DNA strands

The enzyme controlled chemical reactions synthesize the nucleic acids in living cells. DNA polymerases are the enzymes that form the sugar phosphate bond (the phosphodiester bond) between adjacent nucleotides in a nucleic acid chain. A variety of polymerases have been synthesized, isolated and purified then used in the synthesis of DNA in a cell free systems (produced by disturbing cells). The DNA polymerase could catalyze the synthesis of DNA provided:

1. The 5'-triphosphates from the 4-nucleic acids are present. These triphosphates are dATP, dGTP, dTTP, dCTP and their corresponding bases are adenine, guanine, thymine, and cytosine respectively. The triphosphate structures are presented in (Fig. 9.7).
2. Availability of pre-existing single strand of DNA to be replicated should be separated as **template** strand.
3. The primer segment of nucleic acid could be very short. Since, DNA polymerase is not capable of initiating the synthesis, the presence of primer chain with free hydroxyl group (3'-OH) is an absolute requirement.

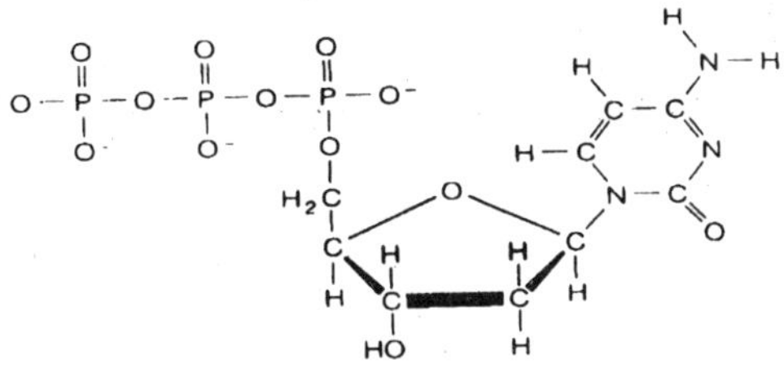

Deoxycytidine 5'-triphosphate

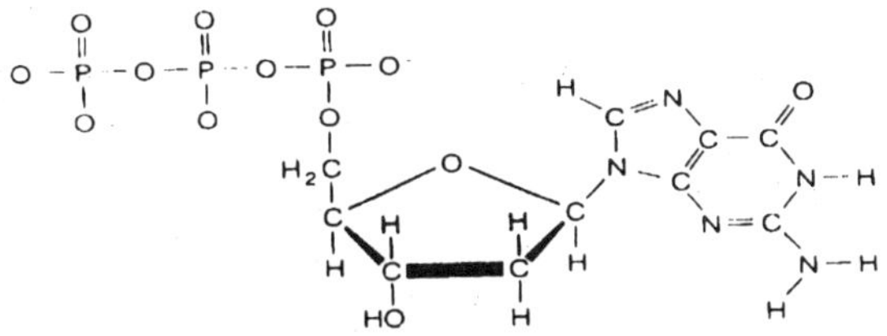

Deoxyguanosine 5'-triphosphate

Fig. 9.7 : Two deoxynucleoside triphosphates used in DNA synthesis

The reaction, the DNA polymerase catalyzes, is the formation of phosphodiester bond between the free priming hydroxyl group of the primer and the inner most phosphate atom of nucleotide triphosphate that is to be incorporated at the position of new primer terminus. Thus, the process can be summarized as DNA synthesis to proceed by the elongation of primer chain always in 5'→3' direction. The recognition of base pair is dependent on the complement nucleotide available in the template chain. The incorporation of nucleotide at the primer terminus is catalyzed by DNA polymerase only when the correct base pair is present. The same DNA polymerase may affect the addition of all the 4-deoxyribonucleoside phosphate to the 3'-OH terminus of growing strand.

Two DNA polymerases have been reported to be needed for DNA replication in *E. coli*. They are named as DNA-*E. coli polymerase I*, often written as *pol I* and DNA polymerase III (*pol III*). Out of these, polymerase III is the major replication enzyme whereas *pol I* plays secondary role. The eukaryotic DNA polymerase responsible for replication of chromosomal DNA is referred as **polymerase-α.** Most of the DNA polymerases are capable of activities like breaking of phosphodiester bond in sugar phosphate back bone. These activities are also known as nuclease activities. The enzyme possessing this activities are of two types.

1. Exonucleases: which remove nucleic acid only from the end of chain.

2. Endonucleases: which break bond within the DNA chain.

In *E. coli* DNA *pol I* and DNA *pol III* act as exonucleases selectively at 3'-terminals. This is referred as a 3'→5' exonuclease activity, which provides for a built in device for correcting rare errors in polymerization. Occasionally, it is possible that polymerase may add an unmatched nucleotide which is not capable of forming correct pair. The presence of such nucleoitide activates 3'→5' exonuclease, which cleaves and removes unwanted unpaired nucleotide from the 3'-OH end of the growing chain. This nuclease activity is known as proof reading which is competent to look back at the distance of one pair. The properties of DNA polymerase that it could initiate the synthesis along the template strand only in 3'→5' direction and secondly, its inability to initiate new chains, impose constraint in replication.

9.4.4. DNA synthesis proceeds in 5'→ 3' direction

About all the known **DNA polymerases** it is true that they can add nucleotide only to the 3'-OH group. Thus if two strands of daughter start growing, it is obvious that each of them needs 3'-OH terminal. However, that two strands of DNA are antiparallal thus, termination in a free 3'-OH group is only possible for one of the growing strands and other must terminate in a free 5' end. This topological reference replication in a single fork, both strands should grow together in 5'→3' direction. The growth along the parental strand should be antiparallel. In order to 5'-3' oriented growth one of the parental strand is replicated in small precursor fragments averaging approximately 2,000 nucleotides. This strand in general is a bottom strand and its synthesis has been initiated only at intervals, which results to cause single stranded region of parental strand to be present on one side of the replication fork. The 3'-OH terminals of continuously replicating strands proceed to be ahead of discontinuous strand hence referred as **leading strand** while former one as **lagging strand** (Fig. 9.8).

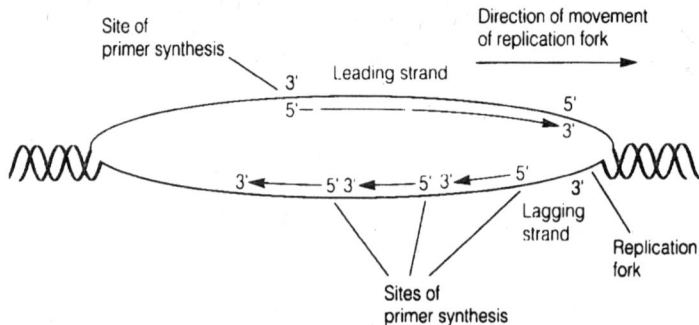

Fig. 9.8 : During DNA replication the leading strand is synthesized as continuous long polynucleotide chain, but the lagging strand, in bottom, is synthesized in short fragments

9.4.5. RNA as an initiator of new DNA strand

Since, DNA polymerases are not capable of initiating synthesis, therefore a free 3'-OH is needed. In most organism special RNA polymerase accomplishes the initiation. RNA is a single strand nucleic acid comprises of four types of nucleosides joined together in 3'→5' direction by phosphodiester bonds. The same bonds as discussed for DNA. In RNA synthesis, a DNA strand serves as template to form complementary strand in which DNA bases paired those which correspond to RNA. The process of complementary RNA strand synthesis is catalyzed by **RNA polymerase**. A synthesis catalyzed by enzyme called RNA polymerase which differs from DNA polymerase in that they can initiate the synthesis of RNA without needing the primer. The elongation of short stretch of RNA initiates the synthesis of DNA usually this counts for 10 to 50 nucleotides length which remains associated with the DNA template while the RNA polymerase dissociates from the DNA. This short stretch of RNA provides a primer over which DNA polymerase can subsequently add deoxy-nucleotides. The DNA primer producing RNA polymerase is called **primase**. Thus, the precursor fragment (Fig. 9.9) during the synthesis of lagging can be depicted by the following structure.

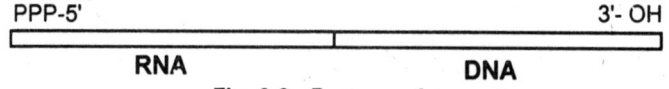

Fig. 9.9 : Precursor fragment

9.4.5.1. Precursor fragment

The precursor fragment finally combined to produce a continuous strand of DNA where no RNA sequence is present. This indicates that assembly of lagging strand must require the selective removal of RNA primer via its replacement by an appropriate DNA sequence. This is performed by DNA polymerase I whereas joining together of fragmented DNA is accomplished by **DNA ligase**. The DNA ligase capable of linking adjacent 3'-OH and 5' phosphate group is present at a nick. The process of fragment combination is depicted in figure 9.10.

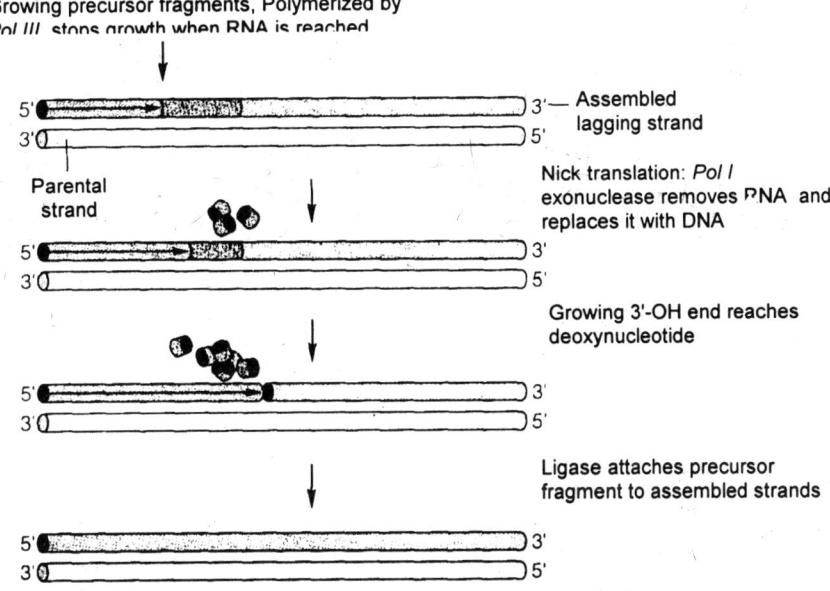

Fig. 9.10 : Sequences of events in joining of the precursor fragments

9.4.5.2. Proteins also participate in DNA replication

DNA replication as discussed is quite complex. During their replication nearly twelve different types of proteins participate in the activity. Polymerase III is an aggregation of nearly 7 polypeptidal chains and the active primer complex include nearly 6 different polypeptides. The replication process in addition to polymerase III complex and primase complex involves at least one type of topoisomerase, proteins which bind and stabilize single stranded combines DNA, the DNA ligase that DNA fragments and polymerase I complex that eliminates RNA primers before lagging strand, fragments joining takes place. The role of some of key enzymes in DNA replication is diagrammatically presented in figure 9.11.

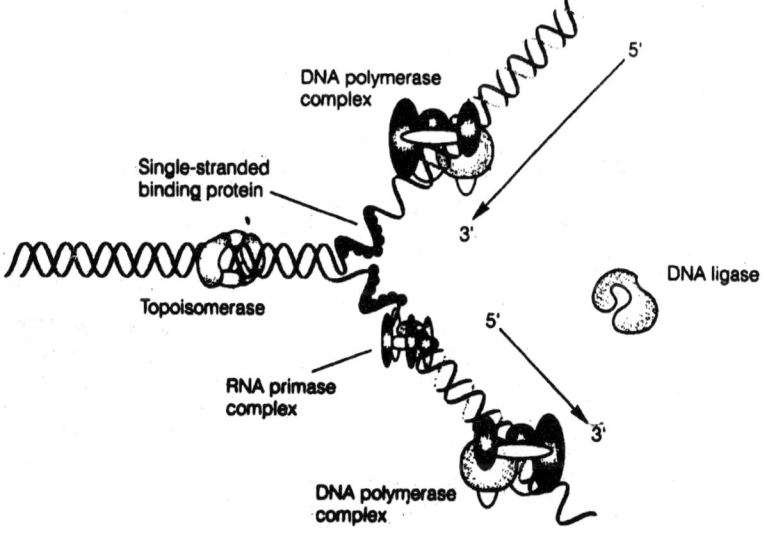

Fig. 9.11 : Role of some enzymes in DNA replication

9.4.5.3. The chemical termination of DNA forms the basis of base sequence determination

If the sequence of bases in a DNA molecule is known a great deal of information about a particular gene fragment could be gathered. Many techniques are available for base sequencing one for the purpose of getting familiar with sequencing technique is being discussed. To obtain the sequence of long stretch of DNA a set of overlapping fragments is constructed and the sequence of bases in each is determined, subsequently all sequences are combined together. The procedure is simple DNA sequences have accumulated at a faster rate. One critical method which is conventionally employed for base sequencing is referred to as di-deoxy sequencing method. It employs synthesis of DNA in the presence of trace amounts of abnormal nucleotides which contain the sugar di-deoxy ribose in place of deoxy ribose (Fig. 9.12)

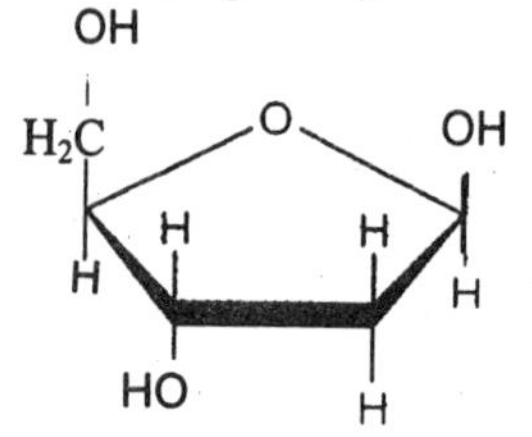

Deoxyribose

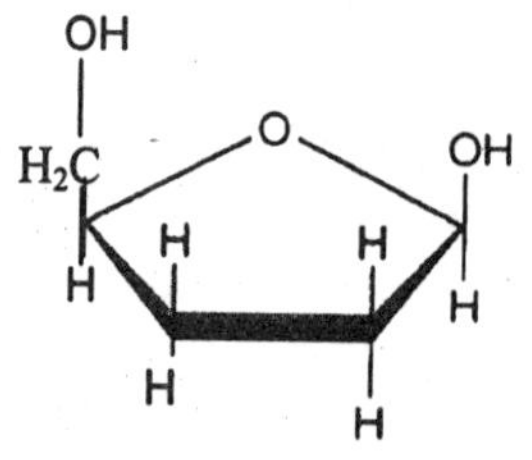

Dideoxyribose

Fig. 9.12 : Structures of normal deoxyribose and dideoxyribose sugars used in DNA sequencing

The sugar lacks the 3'-OH group which is essential for the attachment of the next nucleotide in a growing strand of DNA. Therefore, the incorporation of a di-deoxynucleotide immediately terminates the further synthesis of the strand. The sequence of DNA could be determined using four DNA synthesis reactions each reaction is based on single stranded DNA template that is to be sequenced, a small primer fragment complementary to each stretch of the template, all four deoxyribonucleoside triphosphate and at least one of the nucleosidediphosphate with the di-deoxy sugar form. Each reaction results in a set of newly synthesized DNA fragment that could terminate on random incorporation of di-deoxynucleotide in place of normal deoxy-nucleotide. Thus in each of four reactions the length of each terminated fragment is determined by the position at which polymerase incorporated a di-deoxynucleotide fragment. The gel electrophoresis technique could be utilized for the determination of number of fragments produced and following rule is employed in order to determine the sequence of bases.

If a fragment containing N nucleotides is generated in a reaction carried in the presence of a particular di-deoxynucleotide, then the position N in the newly formed daughter strand is occupied by the base that is present in the di-deoxynucleotide. The numbering is usually done from the 5'-nucleotide of the primer.

In order to exemplify let us consider a case where a 93 base fragment is present in a reaction containing the di-deoxy form of DATP then the 93 base in the daughter generated through DNA synthesis must have adenine (A). Because most native DNA molecules are double stranded therefore it is immaterial whether the sequence of templated strand is determined or that of daughter strand. The sequence of the template strand can be deduced from daughter strand since the strands are complimentary to each other. However, in practice an independent sequence determination is recommended.

9.5. CHEMICAL SYNTHESIS

The role of synthetic chemists in biotechnology has been enlightened with the development of elaborative as well as reliable procedures for chemical synthesis of DNA fragments which could be utilized for construction of long double-stranded DNA of a gene. It is nearly forty years back when Micelson chemically synthesized a simple dinucleotide. However, if the reaction is repeated hundred folds a synthetic DNA could be achieved. This changed, to some extent, when in the late sixties and early seventies the pioneering work of Khorana and associates culminated in the total synthesis of two t-RNA genes. However, Khorana's phosphodiester approach to DNA synthesis was too laborious for most interested groups and only when the modified phosphotriester suggested by the group of Litsinger and associates as well as the phosphoramidite approach described by Caruthers and co-workers, replaced the diester method and the chemical synthesis of DNA became more widely popular and acceptable. Numerous genes have been successfully synthesized and expressed since then.

Numerous strategies have been devised for the chemical synthesis of DNA. A summary of the basic principles involved in the synthesis are presented in table 9.1.

9.5.1. Solid phase method

The best way to synthesize DNA, is by sensible combination of factors listed in table 9.1. However, there is no general answer to the question as to how to obtain synthetic DNA. Most of the DNA syntheses performed now a days are via the phosphotriester or phosphoramidite routes in 3' to 5' direction, and for special requirement of genetic engineering and gene synthesis in particular (small amounts). The synthesis of small oligonucleotides of less than Ca 50 oligonucleotides could be quite conveniently be done with conventional manual procedures, i.e. by using beads as solid support in a syringe or a manual synthesizer. For higher demands reliable auto-synthesizer which are also called as **'gene machines'** could be used. These machines produce, only a crude mixture of short, single-stranded DNA that is chemically modified and biologically dead, they should be classified as 'synthesis machines', 'synthesis automats', 'auto synthesizer' or just the synthesizer. All these systems utilize solid supports in a granulated form (beads, fibers, etc.) placed into a reaction vessel, preferably a column-type. Automation of the synthesizer is then achieved by a suitable solvents and reagent delivery system.

Table 9.1 : Various strategies employed in the synthesis of DNA

Chemistry	Synthesis	Reaction vessel	Phase	Solid phase
diester	5'-3'	flask	homogeneous (on solution)	beads
triester	3'-5'	syringe	heterogeneous (on polymer)	fibers
phosphate (including phosphoramidite)	bireactional	funnel (manual synthesizer column) autosynthesizer column	heterogeneous (on polymer)	segmental supports - filters; distinct column segment or membranes filled with beads or fibers

9.5.1.1. Process overview

Similar to the polypeptides the DNA strands could be synthesized by sequential addition of activated monomers to a growing chain which is linked to a solid (insoluble support). Protonated doeoxyribonucleoside-3'-phosphor-amidites are used as activated monomers. The process is initiated by 3'-phosphorus atom of incoming unit that joins at 5'-oxygen of growing chain to form a phosphite triester. The 5'-OH of activated primer remains unreactive as it is protected by dimethoxytrityl (DMT) protecting group. Similarly the amino groups of purines and pyrimidines are also protected and anhydrous conditions are maintained throughout. In the second step the phosphite triester is oxidized by iodine to form a phosphotriester containing pentavalent (P). Further the DMT protecting group is removed from 5'-OH of the growing chain utilizing dichloroacetic acid. The DNA chain now is elongated by one unit and is ready for another cycle. The scheme is presented in figure 9.13. Each addition cycle takes nearly 10 min. for completion and elongates more than 98% of the chains.

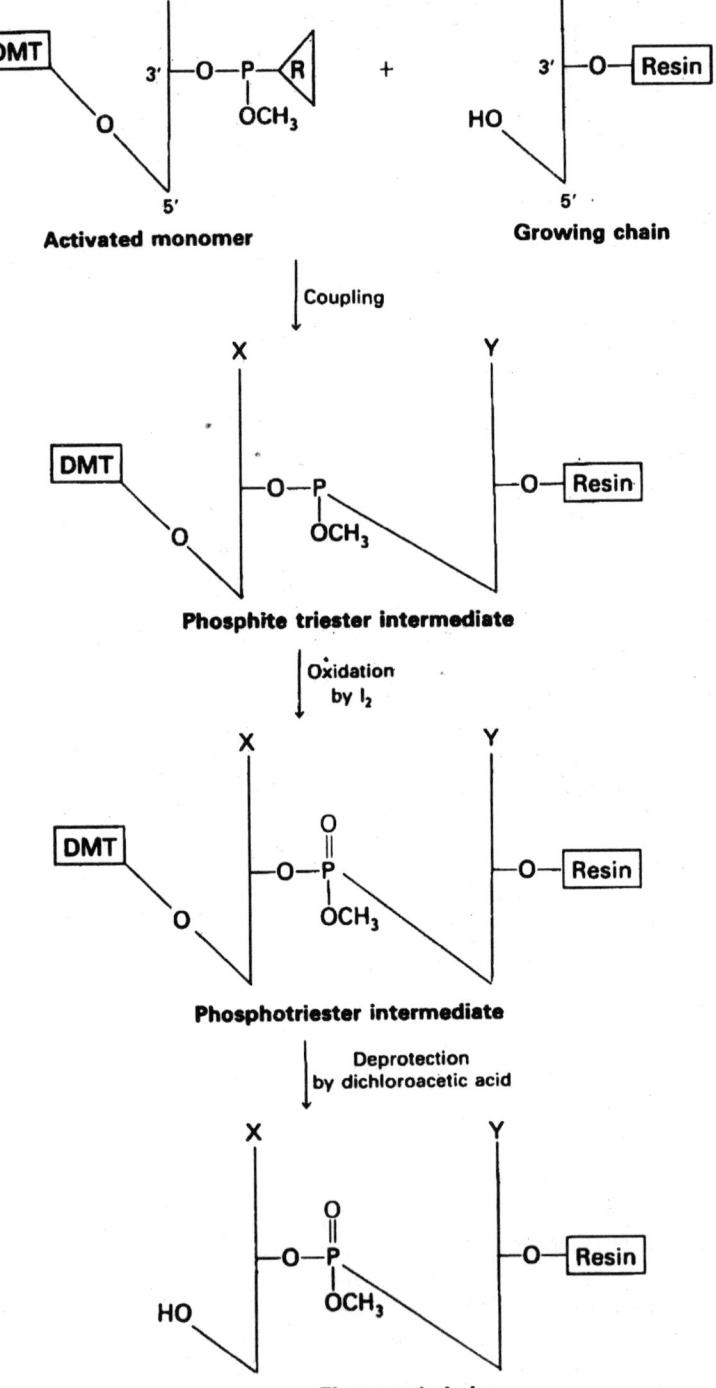

Fig. 9.13 : Schematic presentation of solid phase DNA synthesis

The solid phase approach is the idealistic one for DNA synthesis as it is desired that the product should remain immobilized on the insoluble support until it is finally released. All the reactions occur in a single vessel, and excess soluble reagents could be drained off. Glass beads are generally used as solid supports. After assembly of the desired DNA chain, the methyl group protecting the phosphates are removed by addition of throphenol. The DNA strands are then released from the glass beads by the cleavage of the ester bonds between 3'-OH of the terminal nucleoside and the resin that links it to the glass support using ammonium hydroxide. The base protection imparted by benzoyl and isobutyryl groups is finally withdrawn by heating the DNA in ammonium hydroxide. The sample could then be purified using HPLC and PAGE. The steps involved in the release and purification of the elongated oligonucleotides are schematically presented in figure 9.14.

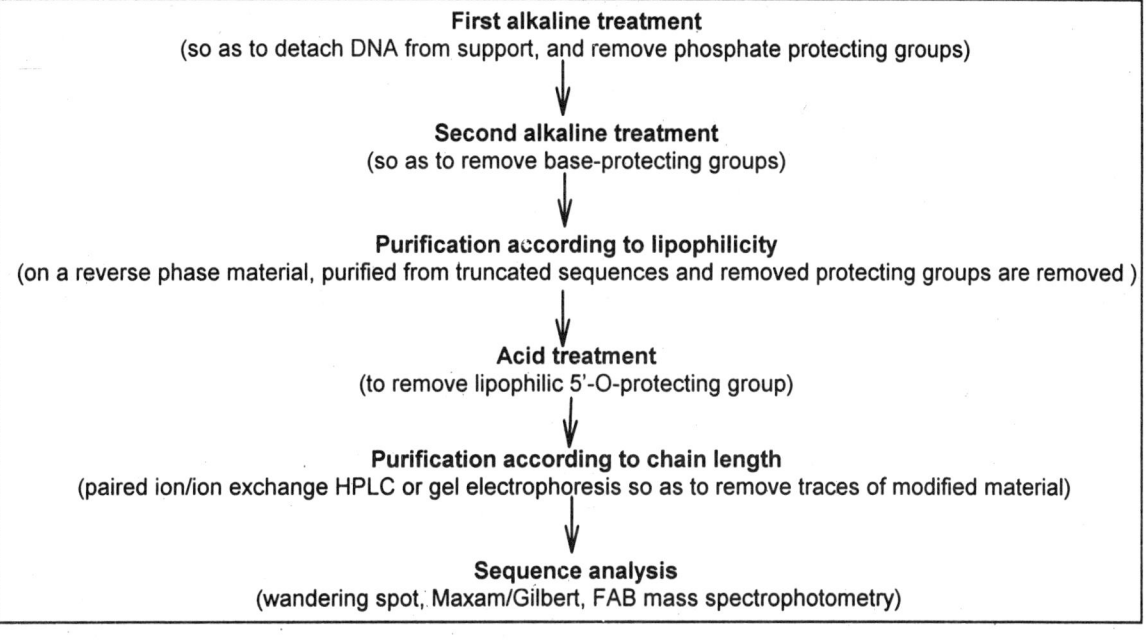

First alkaline treatment
(so as to detach DNA from support, and remove phosphate protecting groups)

Second alkaline treatment
(so as to remove base-protecting groups)

Purification according to lipophilicity
(on a reverse phase material, purified from truncated sequences and removed protecting groups are removed)

Acid treatment
(to remove lipophilic 5'-O-protecting group)

Purification according to chain length
(paired ion/ion exchange HPLC or gel electrophoresis so as to remove traces of modified material)

Sequence analysis
(wandering spot, Maxam/Gilbert, FAB mass spectrophotometry)

Fig. 9.14 : Schematic representation of the most popular chemical method for the DNA synthesis

The introduction of β-cyanoethylphosphoramide and the use of additional base-protecting groups on T and G in the phosphotriester approach allows the utilization of ammonia as the only alkaline deprotection reagent. Chain scission by nucleophilic attack on OH- of phosphorus group is apparently no longer a practical problem, at least in the case of shorter oligonucleotides.

9.5.2. Transcription methods

In some of the synthetic procedures the processes of first deprotection and then subsequently purification of oligonucleotides using polyacrylamide-gel electrophoresis (PAGE) are followed. The method offers the advantage of purification of small quantities, and many samples could be worked up simultaneously on a slab gel. The major disadvantages include the isomers, base-modified sequence, and other impurities which may be formed during chemical synthesis and which could subsequently cause higher rates of false sequence generation during cloning. The exact chemical analysis of the synthesized oligonucleotide is not possible due to the reason that:

1. classical techniques such as elemental analysis and NMR cannot reveal the exact structure of the oligonucleotide.
2. other techniques, such as two-dimensional wandering spot or Maxam/Gilbert-type, chemical degradation sequencing methods are sometimes considered too much time consuming whereas the 'Fast-Atom-Bombardment' mass spectrometry (FAB-Mas) is limited to the oligonucleotides up to thirteen bases in length.

9.6. SPECIAL CHARACTERS OF A DNA

9.6.1. DNA strands can be separated and annealed

DNA molecules have a very important characteristic that owing to helix preservation brought about by weak interaction involving hydrogen bonds and hydrophobic interactions the two strands could possibly be separated by heat treatment or on exposure to alkaline pH. This separation of DNA strands is known as **melting or denaturation** of DNA. The G≡C pair requires more heat as compared to A=T to destabilize the bonds hence melting point of DNA is dependent on the TA/GC ratio.

On cooling following the denaturation, the complementary strands base-pairs and native configuration are restored. The process of restoration of configuration is referred to as renaturation or more frequently annealing. The property established very important base for experimentation, manipulation and engineering of a gene or DNA of our interest. The process of annealing is again dependent on the size of genome, i.e. larger the size relatively more time is taken for annealing. This provides for opportunities to discover repeated sequences in eukaryotic DNA employing repetitive process of melting and annealing.

9.6.2. Hybridization and annealing

The destabilized or separated DNA strands can be stabilized and annealed by complementary RNA. The annealing with RNA molecule having complementary bases to pair with single stranded DNA is called hybrid annealing in which one strand of DNA and other of RNA constitute a hybrid molecule.

Molecular hybridization is a significant method used in the characterization of RNAs. Since the complementary nature is the basis of hybridization a RNA will only hybridize to a DNA from which it was transcribed. Thus the hybridization provides principle on which loaded probes are based. Further denaturation under controlled conditions is used to generate or construct physical map of DNA.

The process of controlled denaturation is referred to as 'Partial Denaturation Mapping'. Partial denaturation is based on the fact that A=T could be dilated using EM as single stranded loops and therefore enables for the measurement of length from loop to the end of DNA molecule.

9.7. RNAs : CLASSES OF CODES AND CONFORMATIONS

Structurally RNA molecules are similar to DNAs except for deoxyribose pentose sugar which is substituted by ribose and out of four bases, base thymine is replaced by uracil. This is important to remember that in cases of RNAs the Chargaff's rules is not applied since RNA molecules consist of only one chain (strand).

9.7.1. Major classes of RNA

Messenger RNA (mRNA), transfer RNA (tRNA) and ribosomal RNA (rRNA), all are essentially involved in the synthesis of protein(s). mRNA carries the transcribed genetic information copied from DNA segment (genes). The information contained in mRNA molecule decides the sequence of amino acid in a protein where as tRNA helps to identify and transport amino acids to ribosomes. The ribosome provides for a molecular scaffold for chemical anchoring of amino acid in a defined sequence.

Though the RNA molecule has a single polynucleotide chain yet it is not a simple construction. Its molecule has extensive region of complement thus hydrogen bonds between GC and AU are formed, as a result molecule folds over itself, forming structure called hair pin loops (Fig. 9.15). Thus it appears like DNA helical structure.

9.6.1.1. tRNA

Transfer RNA or tRNA the molecule actively engaged in protein synthesis is typically 'clover leaf' like in shape due to intrachain pairing of complementary nucleotides in certain region of the tRNA chain. Figure 9.16 presents the structural components of tRNA. Structurally a tRNA molecule could be distinguished consisting of fine distinctive regions.

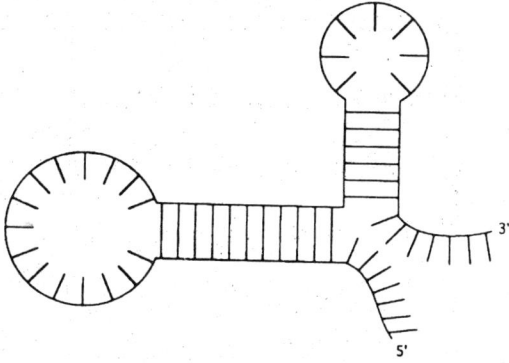

Fig. 9.15 : Structure of RNA

Acceptor region or end terminus region: It consists of four linearly associated nucleotides, of them 3 with the same sequence, i.e. CCA. The 3'-OH hydroxyl group of adenosine is free which subserves as a reaction site for the addition of carboxyl group of amino acids. The amino acid so bound with 3'-OH group of adenosine is transported by tRNA to the ribosome(s) to participate in protein synthesis.

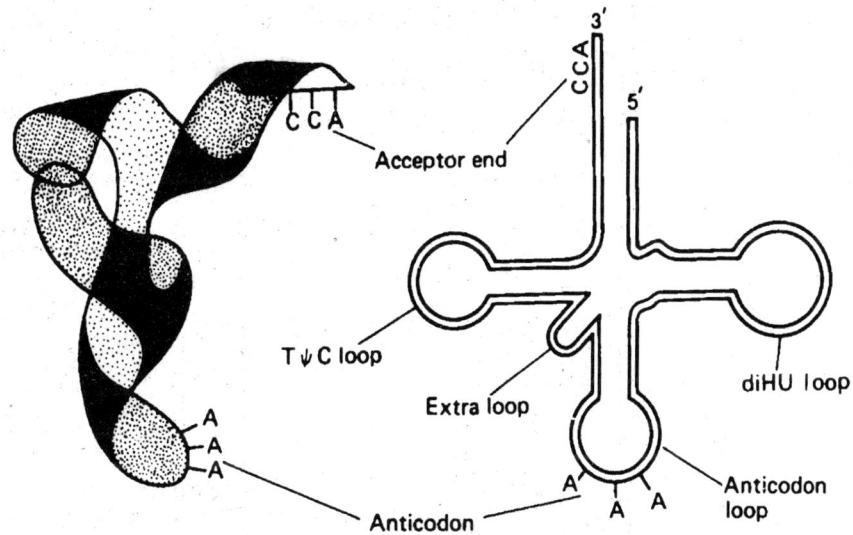

Fig. 9.16 : Secondary (L) and tertiary (R) structure of tRNA

Anticodon loop: It is commonly based on nucleotides with a triplet, specific for each tRNA and referred to as anticodon. tRNA via complementary pairing anchors to the codon of mRNA (Fig. 9.17). This interaction decides about the order of amino acids on polypeptidal chain during assemblage in the ribosomes.

Thymine-pseudouracil loop: It consists of seven nucleotides, with obligatory permanence of pseudouridine residues. It is presumed that pseudouracil involves in binding of tRNA to the ribosome.

Dihydrouridine or DHU loop: It usually consists of nucleotides 8-12 in number among which several DHU residues are necessarily included. DHU residue selectively binds amino-acyl tRNA synthatase, the latter participates in the recognition of an amino acid via its cogeneric tRNA.

Extra loop: An extra loop may be present which varies in shape and nucleotides content and composition from tRNA to tRNA.

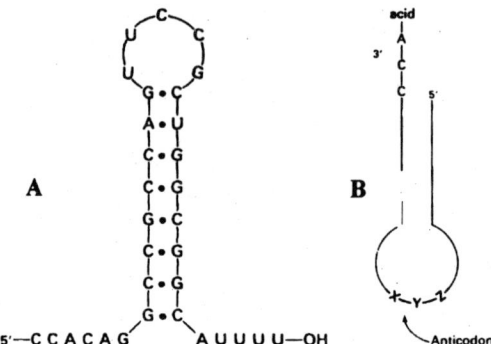

Fig. 9.17 : A. Base sequence of the 3' end of an mRNA;
B. Diagrammatic presentation of an aminoacyl tRNA

9.7.2. RNA and their synthesis

The chemical synthesis of RNA is similar to that utilized for DNA, yet there are some differences as outlined bellow:

1. The RNA molecule produced in transcription derived from a single strand of DNA, and in a DNA in a particular region, only one strand serves as a template for RNA synthesis.

2. The four riboneculeosides 5'-tri phosphate namely adenosine triphosphate (ATP), guanosine triphosphate (GTP) cytidine triphosphate (CTP), and uridine triphosphate (UTP) are used as precursors in the synthesis of RNA. Furthermore, ribose sugar replaces deoxy ribose sugar of RNA and the base urosine replaces thymine (T).

3. The sequence of the DNA template determines the sequence of the RNA strand. Each base added to the growing end of the RNA chain is chosen on the basis of its ability and affinity after the base with which it has to pair.

4. A sugar phosphate bond is formed between 3'- OH group of 1 nucleotide and 5'-triphosphate group of the next nucleotide in line (Fig. 9.18) The nature of the chemical bond remains to be the same as it is in the case of DNA however, the enzyme which brings about ligation is different and named as RNA polymerase rather than DNA polymerase.

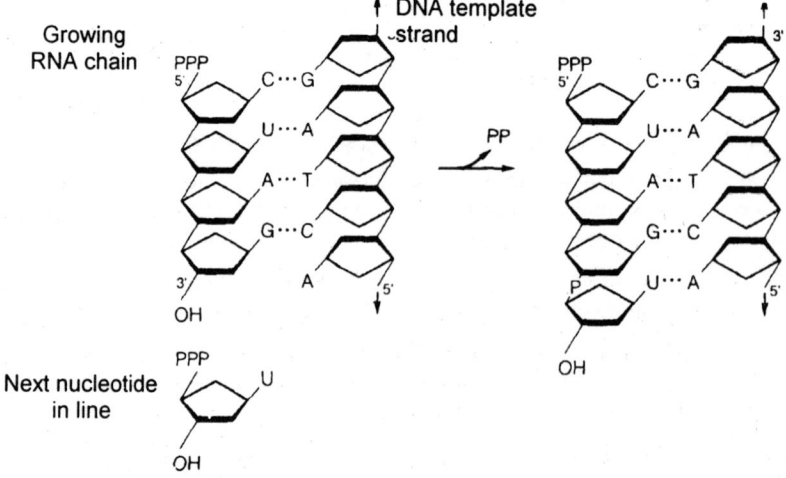

Fig. 9.18 : Polymerization step in RNA synthesis

5. The RNA polymerase can initiate chain growth without a primer.
6. Neucleotides are added only to 3'-OH end of the growing chain. As a result the end 5' of RNA molecule invariably bears a triphosphate group.

The strand of DNA to be transcribed is decided by RNA polymerase. But question arises how does it do so?. How does it recognize the point at which transcription should begin and at what point it should stop?. The overall transcription process involves four discrete stages.

1. **Promoter recognition :** The RNA polymerase selectively binds to DNA at the sites where the DNA has a particular base sequence called promoter. Typical promoters are from 20-200 bases long. Most promoters have certain sequence motifs in common. The strength of the binding of RNA polymerase to different promoters varies greatly, which causes differences in the extent of expression from one gene to another.
2. **Chain initiation :** After the initial binding step, RNA polymerase initiates RNA synthesis at a nearby transcription site. The first nucleoside triphosphate at the site, and the next nucleotide in line is attached to 3' carbon of the ribose, and so forth. Only one of the DNA strands serves as the template for transcription.
3. **Chain elongation :** After the chain initiation, RNA polymerase moves along the DNA template strand, adding nucleotide to the growing RNA chain (Fig. 9.19). Each new nucleotide is added to the 3' end of the chain, and so RNA chains resembles DNA chains in growing in the 5'→3' direction

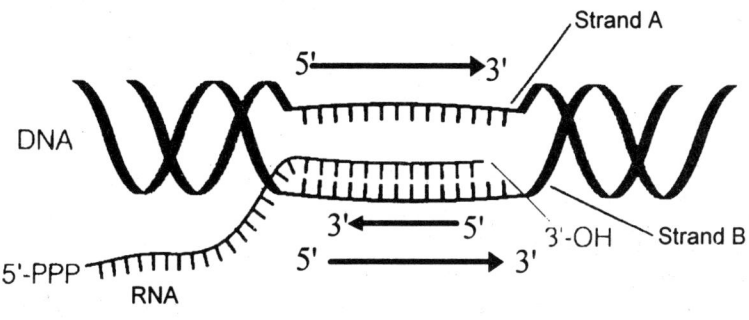

Direction of transcription

Fig. 9.19 : Schematic representation of RNA synthesis

4. **Chain termination :** When the RNA polymerase reaches a transcription-termination sequence in the DNA, the polymerase enzyme dissociates from the DNA and the newly synthesized RNA molecule is released. Two types of termination events are known. Firstly, those that are self terminating and depend only on the transcription-termination sequence in the DNA and secondly, those that require the presence of a termination protein in addition to the transcription-termination sequence. Self termination is the usual case and takes place when the polymerase encounters a particular sequence of bases in the template strand that causes the polymerase to stop.

These stages are dealt in detail under the title protein synthesis emphasizing the significance of various components which play critical role in overall functioning of RNA in the translation of its codes into the protein.

9.7.3. Reverse transcription can copy RNA as cDNA

The source of genetic information is DNA. The DNA contained information is carried by mRNA which subsequently is translated in to the proteins. However, there are instances where RNA is copied into a complementary DNAs by the process **'dubbed' reverse transcription** with the help of enzyme **reverse transcriptase**. This mechanism is used by retroviruses including HIV virus which contains RNA as genetic material. The latter reverse transcribes its DNA which is incorporated or integrated into the genome of the infected host cells. The enzyme reverse transcriptase is an important tool in recombinant (rDNA) technology, particularly in the development of complementary cDNAs (Fig. 9.20) discussed in chapter 10.

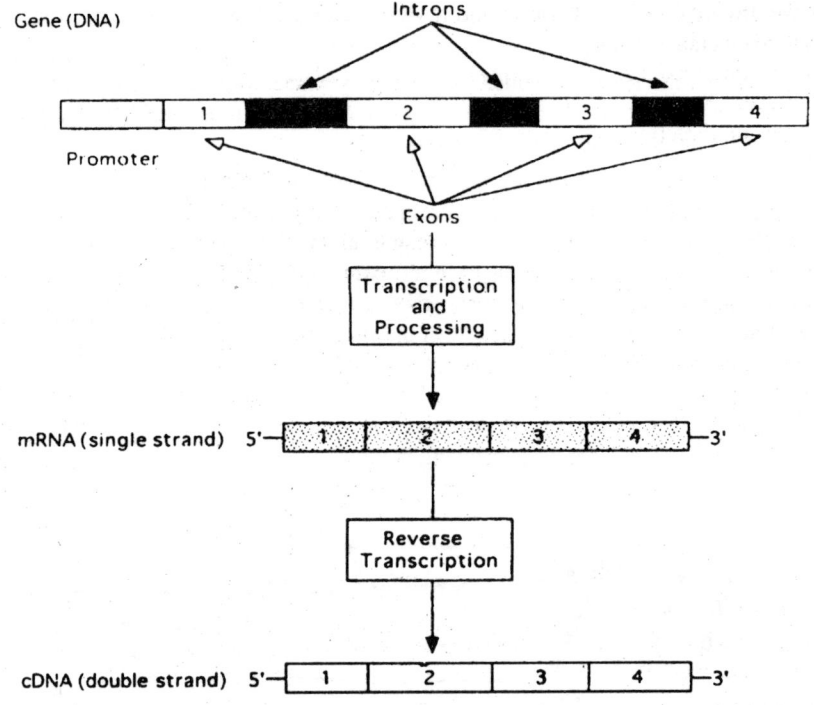

Fig. 9.20 : Relation between a gene; its mRNA and its cDNA

A copy of mRNA is transcribed in the DNA form using **reverse transcriptase** (Fig. 9.21). The cDNA differs from gene counterpart in lacking all the introns. Since mRNAs are highly unstable molecules susceptible to degradation during isolation and storage. The availability of cDNA thus permits the manipulation of coding sequence. However, the process of modification, manipulation is relatively less cumbersome.

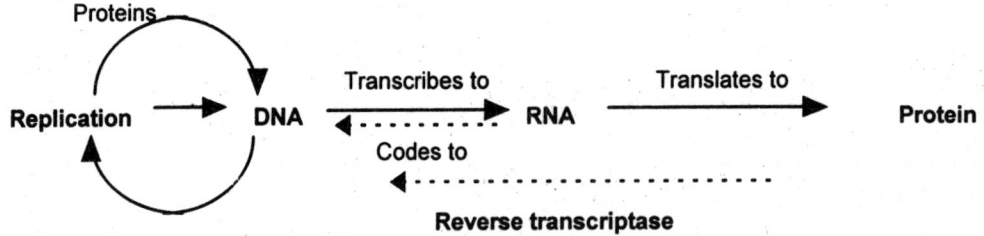

Fig. 9.21 : Transport of genetic information

9.8. GENETIC CODE AND ENGINEERING

Deoxyribonucleic acid (DNA) is a genetic material contained in cells that carry information in the form of codes from cell to cell and parent to offspring. In activated form the information from a gene is copied first into another nucleic acid, referred to as massenger RNA (mRNA) which in turn directs the production of the respective ultimate proteins.

Thus, genetic information are perpetuated through three steps:

1. replication of the DNA and its genetic information by template mechanism;
2. transcription of this genetic information into RNA molecules; and
3. translation of the information involving amino acids in the form of proteins or enzymes.

Thus in molecular biology the word transcription is referred for mRNA synthesis while translation as a synonym for protein synthesis. Transcription is sometimes reversed, means RNA could work as a template to generate back DNA or intermediates. This process is referred as **'reverse transcription'** which may operate in the case of RNA viruses (Retrovirus). Translation of transcribed (RNA contained) information in the form of various proteins is an unidirectional process. It is pertinent to know how DNA codes that information for proteins (which are merely based on sequencing of 20 amino acids).

9.8.1. The genetic code

T.H. Morgen, E.B. Wilson and other suggested in 1910, that the mechanism of hereditary could be related to chromosomal behavior and therefore to the genes contained in them. In 1924 Feulgen showed that the chromosomes contain DNA. Later it was noted that the eukaryotic cells have a constant DNA load which drew attention towards its possible pivotal role in heredity.

Most of the genes code for the proteins. As a principle one gene codes for one polypeptide chain however, some genes only code for RNA such as ribosomal and transfer RNA, hence RNAs are gene expression products.

9.8.1.1. Three nucleotide code for one amino acid : The codon

A genetic unit consisted of 3 nucleotide(s) or a triplet, codes for one amino acid. The information is transformed into the messenger RNA (transcription) which has sequences of nucleotides and nucleotide triplet complementary to DNA from which it is copied. Thus a four letter code is translated into one of 20 amino acids. The code is decoded and read as a group of three bases. Each such triplet corresponds to one amino acid.

By application of permutation process for 4 bases, $4^3 = 64$ various combinations of nucleotides are possible which could code 24 amino acids (Table 9.2). The length of coding portion is dependent on the length of message to be transferred, i.e. number of amino acids required for the sequencing for the synthesis of a peptide/protein. Thus a sequence of 1500 nucleotides shall code for 500 amino acids. The initial amino acid and respective codon decides the starting point. The sequence of the triplet decides the sequence of amino acids in a protein.

Table 9.2 : The genetic code

First position (5'end)		Second Position				Third position (3' end)
		U	C	A	G	
		Phe	Ser	Tyr	Cys	U
U		Phe	Ser	Tyr	Cys	C
		Leu	Ser	Stop	Stop	A
		Leu	Ser	Stop	Trp	G
		Leu	Pro	His	Arg	U
		Leu	Pro	His	Arg	C
C		Leu	Pro	Gln	Arg	A
		Leu	Pro	Gln	Arg	G
		Ile	Thr	Asn	Ser	U
		Ile	Thr	Asn	Ser	C
A		Ile	Thr	Lys	Arg	A
		Met	Thr	Lys	Arg	G
		Val	Ala	Asp	Gly	U
		Val	Ala	Asp	Gly	C
G		Val	Ala	Glu	Gly	A
		Val	Ala	Glu	Gly	G

Amino acid by itself cannot recognize and get connected to its respective codon. It requires an adapter unit for the union which is referred as tRNA (transfer RNA). The latter typically has an amino acid attachment site and another for the recognition of the triplet (codon) in mRNA. This site is referred to as anticodon and its bases pair with codon of mRNA. The translation of the message into proteins occurs in the ribosomes.

9.8.1.2. Deciphering the genetic code

In 1961 when Nirenberg and Mattaci discovered that synthetic polyribonucleotides used as a mRNA stimulate incorporation of amino acids into polypeptide in cell free protein synthesizing system, first RNA used was poly-ribonucleotide (Poly U) in the synthesis of polyphenyl alanine. This concluded that a codon for phenyl alanine is a uridine base (UUU) and this was the first code deciphered.

The cell free protein synthesis system was critically an extract from E. coli from which cell wall was removed by centrifugation. It contained **ribosomes, tRNAs,** synthetase and others required for protein synthesis. The **mRNAs** from *E. coli* are degraded by incubation of extract at 37°C for a few minutes. Poly A stimulated the uptake of lysine (codon AAA) and poly C of proline (codon CCC) in the presence of ATP, GTP and amino acids. Trichloroacetic acid was used for the termination of reaction and to precipitate the proteins. The especial feature of **cell free** protein synthesizer is that synthesis can be halted by the addition of *deoxyribo-nuclease* which destroys the template. The synthesis however could be resumed on addition of a crude fraction of mRNA. The designed system reported to be mRNA responsive.

9.8.1.3. Genetic code and degeneracy

All possible 64 codons are deciphered out of which 61 codons exclusively correspond to amino acids and three represent signal for termination. Since number of amino acid is 20 whereas triplets are several obviously more than one triplet can code for a amino acid. This is referred to as **degeneracy of genetic code**. For example proline is coded by CCD, CCA, CCG, CCC. It is important to notice that invariably in every combination /a codon triplet varies for base at third position, and first two are common and considered to be most important in coding. As a consequence mutation that changes third base goes unnoticed. These mutations may not change amino acid sequence in protein hence termed as **silent mutations**. DNA sequencing studies reveal that almost all possible base combinations (64) are utilized *in vivo*. This minimizes the effect of harmful mutations. Further, it could be realized, rather may prompt a question; Is each codon recognized by a tRNA? Infact they are less in number than number of codon (64). Thus a tRNA could recognize more than one codon (triplet). This may presumably be due to the base that pairs with the third base of the codon (the one which is less important in coding). Genes have to some extent a degree of wobbling, i.e. some movement that allows base to establish hydrogen bond other than the normal complementary.

9.9. MUTATION

As codons on DNA determine the amino acid incorporated into a protein hence change in codons sequence therefore results into change in primary sequence of the protein product. The change in regulatory regions of DNA which are not transcribed or translated can also influence the level, onset of initiation and location of protein expression. Change in DNA so incorporated if not corrected via DNA repairing system of the cell, the altered/mutated gene becomes incorporated into the genome and passed onto generation, i.e. descendants of the mutated cells. The high rate of fidelity replication process minimizes the degree of mutation of DNA in natural course.

An AUG codon representing methionine in protein subjected to single base changes. The various possible mutations are illustrated in table 9.3.

Mutation as such occurs in a randomized way rather spontaneous and is a main cause of genetic disorders and of inherited diseases. The heritable diseases including sickle cell anemia, β-thalassaemia, phenylketonuria and others are caused due to be single base substitution/mutation in DNA encoding for a single protein. Similarly diseases like Alzheimer's, cancer, cystic fibrosis, etc. are the components of genetic disorders brought about by mutations.

Table 9.3 : The effect of genetic mutation on protein expression

Deletion or insertion of a larger number of bases moves the reading frame as shown above
except that a number of amino acids will be removed or added respectively

Correct DNA sequence and protein

!Start									Stop!		
AAT	CCC	ATG	TTA	TGG	TGG	TGG	CTT	TGG	TAA	AAA	TTT
---	---	Met	Leu	Trp	Trp	Trp	leu	Trp	TER	---	---

Point mutation

1. Amino acid change ('missense' mutation)

***	***	***	***	***	TGT	***	***	***	***	***	***
---	---	+++	+++	+++	Cys	+++	+++	+++	+++	---	---

2. No change due to degeneracy: 'DNA polymorphism'

***	***	***	***	***	***	***	CTG	***	***	***	***
---	---	+++	+++	+++	+++	+++	Leu	+++	+++	---	---

3. Early termination ('nonsense' mutation)

***	***	***	TAA	***	***	***	***	***	***	***	***
			TER								

Deletions and insertions

1. Single base insertion:

AAT	CCC	ATC	TTA	ATC	CTC	CTC	CCT	TTC	CTA	AAA	ATT	T??
---	---	Met	Leu	Met	Val	Val	Ala	Leu	Val	Lys	Ile	???

2. Single base deletion:

AAT	CCC	ATG	TTA	TGG	TGT	GGC	TTT	GGT	AAA	AAT	TT?
---	---	Met	Leu	Trp	Cys	Gly	Phe	Gly	Lys	Asn	???

The direction of translation of mRNA and RNAs is 5'→3'. The assembling of polypeptidal chains is sequential starting from the end bearing NH_2 terminus. The starting signal of a protein synthesis, AUG codon has dual function. During initiation it codes for N-formyl methionine whereas in any other position it codes for **normal methionine** (met). The tRNAs for methionine are different. However, in *in-vitro* the initiation codon AUG is not a prime requisite. The termination signal is provided by the codon UAG, UAA or UGA as the ribsosome reaches the termination end of mRNA, the synthesized polypeptidal chain is released. These codons unlike others are not recognized by tRNAs but are recognized by a special protein that is referred to as **releasing protein**.

9.10. MOLECULAR BASIS OF TRANSCRIPTION AND PROTEIN SYNTHESIS

9.10.1. Functional organization

During the active phase of mature cells only a portion of genetic information encoded in the chromatin DNA is used in the transcription as RNA copies. The portion of inactive DNA that makes a part of globular nucleosome of euchromatin is a tightly coiled material which is not capable of transcription. The active portion is an unfolded **linear** nucleosome of heterochromatin which is the actual site of RNA synthesis. In prokaryotes and eukaryotes DNA is an elementary transcription unit and the position which liable for transcription is called transcription. In case of prokaryotic it is referred to as '**operons**'. The transcription length ranges form 300 to 10^8 nucleotides. Transcription is consisted of functionally different **segment** identified to as *informative* and *non-informative.* The informative segment includes structural *cystrons* or *genes*, which carry information about polypeptide chain or non template RNAs like rRNA, tRNA and other RNAs, whereas noninformative section contains nongenetic information and relatively longer than informative transcription section. It has come as a surprise that structural genes could be *continuous* or *discontinuous*, rather interrupted. In many of structural genes especially in the case of eukaryotic the genetic information is recorded in an *intermittent* mode and the section of structural gene that carries information is called **'exons'** while those that carry none are referred to as **'introns'**. In the chromosomal DNA mobile genes or **'transposones'** have been identified which are discrete genetic units that may be transferred from one cell to another and could get inserted into any of multiple sites in the recipient cells DNA. Migration of 'transposones' can be attributed to reverse transcription wherein transcript of mobile gene is generated and used as a template for the insertion of DNA transcript at any other site of chromosome. The exact function of these jumping genes still remains to be explored. It is known, however, that they are capable of producing rearrangements in genome and can effectively bring about functional changes in DNA regions into which they are incorporated. A classical example is the insertion of mobile genes in the vicintity to an 'oncogene', i.e. region of DNA which could induce transformation of normal cell to a tumoral one. and activate oncogene function resulting into tumoral degeneration of tissues. Schematically a functional organization involved in transcription in eukaryotes is presented in figure 9.22.

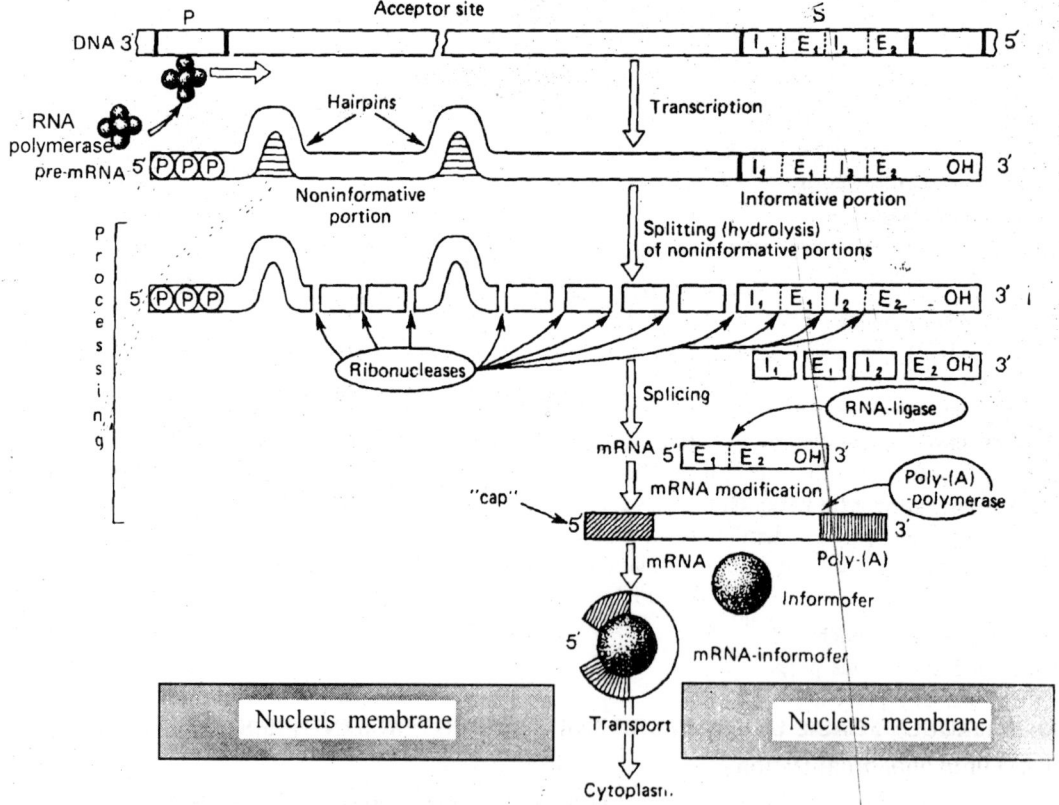

Fig. 9.22 : Schematic representation for transcription and post transcriptional processes in the eukaryotic nucleus

Transcription starts with the involvement of gene portion known as promoter. The transcription enzyme **RNA polymerase** and facilitating proteins are anchored to the promoter from the medium. Next promoter section is the operator of DNA that is capable of binding proteins where the latter acts as transcription regulators. In prokaryotes, these regulations are also termed as repressor. In eukaryotic DNA the transcription section adjacent to promoter is known as **acceptor** or **regulatory** site, which interacts with regulator thus influencing the process of transcription. In the accepted site itself there is a DNA fragment referred to as the enhancer. It facilitates the transcription under coordinated involvement of RNA polymerase.

Structural **cystrons** or **genes** that contain alternating intron and exon regions one adjacent to operator is the acceptor site. A transcription may contain one structure cystron or several and accordingly may be referred to as *mono cystron transcription* or *multi cystron transcription* respectively. At the transcription end invariably every cystron contains a nucleotide sequence which signals for termination of transcription, therefore it is called terminator.

The transcript in the form of RNA is a complementary copy of transcription encoded and extended in a gene from promoter to the terminator end. The various conditions favorable for transcription to proceed are;

1. the DNA section to be transcribed must be untwisted to allow the formation of single-stranded template. Only one DNA strand can serve as a template for RNA synthesis; if both DNA strands are used as a template, then two complementary RNAs carrying information for different proteins would be synthesized during a single transcription;
2. availability of ribonucleoside triphosphates (ATP, GTP, UTP and CTP) for RNA synthesis;
3. availability of a special transcription enzyme, DNA-dependent RNA polymerase, which deforms RNA synthesis on the DNA template.

9.10.2. Mechanism of transcription

The DNA dependent RNA polymerase becomes bound to the DNA promoter sequence which has high affinity to polymerase. The enzyme catalyzes formation of phosphodiester bonds between RNA nucleotides using its core enzyme segment consisted of 4 subunits while the 5th subunit called σ factor can be detached from core enzyme and capable of selecting the site for the transcription by binding with promoter. Thus having been specified by σ factor the coenzymes is added to its α factor and initiates the transcription. It is believed that the separation of DNA strands is brought about by the action of RNA polymerase.

Eukaryotes have polymerases of three kinds namely polymerase I, II and III. These are protein units differing in transcription specificity. Polymerase I is responsible for transcription of rRNA proteins or genes while polymerase III for transcription of tRNA. Polymerase II participates in the synthesis of precursor of mRNA. RNA polymerases make the transcription to proceed in $5' \rightarrow 3'$-direction. This is the reason for 5' end to bear triphosphate and 3' end to bear a free hydroxyl group.

9.10.3. Elongation of transcription

It proceeds as RNA-polymerase moves along the DNA template. Every new nucleotide becomes paired to a complementary base in codogenic DNA template whereas RNA polymerase accelerates the polymerization of nucleotides through phosphodiester bonds formation at a rate of 40-50 nucleotide per second. Obviously within 1 minute about 30 nucleotides long transcript is copied or generated with a protective chemical group cap formed at 5'end. Thus proper transcription and post-transciptional modification proceed simultaneously. The cap is essentially present in all eukaryotic mRNA. The cap is typically *7-methyl guanosine,* linked through a chain considered of these phosphate groups, as $5' \rightarrow 5'$ rather than $5' \rightarrow 3'$ phosphodiester bond to the first nucleotide of mRNA i.e., CH_3-G-P-P-P-mRNA.

9.10.4. Termination

Transcription is terminated when RNA polymerase advances and reaches the termination sequence (codon) and synthesized RNA strand is separated from the template DNA strand. The RNAs are complete copies of DNA containing both (exon) information and non-informative (introns) portion. The introns which could be essential for DNA appear to be of no use to RNA. The primary information so recorded is released of non-informative contents, thus intact informative segment is left with RNA molecules. Therefore primary transcription(s) containing introns are also referred to as RNA precursor which could be mRNA, rRNA or tRNA.

9.10.4.1. Pre mRNA processing

In case of prokaryotes DNA copied as mRNA is immediately available for the translation/expression of respective protein. Every codon transcribed is brought to the translation scaffoldings or machinery. However, this is not the case with eukaryotes where following translation in nucleus, the contents in the form of mRNA are liberated or transferred to cytoplasm to be translated by ribosomes. *Thus primary transcription undergoes maturation and evolves as a translatable message,* maturation involves removal of introns (non informative segment) nonetheless, introns are interspersed within the region of DNA coding for particular gene. Removal of introns is obligatory for the translation of message in the frame of ribosomes. The mechanism of intron removal is known as 'splicing' (9.23).

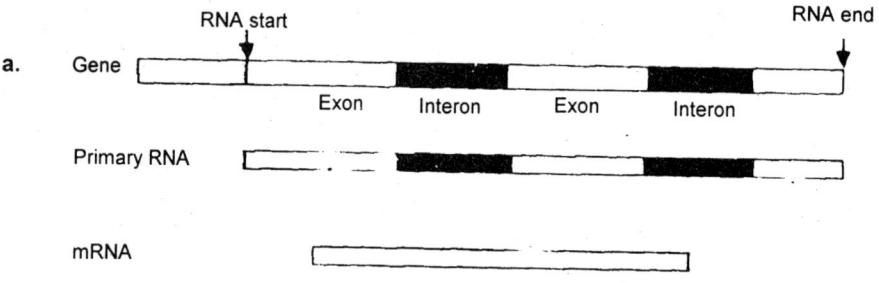

b. Intron-exon junction in human growth hormone (hGH)

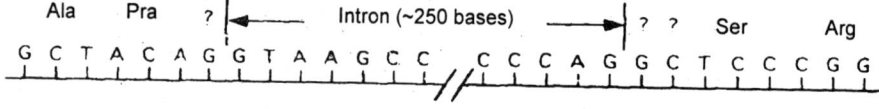

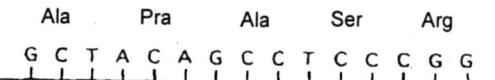

Fig. 9.23 : RNA splicing, a: removal of introns from primary RNA transcript, b: consequences of intron and requirement for removal of translation

It is performed by complex nuclear machinery consisted of RNAs and proteins. Splicing thus results into uninterrupted assembly of exons to produce a continuous run of codons. A single gene may contain multiple introns, some of which may be extremely large contributing thousands of bases to a gene.

The primary transcription of a gene containing multiple introns can be spliced in alternate pattern deriving distinct mRNA. The alternate splicing is utilized in nature and in some cases combinational splicing leads to several distinct messages. A single mRNA splices in two different ways to yield two mRNAs coding for two different proteins with identical amino acid termini but either with calcitonin or CGRP (calcitonin gene related peptide) at the carboxyl terminus (Fig. 9.24). The peptide has been reported to have a key role in differentiation of neurons.

To code for discrete structural and functional domains of a protein there involves more than one exon. For example, in case of myoglobin and hemoglobin central exons code for having binding regions. It is splicing process through which, new proteins evolve via the rearrangement of exons particularly those encoding discrete structural elements, binding sites and catalytic sites. Another example of alternate splicing is seemingly complex that is found to be involved with the derivation of mRNA from the rat muscle troponin gene, where 64 mRNAs are derived from a single gene consisted of 18 axons. The process proceeds through combinational alternate splicing. The function of interon within the gene could not be specified and established as of yet, however, the interons in many cases appear to separate the distinctive coding information for functional domains of a protein. It is supposed that arrangements of information for functional modules separated by stretches of non-coding sequences (introns) in various alternatives shuffles leading to the creation of novel proteins particularly during evolution.

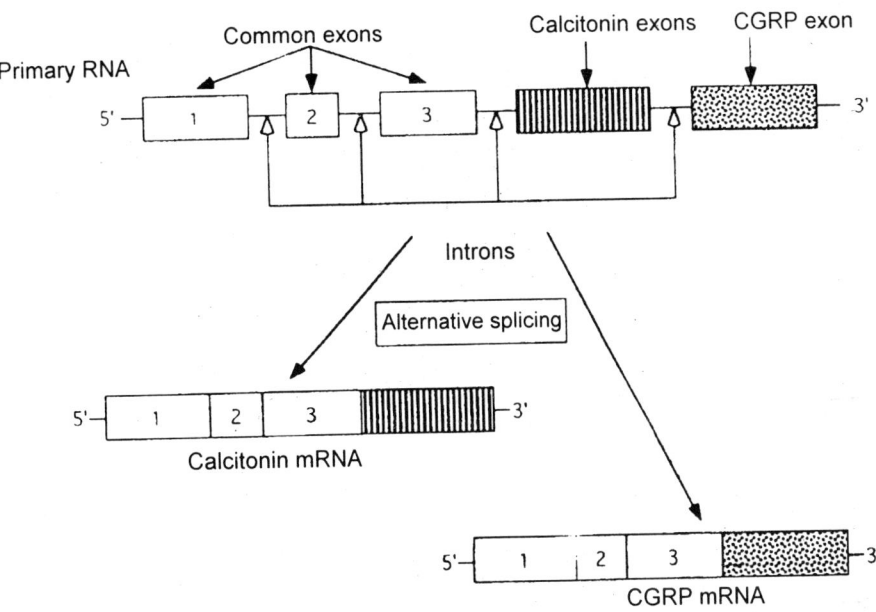

Fig. 9.24 : Alternate splicing of calcitonin gene RNA to produce two different mRNA encodings

Split genes are advantageous for having potential for generating a series of analogous proteins by splicing a nascent RNA transcript in different ways. The precursor of antibody producing cells generates antibody which anchors to the plasma membrane of cell. On activation antibody producing cells splice their nascent RNA transcript in an alternate way to form soluble antibodies in order to make them circulatory rather than static. Thus alternate splicing is a mean of synthesizing a set of proteins which are variations of basic moiety (Fig. 9.25).

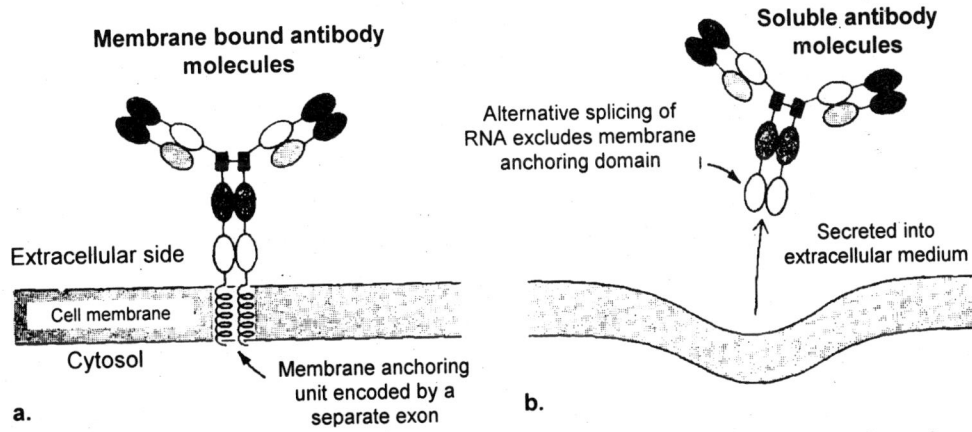

Fig. 9.25 : Alternate splicing of mRNA; a. membrane bound antibody on the surface of a lymphocyte; b. its soluble counterpart

9.10.5. Protein synthesis or translation

When not engaged in the synthesis, the ribosomal unit remains as free exchangeable unit of cytoplasmic pool, dissociation factor that binds to 30 S subunit of ribosomes, separates them. The same factor operates as initiator during 30^S-mRNA binding thus enabling 30^S subunit to participate in a new round of protein synthesis.

tRNA the adapter molecule is an essential for initiation of protein synthesis. The synthesis process starts with the binding of ribosomal binding site on the mRNA molecule (Fig. 9.26). The site contains the codon AUG. mRNA binds with the site in ribosomes which has 3-8 bases that are complementary to sequence at 3' end of 16^S RNA of ribosomes.

The region in the prokaryotes is referred to as **strain** and **Dolgarno sequence**. Once the mRNA template conjugates with ribosomal protein, process of translation starts with the help of tRNA which are special class of molecules having specificity for a particular mRNA. mRNA has specific anticodon complementary to codon on tRNA for specific amino acid. Thus a tRNA typically functions as an adapter molecule and it is a unit for incorporation of amino acids. For each codon on mRNA, there is a distinctive separate tRNA molecule to which amino acids link through covalent bonding, the amino acids which could link with tRNA are specific and directed by codon. In degeneracy, multiple codon code for a amino acid, therefore an amino acid may be linked to a set of tRNAs.

Using complementary codon on mRNA molecule tRNA interacts through base pairing. In addition, at least three proteins initiation factors IF1, IF2, IF3 take part in initiation. These units facilitate the binding of mRNA to ribosomal subunit 30S and GTP. The so formed mRNA-GTP complex, a large subunit of ribosome is added in order to complete the closure of ribosomal subunits. The complex, formed initiates the synthesis of protein and then removed from ribosomes. The energy needed by ribosomal subunits is provided by the hydrolysis of GTP. The initiator complex based upon mRNA-ribosomes-methionyl tRNA then starts elongation. A methionyl tRNA through its anti-codon specially pairs to the AUG codon of mRNA and appears as if suspended or hanged attached to mRNA, whereas its acceptor site is attached to a large ribosomal subunit.

9.11. ELONGATION

The polypeptide synthesis invariably starts with N end and terminates at C end. The addition of amino acids at the polypeptide chain is accomplished in 3 steps.

9.11.1. Step 1:The binding of amino acyl tRNA

In first step tRNA is located onto the right (Fig. 9.26). tRNA is bound to mRNA codons through the anticodons while its acceptor end is linked to the growing peptide. This peptide, which is in the form of peptidal tRNA remains bound to the p-site (donor site) which is a form of protein pocket, associated with large subunit of ribosomes. During first step itself, the second mRNA codon becomes free. This codon could couple to the anticodon of incoming amino acid tRNA. The amino acid of tRNA binds to large ribosomal subunit. Thus first step is completed. During first step energy is provided by breaking the GTP phosphate bonds.

9.11.2. Step 2: Peptide transfer

Its is typically transpeptidation that proceeds in such a way that peptide is transferred from the left side of tRNA onto the amino group of amino acyl tRNA. Thus resulting into peptide bond formation. The peptide bond is established with the help of **peptidal transferase**.

9.11.3. Step 3: Translocation

The third step involves separation of subunits. Peptidal tRNA carrying tripeptide moves along with mRNA to which it is coupled, a distance of codon from the A site to be positioned at the P site. This is referred as to translocation. The process is accompanied by the release of free tRNA from ribosomes. There are elongation factors which assist in protein elongation. Lastly, termination on completion of polypeptide synthesis occurs with the help of stop signals (UAA, UGA and UAG). The tRNA are not capable of binding with termination codons. It is possible that the termination factors probably release the synthesized polypeptide chain.

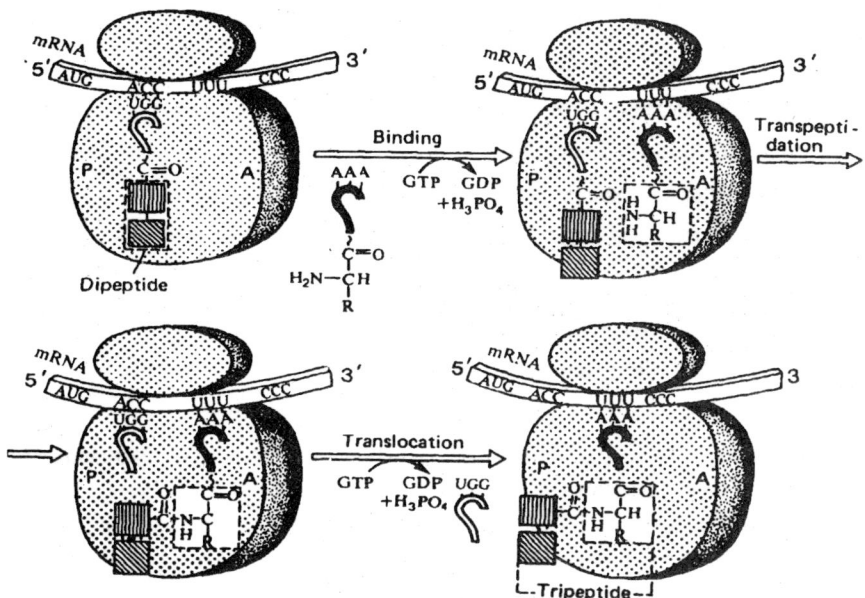

Fig. 9.26 : Schematic representation of protein synthesis

During translation stage the protein molecule starts to fold in order to acquire a three dimensional structure which is completed to its final form following the protein released from the ribosome. S significant part of the synthesized protein remains inside the cell while it is partially exposed to the extracellular fluid and even in some cases may be exported to different parts into the extracellular space. The gland cells liver cells and audder cells are especially active in the secretion of protein. The nascent polypeptide chain passes across the membrane and enters the tubules of endoplasmic reticulum where in the cisterns it becomes concentrated.

The mRNA is stored and subsequently reused during genetic program for assembling the required proteins. However, it is required to be protected from nucleases. The conservation of mRNA is brought about by its binding to cytoplasmic proteins resulting into protein-mRNA complex formation refereed to as informosomes. When the mRNA is demanded for biosynthesis of protein it binds to ribosomal subunit in order to get engaged as well as to participate in the translation. The conservation in particular is utilized by the cells during their development.

The basic knowledge of genetics, its components, their specific behavior and amenability for tailoring for modification or desired engineering offer opportunities for protein modification, recombinant molecule development and immunity related events improvisation and modifications. The application of various structural functionaries of genetics have been discussed in detail under various titles in this book.

SUGGESTED READINGS

Bukhari, A.I., Shapiro, J. and Adhya, S., (1977) **DNA Insertion Elements, Plasmids and Episomes**, Cold Spring Harbor Laboratory.

Carlson, E.A., (1987) **The Gene: A Critical History**, 2nd Ed., Saunders.

Celis, J.E. and Smith, J.D., (1979) **Nonsense Mutations and tRNA Suppressors**, Academic Press.

Friedberg, E.C., (1985) **DNA Repair**, Freeman.

Hartl, D.L., (1995) **Essential Genetics**, Jones and Bartlett Publishers, Sudbury.

Kelley, T. (Ed.), (1988) **Eukaryotic DNA Replication**, Cold Spring Harbor Laboratory.

Kornberg, A., (1990) **DNA Replication**, Freeman.

Lewin, B., (1994) **Genes V**, Oxford University Press, Oxford.

Nirenberg, H., (1963) **Scientific Am.**, March.

Portin, P., (1993) **Quart. Rev. Biol.**, 68, 173-223.

Ross, J., (1989) **Scientific Am.**, April.

Sokal, R.R. and Rohlf, F.J., (1969) **Biometry**, Freeman.

Srb, A., Owen, R. and Edgar, R., (1965) **General Genetics**, Freeman.

Sturterant, A.H. and Beadle, G.W., (1962) **An Introduction to Genetics**, Dover.

Watson, J.D., Hopkins, N.H., Roberts, J.W., Steitz, J.A. and Weiner, A.M., (1987) **Molecular Biology of the Gene**, 4th Ed. (2 Vol.), Benjamin/Cummings.

RECOMBINANT DNA TECHNOLOGY:
Concepts, Methodologies and
Pharmaceutical Applications

10.1. INTRODUCTION

Recombinant DNA technology was introduced way back in earlier 1960's, however, the techniques were employed mostly in the academic investigations related to the basic mechanism's of the cell function. In a few cases they were applied by small biotechnology companies that sought to utilize the procedure for the production of potential therapeutic proteins and drugs, rather than the typical heterocyclic organic chemicals. More recently this technology has emerged as a recognized and powerful tool for facilitating more classical pharmaceutical and drug development research efforts. The advent of classical recombinant DNA technology provided opportunities for large scale production of therapeutics or human derived proteins and peptides. In addition it offers potential for remodelling of protein drugs for site specificity, reduced immunogenecity, stability and improved pharmacokinetics etc.

The reader might be familiar with genetics as it has been discussed at length in previous chapters. Still to prime up the memory and to give a little background of the 'Central Dogma' of Biology, which establishes that information for development, organization and functioning of living systems is stored in discrete units (genes) certainly within the linear deoxyribonucleic acid (DNA) molecule of each cells. At appropriate times, portions of the DNA information are transferred by transcription from the gene into linear ribonucleic acid (RNA) molecules for translation into functionally active proteins (Fig. 10.1).

The basic building blocks of DNA are nucleotides consisted 2-deoxyribose linked through the 1 position to one of the nucleic acid base, guanine (G), thymine (T), cytosine (C), or adenine (A) and linked within a single strand, i.e. the linear DNA molecule through a phosphate ester bond formed between 5' position of deoxyribose of one nucleoside and 3' position of deoxyribose moiety on the adjacent nucleotide. DNA exists as a double helix with one linear strand proceeding in the 5' to3' direction and the other aligned parallel to it but in opposite direction i.e., 3' to 5'. The two strands are held together by the hydrogen bonds in which Cs pair with Gs and Ts pair with As. The resulting DNA forms two complementary strands such that the sequential order of the nucleotides of one of the strands (a gene) can be exactly copied into a messenger RNA (mRNA) molecule (copying of both strands occurs during cell division). RNA also uses four nucleotides (uridine in place of thymidine) that are attached to ribose (instead of deoxyribose) sugars as the backbone. RNA, are single stranded since their synthesis depends upon opening of stranded DNA where RNA polymerase copies one strands through the use of the base pairing principle.

The mechanism of converting linear nucleotides sequence information into linear array of amino acids (proteins) depends upon the recognition of nucleotide triplet (usually AUG for methionine) near 5' end of the mRNA, which encodes the first amino acid (N-terminal). Each amino acid is carried by single t-RNA possessing a specific recognition site triplet (again complementary bases pairing is used). The t-RNA triplet complementary for the next three nucleotides in the mRNA binds and transfers its amino acids. This event continues until a stop codon (e.g. UAG) frame is arrived. The complete translation of mRNA occurs in the ribosomes (a RNA and protein complex) and results in a cellular protein. The protein serves many functions within the cell, ranging from enzymatic machinery of energy metabolism and structural components of membrane to the very specialized function of different cell types. However, it is important that the Central Dogma and the triplet coding systems remain consistent from bacteria to humans; thus, the tools developed over many years of research by microbiologists can be utilized, effectively in designing and engineering of target gene.

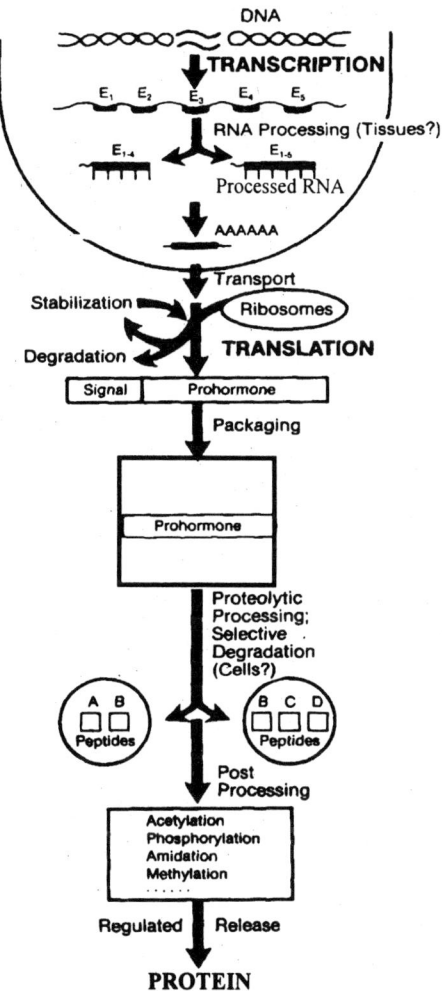

Fig. 10.1 : Genetic regulation cycle within a particular cell

10.1.1. Bacterial impact

An apparent simple impact of the techniques from molecular biology is the ability to insert (using recombinant techniques) a single gene of interest, even from a different species, into bacteria. These transformed bacteria can then serve as small '*biofactories*', since bacteria multiply in number at a fast rate. Thus, these biofactories could effectively be utilized to amplify the expression of an individual product over thousands of times especially over one that occurs endogenously in minute quantities with of original starting material. This product could be cDNA (complementary DNA) or its protein product (if cDNA is used). The second bacteriological procedure that is commonly used is the ability to isolate an individual bacterium (containing the recombinant product of interest, called a clone), from a population by physical separation (spreading out on bacterial agar plates). This is a very powerful tool when compared with classical protein isolation procedures generally used for isolation and identification of the product of interest from a mixture.

10.1.2. Background

The major aim of the chapter is to discuss procedures employed in the engineering of newer arrangements of the genes in the prokaryotes by the movement of the larger blocks of DNA. Parent DNA duplex aligns at region of sequence similarity (homology) and new DNA molecules are formed by exchange of homologous segments this process is called **recombination**. The intermediates in recombination have been isolated and the actions of the enzymes catalyzing the exchange of DNA strands have been delineated. *Transposition* is the movement of a gene from one chromosome to another or from one site to a different one on the same chromosome. *Transposons* are mobile genetic elements that enable a gene to move between non-homologous sites in DNA. General recombination plays a role in the repair of DNA. It is critical when both strands of a duplex are damaged, information for repair must come from another DNA molecules where the recombination provides a template for the synthesis of DNA and to fill up the gap. However, recombination and transposition sometimes lead to generation of newer combination of genes (mutagenes) which highlight their importance in evolution.

In 1964, Robin Holliday proposed a model of general recombination to account for the products of meiosis in fungi (Fig. 10.2). In the scheme proposed two homologous duplexes are aligned. A strand of one duplex and the corresponding strand of the other duplex are nicked by an endonuclease. The end of each nicked strand leaves its own duplex and invades to the other duplex. Strands from different duplexes are then joined to each other to form recombination intermediate that is dynamic in nature. Strand exchange can continue, allowing the crossing over point between duplexes to move, a process called **branch migration**. This combinational intermediate can be cleaved and rejoined in two different ways to form two kinds of recombinant products (G and H in Fig. 10.2).

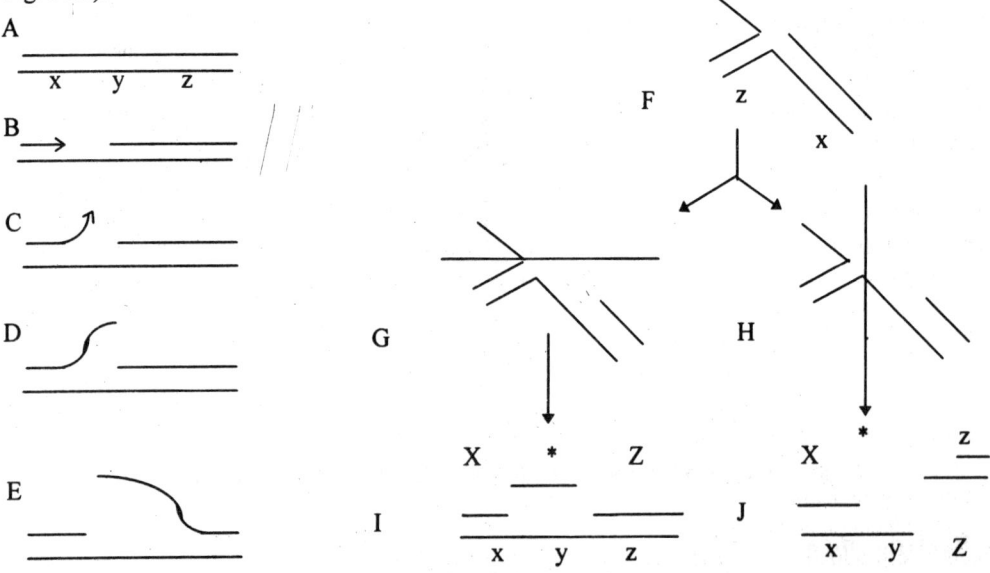

Fig. 10.2 : Robin Holliday model for general recombination

The Holliday model though effectively served stimulating conceptual basis for the studies and understanding of molecular mechanism of recombination however, the intermediates could be observed for their structure and morphology some 15 years later when electron microscopy came into existence and studies were conducted with *E. coli*. These plasmids, i.e., bacterial DNAs, were interestingly noted to readily undergo recombination and were highly resistant to antibiotics. On isolation and structure elucidation, it was found that the plasmid DNA is a typical dimer that could be cleaved by Eco R I endonuclease which specifically cuts the original plasmid giving an overall shapes of a '*chi*'. This further suggested that they are important components of the intermediate recombinations. The contact point in chi forms always divides the structure into pairs of equal length arms. This means that the genome are joined at a region of homology. However, there would be no special relations between the sizes of the arms if the plasmids were joined at unrelated sequence (Fig. 10.3).

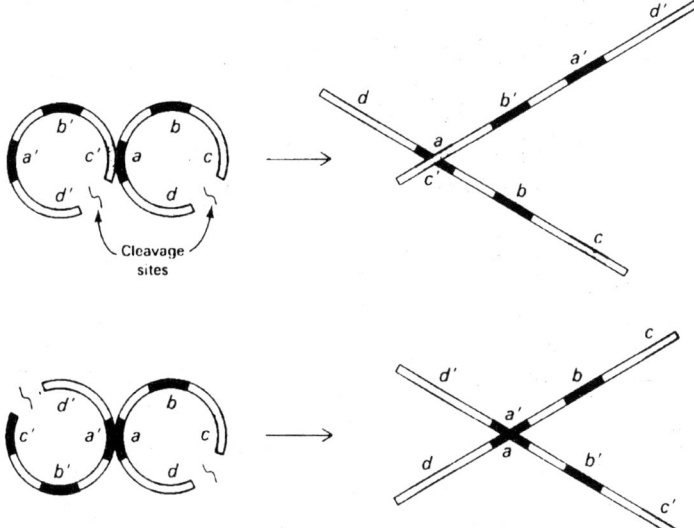

Fig. 10.3 : Expected cleavage pattern for two DNA molecules

Furthermore, it is likely that the compact point occurs with nearly equal probability along the entire plasmid, which shows that pairing can possibly occur at many locations and so the connections at the crossover repairing point can occur at many locations. The four duplexes emerge from a ring of connecting single strand at the junction between the two genomes. The process discussed is called as **general recombination**, because exchange can occur between any pair of homologous sequences on parental DNA molecule.

The most recent advancement in molecular biology techniques is **polymerase chain reaction** (PCR), which has a profound influence on recombinant DNA (rDNA) technology. Concurrent developments of highly efficient and rapid algorithms provided opportunities for safe storage, analysis and comparison of nucleic acid and protein sequences. This organized accumulation of data has led to the formation of widely accessible database which are crucial in rDNA technology. The major techniques and technologies currently used in rDNA applications are:

1. Restriction endonucleases and DNA ligases: Cutting and Rejoining of DNA.
2. Reverse transcriptase: Conversion of mRNA into cDNA.
3. Chemical DNA synthesis: Oligonucleotides.
4. Polymerase chain reaction (PCR): Rapid amplification of specific DNA segments.
5. Vectors for gene isolation and expression.
6. DNA sequencing techniques.
7. Protein overproduction: Appropriate host/vector system.

The introduction is sufficient for the reader to define recombinant DNA as a novel technique for controlled recombination which makes it possible to achieve the target in a shorter period and also to break barrier between totally incompatible genomes. It is a method of bringing together and joining pieces of DNA from unrelated organisms (e.g. human and bacterium genome) in order to achieve the aim and benefit of general recombination. Hence it offers the advantageous method by which genes or other segments of large chromosome can be isolated, replicated and studied by nucleic acids sequencing technique (which is otherwise very laborious if one has to search for a gene in the main DNA molecule at random) and electron microscopy. The various general steps involved in the preparation of recombinant DNA could be briefly summarized as:

1. Selection of DNA of interest (commonly referred to as foreign on target or passenger DNA).
2. A cloning vector or vehicle to carry inserted pieces of target DNA.
3. Restriction endonuclease which makes internal cuts at specific sites on DNA.
4. DNA ligase: The enzyme that joins pieces of nucleotides /DNA together.
5. A host to replicate the vector containing foreign DNA. This may be a prokaryotic or eukaryotic cell.
6. Screening test for recombinants produced by insertion of DNA.

10.2. CUTTING AND REJOINING OF DNA

The analysis of DNA remained one of the most cumbersome part for the molecular biologists until the discovery of restriction endonucleases from several bacterial species which provided the tool for the site specific cleavage of DNA. Once cleaved, the fragments of different sizes could be separated electrophoretically, isolated and analyzed. Restriction enzymes are endonucleases which cleave specific sequences within double-stranded DNA stretches. The recognition and cleavage sequence of a routinely used group of endonucleases (called type II enzyme) may be four, five, six or eight bases long and are symmetrical across the two strands of DNA. Figure 10.4. illustrates the cleavage specificity of a widely used six-base-motif-specific endonuclease Eco R I. Now what seems confusing is the nomenclature (Eco R I). The first three letters of the name refer to the bacterium which is the source of the enzyme, for example Eco R I is obtained from *Escherichia coli*, and the subsequent letters denote the specific enzyme (Table 10.1).

Figure 10.4 shows, the cleaved sequence and the two antiparallel strands of DNA, where the number 5' denotes the direction of strands. The recognition sequence of Eco R I, reading in the 5' to 3' direction is GAATTC. The rules of complementary base pairing i.e. A with T and G with C dictate that the complementary strand should be the same however, in 3'→5' direction similar to a palindrone that is read the same in either directions and has a two-fold axis of rotationary symmetry. Eco R I cleaves at every location in the DNA where this sequence motif occurs. The phosphodiester bonds between the G and A on both the strands are hydrolyzed by enzymes, allowing the scission of the DNA fragments created in this cleavage event. Such ends are referred to as 'cohesive' or 'sticky' ends. Hence it is possible for Eco R I generated ends of bacterial DNA and human DNA to combine by base pairing. The cohesive ends involved in such an association can be sealed by another enzyme DNA ligase, which catalyses the formation of phosphodiester bonds on both strands resulting in uninterrupted DNA. However, these ligation points can be again cleaved by Eco R I.

Table 10.1 Some of the microbial restriction endonuclease with their target site

Name	Source	Target sequence
Eco RI	*E. coli* RY13	5'G↓AATTC 3' 3'CTTAA↓G5'
Hae II	*Haemophilus aegyptius*	5'GG↓CC3' 3'CC↓GG5'
HaeIII	*Haemophilus aegyptius*	5'GG↓CC3' 3'CC↓GG5'
Hind III	*Haemophilus influenzae* Rd	5'A↓AGCTT3' 3'TTCGA↓A5'
Hsu I	*Haemophilus suis*	5'↓A AGCTT 3' 3'TTCGA↓A 5'
Pst I	*Providencia stuartii* 164	5'CTGCA↓G3' 3'G↓ACGTC 5'
Sma I	*Serratia marcescens* Sb	5' CCC↓GGG3' 3'GGG↓CCC5'
Sst I	*Streptomyces stanford*	5'GAGCT↓C3' 3'↓C TCGAG5'

With the development of molecular biology and advancement in cell biology techniques for the general recombination, and the methods for the purification of DNA are mow available. These involve gentle disruption (lysis) of cell containing the target DNA from all other molecules such as proteins, polysaccharides and lipids. This is generally achieved by placing the complex mixture (cell lysate) in centrifuge tubes containing a concentrated solution of cesium chloride or sucrose. This is centrifuged at a high speed in an ultracentrifuge for several hours (about 10-12 hr.). Consequently, the nucleic acids get separated forming specific bands in the solution in centrifuge tube, depending upon the density of DNA. These bands can then be removed (piercing the tubes with specially designed syringes) and purified further by chemical methods. The purified DNA is then subjected to endonuclease treatment.

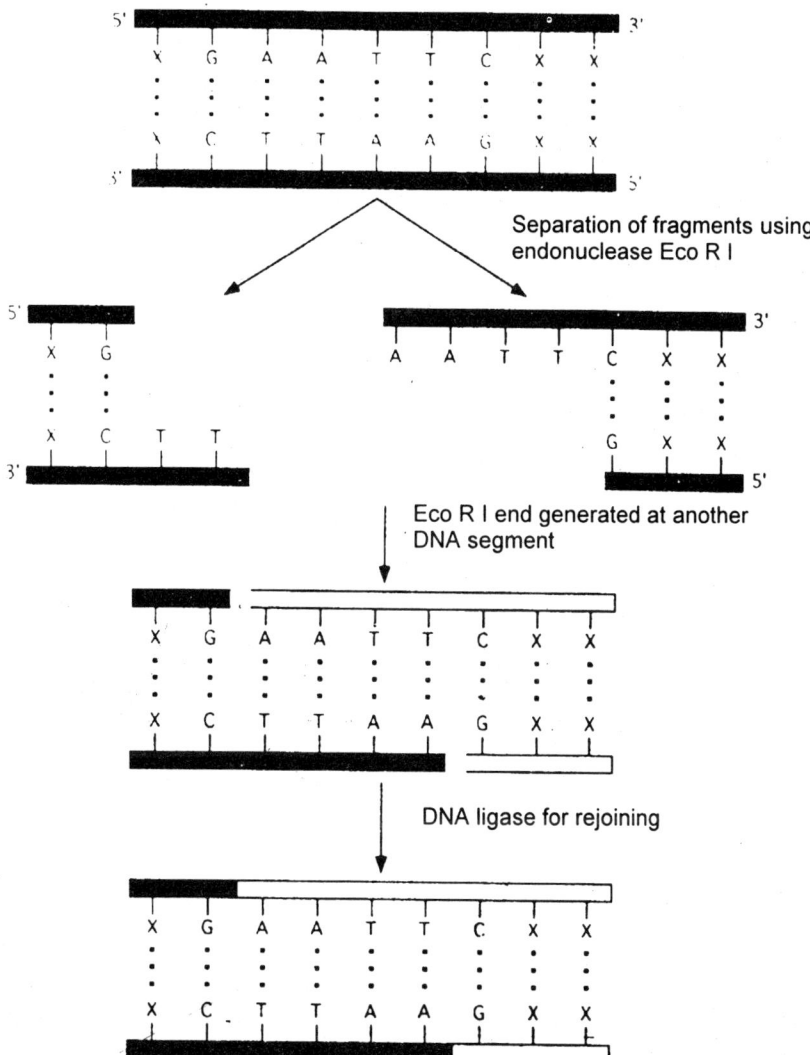

Fig. 10.4 : Cleavage of DNA by restriction endonuclease Eco R I and joining by DNA ligase

After the continual research for nearly two decades, over 700 restriction enzymes recognizing over a hundred unique sequences motifs of DNA have been isolated (some restriction enzymes from different source recognize the same cleavage site). The overhangs produced by different enzymes vary and some restriction enzymes (EcoR I, Sma I) create blunt ends at the cleavage sites. However, DNA ligase is also capable of joining blunt ended DNA under specific reaction condition. Cleavage sites for restriction enzymes occur randomly in the DNA. The frequency of a particular site is dependent on the size of DNA and the size of recognition sequence.

The probability of finding a particular four base run in DNA is 1/256 (1/4 x 1/4 x 1/4 x 1/4) and that of five base run is 1/1024. The probability of occurrence reduces to 1/4096 for a specific six base stretch and to 1/65536 for an eight-base stretch.

Although general trend follows the expected probabilities, sometimes there are wide deviations from expected numbers. Such deviations are common, and are attributed to the variation in the G-C content of the DNA.

Single strand-binding protein (SSB) precipitates in general recombination as well as in DNA replication. The cooperative binding of SSB to single stranded DNA prevents the formation of hairpin loops. SSB stabilizes an unpaired DNA until recA (recombinant A) protein forms a filament around it. Topoisomerase I also plays an important role in recombination by relieving torsional strain produced by winding of one DNA molecule around another during branch migration. An *E. coli* cell normally contains several hundred copies of recA protein. The level of this key enzyme in recombination increases over a hundred fold following damage of DNA. Damage rapidly induces the synthesis of more than fifteen proteins mediating the repair of DNA. This switching on-off of the machinery is called the SOS response (Fig..10.5). Under normal conditions repairing proteins are present at low levels because the synthesis of their messenger RNAs is blocked by a repressor protein called lexA. The essence of SOS response is the cleavage of lex A protein. Single stranded DNA arising from damaged DNA acts as a trigger by binding to recA protein. The ssDNA-recA complex then hydrolyzes an Ala-Gly bond in lexA protein which destroys its capacity to block the transcription of many genes involved in DNA repair. Thus recA protein is multifunctional it is a protease as well as recombinase in nature.

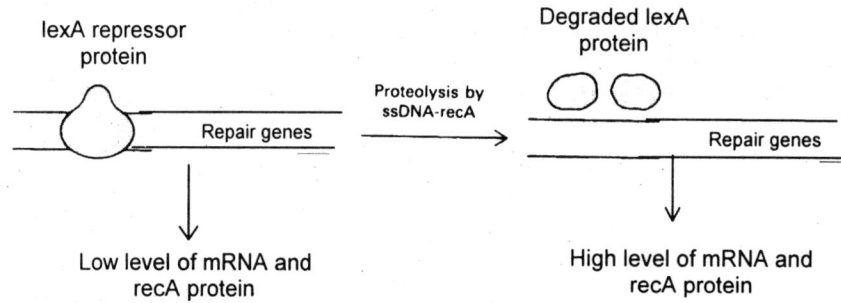

Fig. 10.5 : SOS genes for DNA repair

10.3. MUTAGENESIS

The mutagenesis is an essential requisite employed in any genetic manipulation as well as in the study of gene structure function relationship. The mutants can be classically generated by treating an organism with chemical agents or its exposure to some physical environment, that modifies DNA (mutagens). The method has been extremely successful however, found to be empirical as modification is non-specific, rather it is randomized. This necessitates for strategy which has selectivity. Prior to the development of gene cloning and sequencing methodologies there was no method available to detect the point of mutagenesis and to know whether the mutagenesis occurred is due to single base change, or via an addition or deletion process of DNA.

With the developments in molecular biology related research now the isolation and study of single gene has become not only possible but a routine paving way for precise and defined mutagenesis, as incorporation of special changes in any given base in a cloned DNA sequence is now possible. This is referred as **site directed mutagenesis** *in-vitro*. The technique works as an effective tool in gene manipulations. Mutagenesis as such helps understanding structure function relationship. As a result of modification in gene, the expression of mutant protein(s) with specific changes in regard to constituting amino acids has become a possible reality. The protein mutants facilitate the study relating to elucidation of mechanism of catalysis, substrate specificity or stability of the proteins.

The eukaryotic DNA cloned sequences can easily be isolated and engineered *in vivo* by bacterial genetic method and the same could be attempted *in vitro* by specific enzyme modifications. In order to ascertain the effects of experimentally incorporated changes, on the function and expression of eukaryotic genes, the engineered sequence must be taken out from cloning host and reintroduced into the eukaryotic organism, preferably the one from which they were isolated. It is suggestive that genetic control of eukaryotic specific function must be evaluated or assessed in an eukaryotic environment.

10.3.1. Site directed mutagenesis

The single primer method used for site directed mutagenesis is the simplest method, it involves *in-vitro* priming of DNA synthesis with the help of synthesized oligonucleotide having base which mismatches with the complementary sequence. The DNA selected as a site for mutation must be available in single stranded form which is practically possible through cloning of the gene M-13 based factors. Furthermore, DNA cloned in a plasmid obtained as duplex can easily be converted into a partial single stranded molecule that is suitable for mutagenesis. The synthetic oligonucleotide primer of DNA synthesis, thereby, gets incorporated, resulting into at duplex molecule. With the change of host *E. coli*, the heteroduplex may produce homoduplex with the sequences that of the original wild-type DNA with the mutated base. In order to selectively pick out mutants nucleic acid hybridization using 32-phosphorus radio labelled oligonucleotide as a probe is employed. This enables a quick detection of desired mutant. The DNA sequencing is employed to elucidate any adventitious changes due to mutagenesis. In a variation an oligonucleotide containing preengineered or deleted sequence may be used in the process of mutagenesis.

The single primer method suffers some distinctive deficiencies. The double stranded double duplex molecule generated during the process may get contaminated by a single-stranded non-mutant template DNA uncopied, as well as by partially double stranded molecule. As a result of these contaminations the proportion of mutant progeny generated reduced considerably. To exclude the probability of contamination sucrose gradient centrifugation or gene electrophoresis could be employed effectively. Following transformation, in *in-vivo* synthesis the heteroduplex molecule strands are segregated yielding a mixed population i.e., mutant-non-mutant progeny. This necessitates for mutant progeny purification where cells mismatched repair system may complicate the process. Theoretically, via mismatched repairing an equal number of mutant and non-mutant progeny should be produced. However, in practice mutants are counter selected. Due to this reason no mutant progeny is methyl directed mismatched repair system of *E. coli* which favors repair of non-methylated mutant progeny only.

However, in the case of cell, newly synthesized DNA strands which are unmethylated undergo preferential repair at the points or position of mismatch and prevent process of mutation. Similarly, nonmethylated *in vitro* generated mutant strands are repaired by the cell thereby producing a progeny of wild type. This well identified problem due to mismatch repair can effectively be addressed by using host strains which carry mutN, mutS, mutH capable of preventing methyl directed mismatch repair. With single primer method another problem is of oligonucleotide digestion by 5'→3' exonucleases. As a result if degradation extends beyond the position of single base mismatch then a wild type molecule would be generated. This problem can be circumvented using high quality DNA fragmentation using polymerases which lack 5'→3'exonuclease activity.

10.3.2. Strand selection

It is explicit that a heteroduplex molecule consisting of one mutant and one non-mutant strain invariably may give rise to both mutant and non-mutant progeny upon replication. Therefore, the growth of non-mutant should be suppressed. The suppression of non-mutant requires various strategies.

10.3.2.1. The gapped duplex method

The gapped duplex method is schematically presented in figure 10.6. The target DNA which is selected for mutagenesis is cloned up in a M13 phage vector where from it is recovered in a single stranded form. The vector that contains non-sense mutation can only be grown on a amber suppressing host. A gapped duplex could be generated by annealing the single stranded recombinant DNA template with double stranded denatured DNA of wild-phage origin.

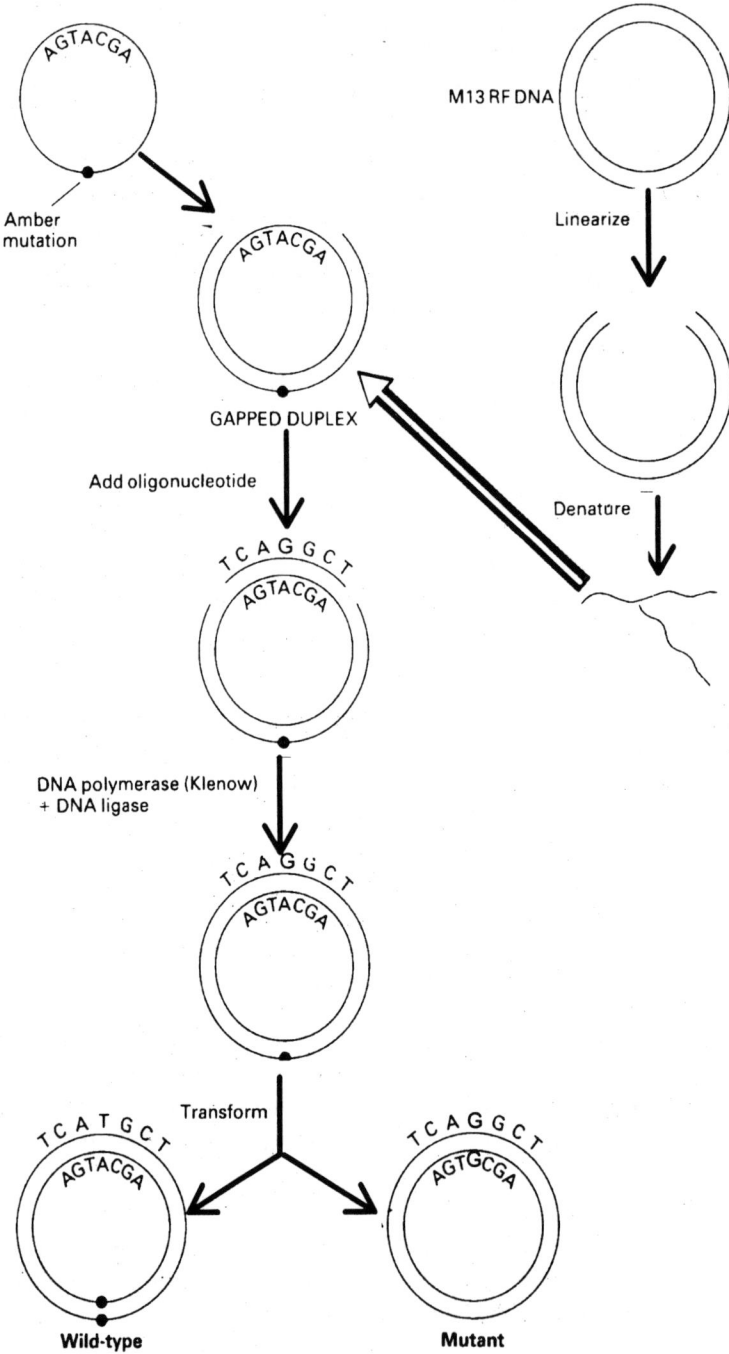

Fig. 10.6 : Site directed mutagenesis the gapped duplex method

The heteroduplex is converted to be fully double stranded form by DNA polymerase and DNA ligase. This could be transformed into an *E. coli*. A specific strain that lacks an amber suppresser is used as a host which allows recovery of only mutant progeny up to 70% level.

10.3.2.2. Coupled priming and cyclic selection

This system of strand selection was first devised by Carter et al. It permits continuous repeats of mutagenesis with recloning. Basically it depends on palindromic sequences between recognition site for **Eco K** and **Eco B** restriction endonucleases. Two primers are used one for the mutagenesis of the site of interest while the other for mutagenesis of Eco K or Eco B strand selected site. A single Eco K restriction site containing special vector system has been developed and utilized. Obviously following mutation, the selection is altered from Eco K to Eco B site as presented in figure 10.7. This suggests that mutant progeny can be selected by growing it in a Eco K restricting host as progeny with an Eco K site in such host cannot survive. If required the Eco B containing mutant can be subjected to second mutagenesis step. A second primer is required to change Eco B site to a EcoK state and an Eco B restricting host is used to clone up the new mutant.

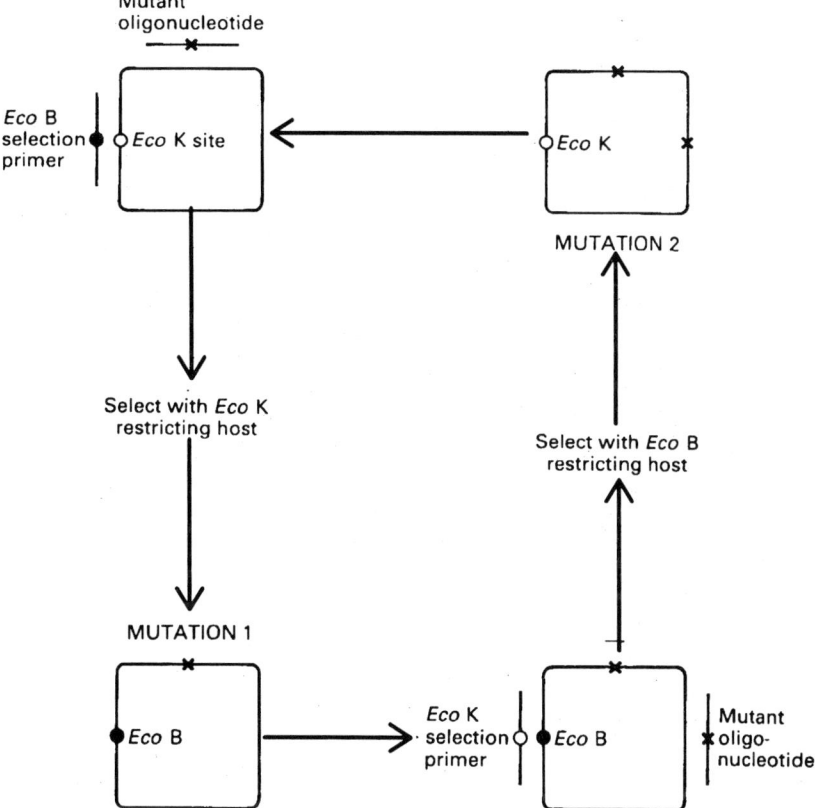

Fig. 10.7 : Cyclic selection of mutagenesis by coupled priming technique

10.3.2.3. The Kunkel method

The method utilizes pregrowth of phages in a specialized host before they are used for mutagenesis. Typically the host used for the purpose is deficient in dUTPase (dUT) and uracil glucocylase. The dUT mutation results in increased intracellular dUTP levels whereas uracil glycosylation allows for the incorporation of deoxyuridine into the DNA replacing thymidine at some positions. Thus, a heteroduplex having uracil in its parental strand

and a mutant strand could be synthesized *in vitro*. In the presence of dTTP it results in to a mutant progeny when plated on a wild type host. The method can also be used for sequential mutation.

***In vitro* methods:** The method discussed so far essentially generates hetero duplex molecules based on a mutant and a non-mutant strand and then selecting the mutant strand of interest *in vivo*. The method is cumbersome, may result in considerable loss of efficiency requiring specific mutant vectors and host strains. Likewise, other methods like gapped-duplex and Primer cycling suffer their own set of limitations. An alternative method has been suggested which appreciably addresses the shortcomings of others. The method employs principle that certain restriction enzymes including Ava I, Ava II, Ban II, Hind II, Nci I, Pst I and Pva I, etc., are unable to cleave phosphorothioate DNA. The mutant oligonucleotide is therefore annealed to single stranded DNA template which is then estimated by DNA polymerase in the presence of thionucleotide. Thus phosphorothioated mutant strand is generated. Then DNA ligase is used to seal up the gap in the mutant strand followed by its interaction with Nui I which selectively cleaves the parental strand. Thus parental strand is partially digested with exonuclease III and subsequently repolymerized (Fig.10.8). The method permits strand selection *in vitro* with high degree of mutation and also allows for desirable deletion and insertions as well. The method does not require specialized host or phage vectors therefore can be used for repeat rounds of mutagenesis.

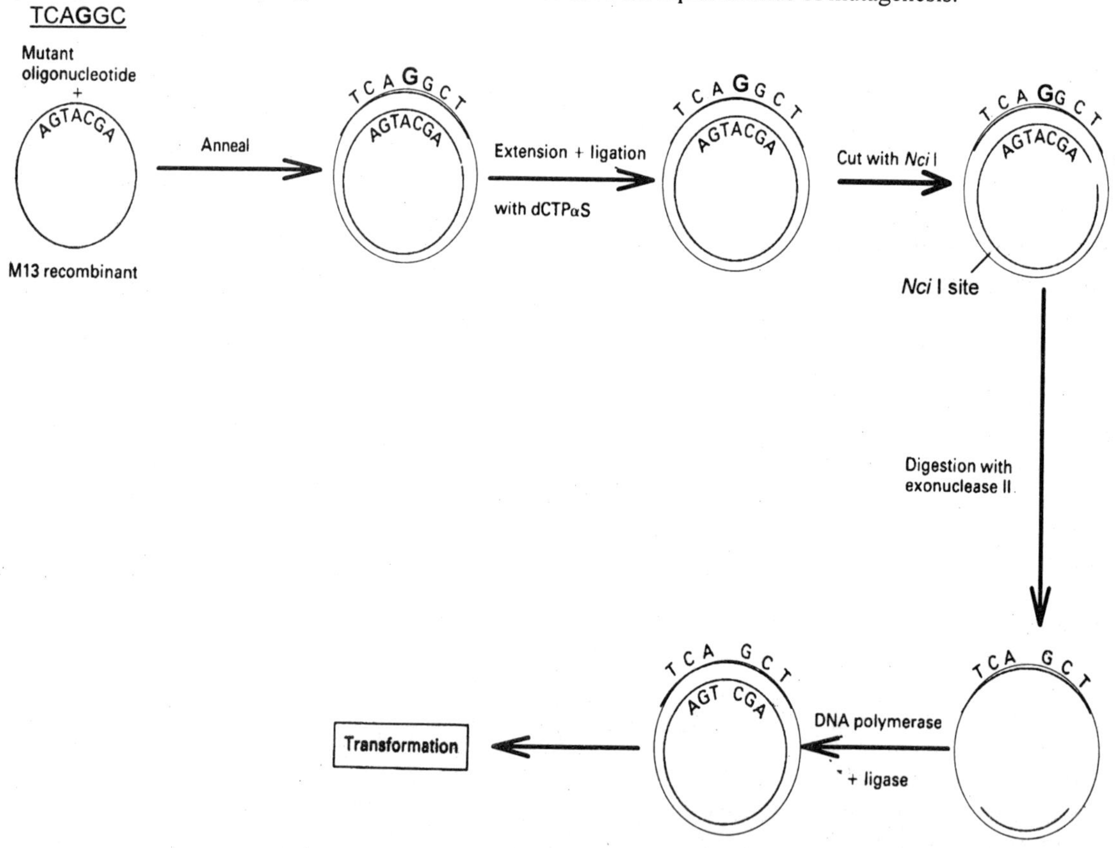

Fig. 10.8 : *In vitro* strand selection of mutants

10.3.3. Mutagenesis based transformation with oligonucleotides

The site directed mutagenesis of a yeast gene by a synthesized oligonucleotide has been discussed by Mocreschell et al. The yeast strain used is unable to grow on fermentable carbohydrates because of CYC-1 gene mutant in it. The mutation as such has been brought about by changing T dinucleotide in a coding sequence to a single residence which effectively results in base substitution along with a frame shift. The CYC-1 mutation corrective oligonucleotide and yeast strain were transformed and revertants obtained were found to be with respective base sequence. The method requires a technique for the selection of revertant a stable mutants and a high concentration of DNA.

10.3.4. Random mutagenesis

Isolation of a series of point mutants and particularly DNA sequences is laborious. Hence to have a random introduction of point mutation at a specifically defined site the enzymatic misincorporation of non-complementary nucleotides is used. This can be brought about during in-vitro enzymatic template dependent DNA synthesis by omission of one of the dNTPs.

Recombinant DNA technique has redefined the classical method of chemical mutagenesis. The segment of DNA to be mutated is cloned in a M13 vector, and a single-stranded DNA is obtained. This is treated with limiting concentration of chemical mutagens. This mutates DNA is then used as a template which while copying depurinated DNA inserts any of the four bases at the site. The double-stranded target DNA is subcloned into a fresh vector for screening and selection of mutants.

10.4. POLYMERASE CHAIN REACTION (PCR) IN GENE AMPLIFICATION

The technology of gene amplification was revolutionized in 1985 by the discovery of a remarkable tool known as polymerase chain reaction (PCR), which is also nick named as people's choice reaction. The PCR is such a powerful tool that it may replace completely the gene cloning in a vector by *in-vitro* process, in the due course of time.

10.4.1. Principle of PCR

During DNA replication, polymerization of the nucleotides occurs via template DNA strands utilizing the enzyme DNA polymerase, however, for the completion of this reaction there is an invariable requirement of the primer strand onto which further addition of nucleotides can be accomplished using DNA polymerase. In the natural process the primer strand is not the DNA strand but it is the RNA molecule synthesized with the help of enzyme RNA polymerase. In the PCR a similar reaction takes place in an 'Eppendorf tubes', in which the addition of the deoxyoligonucleotides (primer strands) and the DNA polymerase enzyme from outside leads to the polymerization. The repetition of the reaction leads to the unlimited supply of DNA molecules. Further the supply of the DNA could be increased by using careful denaturation and renaturation cycles. These cycles are affected by the variation of the temperature. During the denaturation cycle the temperature is raised to 90-98°C so as to separate the two strands of the DNA. Once the two strands are separated the reaction mixture is provided with two primers, which could be further amplified by reducing the temperature to 40-60°C (renaturation cycle) and hence allowing the primers to bind to their complementary strands during the renaturation cycle. The presence of **Taq DNA polymerase** enzyme and all four essential nucleosides triphosphates allows synthesis of the complementary strand in the usual manner. The temperature cycle plays an important role in the continual amplification process only after the discovery and subsequent use of the thermostable DNA polymerases. The most common and the most important is the **Taq DNA polymerase** isolated from *Thermus aquaticus* which grows in hot springs. This enzyme acts best at 72°C and denaturation temperature of 90°C does not destroy the activity of the enzyme. The other thermostable enzymes which have been discovered are **Pflu DNA polymerase** isolated form *Pyrococcus furiosus* and **Vent DNA polymerase** isolated form *Thermococcus litoralis*. These enzymes allow the automation of the entire process as the need for the addition of the DNA polymerase after every denaturation cycle is not required. The computer controlled automatic PCR thermal cycles are now available. In these machines the process is automatically repeated 20-30 times and each renaturation and denaturation cycle is repeated every 1-3 min. Hence, it enables a molecular biologist to avoid the complicated process of vector based cloning and in a short time he can have a billion copies of the sequence. The figure 10.9 shows the diagrammatic representation of these steps up to 2 cycles. Further repetition of these cycles in the similar pattern can lead to a very high yield.

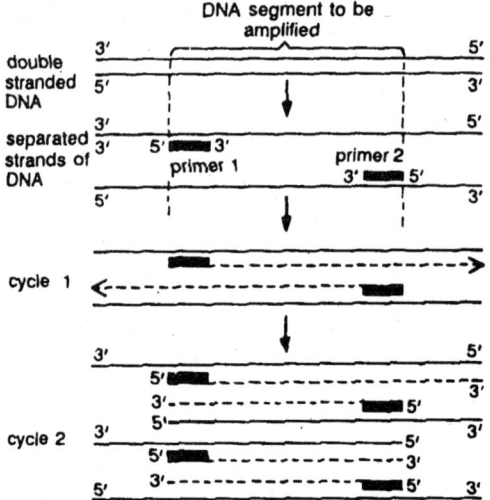

Fig. 10.9 : Major steps involved in the PCR up to 2 cycles

PCR based amplification can effectively reduce the need for the cloning, as only very small quantities (in nanograms = 10^{-9}g) of the initial DNA is required for the process whereas in the cloning process the DNA needed is in micrograms ($1 \mu g = 10^{-6}$g). The other added advantages of the PCR process over the conventional gene cloning are; the biological reagents required in gene cloning process include restriction enzymes, ligases, vectors, bacterial cells which are costly as well as complicated to handle where as in the PCR only the DNA and the polymerase enzymes are to be added; the cloning process could not be automated and requires a highly skilled person to undertake the process whereas the PCR is simple to work with; the time factor required for the PCR is very less (only 4 hr.) as compared to cloning where about 3-4 days are required for the completion of the process.

Recent research in the field of PCR has led to the development of the techniques contributing to the effectiveness of the method to its fullest. Several variations in the process have been suggested which further make the process versatile.

10.4.2. Inverse PCR

The method allows the amplification of those DNA sequences which are away from the primer and not of those which are flanked by the primer. Consider the case, if the border sequences of the DNA segment are not known and those of the vector are known, then the sequences to be amplified may be cloned in a vector and border sequence of the vector may be used as a primer in such a way that the polymerization proceeds in reverse direction, i.e., away from the vector sequence flanked by the primer and towards the sequence of the inserted segment.

10.4.3. Anchored PCR

The PCR methodology as well as the inverse PCR require the utilization of two primers representing the sequence lying at the ends of the sequence to be amplified. However, the limitation of the knowledge about the sequence to only one end leads to the development of the newer technique named as **anchored PCR**. In this technique only one primer may be used instead of the two. Only one strand may be copied first, after which a polyG tail is attached at the end of the newly synthesized stand. This newly synthesized strand with the poly G tail at its 3'end will serve as the template for the daughter strands synthesis utilizing an anchor primer with which a poly C sequence to complement to poly G of the template is linked. In the next cycle both the original primers and the anchored primer are used.

10.5. ISOLATION AND AMPLIFICATION OF GENES : GENE CLONING

A very small fragment of total DNA comprises for an individual mammalian gene e.g., a gene occupying 10,000 base pairs compresses a mere 3×10^{-5} fraction of human genome. Hence, if the fragmentation of human genomic DNA is brought to a conversion of 10,000 base pair fragment, only one fragment of 3,00,000 would contain a gene of interest. This highlights the necessity of techniques for identification and amplification of genes so as to study and utilize them (gene cloning) effectively.

Figure 10.10 depicts the process of cloning a hypothetical mammalian gene contained on a EcoRI fragment. Initially DNA is digested with Eco RI and the resulting fragments are ligated to the DNA of a 'cloning vector' and hence producing the DNA molecule. Vectors are DNA molecules which are capable of replication to very high copy numbers when single copy is introduced into their host cell. They are either autonomously replicating circular DNA molecules known as plasmids or are DNA's of bacteria viruses (bacteriophages) which replicate to high numbers. Segments of foreign DNA legated to the vectors are amplified along with the vector sequencing when introduced into their host, which, in the most of the cases is *E. coli*. The bacteria harboring the vector containing the foreign gene of interest could be very well identified using labelled oligonucleotide complementary to the gene. However, when the genes whose DNA sequences are unknown, oligonucleotides are designed on the basis of inferences from the known sequence of protein encoded by the gene.

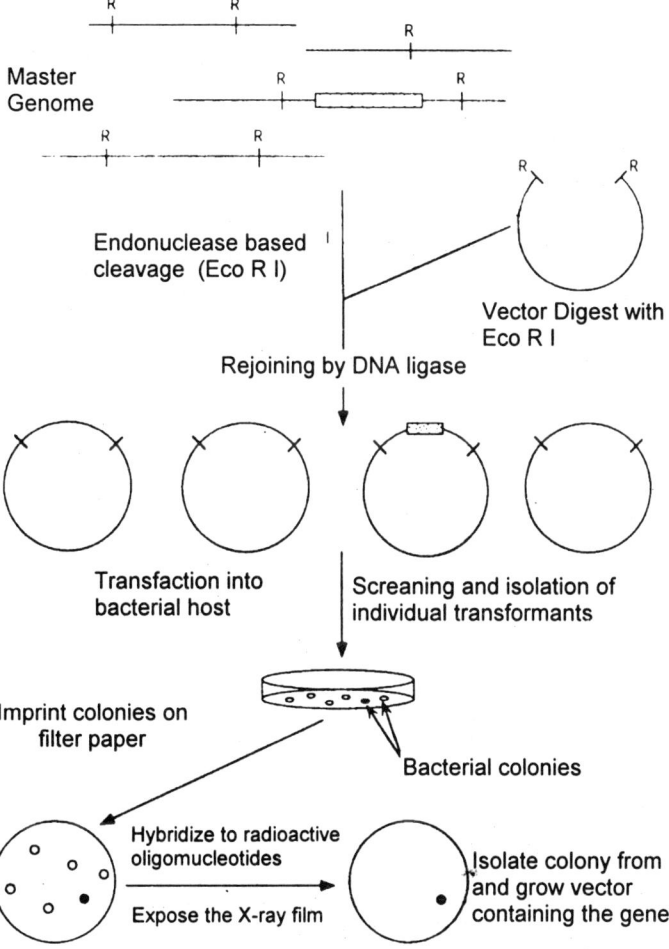

Fig. 10.10 : Isolation of single gene form a large genome

10.5.1. Principle of gene cloning

The basic principle and techniques that comprise the production of the recombinant proteins include isolation of a gene from one cell, placing the gene in a different cell and fermenting a culture of the recombinant cells to produce the desired protein. Each protein is specified by only one genome. Each protein is produced by synthetic machinery in the cell which is able to interpret a set of coded instructions contained in a unique messenger RNA (mRNA) molecule which in turn is a complementary copy of information permanently stored in an inheritance unit, the gene, or DNA of the cell.

DNA cloning procedure has four different essential steps:

1. Method for generating DNA fragment.
2. Reaction which joins foreign DNA to the vector.
3. A means of introducing the artificial recombinant into the host cells in which it can replicate.
4. Method of selecting or screening a clone of the recipient cells that has acquired the recombinant.

A generalized scheme of DNA cloning in *E. coli* is presented in figure 10.11.

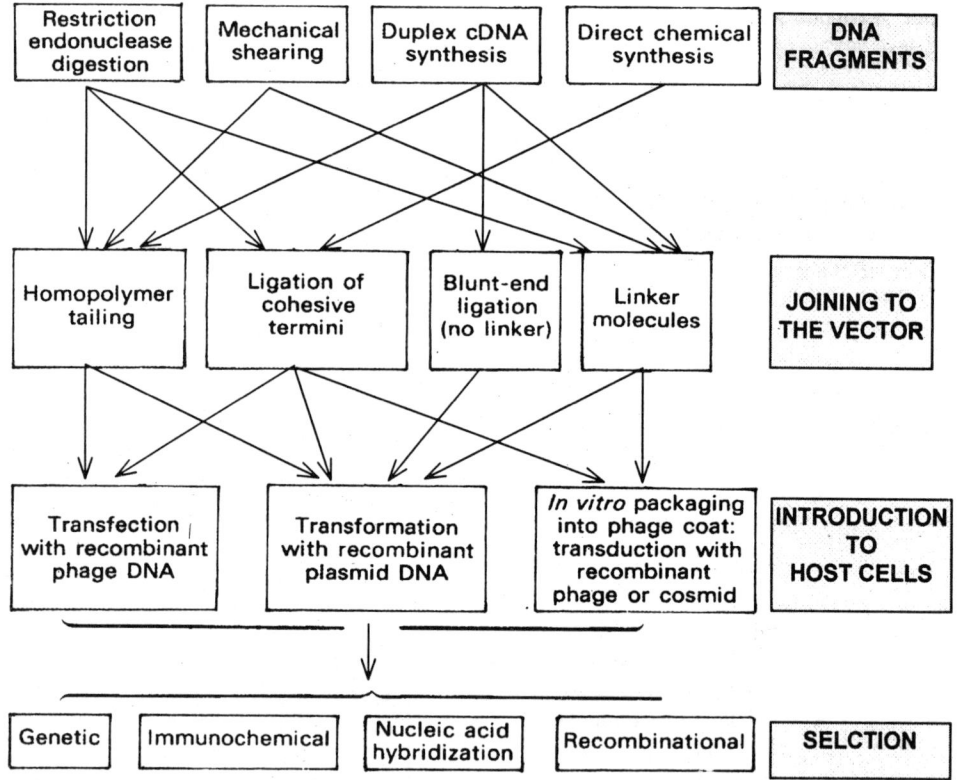

Fig. 10.11 : Generalized scheme of DNA cloning in *E. coli*

In the preceding paragraphs DNA cutting and joining have been described and the properties of several phages and plasmid vectors have also been discussed together with the factors governing the choice between the various cutting and joining methods and different vectors molecules.

The choice depends upon the type of expression system required, i.e., cDNA or genomic DNA clones. A consideration has to be taken if the frequency of the desired sequence in the starting material has to be increased by a prior enrichment. Alternatively a comparison from the gene libraries could be made in which the desired sequence has not been enriched. The latter is termed as *shotgun* approach.

10.5.2. Genomic DNA libraries

10.5.2.1. Construction

Gene libraries can be prepared from fragmented genomic DNA (genomic libraries) synthesized from cellular mRNA. The latter libraries will contain only gene sequence expressed in one cell type or tissue. The choice of the screening of the library is essentially based on whether the tissue or cell source of the protein is known. If a cell line produces readily detectable amounts of the protein or biological activity, a cDNA library derived from mRNA isolated from the cell line is the best line of attack.

When the source of the protein is either unknown or is suspected to be synthesized by a small subset of the cells in a tissue, genomic library screening is the best course of action. Hybridization probe and gene expression screening could be utilized for this purpose. In every event, genomic clones must be considered as an intermediate step towards the final isolation of a cDNA clone since it is this cDNA sequence which will be used for the eventual large-scale expression of the encoded protein. These libraries are of particular importance in the recombinant based production of proteins as they provide an easy opportunity for selection of the gene of interest.

10.5.2.2. Preparation

Methodologies for the preparation of the genomic libraries are well established in the literature. Genomic libraries derived from many commonly used animal species are available within the scientific community. Generally the genomic libraries could be constructed in bacteriophage λ cloning vectors in order to obtain enough independent recombinant to be confident of having a complete genome representation in the library (8.1×10^5 recombinants yields a 99% probability of the presence of any one sequence in a mammalian genomic library of 17 Kb fragments). The method involves insertion of genomic DNA fragments into a restriction site in the vector, replacing a segment of vector DNA. The recombinants are packaged into the phage particles in *in-vitro* and then transfected into *E. coli*.

An alternative system for cloning genomic DNA fragments uses a cosmid vectors. These vectors contain the COS sites of bacteriophage λ necessary for packaging and plasmid sequences for selection and replication in *E. coli*. DNA fragments are inserted into these vectors and the vectors are packaged into the phage particles *in-vitro*.

10.5.3. Preparation of cDNA libraries

cDNA cloning involves the preparation of a double-stranded DNA copy (dscDNA) of mRNA and its insertion into a plasmid or bacteriophage vector for cloning. The first step of dscDNA synthesis remains to be the most difficult step in the cloning process. By undertaking careful synthetic process large cDNA sequences can be synthesized and converted into the double-stranded molecules. Two basic methods are widely used to obtain dscDNA, both involve priming first-stranded synthesis with reverse transcriptase and oligodT. The first stranded sequence is accomplished by initial denaturation of the mRNA with methyl mercuric hydroxide and then by the addition of RNase inhibitor so as to limit the degradation of mRNA during the reaction. The second-stranded synthesis is accomplished in two ways.

One, the cDNA sequence form a hairpin loop like structure at their 3' end which can act as a primer for the second strand synthesis by DNA polymerase I. This structure can then be cleaved at the single stranded terminal by S1 nuclease to produce a blunt-ended, double-stranded cDNA. Second, the hybrid mRNA/cDNA product of first stranded synthesis is incubated with RNase H and DNA polymerase I such that single-stranded nicks in mRNA, are produced by RNase H action. These are used as primer points for DNA polymerase I activity in a repair sequence. *E. coli* DNA ligase appears not necessary for the completion of a continuous second strand. Insertion of cDNA sequence into plasmid vectors for propagation and cloning is accomplished by either complementary oligonucleotide tailing of the cDNA and vector addition of synthetic restriction site-containing linkers specific to the cDNA.

10.5.4. Isolation of gene sequence from the libraries

The most vexing problem encountered and experimented by all investigators wishing to isolate their genes is choosing the best library screening methods. No single method can give full assurance of successful gene isolation in a reasonable period of time since all have potential pitfalls and limitations. The choice can only be made on the basis of assaying the quality of the resource at hand and the nature of the protein being stalked or stored.

10.5.4.1. Protein sequence-based oligonucleotide probe screening

Protein microsequencing techniques using gas phase reaction can provide extensive amino acid sequence information from even microgram quantities of protein. It is possible to predict the nucleotide sequence of the gene encoding these amino acid sequence. Sometimes, a region of this predicted sequence will have ambiguities nevertheless all possible combinations of nucleotide sequence can be synthesized. This mixture of oligo-nucleotides can then be end-labelled with P^{32} and used for *in-situ* hybridization of phage plaques or bacterial colonies. The GC content of the individual oligonucleotides within a group can vary widely, presenting some difficulty in choosing hybridization conditions that are both stringent enough to ensure specificity of hybridization and relaxed enough to ensure hybridization of the lowest GC content oligonucleotide sequence.

10.5.5. Plasmids as cloning vectors

The most widely used cloning vehicles are the plasmids. They are defined as genetically homogeneous constant monomeric units, and have the ability to replicate independently of the chromosome. The basic properties which make them highly acceptable as best possible vector systems are that they are the replicons which are stably inherited in the extrachromosomal state, i.e. they don't require extrachromosomal nucleic acid molecules to replicate. The definition includes the prophages of the temperate phages e.g., P1, which are maintained in extrachromosomal state where as the λ phages are maintained through integration into the host chromosome.

The plasmids exist as double stranded circular DNA molecules in most of the cases where both the strands of DNA are intact circles, the molecules are referred to as covalently closed circles or CCC DNA. However, if one strand is intact then the molecules are referred as open circle or OC DNA. Recently a number of linear plasmids have been described in bacteria such as *Streptomyces* and the spirochete *Borrelia*. Although linear plasmids have not been isolated from *E. coli* this does not mean that they do not exist. In the case of *Streptomyces*, only linear plasmids could be detected by means of recently developed techniques of orthogonal-field-alteration gel electrophoresis. Plasmids are widely distributed throughout the prokaryotes and they vary in sizes from less than 1×10^6 Dalton to greater than 200×10^6 Dalton. The phenotype traits expressed by these plasmids are listed in table 10.2 which could be used for their identification, separation and purification.

Table 10.2 : Phenotypic traits exhibited by plasmid carried genes

Phenotypic traits	Phenotypic traits
Antibiotic resistance	Antibiotic production
Degradation of aromatic compounds	Haemolysin
Sugar fermentation	Enterotoxin production
Heavy metals resistance	Bacteriocin production
Induction of plant tumors	Hydrogen sulfide production

The categorization of plasmid could be made in two major types i.e., conjugate and non-conjugate-dependent upon whether or not they carry a set of transfer gene called the *tra* gene, that promotes the bacterial conjugation. They could also be classified on the basis of their being maintained as multiple copied per cell (relaxed plasmids) or as a limited number of copies per cell (stringent plasmids).

A large number of methods are available for isolation of pure plasmid DNA from cleared lysates. The classical method devised by Radloff et al., in 1967 is described. This method involves isopycnic centrifugation of cleared lysates in a solution of CsCl containing ethidium bromide (EtBr). EtBr intercalates between the DNA base pairs, and in so doing causes the DNA to unwind. A CCC DNA molecule such as a plasmid has no free ends therefore can only unwind to limited extent, thus limiting the amount of EtBr bound. A linear DNA molecule has no such constraints and therefore binds more of the EtBr molecules. Due to the reason that density of EtBr/DNA complex decreases as more of EtBr is bound, and because more EtBr can be bound to a linear molecule than a covalent circle, the covalent circle has a high density at saturating concentrations of EtBrs. Thus, by density gradient centrifugation these covalent circles could be separated from linear DNA.

The properties which are desirable for a plasmid as a cloning vehicles include:

1. Low molecular weight
2. Ability to confer readily selectable phenotypic trait on host cells.
3. Single sites for a large number of restriction endonucleases, preferably in gene with a readily scorable phenotype.

The plasmids could either be of natural origin or be constructed. The term 'natural' is used loosely in this context to describe plasmids which are not constructed *in vitro* for the sole purpose of cloning. Various natural plasmids with their properties are listed in table 10.3.

Table 10.3 : Properties of some plasmids of natural origin

Plasmid	Size (M dal.)	Single sites for endonucleases	Markers for selecting transformants
pSC101	5.8	Xho I, EcoRI, Hind III, Sal I	Tetracycline resistance
Col R I	4.2	Eco RI	Immunity to colicin EI
RSF 2124	74	EcoRI Bam HI	Ampicillin resistance

For example, the plasmid pSC101, DNA and DNA to be inserted are digested with EcoR1 and treated with DNA ligases. The ligated molecules are then used to transform a suitable recipient to tetracycline resistance. The pSC101 is most frequently used cloning vehicle. The examples for its uses include-

1. Expression of *Staphylococcus* plasmid gene in *E. coli.*
2. Cloning of *Xenopus* DNA in *E. coli.*

A simple method for insertion of foreign gene into the plasmid genome is presented in figure 10.12

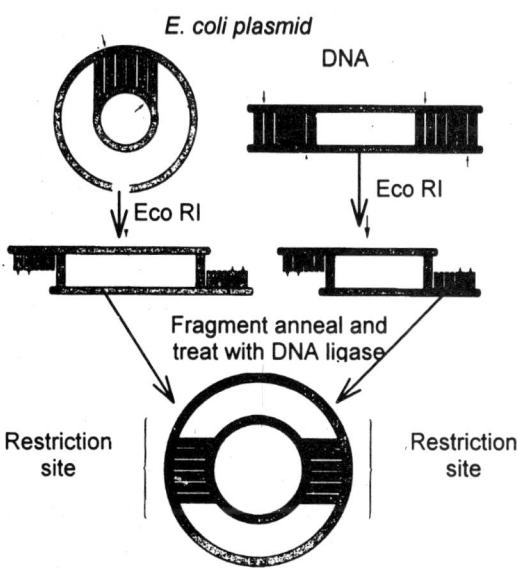

Fig. 10.12 : Insertion of foreign gene in the plasmid

10.5.5.1. New Cloning Vehicles pBR322

Although pSC101, Col E1, and RSF 2124 can be used to clone DNA; they suffer from some disadvantages. Hence, considerable efforts have been expanded on constructing *in vitro* superior cloning vehicles. The most versatile vector is pBR322. The plasmid pBR322 essentially contains the Ap^R and Tc^R gene of RSF2124 and pSC101 respectively combined with replication of pMB1 and a Col E1 like plasmid.

Plasmid pBR322 is the most widely used cloning vehicle. In addition, it has been widely used as a model system for study of prokaryotic transcription and translation as well as investigation of the effects of topological changes in DNA conformation.

10.5.6. Bacteriophage λ as a vectors for cloning in *E. coli*

Bacterophage λ is a genetically complex but very extensively studied vector of *E. coli*. The DNA of phage λ, is in the form in which it is isolated from phage particle, it is typically a linear duplex molecule of about 48.5 kb pairs. In the DNA sequence each ends are short single-stranded 5'-projection of 12 nucleotides, which are complementary in sequence and through which the DNA adapts a circular structure when it is injected into its host cells, i.e. λ DNA naturally has cohesive termini associated to form COS site. The steps of replication of the λ phage are highlighted in figure 10.13.

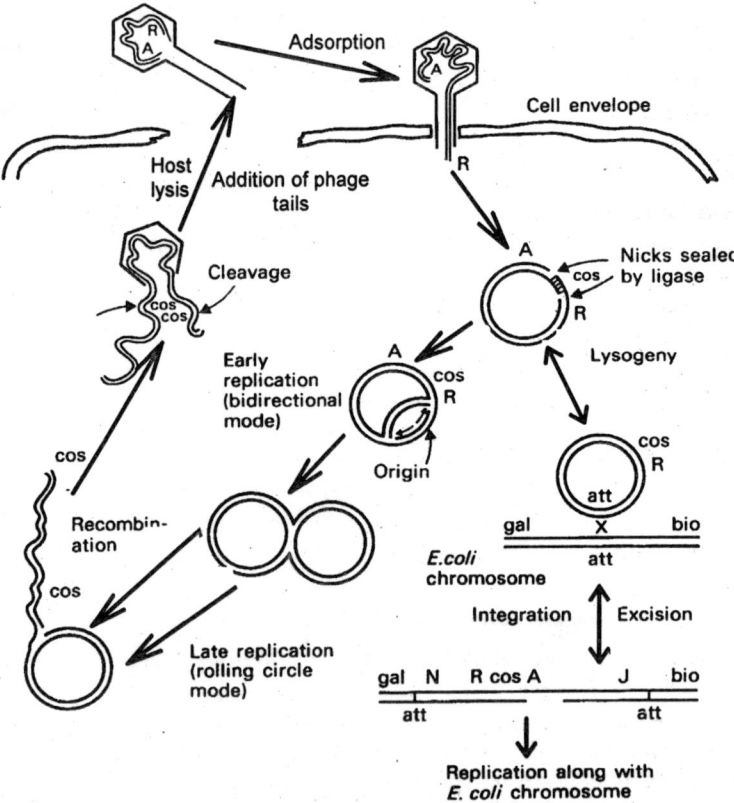

Fig. 10.13 : Replication of the phage λ DNA in lytic and lysogenic cycles

10.5.6.1. Modified phage λ replacement vector

As with plasmid vectors, improved phage and vector diverses have been developed in many laboratories. These are well aimed modifications as:

1. To increase the capacity of foreign DNA fragment, preferably for fragments generated by any one of the several restriction enzymes;
2. To devise methods for positively selecting recombinant formation;
3. To allow RNA probes to conveniently prepared by transcription of foreign DNA insert. This facilitates the screening of libraries in chromosome walking procedures. As an example of a vector with this property is λZAP;
4. To develop vectors for the insertion of eukaryotic cDNA such that expression of the cDNA in the form of a fusion polypeptides with β-galactosidase, is driven by *E coli*. This form of expression vector is useful in antibody screening. An example of this is vector λ gtll.

10.5.7. Role of DNA ligases

The vectors used in the rDNA experiment, can be prepared by splicing and cleaving vector DNA at a single specific site with a restriction enzyme. For example, the plasmid pSC101 (a 9.9 kb double helical circular DNA molecule) is split at a unique site by the EcoRI restriction enzymes. The staggered cut made by this enzyme produces complementary single-stranded ends, which have specific affinity for each other and hence are known as cohesive ends. Any DNA fragment can be inserted into this plasmid if it has the same cohesive ends. Such a fragment can be prepared from a larger piece of DNA by using the same restriction enzymes as was used to open the plasmid DNA. The single stranded ends of fragments are then complementary to those of the cut plasmid. The DNA fragments and the cut plasmid can be annealed and then joined by DNA ligase, which catalyzes the formation of phospodiester bonds between the two DNA chains. The DNA ligase requires a free OH group at the 3' end of one DNA chain and a phosphate group at the 5' end of the other. Furthermore, the chain joined by ligase must belong to double-helical DNA molecule. An energy source, such as ATP or NAD^+ is required for the joining reaction.

The cohesive end joining method for DNA molecule can be made general by using a short, chemically synthesized DNA that can be cleaved by restriction enzymes. First, the linker is covalently joined to two ends of a DNA fragment of vector. For example, the 5' end of a decameric linker and a DNA molecule is phosphorylated by polynucleotide kinase and then joined by ligase from T4 phage. This ligase can form a covalent bond between blunt ended (flush-ended) double helical DNA molecule. The cohesive ends are produced when the terminal extensions are cut by an appropriate restriction enzyme. Thus cohesive ends corresponding to a particular restriction enzymes can be added virtually to any DNA molecule.

10.6. GENE EXPRESSION AND PROTEIN PRODUCTION

The major interest of all the techniques discussed till now is to utilize the expressed protein products of the isolated genes for analysis and clinical application. This process of production of protein from its gene is termed as 'expression' and the DNA components used for expression are termed as **expression vectors**. However, the production of protein of interest occurs in a host cell which is compatible for the maintenance and/or replication of expression vector. Jointly, the host cell and the expression vector are termed as an **expression system**.

It has been previously highlighted that the central 'Dogma' of life is the triplet genetic code and it is universal for all the cells from simple bacteria to plant and humans. Hence if proper regulatory signals recognized by particular cell types are attached to any cell will be capable of translating the message transcribed from a human gene or cDNA i.e., producing appropriate protein. Hence this provides an excellent opportunity for the production of human protein in any cell type for which vector systems are available. The choice of particular vector system is determined by various factors such as the application for which protein is expressed, properties of the protein and the economics of production in the cases where large quantities are desirable.

10.6.1. Choice of expression systems

The large scale production systems of gene products have been developed based on both prokaryotic and eukaryotic cells. In essence, all these systems involve the *in vitro* construction of a DNA sequence containing a promoter of transcription upstream of the desired coding sequence, a terminator of transcription downstream, and a translation initiator either provided by the coding sequence or inserted during construction process. The transcription units could then be inserted into an appropriate DNA vector which will allow either extrachromosomal replication of the DNA or integration of DNA into the host chromosome. Selectable marker genes are included to allow isolation of transformed cells and maintain the introduced DNA. There are many factors which are responsible for the selection of an appropriate expression system to be used for a particular protein. In general high-volume products such as insulin must be made in easily fermentable microorganisms such as yeasts or bacteria, and low volume proteins can be made in higher eukaryotic systems such as mammalian cells.

The most important consideration in the choice of host expression system is the complexity of protein to be produced. Most of the extracellular proteins are held in their active configuration by the disulfide bonds. In small proteins as many as twenty or more such bonds can occur. Although the polypeptide chain alone can define its active conformation and will thus self-assemble, however, where multiple disulfide bond formation is required, the efficient assembly of the protein may only be possible during the sequential process of protein secretion into the oxidizing environment either through endoplasmic reticulum lumen (eukaryotes) or on the periplasmic spaces or medium (prokaryotes).

Till date no such prokaryotic system has been developed for the production of heterogeneous products. Mostly the eukaryotic systems such as yeast or mammalian cells are utilized. The best example is the production of t-PA (tissue plasminogen activator), it could be successfully expressed by the bacterial cells but the expression was found to be inactive. However, the one obtained from mammalian cells is quite active in nature. Another structural consideration to be looked for is the presence of oligosaccharide side chains, such as r-carboxylated glutamic acid residues, or β-OH-aspartic acid. These secondary modifications have a critical effect on the *in vivo* performance of the protein. Mammalian cell-systems express glycosylate heterologous proteins efficiently and probably correctly, which is not possible in bacteria.

The last but not the least consideration in the choice of the expression system for the protein is the requirement for cleavage of primary translation product either to activate the product or to remove N-terminal signal sequence. Insulin in particular requires the removal of an internal domain (the C-peptide) for activation. The two active polypeptides can be synthesized independently in the bacteria, purified and then renatured under controlled conditions. Alternatively, the polypeptide chain can be engineered to built in site for chemical or enzymatic removal of C-peptide.

10.6.2. Expression vectors

The protein production by rDNA approach is accomplished through the use of expression vectors which are an assembly of covalently linked segments of DNA each performing a specific function. The three basic components of expression vectors are:

1. DNA regions which permit the replications of the vectors in the bacterial host cells used in vector assembly and also allow the selection of the host cells containing the vector;
2. DNA regions which confer selectivity on the bacterial host wherein the vector was assembled;
3. The gene or cDNA to be expressed, linked to an appropriate transcription and translational control elements capable of functioning in the expression hosts.

E. coli bacterium propagation is accounted for the construction of majority of the expression vectors. Large amounts of vector DNAs are extracted from *E. coli* cultured and introduced into chosen host cells. Hence, vectors assembled by the manipulation of DNA by restriction nuclease and ligases are introduced in naked DNA form into *E. coli* rendered components to accept extraneous DNA. This is known as 'transformation' process. After the entry of vector in *E. coli* cells, it has to be replicated and maintained so as to avoid its loss due to the dilution that accompanies rounds of cell division. The presence of DNA sequence on the vector functioning as the origin of replication, permits the vector to replicate in the host cells. Figure 10.14 shows the components of a typical expression vector.

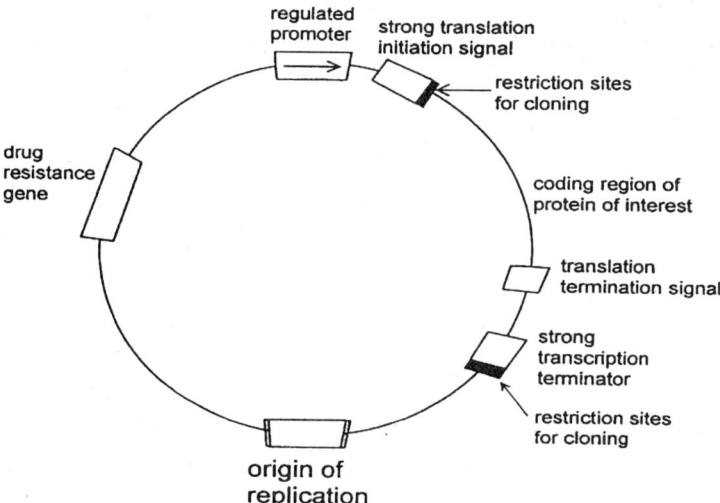

Fig 10.14 : Components of a typical expression vector

When the cells are transformed with naked vector DNA, only a fraction, i.e. 10% of cells takes up DNA. Hence, originates the need for the separation of these cells from the non-receiving ones. This is undertaken using the selectable property encoded by the vectors such as resistance to antibiotics like tetracycline, ampicillin, etc. This will lead to the death of nontransformed cells on exposure with antibiotics. Hence the transformed bacterial cells can be easily isolated, grown and the vector DNA is prepared from them for introduction into the expression host cells of choice.

The second major component responsible for an expression vector comprises of DNA sequences required for selection, maintenance and copy-number amplification of the vector in the host cell where in protein expression is desired. This region is not required for expression of *E. coli*. The third component of an expression vector is the expression cassette comprising of the DNA (either cDNA or gene) encoding the protein to be produced and the sequences required to direct the transcription, RNA processing and translation of the RNA. The coding sequence is proceeded by a promoter sequence which is capable of directing transcription in the chosen host cell and is followed by sequence involved in RNA processing, and transcription termination.

10.6.3. Expression hosts

The preceding discussion highlighted that the universality of genetic code has made possible the production of a protein in any cell type whose biology is understood and for which vectors and method for transformation exists. In most of the cases being utilized in biotechnological industry, proteins of biological interest are expressed in bacteria, yeast and other fungi, insect cells and mammalian cells. However, some newer studies indicated that intact oocytes delivered from frog *xenopus* are amenable for use in expression of mRNAs or genes introduced into them by microinjection. But still the system has not found acceptable utility in large scale production of proteins. Recent advances in the use of transgenic animals for secreting therapeutic proteins in milk are exciting extension of the expression in mammalian cells, that circumvent the need to culture engineered mammalian cells.

There are two factors which play role in the choice of host/vector system are :

1. The ability to produce the protein in a form acceptable for the particular application.
2. Economics of production which should include not only the cost of growing the engineered cells but also the down stream purification techniques necessitated by the characteristics of the production system.

Some of the commonly used expression systems currently in use and their advantages and disadvantages are summed up in table 10.4.

Table 10.4 : Expression systems and characteristics

Expression system	Prototype	Advantages	Limitations
Bacterial	E. Coli	Inexpensive media rapid high-density growth high protein yield secretion	No post-translational modifications endotoxins insolubility
Fungal	S. cerevisiae	Inexpensive media	limited post-translational modifications
		high-density growth	different post-translational modifications
		some post-translational modifications	lower protein yield
Insect	SF9 cells, Baculovirus	High protein yields	Different post-translational modifications
		many post-translational modifications	expensive media and growth
		secretion	lytic not continuous
Mammalian	Chinese hamster ovary cells	Correct post-translational modifications	Expensive media and growth
		secretion	slow growth
		authenticity of product	mammalian pathogens

Amongst all these, bacteria offer the greatest economy of growth. The bacteria have always been the first choice for a protein production in active form, or if the protein is needed as antigenic material where activity is not an issue of concern. However, these offer the major disadvantage of aggregation of these proteins into the amorphous entity called the 'inclusion body'. The disulfide bonds present in many proteins of interest are form in the bacterial cytoplasm. Therefore, it is necessary to extract the protein present in a denatured form and refold it into an active form. The conditions for refolding process vary with each protein and are often laborious. Many of the folding problems can be resolved by inducing the bacterial host to secrete the protein into the extracellular spaces or the bacterial periplasm by attaching the secretion signal from a normally secreted bacterial protein to the amino terminus of the protein to be secreted. Another limitations with bacterial expression system is the inability of bacteria to perform many post-translational modifications which are normally present in mammalian proteins. Furthermore, the assembly of proteins composed of multiple subunits (e.g. antibodies) does not occur in bacterial cells. The characteristics for ideal expression system could be summarized as:

1. Rapid growth rate, high cell densities, i.e. high biomass production.
2. Low-cost medium: Little or no expensive nutrients such as animal sera.
3. High production rates per cell.
4. Low vector copy number/high production: No selection for high copy number.
5. Stable under cultivation.
6. Production in absence of cell growth.
7. No toxic substance for maintenance of the vector.
8. Safety.

10.6.4. Various types of expression systems

There are three major expression host systems in use. These are mammalian cells, yeast cells and E. coli. Many other are still under development.

10.6.4.1. Bacterial expression systems

The bacterial based expression systems could be classified as :
  a. intracellular expression systems
  b. extracellular expression systems

10.6.4.1.1. Intracellular expression systems

E. coli is the bacterium of choice as the expression host for most of the intracellular bacterial expressions due to the reason that its genetics has been elucidatively and extensively studied. Several therapeutically active proteins like interferons, insulin growth hormone are being successfully produced by this system. The expression system is usually designed such that the transcription unit is inducible and the organism could be grown to high density in the absence of product formation. Induction then rapidly produces large amount of the product (up to 40% of total cell protein can be achieved), which accumulates in dense inclusion bodies, essentially containing a precipitate of the product, which makes the purification simpler. Most of the work undertaken on the promoter system has been associated with the Trp promoter inducible by tryptophan depletion, the Pl promoter from bacteriophage λ, using a temperature sensitive repressor so that induction is achieved by temperature modulation, and the Tac promoter, a fusion of Trp promoter sequence with Lac operator so that induction is achieved by adding isopropylthiogalactoside (IGTG). The Trp promoter is the best available system because of its promoter strength and the physiological conditions under which it is induced. The Pl promoter system works effectively but the temperature shift needed to induce this system can induce several proteases which may cause product instability.

The primary translational product of this type of expression is intended to be the final one, however, some proteins require engineering of the encoding sequence so as to remove 5' non-coding sequence and any secretory leader signal sequence. The major problem encountered here is the removal of an N-terminal methionine residue in recombinant protein, not present in natural protein, which can potentially induce immunological reactions in clinical use if allowed to remain.

10.6.4.1.2. Extracellular expression systems

The intracellular synthesis of the peptides does not promote di-sulfide bond formation, and yet many clinically useful proteins such as the serine proteases of the coagulation and fibrinolytic pathways contain many multiple disulfide bonds, which are critical determinants of the activity. However, much attention is being focused on the secretion of product from the bacterial systems. In these systems, the coding sequence of the mature protein is ligated to an N-terminal secretory leader segment like β-lactamase, lamB, ompF, phoA and lpp. All of these can direct the secretion of the product into the periplasmic space. High specific activities have been found in secreted product, employing correct folding of the polypeptide, but very low expressions are at present reported.

Some bacterial species such as *Bacillus* and *Pseudomonas* secrete substantial amounts of protein into the medium. Harnessing of these secretory mechanisms would be an attractive future strategy.

10.6.4.2. Yeast expression systems

During the recent years of scientific development yeast has emerged as a most promising system for expression of foreign proteins. Yeasts offer various advantages. The most advantageous factor is the ability to culture in high-density, large-scale yeast fermentation for which the growth characteristics have been extensively investigated and are well established. Yeast has another capability of producing the proteins following similar mechanism as operate to that in the mammalian cells. These mechanisms could be utilized for expression of foreign proteins in large quantities in highly active forms. Yeasts cells also glycosylate secreted proteins using the same signal sequences in the polypeptide backbone as mammalian cells.

One other advantage offered by the yeast cells is that they secrete a relatively small percentage of its total cellular proteins into the medium, facilitating separation and purification of desired product. Furthermore, yeast cells don't produce endotoxins and are non-pathogenic to man, which should simplify the acceptance of human pharmaceutical products synthesized and expressed in yeast. The development of yeast as an expression host has led to the development of various expressions and secretory vectors for the introduction and maintenance of genes in the yeast. These are:

10.6.4.2.1. Vector System

Expression vector for yeast can either integrate into the genome or may remain in a stable extrachromosomal configuration. Since yeast expression plasmid can be maintained at a relatively high copy number, 20-200 copies per cell, they have become the most frequently used expression vectors. A typical yeast/bacterial shuttle vector of yeast originated replication, which is usually the DNA segments encoding the origin of the yeast 2μ circles, or a chromosomal replication origin (e.g. ARS1) and a yeast selectable marker such as the gene coding for URA3, LEU2 or TRYP1.

10.6.4.2.2. Expression systems

Two types of yeasts trasncriptional promoters have been used to express high levels of foreign proteins in yeast. The inducible promoters are employed wherever the foreign proteins are expected to be toxic to the cell growth. For example, the inorganic phosphate repressible acid phosphatase and the glucose repressible invertase promoters which are induced when inorganic phosphate or glucose respectively, are depleted from the medium. The other classes of the promoter are actively constituted in the cell and include the glycolytic promoter glyceraldehyde,3-phosphate dehydrogenase (GPD 4) triose phosphate isomerase (TP1) and 3-phosphoglycerate kinase (PGK).

Furthermore, it has also been reported that efficient transcription is important for the high level expression. Mutation affecting transcription, termination of cycl-512 gene resulted in a dramatic decrease in transcript level. However, introduction of a yeast termination sequence from invertase SVC2 gene at the 3' end of the transcriptional unit had no effect on the expression of calf prochymosin in yeast. Another factor which may be important for high level expression of foreign proteins in yeast and human cells as it might affect translational efficiency too is the difference in codon usage between yeast and mammalian systems.

10.6.4.2.3. Secretion system

Yeast has been successfully utilized for the intracellular expression of heterologous proteins but some proteins have been synthesized intracellularly as inactive products. One explanation for the observed lack of activity of the cytoplasmically expressed proteins is that they require processing via the secretory pathways to assume the correct active conformation. Hence, lot of efforts have been directed towards the development of the secretion vectors using a variety of different leader sequences.

In several cases such as the interferons, the natural human signal sequences have been found to be efficiently recognized and processed by yeast cells. However, for the other proteins such as α-1-antitrypsin, the natural leader is not efficiently recognized by the yeast cells, resulting in the accumulation of the unprocessed pre-protein. As an alternative to the use of natural leader sequences, yeast derived secretory leaders have been substituted, resulting in increased secretion efficiency and higher yield of the secretory products. As the technology for developing high level expression and secretion systems for yeast becomes increasingly available the promise of yeast as an alternative host for the production of foreign proteins is being met with development of system for production of the yeast-derived hepatitis-B-vaccine. The approach will be discussed in the succeeding paragraphs.

10.6.4.3. Mammalian cell expression systems

The complex nature of many proteins of therapeutic potential requires their expression in the mammalian cell systems. There are many advantages of producing the proteins in the mammalian cells systems like:

a) Expressed proteins obtained are glycosylated similar to their natural counterparts.

b) Expressed proteins and other products obtained are properly folded and contain proper disulfide bonds.

c) Expressed proteins are secreted into the medium so as to facilitate purification.

d) Very large proteins (greater than 100 kDa) have not successfully produced by the microbial system, whereas these can be effectively produced using the mammalian system.

The major problem with the production of the pharmaceuticals in the mammalian system is the high production cost of the mammalian cell culture. Hence, the production of the pharmaceuticals using the mammalian systems is limited only to the proteins which are required in very small quantities, larger in size and could not be produced by the microbial cultures. However, several systems have been developed and utilized for the production of high level proteins in the mammalian cultures. Some of them are:

10.6.4.3.1. Lytic viral vector system

SV40 virus is the most extensively studied lytic viral vector system. This is due to availability of the informations regarding the replication and expression modes of the SV40 in different host cells. Foreign DNA may be substituted into early and the late regions of SV40 and the virus propagates in presence of the helper virus. More recently, the availability of the monkey kidney cell lines expressing early regions of SV40 (COS cells) has allowed the generation of helper free recombinant virus. Although these SV40 viral systems have been successfully used in the expression of several proteins like human growth hormone, hepatitis surface antigen etc., several limitations for the system still exist. Firstly, the SV40 chromosome is small in size so the genes larger than 2.5 kilobases become very difficult to propagate. Secondly, most efficient viruses result from the mixed viral infections and in some cases the helper virus predominantly replicates over the recombinant during continued viral propagation. Thirdly, the virus lyses the host cells such that the expressed protein has to be recovered before the lysis of the membrane. Another lytic vector system with a limited success is the human adenovirus. Apart form the already mentioned limitations the adenovirus also cannot be used as the lytic viral vectors due to a very short lytic cycle. Adenovirus-infected cells lyse 20-24 h post infection and hence very little time is available to accumulate product before the cell lysis.

10.6.4.3.2. Non-lytic viral vectors

RNA and DNA viruses are primarily the two classes of the non-lytic viral vectors, which have been used to express heterologous genes. RNA tumor viruses (retroviruse) have been used to transfer DNA into heterologous cells. The advantages offered by these viruses include:

a) The ability to transduce the gene in a variety of cell types and variety of cell species;

b) Some of these reteroviruses integrate in the host chromosome and DNA is very stable;

c) The efficient transfer of the host cells can approach 100%;

d) High titer recombinant virus stocks can be prepared.

However, the expression of the protein from the retroviral-based vectors has been low and problems with RNA splicing have hampered the usefulness of this vector system. The prototype of DNA based non-lytic viral vector is Bovine Papilloma Virus (BPV), which is a small DNA virus that morphologically transforms a variety of cells. Vectors containing the entire BPV genome or 5.5Kb subgenomic transforming fragments are in many cases stable as multicopy (20-100 copies/cell) extrachromosomal elements in transformed cells. Many of the secreted proteins, such as β-interferon and human growth hormone have been successfully expressed by BPV.

10.6.5. Summarized steps in cloning DNA

Various steps involved in the gene cloning are discussed below and presented in figure 10.15.

10.6.5.1. Step I :Construction of a recombinant molecule

A DNA fragment of interest is covalently joined to a DNA vector. The essential feature of a vector is that it can replicate autonomously in an appropriate host. Plasmids (naturally occurring circles of DNA that act as accessory chromosomes) and α phages (a virus) are choice vectors for cloning in *E. coli.*

10.6.5.2. Step II :Introduction in host cells

Many bacterial and eukaryotic cells take up naked DNA molecule from the medium. The efficiency of uptake is quite low, however an appreciable proportion of cells can be transformed under appropriate experimental conditions. Mutant bacteria that do not rapidly degrade foreign DNA are often used as host cells. DNA molecules can also be injected into many animal and plant cells. Alternatively, target cells can be infected with virus particles assembled to harbor the recombinant DNA molecule.

10.6.5.3. Step III :Selection

The next step is to determine which cells harbor the recombinant DNA molecule containing the gene of interest. The desired cells can be selected by the presence of either of the vector or of the target gene itself.

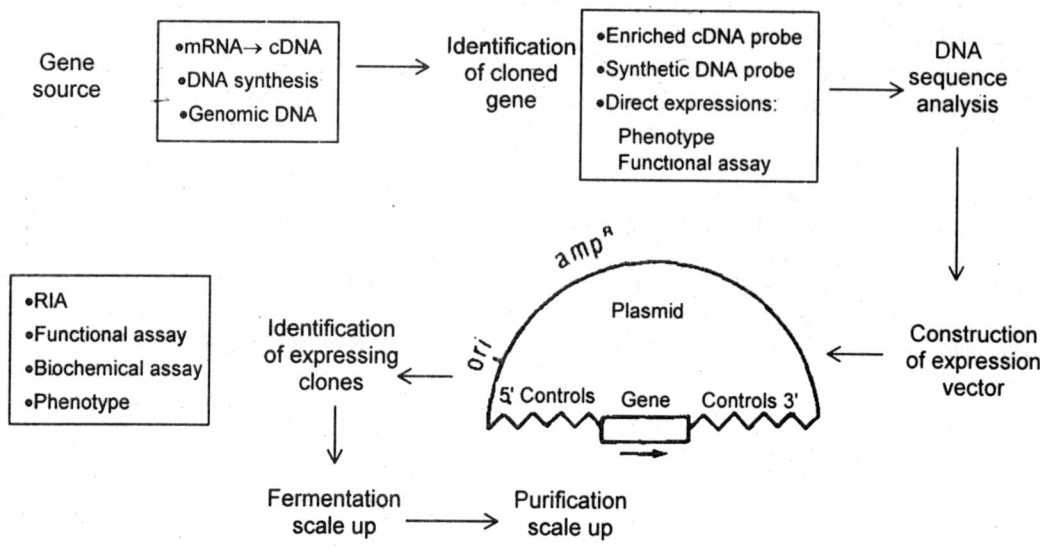

Fig. 10.15 : Summary of cloning of DNA

10.7. CLONING OF A EUKARYOTE GENE

Most of the genes from the higher eukaryotes are quite large, extending over hundreds and thousands of base pairs. Much of the length is made up of introns, which are excised from the mRNA in processing. However, the larger DNA could still be cloned, expression of the gene product in bacterial cells would be impossible because bacterial cells are incapable of RNA splicing. Hence, whenever, a gene it is quite large is difficult to clone and express it directly. It is desirable to clone the coding sequence present in the mRNA to determine the base sequence and to study the polypeptide gene product. Figure 10.16 highlights the method for direct cloning of an eukaryotic coding sequence from the cell in which mRNA is present.

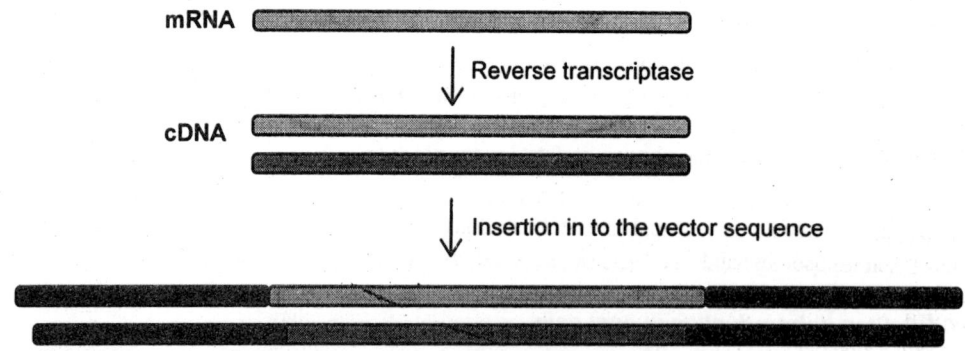

Fig. 10.16 : Cloning of eukaryotic gene

This mRNA can be used to clone a cDNA using a reverse transcriptase, which utilizes single stranded RNA molecule as a template to synthesize a double stranded DNA copy referred to as complememtary DNA (cDNA). The mRNA contains the complete gene sequence with all introns removed, the corresponding cDNA contains uninterrupted coding sequence. The sequence is not identical with the original gene as all the introns are removed, however, the sequence corresponding the protein production is still there. Thus the cDNA could be the tool of choice for cloning of larger genes so as to express a gene product. Further, the cDNA could be linked to a vector sequence and expressed within the host accomplishing the classical techniques.

10.8. APPLICATIONS OF RECOMBINANT DNA TECHNOLOGY

Proteins form the basis of life. Genes are responsible for the expression of the proteins. Traditionally proteins play an important role as they form the intemediaries between gene and phenotypes. These proteins could be effectively isolated and purified from cell extract and studied for their properties *in-vitro*. However, the behavior of a purified protein in the test tube (*in-vitro* biochemistry) could be different from that of the same protein in complex environment of the cell. Furthermore, many key cellular proteins are synthesized transiently (at a particular time/intermeditary) and in very low concentrations viz., proteins involved in the cell division, lymphokines, etc. As described in the previous section that using the recombinant technology it is possible to produce any protein in sufficient quantity for its elucidative study. Some of the proteins successfully produced and studied for their activity are listed in table 10.5. Furthermore, by utilization of recombinant DNA technology, many proteins could be produced for their commercial values as pharmaceuticals. Their current status is listed in table 10.6.

Table 10.5: Recombinant proteins approved for clinical use

Name of the proteins	Applicability
Human insulin	Diabetes
Interferon-α2	Hairy cell leukemia and genital warts
Tissue plasminogen activator	Coronary thrombolysis
Human growth hormone	Pituitary dwarfism
Erythropoietin	Anemia associated with renal failure
Interleukin-2	Cancer
hepatitis B surface antigen	Vaccination

Table 10.6 : Current status of some recombinant products

Product	Expression system	Clinical indication	Status
Human insulin	E.coli	Juvenile-onset diabetes	Already in market.
Human somatotrophin	E.coli	Pituitary dwarfism	Already in market.
Interferon-α2	E.coli and yeast	Hairy cell leukemia and prophylaxis of common cold	Already in market.
Interferon-γ	E.coli	Treatment of cancer and treatment of viral diseases	In final clinical trials
Relaxin	E.coli	Facilitates child birth	Animal trials have proven successful and is under human trials
Interleukin-2	E.coli and animal cells	Treatment of cancer	In market.
Tissue plasminogen activator	E.coli yeast and animal cells	Thrombosis	In market
Erythropoeitin	Mammalian cells	Treatment of anemia	In market
Hepatitis B surface antigen	Yeast and mammalian cells	Vaccination	Now in market
Factor VIII	Mammalian cells	Treatment of hemophilia	In trials
Human serum albumin	Yeast	Plasma replacement therapy	In trials

Recombinant DNA technology has become a well known foremost tool in biotechnology. It offers a number of distinctive advantages. The applications of this technology in a more systematic way is dealt in successive paragraphs.

10.8.1. Novel proteins generation

The utilization of recombinant DNA technology is not only restricted to the introduction of the intact genes of the eukaryotes origin into microbes. However, the genes of completely novel proteins could also be constructed.

The simplest example of the generation of the novel protein involves the redesigning enzyme structure by site directed mutagenesis. The approach has been utilized by Winter and associates (Winter et.al. 1982; Wilkinson et al. 1984). A detailed knowledge of structure of enzyme tyrosyl-tRNA synthetase obtained from *Bacillus stearothermophilus*, helped them to predict point mutations in the gene which increased the enzyme affinity for the substrate ATP.

These changes were introduced and in one case, a single amino acid change could improve the affinity for ATP by a factor of 100. Furthermore, the approach helped in increasing the stability of enzyme. Similarly the thermostability of T4 lysozyme could be increased by introduction of disulfide bonds. The functional promise of gene manipulation coupled with the technique of site-directed mutagenesis was proved by works on subtilisin. Most of the properties like catalysis, substrate specificity, pH and stability to oxidative, thermal and alkaline inactivation were altered. To exemplify, a variant was constructed which was more than 1000 fold resistant to oxidation inactivation than was the wild-type enzyme. This was achieved by replacing a critical methionine residue with alanine. In a similar kind of modification, the replacement of methionine with valine generated an oxidation-resistant variant of α_1-antitrypsin.

A standard technique in conventional medicinal chemistry is to identify, a chemical entity with a desirable pharmacological effect and then to construct analogs and determine if any of them have improved therapeutic properties. A similar technique can be applied to proteins by means of recombinant DNA technology. As in the case of neutral solutions of insulin, it is mostly assembled as zinc-containing hexamers. This may adversely affect its absorption, however, by making single amino acid substitution it is possible to generate insulin which is monomeric at pharmacological concentrations. Hence, the biological efficacy is preserved as well as a three times faster absorption is observed. Thus, by deliberately introducing sequence variations into a protein with multiple biological activities, novel proteins which retain only one or few of these activity may be obtained. Some of the novel proteins which have stormed the pharmaceutical market with the lesser cost and efficacy of production after the utilization of recombinant techniques are:

10.8.1.1 Insulin

Insulin, the secretion from β-cells of islets of Langerhans in pancreas is a peptide hormone responsible for the decrease in blood sugar level. However, an alteration in the secretion of hormone leads to the development of disorder known as Diabetes mallietus. Further, diabetes may either be insulin dependent (nonjuvenile) or insulin independent (juvenile). Although both the diseases arise from malfunctioning in insulin secretion, however, the latter arises due to malfunctioning in the gene related to encoding and hence production of insulin, while the former is due to improper secretion of insulin.

Insulin was for the first time applied to a diabetic nine year old boy in 1922 with success. It was immediately set on for production by Eli-Lilly in 1923 and animal insulin (from pancreas) was marketed. Since then the production of insulin has been a tremendous trend. Insulin is composed of two polypeptides chains A and B linked via disulfide bonds. These two chains are derived from preproinsulin which is synthesized in beta cells of islets of langerhans. The preproinsulin is composed of 109 amino acids, out of which the first 23 amino acids are delinked after it passes through the cell membrane of the synthesizing cells leaving proinsulin. The proinsulin folds up so as to bring first and the last chain together and the central portion of the molecule is cut by the enzymes so as to leave insulin (Fig. 10.17).

Most of the mammalian genes are mosaics of introns and exons. These genes can be easily cloned. These interrupted genes cannot be expressed by bacteria, which lack the machinery to splice introns out of primary transcripts. The difficulty has been effectively circumvented by making bacteria to take up recombinant DNA that is a complementary to mRNA. The best possible example in this context is the production of proinsulin. Proinsulin can further be converted to give insulin. Indeed, much of the insulin used today by millions of diabetics is produced by bacteria especially *E. coli*. Proinsulin or insulin can be synthesized by bacteria harboring plasmid that contains DNA complementary to mRNA that carries transcript for proinsulin. Figure 10.18 describes the process for its production.

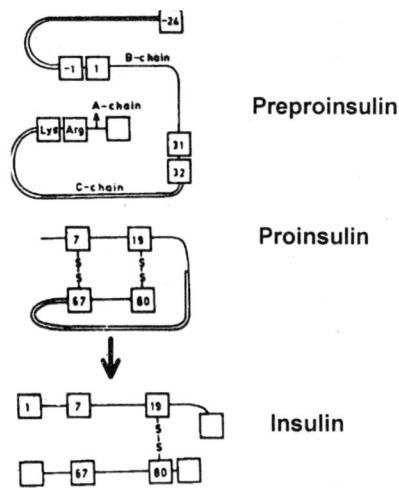

Fig. 10.17 : Biosynthesis of insulin in human body via proinsulin

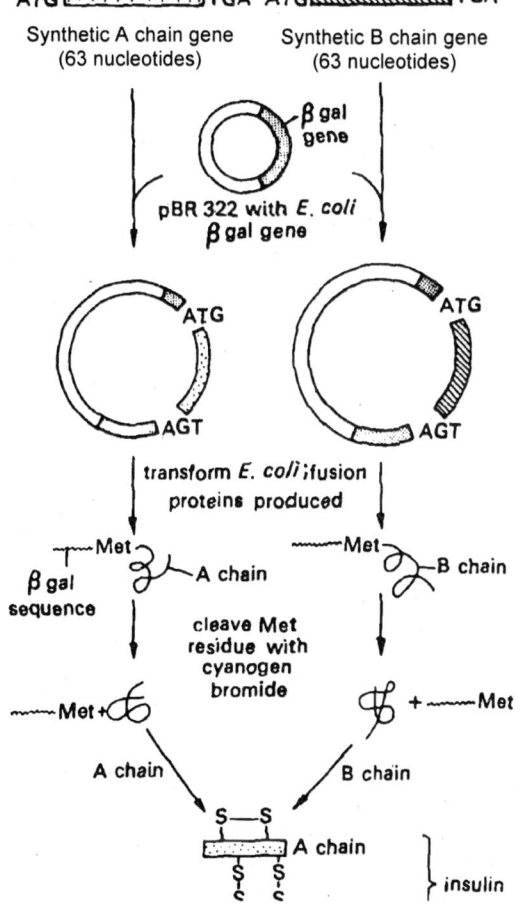

Fig. 10.18 : Synthesis of proinsulin a precursor of insulin by recombinant DNA technology

The key substance responsible for the formation of complementary DNA (cDNA) is the enzyme reverse transcriptase. The retroviruses use this enzyme to form DNA-RNA hybrid in the replication of their genomic RNA. Reverse transcriptase synthesizes a DNA strand complementary to RNA template, if it could be provided with a primer that is base paired to the RNA and which also contain a free 3'OH group. This enzyme synthesizes DNA from mRNA by providing an oligo-dT primer that pairs, with the poly-A-sequence at the 3' end of most eukaryotic mRNA molecules. The rest of cDNA strand is then synthesized in the presence of four deoxyribonucleoside triphosphates. cDNA molecules can be inserted into vectors that favor their efficient harboring in hosts such as E. coli. Such plasmids or phages are called as expression vectors. To maximize transcription, the cDNA is inserted into the vector in the correct reading frame near a strong bacterial promoter.

In addition, these vectors answer efficient translation by encoding a ribosome-binding site on the mRNA near the initiation codon. cDNA clones can be screened on the basis of their capacity to direct the synthesis of a foreign protein in the bacteria. The immunochemical screening approach can be applied whenever a protein is expressed and corresponding antibody is available. The human insulin manufactured by bacteria has already proven to be effective in controlling the pathologies, and has gained a substantial share of the world market.

10.8.1.2. Production of lymphokines (interferons)

In the year 1957 Alec Issacs and Jean Lindermann discovered a wonder molecule named as Interferon with an intention that the molecule will interfere with viral replication without endangering cellular metabolism as well it may serve as potential antiviral agent. However, the major problem encountered, was the quantity of production. The problem was overcome after its production using recombinant DNA based technique utilizing cloned interferon gene in E. coli in later 1970's. Interferons are the set of small proteins which are secreted by cell in response to viral infections. In laboratory, interferon can be produced by simple sensitization of lymphocyte when exposed to particular antigen as well as by treating the cells with double stranded RNA. Their molecular weight ranges between 20,000 to 30,000 Dalton. The interferons are broadly grouped into three types based upon physico-chemical and antigenic properties: Interferon α (Int-α), Interferon β (Int-β), Interferon γ (Int-γ). Interferon α was introduced in market by two major companies in 1986. The first and the most extensively studied interferon by far and large is the one obtained from WBC from human blood on exposing them to sendai virus. These interferons may be absorbed over the adjoining cells wherein they induce chromosome number 21 so as to produce unknown protein that binds mRNA molecule specified by cell. However, in the cell in which interferons are produced, the viral replication is hardly affected. Monoclonal antibody based technique could be utilized to further purify it from culture. Interferons form a class of powerful antiviral agents (effective at concentration of 10^{-12} to 10^{-14} moles/liter). However, interferon does not prevent the virus from infecting the cells but inhibits its intracellular replication. Furthermore, one of the major problems underlying cancer growth is a breakdown of communication between cells, these cytokines and lymphokines help to establish a better immune coordination and response against a tumor cell. Recombinant DNA technology has served as a useful tool in the production of these lymphokines/cytokines (interferon). American scientists Gilbert and Weissman cloned the gene in colon *Bacilli* so as to produce the human interferon. Similarly, the work was undertaken in Israel (Weizman Institute), France (Pasteure Institute). At the same time the nucleotide sequences of genes of IFN α and IFN-β were determined. Both IFN -α and IFN-β obtained from leukocyte interferon and fibroplastic interferon respectively had quite a similar structure and 14 different gene coding for human INF-α have been reported. Interferons act against the viral infections by limiting the viral replication and hence preventing the cells from lysis. Figure 10.19 shows the mechanism of action as well as the natural production of interferons inside the body leading to prevention against viral infection. Furthermore the induction of viral attack based release of interferon could be exploited as a strategy in utilization of retrovirus (RNA based) so as to generate interferons inside the body and thence strengthen the immune system.

The synthesis of interferon based on molecular biology was successful when DNA sequence coding for human leukocyte interferon (Leif-D) was attached to the yeast's alcohol dehydrogenase gene in a plasmid and was introduced into cells of *Saccharomyces cerevisiae*. These yeast cells could synthesize about one million molecules of interferon (on a per cell basis). In *E. coli* the plasmid could also successfully replicate, however, the production is relatively slow in *E. coli* because in yeast it is easy to grow and replicate glycoprotein derived from mammalian cells. In yeast the mechanism of glycosylation (addition of carbohydrate group) is similar to that in animal cell (Fig. 10.19).

Intron A and Alferon M (Interferon α-n3) were approved for use in treatment of genital warts in June 1988 and October 1989, respectively. Referon A and Intron A were granted approval for use in treatment of AIDS related Kaposi's sarcoma November 1988. Schering Plough is seeking to further extend the use of Intron-A and has recently received approval for use in the treatment of chronic hepatitis B and non-A and non-B hepatitis. In 1990, the first γ-interferon was approved by FDA. Interferon-γ-1b (Actimmune) manufactured by Genetech and is indicated for reducing the frequency and security of interferon associated with the chronic granulomatous disease. The production strategies of these molecules are protected under the patent rights. The interferons are only one type of lymphokines being developed via biotechnology and especially recombinant technology.

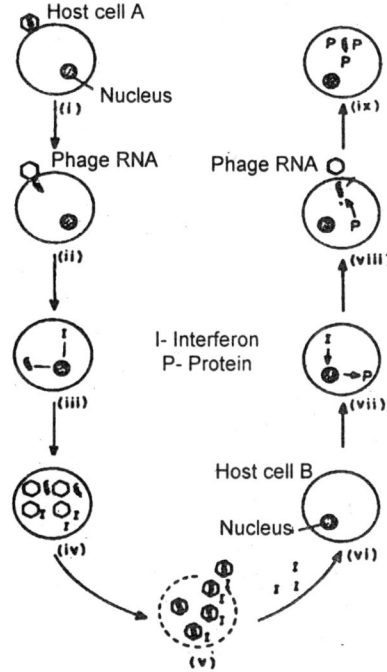

Fig. 10.19 : Production strategy of interferon

10.8.1.3. Growth hormone

Human growth hormone is secreted from the anterior lobe (neurohypophysis) of the pituitary gland and is responsible for regulating and monitoring the growth throughout the body, The human growth hormone (hGH) is a protein with 191 amino acid residues and a molecular weight of 22,000 D (22k-hGH). A minor component of the growth hormone constitutes for a weight of 20,000 D and is only 5% of its more abundant form. It is formed by depletion of 15 amino acids from the original molecule.

The lack of growth hormone in the growing infant leads to an overall dwarfness and an underdeveloped brain as well as the organs. The hormone is supplemented from outside in the hypopituitary children. In initial days the growth hormone was obtained from the animals or human cadavers. However, the development of rDNA technology has held the promise to supplement the overall shortage of the hormone.

The major problem of biosynthetic production of proteins has been to obtain the product without an amino terminal extension, in particular the amino acid methionine encoded by the translation initiation codon AUG. Hence, it has been the aim to produce the human growth hormone identical to the authentic source. Various possible approaches for the protein modification are listed in table 10.7. Out of these three processes the third one, in which the amino extension is removed by the exopeptidase is thought to be high yielding. In the method purified amino extended hGH is converted enzymatically to mature B-hGH after lysis and purification followed by enzymatic treatment.

Cloning: A gene encoding hGH in addition to 13 amino acids of signal sequence has to be constructed by combination of a hGH cDNA fragment (encoding amino acids 24-191) which could be isolated from a human pituitary cDNA library using rat GH cDNA as a probe, with a hGH gene fragment (encoding amino acid 13 to 23), isolated from a human placenta λ library. Further, by the utilization of exonucleases, the 3'→5' activity contained in the Klenow fragment of DNA-polymerase I the DNA coding for the 13 extra amino acids of signal sequence have to be removed (Fig. 10.20).

Table 10.7 : Strategies in growth hormone production

Protein modification	Protein maturation
Single peptide	Enzyme system of E. coli
Amino extension	Specific cleavage site for endopeptidase
Amino extension	Amino extension removed by an exopeptidase

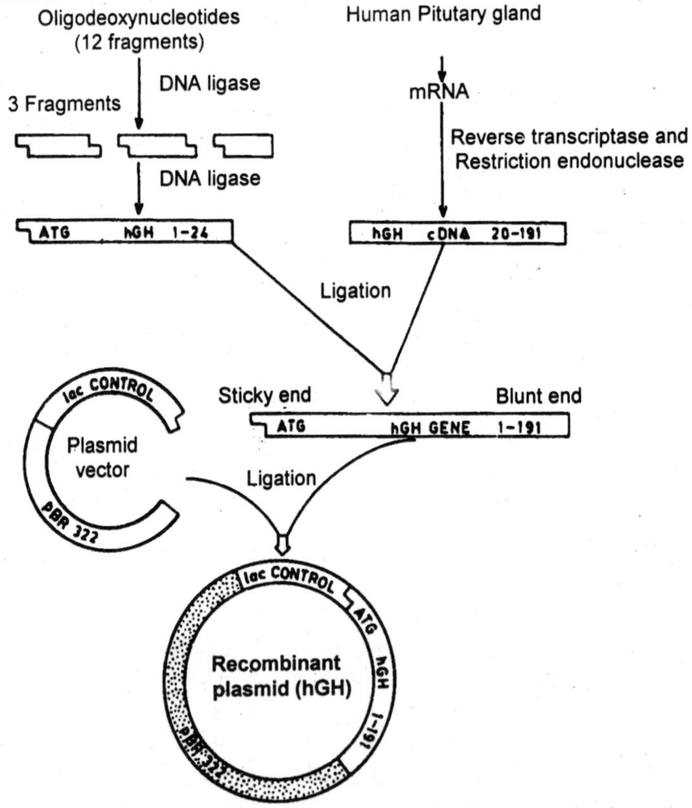

Fig. 10.20 : Strategy in cloning of the growth hormone gene

In order to obtain transcription and translation, the above mentioned DNA fragment is attached to a synthetic constitutive promoter. Furthermore, the transcription terminator from the phage λ was inserted after hGH coding sequence. Several clones were constructed to obtain hGH forms with different amino extension (λ-hGH's). The genetic material was inserted in the non-conjugative plasmid pAT153. The *E. coli* MC1061 was used as host. These expression systems when used for large scale fermentation, have to be genetically stable and should possess a high expression levels of amino extended hGH. The production of human growth hormone using the recombinant based method has improvised effectively the production with increasing yield as well as decreasing the overall cost of production.

10.8.1.4. Erythropoietin

The first potential molecule recognized as biotech's first billion dollar drug is recombinant derived erythropoietin. Erythropoietin was granted FDA approval in 1989 for the indications of anemia in renal failure patient under dialysis patients. Chemically, erythropoietin is a glycoprotein hormone. In normal course it is produced in kidneys and is responsible for the regulation of red blood cells production and it works via erythropoietin specific receptors situated in the erythroid progenitor cells in the bone marrow. Its production is stimulated under renal hypoxia, a direct result of anemia. However, in the patients with chronic renal failure, blood flow to the kidney is continuously decreased, resulting in an incomplete erythropoietin response to anemia and a persistent hypoxic state.

Earlier to 1983 it was being obtained from the sheep plasma or human urine. In 1983 the gene coding for the hormone was identified. This gene was then incorporated into the host chromosome of the Chinese hamster ovary cells and allowed replicate and subsequently express erythropoietin on production scale. The recombinant DNA technology has offered this way out in the production of erythropoietin. The molecule obtained from the earlier sources like sheep, etc. was very costly whereas the development of the recombinant technology has offered a cost effective method for the production and has further improvised its synthesis. Now the peptide is produced effectively by cloning of the production gene in the *E. coli* expression host using the SV40 viruses as the vectors.

It was commercially named as Epogen and the human clinical trials were conducted in 1986 for the treatment of anemia due to end-stage renal disease. An overall increase in the red blood cell production without requiring for the lack of transfusion has been recorded. The normalization of hemoglobin level has proven potential of recombinant DNA technology based erythropoietin (Epogen). Some of the important issues related to the safety of the drug have been considered. It was found that it is fairly safe enough to administer. Furthermore, it was realized that the AIDS patients undergoing treatment with azidothymidine (AZT or zodovidine) could effectively be given erythropoietin so as to reduce the number of blood transfusions. Its production is protected under the patent with Ortho Biotech (USA).

10.8.1.5. Thrombolytics and factor VIII

Recombinant technology was once again in highlight particularly in pharmaceutical market in November 1987 on introduction of recombinant DNA technology based tissue plasminogen activator commercially named as Activase (Genetech, USA). The primary indication for its utilization is in the treatment of myocardial infarction. However, it could not become a cost effective drug as the tissue plasminogen activators (tPA) when compared with other thrombolytics.

All available thrombolytics act through the conversion of plasminogen to plasmin, the enzyme that degrades the fibrin clot. This leads to a 'lytic state' which may subsequently lead to excessive bleeding. Efforts have been put forward to avoid the lytic state by producing a clot-specific agent that would not generate plasmin activity outside the fibrin clot.

A number of tissues secrete protease that enzymatically activates plasminogen. The gene coding for tissue plasminogen activator has been cloned into vectors and expressed to produce recombinant tPA. It is supposed to have two advantages; one is the lack of antigenicity and another is clot specificity. An explanation for the latter may be attributed to its binding to a clot specific agent which may also dissolve homeostatic plugs. Trial results demonstrated an overall advantage in reperfusion of tPA when treatment was begun at an average delay of 48 hours after chests pain. In the case of therapy, beginning during the first 4 hours, the difference was not statistically evident.

10.8.1.6. Cytokines

It was in mid 1960s when activity of cytokines was recognized. In culture supernatants of allogenic lymphocytes, some biologically active components capable of regulating, proliferation, differentiation, and maturation of various lymphoidal cells as well as accessory cells soon after their production by cultured lymphoid via antigenic stimulation were discovered. However, isolation of cytokines from a mixture is a cumbersome process where cytokines are in subnanomolar concentrations, i.e. 10^{-10} or 10^{-15} M. The recombinant technology or gene cloning process circumvented the process related problems and could express autocoids selectivity as single bioactive cellular products.

The gene responsible for cytokine(s) production could be cloned. The general approach is based on generation of cDNA library from appropriate cytokine producing cell lines. Subsequently, the gene of interest could be transfected to monkey kidney cell lines which contains an integrated SV40 genome. When an expression plasmid consisting of SV40 replication component and a cytokine gene, transfects COS cells, the plasmid replication proceeds massively allowing COS to express high concentration of the respective cytokines. Identification of the COS line selectively expressing a desired cytokine could be made employing some suitable biological assays. Thus, cytokine responsive cells when added to supernatant of COS cell lines expressing cytokines, a biological response is generated which could quantitatively be recorded. Monoclonal antibodies, alternatively can be used to identify cytokine(s) in COS cell culture using an ELISA or RIA.

10.8.2. Novel route to small molecules

10.8.2.1. Indigo and ascorbic acid

Recombinant DNA technology not only offers method for production of proteins but also provides newer way for making low molecular weight compounds. The most simplest example is the synthesis of blue dye indigo. The compound is not normally produced by microbes. However, the cloning of a single gene from *Pseudomonas putida*, for encoding naphthalene deoxygenase, resulted in generation of an *E. coli* strain that synthesizes indigo in medium containing tryptophan (Fig. 10.21). Similarly vitamin C (ascorbic acid) could be produced. The conventional process involves one micro-biological and 4 chemical steps to produce ascorbic acid where glucose is used as a starting material (Fig. 10.22). The complicated method could be modified using cloned gene technology. The cloning of the gene that encodes for 2,5 diketogluconic acid reductase in *Erwina*, can further simplify the method to be a single microbiological or single chemical step based process.

10.8.2.2. Aminotransferase

Bioconversions (or biotransformations) are processes in which micro-organisms convert a compound to a structurally related product. They comprise of only one or small number of enzymatic reactions, contrary to the multireaction sequences that operate in fermentation. Although hundreds of different bioconversions have been described, there are only a few which are used commercially. Chemical approaches are too costly or difficult especially in cases where stereoselectivity is required. A key feature of bioconversions is that they are easy to scale up, since the only parameter of interest is the level of the enzyme mediating the transformation. This makes bioconversion an obvious candidate for application of recombinant DNA technology. This can be utilized for reconsideration of economical process. The level of aspartate amino transferase in wild type *E. coli* is too low to make the organism of much practical use for L-amino acid synthesis from keto acid. Cloning of the relevant gene tends enzyme levels to be raised over 20% of the total soluble protein and as a result bioconversion becomes feasible. Once the gene is cloned, it becomes possible to use site directed mutagenesis to produce enzyme variants with enhanced thermostability or altered substrate profile.

10.8.2.3. Actinorhodin

Just as the novel proteins can be produced by recombinant technology so can be the novel small molecules. The *Streptomyces coelicolor* gene cluster encoding for enzyme responsible for the biosynthesis of the isochromanequinone antibiotic actinorhodin has been cloned.

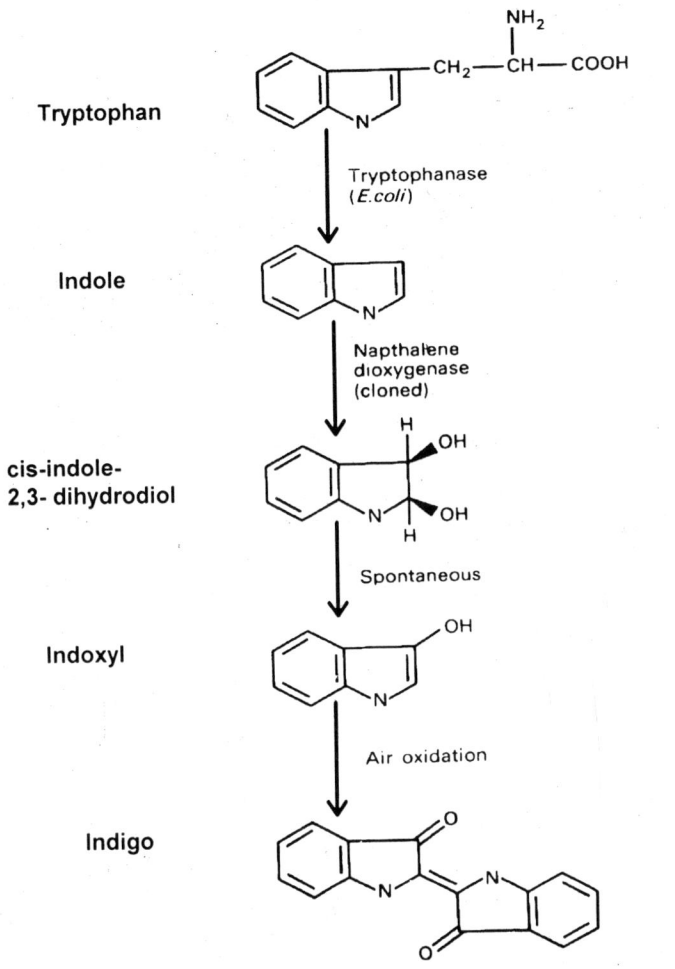

Fig. 10.21 : Proposed pathway for indigo biosynthesis by *E. coli* carrying the cloned gene for nepthalene deoxygenase

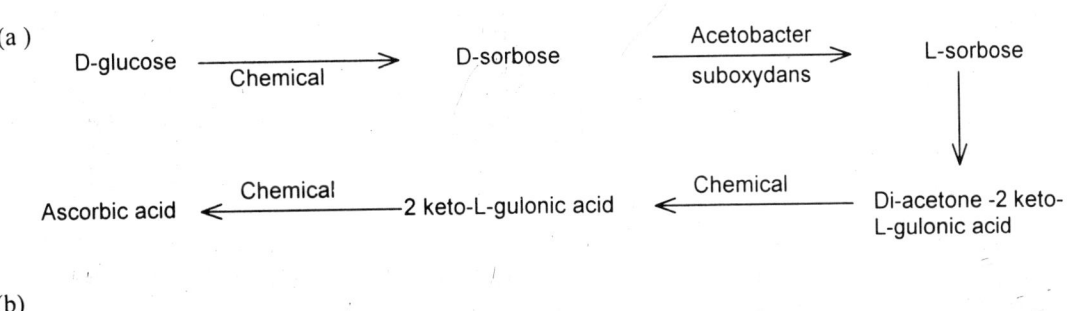

Fig 10.22 : Simplified route to vitamin C (ascorbic acid) developed by cloning in the *Corynebacterium* gene for 2,5-diketogluconic acid reductase (a) Classical route to vitamin C (b) the simplified route

When the cloned genes were introduced into a variety of other *Streptomyces spp.* producing different isochromanequinones, at least three new antibiotics were detected. Clearly actinorhodin, or one of its precursors, is a novel metabolite in these other *Streptomyces spp.* and it is subjected to further enzymatic modifications.

The utilization of rDNA technology in the production of low molecular weight compounds is not only restricted to the bacteria, but the plant cells can also be manipulated. Plant remains a major source of structurally complex, high value small molecules, e.g. atropine, hyoscyamine. When plant cells are infected with *Agrobacterium rhizogenes,* closely related to *A. tumefaciens* they become transformed. These transformed cells form a callus from which hairy root appears. Hairy root cultures can be established which are both rapidly growing as well as productive. Since plasmid transfer is involved in the formation of hairy roots, the system is amenable to further genetic manipulation.

10.8.3. Transgenesis

Gene manipulation to modify germ cells of animals permanently is called transgenesis. The typical example of transgenesis in animals is the production of 'super mice' which are extra-large as a result of the over production of growth hormone. The 'super mice' is not of much industrial or commercial value but they have a great academic value.

The greatest technical advancement of recent biology is to introduce genes into the germline of mammals. As a result the gene manipulation is inherited by offspring of these animals. All cells of these offsprings inherit the introduced gene as part of their genetic make-up. Such animals are said to be transgenic. The whole animal thus becomes an ultimate assay system for manipulated genes which govern complex biological processes. Furthermore, the transgenic animals provide exciting possibility for expressing useful recombinant proteins and for generating precise animal models of human genetic disorders.

10.8.3.1. Methods for production of transgenic mammals

A large number of methods are available for introduction of foreign DNA into the germline of mammals. A generalized method is shown in figure 10.23.

Basically the method entails for the facilities and technique for removing fertilized eggs or early embryos, culturing them briefly *in vitro* and then returning them to foster mothers where further embryogenesis could proceed. In this way the cells from different embryos could be mixed, i.e. chimera production and pluripotent cells such as ES cells introduction into developing embryos, for microinjecting DNA and for transfections by retroviruses.

10.8.3.1.1. Microinjection of DNA

The microinjection was used to introduce DNA into mouse embryos. As described earlier SV40 DNA was deposited in embryo at the preimplantation blastocystic (4 to 40 cell) stage. These embryos were implanted into the uteri of foster mothers and allowed to develop. Some cells of the embryo got incorporated DNA within their chromosome, but the adult animals which resulted were mosaics, with only a proportion of the cells in a tissue containing integrated DNA. However, integration into some germlines cells did occur and genetically defined substrains could be obtained in the next generation. Moreover, in the later experiments viral DNA (cloned proviral Moleney murine leukaemia virus DNA) was injected into the cytoplasm of one cell embryos (zygotes) such embryos developed into adults carried a single inserted copy of the viral DNA invariably in every cell.

The procedure which has altogether revolutionized transgenic mouse production, is essentially based on the direct microinjection of DNA into one of the pronuclei of the newly fertilized egg. The process is shown in figure 10.24. The male pronucleus contained in the sperm larger than the female pronucleus is usually chosen for microinjection. Typically in the process of microinjection about 2pl of DNA-containing solution is introduced. The two pronuclei subsequently fuse to form the diploid, zygote nucleus of the fertilized egg. The injected embryos are further cultured *in vitro* up to morulae or blastocytes stage and then transferred to the pseudopregnant foster mothers. In such transgenic mice the foreign DNA must have been integrate into one of the host chromosomes at an early stage of embryo development.

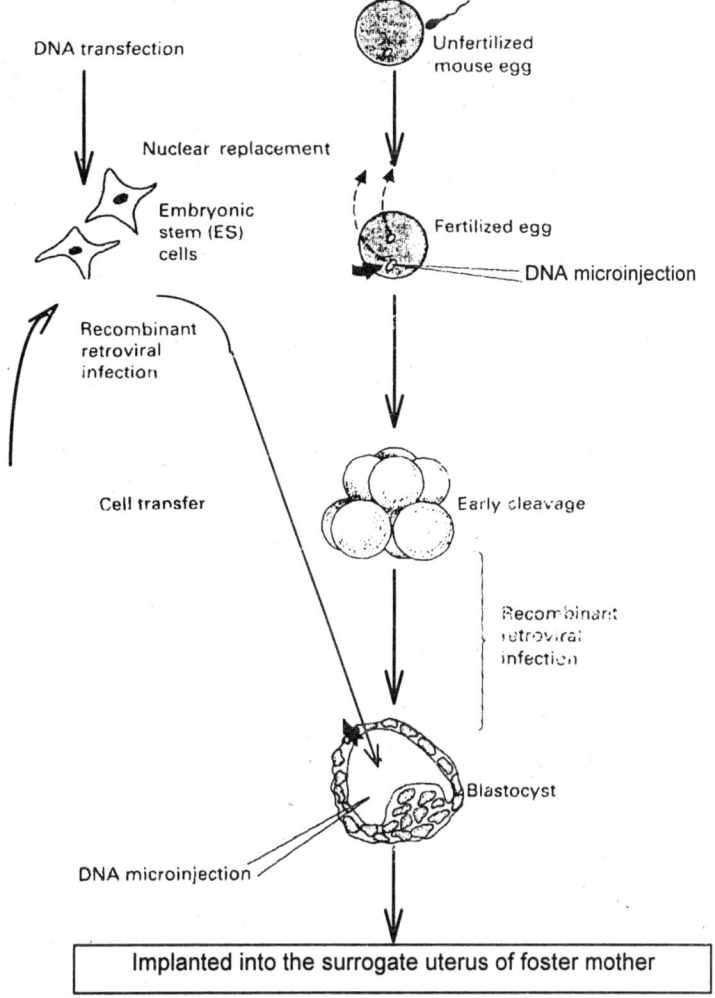

Fig. 10.23 : Schematic representation of the mythology in production of transgenic mice

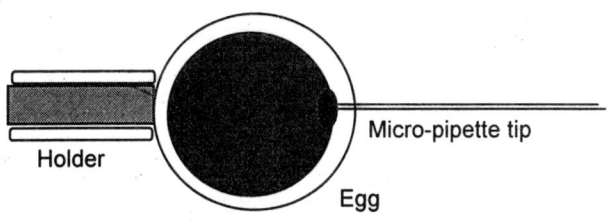

Fig. 10.24: DNA microinjection

10.8.3.1.2. Retroviruses and ES cells

The proviral DNA of retroviruses integrate through a special and precise mechanism into the genome of the infected cells. Only a single proviral copy is integrated at a given chromosomal site. The chromosomal site is 'random' but the junctions of proviral DNA are precise with respect to viral sequences. Infection of pre-implanted embryos by natural or recombinant retroviruses can lead to germ-line integration and hence transgenic animals. An advantage of this method is its technical simplicity, eight cell embryos with the zone pellucida removed and exposed to concentrated virus stock and then transferred to the foster mothers. However, it has the limitation that additional steps are required for construction of recombinant viruses, size limitation of foreign DNA and mosaicism of founder animal because infection occurs after cell division, begins hence possible interference of proviral LTR sequences with the expression of foreign gene may occur.

The major problem encountered in the production of transgenic mice is that transgene integrates randomly within the genome. To overcome the problems a newer strategy has been devised by researchers known as gene-targeting technique in which the specific DNA sequence in chromosome is introduced with cloned gene by homologous recombination. The desired gene is targeted to specific sites within the germ line of a mouse by introduction of cloned DNA into embryonic stem cells (ES cells).

These special cells, derived from the inner cell mass of a mouse blastocyst, are undifferentiated (pluripotent) cells that can differentiate in a variety of directions, generating distinct cellular lineages (e.g. germ cells, myocardium, blood vessels, myoblasts, nerve cells). The cloned DNAs containing a desired gene can be introduced into ES cells in culture by transfection, mircoinjection or retroviral infection technology. The DNA will pair with the chromosomal DNA in some of the ES cells and is then inserted by homologous recombination. The ES cells are then screened and selected. The altered ES cells are colonially expanded in cell culture and injected back into the blastocoelic cavity of a preimplanted mouse embryo where it develops into a transgenic mice.

10.8.3.2. A case with transgenic mice (The mouse metallothioneine gene promoter)

The mouse metallothioneine-I (MMI) gene encodes a small cystein-rock polypeptide that binds heavy metals and is thought to be involved in zinc homeostasis and detoxification of heavy metals. The most abundant tissue containing the protein is liver. Synthesis of this protein is induced by heavy metals and glucocorticoidal hormone. The regulation occurs at transcription levels.

Brinster et al., (1981) constructed plasmids in which the MMT gene promoter and upstream sequences had been fused to the coding region of the herpes simplex virus TK gene. The thymidine kinase (TK) enzyme can be assayed readily which provides a convenient 'reporter' of MMT promoter function. The fused MTK (Metallothionein-thymidine kinase) gene was injected into the pronucleus of newly fertilized eggs which were then incubated in vitro in the presence or absence of cadmium ions. The thymidine kinase activity was found to be induced by heavy metals. By making a range of deletious mouse sequence upstream of the MMT promoter sequence, the minimum region necessary for inducibility was localized to a stretch of DNA 40-180 nucleotides up stream of the transcription initiation site. Additional sequences that potentate both basal and induced activities extended to at least 600 base pairs upstream of the transcription site. The same MK fusion gene was injected into the embryos which were raised to transgenic adults. Most of these mice expressed the MK gene and these mice were found to contain 1 to 150 copies of the gene. The receptor activity was inducible by cadmium ions and showed a tissue distribution very similar to that of metallothionein itself Therefore these experiments showed that DNA sequence necessary for heavy metal induction and tissue specific expression can be functionally dissected in eggs and transgenic mice. For unknown reasons there was no response to glucocorticoid in either the egg or transgenic mouse experiments.

As expected, the transgenic mice transmitted the MK gene to their progeny. The gene was inherited as they were integrated into single chromosome. However, when the reporter activity was assayed in these offspring the amount of expression recorded was different from parent.

10.8.4. Vaccine production

Vaccines are prepared so as to generate humoral and/or cell-mediated immunity which prevents the development of disease upon exposure to the corresponding pathogens. This is achieved by presenting pertinent antigenic determinants to the immune system in a fashion which mimics a natural infection. Conventional viral vaccines consist of inactivated virulent strains or live-attenuated strains but they are not without any problems. There always exists a danger of vaccine related diseases when using inactivated viruses, since replicating competent viruses may remain in the inoculum. Outbreak of foot-and-mouth disease in Europe have been attributed to this cause. Finally the attenuated virus strains have the potential to revert to a **virulent phenotype** upon replication in the vaccine. This occurs about once or twice in every million people who receive live polio vaccines. Recombinant DNA technology offers some interesting solutions to these problems.

The heterogeneous genes can be easily expressed in various prokaryotic and eukaryotic systems. This makes the production of purified immunogenic material for the production of subunit vaccine more easier. A whole series of immunologically useful genes have been cloned and expressed, however, the results have been disappointing. For example, polypeptides of foot-and-mouth disease virus, only VP1 has shown to have immunizing activity. However, the polypeptide VP1 produced by recombinant method was found to be a poor antigen. The hepatitis B vaccine, which is commercially available differs in this respect, as it expresses the surface antigen in yeast. A similar phenomenon is seen with Ty vector carrying a gene for HIV coat protein. These subunit vaccines have another disadvantage, i.e. being inert they do not multiply in the vaccine thus unable to generate effective cellular immune response. An effective approach in vaccine preparation is to make use of an animal virus as a vector to express immunologically active proteins. Vaccinia virus and the retroviruses are the most suitable candidates for this approach.

10.8.4.1. Vaccinia virus

Vaccinia is the strongest candidate because of successful history as an immunizing agent. Vaccinia virus was the immunogen, used to accomplish global eradication of small pox. The advantageous properties which contribute to its success as live vaccine are stability in the freeze-dried preparation, low production cost and its subdermal route of administration.

Smith et al., (1983) adapted an interesting strategy for expressing hepatitis B virus surface antigen (Hbs Ag) in vaccinia. The fragments of vaccinia DNA were cloned in E. coli plasmid vector that contained a non-functional vaccinia thymidine kinase gene. This gene had been rendered active on insertion of a vaccinia DNA fragment containing a promoter in the correct orientation. This chimeric HbsAg gene was then inserted into vaccinia DNA by homologous recombination. Monkey cells were infected with the wild type of vaccinia and simultaneously the recombinant E. coli plasmid. Homologous recombination could replace the functional TK gene sequence which included the HbsAg chimeric gene. Such a virus would TK⁻ and would be selectable on the basis of resistance to brominated uridium deoxyribose (BUDR). When cells were infected with such TK virus, they were found to synthesize HbsAg and secrete it into the culture medium. Vaccinated rabbits rapidly produced high titer of antibody to HbsAg. A similar strategy (Fig. 10.25) was then used to construct an infectious recombinant vaccinia virus which expresses the influenza hemagglutinin gene and induces resistance to influenza virus infection in hamsters.

Subsequently recombinant vaccinia virus expressing other important genes have been constructed, influencing AIDS envelope gene, HTLV-III envelope and hepatitis B virus surface antigen. The prospects of using recombinant vaccinia virus for immunization of human population have received considerable attention. A heat-stable polyvalent vaccinia could simultaneously provide immunity to several diseases that require only one inoculation which may be both feasible and economical, using a live vector such as vaccinia. It has been possible to construct an infectious vaccinia recombinant which expresses multiple foreign antigen. Other vector systems based on *Mycobacterium*, *Salmonella typhimurium*, adenoviruses and herpes virus, including *Varicella zoster* have been proposed as live, possible polyvalent, vaccines. A possible limitation of such live polyvalent vaccines is, existing immunity within the target population, not only to a potential vector, but to any of the expressed antigen.

The recombination technology is being employed by most of the researchers world wide to exploit its potential for development of AIDS vaccine. Several recombinant vaccines for human immunodeficiency viruses are presently being developed and assessed in volunteers as potential vaccines for AIDS. Other animal models include the β-subunit of cholera toxin, the endotoxin of *E.coli*, the cirumsporozoite protein of malaria parasite and glycoprotein membrane antigen for *Epstein Barr Virus*. Animals immunized with these recombinant vaccines have in some cases mounted a protective immune response to a subsequent challenge with live pathogen. One most important disadvantage of recombinant protein or glycoprotein vaccines is that they are processed as exogenous antigens and therefore do not tend to induce activation of class I MHC-restricted T cells.

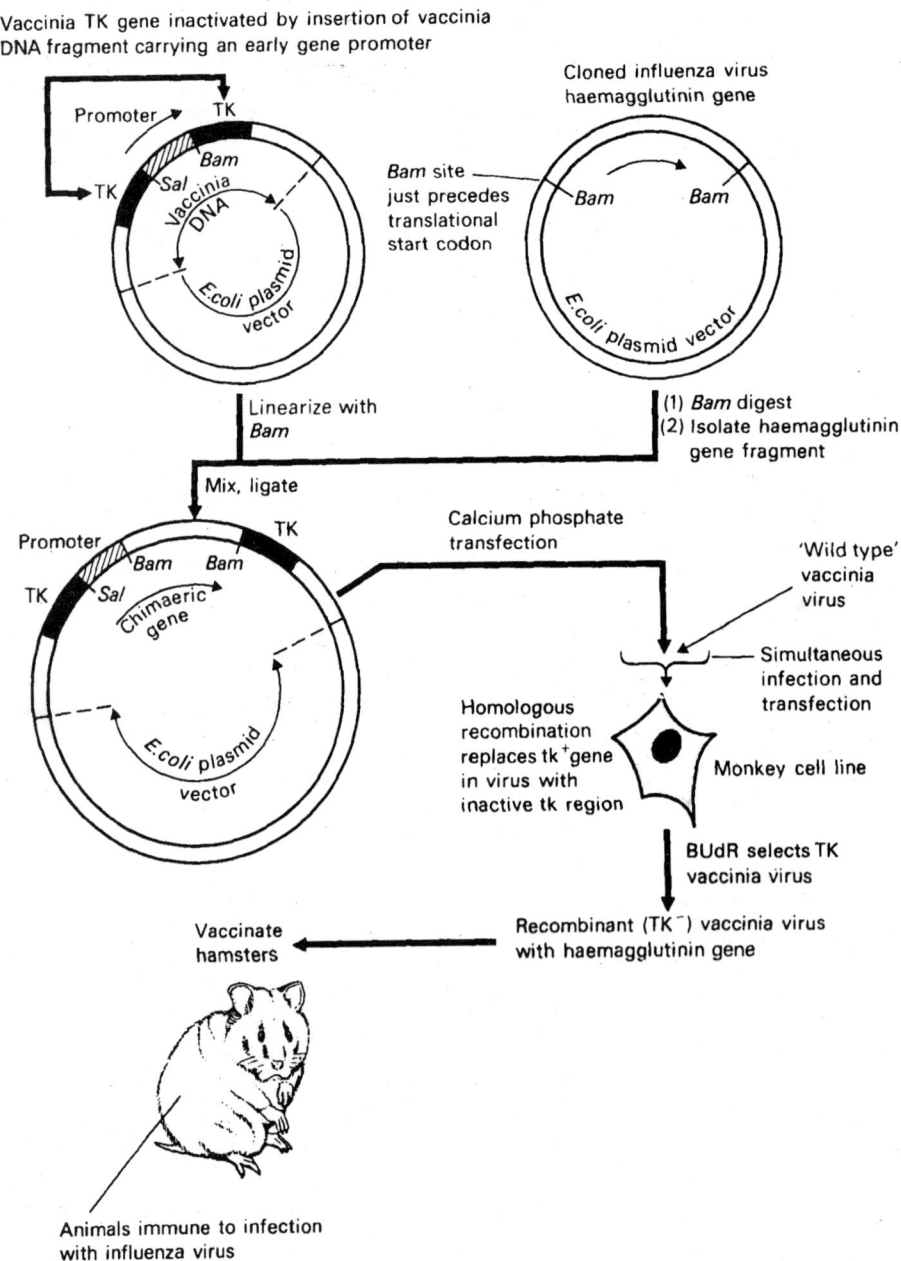

Fig. 10.25 : Production of vaccinia virus using the recombinant DNA technology

10.8.4.2. Recombinant retroviruses

Retroviruses are having some of very important properties to be utilized as viral vectors. This is due to the following reasons:

1. They cover a wide host range, including avian, mammalian and other animal hosts;
2. The infected cells do not die but they produce a large amount of viruses over an indefinite period;
3. Strong promoters harnessed to the foreign gene could drive faster viral gene expression;
4. The promoter can be switched on and off experimentally in the case of murine mammaliar. tumor virus.

RNA genomes are present in these retroviruses. These virus particles actually contain two copies of viral RNA. This RNA genome has many similarities with the eukaryotic mRNA like it has poly(A) sequence of approximately 200 residues at 3' terminus and a typical cap structure at the 5' terminus. The detailed retrovirus replication cycle is present in figure 10.26.

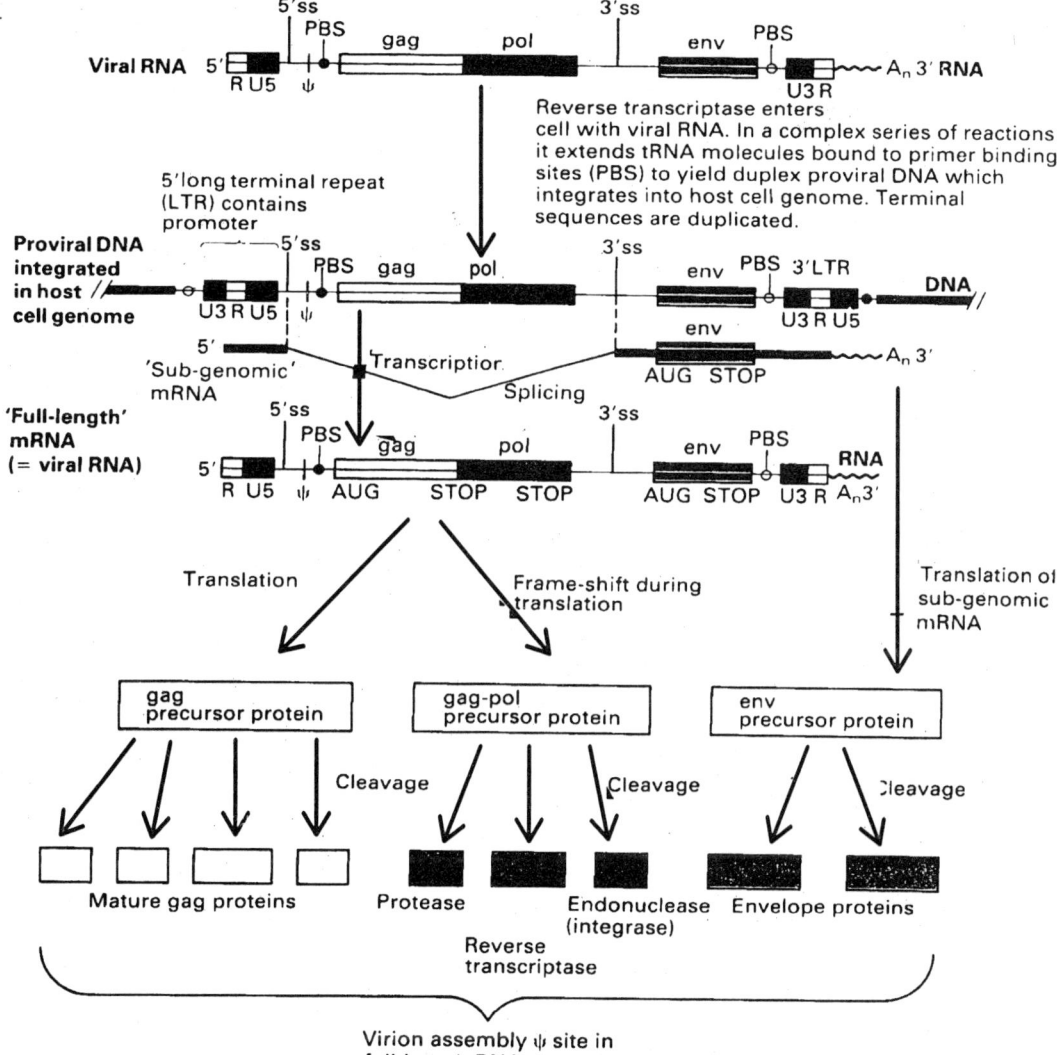

Fig. 10.26 : Retroviral replication cycle in brief

The figure 10.26 gives a clear representation of main points for the application of retrovirus as a vector. The steps in brief are:

1. On entrance of viral RNA into the cell, it is accompanied by reverse trancriptase and integrase which are packaged into the virion;
2. The reverse transcriptase then engages in a complex series of cDNA synthesis reactions which lead to the production of double-stranded DNA copy of viral RNA;
3. This DNA copy, known as proviral DNA, is slightly longer than the RNA from which it was derived because terminal sequences are duplicated in the process of converting it to double-stranded form;
4. The proviral DNA circularize and through the action of the integrase protein, inserts into the host genome;
5. Usually only a single copy of proviral DNA integrates per cell, the site of integration in the genome is 'random' and the proviral DNA integrates such that it is bound by the long terminal repeat also known as LTR; the sequence which includes a strong promoter for RNA polymerase II;
6. The proviral genome contains three genes: **gag, pol and env**;
7. These are transcribed and translated into precursor proteins which are subjected to proteolytic cleavages to produce mature proteins;

10.8.4.2.1. Strategies of vector construction

Certain species of retroviruses are thought to be oncogenic (cancer causing). These viral oncogenes are derived from cellular genes and are often the result of obvious gene fusion with viral gene. As a result such oncogenin viruses have lost essential viral gene function leading to defective viruses which could replicate in a mixed infection with a helper virus which subsidizes the lost functions. Such oncogenin viruses demonstrate the natural ability of retroviruses to act as vectors.

The retrovirus vectors are constructed by starting with the cloning of DNA of the virus. The necessary factors playing the role are the cis-acting sequences in the genome which are essential in replication and packaging, and the LTRs which are essential for efficient transcription of proviral DNA as well as for generating the 3' end of the full-length transcripts. The **gag, pol and env,** genes are dispensable because their function can be provided from another proviral DNA.

10.8.4.2.2. Generation of infectious recombinant retroviruses

Retroviral vectors have been developed by the replacement of some regions of proviral DNA by foreign DNA. It is common to insert a selectable marker gene such a **neo**, along with the non-selective gene of interest. Many arrangements could be attempted like the LTR when used to drive expression then the inserted gene is most simply expressed if its ATG is in similar location to that of the **gag** gene which it replaces. Alternatively, the foreign gene may be driven by its own accompanying promoter.

The construction of such recombinant takes place in *E. coli* using proviral DNA sequence carried by *E. coli* plasmid vector. Infectious recombinant virus can then be generated by using standard calcium phosphate-mediated transfusion of suitable animal cell line. The missing functions of the recombinant retroviruses are most simply provided by co-infection with non-defective helper virus DNA. Retroviruses can be used to reduce the size of gene inserts containing introns.

10.8.4.3. AIDS (Acquired immuno-deficiency syndrome) vaccine development

AIDS is one of the deadliest disease of this century. In the year 1984, Robert Gallo's group of National Cancer Institute, USA, identified a retrovirus that they called as HTLV-III for human T-cell lymphotroph virus type III. The virus was independently identified by Jay Francisco who called it as ARV (AIDS-related virus). In 1983 Luc Montagine's group at Pasteur Institute isolated a retrovirus from a patient manifesting persistent generalized lymphadenopathy and called it as LAV for lymphadenopathy associated virus. Subsequently the studies revealed that all the three isolated strains of virus were the same and in 1986 the international committee accepted it as human immunodeficiency virus (HIV). Following the discovery of an antigenic variant in 1986 the original virus was designated as HIV-1 and variant was designated as HIV-2. Both HIV-1 and HIV-2 were genetically related to the simian immunodeficiency viruses (SIVs), which were found in African primates.

The precedent literature reveals that the development of a vaccine requires a in-depth knowledge of infecting agent and the immune system. Similarly, AIDS vaccine development offers a major challenge that the human trials are not easily possible and the animal models responding to AIDS infection are chimpanzee and pig-tail macaque monkey which are not easily available. Although in the former the alteration in immune response is not found, yet it is one of the major animal model suitable for AIDS vaccine testing. Furthermore, the AIDS virus mutates and there is a change in the surface glycoproteins hence allowing it to evade the immune response. Such an antigen shift presents one of the major obstacle in the development of AIDS vaccine. Se eral strategies for the development of AIDS vaccine have come up during all the research undertaken by scientists. These strategies are based on Inactivated Whole Virus (inactivating HIV-1 and SIV by irradiation and treatment with formaldehyde), Attenuated Viruses (by growing the live viruses under unusual culture conditions that force the virus to mutate and to survive in the new condition).

Anti idiotype antibodies (when such antibodies specific for the paratope are administered, an animal makes antibody to the binding site on the anti- idiotype antibody, which will bind to the original antigen), have been generated employing recombinant techniques. The other techniques have been discussed at length elsewhere in this book. However, in recombinant technology there are three approaches which have been reported with promise.

10.8.4.3.1. Recombinant virus vectors carrying HIV genes

The approach has proven useful in the preparation of AIDS vaccine. As discussed earlier the vaccinia virus could be developed with a foreign gene, i.e. containing genes from HIV-1. Similarly, Sabin polio virus both live and attenuated could also be engineered with the gene form HIV-1 and hence could successfully be utilized as HIV vaccines. However, the recombinant virus is attenuated (not inactivated), it is able to infect host cells and hence therefore be expected to induce CTL response.

Vaccinia virus, is quite a large in size and could be engineered to carry several dozen foreign genes, without, impairing its capacity to infect host cells and to replicate in them. A genetically engineered vaccinia virus could be prepared as described previously. They could be administered simply by dermal scratching, and the virus causes a limited localized infection. Further, the foreign gene is expressed by vaccinia and if it is a viral envelope protein then it is inserted into the membrane of the infected host cell and there stimulates the T cell-mediated immunity. An infection in host cells near the site of scarification was found when vaccinia virus carrying gp160 was induced further. The glycosylation and cleavage of gp160 results in gp120 and gp41 proteins which get incorporated in to host cell membrane. The trials of these types of vaccines are underway in various laboratories round the world.

10.8.4.3.2. Synthetic crown-sequence peptides

It has been demonstrated in chimpanzee that they were protected from HIV infections due to the formation of antibodies for V3 loop glycoprotein 120 (gp120). Furthermore, the principle neutralizing epitope of HIV overlaps with V3 loop of gp120 and antibodies generated against V3 loop could effectively present chimpanzee from HIV infections. However, there is a high level of variation in the V3 loop, but the antibody neutralization is always strain specific. The so called crown sequence (amino acid sequence) V3 loop is conserved to a considerable degree. Synthetic peptides of different HIV crown sequence, including the MN sequences (which is found nearly 30% in not the American HIV isolates) have been prepared, and tested for their ability to activate T-cells proliferation and cytotoxicity *in vitro*. The synthetic peptides appear to activate a population of T_H cells and to induce some cytotoxicity.

10.8.4.3.3. Cloned CD4 and immunoadhesion

An other approach tried by some laboratories is to clone CD4 and use it as a vaccine in an effort to block HIV infection. The concept behind was that gp120 of HIV have high affinity for CD4 and hence if more of soluble CD4 are added, it may bind effectively to gp120 on HIV and thus could block viral binding to the host cells.

The *in vitro* studies have revealed that soluble cloned CD4 can indeed inhibit HIV binding and infection of T cells and can also inhibit syncytia formations. The major problem with soluble CD4 vaccine in humans is that CD4 has a half life of only 30-120 minutes in serum and there is the necessity for regular injection. D.J. Copon and associates reported that the problem could be effectively overcome by linking CD4 gene to the constant-region gene of human IgG 1. The newly formed CD4 immunoglobulin encoded by recombinant gene, is called as immunoadhesion, exhibits the high-affinity binding of gp120 characterization of CD4, but it has the longer serum half life characteristics of IgG 1. The half life of this immunoadhesion was reported to be nearly 21 days.

Whether recombinant vaccinia viruses will ever be utilized for human vaccination remains to be seen. The following arguments have been put forward against them:

1. Recombinant vaccinia viruses are often less virulent than wild-type vaccinia, but too little is known about the mechanism of the attenuation.
2. Vaccinia virus has a broad host range and transmission might occur from man to animal and back again. Therefore the deliberate spreading of the recombinant virus could be viewed as particularly undesirable.

The fact that the present human population contains individuals who have been vaccinated against small pox may render recombinant vaccinia ineffective.

10.8.5. Cloning of hemoglobin in *E. coli*

This provides for the basis of probiotics where surrogate prokaryotes are utilized *ex-vivo*, for the expression of hemoglobin a human blood protein. Essentially it involves isolation of total RNA from human erythrocytes followed by mRNA which is purified then used as a template for reverse transcriptase reaction in order to synthesize first cDNA strand using random primers. Fragments of α and β genes are obtained through PCR amplification using respective pairs of primers. PCR derived products are then purified and ligated with plasmid pTy-Blue. The ligation products are then transformed into competent cells of XL-1Blue. Clones of interest were identified and screened by PCR amplification followed by digestion with restriction endonucleases. DNA sequences are then applied to select identical sequences. The α and β genes are then cut from plasmid PT-7-Blue and ligated with various expression plasmids i.e., pET-21B, pBV220 and pDOGC. The plasmid transferred *E. coli* cells are used in the expression of α and β genes.

If this *E. coli* based system is utilized for *in vivo* expression of hemoglobin then the problem of artificial blood production could be resolved. It could be proposed that the *E. coli* expressing the hemoglobin gene could be denatured surfacially to be nonimmunogenic, its injection will lead to the production of hemoglobin within its envelope which could serve the purpose of artificial blood.

10.8.6. Cloning of human artificial receptor for drug design and testing

The recombinant DNA technology has offered unique assay tools, humanized antibodies, newer insight into the disease mechanism, novel functional assays, including cloned and expressed human receptors and transgenic animals.

Cloning of human receptors for neurotransmitters and expressing them in suitable host cells makes it possible to discover the strategies for successful targeting of drugs to single human proteins. Recent research has presented evidences that some of the human receptors like $5-HT_{1D}$ and $5-HT_2$ receptors could be successfully expressed in non-human, non-neuronal cell lines (mouse fibroblasts cells). These human receptors expressed in mouse cells have the pharmacological profile of human, and not of the mouse receptor, which substantiate that it is the primary structure itself, and not the environment, that dictates properties. However, the non-mammalian systems offer greater potential efficiency for better screening. Recently, one of the research groups exploited the signal transduction system used by the G-proteins coupled pheromone receptors in the yeast (*Saccharomyces cerevisiae*) so as to develop a host in which responses against binding to a transfected receptor could be measured colorimetrically. These artificial receptors were prepared by cotransfection of a modified human β_2-adreno receptor gene, under the control of the galactose-inducible GAL1 promoter with mammalian G-protein subunit Gs α into the strain of yeast in which a pheromone-responsive FUS1 gene promoter had been fused with a reporter gene (β-galactosidase) and suitably integrated into the genome (Fig.10.27).

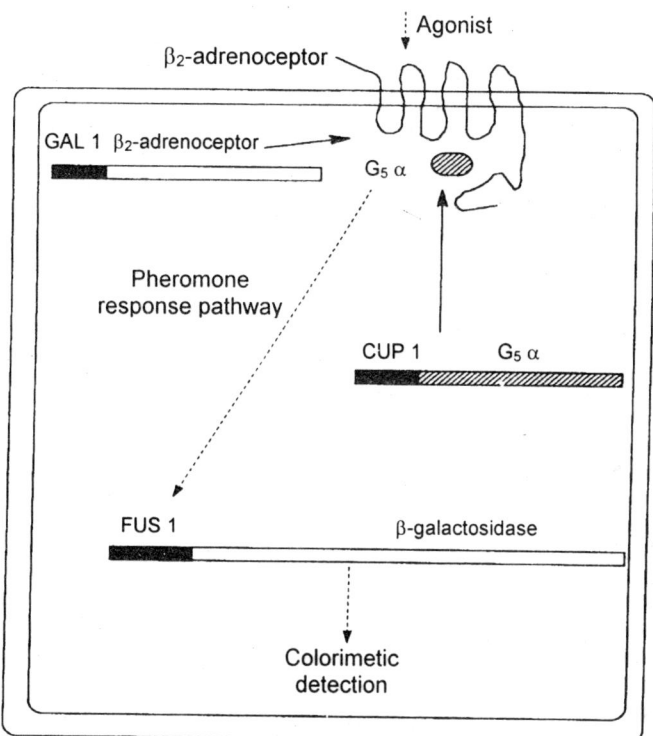

Fig. 10.27 : Super expression of human β_2-adenoreceptors and signal transduction system in yeast

Another similar approach for the utilization of artificial receptors in analyzing drug response is based on antibody technology. Library of antibody genes collected from the immunized mouse B cell can be prepared using the polymerase chain reaction, antibodies expressed on the surface of bacteriophage are isolated rather purified using exclusion affinity chromatography wherein minor coat proteins immobilized onto appropriate support is used as affinity media which selectively sort out the antibodies by their affinity retention. The retained antibodies would subsequently be liberated using exclusion buffer as eluting fluid. The potential exists for creating antibodies with newer properties **without human or animal immunization**.

Gene cloning technology has offered many other interesting applications in the receptors research. These are:

1. Cloning and DNA sequencing reveals that the closest relative of the particular receptors may often be receptors in the same structural suprafamily but for a different neurotransmitter. The implication of this technology in the pharmaceutical research is still to be exploited.

2. Cloning techniques have not only proved useful in revealing difference receptor subtypes, but also opening up various parts of intracellular signaling systems as possible targets for selective drug action. This is because the major enzymes involved in the formation and destruction of the second messenger have been shown to exist as different subtypes which also may have isomeric forms. This effect has opened the possibility of drugs acting selectively on the tissues containing particular subtypes, for example phosphodiestertase or protein kinase, although selective permeability may possibly be achieved.

10.8.7. Diagnostic aids using rDNA

Human genetic disorders arise due to alteration in the DNA sequence of the coding or control regions of a gene due to mutations. These mutations finally result in an inappropriate expression or non-expression of functional gene product. The mutation could be either germline or heritable and thus be studied by analysis of family members, or can arise semantically and be studied by comparing affected cells and non mutated ones. The diagnosis of these diseases occurring from the somatic mutations, or the determination of carrier status for recessive heritable disorders, can thus be approached by analyzing DNA. The DNA level diagnosis requires methodology that permits specific analysis of the potential mutant sites or regions well identified and characteristically specific as compared against the entire background of genomic sequence.

The DNA for analysis could be extracted from the tissues or can be amplified from the smaller tissue samples by polymerase chain reaction (PCR). Methods for analysis include the complex steps of digestion of DNA with restriction endonucleases, operation of DNA fragments by size using agarose or polyacrylamide gel electrophoresis and detection of specific fragments containing complementary sequences by hybridization with a nucleic acid probe for that sequence. The heritable diseases, the inheritance of that chromosomal region is determined in family studies by analysis of the linkage of the disease to the DNA marker for that chromosomal region. However, for the somatic disorders, such as some tumors, the genetic structure of tumor tissue is compared with that of the normal somatic cells..

10.8.7.1. Method

Various methods which have been utilized recently in DNA analysis are:

10.8.7.1.1. Hybridization of nucleic acids

The most important basis of DNA analysis is the ability of single-stranded nucleic acids to form stable duplexes with complementary sequences. The method is highly specific in nature and hence allows for analysis of that small fraction of the genome which may contain a disease-causing mutation, within the complexity of the complete genome for which the haploid size is approximately 3×10^9 base pairs of DNA. There are two important features of the process:

1. the two sequences involved in duplex formation must be complementary;
2. the stability of the resultant double stranded structure is determined by complement affinity.

All the major diagnostic techniques involve the utilization of nucleic acid probes that detect single complementary or unique DNA sequence that occurs once per haploid genome. The probe is in the form of a short DNA or RNA sequence that is labelled with a radioisotope, a fluorescent tag, or some reporter group. The labelled probe binds its complementary sequence in the DNA being analyzed (the target) by formation of sequence specific, base-paired duplex between the probe and the corresponding genomic sequence. The existence of that duplex is then determined by assaying the reporter group.

Hybridization in most of the technique is carried out with target DNA denatured and bound to the membrane. If the DNA is bound after having been separated electrophoretically, the process is referred to as Southern blot (Fig. 10.28). Denatured DNA can also be applied to the membrane as circular dots (dot blot) or as elongated dots (slot blot).

10.8.7.1.2. Southern blotting

In order to determine the sequences of DNA restriction fragments which are transcribed in RNA or be able to map hybridization to restriction fragments the technique named as Southern blot is used. The method was devised by scientist Southern in 1975. Since this has been extended to the analysis of RNA and proteins, the respective methods have acquired the terms Northern and Western blotting.

The basis of these blotting techniques is to transfer the macromolecules from the gel, through which they have been electro-phoretically separated on the surface of a membrane. Once transferred the macromolecules can be immobilized or fixed more or less permanently on the membrane. The membrane is relatively easy to handle and can be subjected to a variety of analytical techniques. And is widely used in the detection and analysis of nucleic acids.

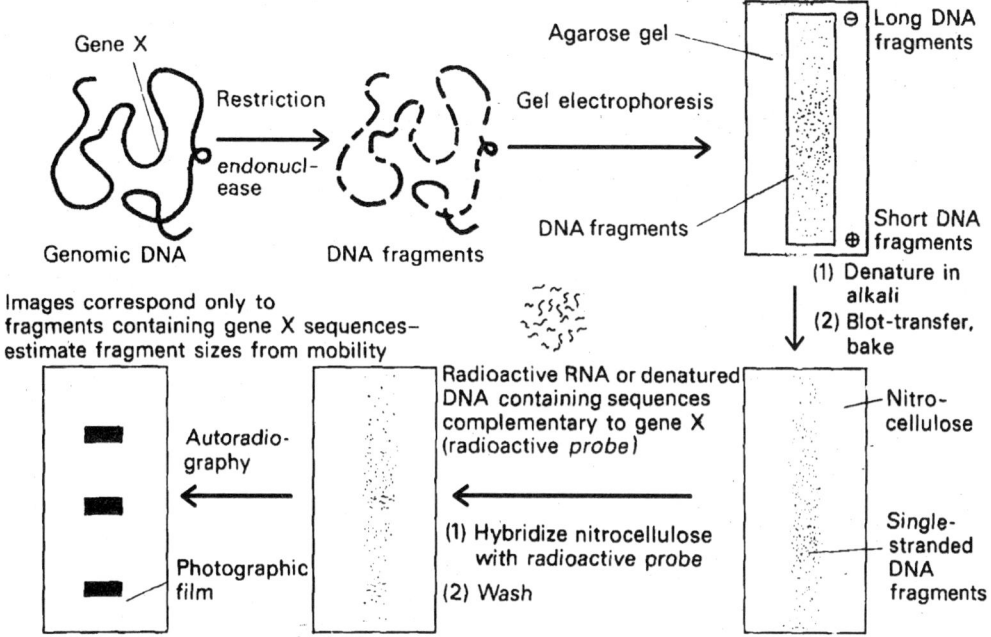

Fig. 10.28 : Southern blot technique for the mapping of the gene sequence

A prototype for this method is shown in figure 10.28. DNA restriction fragments on an agrosee gel are denatured into single stranded form by alkali treatment, and the gel is then laid on the top of the buffer saturated filter paper. The top of the surface of the gel is covered with a nitrocellulosic filter membrane and this membrane is itself overlaid with a dry filter paper. Further, many layers of the dry filter paper or the absorbent tissue are stocked on it. Drawn by the capillary action, the buffer passes through the gel accompanying the progressive wetting of the dry filter and in so doing, elutes out the denatured DNA from the gel. When the single stranded DNA comes in contact with the nitrocellulose it binds therein. This blotting takes several hours to complete and then results in transfer of DNA from the gel to the membrane so as to give a special pattern of band on the surface. The stack can then be dissembled and the DNA is permanently immobilized by baking of the membrane at 80°C in vacuum. The filter is then kept in the solution of the radioactive RNA through which the formation of the complementary bands takes place, which could be analyzed further for the final strand sequence of the initial DNA.

10.8.7.1.3. Direct sequence variation

Restriction endonucleases are the enzymes that cut both strands of DNA at a specific nucleotide sequence. The recognized sequence is typically in form of four to eight base pairs in size. The cut segments could be separated using size electrophoresis in agarose or polyacrylamide gel. In the case of complex genomes, there are too many individual DNA fragments to be resolved, but 9 fragments containing a particular sequence can be identified by Southern blotting using a nucleic acid probe for that sequence. The samples of genomic DNA from different individuals are digested with a particular restriction enzyme, separated electrophoretically, transferred to a membrane, and hybridized to a nucleic acid probe (for which the sequence is unique in the genome). The size of the fragments that the probe detects may however vary. The size of the restriction fragments that are detected depend on the probe-enzyme combination and may result because of a polymorphism affecting the recognition of sequence for that particular enzyme, a small insertion or deletion, a variable number of tandem repeat elements (VNTRs) or chromosomal rearrangements. This polymorphism is detected by different lengths of DNA fragments generated by enzyme cuts at or adjacent to the polymorphic site, they are termed as enzyme cut at or adjacent to polymorphic sAe, they have been termed **restriction fragment length polymorphism**

(RFLPs). In some cases these RFLPs are disease-related, as in sickle cell anemia, where the coding change from GAG to GTG in codon 6 of β-globin changes the recognition sequence for restriction enzyme CvnI.

10.8.7.1.4. Polymerase chain reaction and sequence variation

The ability to amplify specific segment of DNA by the polymerase chain reaction (PCR) has changed ways in applicative molecular biology. As PCR produces large amounts of specific DNA fragments from small amounts of complex template, it can be used to detect point mutations, deleterious and sequence polymorphism. The polymerase chain reaction is used to amplify DNA that lies between two regress of known sequence, DNA polymerase cannot synthesize DNA starting anywhere or on a template; they must extend the free 3' end at a duplex region. Hence two oligonucleotides (amplimers) are used as primers for a DNA synthesis reaction performed *in vitro*. The sequences are chosen so that the oligonucleotides are complementary to the sequences chosen on opposite strand of DNA and oriented so that when the amplimer binds to the template, their 3' end points towards the segment of DNA to be amplified.

The utilization of temperature variations cycle involves:

1. template denaturation;
2. primer annealing to template;
3. synthesis of DNA polymerase extending from the annealed primers result in to the accumulation of a specific double-stranded DNA fragment. The product of one round of amplification serves as template for the next, each successive cycle doubles the amount of the amplified fragments.

The PCR, is used to amplify a specific sequence from patients genomic DNA that may contain a known mutation. This amplified sequence is then analyzed for its size by electrophoresis or its sequence content by hybridization or direct sequencing. Only a small amount of the template DNA is required for the amplification. The adequate samples can be obtained by amniocentesis, chorionin villus sampling, or a simple mouth rinse. The speed of analysis is enhanced spectacularly.

10.8.8. Gene probes

Gene probes are used to find genes of particular interest. The gene is accomplished by using molecular hybridization technique, exploiting the typical characteristics of DNA that its two strands can be dissociated and reassociated *in-vitro*. Thus, one can identify the gene of interest by constructing a DNA with identical sequence which will anneal only to the target gene but not to the rest of the DNA. Similarly, using the enzyme RNA-dependent-DNA-polymerase, cDNAs were synthesized from mRNA isolated from mammalian cells. The DNA probe is schematically represented in figure 10.29.

MAbs and cDNAs have been used as bioprobes to identify the specific cytochrome p-450 responsible for xenobiotic and endobiotic metabolism. MAbs are specific to each epitope of p-450 and can phenotype, and quantify the levels of expression of individual p-450 forms. They also determine the contribution of individual p-450 to metabolism for reaction phenotyping. MAbs inhibitory to enzyme activity can determine the contribution of the MAb specific p-450 to the total reaction of an individual substrate in a tissue preparation such as microsomes. Inhibitory MAbs can also be added to the tissue preparation at saturating levels and inhibition can be observed. In addition to examine inter-tissue differences, interspecies comparisons can be made with activity inhibition experiments for different animal species. While MAbs can be used as probes for the detection of p-450 proteins, p-450 cDNAs isolated from cDNA libraries can also be used as probes for the detection of mRNA transcripts of p-450 genes in different human organs and tissues. The DNA fragments present in cells can be amplified by specific polymerase chain reactions.

Many of the techniques of gene manipulation depend on the hybridization of a nucleic acid probe to a target DNA/RNA sequence. In many probe applications a certain degree of resolution is necessary as an information about the relative position of a nucleic acid fragment. Since very small amounts of material are normally available and the sequence of interest may present at low abundance, there usually required a high sensitivity.

The choice for labelling the probe is a trade-off between sensitivity and resolution, in combination with other factors such as probe stability, safety and ease of use.

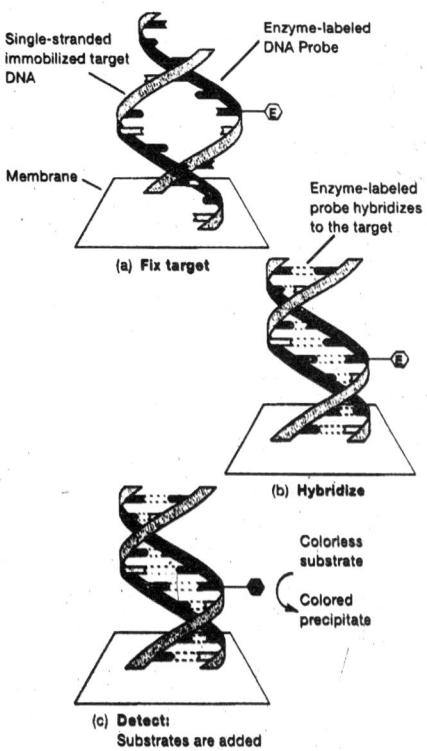

Fig. 10.29 : DNA probes; a. single stranded target nucleic acid is bound to a membrane; b. the probe is added to the membrane; c. detection

10.8.8.1. Radioactive labels

These are most widely used labelling components. Autoradiography is usually used to detect probes which have been hybridized to the target DNA along with the positional information. Radionucleotides used for labelling probes are ^{32}P, ^{33}S, ^{125}I and ^{3}H with a detecting limit of 50, 400, 100 and 8000 dpm/cm^2 respectively. Detection of probes is accomplished usually by an intensifying screen or by fluorography. The disadvantages of radiolabelled probes are two fold. First, the radioisotopes have short half life and hence, fresh preparation of probes is must. Second, worker's incompliance towards radioactivity in diagnostic laboratories. The utilization of the method is schematically presented in figure 10.30.

10.8.8.2. Non-radioactive labels

These labels for probes are available in limited number, but the only one in extensive use is biotin. Biotin can be incorporated in to poly-nucleotides enzymatically using biotinylated nucleotides as the substrate. An alternative labelling method is to use a photoactivatable analogue of biotin. Upon brief irradiation with visible light, stable linkages are formed with both single- or double-stranded nucleic acids. Biotin labelled probes are detected via glycoproteins, avidin or streptavidin through a variety of signal generating systems. The major disadvantage of biotin and of the other non-radioactive labels, is low sensitivity compared to conventional radioactive labels. Recently, in order to increase the sensitivity of currently available non-radioactive labelling techniques, a method called the **polymerase chain reaction**, has been introduced for amplifying DNA *in vitro* it eliminates the requirement of very sensitive systems. Some of these non-labelled systems are exemplified by Southern blots, Northern blots, dot blots, colony/plaque blots, S1/RNase mapping, etc.

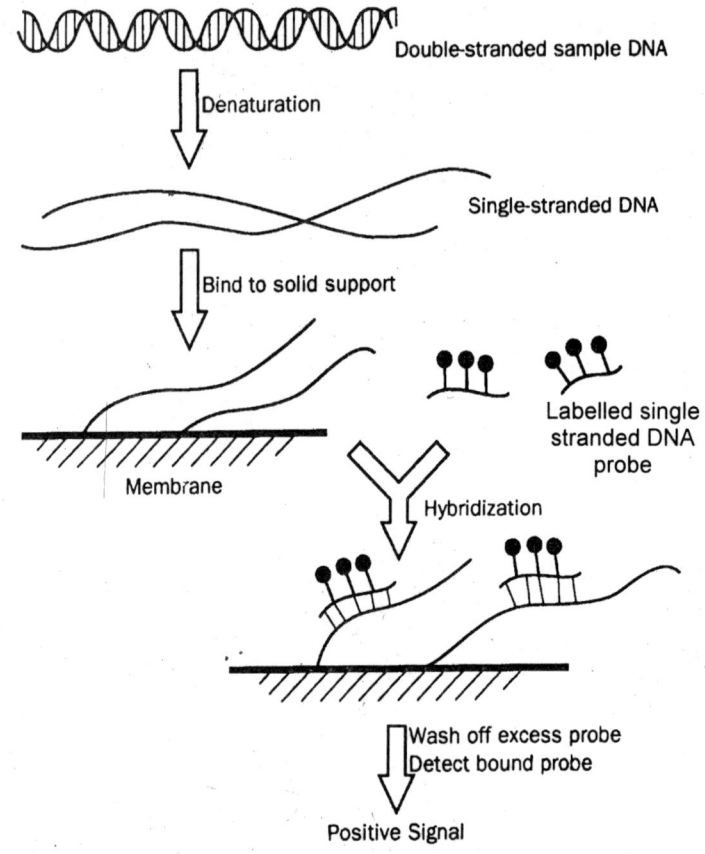

Fig. 10.30 : Radiolabelled DNA probes

10.8.8.3. Application of probes

Nucleic acid probes have been exploited for a number of biotechnological aspects. For the purpose of description, they are discussed here for three basic applications:

1. Detection of micro-organisms in clinical specimens. The sequences detected are usually large (i.e., an entire gene or cluster of genes) and mismatching between the target and probe sequences can be corrected.
2. Detection of changes to specific sequence, most commonly found in clinical genetics. These changes can include deletions or re-arrangements in the test to DNA or to the level of single base changes.
3. Detection of size distribution of DNA fragments bearing repetitive DNA sequences, most commonly found in forensic practice. This technique is referred to as **DNA finger printing**.

These three basic applications of nucleic acid probes can be exploited for a series of therapeutic, diagnostic and clinical purposes. In this chapter, they are dealt in brief.

10.8.8.4. Probes as diagnostic and clinical agents

10.8.8.4.1. Detection of sequences at the gross level

Labelled hybridization probes have been applied to determine a particular nucleic acid sequence. The greatest potential of this aspect has been realized in clinical microbiology for detecting specific nucleic acid sequences of the infectious bacteria pathogenic to gastrointestinal tract. Hybridization of the test sample with a battery of probes is more suitable technology than conventional diagnostic practice. Hybridization technology for the diagnosis of infectious disease has been found effective for the following reasons.

First: It is useful in curtailing the requirement of microbe cultivation, if sufficient of the infectious agent is present. The polymerase chain reaction is suitable as the isolation and identification of pathogenic species is not required vis-à-vis, detection time reduces considerably.

Second: It can be used, when the target organism cannot be cultured, as with viral infections. The method will work with infections having rising titer of respective antibody and also with latent infections, when no antibody may be present.

Third: The hybridization may identify all the serotypes of an infectious organism without requiring the presence a single antibody.

An important diagnostic tool is *in-situ* hybridization technique, useful for detection of viral pathogens that correlates the cytopathology of traditional staining methods with nonradioactive probes. Hybridization as a diagnostic tool is not restricted to clinical microbiology it is extended to the plant pathology, and microbial ecology as well.

10.8.8.5. The detection of genetic disorders

It has been recognized that genetic diseases in man result from single recessive mutations, attributed either to defective or absent protein product or to the nature of mutations. From most of the genetic diseases, the inherited hemoglobin disorder has been the most extensively studied at the DNA level. Antenatal diagnosis of hemoglobinopathies by rDNA techniques is a prototype for other genetic disorders. In clinical genetics, the most important hemoglobinopathies are sickle cell anemia and the thalassaemia.

10.8.8.5.1. Fetal DNA analysis

It has been established that if a mutation either removes or produces a restriction enzyme site in genomic DNA, this can be used as a marker in treating the presence of defect or otherwise absence of it. The mutation from GAG to GTG in sickle-cell anemia eliminates a restriction site for the enzyme Dde I (CTNAG) or the enzyme Mst II (CCTNAC 3). The mutation can therefore be detected by digesting mutant and normal DNA with the restriction enzyme while performing a Southern blot (detection of gel fractionated DNA molecules following transfer to a membrane)for fragmentation and subsequent hybridization with a cloned β-globulin DNA probe. This approach, is suitable for restriction site altered disorders. This can also be exploited where a major deletion or rearrangement alters the restriction pattern. There are many polymorphic restriction sites scattered throughout the β-globin gene cluster, which can be used as linkage markers for antenatal diagnosis, i.e., the close physical linkage with a β-globin gene suggests that the polymorphic site will trace the inheritance of that gene.

Recently, a direct approach to analyze point mutations has been devised based on oligonucleotide probes. Radiolabelled oligonucleotides were used to probe Southern blots, out of which one was complementary to normal β-globin gene(β^A) and other to the sickle cell β-globin gene (β^S). The DNA from normal homozygotes only hybridized with the β^A probe, whereas DNA from sickle cell homozygotes only hybridized selectively with the β^S probe. DNA of heterozygotes however, hybridized with either probes. Thus, these probes can discriminate between a fully complementary DNA and one containing a single mismatched base. Similar performances have been recorded with a point mutation in the α-anti-trypsin gene which is implicated in pulmonary emphysema.

10.8.8.5.2. DNA Finger Printing

DNA probes hybridize to a number of polymorphic loci have been developed known as hypervariable regions (HVRs) or variable number tandem repeats, contained in the human genome. Polymorphism at such loci is the result of variations in the number of tandem of repeats of a short core sequence. DNA probes at low stringency hybridize simultaneously to a number of these loci to produce individual specific fingerprints. The technique has been exploited in forensic applications. Several DNA probes have been described including those for myoglobin, insulin, inter-δ and α-globin Z' HRVs. Recently bacteriophage DNA has also been investigated for its potential to produce individual specific finger prints. DNA finger printing is not restricted to human DNA, it may be extended to cats, dogs, birds and other animals where it has been used to confirm cell line identity in a cell lines collection.

Among the forensic applications are investigations of identity, rape, murder and other offensive acts of particular value, suitable high molecular weight DNA can be isolated from such stains as blood and semen made on clothing several years previously. Also, sperm nuclei can be separated from the vaginal cellular debris, present in semen, contaminated vaginal swabs taken from raped victims. The DNA fingerprints of a family were obtained with DNA probes and were found to be instrumental in resolving an immigration dispute.

10.8.8.6. Probes as therapeutic agents

Oligonucleotide probes have been synthesized complementary to part of the 3'-5'nucleotide sequence present at the 5'end of all mRNAs of the blood parasite *Trypanosoma brucei*. Acridine linked antimessenger oligonucleotides were tested on cultured trypanosomes and had lethal effects, which were not seen with the unmodified oligonucleotide or with an acridine linked oligomer not complementary to mRNA. This concept has been put forward for the development of new trapanocidal drugs of high specificity and efficiency.

10.8.9. Role of recombinant DNA technology in gene delivery and correction of genetic disorders

One of the major advantage offered by the recombinant DNA technology to medicinal science is the correction of genetic disorders arising due to hereditary or mutational changes. The correction of the genetic disorder by the utilization of the rDNA technology could be either direct or indirect.

10.8.9.1. Direct correction (Germline)

It is one of the most tedious ways of correction of gene, however with the advancement in the delivery technology it could be applicable. With the utilization of various intracellular target oriented drug delivery systems like cation liposomes the aim seems to be achievable. Many other delivery systems are also applicable in similar correction. The interested readers are suggested to refer chapter 11.

The major disadvantage of these types of the gene correction systems is that one has to rely on probability that the injected carrier containing the corrected gene will present the DNA to the specific cell lines and the DNA will then be incorporated inside the genetic material of each cell as well as would be replication, competent.

10.8.9.2. Indirect method (Somatic delivery)

This method of gene correction is quite simple and highly applicable. The genetic disorder arisen in the particular patient is characterized to the molecular level in regard to the defected gene and its protein expression. By utilization of the recombinant technology the gene could be cloned in the expression hosts of either bacterial or mammalian origin. Then these expression systems are implanted into the body where they express the desired protein of the quantity required. These cells could be either implanted in the body cavities in the form of non-immunogenic biodegradable implants or be directly injected into the blood in the form of long circulating bioreactors producing the desired enzyme. They are also termed as **artificial bioprotheses**. For further details the reader may refer chapter 11.

10.8.10. Chimeric monoclonal antibodies

The recombinant technique has been suggested as of great significance in engineering of chimeric MAbs endowed with specificity and avidity. The approach utilizes the cloning technology for a designed DNA construct based on a promoter, a leader and a variable region sequence derived from mouse antibody gene and the constant region exones from a antibody gene. The antibody encoded by such a recombination appears to be a mouse-human chimera commonly referred to as **humanized antibody**. The production of such antibodies is represented in figure 10.31.

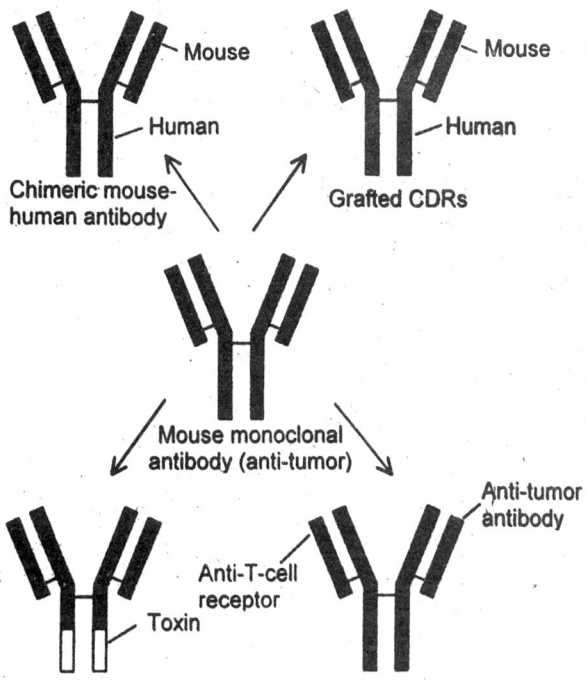

Fig. 10.31 : Production of chimeric monoclonal antibodies

The variable region derived from mouse DNA confers antigenic specificity of which the isotypes determined by constant region are derived from the human DNA. Since the constant region of such a system is encoded by human genes, these chimeric constructs contain limited number of mouse antigenic determinants hence as far as immunogenicity is concerned, it is far less as compared to mouse MAbs when administered to humans. Additionally, the chimeric antibody retains the biological effector functions of human antibody, therefore, more likely to trigger complement activation or Fc receptor binding. Because, the variable region of these engineered antibodies is from mouse they can also induce an antigenic response in humans. The chimeric systems only based on complementarity determining regions (CDRs) have been developed (Fig. 10.32). This novel alternative approach involves the grafting of CDRs from mouse antibodies together with human frame work regions in order to fabricate a variable region that classically retains the human β strain frame work with only the hyper variable loop of mouse origin. The antibodies so designed are relatively less immunogenic in humans as compared to humanized antibodies which contain the entire mouse variable region. Since the antigen-binding site is constituted by the hyper variable loop, at times CDR-grafted antibody could also bind to antigen. Often a reduced binding affinity however, has been demonstrated by CDR-grafted antibodies. The problem can be corrected with improved antibody affinity. Number of clinical trials have been conducted on CDR-grafted antibodies demonstrating marked clinical remission in some patients with non-Hodgkin's lymphoma when they are administered with CDR-grafted antibody specific for cell membrane antigen presented by the lymphoma cells.

The chimeric concept can judiciously be employed to engineer an antibody possessing a constant region with a desired biological effector function. For instance, the γ_1 constant region particularly in humans has been found to be effective in mediating complement lysis. By engineering antibodies equipped with γ_1 constant region it is anticipated that a complement mediated destruction of tumor cells can be negotiated. Similarly, the terminal constant region domain can be replaced with a toxin resulting into a chimera which is most commonly referred to as immunotoxins and as they lack the terminal domain of the Fc, their binding Fc receptor is blocked.

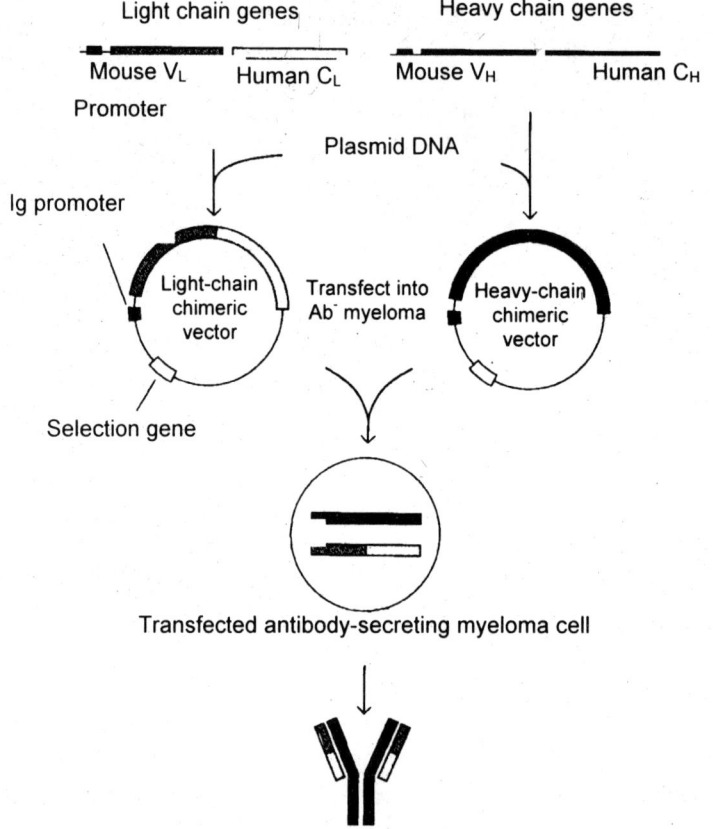

Fig. 10.32 : Engineering of monoclonal antibodies using recombinant principle

Some of the CDR cloned antibodies are presently being assessed at all levels as indicated in table 10.8.

Table 10.8: Therapeutic uses for CDR grafted antibodies

Target antigen	Clinical Potential
CDw52 (surface molecules on leukocytes)	Lymphomas; systemic vasculitis; rheumatoid arthritis
CD3 (T-cell marker)	Organ transplantation
CD4 (T-cell marker)	Organ transplantation; rheumatoid arthritis; Crohn's disease
Receptor for interleukin 2	Leukemia's and lymphomas; organ transplantation; graft-vs-host disease
Tumor necrosis factor α	Septic shock
Human immunodeficiency virus (HIV)	AIDS
Rous sarcoma virus (RSV)	Respiratory syncytial virus infection
Herpes simplex virus (HSV)	Neonatal; ocular and genital herpes infections
Receptor for human epidermal growth factor (EGF)	Cancer
Placental alkaline phosphatase	Cancer
Carcenoembryonic antigen (CEA)	Cancer

10.8.11. New genes inserted into eukaryotic cells

Bacteria are the ideal hosts for the amplification of DNA molecules. They can also serve as factories for the production of a wide range of prokaryotic and eukaryotic proteins. However, post translational modifications such as specific cleavage of polypeptides and attachment of carbohydrate units are not carried out by bacteria, because they lack the necessary enzymes. Hence many eukaryotic genes can be correctly expressed in eukaryotic host cells only. Another factor motivating the introduction of recombinant DNA molecules into host cells of higher organisms is to gain insight how their genes are organized and expressed.

Recombinant DNA molecules can be introduced into animal cells in several ways.

1. Foreign DNA molecules are precipitated by calcium phosphate are taken up by animal cells. A small fraction of the imparted DNA becomes stable integrated into chromosomal DNA. However, the efficiency of incorporation may be low but the method seems useful because it is easy to apply.
2. DNA is injected into the cells. A fine tipped (0.1 µm diameter) glass micropipette containing a solution of a foreign DNA is inserted into a nucleus. A skilled investigator can inject hundreds of cell per hour.
3. Viruses can be used to bring new genes into animal cells. The most effective vectors are retroviruses (RNA tumor viruses) (Refer Chap. 11). Foreign genes have been efficiently introduced into mammalian cells by infecting them with vectors derived from Moloney murine leukemia virus, which can accept inserts as along as they are up to 6 kb.

10.8.11.1. Production of novel plants

The recombinant DNA principles have been extensively used in the designing of the novel agricultural plants which are high yielding and pest resistant. The cloning of the gene from the wild pest resistant varieties has been used as the basis of the concept.

10.8.11.2 Strain improvement for fermentation

The recombinant DNA technology has been extensively for the improvement of the strains of the microbes used in the production the fermented products. A complete overview of the process is mentioned in the chapter dealing with general fermentation technology (Chapter 5). Interested readers may refer the chapter for details.

10.8.12. Genetically engineered insect pathogens as novel pesticides

A number of infectious microbes have been reported to have association with the crop pests. However, till date a few reports have been focused with this intention. Amongst the most exploited ones are the viruses of genus *Baculovirus* and bacterial genus *Bacillus* (especially species *thuringiensis)* are the most prominent. Genus *Baculovirus* (family Baculoviridae) has several qualities that are described in biological insect control agents/ The most versatile advantage offered by the genus is that it is not pathogenic to vertebrates or plants. Polyhydrin is the protein identified for its efficacy, which is the product of a single gene. The protein leads to the formation of the occlusion body which make the embedded virion stable so as to stay for years together within the soil and endure traditional insecticide application equipment. This suggests that the natural virus will act as insecticide, however, this is not true due to the major problem of speed of action which the virus takes for action, as compared to its normal counterparts like synthetic pesticides. In order to increase speed-of-killing the scientist have begun inserting into the *bacoulovirus* genome, a foreign genome, expressing a toxin for initiation of the pesticidal action at a faster rate. The *baculovirus* genome does not offer a big hurdle in the insertion of the genome and hence a faster offcourse sustainable action could be imparted to the baculoviruses making them effective as novel pesticides.

10.8.13. Cloned CD4 toxin

Recombinant CD4 (rCD4) has been proven to be an effective carrier for toxin. rCD4 has cell specificity and affinity fairly comparable antibodies do. rCD4 has been chosen for its high affinity for HIV envelop gp120 (discussed **earlier**). rCD4 exhibits same high affinity as exhibited by natural CD4 towards gp120 and it can potentially target the coupled antiviral drugs to HIV infected cells.

The loss of CD4 + cells in HIV patients is partly due to interaction of gp120 in the membrane of infected **cells** with CD4 molecules or non-infected cells. This leads to cell membrane fusion and syncytium formation **and** implies that rCD4 carrier will have an additional intrinsic therapeutic effects. A recombinant protein, **containing** the HIV-binding portion of human CD4 molecules was linked to active regions of *Pseudomaons* **exotoxin** A(PE-A) and displayed selective toxicity towards the cells expressing gp120. A combination of this **CD4-PE-A** and reverse transcriptase inhibitors results in highly synergistic effects and led to a complete **elimination** of infectious HIV-1 from humans T-cell-lines *in-vitro*. Major problem may be encountered is the **Immunogenecity** of the rCD4 products as well as in harmful effects caused by interaction with elements of the **immune** system. Furthermore, destruction of HIV-infected cells and the sudden release of the particles may lead to a massive infections of previously uninfected (CD4-positive) cells.

10.8.14. Production of glutamine synthetase by gene amplification in chinese hamster

Gene amplification as an eukaryotic phenomenon was considered to be a rare and unimportant until the demonstration of the amplification of the enzyme dehydrofolate reductase (dhfr) in methotrexate resistant cell lines. Subsequently gene amplification has been shown to be a common eukaryotic phenomenon which has lead to the development of many cell lines, over, producing enzymes and proteins in response to growth in other toxic metabolites. The amino acid glutamine is an extremely important metabolite. It is used for production of proteins as an energy source and as a nitrogen donor, as well as taking part in homeostatic processes such as pH regulation. Many cells require the addition of glutamine to the culture media and even though it is not classed as an essential amino acid. Most of the eukaryotic cells contain a gene coding the glutamine synthetase which produces glutamine from glutamic acid. The principle involved in the production of glutamine synthetase is that by utilization of sulphoximine (MSX), an irreversible inhibitor of glutamine synthetase, a newer mutant cell line could be created which over produces glutamine synthetase. This over production is due to amplification of genomic DNA sequence of at least 100kbp containing the coding sequence for the for GS gene.

10.9. FUTURE PERSPECTIVES

The possible application of recombinant technology in the context of neurotransmitter action elucidation, aging diseases and control of phenotypic expression will certainly lead to a better understanding of system complexities. Genetic engineering particularly based on recombinant technology will certainly open up highly explorable, conceptually simple, however amazing vistas of future. The possibilities of master genome insertion into evacuated germline cells and their subsequent culturing into foster mother created the real wonder of the century known to us all as 'dolly sheep' a typical land mark example of gene cloning technology. The successful experimentation is exciting on realization as it has all potentials and promises to turn fantasies into the realities. Dwelling in to the concept it would not be surprising if the principle be utilized in the genesis cloned offspring, of crime commiter, crime sufferer, which could subsequently be utilized to unravel the intriguing mysteries. The recombinant technology together with organ culturing techniques has been used to produce cloned organs. Probably this will greatly resolve the problem associated with the availability of organs for implantation. The other problems related to organ transplantation like tissue rejection etc. shall be resolved as these organs shall be autologous in immunity sense. It is also likely to be that future will be the time of recombinant technology based molecules shall they be therapeutic proteins or novel small molecules is immaterial, however, the reproducibility cost effectiveness and defined characteristics of product will certainly lend them to be acceptable versions. If so comes to be true, a time will come when rearing of animals will be for the purpose of medicinal production, where they shall serve as walking mini pharmaceutical units ready for expression (production).

With the advent in modern genetics and development of new procedures, it is now possible to have a further insight into the specific mechanism related to cellular functions. A recent report presents that with the help of *in situ* hybridization, the unprocessed complex RNA containing both exons and introns in the nucleus with an intron-specific probe could be detected. These molecules exist immediately after transcription of the gene. Therefore, it is possible that transcriptional activity could be detected in individual cells with the help of histochemistry based on *in situ* hybridization. This provides for possible extension to the studies which were performed upto steady state cytoplasmic RNA levels. Additionally, it may provide for successful exploration of receptor activities as well as enzymatic regulation at the cellular levels. The results of continual researches in molecular genetic technologies have been infused into invariably all scientific disciplines and answered fundamental biological questions in most convincing manner. The DNA hypersensitivity sites to determine potential regulatory regions on a gene, determining domains within each gene that are receptors for DNA binding proteins which control gene functions, and PCR, constitute some of the leading examples of recombinant DNA technology application potentials.

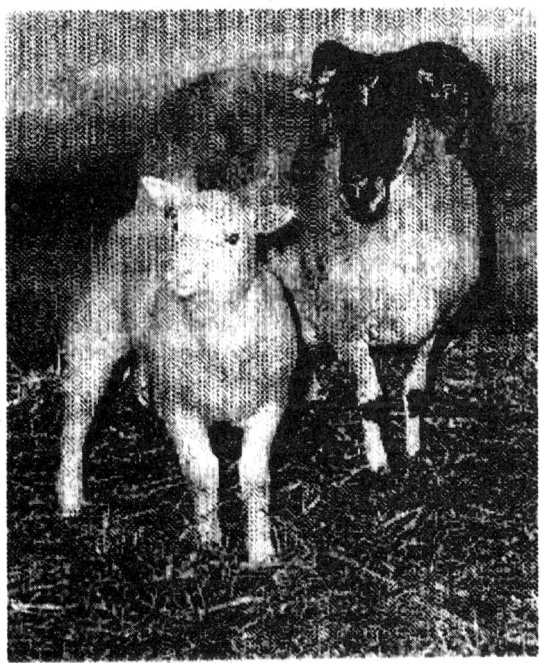

Fig 10.33 : Dolly sheep and its surrogate mother

SUGGESTED READINGS

Alwine, J.C., Kemp, D.J, Parker, B., Reiser, J., Renart, J., Stark, G.R. and Wahl, g.M. (1979) *Detection of specific RNAs or specific fragments of DNA by fractionation in gel and transfer to diazobenzyloxymethyl paper*, **Methods Enzymology**, 68, 220-242.

Anderson, S., Gart, M.J., Magol, L. and Young, I.g., (1980), **Nucleic Acids Res.**, 8,1731-1743.

Anderson, S., Marks, C.B., Lazarus, R., Miller, J., Stafford, K., Seymour, J., Light, D., Rastetter, W. and Estel, D., 91985) **Science**, 230, 144-149.

Backman, K. and Ptashne, M., (1978) **Cell**, 13, 65-71.

Blocker, H. and Frank, R., *Synthetic Genes*. In : **Biotechnology Potentials and Limitations**, S. Silver (Ed.), Springer-Verlag, Berlin, 41-55.

Brod, P., (1979), **Plasmids**, Freeman and Co., San Francisco.

Dugaiczyk, A., Boyer, H.W. and Goodman, H.M., (1975) **J. Mol. Biol.**, 96, 171-184.

Erlich, H.A., (Ed.), (1989), **PCR Technology: Principles and Application for DNA amplifications**, Stockhom Press, New York.

Glover, D., (Ed.), (1985) **DNA Cloning: A Practical Approach**, Vol. 2, IRL Press, Oxford.

Gupta, P.K., (1997), **Essentials of Biotechnology**, Rastogi Publications, Meerut, India.

Hochfeld, W.L., (1994) **Building Blocks Biotechnology Reagents and Consumables**, Interpharm Press, Inc., Buffalo Grove, IL.

Hoyer, L.W. and Dorhan, W.N., (Eds.), (1991) **Recombinant Technology inHemostasis and Thrombosis**, Plenum Press, New York.

Kay, R.M., Kaufamn, R., Schendel, P., Turner, K., Kamen, P., (1986), *Cloning and Expressing Genes for Clinically useful Proteins*. In : **Biotechnology Potentials and Limitations**, S. Silver (Ed.), Springer-Verlag, Berlin, 19-41.

Old, R.W., Primros, S.B., (1989) *Principles of Gene manipulation*. In: **Introduction to Genetic Engineering**, Blackwell Scientific Publications, Oxford, London.

Paoletti, E., Perkus, M.E., Piccini, A., Lipinskas, B.R., Merca, S.R., *Modern Approach to Liver Vaccines: Recombinant Proviruses* In : **Biotechnology Potentials and Limitations**, S. Silver (Ed.), Springer-Verlag, Berlin.

Pezzuto, J.M., Johnson, M.E., Manesse. H.R.. Jr.. (1993) **Biotechnology and Pharmacy**, Chappman and Hall, New York.

Prokop, A., Bajpai, R.K. and Ho.c. (Eds.), (1991) **Recombinant DNA Technology and Applications**, Mc Graw hill, Hew York.

Stewart, C., (1997), **Nature**, 385, 769-771.

Stlow, J.K. and Mollaender, A., (Eds.), (1980), **Genetic Engineering**, vol. 2, Plenum Press, New York.

Wilmut, I., Schnwike, A.E., Mc Whir, J., Kind, A.J. and Campbell, K.H.S., (1997) **Nature**, 385, 810-813.

DRUG DELIVERY SYSTEMS
IN GENE THERAPY

11.1. INTRODUCTION

The ability to transfect genes into cells and to cause their expression is leading to the practical emergence of human gene therapy, wherein, functionally active genes are putatively inserted into the (somatic) cells of a person requiring the expression of a given protein. A novel adaptation of gene therapy is the transfection of cells with non-resident genes in order to accomplish *in situ* expression of a pharmacologically beneficial protein or create a site for further therapeutic intervention. In other words, genes would act like "drugs", generating a product with a specific pharmacological effect. In simple terms, gene therapy involves insertion of genetic material into a patient's cells to make them capable of producing therapeutic protein.

Today's gene therapy has gone beyond the original definition of gene therapy (Roomer and Friedman, 1992). *Gene therapy* has given an opportunity to *fight the cause* of a disease *rather than its symptoms*. Over 45,000 human diseases have been identified related directly to the genetic disorders (MuKusick,1988). Until recently, approaches to the treatment of genetic disorders were by employing substitution therapy, e.g., enzyme storage disease(s), cystic fibrosis (CF), etc., or more rationally to replace a missing protein. In contrast, gene therapy paves way to either *replace the missing or defective gene at the origin or arrest undesired gene expression (viral and oncogene expression) at the origin.*

Gene medicines are generally based on gene expression system that contains a therapeutic gene and a delivery system. A gene delivery system controls the distribution and access of a gene expression unit to the target tissue, its recognition by cell-surface receptors and its intracellular trafficking (Tomlinson and Rollond, 1996).

With the advent of gene manipulation by biotechnological techniques it has now become feasible to splice and insert human gene into viral or bacterial genome while the latter is referred as vector. The technique is essentially based on recombinant DNA technology which allows the isolation of genes and their subsequent utilization in the production of respective proteins, as well as to engineer them to be a corrective gene system. It is interesting to note that therapeutic protein expressions have their mode of action by being in the blood stream and exercising their effect from there. This remains to be a constraint in effective delivery, i.e. cell specific gene or genome delivery. Hence gene(s) could effectively be delivered to the somatic cells or germ-line.

11.1.1. Genes

Before going into the details of gene therapy, we will look into the aspects associated with this in brief. Humans have certain things in common as compared to other species. However, no two person are same. This is all based on genetics. Now what is this genetics? Genetics is the study of biologically inherited traits, including traits that are influenced in part by the environment. Inherited traits are determined by elements of heredity. These particular heredity elements are called **genes**, that are transmitted from parents to offspring in reproduction. Genes can also be defined as a sequence that codes for a functional product.

Bacterial genetics which forms the basis of molecular genetics is something very interesting. However, discussing it in depth would be out of the scope of this book. Hence it is discussed here in brief. In early 1900s, there was a misunderstanding of genotypic changes which is arising in a single cell as to phenotypic adaptations where in reversible changes in all the cells of a population occurs. It was in the 1940s that the speed of genotypic change in bacterial cultures in a new environment was realized. This discovery of gene transfer in bacteria has paved way for many developments.

It is now clear that any heritable change in a gene is brought about by **mutation**. A mutation can be defined as any change in the base sequence of the DNA. Some mutations are **silent**, i.e., without demonstrable phenotypic while some are **wild type**. The changes in various kinds of mutations can be precisely identified in terms of base sequences in DNA and amino acid sequences in the protein. The DNA changes include **nucleotide replacements, deletions, insertions** and **rearrangements**. Replacement may be **transition**, where a purine is replaced by a purine and a pyrimidine by a pyrimidine or **transversion**, where a purine is replaced by a pyrimidine and vice-versa.

Nucleotide replacements, single-nucleotide deletions (microdeletion) and large insertions are point mutations, i.e., they all give wild-type recombinants with each other, and they undergo true reversion through appropriate replacements, insertions or deletions. However, large deletions lead to wild-type recombinants with other strains that can replace the entire deleted region and they do not revert. This genetic stability has made them useful in metabolic and genetic studies where reversions would interfere.

Consequences of mutations has an effect on the coding properties of the DNA. Among the replacements, **missense mutations** cause the substitution of one amino acid for another; the protein may remain functional provided there is no marked effect of substitution on its tertiary structure. In case of **nonsense** (terminator) mutations, premature termination in the growth of the peptide chain occurs almost destroying its function. Larger deletions destroy the function except when they remove small unessential parts of proteins. Deletions at the boundary between two genes, if in frame, cause the two polypeptide chains to be synthesized as a single chain (**gene fusion**), with partial retention of one or both functions. A shift of the reading frame causes the production of a jumbled distal sequence resulting in loss of function which can be corrected by another shift in the opposite direction provided the jumbled region is small and not in a critical position. Insertions, usually caused by transposons or prophages, frequently destroy the function of the protein and affect the expression of distal genes (for further details regarding mutation refer to chapter 9). The procedure for introducing mutations into specific genes is called **gene targeting**. The specificity of gene targeting comes from the DNA sequence homology needed for homologous recombination.

11.1.2. Plasmids

Plasmids are a highly diverse group of extrachromosomal genetic elements which are circular in shape with double-stranded DNA molecule with the capacity for autonomous replication in cells. Plasmids may be regarded as symbionts of bacteria. In general, the chromosome carries all the genes essential for growth, whereas plasmids carry **optional genes** that confer additional properties. Hence, cells that have lost their plasmids are still viable. Bacterial properties that depend on plasmids may fluctuate easily. The genetic composition of the plasmids fluctuates, in part because the genes that affect the host phenotype are present in highly mobile segments of DNA, called **transposons**, and these also code for an enzyme that mediates their loss or their transfer between plasmids or between a plasmid and the chromosome.

11.1.3. Gene manipulation

The classic foundation of genetic studies in past few decades is the technique of gene transfer in bacteria to produce recombinants between different mutations. In a more recent development, the recombination of DNA into plasmids and phages *in vitro* has made it possible to transfer genes of any origin into bacteria.

11.1.4. Molecular cloning (recombinant DNA)

The basic principle of molecular cloning is to insert a DNA segment into a small replicon (a vector), generating a recombinant (chimeric) vector capable of replicating in cells. The vector must have all the genes essential for its replication along with transcription and translation control signals recognized within the cells.

The *in vitro* splicing of DNA into a bacterial replicon followed by multiplication in cells is carried by a procedure which uses the enzyme **restriction endonucleases** that makes staggered cuts, leaving overlapping ends. After separation, these complementary (cohesive) ends can be made to pair by annealing and they can then be covalently linked by polynucleotide ligase. A given restriction enzyme produces the same self complementary ends in all its products. Hence, in a mixture of purified vector and some other DNA, both cut with the same enzyme, will yield both the reconstituted original vector and recombinants (for further details regarding recombinant DNA refer to chapter 10).

11.1.5. Reverse genetics

Genetics has traditionally relied on mutation to provide the raw material needed for analysis. The usual procedure has been to use a mutant gene and phenotype to identify the wild type allele of the gene and its normal function. However, this approach has certain limitations. For example, it may prove difficult or impossible to isolate mutations in genes that duplicate the functions of other genes or that are essential for the viability of the organism.

Reverse genetics is a procedure by which certain problems can be solved. The procedure is so called because it reverses the usual flow of study. Instead of starting with a mutant phenotype and trying to identify the wild type gene, reverse genetics starts by making a mutant gene and studying the resulting phenotype. Using recombinant DNA technology, wild type genes are cloned, intentionally mutated in specific ways, and introduced back into the organism to study the phenotypic effects of the mutations. Because the position and molecular nature of each mutation is precisely defined, a very fine level of resolution is possible in defining promoter and enhanced sequences that are necessary for transcription, RNA splicing, particular amino acids that are essential for protein function and so on.

11.1.6. Vectors

Bacterial vectors are derived from plasmids or from phage genome. Both have been severely reduced in size so that they can accommodate large foreign segments while retaining the genes required for autonomous replication. The cyclic replicons of nonconjugative plasmids are excellent vectors because they can accommodate variable amounts of foreign DNA, are easy to purify, have selectable genes, and can be made to reproduce to large numbers in a cell.

The host range has been extended to **eukaryotic vectors**, using plasmids or DNA from viruses. Vectors capable of replicating in both bacteria and eukaryotic cells (shuttle vectors) are created by fusing two replicons, one bacterial, the other eukaryotic. Shuttle vectors are useful for many application, especially those in which they are studied in animal cells but amplified in bacteria or yeast. While many vectors are designed merely to clone and amplify the foreign DNA, some are made to obtain large amounts of the protein specified by the inserted gene. These vectors are named as **expression vectors**. In these vectors, the inserted gene is under the control of a promoter and a ribosome-binding site suitable for expression in the host cells.

The introduction of DNA cloning has revolutionized the study of many fields in biology. A possible application in humans is **gene therapy**, introducing a cloned gene into somatic cells or into germline cells to compensate for a defective gene.

11.2. APPROACHES FOR GENE THERAPY

Various approaches have been tried for effective transfer of genes to appropriate target site. These approaches broadly fall into four categories. They are:

1. Gene modification
   a. Replacement therapy
   b. Corrective gene therapy
2. Gene transfer
   a. Physical (Microinjection, Gene gun, 'naked DNA', EPD, Electroporation, etc.)
   b. Chemical (Liposomes, Cationic liposomes, Oligonucleotides, etc.)
   c. Biological (Viral vectors, mammalian artificial chromosomes, etc.)
3. Gene transfer in specific cell lines
   a. Somatic gene therapy
   b. Germline gene therapy
4. Eugenic approach (gene insertion)

11.2.1. Gene modification

Before discussing different approaches to gene therapy, we should be clear what our ultimate goal is, replacement therapy or corrective gene therapy. In **replacement therapy**, a defective gene is inserted somewhere in the genome so that its product could replace that of a defective gene. This approach may be suitable for recessive disorders, which are marked by deficiency of an enzyme or other proteins. Though the gene functions in the genome providing an appropriate regulatory sequence, this approach may not be successful in treating dominant disorders associated with the production of an abnormal gene product which interferes with the product of a normal gene. On the other hand, **corrective gene therapy**, requires replacement of a mutant gene or a part of it with a normal sequence. This can be achieved by using recombinant technology. Another form of corrective therapy involves the suppression of a particular mutation by a transfer RNA that is introduced into a cell.

11.2.2. Gene transfer

Gene transfer can be used for improvement of a specific disease. For example, introducing a growth hormone gene to increase the height. This gene transfer into cells can be brought about by physical, chemical and biological methods.

11.2.3. Gene transfer to specific cell lines

Somatic gene therapy, which has emerged as a new approach for the treatment of a variety of genetic and acquired diseases, involves the insertion of genes into specific somatic cells. If all goes well, they function during the lifetime of an individual and hence correct a genetic disease. Though it sounds well, it presents a number of practical problems.

On the other hand, injection or insertion of genes into germ cells, i.e. into fertilized eggs is known as **germline therapy** which differs from somatic cell therapy. Here, the inserted genes would be passed on to future generations too.

11.2.4. Eugenic approach (gene insertion)

Eugenic approach is brought about by inserting genes to alter or improve complex traits of a person. For example, intelligence. However, it is far beyond the current technological feasibility.

11.3. PROBLEMS ASSOCIATED WITH GENE THERAPY (SAFETY CONSIDERATIONS)

Human gene therapy has progressed from speculation to reality within a short span. The first clinical gene transfer (albeit only a marker gene NeoR/TIL) in an approved protocol was attempted successfully on 22 May, 1989, at National Institute of Health, Bethesda, MD for malignant melanoma. The first federally approved gene therapy protocol, for correction of adenosine deaminase (ADA) deficiency, began on 14 September 1990, at

National Institute of Health, Bethesda, MD. In spite of wide application they too have problems when brought in practice. For example, the problems encountered in attempting to correct a single gene disorder like β-thalassaemia, with an objective to replace the product of a defective or missing β globulin gene with that of a normal β gene. Now the question arises what is our target cell for insertion of the normal gene? And would the 'new' genes function properly in recipient cells? To cure a genetic blood disorder like thalassaemia, a 'good' gene must be inserted into hemopoietic stem cells, the self-sustaining cell population from which are derived all the formed elements of the blood. First, we can't identify the human stem cells, as they can only be assayed in murine systems. Secondly, till now no efficient method is discovered or available using which successful introduction of corrective gene could be affected. Another problem which comes across is the safety in transferring genes into foreign cells. But the most worrying part is the possibility that the 'new' gene might activate an oncogene and may give rise to neoplastic change in a particular cell population.

Besides the medical concerns, there are a number of philosophical, ethical and theological concerns. Though there is a general consensus that somatic cell gene therapy for the purpose of treating a serious disease is an ethical therapeutic option, considerable controversy exists as to whether or not germline gene therapy would be ethical.

11.4. IMMUNOLOGICAL PROBLEMS FOLLOWING GENE THERAPY

The major problem of human gene transfer therapy is, regardless of the route of gene transfer, it elicits an immune response in the recipient. However, there is very little information available about the antigenic properties of 'foreign' proteins of this type. A number of genetic disorders have been corrected successfully using bone marrow transplantation. But, this is always followed by the administration of drug that suppresses the immune system and therefore the antigenic properties of the newly introduced protein may well be masked. Again, the mounting amount of immune response varies from patient to patient, e.g. about 15% of patients with hemophilia A develop inhibitors, antibodies against factor VIII. Interestingly, only about 1% of patients who receive blood products to correct the defect in hemophilia B make antibodies. One reason may be the type of cell in which the foreign antigen is presented to the patient, and the other may be due to mutation.

11.5. PRE-REQUISITES FOR HUMAN GENE THERAPY

Before the patient is being subjected to gene therapy, several, essential prerequisites are to be fulfilled. They are:

1. It must be possible to isolate the appropriate gene and to define its major regulatory regions.
2. Identification and harvesting of appropriate target cells and development of safe and efficient vectors with which the new gene could be introduced.
3. Clear evidence of experimental details on the adequate functioning of the inserted gene, life span of the recipient cell and that no untoward effect exists, should be ensured.
4. Last but not the least, the patient or their family must be fully counseled.

11.6. CANDIDATE DISEASES FOR GENE THERAPY

In general, genetic diseases in which genetic factors play an important role can be classified as below:

- Single gene disorders
- Chromosomal disorders
- Congenital malformation and common diseases
- Multifunctional inheritance
- Cytoplasmic inheritance
- Somatic cell mutations.

For gene therapy, it is wiser to initially focus on a genetic disease in which corrected cells might have a selective growth advantage in patients (Anderson, 1984). In other words, a disease wherein mutation is involved in DNA metabolism so that cell division is inhibited by the defect. Three diseases fall under this category: ADA deficiency, PNP (purine nucleoside phosphorylase) deficiency and HGRPT (hypoxanthine-guanine phosphoribosyl transferase) deficiency, also known as Lesh-Nyhan disease. These diseases are due to deficiencies of enzymes produced by house keeping genes (genes that are expressed at a relatively low level in most cells), which are 'on' in most cells and do not require very precise regulation. In spite of various problems, i.e. the requirement of a tight regulation in terms of tissues as well as in their level of expression. The first target for gene replacement therapy was globulin.

As each biological target will require a unique gene delivery and gene expression system, many of the principles and methods established in development of advanced drug delivery systems can be applied to the design and preparation of synthetic gene delivery system. The delivery of gene(s) generally falls under two category *ex vivo* and *in vivo* approaches. The former involves the use of either viral or non-viral systems to insert genes into cells that have been removed from patients, followed by reimplantation of these transduced or transfected cells back into the patient (Culver and Blaese, 1994). While, the latter involves the administration of genes directly into the patients. Under this, two major methods have been proposed.

(a) Viral-mediated gene transfer

(b) Non-viral-mediated gene transfer

The natural ability of several viruses to infect cells efficiently leads investigators to make use of the same in *in vivo* viral-mediated gene delivery. Such viruses include retrovirus, adenovirus (AV), adeno-associated virus (AAV) and herpes simplex-1 virus (HSV-1) (Miller, 1992; Kay et al., 1993; Rosefeld et al., 1992; Glorioso et al., 1994).

In addition to viral mediated gene delivery, non-viral mediated gene delivery have also shown promising results and has emerged as an alternative. Cationic liposomes, polymer based gene delivery, peptide-based gene delivery are to cite a few.

11.7. VIRAL MEDIATED GENE DELIVERY

Gene delivery has become quite easy with the availability of several viral and non-viral delivery systems. Various viruses used as carrier include Moloney murine leukemia virus (MoMLV) and the human immunodeficiency virus (HIV), adenoviruses (AV), adeno-associated virus (AAV), herpes simplex virus (HSV), Epstein Barr virus (EBV), Sindbis virus, bovine, human papilloma viruses (BPV and HPV), hepatitis B virus (HBV), vaccinia virus and polyoma virus. The delivery and the mechanism involved depends on the viral encoded proteins.

11.7.1. Retroviral vectors

Principally, retroviral vector actively introduces genetic sequence into the host cell vis-à-vis proliferate in helper cell line for its own cloning. Characteristically, it offers a number of advantages in effective gene delivery to the cell.

1. It provides for official entry of genetic material into a wide variety of cells.

2. It is well understood with simple molecular biology.

3. Integrates into host genome.

4. It has a potential control over the range of cells to be infected.

5. It is capable of gene expression.

6. It could carry upto 8 kb of coding information.

7. Above all, it establishes one way, non-replicative infection of target cells.

Mammalian retrovirus vectors commonly used for gene transfer are classified on the basis of their host range as they could be **ecotropic**, which only infect murine cells, or **amphotropic**, which infect both murine and non-murine cells.

The main features of the genome of a typical retrovirus are as shown in the figure 11.1. Retroviruses which are RNA viruses, pass through a DNA stage after infection and integrate into the host genome to form provirus (Fig.11.1).

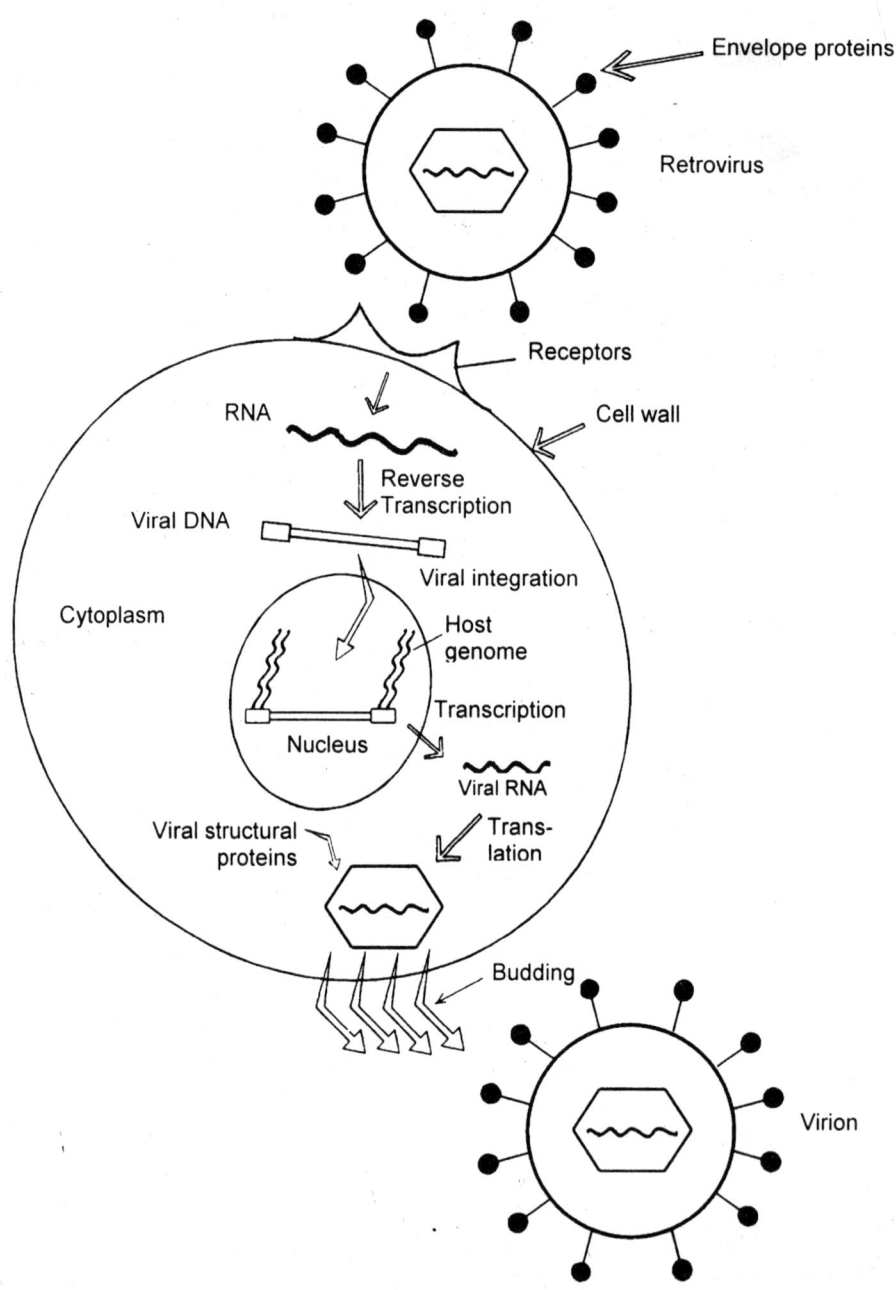

Fig. 11.1 : Life cycle of a retrovirus

This provirus can be characterized for its protein coding region (transacting) and the sequences corresponding to the replication, transcription and integration signals (Fig.11.2). Cell lines which make transacting viral proteins but no functional viral particles can be constructed using the "helper" gene sequences coding for the canonical retroviral *gag, pol* and *env* proteins, linked by appropriate promoters and polyadenylation signals, but devoid of packaging sequences (Fig.11.2).

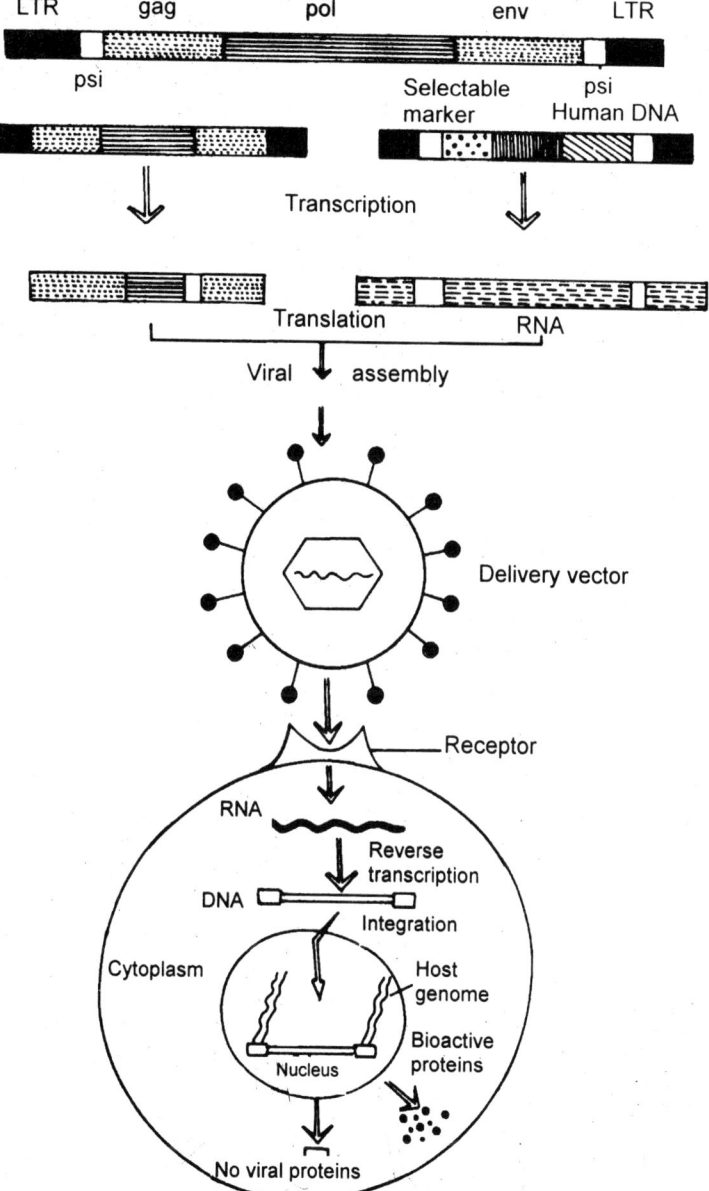

Fig. 11.2 : Generation of a retrovirus vector and its delivery

The viral genome needed for the infection, integration and transcriptional control of the genome is all contained in the long terminal repeat sequences (LTR's), which in turn are preserved together with packaging sequences (psi). At the same time, viral sequences of which the function can be supplied in *trans*, are taken out. Thus, the *gag* sequences which encode internal structural proteins of the virion core, *pol* genes which encode reverse transcriptase and *env* genes which encode the envelop glycoproteins are all deleted and replaced by a dominant selectable marker and the gene that we wish to transfer. Virus is continuously produced by the helper cell and can be harvested from tissue culture supernatant for infection of target cells.

The "helper cells", which provide complementing functions to retroviral vectors (Fig. 11.2), are then introduced into helper cells. This modified cells, called "helper cells" are replication-deficient virus which can supply the missing viral proteins to form a new virion. They produce viral particles which are microscopically identical to genuine retroviral particles, but carry a desired foreign gene (Fig. 11.2). These particles which are capable of introducing their RNA genomes into target cells, reverse transcribing them into DNA followed by integration into the cellular genome. The new genetic information thus resides in the target cell and does not propagate further as a virus (Fig. 11.2).

The first human replacement gene therapy using a retrovirus vector was approved for the replacement of a defected, missing, ADA gene in children suffering from severe combined immune deficiency (SCID) (Culver and Balese, 1994). The lymphocytes were harvested transduced or transfected *ex vivo* with a retrovirus vector containing a functional ADA gene and then the lymphocytes were reinfused into the host. Spectacular results were recorded in patients indicating a significantly enhanced ADA levels and as a result improved immune function.

Hepatic genetic deficiencies have been experimentally treated with genes introduced via retroviral vectors (Ledley et al., 1991). A case of hypercholesterolemia in rabbits following *ex-vivo* treatment and reimplantation of hepatocytes with the LDL receptor gene has been reported by Chowdhury et al., (1991). Similarly, human hepatocytes were transfected with the neomycin resistant gene in a retroviral vector followed by eventual transplantation of modified cells into the spleen of mice that suffered SCID.

A major focus of gene therapy in recent days is in the area of human immunodeficiency virus-1 (HIV-1) infection. In the case of this dreaded disease, the HIV-1 gp120 binds selectively and with high affinity to the CD4 receptor, if a high concentration of circulating, soluble CD4 could compete with cellular CD4 for HIV binding, it could intercept circulating HIV-1 virus before it can infect host cells (Morgan et al., 1990). The other strategy involves the introduction of a mutant HIV-1 envelopes which would compete with the wild-type, occupying the CD4 receptor and therefore, inhibit the spread of the wild-type virus (Buchschacher et al., 1992). The third strategy also known as *"suicide"* strategy involves transfection of T-lymphocytes with a HIV-regulated diphtheria toxin A chain gene (Harrison et al., 1992).

The next major area of interest in gene therapy is cancer gene therapy. Studies have suggested that introducing cytokine genes directly into tumor cells, immunize the animals against the tumor (Gansbucher et al., 1990; Golumbek et al., 1991).

Cardiovascular diseases have also been the area of attention for gene therapy. It has been shown in the Yucatan mini pig model that both endothelial cells and vascular smooth muscle cells, when transfected *ex-vivo* with the galactosidase marker gene, could be inserted in predetermined arterial segments using an intravascular catheter. Two to four weeks after treatment, histo-chemical staining showed positive results (Nabel et al., 1989; Plautz et al., 1991).

Another unique application of gene therapy is the use of transfected endothelial cells as 'coating' material for prosthetic devices (Wilson et al., 1989) with the aim to continuous release of thrombolytic agents, e.g. tissue plasminogen activator (tPA) (Dichek et al., 1991). The use of retrovirus is extremely efficient and results in stable insertion of the transfected gene into the host genome.

11.7.2. Adenovirus (AV) vectors

Adenovirus, a non-enveloped double-strained DNA virus in contrast to the retrovirus can be loaded with upto 36 kb DNA segments and can be used for *in vivo* transfection as it can also infect non-replicating cells. The AV gene remains episomal without insertion into the host genome, after gaining cell entry via endocytosis and it subsequently releases into the cytoplasm, which eliminates possible eventuality of insertional mutagenesis, the major obstacle with retroviral vectors (Horwitz, 1990).

Adenoviruses (AV) can infect a wide range of cell types and live AV have been used as vaccines in US military personnel without any major side effects. Two serotypes, Ad5 and Ad2 have been studied extensively. Of the several genes encoded by the adenoviral genome the proteins encoded by the E1 gene are crucial for virus replication and deletion of E1 gene renders the virus replication defective. AV are attractive candidates for gene therapy of lung disorders because of their natural tropism for infecting respiratory epithelium (Crystal, 1994). Unlike retroviruses, they can infect post-mitotic cells and thus their use for gene transfer towards brain is of prime importance (Davidson et al., 1993; Bajocchi et al., 1993).

Recombinant AV vectors have been designed which are replication deficient and contain tissue-specific promoters which restrict the site of transgene expression (Berkmer, 1988). AV vectors are similarly broad in range of infectivity as retroviruses, AV infects the pulmonary epithelium avidly and has been successfully employed in the *in-vivo* transfection of pulmonary epithelial cells with the hα1aT gene and the CFTR gene both in the cotton rat (Rosenfeld et al., 1991;1992).

AV gene constructs have also been employed to correct ornithine deficiency *in-vivo* by transfecting the gene for ornithine transcarbamylase in a mouse model (Stratford-Perricaudet et al., 1990), and to demonstrate lacZ gene expression (β-galactosidase activity) in skeletal and cardiac muscle following intravenous and intra-muscular administration in mice (Stratford-Perricaudet et al., 1992).

Two different methods of AV viral mediated gene transfer are currently under investigation. The first method involves the insertion of gene of interest into deleted AV particles similar to AV approach (Quantivi et al., 1992). The second method involves complexing the DNA to be inserted with transferrine-polylysine and the viral coat of AV is similar to a sendai virus gene transfer approach (Wagner et al., 1992). Using this approach Lemarchand et al., (1993) could successfully transfer genes into blood vessels.

The major concern with AV vectors is similar to other viral vectors, i.e., recombination with wild-type AV, especially in the upper airways, which would lead to the generation of replicating AV with unknown pathogenicity. A significant fraction of the population has developed immunity to AV (Straus, 1984), the latter could affect the efficiency of transfection.

11.7.3. Adenovirus-associated viral (AAV) vectors

AAV is a nonpathogenic human parvovirus which has aroused a lot of interest as a vector for gene therapy. It contains a single strand of DNA of 4.7 kb (Muzyezka, 1992). It has been observed that human AAV infection appears to be non-pathogenic with a majority of the population testing positive for AAV capsid protein antibodies. AAV is a dependovirus and require a helper virus co-infection for viral replication. In the absence of co-infection with a helper virus such as AV, herpes virus or cylomegalovirus, the viral genome integrates into the human genome usually at a specific site, 19q 13.3qter. The biology of AAV vectors is not as well understood as of retrovirus or AV hence, the system is still in its infant stage (Berns and Linden, 1995). In terms of gene therapy, the site-specific insertion of wild-type AAV in chromosome 19 is of great interest. AAV vectors have been used to transfect a human leukemia cell line (Dixit et al., 1991) and a cystic fibrosis cell line (Flotte et al., 1992). They have successfully been applied *in vivo* to transfect a lung lobe with CAT in Sprague-Dawley rats (Flotte et al., 1993).

11.7.4. Herpes simplex virus-1 (HSV-1) vectors

Among the viral vectors, HSV-1 has potentially the largest DNA carrying capacity. It is capable of establishing long term, non-cytopathic relationships with the neurons that it infects. Like AV, HSV-1, infects non-dividing cells (Geller and Breakefield, 1988). In addition, HSV do not generally integrate into the host genome, providing an element of safety as there is little opportunity for insertional mutagenesis of infected cells. However, these viruses contain a genome of much greater complexity (152 kb) than the more familiar retroviral gene transfer vector (10 kb). This puts considerable amount of difficulty in development of these vectors.

Three general strategies have been used to develop HSV for use as gene transfer vector (Fig. 11.3) (Breakefield and DeLuca, 1991):

- The use of a replication-competent virus with a transgene introduced into a non essential part of the viral genome (Palella et al., 1989). However, their limitation being their ability to retain and propagate the cytotoxic property which are not clinically useful.

- The use of small 'Amplicon' vectors containing a herpes virus origin of replication, a virion packaging signal and a transgene of interest (Geller et al., 1990). Except for a few reports, others are not encouraging.

- The incorporation of transgene by recombination into the backbone genome of a replication defective parent HSV mutant (Breakefield and DeLuca, 1991).

HSV vectors are promising vehicle for gene transfer in neural disorder especially the brain cells. Initial studies of the effectiveness of the HSV vector were carried out using a marker gene encoding β galactosidase. This expression of the transgene can be assessed both quantitatively and with a simple histochemical strain.

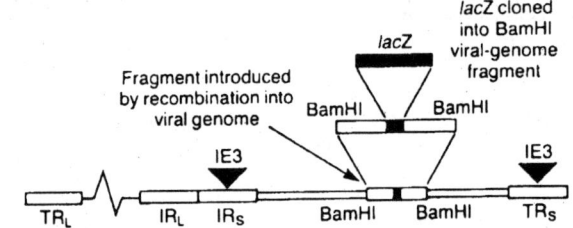

Fig. 11.3 : Construction of a herpes simplex virus (HSV)

11.7.5. Alpha viruses as vectors

Alpha viruses are a group of arthropod-borne Toga viruses that infect many types of host ranging from mosquito to avian and mammalian species (Strauss and Strauss,1994). Alpha viruses genome consists of a single stranded RNA molecule of positive polarity, i.e. a productive infection can be initiated either by infection or by transfection of a cell by the isolated RNA. This strategy of self replication with its highly efficient production of new RNA molecules and protein products, provides the basis for the alpha virus expression vector that have recently been developed (Lijestrom, 1994; Schlesinger, 1993). The genome is divided in such a way that the replicase (Fig. 11.4) is encoded by one open reading frame (ORF) on the genomic RNA while the structural proteins are encoded with second ORF on separate subgenomic species. Manipulation of alpha viruses are brought about by manipulating these subgenomic sequences which do not affect the replication capacity of the system.

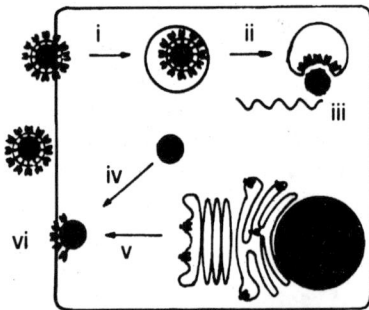

Fig. 11.4 : Life cycle of the alpha virus **(a)** (i) Infection of the cell via the virus by receptor--mediated endocytosis (ii) Nucleocapsid is delivered into the cytoplasm by pH drop in endosome causes fusion between the viral & endosomal membrane (iii) Disruption of nucleocapsid and release of genomic and subgenomic RNA (iv) Formation of cytoplasmic nucleocapsids by binding of capsid protein monomers and genomic RNA (v) Transport of spike protein to the cell surface (vi) Delivery of mature virus particle to the extracellular medium

Alpha virus vectors have established themselves as a basic tool in research and have demonstrated their versatility towards gene delivery. It is also found that these vectors can be used for *in-vivo* application for the development of recombinant vaccines.

Viral replicase will initiate RNA synthesis from any subgenomic promoter on a minus-strand molecule thus making it possible to express a foreign sequence packed in infectious viral RNA simply by adding a second transcription unit either upstream or downstream from the structural gene (Fig. 11.5). However, they are found to be unstable upon extensive passaging with an additional drawback towards *in vivo* application wherein new virions are also formed. Thus, the preferable strategy is to replace the structural gene with foreign sequences. This does not affect the intracellular replication of RNA molecule and high level of expression ranging upto 50% of total cell protein can be achieved.

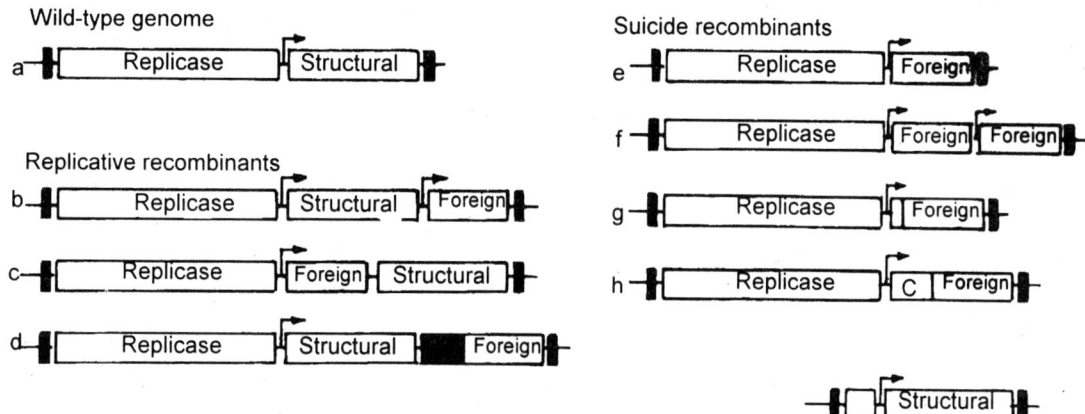

Fig. 11.5. : Types of alphavirus **(a)** Genomic RNA; **(b-d)** replicative forms of rRNA that produce virus upon transfection into cells; **(e-h)** suicidal forms; **(i)** helper vector with majority of the replicase region deleted, including packaging sequence

Delivery of recombinant RNA (rRNA) into the cell can be negotiated in a number of ways. Among which the most simple and efficient method to transfect RNA, is to transcribe *in vitro* using electroporation or lipofection (Fig. 11.6a) (Ligestrom and Garoff, 1994).

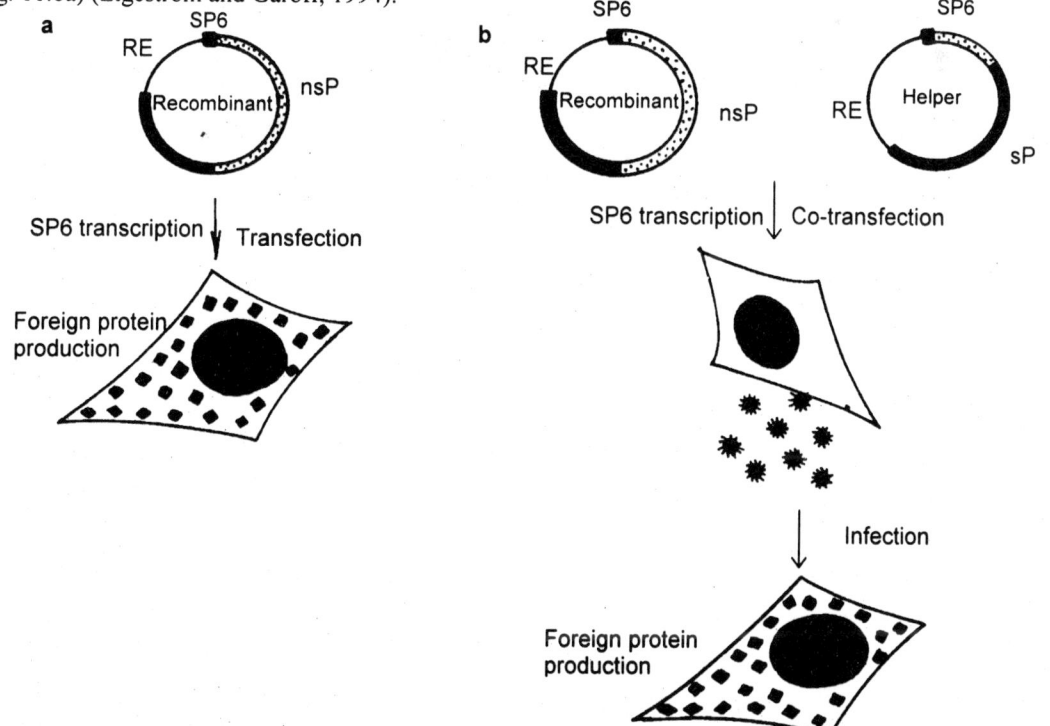

Fig. 11.6 : Strategies for expressing foreign sequences with alpha virus vectors

T-ansfection efficiencies of up to 100% can be achieved under *in vitro* cell culture conditions. However, it is a cumbersome process when different cell types are used especially in *in vivo* application. Therefore, a preferable mode of delivery is to make use of the very broad host-range of these viruses for infecting cells. Helper vectors that allow rRNA to be packed into infectious virus particle have been developed (Fig.11.6b) with high titer values (10^9-10^{16}/ml).

Although several alpha viruses are pathogenic, the two viruses used as vector i.e., SFV and SIN are avirulent in human (Strauss and Strauss, 1994). For safety and economic reasons a novel strategy involving a layered DNA-RNA vector system has been developed (Fig.11.7). This system is independent of helper vectors. Recombinant alpha virus expression-cassette cDNA is controlled by a eukaryotic promoter, such as the cytomegalovirus early promoter (pCMV). This plasmid-DNA construct can be delivered directly into the cell by DNA transfection method. Here, in the cell nucleus, RNA polymerase transcribes the complete unit into RNA which is transported to the cytoplasm. This results in obtaining a positive polarity and the RNA is translated to form the viral replicase, which takes over the replica of the whole molecule in the same manner as during normal replication of alpha virus RNA molecule.

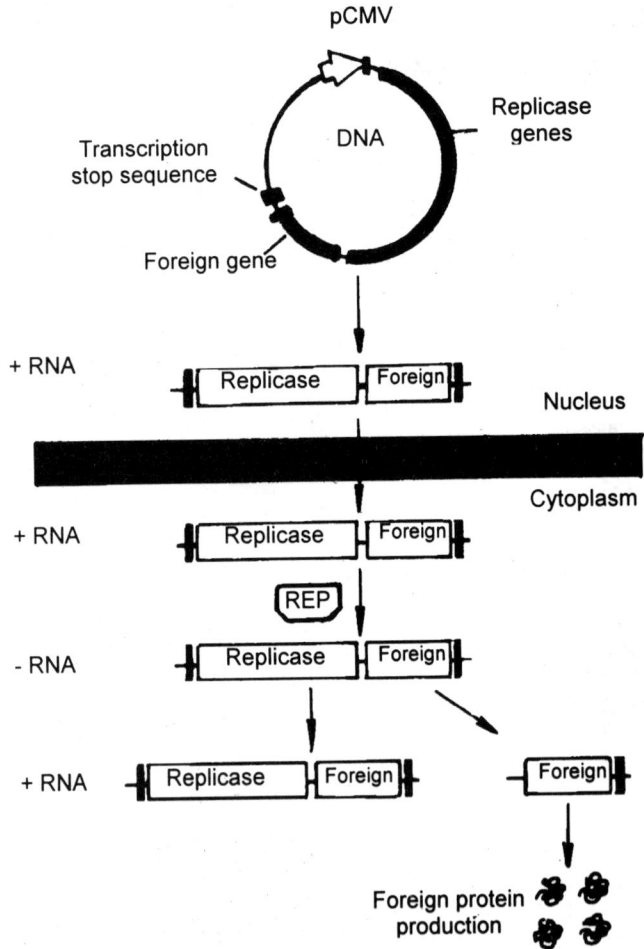

Fig. 11.7 : Layered DNA-RNA vector system

Alpha virus vectors have been successfully used to study the structure and function of protein and for protein production. It has been found to be a useful tool in targeting of transient, high level protein expression to desired areas. They have also found place in development of recombinant vaccines (Berglund et al., 1996).

11.7.6. Epstein Barr virus (EBV)

Long term gene expressions are required for certain applications which do not involve the integration of transferred DNA. For this, persistent gene expression and episomal maintenance are required. An ideal-long term expression system bears the following features :

- Nuclear retention by attachment of DNA to the nuclear matrix.
- Autonomous replication
- Enhanced gene expression
- Prevention of plasmid degradation
- Efficient delivery into the nucleus

These features can be brought about by using parts of viral systems. One such viral system is the Epstein Barr Virus (EBV) which can be used to provide autonomous replication and nuclear retention. EBNA1 protein that interacts with the EBV origin of replication (*ori*P) provides such a function. Mammalian artificial chromosomes are also reported to provide such features.

11.7.7. Suicide gene

In the present scenario none of the DNA delivery system existing could mediate a transfection into all the cells *in-vivo*. This is a major drawback in cases like cancer where the treatment requires 100% selective delivery of therapeutic genes to tumor cells. By using the suicidal gene strategy, a bystander effect could be produced, where 100% DNA delivery to cells is otherwise not necessary. Instead, in these systems, a small portion of the tumor cells (1-10%), expresses a suicide gene product. The system which is now present in a population of 1-10%, expresses a suicide product which transmits its toxic effect to the neighboring tumor cells, which originally do not possess the suicide gene. In this way, 100% killing of tumor cells is achieved. The strategy mostly involves the use of herpes simplex virus-thymidine kinase (HSV-TK) and cytosine deaminase. The use of HSV-TK was first reported for the treatment of brain tumors. In this approach, Ganciclovir, a drug that when administered intravenously following the administration of HSV-TK gene reaches the tumor cells, interacts only with HSV-TK enzyme and produces toxicity to cells expressing HSV-TK. The selective toxicity attributes to HSV-TK expressed enzyme that converts ganciclovir into nucleotide-like precursors which block DNA synthesis and kill cells. This toxic effect is diffused to the surrounding tumor cells, which originally do not express HSV-TK, ultimately killing them.

One another example of suicide gene involves the use of a nontoxic prodrug 5-fluorocytosine (5-FCyt). The strategy involves the use of tumor-specific promoters to express the cytosine deaminase gene. The prodrug is converted into the toxic 5-fluorouracil (5-FU) with the help of cytosine deaminase. This can be well explained by taking carcinoembryonic antigen (CEA) promoter as an example. CEA promoter are active in human colorectal carcinoma cells while they are totally inactive in normal colorectal cells. Once the vector carrying the cytosine deaminase gene is expressed by CEA promoter into the colorectal carcinoma cells, on administration of the prodrug 5-FCyt, 5-FU is produced by only those cells that express cytosine deaminase. The highly diffusible 5-FU diffuses to the surrounding tumor cells and kills them.

11.8. NON-VIRAL MEDIATED-GENE THERAPY

At present, majority of the approved clinical trials on gene therapy in human subjects have involved viral transfection using viral vector mediated transfer (Fig. 11.8). In the recent past, non-viral gene medicines have emerged as potentially safe and effective gene therapy method for a wide variety of acquired and genetic diseases.

11.8.1. Disadvantages of viral mediated gene therapy

1. Retroviral vectors are not capable of replication although they infect and introduce the provirus into the target.
2. Retroviral vectors function as single hit gene transfer systems.

3. Retroviral vectors can only infect dividing cells.
4. The transgenes inserted by retroviral vector do not remain transcriptionally active thus possessing a "viral shut down" problem.
5. Difficulty in targeting to certain cells.
6. Requirement for a packaging cell line.
7. They possess a low DNA transfer.
8. Size limitation of DNA constructs.
9. Production of high titer viral vectors is difficult.
10. No assurance for completely free replication-competent virus.
11. Severe immunogenic reactions and safety concerns.
12. Toxic side effects.
13. Possibility of insertional mutation.
14. Possible triggering of oncogene(s) or desirable tumor suppresser gene(s).
15. Above all, the possibility to revert back or to retain an infectious form.

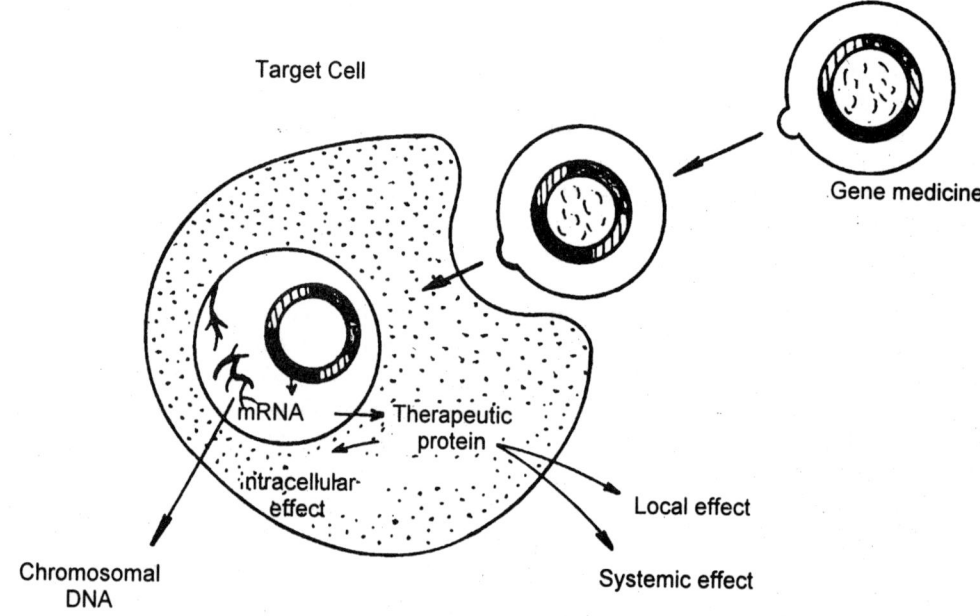

Fig. 11.8 : Mode of action of non-viral gene delivery system

11.8.2. Interstitial administration of tissue-specific gene medicines

Interstitial administration of plasmid-gene expression systems using needle-free jet injection devices, e.g. *'gene guns'* or *'golden guns'* and *'hypospray'* or by direct injection have been reported to be taken by a variety of cells *in vivo* (Hickman et al., 1994; Manthrope et al., 1993; Sikes et al., 1994; Raz et al., 1994). These gene guns (Fig.11.9) are said to utilize tissue bombardment with gold or tungsten microparticles coated with a DNA plasmid-based gene expression system. Ballistic methods that use particle-mediated or 'gene gun' technology have shown up to 100 fold greater gene expression levels both in *ex vivo* and *in vivo* in comparison to cationic lipid delivery or other non viral gene delivery systems. This method has been successfully used to deliver DNA *in vivo* into liver, skin, pancreas, muscle, spleen, and tumors. Expression of reporter genes (e.g. firefly luciferase and β-galactosidase) or therapeutic genes (human growth hormone) have also been reported (Cheng et al., 1993; Eisenbrann et al., 1993; Andree et al., 1994). 'Hypospray' devices which do not require non-biodegradable microparticles have been used for the *in-vivo* administration to mouse skin either as a skin-specific gene expression system (driven by human keratin K6 promoter) or as a non-tissue-specific construct (driven by a viral CMV promoter), both the systems contained a β-galactosidase reporter gene (β-gal) (Selheyer et al., 1993; Furth et al., 1992; Ledley et al., 1994). These studies concluded that there was a significantly increased level of gene expression as compared to the administration of the same in the form of saline suspensions.

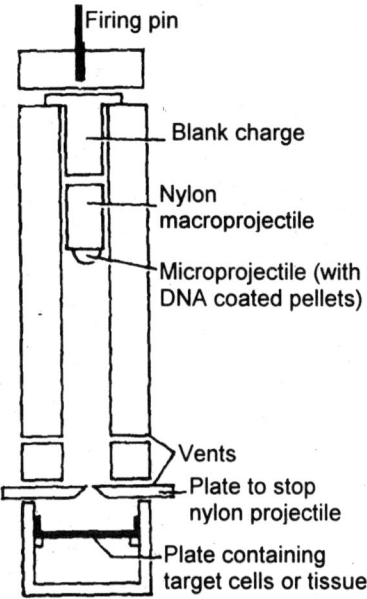

Fig. 11.9 : Diagrammatic presentation of a gene gun

Interstitial administration of plasmid-based gene expression have shown low levels of gene expression with the exception of such systems for vaccination purposes (Ulmer et al., 1993; Davis et al., 1993). Such results have led to design a number of approaches for enhancing the location and amount of genes to the nuclei of target cells. These approaches include (Felgner and Ringold, 1989; Felgner et al., 1987; Wu et al., 1991):

1. Cationic lipids.
2. Charged synthetic polymers.
3. Peptides that act in a non-specific manner.
4. Peptide and carbohydrate-based targeting ligand.

11.8.3. Liposome-mediated delivery

Liposomes have been well studied for the delivery of drugs to specific site in a controllable manner. Nicolau and co-workers in 1983 demonstrated the delivery of prepro-insulin gene to the liver of rats. The DNA plasmids were encapsulated in lactosylceramide based liposomes which were then administered intravenously. Intra-cellular trafficking of DNA following endocytosis by cells have also been demonstrated using pH-sensitive liposomes and proteoliposomes (Wang and Huang, 1987; Nicalou and Cudd 1989; Kato et al., 1991).

pH-sensitive liposomes are known to fuse with the lipid membranes in the acidic environment of the endosomes, thereby facilitating the endosomal release of encapsulated gene expression systems into the cytoplasm of transfected cells. The limiting step however, is the transfer of encapsulated plasmid DNA from the endosomal compartment to the nucleus of the target cell. Thus, an attempt was made to facilitate the translocation of encapsulated gene expression systems to the nucleus by incorporating a nuclear localization (specific) peptide into the expression system. However, the same did not turn fruitful (Legendre and Szoka 1992). At the same time, it was found that addition of a lysosomotrophic agent like chloroquine, which raises the acidic pH of the endosomes, obviates the fusing efficiency of the liposome with endosomal membrane and consequently reduces the probability of gene transfer to the nucleus.

Proteoliposomes (Chimerasomes) have been shown to transfer genes effectively. But the difficulty in their purification and characterization have limited their use. Proteoliposomes containing sendai virus glycoproteins, however could mediate the cellular entry and fusion of the liposomes with the endosomal membrane (Kato et al., 1991; Gould-Fogerite et al., 1989).

11.8.4. Cationic liposomes

The use of cationic liposomes to deliver antisense constructs is only emerging at this point. Cationic lipids have been used to reduce the net negative surface charge on DNA plasmid-based gene expression systems in order to reduce charge-charge repulsion at the surface of biological membranes. Such lipids have been reported to form a stable complex with the gene expression system (Felgner and Rigold 1989; Gao and Huang 1991; Felgner et al., 1994; Mc Lachlan et al., 1994; Staedel et al., 1994; Rojanasakul 1996).

Cationic liposomes as the name indicates consist mainly of a positively charged lipid. "Lipofection" a novel and highly efficient DNA transfection system based on lipofectins was introduced in 1987 (Felgner et al., 1987). The lipofection system consisted of the positively charged quaternary amino lipid N-[1-(2,3-di-oleyloxy) propyl]-N,N,N-trimethylammonium chloride (DOTMA) in a 1:1 weight mixture with dioleylphosphatidyl choline (DOPE). As DOPE can fuse with endosomal membrane, it is generally included to effect the endosomal release of a gene expression system. DNA on mixing with cationic liposomes produces a condensed DNA along with a tubular structure and liposome aggregate. The mechanism by which DNA-cationic liposome complex delivers the DNA is understood to be as follows (Fig.11.10). The complex first interacts with the cell membrane, followed by endocytosis and finally disruption of endosomes. These lipid-based transfective agents have been employed successfully for genetic loading of a variety of cell lines *in vitro* and *in vivo*. Luciferase mRNA was transfected into NIH 3T3 cells using the DOTMA-DOPE liposome complex. Lipophilic polylysines, i.e. lipopolylysine (LPLL) mediated gene delivery has been reported (Zhao and Huang 1991). LPLL when mixed with DOPE followed by sonication readily forms unilamellar liposomes, which could effectively negotiate the transfer of gene into cell line(s).

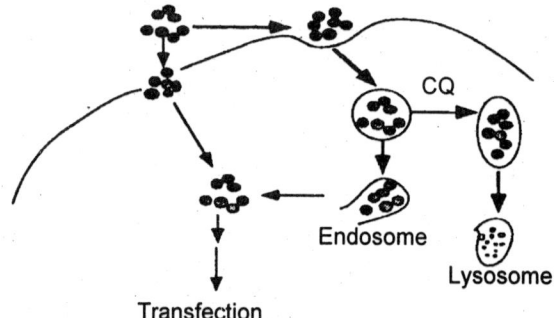

Fig. 11.10 : A model for gene delivery mediated by cationic liposomes

D-Chol, nothing but 3β-[N-(N',N'-dimethylaminoethane)carbamoyl] cholesterol along with DOPE, a cationic liposome has been reported for efficient delivery of nucleic acids (Li et al., 1996).

The use of *cationic liposomes* as synthetic viral vectors for the delivery of gene has numerous therapeutic, toxicological and technological attributes.

1. Complexation of cationic lipid and DNA is quantitative and needs separation of unencapsulated DNA.
2. Production of such complexes is rapid, highly reproducible and involves only one step.
3. DNA vectors directly complex with cationic lipid. There is no need for virus production or screening.
4. Due to the net negative charge, transfection is spontaneous.
5. The DOPE component of cationic liposomes is responsible for the escape of complex from the endosomal compartment into the cytosol.
6. Cationic liposomes are non immunogenic.

11.8.5. Reconstituted sendai virus envelopes (RSVE)

It is a unilamellar proteoliposome, which incorporates the fusogenic protein(s) of the sendai virus (an enveloped virus of the paramyxovirus family) (Fig.11.11). The vesicles are known as reconstituted sendai virus envelopes (RSVE). The potential of RSVE to deliver encapsulated materials intravascularly have been reported (Ardizzoni et al., 1988; Gitman et al., 1985; Bartzatt 1987; 1988; Bagai and Sarkar, 1993; 1994).

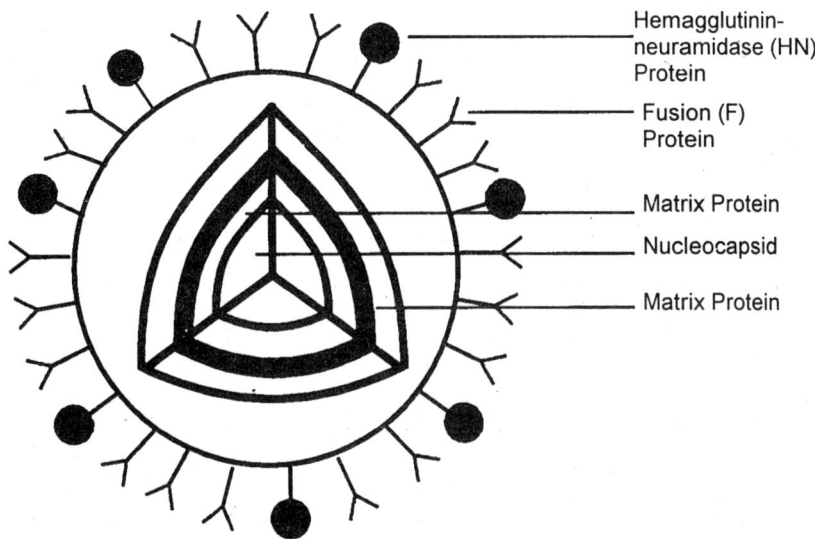

Fig. 11.11 : Structure of a sendai virus particle

In general, the encapsulation of the genetic material into the sendai virus is accomplished as follows:

Two types of proteins (Haemagglutinin (HN) and fusion (F) protein) are inserted into the sendai virus in which the nucleocapsid is encapsulated within the lipid membrane or envelope (Fig.11.12). HN, mediates viral attachment to cell surfaces, while its neuraminidase activity prevents unproductive binding to cell receptors. The other protein is the F protein which as the name suggests is a fusion protein involved in fusion of the virus envelope to the plasma membrane of the cell. Fusion of the RSVE results in microinjection of the viral genome into the cell cytoplasm, where it is replicated in a productive infective manner or phase.

11.8.6. Synthetic retrotransposon vectors

11.8.6.1. Transposable elements

Cells contain a variety of transposable elements that can become inserted at many places in the bacterial chromosome, and can be excised by site-specific recombination. The important feature is that after transposing with high frequency at a given set of conditions, they become quite stable under others. Transposable elements are of important value especially in transfer of drug resistant genes to other bacteria.

Transposable elements are not replicons, but they are usually duplicated, leaving the original element intact while inserting a copy elsewhere and thereby increasing the total number in the cell. In this transfer, **transposase**, an enzyme specified by a gene of the element itself interacts with its ends and with target sequences in the recipient DNA. The enzymes of different transposable elements recognize different targets, which differ in abundance.

Insertion sequences(ISs), the simplest transposable elements, were discovered as mutagens, whose trans-position into a gene usually inactivates it. The ISs are short (150-1500 base pairs), with inverted repeats of 15 to 40 base pairs at the ends. Large ISs contain the gene for the transposase. **Transposons** are larger and contain additional genes, often for antibiotic resistance.

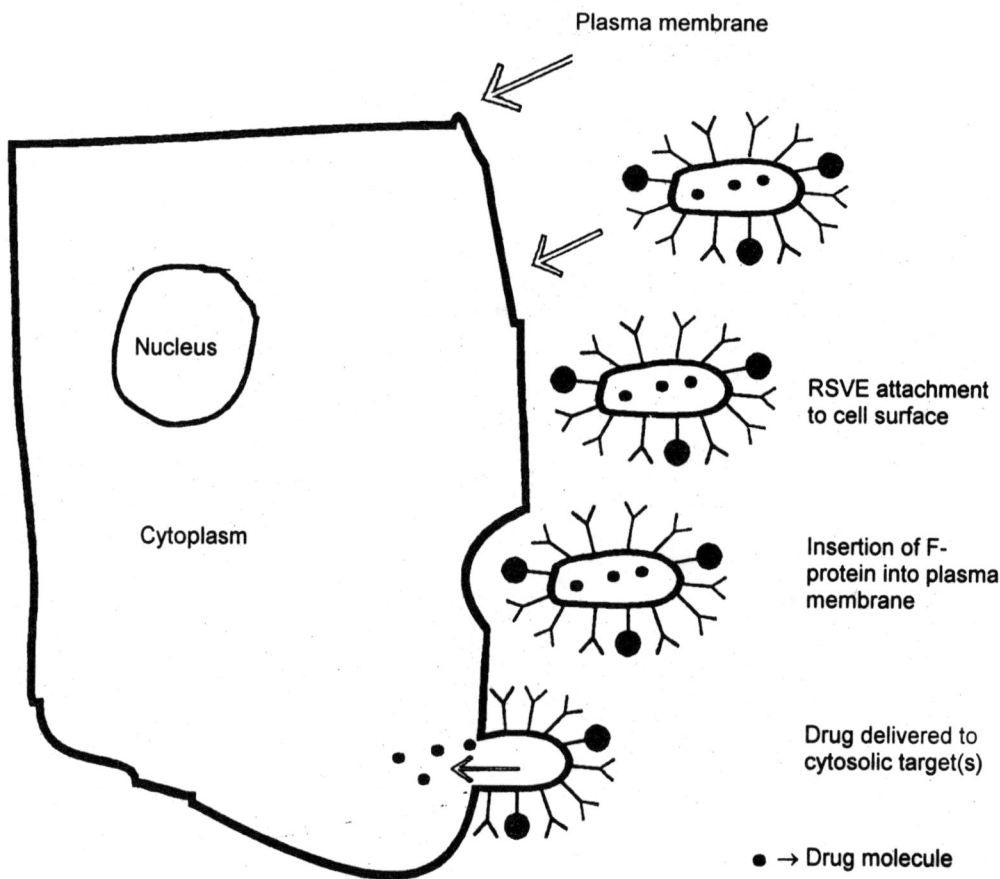

Fig. 11.12 : RSVE - mediated drug delivery

The prokaryotic transposons can be categorized under three classes. **Class I** are bounded by two ISs (e.g., Tn10, a gene for tetracycline resistance), while **class II** are bounded by two short repeats, 30 to 40 base pairs long instead of terminal ISs (e.g., Tn3, with a gene for ampicillin resistance). While **class III** transposons are phages.

11.8.6.2. Mechanisms of transposition

Some transposons (e.g., Tn7) can integrate essentially at a single site, causing the appearance of hot spots for transposition. While some others (e.g., Tn10) integrate at many sites which are related in sequence. Finally, others (e.g., IS1) integrate almost anywhere, although they prefer certain sequences.

Transposition can give rise to **simple insertions** or to **cointegrates**. In simple insertion, a conservative transposition displaces the transposon from its location to a new location without replication. While in cointegrate formation, each strand of the transposon is copied, resulting in two complete copies separated by a lost chromosome segment and integrated in direct orientation.

11.8.6.3. Consequences of transposition

Transposons may have positive functional consequences for the host cells by introducing new genes. They may also inactivate a host gene, by interrupting a coding sequence, or by terminating transcription or translation upstream. However, the gene can be reactivated by precise excision of the transposon. Finally, transposons can activate neighboring genes by initiating transcription. In this function some transposons act as switches for adjacent genes (**gene switches**) by reversible recombination between inverted repeats. In one direction, they initiate transcription, in the other, they fail to initiate it or terminate it.

Today's gene therapy vectors are either viral or nonviral. Among the viral vectors, retroviral vectors have been studied widely for their ability that a single copy of the gene is precisely and permanently integrated into an active region of host chromatin. In retroviral vectoring systems, the viral genome is split into its *cis*-acting sequences (the vector), and its *trans*-acting viral structural genes (latter inserted into vector produced cells). The shortcoming in this approach is that the *cis* and *trans*-acting sequences often recombine during propagation of the vector, resulting in replication-competent retrovirus (RCR). To overcome such shortcomings of this most popular form of gene therapy, some improvements have been suggested. The first is substituting synthetic components for viral ones, starting with the vector and proceeding towards a synthetic gene delivery particle (Hodgon, 1995). In addition, some retroelements can be used for site-specific integration or cell-specific transcription targeting (Kirchner et al., 1995).

Retroelements include retroviruses, defective retroviruses, retrotransposons, short interspersed repetitive elements (SINES) and pseudogenes. Retroelements are major structural components of the genome, wherein they have both positive (evolutionary) and negative (insertional mutagenesis) effects. In addition, they are also known to regulate the expression of cellular genes at instances (Mc Donald, 1993). Among the retroelements studied as transcriptional promoters, murine leukemia viruses (MLVs) are the only retrovectors studied clinically. However, another emerging candidate of this class is the virus-like 30s (VL30) retrotransposon found in vertebrates. These retrotransposon resembles retrovirus in structure but contains no retroviral structural gene (Hodgson et al., 1983). They do not have any sequence similarity to retrovirals. But they can co-pack into the retroviral virions and are transferred to the recipient cells along with the retroviral genome (Besmer et al., 1979). They are then converted into DNA via retroviral **reverse transcriptase** and then integrated into the human genome from where they are transcribed. Thus, VL30 can be used to transmit DNA efficiently.

The minimal *cis* acting synthetic retrotransposon vectors have been synthesized by comparing the sequences of the two types of retrovectors (VL30s and MLV) and identifying the most essential ones such as LTR boundaries, adjoining primer binding sites, and putative packaging. Synthetic oligonucleotide primers were used to gene-amplify the LTRs of a VL30 element (NVL-3) together with essential and non-essential *cis*-acting sequences with convenient linking and gene insertion sites. They are then synthesized using the polymerase chain reaction (PCR), the LTR blocks are isolated from agarose gels (to eliminate primers and spurious products), digested with the appropriate restriction endonucleases at the joining region, re-purified on agarose gels, ligated at common restriction sites to create cohesive termini, digested at the distal termini and finally ligated to a compatible plasmid (pGEM3) (Chakraborty et al., 1993). The so formed synthetic retrotransposon vectors were found to be biologically active in the sense that they transmit via retrovirus particles, integrate properly, and express their gene(s) as RNA and protein.

11.8.7. Oligonucleotide carrier systems

Introduction of a potent gene inhibitor is equally important to that of introducing a missing gene or to correct a mutant gene. These are especially required in cases like neoplastic infections and some inherited diseases (Cohen, 1991). Various "antisense" strategies have been developed.

"Antisense" compounds/oligonucleotides are short synthetic strands of nucleic acid which bind to DNA, mRNA or extracellular proteins in a complementary fashion and arrest protein synthesis by inhibiting transcription or translation (Inouye, 1988; Miller and Ts'O, 1988; Stein and Coher, 1988).

Three basic approaches have been explored in this area.

1. Antisense oligonucleotides bind to mRNA and block translation. This approach was used to inhibit translation of HIV *tat* RNA (Stevenson and Iversen 1989).

2. Triple-helix-forming oligonucleotides which binds in a sequence-specific masses in the manor groove of duplex DNA (Show et al., 1991).

3. Oligonucleotides which bind to extracellular proteins and inhibit their enzymatic activity (Wang et al., 1993).

The rapid degradation *in vivo* by 3'-exonuclease digestion (Tidd and Warenius 1989) limits the use of natural oligodeoxynucleotides. Therefore, nuclease resistant oligonucleotides were synthesized modifying the phosphodiester backbone. Among them, the widely investigated ones are phosphorothioates (anionic) and methylphosphonate analogs (nonionic) (Goodchild 1990).

Basic structure of a chemically modified oligonucleotide (see Goodchild 1990)

The major problem of oligonucleotide delivery is their limited access to the intracellular (and intranuclear) space. Chemical means to overcome cell exclusion, e.g. the design of more lipophilic compounds, are limited as they may compromise the selectivity and binding affinity for the intended target DNA or RNA. Such problems can be undermined by employing intracellular carrier systems.

Both cellular as well as intranuclear delivery of an antisense oligonucleotide hybridized to ICAM-1 was found to be increased in the presence of a cationic liposome carrier (Lipofectin®).

11.8.8. Self-organized DNA-photonic nanostructures

Many techniques have been developed for the synthesis and modification of nucleic acids for their potential uses in clinical diagnostics, "DNA probes" and as therapeutic agents "antisense DNA". Synthetic nucleic acids are generally referred to as "oligonucleotides". These synthetic nucleic acids have inherent recognition properties and can be easily functionalized. They are ideal candidates for creating molecular photonic and electronic mechanisms. Oligonucleotides incorporated with simple electronic/photonic mechanisms which could self-assemble into organized structures have been studied. This involved fluorophore labelled oligonucleotides which carry out an efficient Forster non-radiative energy transfer process (Heller et al., 1983; Heller and Morrison 1985; Heller and Jablonski 1987).

Forster non-radiative energy transfer is the process by which a fluorescent donor (D) group excited at one wavelength transfers its absorbed energy via resonant dipole coupling process to a suitable fluorescent acceptor (A) which emits it at a second wavelength (Lakowicz, 1983). It has been demonstrated that when two fluorophore labelled oligonulceotides are designed to bind (hybridize) to adjacent positions of a complementary target nucleic acid strand, they produce efficient fluorescent energy transfer (Fig. 11.13). Since these functional molecular components can be programmed, via their nucleotide sequence, they can be designed to self-assemble and organize into large and more complex but defined nano structures.

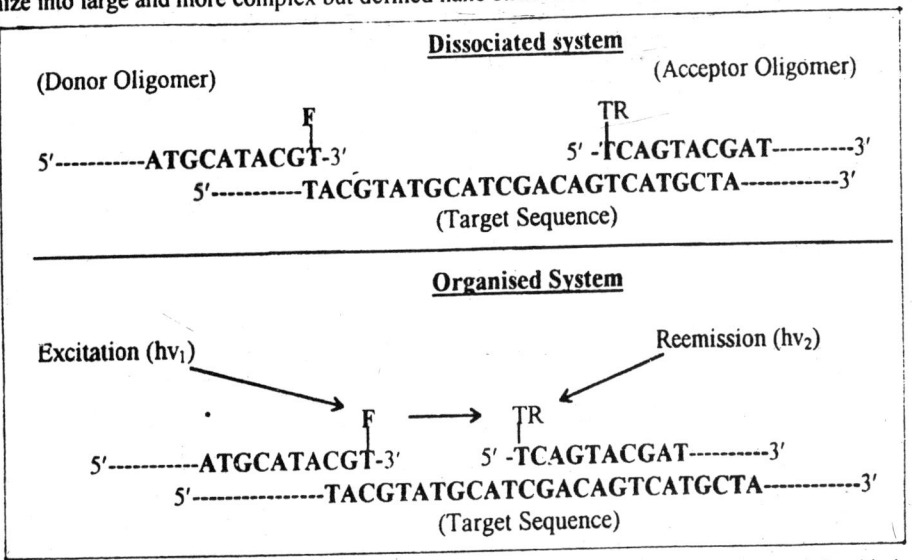

Fig. 11.13 : Scheme illustrating how two fluorophore-labelled oligonucleotides are designed to bind or hybridize to adjacent positions on a complementary target nucleic acid strand F-fluorescein donor group, TR-Texas Red

11.8.9. Polymer-based gene delivery systems

Similar to cationic lipids, cationic polymers, such as polybrene and DEAE-dextran, have been studied in the past for transfecting cells *in vitro*. However, their use was limited *in vitro*, for their low efficiency, cytotoxicity and non-biodegradability (Ishikawa and Homey 1992; Kawai and Nishizawa 1984). Recently, non-linear polycationic polymers have been synthesized and proposed for non-viral gene delivery (Haensler and Szoka 1993).

Intramuscular administration of plasmid-based gene expression system results in lower uptake of plasmids from an isotonic saline formulation leading to varying levels of therapeutic protein expression *in vivo* (Manthorpe et al., 1993; Levy et al., 1994). To overcome such problems, an interactive polymeric gene delivery system that enhances the delivery of genes to muscle cells has been reported (Mumper et al., 1995). This system offers opportunities for the treatment of both muscle and peripheral nerve disorders.

The polymeric gene delivery system using interactive polymers like polyvinylpyrrolidone (PVP) and polyvinyl alcohol (PVA) and other polyvinyl derivatives have been said to interact with a DNA plasmid via hydrogen bonding and hydrophobic interactions. Among this class of polymers, PVP and PVA interact with plasmids through hydrogen bonding (Mumper et al., 1995). This type of interaction results in protecting the plasmids from nucleases born destruction probably via hydrophobic coating of the plasmid. PVP based gene formulations are hypo-osmotic thus resulting in an improved dispersion of plasmids through the extracellular matrix of the muscle tissue. This might be due to increasing intracellular space, under osmotic effect.

The function of administered genes within muscle cells can be controlled using muscle-specific gene expression systems. An *in vivo* pulsatile production of proteins may be beneficial for certain therapeutic applications. This type of *in vitro* and *in vivo* pulsatile production of proteins can be achieved using 'gene switches' which are activated by low molecular weight drugs (Wang et al., 1994). 'Gene switches' are nothing but modified receptors which do not bind to their respective hormone or other endogenous hormones, but selectively bind with antagonistic drugs that act as agonists at low doses (Wang et al., 1994). The mode of action of these gene switch is depicted in figure 11.14. These gene switches are constitutively expressed within the target cells and are designed to be part of a gene expression system. This gene expression system contains both the gene switch and a therapeutic gene.

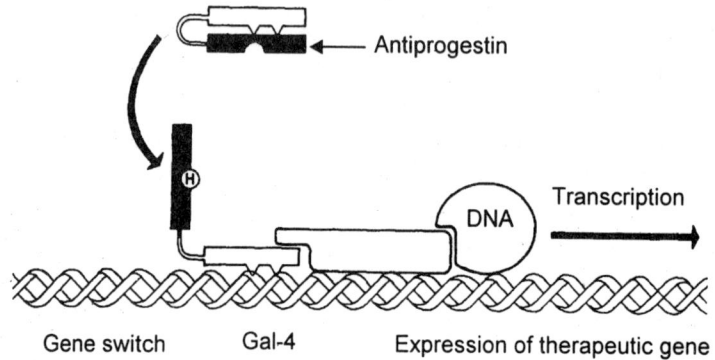

Fig. 11.14 : Mode of action of an antiprogestin-activated gene switch

Starburst™ polyamidoamine (PAMAM) dendrimers are a new type of synthetic polymer characterized by a branched spherical shape and a high density surface charge. These high density surface charges help bind to various forms of nucleic acid on the basis of electrostatic interactions. This ability has been investigated for the effective delivery of 'antisense oligonucleotides' and 'antisense expression plasmids' (Bielinska et al., 1996).

Starburst™ polyamidoamine (PAMAM) dendrimers are a new class of highly branched spherical polymers that are highly soluble in aqueous solution and have a unique surface of primary amino groups (Latallo, et al., 1996). They can be precisely synthesized and produced in large quantities similar to that of proteins. These molecules fall in the size range of 10 to 100 Å. These well defined structures of these molecules with their large number of surface primary amino groups is able to interact on an electrostatic charge basis with biologically relevant polyions, such as nucleic acids, antibodies, contrast agents, etc.

Gene expression systems encoding reporter genes have been complexed with different generations of dendrimers (Polyamidoamine cascade polymers, known as Starburst™ dendrimers) (Tomalia et al., 1990; Service, 1991). These dendrimers are said to condense DNA through electrostatic interaction of their terminal amines with the phosphate groups of DNA molecules. Such complexes are said to control the efficiency of delivery.

Investigations have been conducted using Starburst™ dendrimers as a carrier to enhance transfer of DNA into mammalian cell lines. The efficiency of this was confirmed using well defined analytical techniques e.g., based on the reporter gene systems like firefly luciferase and bacterial β-galactosidase.

11.8.10. Peptide-based gene delivery system

The site-specific delivery of gene expression system to target cells involved the use of ligands that recognize cell-surface receptors and use them for receptor-mediated cell entry. A current limitation for efficient gene delivery via both non-specific and receptor mediated gene transfer is the effective elimination of a gene expression system by endocytic vesicles. Poly-L-lysine, a cationic carrier, has been studied by many workers (Wilson et al., 1992; Wagner et al., 1991) as a carrier for delivery of DNA via endocytic pathway. In order to impart tissue selectivity, the carrier was covalently coupled to a receptor selective targeting molecule such as asialoorosomucoid, a galactose-terminal asialoglycoprotein targeted to the hepatocyte asialoglycoprotein receptor, to human transferrin or antithrombomoulin antibody 34A. The release of viral genome from endosomes by either disruption or by fusion with endosomal membranes was first reported by Curiel et al. (1991) and Cotton et al. (1992), wherein replication-defective adenoviral particles were added to DNA/transferrin-poly-L-lysine complexes. To reduce the risk of immunogenicity associated to polypeptides, in particular polylysine, a novel synthetic condensing peptide with a shorter amino acid sequence has been reported (Tomlinson and Rollond-1996). It has been reported that these peptides form an α-helices with a hydrophobic face with strong apolar amino acids, while the hydrophilic face is dominated by negatively charged glutamic acid residues. The haemolytic activity of these novel fusogenic peptides was shown to be pH dependent. Haemolysis was said to occur in acidic pH and not in physiologic pH.

Synthetic amphipathic peptide (GALA) covalently bound to dendrimers through a disulfide bond exemplifies the approach which was studied for effective gene transfer (Haensler and Szoka 1993).

11.8.11. Electronic pulse delivery (EPD)

The EPD technology has demonstrated a great potential in gene therapy applications, namely by transferring DNA, RNA and proteins into living cells for therapeutic purposes. In order to achieve effective gene therapy, the therapeutic gene needs to be introduced permanently, stable, functionally and heritably into the target cells to provide permanent new genetic functionality and heritably into the target cells. The EPD technology which meets the above criteria can be used as an effective, efficient and safe means of delivery system. The target cells suitable for EPD delivery include haematopoietic stem cells (HSCs), hepatocytes, fibroblasts and myoblasts and for protein and gene therapy.

The major challenge that comes across in gene therapy is delivering therapeutic genes into non-dividing cells, such as the hematopoietic stem cells. These cells are ideal target cells for gene therapy as their survival period is long and are capable of renewing themselves and producing new progenitors and mature blood cells. However, retroviral vector mediated delivery to these cells are problematic as they are quiescent. This can be overcome by using EPD technology.

EPD is a sophisticated method which subjects the targeted cells to a precisely controlled pulses of electric field in a computer controlled molecular transfer system (Zhao 1995). The EPD system consists of a controller and a reaction chamber. The controller, driven by an EPD computer accurately controls the output of electronic pulses which in turn are controlled by different parameters. The reaction chamber where the DNA\transfer takes place holds the target cells and therapeutic gene as a mixture. The target cells and the transfer material are placed in a reaction chamber with a movable conductive probe isolated from the cell/DNA solution.

EPD has been confused sometimes which electroporation procedure. In electroporation, the target cells are damaged after which the molecular transfer takes place. Furthermore, electroporation often applies a significant · electric current through the cells. In contrast, EPD technology limits the electric current and needs no contact by electrode(s) to the mixture of genes and the target cells.

Advantages of EPD technology
1. Using this technology, large molecules can be transferred into target cells (e.g. DNA construct $\approx$ 15 kb).
2. EPD inserts only the therapeutic genes into the target cells without the involvement of any other molecules.
3. It has no toxic effect on the target cells and is completely free from other potential hazards.
4. It has a good cell viability reserve.
5. EPD technology has remarkable transfer efficiency (ranging 80-90% transfer)
6. It gives a wide spectrum to select device parameters for different transferring applications.
7. It can be operated in a batch or continuous process.
8. The time taken by this method for transfer is very short (from few seconds to a minute). This renders the time required by the target cell to remain *ex vivo* or *in vitro*. (Zhao et al., 1990;1993; Hoeben et al., 1992; Palemer et al., 1989; 1991; Lu et al., 1993) to be minimum.

11.8.12. Electroporation

A physical method which involves the use of non-viral delivery system is **electroporation**. In this process, DNA is transferred into cells in suspension by applying pulses of high-voltage electricity that creates pores in cell membranes.

Electroporation is one of the several physical methods used for gene transfer (Grierson, 1991). Electroporation method of gene transfer involves the use of short electrical impulses of high field strength. The generated impulses of high field strength. The generated impulses increase the permeability of protoplast membrane thereby facilitating the entry of DNA molecules into the cells. The pulse required for an efficient transfer of the DNA by electroporation is generated by discharging a capacitor across the electrodes from a specially generated electroporation chamber. The generated pulse may be either a high voltage (1.5 kV) rectangular wave pulse for a short duration or a low voltage (350 V) pulse for a longer duration (Fig. 11.15).

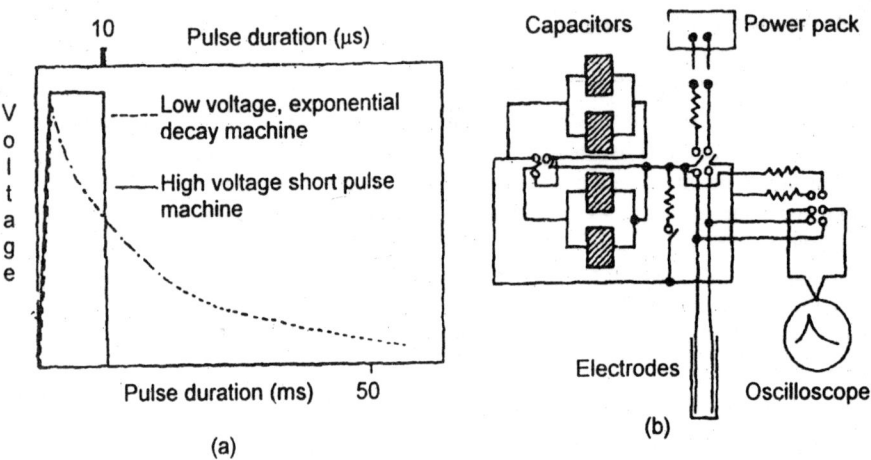

(a)

(b)

Fig. 11.15 : a. Characteristic output from a electroporation device; b. circuit diagram of a electroporation unit

DNA transfer is carried out by suspending the protoplast containing vector DNA in a ionic solution between the electrodes. Using electroporation method, successful transfer of genes was achieved with the protoplasts of tobacco, petunia, maize, rice, etc.

11.8.13. Aquasomes as gene carriers

A self-assembled molecular carrier "Aquasomes" (Kossovsky et al., 1996) formed with preformed carbon ceramic nanoparticles and self-assembled calcium phosphate dihydrate particles with a glassy carbohydrate coating can be studied for the delivery of genes (Kossovsky et al., 1995). *In vitro* studies have been carried out by immobilizing DNase, a therapeutic enzyme used in the treatment of cystic fibrosis, on to a ceramic carbon nanocrystalline particulate core coated with pyridoxal-5-pyrophosphate (Hnatyszyn, 1995). A marked retention of biological activity was observed with surface immobilized DNase on the solid phase of a colloidal calcium-phosphate nanoparticle coated with a polyhydroxyl oligomeric films. Kossovsky (1996) has envisioned a model for how the synthetic product of self-assembling chemistry using non-covalent forces comprising a ceramic nanocrystalline core with a polyhydroxyoligomeric film coating will appear (Fig. 11.16).

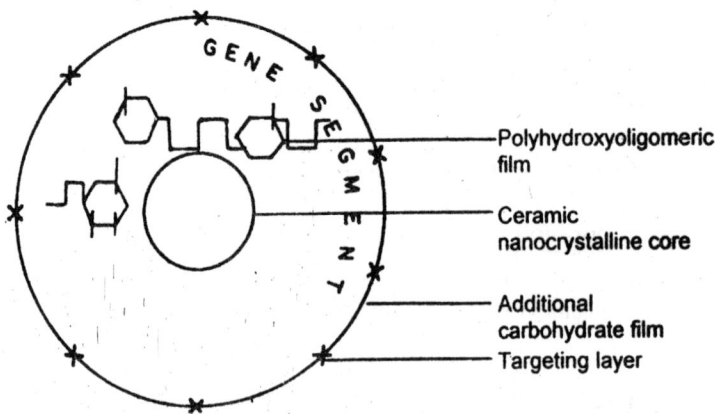

Fig. 11.16 : Aquasomes for gene therapy

11.8.14. Proton sponge

Any vector used to deliver a DNA to the nucleus completes the task either by cell membrane rupture mechanisms or by nuclear targeting. This membrane rupture occurs either directly at the cell surface or after endocytosis. In both the cases, the viral fusogenic protein undergoes a major conformational change induced either by binding to a cell surface receptor or by the acidic nature of the endosomal compartment. Use of different cationic vectors, i.e. cationic lipids and cationic polymers puts us to the question the buffering capacity of a vector under physiological conditions and its transfection potentials.

Understanding this chemistry, several non-permanent polycations like lipopolyamines, and polyethylenimines with substantial buffering capacity below physiological pH have been studied as efficient transfection agents. These agents can transfect efficiently without any addition of lysosomotropic bases or cell transfecting agents or membrane disrupting agents. These agents/vectors have been shown to deliver genes as well as oligonucleotides (Demenix and Behr 1996).

A number of synthetic macromolecular compounds with high amine group densities were studied. These cationic compounds could be able to compact the DNA, but owing to the repulsion between like charges existing close to each other they are not fully protonated at physiological pH.

Structure of polyethyleneimine

A constitutive candidate for the development of proton sponge system was the commercially available polymer polyethylenimine (PEI). One in every three atoms of the polymer is an amine group therefore the system demonstrates variability in protonation level which increases between pH 7 to 5.

The mechanism involved in the gene transfer using polycation/DNA complex is as depicted in Fig. 11.17. The polycation/DNA complex probably enters the cell via spontaneous endocytosis. This positive charge covered complex when interacts with the cell membrane produces a high local concentration of PEI in the endosome. During such intracellular trafficking, the buffering capacity of the PEI not only tends to inhibit the lysosomal nuclease, which have an optimal acidic pH, but also alters the osmolarity of the vesicle. Thus, proton accumulation is brought about by endosomal ATPase which leads to the influx of chloride anions. This will result in swelling of the polymer by internal charge repulsion and osmotic swelling of the endosome finally leading to the rupture of the endosome followed by the liberation of PEI. This rapid liberation of PEI-DNA complex is of importance in gene therapy.

11.8.15. Miscellaneous approaches

A synthetic lipophilic polylysine-phosphatidylethanolamine conjugate ("lipopolylysine") has been used successfully as transfecting agent. A non-viral delivery system involving a chemical method of calcium phosphate or DEAE-dextran conjugate formation that mediated gene transfer has been reported.

Other approaches include, insulin as a receptor-specific carrier, linked to positively charged N-acylurea, albumin, plasmid packed with a polylysine-asialoorosomucoid conjugate. An albuminemia in Nagase rats by hepatic transfection of the structural human gene which resulted in albumin secretion was demonstrated on similar lines.

The ambiguous transferrin receptor may serve as a target part for more generalized gene delivery using polylysine-transferrin conjugate. This concept is generally utilized in achieving high level of iron by rapidly dividing neoplastic cells. In place of "forced" cell entry by cationic liposomes, a method involving the physiologic pathway of endocytosis may be utilized in effective targeting. This method also has the disadvantage that it is enzymatically degraded during endolysosomal pathway. Accordingly, augmentation of gene expression was accomplished using chloroquine to suppress lysosomal degradation. An escape mechanism from the endolysosomal compartment was designed by some workers by hybridizing polylysine-DNA complex and AV. Here, AV makes the complex capable to escape endolysosomal degradation.

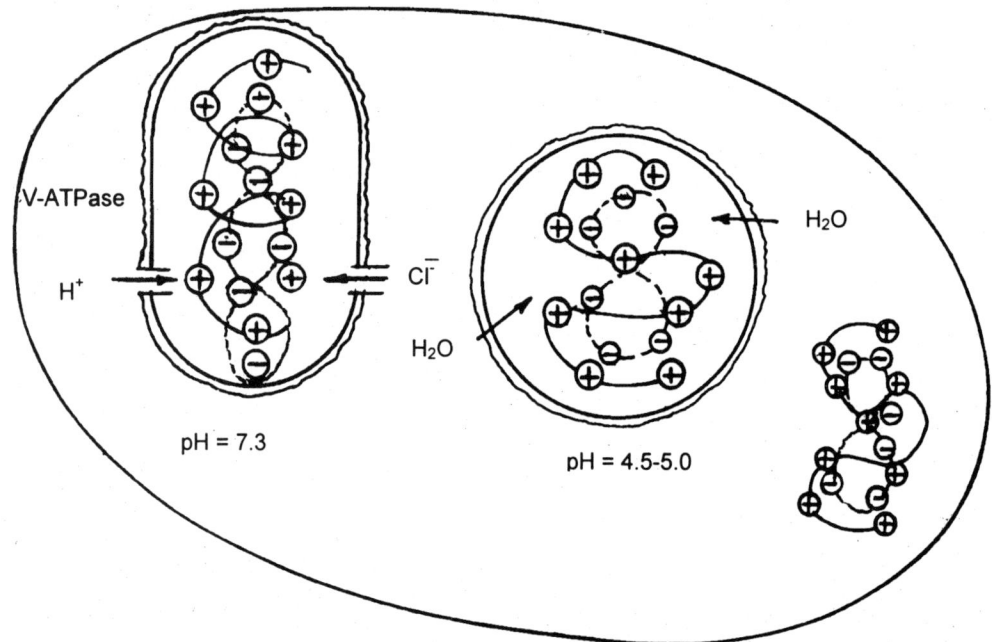

Fig. 11.17 : Proton sponge hypothesis; H^+ and Cl^- enter into the endosomes leading to osmotic swelling and finally to endosome rupture

11.8.15.1. Targeted modification of human genes

Targeted modification of genes by exogenous DNA has gained wide attention in recent years especially in the alteration of the human genome. This, in particular is a site directed approach for the replacement of defective genes. The theme behind this is the "Nature's" way of mixing the gene, i.e. the exogenous DNA should contain a region with the same nucleotide sequence as of the target gene, whereby homologous recombination occurs. Depending on the arrangement of the incoming sequences relative to the target the recombination even could either introduce new sequences into the recipient chromosome by a single crossover, or substitute sequences by gene conversion or double crossover events.

The recent advances in this field include, linearized plasmids with restriction enzymes to produce a double strand break within the region homologous to the gene target.

11.8.15.2. Transgenic approaches

Experiments have been carried out in developing the transgenic animal as a model for studying gene regulation. The DNA is introduced into fertilized eggs and subsequently integrated into both somatic cells and germ cells. For example, the introduction of metallothionine/growth hormone fusion genes into mice stimulates the production of growth hormone in tissues that normally synthesizes metallothionine. Induction of metallothionine promoters with metals have caused treated mice to grow to about twice their normal size. A number of genetic diseases in mice, including thalassaemia have been treated using tissue-specific expression from a variety of human genes.

11.8.15.3. Gene therapy with engineered stem cells

Gene therapy for the treatment of disorders involving blood cells can be cured by this method. In this approach, hematopoietic stem cells are removed from an affected individual and transfected with functional genes. The engineered stem cells are then reinjected into the individual. This method has been studied with individuals suffering from serve combined immunodeficiency disease (SCID) resulting from a defective gene encoding adenosine deaminase (ADA).

11.9. DISEASES AND GENE THERAPY

Diseases wherein gene therapy has been focused upon include -
- Cystic fibrosis
- Thalassaemia
- Malignant melanoma
- Pediatric AML
- Neuroblastoma
- Adenosine deaminase deficiency SCID
- Hemophilia B
- Chronic myleogenous leukemia
- Hepatitis B
- Hypercholesterolemia
- Diabetes
- Cardiovascular diseases
- Phenylketonuria
- Acquired immunodeficiency syndrome (AIDS)

The basis of gene therapy of a few above mentioned diseases has been discussed below in brief.

11.9.1. Gene therapy for insulin-dependent diabetes mellitus

Diabetes can be classified into Type-1 or insulin dependent diabetes mellitus (IDDM) and Type-2 or non-insulin dependent diabetes mellitus (NIDDM). Among the two, IDDM is an autoimmune disease which is produced as a result of the destruction of insulin-producing β-cells of the pancreas. At present, careful monitoring of blood glucose levels, multiple injections of insulin, diet control and exercise regimens are the treatment provided for IDDM. This leads to the exploration of gene therapy for this disease.

As the β-cells are destroyed in IDDM, any attempt to reconstitute insulin gene expression must be directed to an ectopic organ. The liver fits in as the right target, as it is the principal effector organ in maintaining blood glucose homeostasis and ketogenesis. A somatic gene therapy has been attempted. The results observed were encouraging (Kolodka et al., 1995). A recombinant retroviral vector, LX/rINS, encoding the complete sequence for rat pre-proinsulin 1cDNA under the transcriptional control of the viral LTR promoter was constructed and used to transduce rat hepatocytes in-vivo (Ullrich et al., 1977).

11.9.2. Gene therapy for hemophilia B

Hemophilia B is a X-linked blood coagulation disorder resulting from a deficiency of factor IX production which ultimately leads to severe bleeding. Normally, the treatment for this is protein replacement therapy. Due to the short half-life of factor IX in the circulation, the goal is not achieved. To overcome this problem and to provide an effective therapy, recombinant retroviral and adenoviral vectors encoding canine factor IX to transduce the hepatocytes to hemophilia B in dogs have been studied (Kay et al., 1993; 1994). An infusion of amphotropic retroviral vector encoding the canine factor IXcDNA under the transcriptional control of the viral LTR (LX-CFIX) was administered into the portal vasculature of hemophilia B dogs. An increase in plasma factor IX concentration was observed (Evan et al., 1989).

11.9.3. Gene therapy for cystic fibrosis (CF)

Cystic fibrosis is a complex, multi-system disease which is inherited in an autosomal recessive pattern. The goal of gene therapy in young children is to prevent the generation of infectious lung disease, whereas the realistic goal in CF patients with established lung disease is to prevent a further loss of lung function. CF is due to a mutation in the CFTR gene, which perturbs the salt and water composition of secretions, slows the mucocilliary clearance of airways and promotes infection. However, this does not explain the predilection for infection in CF with *Staphylococcus aureus* and *Pseudomonas aeruginosa*. CF is dominated by involvement of the respiratory tract which is characterized by airway obstruction caused by accumulation of thick purulent secretions and progressive deterioration of lung functions. Majority of the patients acquire bronchopulmonary infections due to *Pseudomonas aeruginosa*. The current therapy involves the use of antibiotics and approaches to improve mucous clearance.

A large number of studies have established that many gene transfer vectors are highly efficient *in vitro*. It has been found that transformed and primary cultures of human airway epithelia in non-polarized and polarized culture conditions have been relatively easy to transduce with the help of adenoviral vectors containing CFTR, with correction of the CF Cl^- transport defect (Zabner et al. 1994). Figure 11.18 depicts the relationships between gene transfer efficiency and correction of CF airway epithelial chloride ion (Cl^-) and sodium ion (Na^+) transport defects.

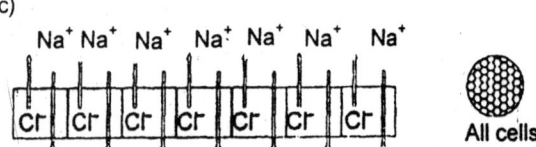

Fig. 11.18 : Gene transfer and correction of CF airway

Step (a) shows airway epithelium in the untreated state (CF), it is also clear that there is a reduced Cl^- secretion and accelerated Na^+ absorption reflecting the absence of CFTR. **Step (b)** shows the CF epithelium that has been "treated" (shaded cells) with a gene transfer vector that corrects about 10% of the cells. It is also noticed that inspite of the CFTR Cl^- channel, function is confined to a 'single' cell, the Cl^- channel exit path is sufficiently 'large' to accommodate flow into the corrected cell from neighboring non-corrected cells to mediate a 'normal' rate of Cl^- secretion. **Step (c)** shows correction of all cells by a gene transfer vector. Here, both the defective Cl^- secretion and the accelerated Na^+ absorption are normalized

The efficiency of adenoviral vectors has shown substantial variation *in-vivo*. However, adenoviral gene transfer efficiency to the uninjured airway of primates and man appears to be very low.

New generation modalities in the treatment of CF utilize recombinant human deoxyribonuclease I (rhDNase) which reduces the viscoelasticity of respiratory tract (Shak et al., 1990). A plasmid encoding for chloramphenicol acetyl transferase (pRSV2-CAT) complexed with Lipofectin liposomes has demonstrated for its *in vivo* functioning by Brigham et al., in 1989. Similarly, delivery of CFTR to the respiratory tract using cationic liposomes have also been reported (Logan et al., 1995). For a detailed review refer Schreier and Swayer 1996.

Inspite of the wide advantages there are certain problems posed for CF gene therapy. The preeminent problem for CF gene therapy is the functional efficiency of the system *in vivo*. The second problem is the safety profiles of the various vectors that continue to be uncovered both in *in vitro* studies and in clinical trials. Certain vectors like adenoviral vectors can slow the cell cycle and induce apoptosis. Novel cationic lipid formulations appear to be more inflammatory in lungs. In addition the amount of liposomal lipid delivered to the lung and surfactant metabolism in pulmonary surface liquids will have to be evaluated.

11.9.4. Gene therapy for cardiovascular disease

Cardiovascular disease is the commonest cause of mortality in the recent past. Over 7 million individuals suffer from cardiovascular ailments every year around the globe. Although significant progress has been made in the areas of treatment and prevention of persisting various cardiac diseases, still cardiovascular diseases remain the leading public-health problem. In spite of many recent advances there are still diseases which are not having an effective therapy, familial hypercholesterolemia (FH) and retenosis after angioplasty are a few to note.

Table 11.1 : Various gene transfer techniques applicable in cardiovascular diseases

Viral mediated methods	Retrovirus, sendai virus, adenovirus
Lipid-mediated methods	Liposomes, cationic liposomes
Other methods	Microinjection, mechanical (high energy microparticle bombardment), implantation (myoblast)

Research have been diversified towards the use of gene as a medicine for different ailments. Gene therapy towards cardiovascular diseases can be brought about by gene transfer which can be carried by three methods of gene modification, gene replacement, gene correction and gene augmentation. Among them gene augmentation is the most promising technique for modifying targeted cells in cardiovascular therapy.

Table 11.2 : Disease and suitable target gene for the treatment of cardiovascular disease

Indication	Target gene
Systemic gene therapy	
Familial hypercholesterolemia	Low density lipoprotein receptor
Atherosclerosis	High density lipoprotein
Hypercoagulable states	Tissue-plaminogen
Refractory diabetes mellitus	Insulin
Local gene therapy	
Restenosis after angioplasty	Cell-cycle regulatory gene
Transplant rejection	Leukocyte adhesion molecule
Transplant vasculopathy	Cytokine
Myocardial infarction	Fibroblast growth factor Transforming
Cardiac remodeling; Angiogenesis	growth factor β
Myocarditis	Cytokine
Congenital heart disease	Myocyte differentiation factors
Glomerular diseases	Cytokine, cell-cycle regulatory gene
Aortic aneurisms	Protease

Gene-transfer techniques appropriate for cardiovascular applications include:-

a. Viral-vector-mediated gene transfer. Example retrovirus, adenovirus, and sendai virus.

b. Liposomal gene transfer. Example cationic liposomes.

c. Re-implantation of cells modified *in vitro*

The application of gene in cardiovascular therapy includes the treatment of vascular diseases, cardiac diseases, metabolic disorder, hereditary coagulation disorders and auto-immune diseases. The vascular wall, heart, liver, kidney and muscle have been target organs for cardiovascular gene therapy. Figure 11.19, shows the mechanism by which *in vivo* gene transfer using sendai virus -liposome vesicle complex can be affected.

There has been little experience of *in vivo* gene transfer to the heart. Direct injection of DNA is the only way of gene transfer into the heart to date. Lin et al., first reported the expression of β-Gal in cardiomyocytes *in vivo* for at least four weeks after direct injection in the left ventricle.

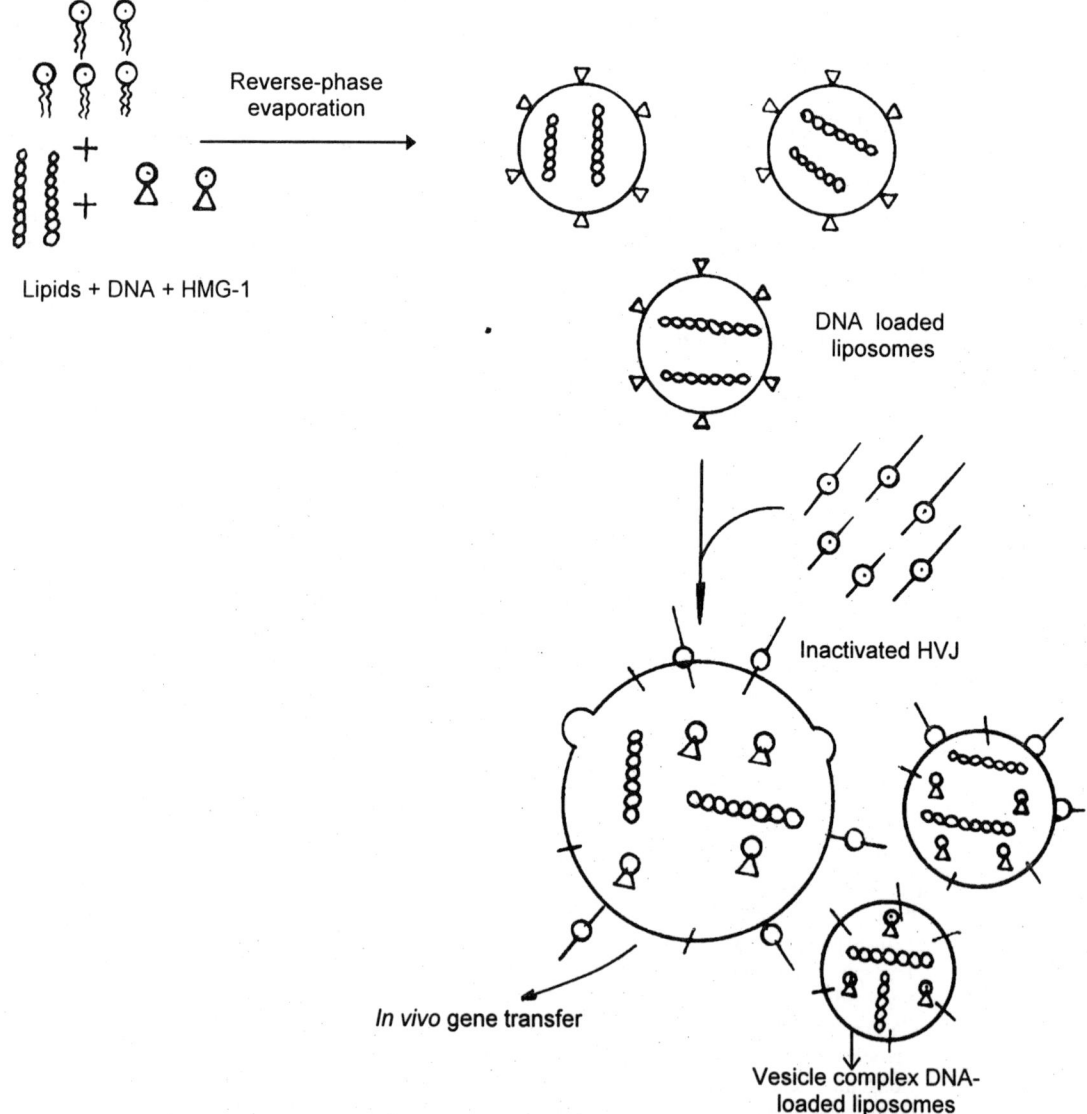

Fig. 11.19 : *In vivo* gene transfer using sendai virus-liposome vesicle complex

11.9.5. Gene therapy of nervous system disorders

Gene therapy has been in the light during the recent past as a means of therapeutic approach for various diseases. The candidate diseases include CF, cancer, HIV infection, various hormonal and enzyme disorders, etc. However, disorders of the central nervous system (CNS) though of prime importance have not gained the due attention of researchers for the reason being a structurally and functionally complicated organ. In addition, the CNS involves differentiated cells which have different functions and different anatomical connections. Similarly the neurons are also much complicated both functionally and anatomically. In case of other candidate diseases gene therapy was possible for the reason being relatively easy in *in vitro* gene n anipulation and the source for *in vitro* gene manipulation were simulated easily.

Despite these difficulties, a number of neurological disorders have emerged as promising. gene therapy models. This advancement offered the realization that gene therapy for certain disorders, may not require the brain cells. Instead "surrogate" cells, such as autologous fibroblast, may be useful for delivery of therapeutic gene products after gene manipulation and transplantation to the brain (Gage et al., 1987). A second factor which has been helpful in achieving effective gene transfer is the availability of the new class of gene transfer vectors, capable of transferring the gene directly into neurons and glia *in vivo*. The genetic modification of cultured cells are made with retroviral vectors followed by grafting the cells into living animals.

Alzheimer's disease, a neurodegenerative disorder in which there is a progressive loss of cholinergic neurons in the basal forebrain, with associated profound cognitive impairment. Treatment of this disease involves the delivery of nerve growth factor (NGF) which prevents the neuronal loss in addition to ameliorating deficits in learning and memory associated cells. The intracerebral transplantation of genetically modified fibroblasts has been applied to an animal model wherein a sparingly small amount of cholinergic neurons has been observed to produce NGF (Rosenberg et al., 1988).

Parkinson's disease, a disorder in which degeneration of dopaminergic neurons of the nigrostriatal pathways associated with a severe impairment of voluntary movement. Studies involving grafts of fetal substantia nigra dopamine neurons into the dopamine-depleted brain indicated that delivery of dopamine from grafted cells could lessen the movement disturbances (Lindwell et al, 1989; Fahn, 1992; Widner et al., 1992; Freed et al., 1992). These studies led to the suggestion that non-neural cells that have been genetically modified to produce dopamine or the dopamine precursor L-DOPA, might also be effective.

While the intracerebral transplantation of genetically modified cells may be suitable for some disorders, other disorders will almost certainly require the delivery of genetic material directly into resident brain cells. For this purpose, considerable effort has been devoted to the development of viral mutants to serve as vectors for introducing genetic material into the brains. The first candidate for such a function has been derivative of neurotropic viruses, such as the herpes simplex viruses (Breakefield and DeLuca, 1991).

Initial studies have clearly indicated that herpes virus vectors can be used to infect neurons and glia both *in vitro* and *in vivo*. Lesch-Nyhan disease, one of the first neurogenic disorders chosen as a model for gene therapy (Wills et al., 1984; Miller et al., 1983;1984; Friedmann, 1985), which was the first disease model to be tackled with a herpes-virus vector. Lesch-Nyhan disease is an inborn error of metabolism resulting from deficiency of the purine-salvage-pathway enzyme hypoxanthine-guanine phosphoribosyl-transferases (HPRT) and several prominent neurological abnormalities, including involuntary movements, retardation and self-mutilation (Seegmiller et al., 1967). The herpes-virus vectors are promising vehicles for direct gene transfer into brain cells. However, there are a number of problems with these vectors which remain to be circumvented.

More recently, adenovirus vectors have also been shown to be potentially useful vehicles for gene transfer into the brain. Transgenes introduced by recombination into the genomes of adenoviral mutants can be expressed in a wide variety of recipient cell types, including neurons, glia and ependymal cells lining the centricles (Le Gal La Salle et al., 1993; Bajacchi et al., 1993; Davidson et al., 1993; Akh et al., 1993).

Gene transfer into peripheral organs for correction of CNS diseases is also in focus. One such example is the inborn error of amino acid metabolism involving phenylketonuria, which is mainly due to a defect in hepatic phenylalanine hydroxylase. In spite of this enzyme being expressed predominantly from the liver, the major clinical manifestations of the disease are attributable to the accumulation of toxins which impair neural function. Similarly, some of the lysosomal storage disorders which dispose in neurophathological changes might respond to genetic modification of bone-marrow stem cells, since these cells are thought to give rise to migratory macrophages that can populate the brain (Hoogerbrugge et al., 1988).

A number of different approaches, including the intracerebral transplantation of genetically modified cells, the direct intracerebral introduction of gene transfer vectors and genetic alterations targeted to peripheral organs, are being actively pursued in animal studies as models for gene therapy of neurological disease (Table 11.3).

Table 11.3 : Gene therapy models for neurological disorders

Disorder	Transgene	Method
Neurodegenerative disorders		
Alzheimer's disease	NGF or other tropic	Surrogate cells grafted to basal forebrain or cortex
Parkinson's disease	factors	Direct delivery of vector to basal forebrain or cortex
Genetic Disorders	Tyrosine hydroxylase	Surrogate cells grafted to the basal ganglia
Phenylketonuria	Phenyalanine hydroxylase	Direct delivery of vector to basal ganglia
	HRPT	or midbrain
Lesch-Nhyan disease		Transplants of genetically modified hepatocytes
Lysosomal storage disease	Lysosomal enzymes	Direct delivery of vector to liver
		Surrogate cells grafted to brain
		Direct delivery of vector to brain
		Transplants of genetically modified bone marrow cells

Each of these approach has its own merits and demerits which render it useful under different circumstances. Further, studies will be necessary to characterize the long-term viability of the transplanted cells or vectors, the stability of gene expression, immunological responses are the potentials for inducing direct or indirect neuro-pathological changes.

11.9.6. Gene therapy for cancer

Cancer is a disorder of the genetic make-up of somatic cells which results in a clone of cells with an abnormal pattern of growth control. Human genome contains both normal genes and oncogenes. When an ideal (favorable for growth) condition is created inside the body, oncogenes are multiplied and ultimately result in tumor formation.

Conventional cancer treatment with chemotherapy, radiotherapy and surgery aims at destroying the tumor, leaving as much as possible of the normal host tissue intact. With regard to chemotherapy, a curative dose is ultimately a toxic dose, while the same in low doses develops resistant tumors. While the problem with both surgery and radiotherapy is tumor invasion and spread outside areas that are directly accessible to these treatments. In addition, the growth of tumor is observed at adjacent areas other than the main region.

Biological approaches to the treatment of cancer were realized under certain circumstances wherein not only the tumor cells are recognized by the host immune responses but also by the effective destructive mechanism (Mestrangelo et al., 1988). Isolation of genes encoding cytokines which are involved in the control of immune system has been produced in sufficient quantities such as interferons and **interleukins**. The cytokines have shown sufficient action against certain types of tumors. However, their mechanism of action is not clear.

The present research is focused upon human genome mapping by which a comparison between the genetic constitution of cells exhibiting abnormal growth pattern against their normal growth pattern can be appreciated. Analysis of oncogenes and tumor suppresser genes will, almost certainly, reveal targets for therapy at the molecular level. Gene manipulation has become easier with the help of homologous recombination, retroviral and other gene transferring vectors and antisense technology along with powerful analytical tools such as the polymerase chain reaction (PCR) will be helpful in manipulating and monitoring cell cultures.

It has been demonstrated that a major difference between normal and cancer cells is the decrease or functional impairment of major histocompatibility complex (MHC) on the surface of tumor cells. The importance of this observation has been undenied by the fact that tumor cells transfected with MHC class I can not only prevent tumor spread when administered as a prophylactic vaccine, but also induce metastatic remission in established disease in a number of murine model which includes lymphoma, carcinomas and melanomas. With this knowledge it is now possible to prepare and transfect cell lines with known retroviral vectors carrying genes for MHC class I molecules.

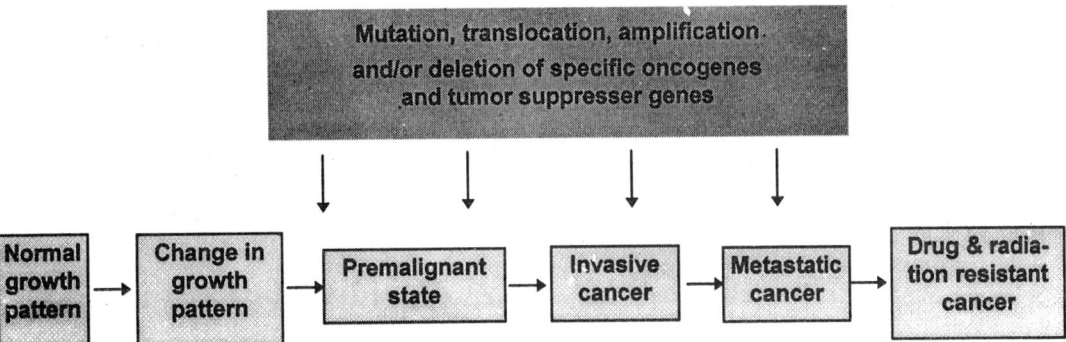

Fig. 11.20 : Development of malignant cells

11.9.7. Gene therapy for AIDS

Acquired immunodeficiency syndrome (AIDS), a fatal retroviral-disease caused by the human immuno-deficiency virus (HIV) and the cure for them has become the core concern of scientist. The disease is said to be caused by a RNA virus which made the researchers to focus on an agent that would inhibit the *in vitro* multiplication of the virus. This leads to two different approaches. One towards finding a nucleoside candidate and the other to target at an enzyme (reverse transcriptase, RT), known to be present in RNA viruses.

Human Immuodeficiency Virus type-1 (HIV-1) has circumvented most conventional anti-viral strategies in large through its rapid rate of replication and resultant genetic heterogeneity. However, ribozyme engineering coupled with gene therapy applications offers one potential strategy for countering HIV-1 infection *in vivo*.

"Hairpin ribozyme" an enzymatic RNA molecule was first isolated from the negative strand satellite RNA (or viroid) plant pathogen, Tobacco Ringspot Virus {[-]s TRSV} (Hampel and Tritz, 1989). The ribozyme complex consists of a 50 nucleotide (nt) catalytic domain with a 14 nt substrate binding region (Hampel et al., 1990). These two domains fold and anneal into a loop resembling a hairpin and is utilized during rolling circle replication of the small RNA genome (Bass and Weintrab 1988). The 14nt tail region of the hairpin binds through complementary base-pairing with the substrate resulting in the formation of two adjacent helical structures. This helix acts as a handle-bar forming a bulge in the center of the substrate strand which is cleaved by the 50nt catalytic domain of the ribozyme (Akhtar et al., 1995). Mutagenesis studies have identified N*GUC sequence as the cleavage site (*-cleavage site) on the substrate. These minimal requirements for ribozyme binding and cleavage made the synthesis or genetically engineered base-pair with any other heterologous RNA region surrounding the N*GUC sequence possible (Breaker and Joyce, 1994). As this reaction was found to occur at near physiological condition *in vitro*, their potential uses have been studied against infectious agents (Ojwang et al., 1992).

11.10. PROBLEMS AND PROSPECTIVES

The advent of recombinant DNA technology and the availability of a wide array of gene cloning techniques have had a dramatic impact on the conduct of research in biology and medicine. Genetic information in the form of expressed sequence tags (ESTs) and whole genome sequence are filling computer data banks faster than ever and never has gene cloning found more prominence in biology than now. With the brute force approach of positional cloning, it is now possible to identify a disease related gene without any knowledge of its biochemical function. The difference between basic and applied research is disappearing fast and the results of basic research are finding immediate biotechnological applications.

The ultimate goal of human gene therapy is to replace a defective gene with a normal one via targeted insertion into the genome by homologous recombination. Such a strategy, referred to as gene replacement therapy, would not only permit physiological regulation of the transgene but also eliminate the possibility of intestinal inactivation of other cellular genes, which happens during random integration of the foreign gene.

Gene therapy will have a major impact on the health care of our population only when vectors are developed that can safely and efficiently be injected directly into patients as drugs like insulin are now. Vectors need to be engineered that will target specific cell types, insert their genetic information's to a safe site in the genome, and be regulated by normal physiological signals. When efficient vectors of this type are produced, retroviral, viral, synthetic or a combination of all three-then gene therapy will probably have a profound impact on the practice of medicine.

The viral and non viral gene delivery strategies have been fairly successful in cell culture systems and animal models but the therapeutic success of clinical trials in human still remains questionable. Two types of clinical trials are being conducted in humans using these vectors; gene marking and therapeutic studies. Gene marking involves areas in which potential therapeutic application are involved such as hematopoietic stem cells, T cells, etc., which are removed from the patient, cultured and transfected with vectors encoding gene markers which are again reintroduced into the patient. The presence of gene markers are examined time to time by recovering the cells and are observed for the presence of marker gene.

Cell-marking studies are used to detect residual cancer cells in the marrow infused patients during autologous bone marrow transplantation. In general therapeutic trials are aimed at transfer of therapeutic genes into patients for treatment of specific genetic disorders and cancer. Some results of therapeutic clinical trials are now available. Some examples, the successful *ex-vivo* human gene transfer studies of adenosine deaminase (ADA) gene transfected T cells or cord blood cells in SCID, transfer of autologous hepatocytes encoding low-density lipoprotein (LDL), etc. Similarly, the successful *in vivo* gene transfer of CFTR, human leukocyte antigen (HLA-B7) and β2-microglobulin gene transfer are to cite a few.

In addition to the treatment of genetic disorders, the gene transfer techniques have also been applied extensively in the treatment of cancer and other acquired disorders. The corrective gene therapy is aimed at introducing wild type tumor suppresser genes or genes encoding dominant negative mutants of oncogenes that are mutated in the tumor cells. The major limitation of this approach has been the difficulty in delivering the corrective gene into every tumor cell. Despite promising results obtained in animals, there is no convincing evidence that any of the gene therapy protocols actually led to regression of tumors in humans. Thus, it is clear that the move from animal to man is not going to be easy. None of the clinical trials conducted so far could convincingly demonstrate the therapeutic benefit of gene therapy and has not been as effective as expected. While nobody has taken into consideration the long term potential of human gene therapy, it is now clear that the current gene transfer techniques are largely inadequate to promote sustained, high level expression of foreign genes *in vivo*. Hence, to bring about gene therapy in reality, research towards understanding the pathophysiology of diseases as the mechanism of gene regulation *in vivo* are to be well understood.

With the explosive increase in the availability of information on human genome, several genetic disorders would become candidates for gene therapy. The field is still at its infancy and relevant. The need of the hour is to initiate more studies in different systems on the various aspects mentioned earlier. In spite of the various drawbacks, gene therapy has witnessed a rapid growth towards the end of this century and hopefully the progress would continue.

SUGGESTED READINGS

Akhtar, S., James, H. and Gibson, I., (1995) **Nature Medicine**, 1, 300-302.

Akli, S., Caillaud, C., Vigne, E., Stratford-Perricaudet, L.D., Poenaru, L., Perricaudet, M., Kahn, A. and Peschanski, M.R., (1993) **Nature Genet.**, 3, 224-228.

Anderson, W.F., (1984) **Science**, 226, 401.

Andree, C., Swain, W.F., Page, C.P., Macklin, M.D., Slama, J., Hatazis, D. and Erikson, E., (1994) **Proc. Natl. Acad. Sci. USA**, 91, 12188-12192.

Ardizzoni, S.C., Michaels, A. and Arendas, G.W., (1988) **Science,** 239, 183-188.

Bagai, S. and Sarkar, D.P., (1993) **Biochem. Biophys. Acta**, 1152, 15-25.

Bagai, S. and Sarkar, D.P., (1994) **J. Biol. Chem.**, 268, 1966-1972.

Bajocchi, G., Feldman, S., H., Crystal, R.G. and Mastrangeli, A., (1993) **Nature Genet.**, 3, 229-234.

Bartzatt, R., (1987) **Med. Sci. Res. Biochem.**, 15(13-1),791.

Bartzatt, R., (1988) **Biotechnol. Appl. Biochem.**, 11(1), 133-135.

Bass, B. and Weintrab, H., (1988) **Cell**, 55, 1089-1098.

Bennet, C.F., Chiang, M.Y., Chan, H. and Grimm, S., (1993) **J. Liposome Res.**, 3, 85-102.

Bennet, C.F., Chiang, M.Y., Chan, H., Shoemaker, J.E.E. and Mirabelli, C.K., (1992) **Mol. Pharmacol.**, 41, 1023-1033. .

Berglund, P., Tublekas, I. and Liljestrom, P., (1996) **Trends Biotechnol.**, 14, 130-134.

Berkner, K.L., (1988) **Biotechniques**, 6, 616-629.

Berns, K.I. and Linden, R.M., (1995) **Bioessays**, 17, 237-245.

Besmer, P., Olshevsky, U., Baltimore, D., Dolberg, D. and Fan, H.J., (1979), **J. Virol.**, 29,1168-76.

Bielinska, A., Kukowska-Latallo, J.F., Johnson, J., Tomalia, D.A. and Baker, J.R. Jr., (1996) **Nucleic Acids Res.**, 24, 2176-2182.

Breakefield, X.O. and De Luca, N.A., (1991) **N. Biol.**, 3, 203-218.

Breaker, R.R. and Joyce, G.F. (1994) **Trends Biotechnol.**, 12, 268-275.

Bringham, K.L., Meyrick, B.O., Christman, B.W., Magnuson, M., King, G. and Berry, L.C. Jr., (1989), **Am. J. Med. Sci.**, 298, 278-281.

Buchschacher, G.L., Free, E.O. and Panganiban, A.T., (1992) **Hum. Gene Ther.**, 3, 391-397.

Chakraborty, A.K., Zink, M.A., Hodgson, C.P., (1993, **FASEB J.**, 7, 971-975.

Cheng, L.,Zielhoffer, P.R. and Yang, N.S., (1993) **Proc. Natl. Acad. Sci. USA**, 90, 4455-4459.

Chowdhury, J.R., Grossman, M., Guptam S., Chowdhury, N.R., Baker, J.R. and Wilson, J.M., (1991) **Science**, 254, 1802-1805.

Cohen, J.S., (1991) **Pharmacol. Ther.**, 52, 211-225.

Cotton, M., Wagner, E., Zatloukai, K., Philips, S, Curiel, D.T. and Brinstiel, M.L., (1992) **Proc. Natl. Acad. Sci. USA**, 89, 6094-6098.

Crystal, R.G., (1994) **Nature Genet.** 8, 42-51.

Culver, K.M. and Blaese, R.M., (1994) *Gene therapy for adenosine deaminase deficiency and malignant solid tumor*, In: **Gene Therapeutics: Methods and Applications of Direct Gene Transfer**, J.A. Wolff (Ed.), Birjhauser, Boston, pp. 263-280.

Curiel, D.T., Agarwal, S., Wagner, E. and Cotton, M., (1991) **Proc. Natl. Acad. Sci. USA, 88**, 8850-8854.

Curiel, K.M., Agarwal, S., Romer, M.U., Wagner, E., Cotton, M., Birnstiel, M.L. and Boucher, R.C., (1992) **Am. J. Respir. Cell Mol. Biol.**, 6, 247-252.

Davidson, B.L., Allen, E.D., Kozarsky, K.F., Wilson, J.M. and Roessler, B.J., (1993) **Nature Genet.,** 3, 219-223.

Davis, H.L., Micher, M.L. and Whalen, R.G., (1993) **Hum. Mol. Genet.,** 2, 1847-1851.

Demenix, B.A. and Behr, J.P. (1996) In: **Artificial Self-Assembling Systems for Gene Delivery,** P.L. Felgner, M.J. Heller, P.Lehn, J.P. Behr, F.C. Szoka, Jr. (Eds.), Conference Proceedings Series, American Chemical Society, Washington, DC, p146-151.

Dichek, D.A., Nussbaum, O., Degen, S.J.F. and Anderson, W.F., (1991) **Blood,** 77, 533-541.

Dixit, M., Webb, M.S., Smart, W.C. and Ohi, S., (1991) **Gene,** 104, 253-257.

Earl, R.T., (1989) Drug Delivery and Targeting Systems Latest Advances, Conference documentation, Organized by IBC Technical Services Ltd.

Eisenbraun, M.D., Fullwer, D.H. and Haynes, J.R., (1993) **DNA Cell Biol.,** 12, 791-797.

Evans, J.P., Brinkhous, K.M., Brager, G.D., Reisner, H.M. and High, K.A., (1989) **Proc. Natl. Acad. Sci. USA** 86, 10095-10098.

Fahn, S., (1992) **N. Engl. J. Med.,** 327, 1589-1590.

Felgner, O.L., Gadek, T.R., Holm, M., Roman, R., Chan, H.W., Wenz, M., Northrop, J.P., Ringold, R.M. and Danielsen, M. (1987), **Proc. Nalt. Acad. Sci. USA,** 84, 7413-7417.

Felgner, P.L. and Ringold, G.M., (1989) **Nature,** 337, 387-388.

Flotte, T.R., Solow, R., Owens, R.A., Afinoe, S., Zeittine, P.L. and Carter, B.J., (1992) **Am. J. Respir. Cell Mol. Biol.,** 7, 349-356.

Freed, C.R., Reeze, R.E., Rosenberg, N.L., Schenck, S.A., Krick, E., Qi, J.X., Lone, T., Zhang, Y.B., Sindyer, J.A., Wells, T.H., Raning, L.O., Thompson, L., Mazziota, J.C., Huang, S.C., Grafton, S.T., Brooks, D., Sawle, G., Schroter, G. and Ansari, A.A., (1992) **N. Engl. J. Med.,** 327, 1549-1555.

Friedmann, T., (1985) **HPRT Gene Transfer as a Model for Gene Therapy,** Plenum Press.

Furth, P.A., Shamy, A., Wall, R.J. and Hennighausen, L., (1992) **Anal. Biochem.,** 20, 365-368.

Gage, F.H., Wolff, J.A., Rosenberg, M.B., Xu, L., Lee, J-K., Shults, C. and Friedmann, T., **(1987), Neurosciences,** 23, 795-807.

Gansbacjer, B., Zier, K., Baniels, B., Cronin, K., Bannerji, R. and Gilboa, E., (1990) **J. Exp. Med.,** 172, 1217-1224.

Gao, X.A. and Huang, L., (1991) **Biochim. Biophys. Res. Commun.,** 179, 280-285.

Geller, A.I. and Breakefield, X.O., (1988) **Science,** 241, 1667-1669.

Geller, A.I., Keyomarsi, K., Bryan, J. and Pardee, A.B., (1990) **Proc. Natl. Acad. Sci. USA,** 87, 8590-8594.

Gitaman, A.G., Graessmann, A. and Loyter, A., (1985) **Proc. Nalt. Acad. Sci. USA,** 82(21), 7309-7313.

Golumbek, P.T., Lazenby, A.J., Levitsky, H.I., Jaffee, L.M., Karasuyama, H., Maker, M. and Pardoll, D.M., (1991) **Science,** 254, 713-716.

Goodchild, J., (1990) **Bioconjugate Chem.,** 1, 165-187.

Gould-Forgeite, S., Mazurkiewicz, J.E., Raska, K., Voelkerding,K., Lehman, J.M. and Mannino,R.J., (1989) **Gene,** 84, 429-438.

Grierson, D., (1991) *Plant Genetic Engineering,* In: **Plant Biotechnology,** Vo.I, Blackie, Glasgow.

Hampel, A. and Tritz, R., (1989) **Biochemistry,** 28, 4919-4933.

Hampel, A., Tritz, R. and Cruz, P., (1990) **Nucleic Acid Res.,** 18, 299-304.

Hanensler, J. and Szoka, F.C. Jr., (1993) **Bioconjugate Chem.,** 4, 372-279.

Harrison, G.S., Long, C.J., Curiel, T.J., Maxwell, F. and Maxwell, I.H., (1992) **Hum. Gene Ther.,** 3, 461-469.

Heller, M.J. and Jablonski, E.J., (1987) European Patent Application No. 0229 943.

Heller, M.J. and Morrison, L., (1985) In: **Rapid Detection and Identification of Infectious Agents**, D. Kingsbury and S. Falkow (Eds.), Academic Press, New York, p345-356.

Heller, M.J., Morrison, L.E., Prevatt, W.D. amd Akin, C., European Patent Application No. 070 685, 1983.

Hickman, M.A., Malone, R.W., Lehmann, K., Sih, T.R., Knoell, D., Szoka, F.C. Jr., Walzem, R., Carlson, D.M. and Powell, J.S., (1994) **Hum. Gene Ther.**, 5, 1477-1483.

Hnatyszyn, H.J., (1995) Ph.D. Thesis, University of California, Los Angeles,.

Hodgson, C.P., (1995) **Bio/Technology**, 11, 222-225.

Hodgson, C.P., Elder, P.K., Ono, T., Foster, D.N., Getz, M.J., (1983) **Mol. Cell Biol.**, 3, 2221-2231.

Hoeben R.C., Valerio, D., Van der Eb, A.J. and Van Ormondt, H., (1992) **Clin. Rev. Oncol. Hematol.**, 13, 33-54.

Hoogerbrugge, P.M., Suzuki, K., Poorthuis, B.J.H.M., Kobayashi, T., Wagemaker, G. and van Bekkum, D.W., (1988) **Science** 239, 1035-1038.

Horwitz, M..S., (1990) *Adenovirus and their replication.* In: **Virology**, Fields, B.N. Knipe, D.M. ((Eds.), Vol. 2, Raven Press, New York, pp. 1679-1721.

Huckett, B., Ariatti, M. and Hawtrey, A.O., (1990) **Biochem. Pharmacol.**, 40, 253-263.

Inouye, M., (1988) **Gene**, 72, 25-34.

Kato, K., Kaneda, Y., Sakurari, M., Nakanishi, M. and Okada, Y., (1991) **J. Biol. Chem.**, 266, 22071-22074.

Kay, M.A., Landen, C.N., Rottenberg, S.R., Taylor, L.A., Leland, F., Wielle, S., Fang, B., Bellinger, D., Finegold, M., Thompson, A.R., Read. M.S. Brinkhous, K.M. and Woo, S.L.C., (1974) **Proc. Natl. Acad. Sci. USA**, 91, 2353-2357.

Kay, M.A., Rothenberg, S., Landen, C.N., Bellinger, D.A., Leland, F., Toman, C., Finegold, M., Thompson, A.R., Read, M.S., Brinkhous, K.M. and Woo, S.L.C., (1993) **Science**, 262, 117-119.

Kolodka, T.M., Finegold, M., Moss, L. and Woo, S.L.C., (1995) **Proc. Natl. Acad. Sci. USA**, 92, 3293-3297.

Kossovsky, N., (1995) Presented at the Cambridge Healthtech Institute Conference on *Artificial Self-Assembling Systems for Gene Transfer*, Boston, M.A., September 1995.

Kossovsky, N., (1996) In: **Artificial Self-Assembling Systems for Gene Delivery**, P.L. Felgner, M.J. Heller, P.Lehn, J.P. Behr, F.C. Szoka, Jr. (Eds.), Conference Proceedings Series, American Chemical Society, Washington, DC. p 152-168.

Kossovsky, N., Gelman, A., Rajguru, S., Nguyen, R., Sponsler, E., Hnatyszyn, H.J., Chow, L., Chung, A., Torrer, M., Zemanovich, J., Crowder, J., Barnajian, P., Ly, K., Philipose, J., Ammons, D., Anderson, D., Anderson, S., Goodwin, C., Soliemanzadeh, P., Yao, G. and Wei K., (1996) **J. Control. Rel.**, 39, 383-388.

Krichner, J. Connolly, C.M., Sandmeyer, S.B., (1995) **Science,** 267, 1488-91.

Kukowska-Latallo, J.F., Billinska, A.U., Johnson, J., Spindler, R., Tomalia, D.A. and Baker, J.R. Jr., (1996) **Proc. Natl. Acad. Sci. USA**, 93, 4897-4902.

Lakowicz, J.R., (1983) In: **Principles of Fluorescent Spectroscopy**, Plenum Press, New York, p305-337.

Le Gal La Salle, G., Berrard, J.J.R., Ridoux, V., Stratford-Perricaudet, L.D., Perricaudet, M. and Mallet, J., (1993) **Science**, 259, 988-990.

Ledley, F.D., O'Malley, B.W. Jr., Borchardt, J. Roop, D., Rolland, A.and Tomlinson, E., (1994) **J. Cell Biochem.**, 18A, 226,

Ledley, F.D., Woo, S.L., Ferry, G.D., Whisennand, H.H., Brandt, M.L., Darlington, G.J., Demmler, G.J., Finegold, M.J., Pokorny, W.J. and Rosenblatt, H., (1991) **Hum. Gene Ther.**, 2, 331-358.

Legendre,J.Y. and Szako, F.C., Jr., (1992) **Pharm. Res.**, 9, 1235-1242.

Lemarchand, P., Jones, M., Yamada, I. and Crystal, R.G., (1993) **Circ. Res.**, 72, 1132-1138.

Levy, M.Y., Meyer, K.B., Barron, L. and Szoka, F.C., Jr., (1994) **Pharm. Res.**, 11, 317.

Li, S., Gao, X., Son, K., Sorgi, F., Hofland, H. and Huang, L., (1996) **J. Control. Rel.**, 39, 373-381.

Liljestrom, P. and Garoff, H., (1994) In: **Current Protocols in Molecular Biology** (Ausubel, F.M. et al., Eds.), pp. 16.20.1-16.20.16., Greene Publishing Associates and Wiley Interscience.

Liljestrom, P., (1994) **Curr. Opin. Biotechnol.**, 5, 495-500.

Lindvall, O., Brundin, P., Widner, H., Rehncrone, S., Gustavii, B., Frackowiak, R., Leenders, K., Sawle, G., Rothwell, J., Marsden, D. and Bjorklund, A., (1989) **Science**, 247, 574-577.

Logan, J.J., Bebok, Z., Walker, L.C., Peng, S., Felgner, P.L., Siegal, G.P., Frizzell, R.A., Dong, J., Howard,M., Matalon, S., Lindsey, J.R., Du Vall, M., Sorscher, E.J., (1995) **Gene Ther.**, 2, 38-49.

Lu, D.R., Zhou, J.M., Zheng, B., Qiu, X.F., Xue, J.L., Wang, J.M., Meng, P.L., Han, F.L., Ming, B.H., Wang, X.P., Wang, J.B., Liang, J.J. and Jiang, Z.S., (1993) **Sci. China**, 36, 1342-1351.

Manthorpe, M., Cornefert-Jensen, F., Hartikka, J., Felgner, J., Rundell, A., Margalith, M., and Dwarki, V., (1993) **Hum. Gen. Ther.**, 4, 419-431.

Markowitz, D., Goff, S. and Bank, A., (1988) **Virology**, 167, 400-406.

Mastrangelo, M.J., Schultz, S., Kane, M. and Berd, D., (1988) **Semi. Oncol.**, 15, 589-594.

Mc Lachlan, G., Davidson, H., Davison, D., Dickinoson, P., Dorin, J. and Porteous, D., (1994) **Biochemic.**, 11, 19-21.

McDonald, J.F., (1993) **Curr. Opin. Genet. Dev.**, 3, 855-864.

McKusick, V.A., (1988) **Mendelian Inheritance in Man**, 8th Ed, Johns Hopkins University Press, Baltimore, MD.

Miiler, A.D. and Buttimore, C., (1986) **Mol. Cell Biol.**, 6, 2895-2902.

Miller, A.D., Eckner, R.J., Jolly, D.J., Friedmann, T. and Verma, I.M., (1984) **Science**, 225, 630-632.

Miller, A.D., Jolly, D.J., Friedmann, T. and Verma, I.M., (1983) **Proc. Natl. Acad. Sci. USA**, 80, 4709-4713.

Millers, P.S. and Ts'O, P.O.P., (1988) **Annu. Rep. Med. Chem.**, 23, 295-304.

Morgan, R., Looney, D.J., Muenchau, D.D., Wong-Staal, F., Gallo, R.C. and Anderson, W.F., (1990) **Res. Hum. Retrovir.**, 6, 183-191.

Mumper, R.J., Barron, M.K., Anwer, K., Lessard, R.L., Liu, Q., Nitta, H., Alila, H. and Rollond, A.P., (1995) **Pharm. Res.**, 12, 80.

Muzyezker, N., (1992) **Curr. Top. Microbiol. Immunol.**, 158, 97-129.

Nabel, E.G., Plautz, G., Boyce, F.M., Stanley, J.C. and Nabel, G.J., (1989) **Science**, 244, 1342-1344.

Nicolau, C. and Cudd, A., (1989) **Crit. Rev. Ther. Drug Carrier Syst.**, 6, 239-271.

Nicolau, C., Le Pape, A., Soirano, P., Fargette, F. and Jubel, M.F., (1983) **Proc. Natl. Acad. Sci. USA**, 80, 1068-1072.

Palella, T.D., Hidaka, Y., Silverman, L. J., Levine, M., Glorioso, J. and Kelley, W.N., (1989) **Gene**, 80, 137-144.

Palmer, T.D., Rosman, G.J., Obsborne, W.R.A. and Miller, A.D., (1991) **Proc. Natl. Acad. Sci. USA**, 88, 1330-1334.

Palmer, T.D., Thompson, A.R. and Miller, A.D., (1989) **Blood**, 73, 438-445.

Plautz, G., Nabel, E.G. and Nabel, G.J., (1991) **Circulation**, 83, 578-583.

Quantin, B., Perricaudet, L.D., Tajbakhsh, S. and Mandel, J.L., (1992) **Proc. Natl. Acad. Sci. USA**, 89, 2581-2584.

Raz, E., Carson, D.A., Parker, S.E., Parr, T.B., Abai, A.M., Aichinger, G., Gromkowski, S.H., Singh, M., Lew, D., Yankauchas, M.A., Baird, A.M. and Rhodes, G.H., (1994) **Proc. Natl. Acad. Sci. USA**, 91, 9519-9523.

Rojanasakul, Y., (1996) **Adv. Drug Deliv. Rev.**, 18, 115-131.

Romer, K. and Friedmann, T., (1992) **Eur. J. Biochem.**, 208, 211-225.

Rosenberg, M.B., Friedmann, T., Robertson, R.C., Tuszynski, M., Wolff, J.A., Breadkfield, X.O. and Gage F.H., (1988) **Science**, 242, 1575-1578.

Rosenfeld, M.A., Siegfried,W., Yoshimura, K., Yoneyama, K., Fukayama, M., Stier, L.E., Pakko, P.K., Gilardi, P., Stratford-Perricaudet, L.D., Perricaudet, M., Jallat, S., Pavirani, A., Lecacq, J.P.and Crystal, R.G., (1991) **Science**, 252, 431-434.

Rosenfeld, M.A., Yoshimura, K., Trapnell, B.C., Yoneyama, K., Rosenthal, E.R., Dalemans, W., Fukayama, M., Bargon, J., Stier, L.E., Straford-Prericaudet, L.D., Perrocaudet, M., Gaggino, W.B., Pavirani, A., Lecocq, J.P. and Crystal, R.G., (1992) **Cell**, 668, 143-155.

Schlesinger, S., (1993) **Trends Biotechnol.**, 11, 18-22.

Scjreoer. J. and Sawuyer. S., (1996) **Adv. Drug Del. Rev.**, 19, 73-87.

Seegmiller, J.E., Rosenbloom, F.M. and Kelly, W.N., (1967) **Science**, 155, 1682-1684.

Selheyer, K., Bickenbach, J.R., Rothnagel, J.A., Bundman, D., Longley, M.A., Krieg, T., Roche, N.S., Roberts, A.B. and Roop, D.R., (1993) **Proc. Natl. Acad. Sci. USA**, 90, 5237-5241.

Service, R.F. (1995), *Science* 267, 458-459.

Shak, S., Caponm, D.J., Hellniss, R., Massters, S.A. and Baker, C.L., (1990) **Proc. Natl. Acad. Sci. USA**, 87, 9188-9192.

Shaw, J.P., Milligan, J.F., Krawczyk, S.H. and Mateucci, M., (1991) **J. Am. Chem. Soc.**, 113, 7765-7766.

Sikes, M., O'Malley, B.W., Jr., Finegold, M.J. and Ledley, F.D., (1994) **Hum. Gene Ther.**, 5, 837-844.

Staedel, C., Remy, J.S., Hua, Z. Broker, T.R., Chow, L.T. and Behr, J.P. (1994), **J. Invest. Dermatol.** 102, 768-772.

Starford-Perricaudet, L.D., Makeh, L., Perricaudet, M. and Briand, P., (1992) **J. Clin. Invest.**, 90 , 626-630.

Stein, C.A. and Cohen, J.S., (1988) **Cancer Res.**, 48, 2659-2668.

Stevenson, M. and Iversen, P.L., (1989) **J. Gene Vinol.**, 70, 2673-2682.

Strarford-Perricaudet, L.D., Levrero, M., Chasse, J.F., Perricaudet, M. and Briand, P., (1990) **Hum. Gene Ther.**, 1, 241-256.

Straus, S.E., (1984) *Adenovirus infections in humans.* In: **The Adenovirus**, H.S. Ginsberg (Ed.), Plenum Press, NewYork, pp. 451-496.

Strauss, J.H. and Strauss, E.G., (1994) **Microbiol. Rev.**, 58, 491-562.

Tidd, D.M. and Warenius, H.M., (1989) **Br. J. Cancer**, 60, 343-350.

Tomalia, D.A., Naylor, A.M. and Goddard, W.A., (1990) **Angew. Chem. Int. Ed. Engl.**, 29, 138-175.

Tomlinson, E. and Rolland, A.P., (1996) **J. Control. Rel.**, 39, 357-372.

Ullrich, A., Shine, K.J., Chirgwin, J., Pictet, R., Tischer, E., Rutter, W.J. and Goodman, H.M., (1977) **Science**, 196, 1313-1319.

Ulmer, J.B., Donnelly, J.J., Parker, S.E., Rhodes, G.H., Felgner, P.L., Dwarki, V.J., Gromkowski, S.H., Deck, R.R., Dewitt, C.M., Friedman, A., Hawe, L.A., Oeander, K.R., Martinez, D., Perry, H.C., Shiver, J.W., Montgomery, D.L. and Liu, M.A., (1993) **Science**, 149, 1745-1749.

Varmus, H., (1988) **Science**, 240, 1427-1435.

Wagner, E., Cotton, M., Foisner, R. and Birnstiel, M.L., (1991) **Proc. Natl. Acad. Sci. USA**, 88, 42545-4259.

Wagner, E., Zatloukal, K., Cotton, M., Kirlappos, H., Mechtler, K., Curiel, D.T. and Birnstiel, M.L., (1992) **Proc. Natl. Acad. Sci. USA,** 89, 6099-6103.

Wang, C.Y. and Huang, L., (1987) **Proc. Natl. Acad. Sci. USA,** 84, 7851-7855.

Wang, K.Y., McCurdy, S., Shea, R.G., Swaminathan, S. and Bolton, P.H., (1993) **Biochemistry,** 32, 1899-1904.

Wang, Y., O'Malley, B.W. Jr., Tsai, S.Y. and O'Malley, B.W., (1994) **Proc. Natl. Acad. Sci. USA,** 91, 8180-8184.

Widner, H., Tetrud, J., Rehncrone, S., Snow, B., Brundin, P., Gustavii, B., Bjorklund, A., Lindvall, O. and Langston, J.W., (1992) **N. Engl. J. Med.,** 327, 1556-1562.

Willis, R.C. W., Jolly, D.J., Miller, A.D., Plent, M.M., Esty, A.C., Anderson, P.J., Chang, H.C., Jones. O.W., Seegmiller, J.E. and Friedmann, T., (1984) **J. Biol. Chem.,** 259, 7842-7829.

Wilson, J.M., Birniyi, L.K., Salomon, R.N., Libby, P., Callow, A.D. and Mulligan, R.C., (1989) **Science,** 244, 1344-1346.

Wilson, J.M., Grossman, M., Wu, C.H., Chowdhury, N.R., Wu, G.Y. and Chowdhury, J.R., (1992) **J. Biochem.,** 167, 963-967.

Zhao, X., (1995) **Adv. Drug. Del. Rev.,** 17, 257-262.

Zhao, X., Batten, B. and Singh, B., (1990) **Oncogene,** 5, 1727-1730.

Zhao, X., Klibanov, A.L. and Huang, L., (1991) **Biochim. Biophys. Acta,** 1065, 8-14.

Zhao, X., Zhange, P.J. and Wong, T.K., (1993) **Mol. Marine Biol. Biotech.,** 2, 63-69.

BASIC IMMUNOLOGY

12.1. INTRODUCTION

Our environment contains a large variety of invading, pathogenic microbes/ micro-organisms against which an effective, protective cover is given by the immune system. The immune system is a remarkably adaptive defense system which is able to generate a variety of cells and molecules capable of specifically recognizing and eliminating a variety of limitless foreign invaders into the system. On the basis of their function, the immune system can be divided into recognition and response. The immune system is capable of recognizing and distinguishing one foreign pathogen from the other. Once it recognizes the foreign organism/invaders it works out effectively to either eliminate or neutralize them.

The term **immune** is derived from the Latin word *immunis* meaning *exempt from charges* (i.e. taxes and expenses). Although the concept of immunity existed since 430 BC when Thucydides, described about plague in Athens, wherein he wrote that only people who recovered after a plague infection could nurse the sick as they would not harbor the disease for a second time, it was almost two thousand years for making it medically acceptable and successful. The first recorded crude attempt to protect against variola (smallpox) was made in ancient China and in West Asia by inoculation using vesicle fluid from persons with mild forms of smallpox (variolation) or by seeking personal contact with diseased individuals. It was in 1718 that Lady Mary Wortley Montageu introduced the process of **variolation**/inoculation with unmodified smallpox virus. In 1798, Edward Jenner an English Physician introduced vaccination against smallpox by means of using cowpox. The term **Vaccination**, in Latin *Vacca* means *cow*, was introduced in place of variolation. It was not until Louis Pasteur and his team brought into picture the use of **attenuated strains of micro-organisms** for vaccination almost a entury after Jenners study. Then came the "Cellular immunity" theory, "Humoral" theory, and Ehrlich's "side-chain" theory. The history behind these theories are not dealt here in as it is beyond the limits of this book.

Immunity can be broadly classified into natural and acquired. They can be further classified into active and passive which are again sub-classified into natural and acquired (Fig. 12.1).

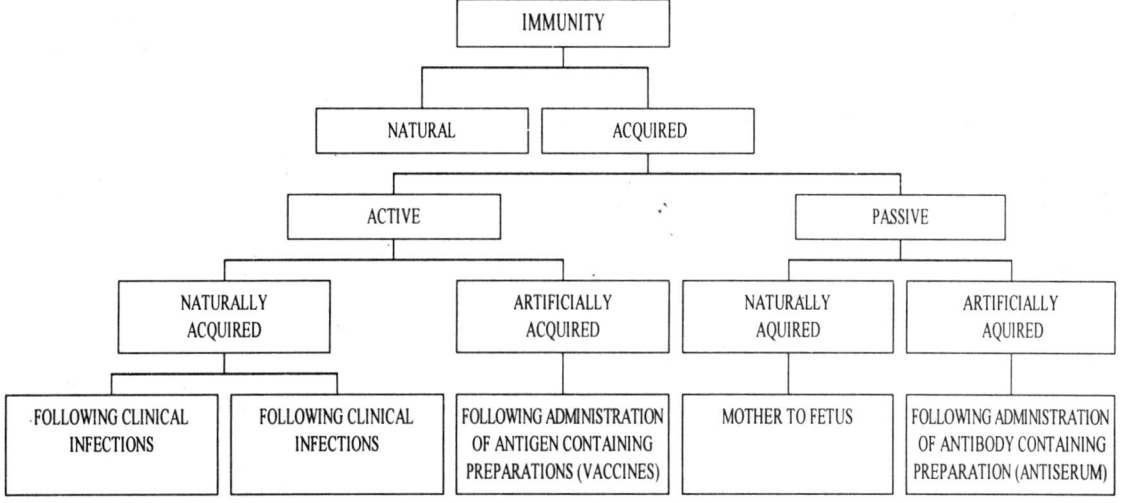

Fig. 12.1 : Classification of immunity

12.2. NATURAL IMMUNITY

It is resistance to a disease *possessed* by an individual. Putting into a nut shell- constitutional make up. Nature has given certain individuals, species and races some advantage, i.e. by providing them immunity against certain diseases. For example, some individuals are more resistant to certain infections than others. Similarly plague a dreaded disease which attacks man does not harm fowls. Again, among races there are differences, Negroes are highly resistant to yellow fever while the whites are highly susceptible.

12.3. ACQUIRED IMMUNITY

Only with the cover of natural immunity it is difficult to survive. Hence, immunity is provided by wither stimulating an individuals antibody production or by introducing antibodies acquired from a person or an animal. In short, acquired immunity is *developed* during a persons lifetime; it is not inherited. Immunity can be acquired *actively* or *passively*. This active or passive, acquired immunity may be either natural or acquired.

12.3.1. Naturally acquired active immunity

Naturally acquired immunity is a developed immunity, which is acquired when a person is exposed to natural infection by pathogens or to some antigens in the day-to-day life. Following the exposure, the immune system responds by producing specialized lymphocytes and special protein called *antibodies*. Immunity of this kind lasts long in most cases. Immunity developed following clinical and sub-clinical infections also fall under this category.

12.3.2. Artificially acquired active immunity

Artificially acquired active immunity results following the stimulation of antibody production by introducing specially prepared antigens called vaccines into the body by safe means. This can also be termed as *Vaccination* or *active immunization*. Vaccines are consisted of inactivated bacterial toxins (toxoids), killed micro-organism or living but attenuated (weakened) micro-organism. These substances are subjected to treatment wherein they lose their toxicity or the ability to cause a disease but still capable of stimulating the immune system.

Table 12.1 : Comparison between active and passive immunity

Active	Passive
Developed immunity	Produced immunity
Develops slowly and long lasting	Relatively fast and short lived
A booster dose, if required can be given to give life long immunity	A booster dose also doesn't help in maintaining it for long
It is mainly to prevent a disease and is administered before infection	Generally, after the subject has been exposed to an infection.
Given in long term prophylaxis	Given in short term prophylaxis and therapeutically
Antigens are administered	Antibodies are administered

12.3.3. Naturally acquired passive immunity

Similar to active immunity this is a *produced* immunity. This involves the natural transfer of antibodies from a mother to fetus via placenta and thus providing immunity to the new born from few days to few months. Here, the fetus is immune to those diseases for which the mother is immune, but for a short period. For example, if the mother is immune to diseases like diphtheria, chicken pox, polio etc., the new born is also immune but not more than for a period of six months. Similarly, certain amount of immunity is provided through breast feeding. Certain antibodies are capable of passing from the mother to the infant via the breast milk.

12.3.4. Artificially acquired passive immunity

We have seen earlier that by administering antigens, we can produce artificial-active immunity which lasts long. However, here, we are administering antibodies for stimulation of immune response. These antibodies are either produced in animals or in human and then administered to the subject. The antibodies are found in the serum of the immune animal or human and hence the term S*erum* or *sera* or *antisera* is frequently used.

Looking back into the characteristics of immune system, it can be divided into two types, namely the **innate immune system** and the **adaptive immune system**. The first line of defense is provided by the innate immune system. If this first line defense fails, then the adaptive system fall in action. While the innate immune system checks out potential pathogens even before they could establish an infection. The adaptive system produces a specific reaction to each infectious agent which normally eradicates that agent. In addition, the latter remembers that particular infectious agent and recalls whenever they come across next time, thus preventing from cause of a disease.

12.4. THE INNATE IMMUNE SYSTEM

Intact skin acts as an effective barrier to most organism. This is very clear from patients suffering from burns. Here, the prime entry of infection is via the damaged skin. Most infections enter the body via the epithelial surface of the nasopharynx, gut, lungs and genito-urinary tract. A variety of physical and biochemical defense mechanisms exist in these areas and protect them from most infections (Fig.12.2). Lysozyme an enzyme widely distributed in different secretions and capable of splitting a bond found in the cell wall of many bacteria, is a very good example.

12.4.1. Endocytes and phagocytes

If an organism penetrates an epithelial surface, a special type of innate defense mechanism also comes into action that is the infestation of extracellular macromolecules. This is brought in either by endocytosis or phagocytosis. Endocytosis is a mechanism where in the macromolecules contain within the extracellular tissue

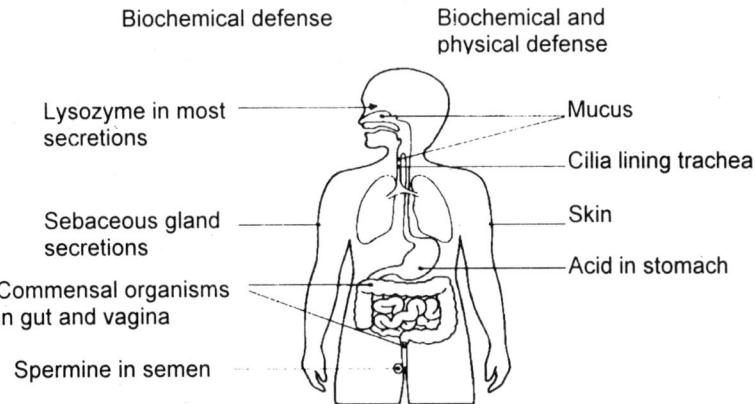

Biochemical defense

Biochemical and physical defense

Lysozyme in most secretions

Mucus

Cilia lining trachea

Sebaceous gland secretions

Skin

Acid in stomach

Commensal organisms in gut and vagina

Spermine in semen

Fig. 12.2 : Physical and biochemical defense

fluids are internalized by either of the two processes: *pinocytosis or receptor-mediated endocytosis* (Fig. 12.3). Internalization of macromolecules through non-specific membrane is known as pinocytosis. This process depends upon the concentration of the macromolecules. In receptor-mediated endocytosis, macromolecules are selectively internalized after binding to specific membrane receptors.

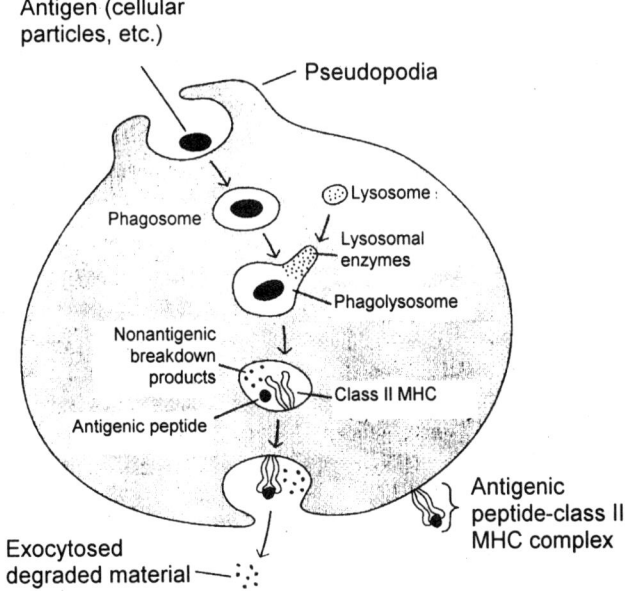

Antigen (cellular particles, etc.)

Pseudopodia

Phagosome

Lysosome

Lysosomal enzymes

Phagolysosome

Nonantigenic breakdown products

Class II MHC

Antigenic peptide

Antigenic peptide-class II MHC complex

Exocytosed degraded material

Fig. 12.3 : Phagocytosis and processing of exogenous antigens by macrophages

The organism which penetrates an epithelial surface is encountered by phagocytic cells of the reticulo-endothelial system (Fig.12.4). The specialized phagocyte cells are derived form bone marrow of stem cells and include neutrophils, monocytes and tissue macrophages. The function of phagocytes is to engulf particles, internalize them and destroy them.

12.4.2. Natural killer (NK) cells and soluble factors

NK cells are leukocytes capable of recognizing cell surface changes on virally-infected cells. The NK cells bind to these target cells and kill them. Interferons, a group of proteins produced by virus infected cells and sometimes by lymphocytes activate the NK cells.

Among a variety of soluble factors, lysozyme a hydrolytic enzyme found in mucous secretions cleaves the peptidoglycan layer of the bacterial cell wall. Interferons are produced at the early stages of infection and act as first line of resistance against many viruses. In addition as discussed above, they stimulate NK cells.

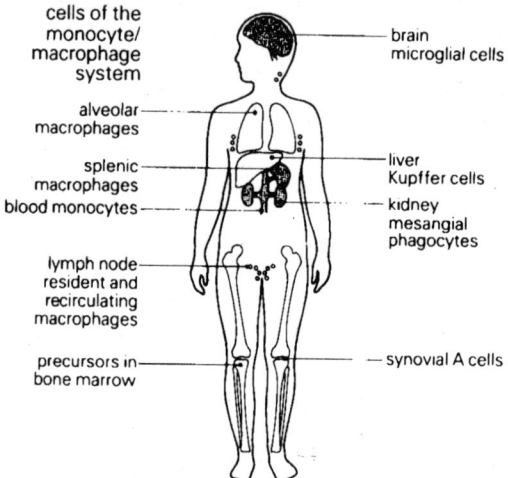

Fig. 12.4 : Phagocytes of reticuloendothelial system

The serum concentration of a number of proteins increases rapidly during infection. These proteins are called acute phase proteins. An example of this is the C reactive protein (they bind to the C protein of *pneumococci*). Bacteria bound by C-reactive protein promote the binding of complement (a group of serum protein that circulate in an inactive proenzyme state), facilitating the uptake of phagocytes. This process is termed as *opsonization..* The complement system is spontaneously activated by the surface of the micro-organism by the alternative complement pathway. Followed by this is either opsonization leading to phagocyte or attract the phagocytes to the site of infection. In addition to this, the complement system has an intrinsic ability to lyse the cell membrane of many bacterial species (Fig. 12.5).

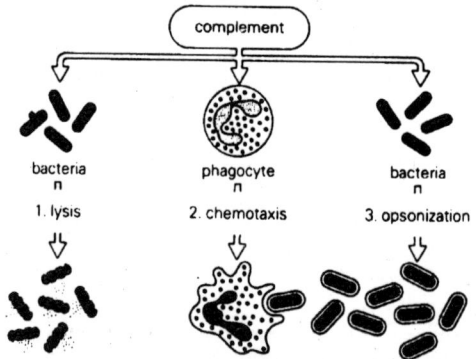

Fig. 12.5 : Schematic representation depicting the function of a complement system

12.4.3. Inflammatory response

Inflammation is the body's reaction to an injury or to an invasion by an infectious agent. Inflammation is manifested by :

1. An increase in blood·supply to the infected area.
2. Increase in capillary permeability caused by retraction of endothelial cells.
3. Influx of phagocytic cells.

The increase in capillary permeability permits larger molecules to traverse across the endothelium and thus allows the soluble mediators to reach the site of infection. similarly, the migration of leukocytes out of the capillaries into the surrounding tissues, makes them move towards the site of infection by the process of chemotaxis (the process by which phagocytes are attracted to site of inflammation).

12.5. ADAPTIVE/ACQUIRED/SPECIFIC IMMUNITY

Adaptive or specific immunity of the immune system is based upon the presence of a functional immune system that is capable of specifically recognizing one particular antigen and selectively eliminating foreign micro-organism. The main features which characterize all immune responses by acquired immune system include specificity, diversity, memory and self or non-self recognition. Acquired immunity does not occur independently of innate immunity, i.e. it does not act in isolation. Cells of the phagocytic system, mostly the macrophages, are involved in activation of the specific immune response.

The question arises how can a lymphocyte recognize a particular antigen among thousands of them and how adequate response is brought in? The answer is by *clonal selection.*

12.6. ANTIBODY CLONAL SELECTION

Antigens recognize the small number of cells and bind to them. There in, they proliferate to produce sufficient cells to mount an adequate immune response, that is the antigen selects the specific clone of antigen binding cells (Fig.12.6). This process occurs both for the B and T lymphocytes.

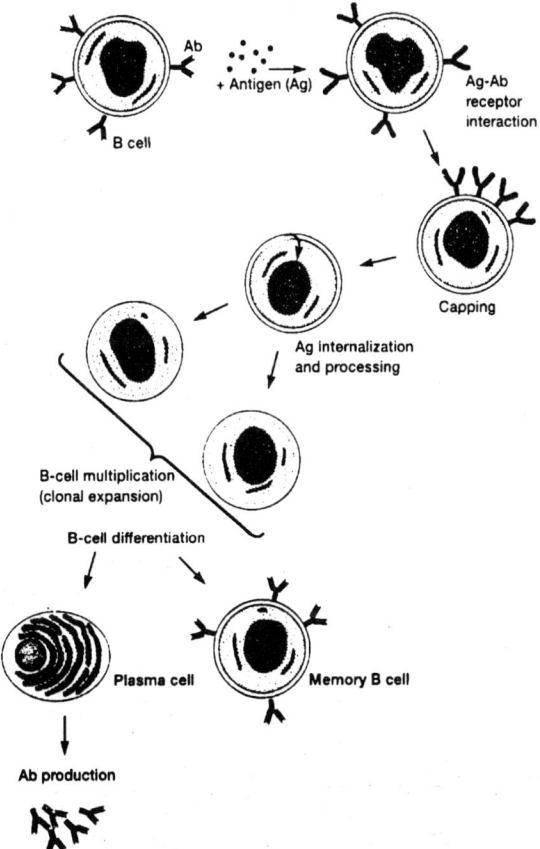

Fig. 12.6 : Antibody clonal selection

12.7. THE CELLS OF THE IMMUNE SYSTEM

Generation of an effective immune response involves a number of organs and several; different cell types which can accurately and specifically recognize non-self antigens on micro-organism and to eliminate those organism. Two major groups of cells fall under this category:

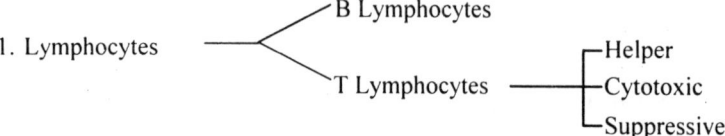

1. Lymphocytes
   - B Lymphocytes
   - T Lymphocytes
     - Helper
     - Cytotoxic
     - Suppressive

2. Antigen presenting cells (APC)

Among the two different kinds of lymphocytes, T cells differentiate initially in the thymus whilst B cells differentiate in fetal liver, spleen and in bone marrow. In addition to these cells, non-B or non-T cells or third population cells/null cells are also present. Further, a number of auxiliary cells are involved in generating immunity against invading organism.

12.7.1. Lymphoidal cells

12.7.1.1. B lymphocytes or B cells

Classically, the B lymphocytes are defined by the presence of endogenously produced immunoglobulins (antibody). That is the B cell receptor is an antibody molecule, a membrane-bound glycoprotein. They mature in the bone marrow and leave the marrow with a unique antigen-binding receptor on the membrane (Fig. 12.7).

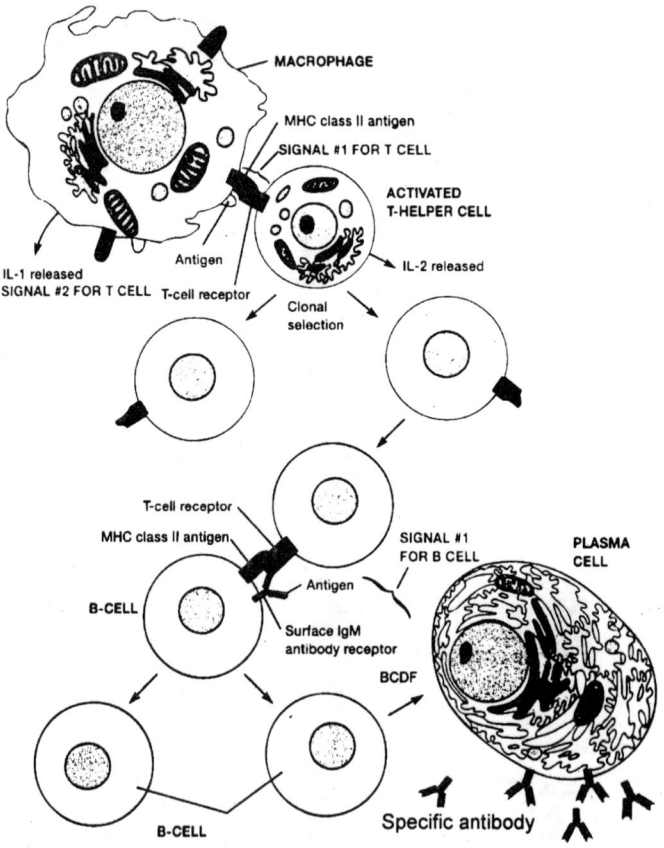

Fig. 12.7 : T-dependent antigen triggering of a B cell

They constitute about 5-15% of the circulating lymphoidal pool. They are detected on the surface of mature cells by staining cell suspension with fluorescent labeled, specific antibodies. When a virgin B cell first encounters the antigen, the cell begins to divide rapidly. They differentiate themselves into memory B cells and plasma cells or effector cells. The memory B cells have a longer life span and resemble their parent in their function. Plasma cells do not produce membrane-bound antibody instead they produce the antibody in a form that can be secreted. They are short living cells, secreting enormous amount of one of the five classes of antibody within their life span. These secreted antibodies are the major effector molecules of humoral immunity. The human peripheral blood B lymphocytes express both surface Ig M and Ig D antibodies. Very few cells express surface Ig G, Ig A or Ig E in the circulation.

12.7.1.2. T-Lymphocytes or T cells

The name originated from their site of maturation namely the thymus (Fig.12.8). Like B cells, they have structurally distinct antigen binding receptor site. T cells can be distinguished from B cells, as the former has a different surface proteins which can bind to sheep erythrocytes. T cell receptors can recognize antigens only when they are associated with self-molecule encoded by genes within the major histocompatibility complex (MHC). This is the basic difference between humoral and cell-mediated immunity.

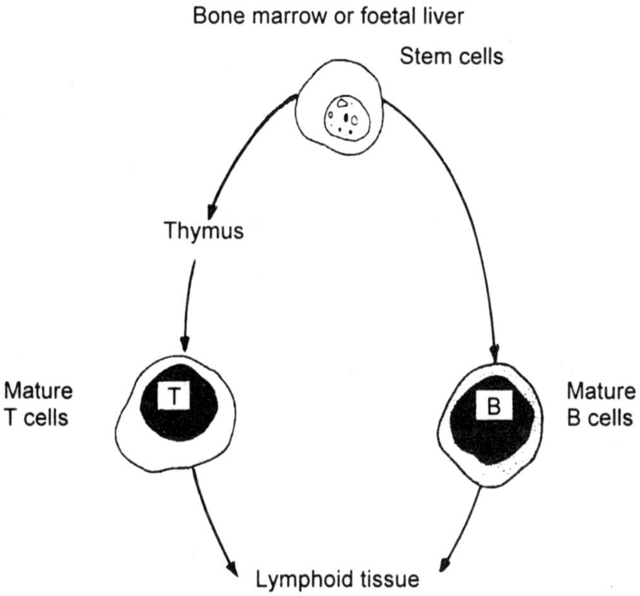

Fig. 12.8 : Difference between B and T cell production

The T cells have two major sub-population namely T helper cells (T_H) and T cytotoxic cells (T_C) while a third, namely the T suppressor cells (T_S) is also said to be in existence.

12.7.1.3. Null cells

The null cells are a group (small) of peripheral-blood lymphocytes which do not bear the necessary membrane proteins to differentiate themselves between B and T lymphocytes. These cells also fail to display antigen-binding receptors as either of the lymphocyte cells. A population, of null cells namely the *natural killer* (NK) cells first described in 1976, constitutes 5-10% of the peripheral-blood lymphocytes. The NK cells produce cytotoxic activity against a wide range of tumor cells in spite of any previous immunization against that particular tumor. These NK cells play an important role in displaying host defense against tumor cells. The defense is said to be created in two different ways; by creating a direct membrane contact with the tumor cells in a non-specific way, i.e. antibody-independent process, secondly by antibody dependent cell-mediated cyto-toxicity wherein NK cells bind to antitumor antibodies present on the surface of tumor cells.

12.7.2. Mononuclear cells

The prime cells of mononuclear phagocytic system are the circulating monocytes and macrophages in the tissues. Macrophages which are dispersed throughout the body can be classified into *fixed macrophages* and *wandering* or *free macrophages*. The fixed macrophages serve different functions in different tissues and their names reflect their location. These cells in the liver are called *Kupffer cells*, *histocytes* in the connective tissue; *alveolar macrophages* in the lungs; *mesangial cells* in the kidney and microglial cells in brain. Generally, the macrophages are in resting stage, but in the course of an immune response, a variety of stimuli activate macrophages.

12.7.2.1. Antigen-presenting cells (APC)

APCs are one among the two types of mononuclear cells. Their role is to present antigen to specific antigen-sensitive lymphocytes. They are primarily found in the skin, lymph nodes, spleen and thymus. The archetypal APC is the Langerhans cell in the skin. These cells have a characteristic *tennis racket* granules termed **Briback granules** (Fig. 12.9).

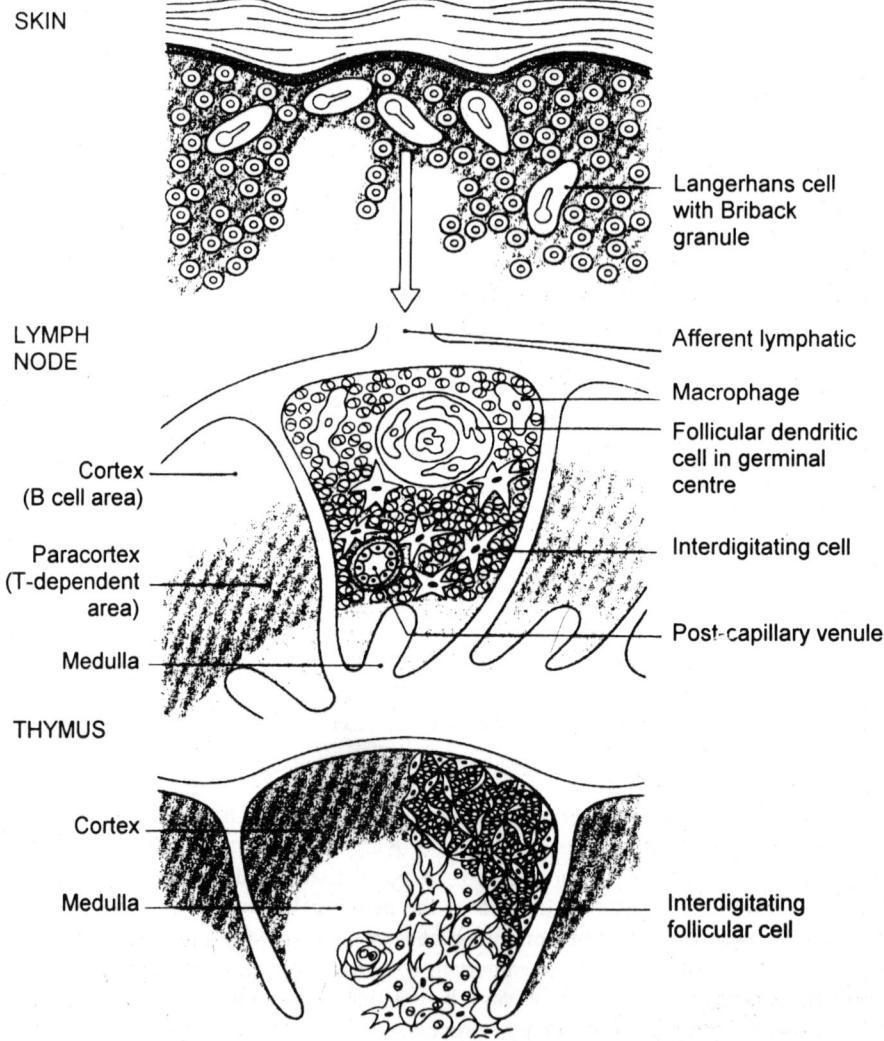

Fig. 12.9 : Antigen presenting cells (APC)

They migrate via the afferent lymphatics as *'veiled cells'* into the paracortex of the draining lymph node (Fig.12.9) and interdigitate with many T cells. This provides as an efficient mechanism to present antigen, carried from the skin, to T cells in the draining lymph nodes. These APCs are rich in class II MHC antigens and are important for presenting antigens to T cells. The other specialized APCs include, the follicular dentritic cells, found in the secondary follicles of the B cell areas of the lymph nodes and spleen.

The other cells of the immune system are polymorphonuclear granulocytes which include neutrophils, eosinophils, basophils, mast cells and platelets.

12.8. ORGANS OF THE IMMUNE SYSTEM

A number of organs are involved in the development of an immune response and they impart different functions.

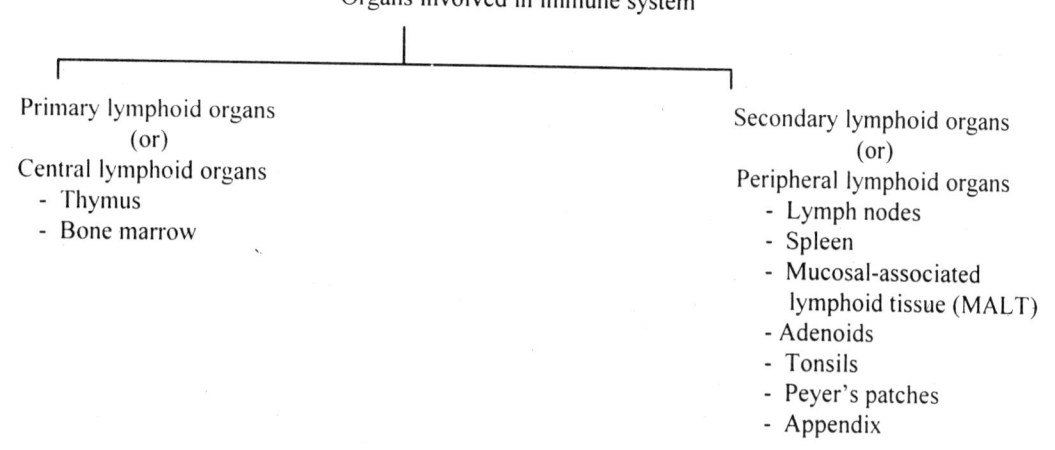

Organs involved in immune system

Primary lymphoid organs
(or)
Central lymphoid organs
- Thymus
- Bone marrow

Secondary lymphoid organs
(or)
Peripheral lymphoid organs
- Lymph nodes
- Spleen
- Mucosal-associated
  lymphoid tissue (MALT)
- Adenoids
- Tonsils
- Peyer's patches
- Appendix

12.9. HUMORAL IMMUNITY

Emil von Behring and Shibasaburo Kitasato in 1890 were the first to present to the World the insights of mechanism involved in immunity. They demonstrated that serum from animals, previously immunized, when administered to non-immunized animals, provided immunization to these animals. Since the immunity was mediated by antibodies contained in body fluids (in early days it was known as *humors*), the kind of immunity was named *humoral immunity*.

Humoral immunity or response is carried by a special group of cells called B cells. These B cells are responsible for the production of antibodies. The humoral response, which involves in the elimination of extracellular pathogens, is well classified by the production of a large number of antibody molecules. B cells which are produced in the bone marrow, mature and migrate into the lymphoidal organ, where they encounter antigen (Fig. 12.10). When an appropriate antigen contacts the antigen receptor antibodies on a B cell, the B cell proliferates into a large clone of cells. This phenomenon is known as clonal selection (discussed in the early part of this chapter). Sometimes, the production of antibodies by a B cell depends on other cells e.g., production of antibodies against T-dependent antigens requires the help of certain macrophages and T cells.

The above discussion makes it clear that humoral immune system involves antibodies that are found in blood plasma and lymph.

12.10. CELL-MEDIATED IMMUNITY

As the name suggests, it is clear that immunity is produced by transfer of some cells. It was observed that immunity against certain organisms, acquired by simple transfer of serum. Later on it was recognized that transfer of certain cells (lymphocytes) could produce immunity. It was Elie Metchnikoff in 1883, who discovered that cells also contribute to the immune system. He observed that some white blood cells were able to engulf the micro-organism and he named these cells as *phagocytes*. The principal cells involved in cell-mediated immunity and their function are given in table 12.2.

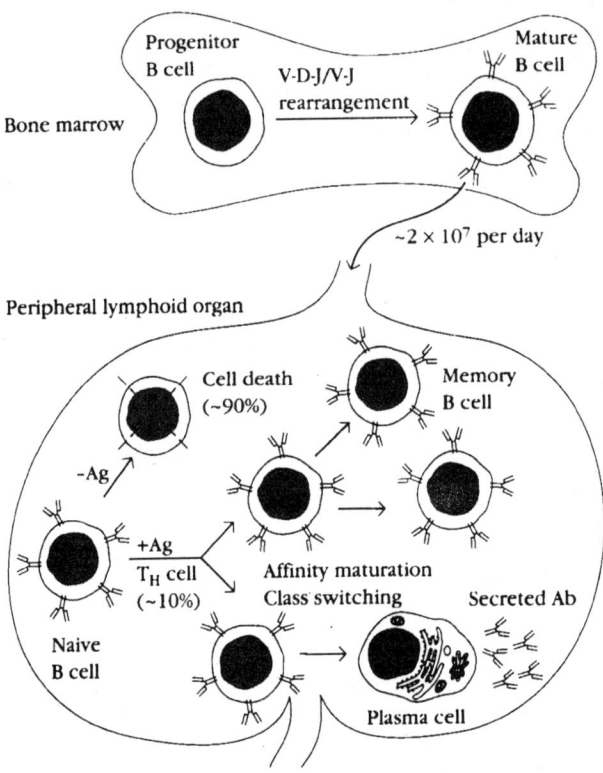

Fig. 12.10 : Schematic presentation: possible fate of B cells

T cells, like B cells, have specificity for a single antigen indicating the presence of T cell receptors which can recognize the antigen (Fig.12.11). However, the response is not on the same line, for the reason being, soluble antigens are unable to stimulate T cells as they cannot bind to T cells. A T cell responds only to those antigens processed by an antigen-presenting cell (APC).

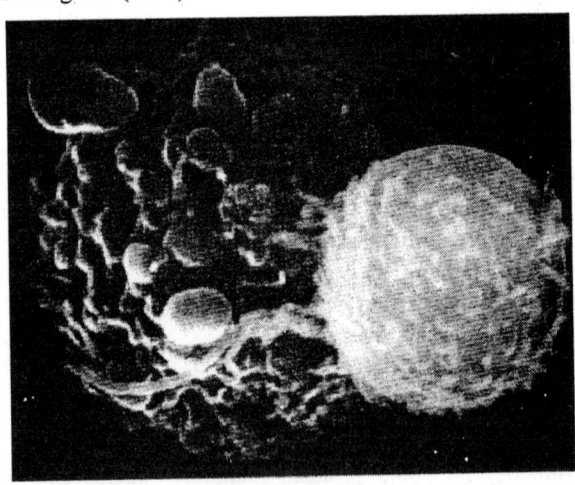

Fig. 12.11 : Killer T-lymphocytes inducing a cancer cell to undergo programmed cell death

As we have discussed earlier in this chapter under B cells the major difference between T cell response and B cell response is that, the T cell recognizes an antigen only when it is in close association with a major histocompatibility complex (MHC) antigen. This type of recognition is known as associative recognition.

Table 12.2 : Different cells involved in cell-mediated immunity and their functions

Cell	Function
Helper T Cell (T_H)	Necessary for B cells activation by T-dependent antigens
Suppressor T cells ((T_S)	Regulates immune response and helps in maintaining immune tolerance
Delayed hypersensitivity T cell (T_D)	Provides protection against infectious agents; causes inflammation in association to tissue transplant rejection
Cytotoxic T cell (T_C)	Destroys target cells on contact
Killer cell (K)	Attacks antibody-coated target cells
Natural Killer cell (NK)	Attacks and destroys target cells

Once the APC is stimulated by an antigen, the cell starts secreting a substance called *interleukin-1* (IL-1), a monokine (secreted by macrophages and biologically active). This biologically active substance in turn activates the T cell, which in turn begins to synthesize interleukin-2 (IL-2). The T cell also synthesizes surface receptors for IL-2. When the receptors bind to the IL-2, the T cells begin to proliferate and differentiate into different effector cells. IL-2 receptors on T cells are present only if the T cell has been stimulated by an antigen (Fig. 12.12).

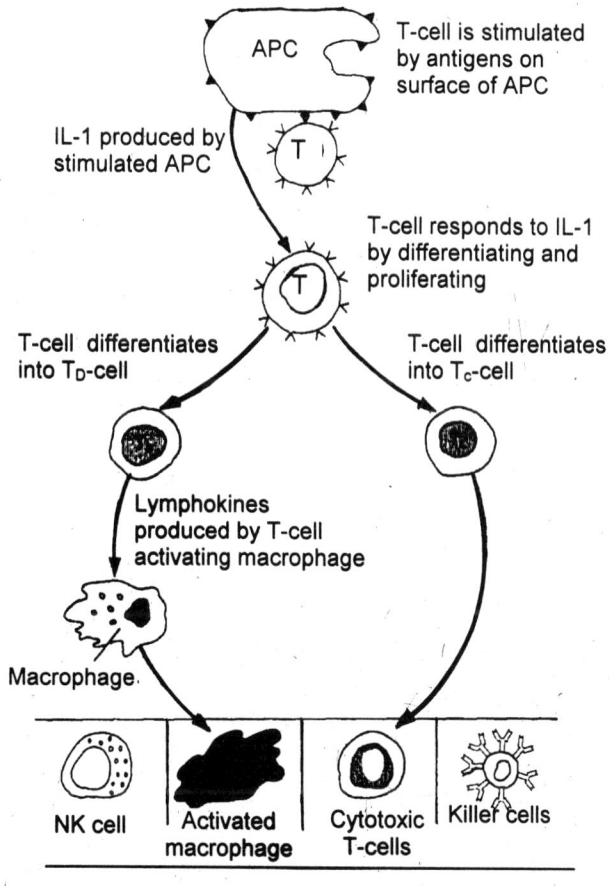

Fig. 12.12 : Cell-mediated immunity

A list of some diseases based on phagocytic, humoral, cell-mediated and combined humoral and cell-mediated deficiencies is given in table 12.3.

Antigens are substances of various chemical natures capable of stimulating the immune system to produce a response specifically directed at the inducing substance and not towards unrelated substance. The molecular properties of antigens and the specificity of the immune response to chemical structures (antigenic determinants), play a central role in understanding the immune system. An antibody directed towards an antigenic determinant of a particular molecule will react only with this determinant or another very similar structure. Even a minor change in the shape or chemical modification in the determinant will markedly alter the ability of the determinant to react with antibody.

Table 12.3 : Immunodeficiency related diseases based on cells involved in immune response

Phagocytic deficiencies	Humoral deficiencies	Cell-mediated deficiencies	Combined Humoral and Cell mediated deficiencies
Congenital agranulocytosis	X-linked agammaglobuli-nemia (XLA)	Di-George syndrome	Reticular dysgenesis
Leukocyte-adhesion deficiency (LAD)	X-linked hyper Ig M (XHM) syndrome	Nude mice	Bare-lymphocyte syndrome
lazy-leukocyte syndrome	Common variable hypogammaglobulinema (CVH)		X-linked SCID
Chronic granulomatus disease (CGD)	Selective immunoglobulin deficiencies		Autosomal recessive SCID
			ADA deficiency SCID
			PNP deficiency SCID
			CB-17 scid mouse
			Wiskott-Aldrich syndrome (WAS)

12.11. IMMUNOLOGIC PROPERTIES OF ANTIGENS

On the basis of the immunological properties of antigen, they can be categorized as immunogenic, antigenic, allerogenic and tolerogenic.

Immunogenic substances are those which are capable of inducing an immune response whether humoral or cell-mediated.

$$\text{B cells + antigen} \longrightarrow \text{plasma cells + memory cells}$$
$$\text{T cells + antigen} \longrightarrow \text{T effector cells + memory cells}$$

All immunogenic substances are said to be antigenic

Antigenic substances are those which have the ability to combine specifically with the final products of a immunogenic response (i.e., antibodies/or cell-surface receptors). In contrast, some small molecules referred to as *haptens* are not capable by themselves of inducing a specific immune response. In simple terms, they lack immunogenicity. In order to induce a immune response, the hapten requires to be attached to a carrier molecule (usually a serum protein such as albumin). Now, the hapten molecule acts as a determinant of antigenic, specificity and is referred to as an *antigenic determinant.*

Allerogenic substances are those which have the ability to induce various types of allergic responses. *Allergens* are immunogens that tend to activate specific types of humoral or cell-mediated responses.

Tolerogenic substances are those which possess the capacity to induce specific immunologic non-responsiveness in either the humoral or cell-mediated branch.

12.12. FACTORS INFLUENCING IMMUNOGENICITY

The following factors are influential in providing an effective protection against infectious agents.

1. The immune system must be able to recognize bacteria, bacterial products, fungi parasites and viruses as immunogens.

2. Immune system usually recognizes a particular macromolecule of an infectious disease generally proteins or polysaccharides.

3. Lipids and nucleic acids do not serve as immunogens.

4. When complexed to proteins or polysaccharides, lipids and nucleic acids serve as immunogens.

5. Soluble proteins or polysaccharides are used as immunogens for study of humoral immunity [e.g., Bovine serum albumin (BSA)].

6. Only proteins serve as immunogens for cell mediated immunity. However, they are not recognized directly, instead, they are processed into small peptides and then presented along in association with major histocompatibility complex (MHC).

7. Immunogenicity is not an intrinsic property of a macromolecule.

8. To elicit an immune response, a molecule must be recognized as non-self by the biological system. This is termed as foreignness.

9. Generally, a substance to be immunogenic should have a molecular weight not less than 5,000 Da.

10. Co-polymers of sufficient size, containing two or more different amino acids are immunogenic while polymers composed of a single amino acid or sugar lack immunogenicity.

11. Macromolecules that cannot be degraded and processed by antigen-presenting cells are poor immunogens.

12. Large, insoluble macromolecules are generally more immunogenic as they are readily phagocytosed and processed.

13. Intermolecular chemical cross-linking, heat aggregation and attachment to insoluble matrices have been used to increase the insolubility of macromolecules and there by the immunogenicity.

14. Genetic constitution of an immunized animal also influences the type of immune response that is manifested.

15. Genes encoding B-cell and T-cell receptors and various proteins involved in immune regulation also play a key role in immune response.

16. The dose of immunogen is important in eliciting a immune response, the dose should be neither high nor low.

17. The route by which the immunogens are administered is also critical. Generally, they are administered by routes other than oral, e.g. intradermal, subcutaneous, intravenous, intramuscular, etc.

18. Use of adjuvants (substances which when mixed with an antigen, serve to enhance immunogenicity of that antigen).

19. Low molecular weight substances are antigenic (e.g., aspirin, penicillin and sulfonamides). This is because they form a covalent bond complex with tissue proteins.

20. Particle size also plays an important role in determining antigenicity. Example, aggregated BSA is more effective as compared to aggregate free BSA.

12.13. ANTIGENIC DETERMINANTS OR EPITOPES

Immunogenic molecules are generally not recognized by immune cells or do they interact with them, but the lymphocytes recognize the discrete site on the macromolecules called epitopes or antigenic determinants. Epitopes are immunologically active regions of an immunogen which bind specifically to membrane receptors of an antigen on lymphocytes or to secreted antibodies. Antigen-lymphocytes interaction involves several levels of antigenic structure depending upon whether they are protein antigens or polysaccharide antigens. In the case of protein antigens, the structure may involve elements of primary, secondary, tertiary and or quaternary structure of the protein. While in the case of polysaccharide antigens, extensive side-chain branching via glycosidic bonds affects the over all three dimensional conformation of the individual epitopes.

T cells and B cells exhibit fundamental differences in an antigen recognition. B cells recognize soluble antigen when it binds to their membrane-bound antibody. Since B cells bind antigen that is free in solution, the epitopes recognized are highly accessible sites on the exposed surface of the immunogens. Such exposed epitopes generally contain hydrophilic amino acids and are often located in bands in the amino acid chain, imparting a greater degree of mobility to these residues. T cells, on the other hand, recognize processed peptides associated with MHC molecules on the surface of antigen presenting cells and alter self-cells. T cells thus exhibit MHC-restricted antigen recognition.

The CD4 sub-population recognizes antigen in association with class II MHC molecules, where as the CD8 sub-population recognizes antigen in association with class I MHC molecules and generally functions as T cytotoxic cells. Thus, T cell epitopes cannot be considered apart from their associated MHC molecules.

12.13.1. Properties of B cell epitopes

Several B cell properties have been generalized from study with immunogens. Using this, the conformation of the epitope recognized by B cell has been determined. They are:

1. The size of a B cell epitope is determined by the size of the antigen binding site on the antibody molecules displayed by these cells.
2. The binding of an antibody to an epitope involves weak non-covalent interactions.
3. The size of the epitope recognized by a B cell is determined by the size, shape and amino acid residues of the antibody's binding site.
4. B cell epitopes in native proteins generally are hydrophilic amino acids on the protein surface.
5. B cell epitope must be accessible in order to be able to bind to an antibody.
6. Amino acid sequences that are hidden within the interior of a protein cannot function as B cell epitopes unless the protein is first denatured.
7. Most antibodies elicited by globular protein antigens bind to the protein only when it is in its native conformation.
8. Epitopes may be composed of sequential continuous residues along the polypeptide chain or non-sequential residues from segments of the chain brought together by the folded conformation of the protein.
9. Sequential and non-sequential epitopes generally behave differently when a protein is fragmented or reduced.
10. B cell epitopes tend to be located in flexible regions of an immunogen and display site mobility. The epitopes on a number of protein antigens (myohemerytherin, insulin, cytochrome C, myoglobulin and hemoglobulin), by comparing with the positions of the known B epitopes, revealed that the major antigenic determinants in these proteins are generally located in the most mobile regions.
11. Complex proteins contain multiple overlapping B cell epitopes.
12. Some epitopes known as immunodominant induce a more pronounced immune response than other epitopes in a particular animal.

12.13.2. Properties of T cell epitopes

1. Gell and Benacerraf in 1959 suggested that there is a qualitative difference between the T cell and the B cell response to protein antigens. They compared the humoral and cell mediated responses to a series of native and denatured protein antigens. They found that primary immunization was with a native protein. In contrast, the secondary cell mediated response discriminate between native and denatured proteins.
2. Oligomeric peptides function as T cell epitopes. The antigen binding cleft of an MHC molecule determines the nature and size of the peptide(s) that it can bind and consequently the maximal size of the T cell epitope. Studies of the binding of the peptides to class I MHC molecules have revealed that peptides of 9 amino acid residues (monomers) bind most strongly; peptides of 8-11 residues also bind but generally with lower affinity than monomers. In the case of class II MHC molecules, peptides of 11-17 amino acid residues are preferentially bound.
3. Antigenic peptides recognized by T cells form trimolecular complexes with a T cell receptor and a MHC molecule. Antigens recognized by T cells must, therefore, possess two distinct interaction sites: one (the epitope) interacts with the T cell receptor, and the other called the agretope, interacts with a MHC molecule. The binding of a peptide to the cleft in a MHC molecule does not appear to have the kind of fine specificity exhibited in the interaction between an antibody and its epitope. Instead, a given MHC molecule can selectively bind a variety of different peptides. For example, the class II MHC molecules designated IA^d can bind peptides from ovalbumin (residues 323 to 329), hemagglutinin (residues 130 to 142), and lambda repressor (residues 12 to 16). These broad, but selective interactions suggest that the agretopes on these various peptides may share some structural features, enabling them to bind to the same MHC molecule.

4. Antigen processing is required to generate peptides that interact specifically with MHC **molecules.** Endogenous antigens and exogenous antigens appear to be processed by different intracellular **pathways.** Endogenous antigens are processed into peptides within the cytoplasm, while the exogenous antigens **are** processed within the endocytic pathway. Processing yields antigenic peptides that associate with class I or class II MHC molecules; the resulting peptide-MHC complexes are then presented on the cell surface **where** they can be recognized by T cells (Fig. 12.13).

5. Antigens recognized by T cells often contain amphipathic peptides. The primary function of the **antigen** processing may be to unfold an antigen and reveal internal regions that are amphipathic (i.e., possessing **both** hydrophilic and hydrophobic amino acid residues). The hydrophobic residues may act as agretope, **interacting** with MHC molecules, and the hydrophilic residues may act as epitopes, interacting with T cell receptors.

6. Immunodominant T cell epitopes are determined in part by the set of MHC molecules expressed by an individual. It has been suggested through various experiments that the MHC plays a significant role in determining each T cell epitopes in a given antigen will be immunodominant in a given individual.

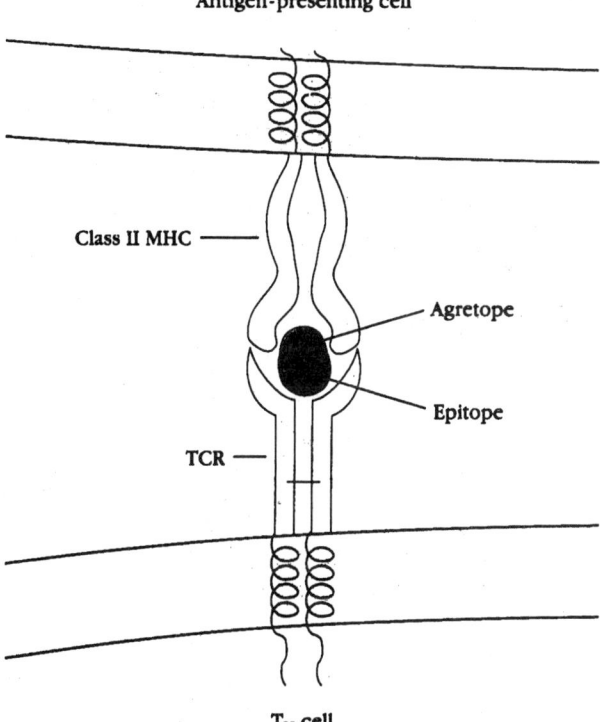

Fig. 12.13 : Schematic diagram of the ternary complex formed between T-cell receptor (TCR), antigen and MHC molecule

12.14. HAPTENS

Landsteiner in the 1920s, chemically defined a system for studying the binding of an individual antibody to a unique epitope on a complex protein antigen. In his approach he coupled small organic molecules called **haptens** to larger protein molecules called carriers. The resulting hapten-carrier conjugate was used to immunize animals. Haptens are small molecules that can bind to antibodies but cannot by themselves function as immunogens. The system developed by Landsteiner does not stimulate a clonal selection alone. However, if multiple copies of a hapten are coupled to a large non-immunogenic homopolymer, the molecule can sometimes behave as an immunogen. Here, the homopolymer provides the requisite size, and the hapten provides the complexity and multivalency. The major advantage of the hapten carrier system is that it provides immunologists with a chemically defined determinant that can be subsequently modified by chemical means to determine the effect of various chemical structures on immune specificity. He also studied specifically, the reaction of the anti-hapten antibodies in the immune serum and that of antibodies to the original carrier epitopes. Landsteiner further tested if an antihapten antibody could bind to other haptens having a slightly different chemical structure. Many biologically important substances, including drugs, peptide hormones and steroid hormones can function as haptens. The home pregnancy test kit, which determines the presence or absence of human chronic gonadotropin (HCG) in a woman's urine, is a classical hapten-inhibition assay.

12.15. MITOGENS

Mitogens are agents that are able to induce cell division in a high percentage of T or B cells. Unlike immunogens, which activate only lymphocytes bearing specific receptors, mitogens activate many clones of T or B cells irrespective of their antigen specificity. Because of this ability, mitogens are known as polyclonal activators. A variety of diverse agents function as mitogens. A number of common mitogens are proteins (called lectins) that are derived from plants and bind sugars. This immediately puts a question in the mind, Are all lectins mitogenic in nature?. The answer is No. Lectin recognizes different glycoproteins on the surface of various cells, including lymphocytes. Their binding often leads to agglutination, or clustering of the cells, followed by cellular activation. Some mitogens preferentially activate B cells, some activate T cells, while some activate both. Three commonly used lectins with mitogenic activity are concanavalin A (Con A), phyto-hemagglutinin (PHA) and pokeweed mitogen. Each of these binds to carbohydrate residues in glycoproteins and are able to cross link glycoproteins on the surface of cells. The lipopolysaccharide (LPS) component of the gram-negative bacterial cell wall functions as a B-cell mitogen, Con A and PHA are T-cell mitogens, while pokeweed mitogen acts as both. Among the group of T cell mitogens, an unusual group of substances, known as *superantigens*, is found to be most potent. These superantigens are said to bind to residues in the V_β domain of the T cell receptor and residues in class II MHC molecules outside of the antigen binding cleft (Fig.12.14).

Antigen-presenting cell

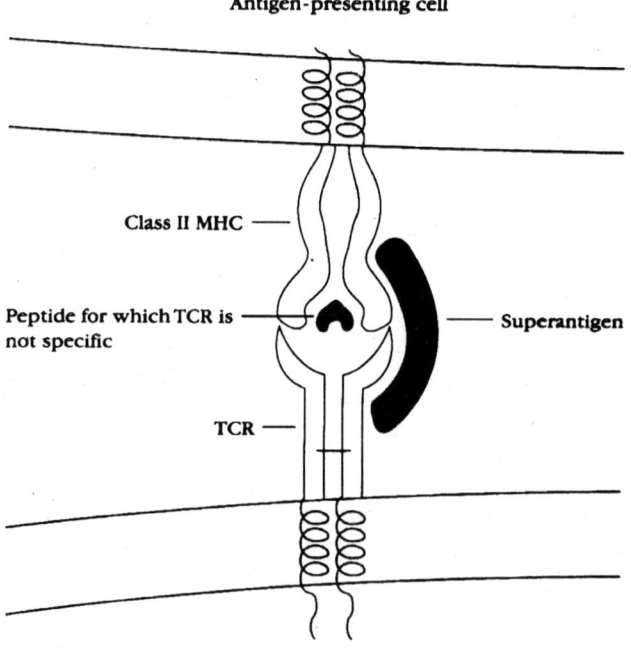

Fig. 12.14 : A ternary complex formed between a T-cell receptor, superantigen and MHC molecule

In this way the superantigen cross-links a T cell to a class II MHC molecule in an antigen-independent manner, resulting in the activation of distinct set of V_β expressing T cells. Staphylococcal enterotoxins (Ses) and toxic-shock syndrome toxin 1 (TSST1) are examples of superantigens. These toxins are said to activate a large number of T_H cells by cross-linking the T cell receptors with any class II MHC molecule expressed on an antigen-presenting cell.

12.16. ANTIBODIES OR IMMUNOGLOBULINS

The immunoglobulins or antibodies are a group of glycoproteins present in the serum and tissue fluids of all animals. Immunoglobulins, function as antibodies, the antigen binding proteins are present on the B cell membrane and are also secreted by plasma cells. The secreted antibodies serve as the effector molecules of humoral immunity and are said to circulate in the blood, searching for and neutralizing or eliminating antigens. Their production is induced when host's lymphoid system comes in contact with immunogenic foreign molecules (antigens) and they bind specifically to the antigen which induces their formation. All immunoglobulins share certain structural features and thus to a significant extent governs the specificity and effective functions of immunoglobulins. Here, the main focus will be on the structure and function of immunoglobulins. It was in 1939 when Tiselius and Kabat subjected the serum of ovalbumin immunized rabbits to electrophoresis, and obtained four fractions; albumin, the alpha (α), beta (β) and the gamma (γ) globulins. While the same serum when reacted with an antigen formed a precipitate. The serum left over after separating the precipitate when subjected to electrophoresis showed a significant drop in the amount of γ globulin fraction, thus it was identified that the γ globulin fraction contained serum antibodies, which they named as *immunoglobulins* (Ig)

12.16.1. Immunoglobulin structure

Porter and Edelman in 1960s first separated the γ globulin fraction of serum into a high molecular weight fractions with a sedimentation constant of 19S and a low molecular weight fraction with a sedimentation constant of 7S with a molecular weight of 1,50,000. They designated this 7S fraction of γ globulins as immunoglobulin (IgG) for their studies.

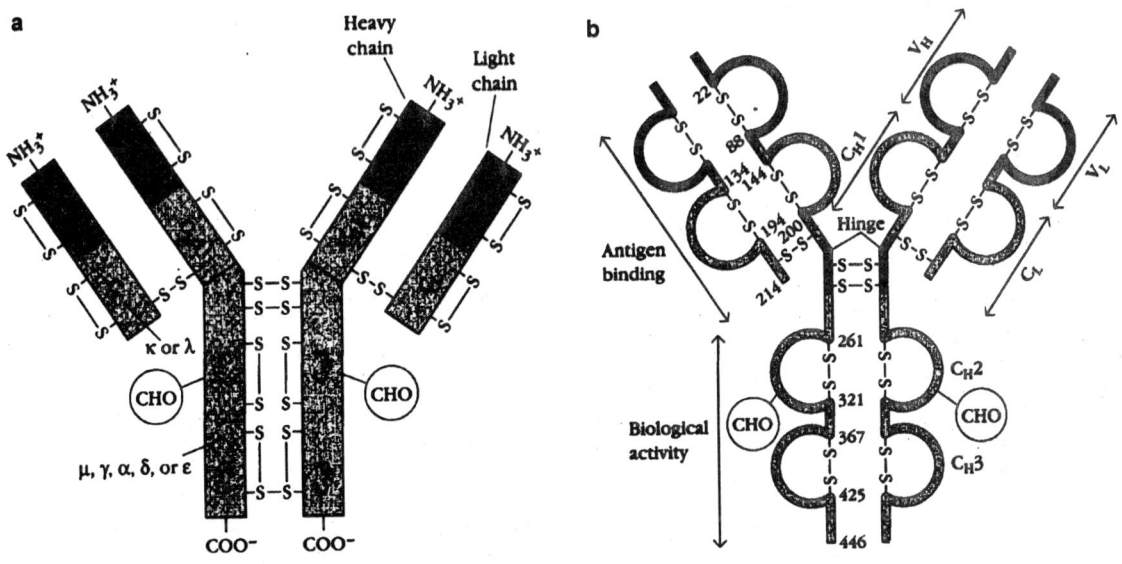

Fig. 12.15 : Primary and secondary structure of immunoglobulins

The chain structure of IgG was first suggested by Edelman and was latter on confirmed by Porter. Their experiments revealed that the 1,50,000 MW IgG was composed of two 50,000 MW polypeptide chains designated as heavy (H) chain and two 25,000 MW chains, designated as light (L) chains.

Porter in 1962 proposed a prototype structure of IgG (12.16). He found that IgG on brief digestion with papain resulted in the formation of fragments. Among the fragments, two were identical (each with 45,000 MW) called **Fab fragments** due to their 'antigen-binding' activity and one fragment, namely the **Fc fragment**, so named because they crystallized during cold storage. However, when another scientist namely Alford Nisonoff found that on digestion with pepsin, IgG produced only a single fragment with molecular weight 1,00,000/ He designated this as **F(ab')₂ fragment** which like Fab could precipitate antigens. However, no Fc fragment could be recovered by him.

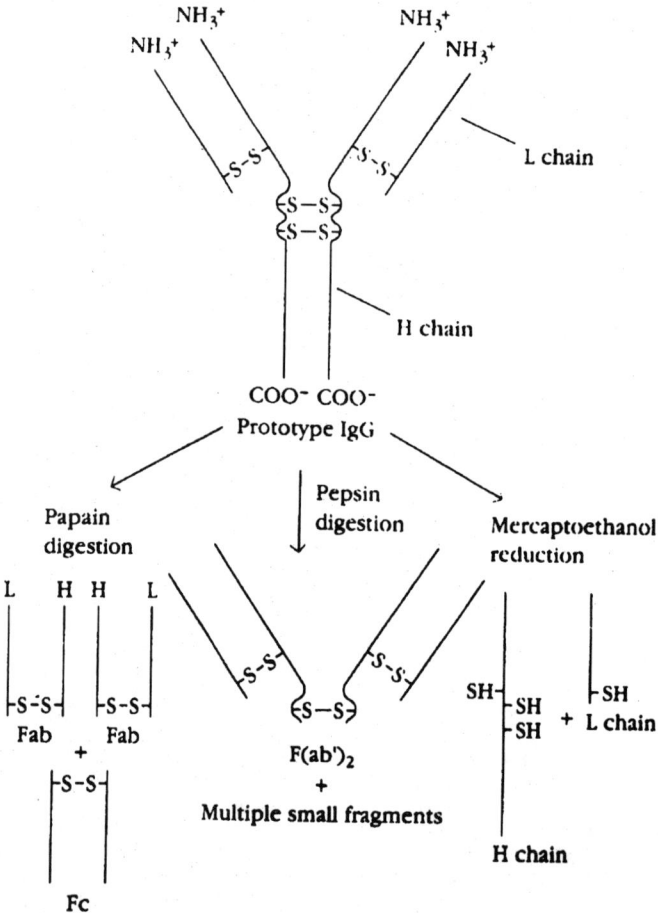

Fig. 12.16 : Prototype structure of IgG

12.16.2. Immunoglobulin sequences

A single antibody has two identical heavy chains and two identical light chains. Immunoglobulins have similar basic structure and similar chemical properties. However, their antigen binding specificity and their exact amino acid sequence differ.

Light chain sequencing: Studies carried out on various amino acid sequences revealed that the amino-terminal half of the amino acid chain varied among different proteins. This region is called **Variable (V)**

region. The carboxyl terminal half of the molecule is called as **Constant (C)** region. The constant region was found to have two basic amino acid sequences named **Kappa(κ)** and **Lambda (λ)** (Fig.12.17). In human being 60% of the light chains are Kappa and 40% Lambda, whereas in mice 95% of the light chains are Kappa while only 5% constitute Lambda. A noteworthy point is that a singly antibody molecule expresses either κ light chains or λ light chains but never both.

Heavy chain sequencing: The heavy chains of antibodies like their counter parts (light chain) showed a variation in their amino terminal which were again designated as variable (V) region. However, the remaining part of the protein revealed five basic amino acid sequence patterns (μ,γ,α,δ and ε) corresponding to five different heavy chain constant (C) regions (Fig.12.15). It is these chains (heavy) which determines the class on antibody, i.e. IgG , IgA, IgM, IgE and IgD. A single antibody molecule has two identical light and heavy chains. However, the light chain may be κ or λ (Table 12.4).

Table 12.4 : Composition of immunoglobulin chain among the five different classes in human

Class	Heavy chain	Light chain	Subclasses
IgG	γ	κ/λ	γ1, γ2, γ3, γ4
IgA	α	κ/λ	α1, α2
IgM	μ	κ/λ	– – – –
IgD	δ	κ/λ	– – – –
IgE	ε	κ/λ	– – – –

12.16.3. Antigenic determinants on immunoglobulins

As we know by now that antibodies are comprising of glycoproteins, which alone can function as a potent immunogen there by inducing an antibody response. The antigen determinants fall into three major categories; isotypic, allotypic and idiotypic determinants, which are located in characteristic portions of the molecule (Fig.12.17).

12.16.4. Isotypic determinants

Isotypic determinants, define constant region determinants that distinguish each heavy chain class and subclass and each light chain type and subtype within a species. Each isotype is said to be encoded by a separate constant region gene and they do not vary within species. A healthy member of a species will express all isotypes in their serum. However, different species inherit different constant region genes, thus expressing different isotypes. Therefore, when an antibody from one species is injected into another species, the isotypic determinants are recognized as foreign and there by inducing antibody response to the foreign antibody. This has generally been used in research to determine the class or subclass antibodies produced during an immune response.

12.16.5. Allotypic determinants

This refers to genetic variation within species. Although all members of a species inherit the same set of isotypic genes, multiple alleles exist for some of the genes. These alleles cause a difference in amino acid sequence. In humans, allotypes have been characterized for all four IgG subclass for one IgA subclasses and for the κ light chain. Antibodies to allotypic determinant can be produced following a blood transfusion or from mother to fetus or by injecting antibodies from one species to another.

12.16.6. Idiotypic determinants

Variation in the variable domain (in particular to the highly variable segments) produces idiotypes. Idiotypes are usually specific for individual antibody clone, but are sometimes shared between different clones. Each individual antigenic determinant of the variable region is referred to an idiotope.

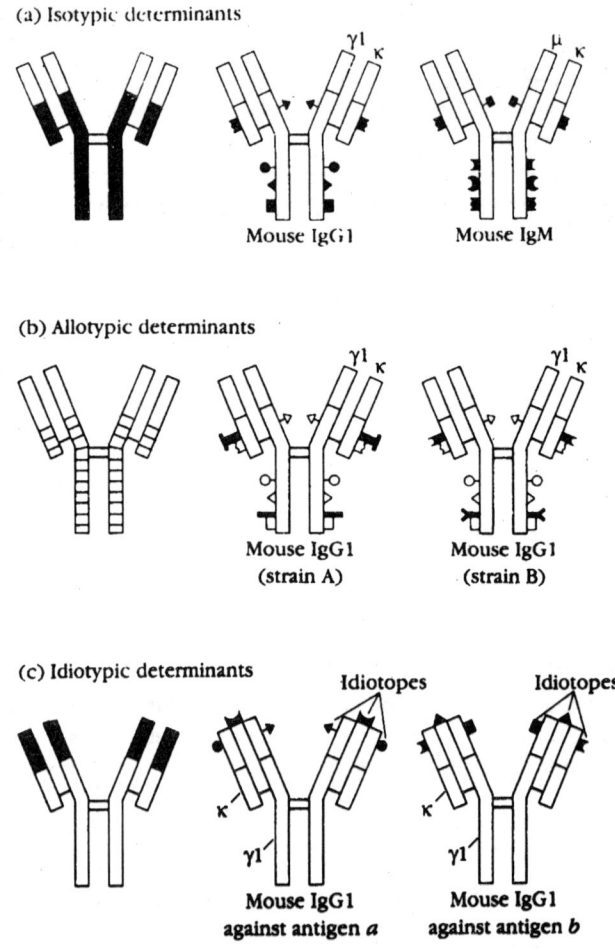

(a) Isotypic determinants

Mouse IgG1   Mouse IgM

(b) Allotypic determinants

Mouse IgG1
(strain A)

Mouse IgG1
(strain B)

(c) Idiotypic determinants

Idiotopes   Idiotopes

Mouse IgG1
against antigen *a*

Mouse IgG1
against antigen *b*

Fig. 12.17 : Antigenic determinants of immunoglobulins

12.17. IMMUNOGLOBULIN CLASSES

In this section, we will be discussing about different immunoglobulin classes which differ from each other uniquely in their size, structure and amino acid sequences in the heavy chain constant region that results in structural and functional differences among different immunoglobulin. Five distinct immunoglobulin classes have been recognized in higher mammals namely IgG, IgA, IgM, IgD and IgE. These five classes typically represent immunoglobulin isotypes.

12.17.1. Immunoglobulin G (IgG)

IgG, the major immunoglobulin isotype in normal human serum constitutes 70-75% of the total serum immunoglobulin. IgG is a monomeric protein with two γ heavy chains and two κ or λ light chains (Fig.12.16). It has a molecular weight of 1,46,000 with a sedimentation coefficient of 7S. The IgG class is distributed evenly between the intra and extravascular pools. It is the major antibody of secondary immune responses and the exclusive-toxin class. There are four IgG subclasses namely IgG1, IgG2, IgG3 and IgG4 numbered in accordance with their order of occurrence in the serum. One important thing to be noted is that no two subclasses are identical. This may be either with reference to the number or the distribution of interchain disulfide linkage. The four subclasses are encoded by different germ-line C_H genes whose DNA sequences are

90-95% homologous. The difference in amino acid sequence in IgG subclasses is directly related to its biological activity. While IgG1, IgG3 and IgG4 could clearly cross the placenta and play an important role in protecting the fetus, IgG2 crosses partially in some cases but not totally. Similarly, the complement activation efficiency also differs; IgG3 is found to be the most effective one followed by IgG1, IgG2 and IgG4 and said to be totally ineffective in activating a complement sequence. The opsonin activity of IgG is attributed .to its binding to Fc receptors on phagocytic cells. Again, the different subclasses have different affinity. IgG1 and IgG3 have a higher affinity to Fc receptors while IgG4 has an intermediate affinity, IgG2 ıs said to have an extremely low affinity.

12.17.2. Immunoglobulin A (IgA)

Immunoglobulin A (IgA), the predominant immunoglobulin in seromucous secretions, constitutes 15-20% of the normal human serum immunoglobulin pool. It is protected from proteolysis by combination with another protein the secretory component IgA is predominantly seen in external secretions such as breast milk, saliva, tears and mucous of the bronchial, genitourinary and digestive tracts. Hence, they are frequently known as **secretory IgA (sIgA). In serum,** IgA exists as a monomer, however, in most cases it is polymeric, i.e. dimers, trimers, etc. The sIgA consists of a dimer or tetramer, a J chain polypeptide and polypeptide chain called secretory component.

The secretory component is a polypeptide with 70,000 MW and produced by epithelial cells of mucous membranes. It consists of five immunoglobulin like domains that bind to the Fc regions of the IgA dimer.

12.17.3. Immunoglobulin M (IgM)

IgM accounts for about 10% of the total serum immunoglobulin with an average serum concentration of 1.5% mg/ml. Unlike IgG or IgA, IgM has a pentameric structure in which individual heavy chains have a molecular weight of approximately 65,000 while the total molecular weight is amounting to 9,70,000. The monomeric units consist of two μ heavy chains and two light chains. The subunits are held together by disulfide bonds between their carboxyl terminal (Cμ4/Cμ4) domains and Cμ3/Cμ3. The subunits are so arranged that their Fc region is in the center of the pentamer. It is believed that IgM has 10 antigen binding sites but they are unable to combine with the antigen with similar efficiency thus making it difficult to demonstrate the presence of 10 sites. In addition to the above, a Fc linked polypeptide called J (joining) chain, which is disulfide bonded to the carboxyl terminal cysteine residue of two of the 10μ chains. It is just added before secretion of the pentamer and it is understood that the J chain appears to be required for polymerization of the monomer. The presence of the J chain allows IgM to bind to receptors on secretory cells, which helps them in transporting across the epithelial linings to the external secretions that bathe mucosal surfaces.

IgM is largely confined to the intravascular pool and is the predominant 'early' antibody frequently directed against antigenic complexes after a primary response. It is also the first to be synthesized by the neonate. Monomeric IgM is expressed as membrane bound antibody on B cells. Because of its pentameric structure, serum IgM has higher valency than others. For example, it takes 100-1000 times as many molecules of IgG as of IgM to achieve the same level of agglutination. Due to its large size, diffusion to the intracellular tissue fluids is very low.

12.17.4. Immunoglobulin D (IgD)

IgD constitutes for less than 1% of the total plasma immunoglobulin with a serum concentration of 30μg/ml. IgD, together with IgM, is the major membrane bound immunoglobulin expressed by mature B cells. Though their exact biological function is not clear they are thought to function in the activation of B cell by an antigen. IgD is more susceptible to proteolysis than any other immunoglobulin class. IgD has a simple disulfide bond between the δ chains and a high content of carbohydrate distributed in multiple oligosaccharide units. One of these units is rich in N-acetyl galactosamine, a sugar which occurs in IgA1 but not in other immunoglobulin.

12.18. ANTIGEN-ANTIBODY REACTIONS

The antigen-antibody reaction, a bimolecular association similar to an enzyme-substrate interaction is with the distinction that it does not lead to an irreversible chemical alteration. The reaction involves various non-covalent interactions between the antigenic determinant or epitope of the antigen and the variable region of the antibody. The non-covalent interactions include:

(1) Hydrogen bonds (2) Ionic bonds
(3) Hydrophobic interactions (4) Van der Waals interactions

Antigenic determinant + $V_{H/L}$ of antibody $\rightarrow$ Antigen-Antibody reaction

Table 12.5 : Summary of immunoglobulin classes

Characteristics	IgG	IgM	IgA	IgD	IgE
Location	Blood, lymph, intestine	Blood, lymph, B- cell surface	Secretions (saliva milk), blood, lymph	B cell surface, blood, lymph	Bound to mast and basophil cells through out the body, blood
% of total serum antibodies	80-85	5-10	15	0.2	0.002
Normal serum level (mg/ml)	3	1.5	2	0.03	0.0003
Molecular weight	1,50,000	9,00,000	3,20,000	1,85,000	2,00,000
Molecular form	Monomer	Pentamer	Dimer	Monomer	Monomer
In vivo serum half life (days)	23	5	6	3	2
Complement fixation	+	+	-	-	-
Placental transfer	+	-	-	-	-
Functions	Enhances phagocytosis toxins and virus neutralization and protection of fetus and new born	First Ab produced in response to initial infection. Especially effective against micro-organism and agglutinating antigens	Localized protection on mucosal surfaces	Unclear, but presence of B cells may indicate function in initiation of immune response	Allergic reactions

The antibody can combine only with antigen which is identical or nearly identical with the inducing antigen and not with unrelated antigens. When a molecule of antibody and antigen is brought together in solution, it interacts with each other by formation of a link between an antigen-antibody site in the immunoglobulin molecule, part of the Fab fragment and other antigenic determinant parts. The molecules which are held together by noncovalent intermolecules are effective only when the antigen-binding site and the antigenic determinant groups are able to make close contact. The better the fit, the closer the contact, stronger is the antigen-antibody bond. The strength of the sum total of non-covalent interactions between a single antigen binding site on an antibody and a single epitope is the **affinity** of the antibody for that epitope. The affinity at one binding site does not always reflect the true strength of the antibody-antigen interaction. When a complex antigen containing multiple, repeating antigenic determinants are mixed with antibodies containing multiple binding sites, the interaction of antibody with antigen at one site will increase the probability of reaction at a second site. The strength of such multiple interactions between a multivalent antibody and antigen is called **avidity**. The avidity of an antibody is a better measure than the affinity of its binding capacity within biological systems.

12.19. CROSS-REACTIVITY

Though antigen-antibody reactions are highly specific, they may cross react at times with an unrelated antigen if it has an identical epitope or if antibody specific for one epitope can bind to another. Cross-reactivity is often observed among polysaccharide antigens that contain similar oligosaccharide residues. For example, ABO blood group antigens have glycoproteins expressed on red blood cells (RBC).

Blood group antibodies + microbial antigen on intestinal bacteria

↓

induce antibody formation lacking in these antigen

↓

with oligosaccharide on RBC

The terminal sugar portion distinguishes the A and B blood group antigens. If an individual is lacking one or both of these antigen will have serum antibodies to the missing antigen(s). Thus, type O individual has both Anti A and Anti B antibody. Similarly, a type A individual has anti B while a B type individual has anti A. Their presence is justified due to cross-reactivity of the blood group antibodies by exposure to cross-reactive microbial antigens present on common intestinal bacteria and not by to exposure to RBC antigens.

The methods used for the detection of antigen-antibody reactions in the laboratory fall in two functional groups.

1. **procedure** designed to elucidate the cytodynamics of antibody formation which involved the study of the behavior of single cells or small populations of cells.
2. **procedure** involving the detection and quantitation of secreted antibodies circulating in the blood or present in the tissue fluids.

In practice, the union of antibody with antigen can be detected at two different levels.

a. Primary interaction

b. Secondary phenomena

Primary interaction is one in which the two reactants unite of which one or other reactant is labeled with a **suitable** marker such as a fluorescent dye or a radioactive isotope. This is the first level detection. The second level detection involves the detection after the primary interaction which develops in the formation of certain changes in the physical state of the complex, resulting in precipitation or agglutination of the components such as serum complement or histamine from mast cells. Reactions of this type are termed as **secondary phenomena**. This type of reaction can be used to identify antigens in the tissues or body fluids.

12.20. PRECIPITIN REACTIONS

The interaction between an antibody and antigen molecule in soluble form, forms a lattice that eventually develops into a visible precipitate. The formation of soluble antigen-antibody complex occurs within minutes while their visual recognition is very slow which often takes a day or two to reach completion. Formation of an antigen-antibody lattice depends on the valency of both the antibody and antigen. The prime requirement is that the antigen must be either bivalent or polyvalent and must possess at least two copies of the same epitope or different epitopes with different antibodies present in polyclonal antisera. A precipitin reaction will not take place with monovalent Fab fragments or monovalent antigens.

12.20.1. Precipitin reactions in fluids

Precipitin reaction, a simple reaction that occurs between antibody and antigen molecules in soluble form can be explained as follows. A quantitative precipitin reaction can be performed by placing a constant amount of antibody in a series of test tubes and by adding a measured amount of antigen to the tubes (Fig. 12.18). The formed precipitate is separated and measured. A precipitin curve is obtained by plotting the amount of precipitate against the antigen concentrations. This is well depicted in figure 12.19. It can be well understood that maximum precipitate occurs when the ratio of antibody to antigen is optimum. This is projected as the **equivalence zone**. As a large multimolecular lattice is formed at the equivalence zone it precipitates out due to their large size. The other two zones are the **antibody excess zone** and **antigen excess zone**. This test is a rapid qualitative **test for determining** the presence of antibody or antigen. This is performed by adding antiserum to small tube **and layering** antigen on top. If the antiserum contains antibodies specific for the test antigen, then the antibody and antigen diffuse towards each other and form a visible band of precipitate at the interface within few minutes (Fig.12.19). This test is of value in detecting and identifying antigens having applications in the typing of streptococci or pneumococci.

12.20.2. Precipitin reactions in gel (or) Immunodiffusion reactions

Precipitin reactions are not found only in fluids but also take place in agar matrix. The diffusion of antibody in antigen bearing agar or vice versa, results into the formation of a visible line of precipitate. This line occurs at the region of equivalence and no visible precipitate forms/occurs in region of antigen excess and antibody excess. These immunodiffusion reactions can be used in determining the relative concentration of antibodies or antigens to compare antigens or to determine the relative purity of an antigen preparation. Immunodiffusion technique can further classified into two techniques which are used commonly.

1. Radial immunodiffusion or Mancini method

2. Double immunodiffusion or Ouchterlony method

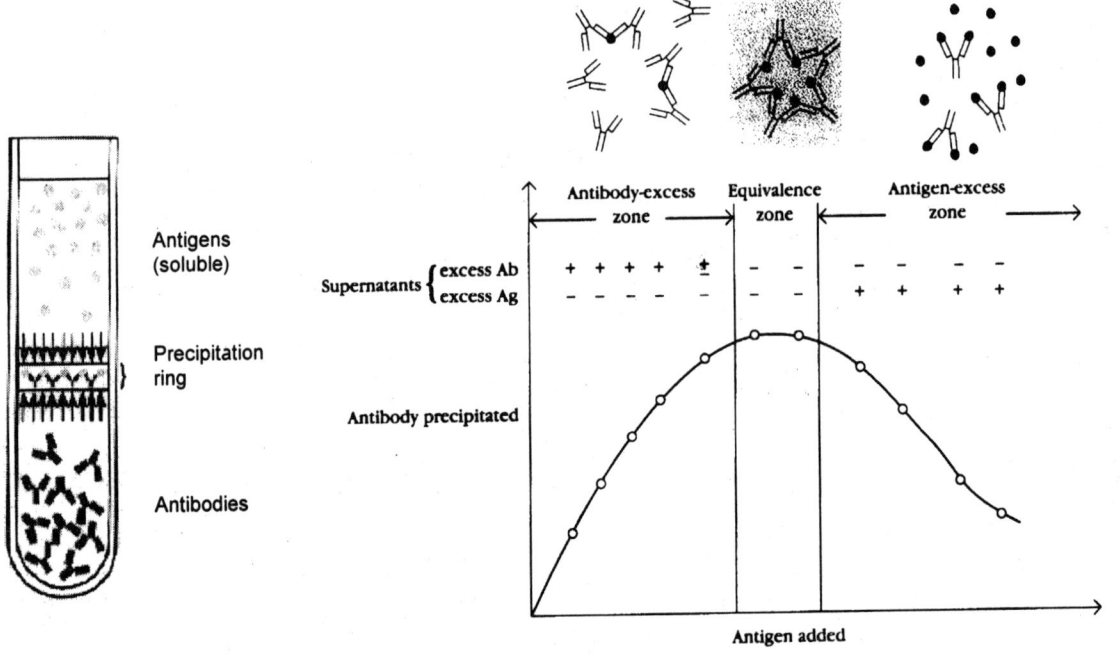

Fig. 12.18 : Immunoprecipitation ring test

Fig. 12.19 : Precipitin curve

12.20.2.1. Radial immunodiffusion or Mancini method

Radial immunodiffusion-method is a simple quantitative assay wherein an antigen sample is placed in a well and allowed to diffuse into agar containing a suitable dilution of an antiserum. A precipitin ring forms at the zone of equivalence. The area of precipitin ring is proportional to the concentration of antigen (Fig.12.20).

Comparing the area with a standard curve, the concentration of antigen can be determined. This technique is widely used to quantitate serum IgM, IgG and IgA by incorporating suitable anti-isotype antibody into the agar. It has gained wide application in determining concentrations of serum complement components. However, the test limits to concentration of antigens above 10 μg/ml.

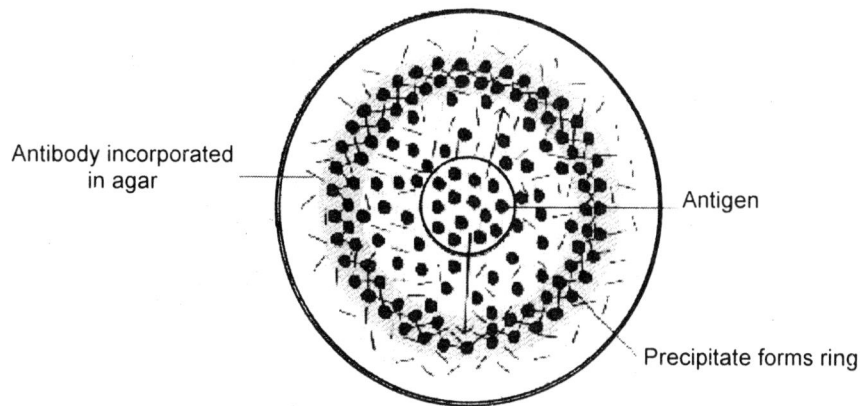

Fig. 12.20 : Diagrammatic presentation of radial immunodiffusion

12.20.2.2. Double immunodiffusion or Ouchterlony method

Unlike, Mancini method, in this method both antigen and antibody are placed in separate wells and both diffuse radially to each other and thereby establish a concentration gradient (Fig.12.21). This method plays as a tool in determining the relationship between antigens and the number of different antigen-antibody systems present. The pattern of precipitate lines that form when two different antigen preparation are placed in adjacent well indicate whether or not they share epitopes.

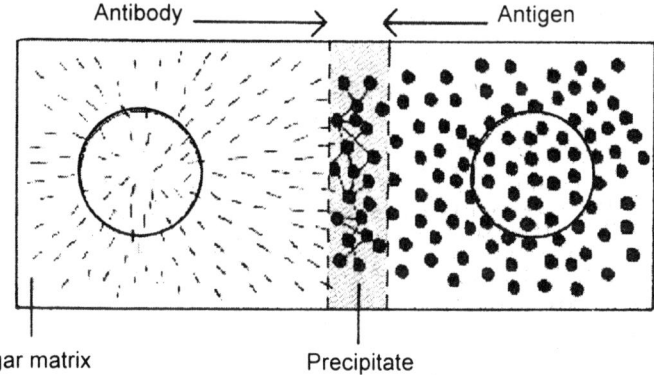

Fig. 12.21 : Diagrammatic presentation of double immunodiffusion method in a gel

This can be explained by an example wherein two antigens share identical epitopes, here, the antiserum will form a single precipitin line with each antigen that will grow towards each other and fuse to form a patterned *identity* (Fig.12.22). However, when the antigens are unrelated, the antiserum will form independent precipitin lines that cross (Fig.12.22) proving *non-identity*. This crossing is possible as the unrelated antigen and antibody do not precipitate and are hence free to diffuse apart.

A third type of identity namely *partial identity* is seen when two antigens share the same epitopes but one or the other has a unique epitope. In this case, the antibodies to the common epitope form a line of identity, but antibodies to the unique epitope(s) diffuse past the precipitating line to form a spur, a precipitin line formed with the unique epitope(s) of the more complex antigen. This test is however not without limitations of which the prime one being the time consuming as it takes around 18-24 h in this case. This can however be overcome by using counter-current electrophoresis.

12.20.3. Immunoelectrophoresis

Immunoelectrophoresis is a qualitative technique that can detect antibody concentration of 3-20 µg/ml. When a large number of different antigens are present in a solution, it is difficult to separate the precipitin bands for each of the antigen-antibody reaction by simple diffusion method as discussed above. In such situations, where, multicomponent analysis is required, electrophoresis could be used effectively. Here, the antigen mixture is first electrophorized and separated by application of a charge. Then troughs are cut into the agar gel parallel to the direction of electric field and to this is added an antiserum. Following this, incubation is carried out in a humid chamber where the antigen and antibody diffuse towards each other leading to the formation of precipitin bands (Fig.12.23).

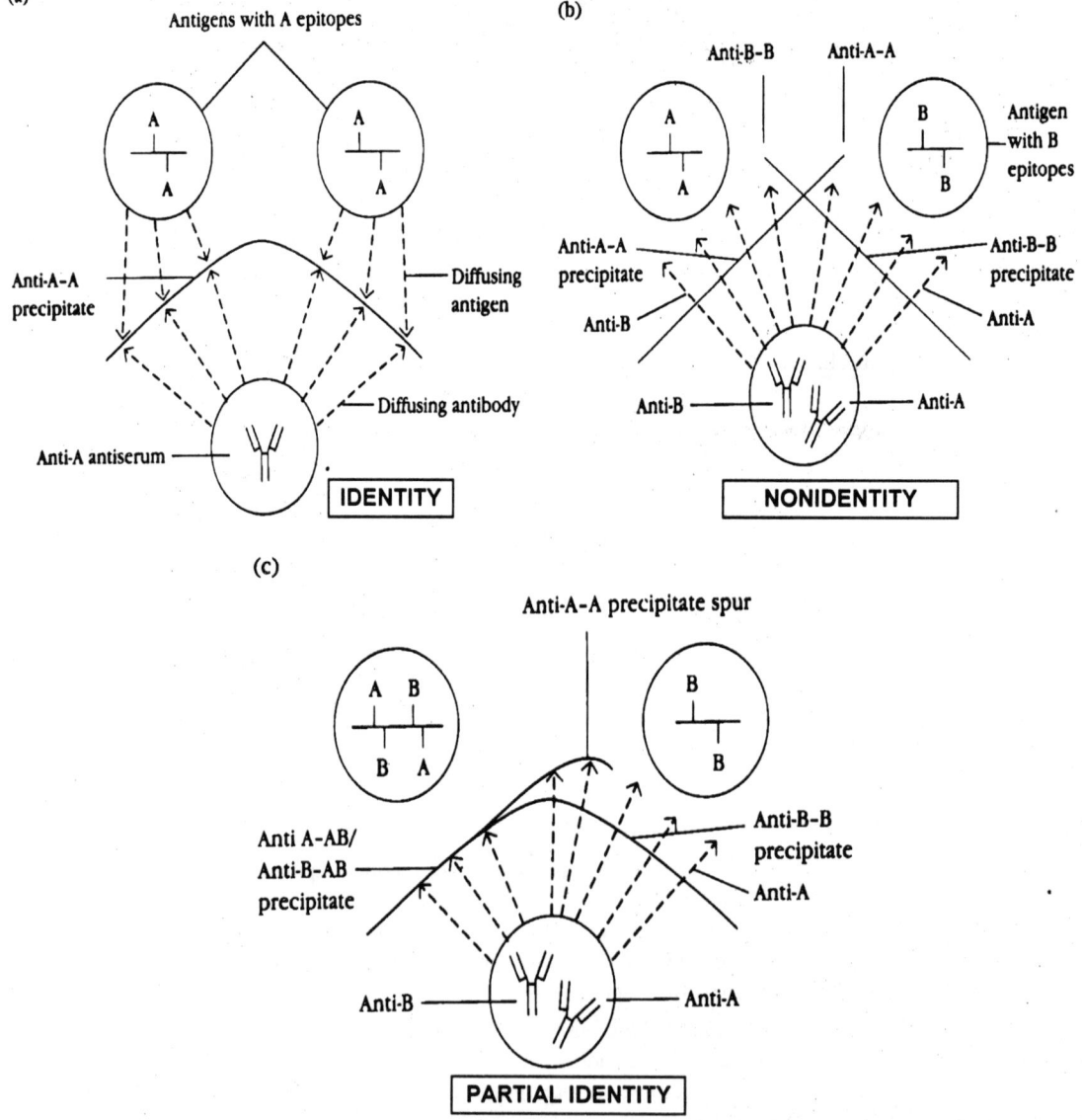

Fig. 12.22 : Diagrammatic presentation of possible precipitin patterns obtained in double immunodiffusion

Immunoelectrophoresis is a technique widely used in detection of serum proteins. It is also helpful in determining whether a patient has an immunodeficiency or not. Other than simple electrophoresis are rocket electrophoresis and two-dimensional electrophoresis.

12.20.4. Rocket electrophoresis

One among the two immunoelectrophoresis which involves application of only negatively charged antigen is subjected to electrophoresis in a gel containing antibody. The name of the technique so derived because of the shape of the precipitate formed due to antigen-antibody interaction which is in a rocket shape. The method is limited to negatively charged antigens only.

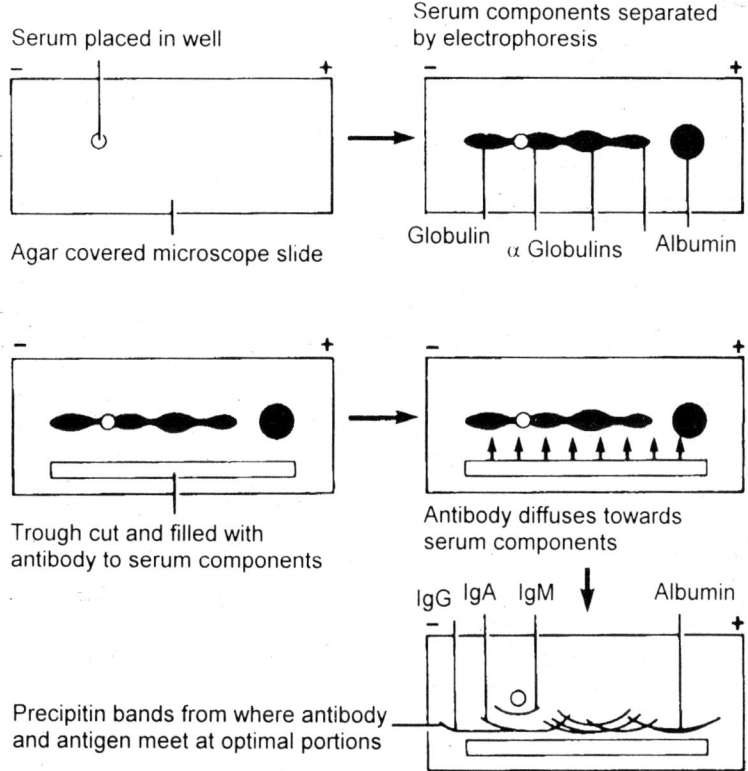

Fig. 12.23 : Diagrammatic presentation of immunoelectorphoresis

12.20.5. Two-dimensional immunoelectrophoresis

A modified version of the rocket electrophoresis is the two-dimensional immunoelectrophoresis. It is of quantitative method for the estimation of the antigen in a complex mixture. In this method, the antigen is separated into its components by electrophoresis. The gel is then laid over another agar gel containing antiserum, and electrophoresis is repeated at right angles to the previously conducted. This appears in the form of precipitin peaks.

12.21. AGGLUTINATION REACTIONS

The agglutination reaction is similar in principle to the precipitation reaction. The interaction between antibody and a particulate antigen results in visible clumping called **agglutination.** In this reaction, the antigen is a part of the surface of some particulate material such as a red cell, bacterium or some inorganic particle which has been coated with antigen. Addition of antibody to a suspension of such particles combines with the surface antigens and links them together to form clearly visible aggregates or agglutinates. However, a practical difficulty in this test is the occasional inhibition of agglutination in the first tube of an antiserum dilution series, agglutination occurring only in those tubes containing more dilute antiserum. This effect of excess antibodies to inhibit agglutination reactions is known as ***prozone effect***, which may be caused by several mechanism. Firstly due to the stabilizing effects of high protein concentration on the particles. The protein coats the particle, increases their net charge and so brings about increased electrostatic repulsion between individual particles, thus opposing the efforts of the antibody molecule to link the particles together. Secondly, when high concentrations of antibodies bind to the antigen but do not induce agglutination. Such antibodies are called *incomplete antibodies*. IgG often represents this class.

12.21.1. Hemagglutination

Agglutination reactions are routinely performed in typing ABO antigens. Here, the red blood cells (RBCs) are mixed on a slide with antisera to the A and B blood group antigens. If the antigen is present on the cells, they agglutinate, forming a visible clump on the slide (Fig.12.24).

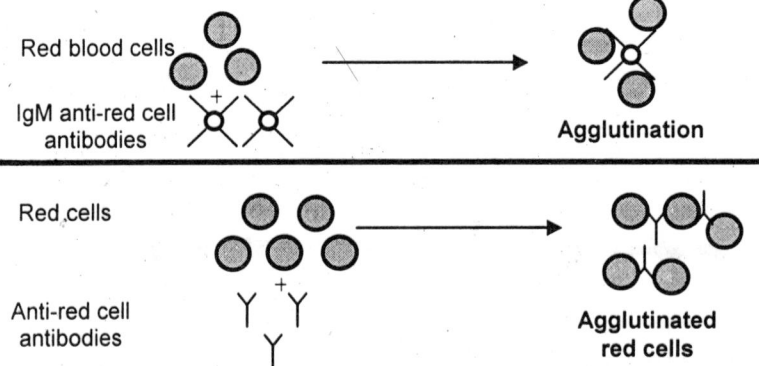

Fig. 12.24 : Diagrammatic presentation of agglutination reaction

12.21.2. Bacterial agglutination

Any bacterial infection could result in to the elicitation of the production of the serum antibodies specific for that particular surface antigen of the bacterial cells. Using agglutination reactions, presence of such antibodies can be detected.. One of the classical application of the agglutination test is the **Widal test** used for the demonstration of the antibodies to *Salmonellae* in serum specimens taken from suspected enteric fever cases. The test is performed by taking serum samples of infected patients and is serially diluted in a series of tubes to which the bacteria is added. The last tube showing the visible agglutination will reflect the sera antibody titer of the patient for that particular bacteria. The *agglutination titer* is defined as the reciprocal of the last serum dilution that elicits a positive agglutination reaction. For example, if the dilution 1/256 shows agglutination but the dilution 1/512 does not, then the agglutination titer of the patient's serum is 256. For some bacteria, high serum titer is obtained up to 1/50,000 and still shows agglutinations. Agglutination reactions also provide a way to type bacteria.

12.21.3. Passive agglutination

Agglutination reactions can be extended to soluble antigens by the technique of passive agglutination. The technique is very simple and sensitive. Here, the soluble antigen is mixed with red blood cells that have been treated with tannic acid or chromium chloride, in order to promote the adsorption of the antigen to the surface of the cells. Serially diluted serum containing antibody is taken into micro titer plate well, to this is added the antigen coated red blood cells. Agglutination is assessed by the size of the characteristic spread pattern of agglutinated RBC at the bottom of the well. Passive agglutination is more sensitive than precipitin reactions which can detect antibody concentrations as low as 0.001 µg/ml.

12.21.4. Agglutination inhibition

Agglutination inhibition is a modification of the agglutination assay and is highly sensitive method by which small quantities of antigen can be detected (0.001-0.01 µg/ml). It is a widely used diagnostic procedure. The presence of antibody in the patients serum is thus detected by its ability to link with virus particles and prevent them from bringing about agglutination of the red cells.

Red cells and inert particles such as polystyrene particles can be coated with various antigens and these coated particles are then used in a variety of diagnostic tests (Fig.12.25). One such test is the test for pregnancy wherein latex coated particles with human chronic gonadotropin (HCG) and antibody to HCG are used. Addition of urine from a pregnant woman, which contains HCG, inhibit agglutination of the latex particles and thus confirm pregnancy. Similarly, thyroid antibody test using thyroglobulin cells or latex particles can be used. Hormone-coated red cells or inert particles are used in many hormonal assay procedures which are based on the inhibition of the antibody-induced agglutination of the hormone coated particles by hormone added to the sample under test. Agglutination inhibition also has wide clinical application in identifying if an individual has got an exposure for a specific type of virus that causes agglutination of red blood cells. Example, the myxoviruses causing influenza and mumps have the property of bringing about agglutination of red blood cells.

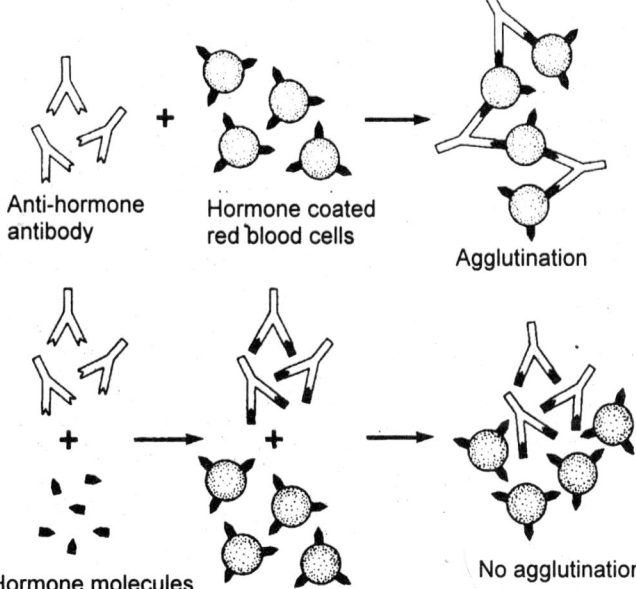

Fig. 12.25 : Diagrammatic presentation of agglutination inhibition

12.22. COMPLEMENT FIXATION

The complement system which comprises of a group of serum proteins plays an important role in immune response. The complement system acts in a cascade fashion, i.e. the activation of one complement results in the activation of the next. The complement system, collectively makes up much of the globulin fraction of serum. These proteins are as such in an inactive state. However, they are activated after the binding of antibodies to antigens and are specifically directed against the target molecules identified by the antibodies. Since the complement activation involves binding of the components to antibody-antigen complexes and to each other with their consequent removal from serum, this event is called **complement fixation.**

Complement activation takes place by two pathways: the classical and alternative pathways. When a complement binds to an antigen-antibody complex, it becomes "fixed" and "used-up". Complement fixation tests are very sensitive and are used to detect extremely small amounts of an antibody for a suspect microorganism. The sequence of complement fixation is well depicted in figure 12.26. A known antigen is mixed with test serum lacking complement (Fig.12.26a). The mixture is kept aside in order to form a complex if any. Now, complement is added to the mixture (Fig. 12.26b). If immune complexes are present, they will fix and the complement is consumed. This is followed by the addition of sensitized indicator cells, usually sheep red blood cells previously coated with complement fixing antibodies are added. Lysis of these indicator cells (Fig.12.26c) results if an immune complex is not formed in the first step (Fig.12.26a) of the test. Absence of lysis shows that specific antibodies are present in the test serum and the complement is consumed by the immune complex.

Wassermann test used in the diagnosis of syphilis is an example of complement fixation test. Currently, it is used in the diagnosis of certain viral, fungal, rickettsial, chlamydial and protozan diseases.

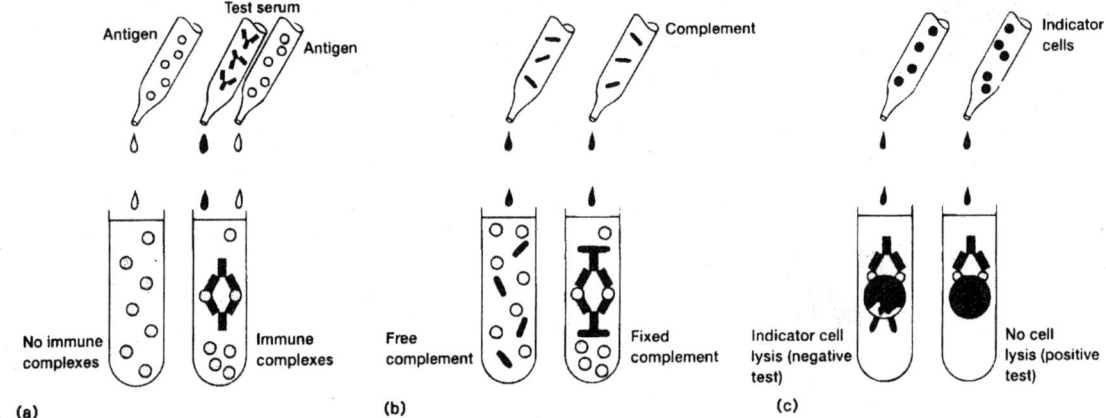

Fig. 12.26 : Diagrammatic presentation of complement fixation test

12.23. NEUTRALIZATION REACTIONS

12.23.1. Toxin neutralization

Neutralization reactions are antigen-antibody reactions that determine whether the activity of a toxin or virus has been neutralized by an antibody. Immunity to a disease like diphtheria depends on the production of specific antibodies that inactivate the toxins produced by the bacteria. This process is known as **toxin neutralization** (Fig.12.27). Once the toxin gets neutralized, the toxin-antibody complex is either unable to attach to receptor sites on host target cells or unable to enter the cell. Antiserum containing neutralizing antibody against a toxin is called **antitoxin**.

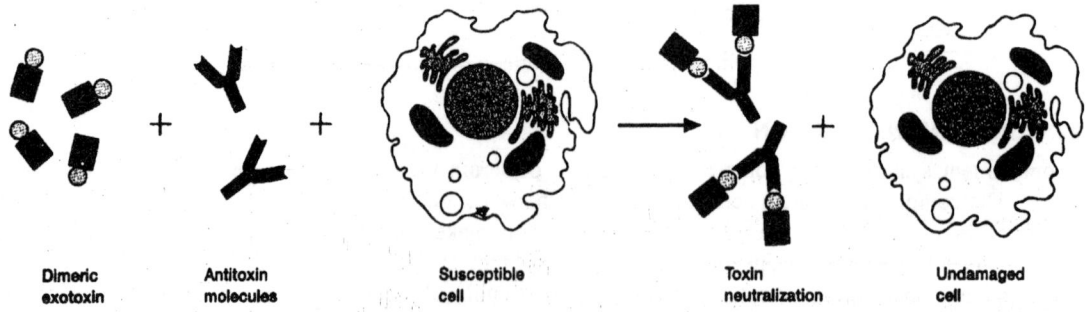

Fig. 12.27 : Diagrammatic presentation of a toxin neutralization by an antitoxin

12.23.2. Viral neutralization

Fixation of classical pathway complement component C4b to the virus aids the neutralization process (Fig.12.28). Antibodies such as IgG, IgM and IgA bind to some virus during their extracellular phase and inactivate them. This antibody-mediated viral inactivation is called **viral neutralization**.

Viral neutralization assays are used to detect viral infections. Serum containing viral antibodies can be introduced into tissue culture cells or embryonated egg cells. Viral neutralization occurs in cases where antibodies against the virus are present and they prevent the virus from infecting the culture cells (Fig.12.28).

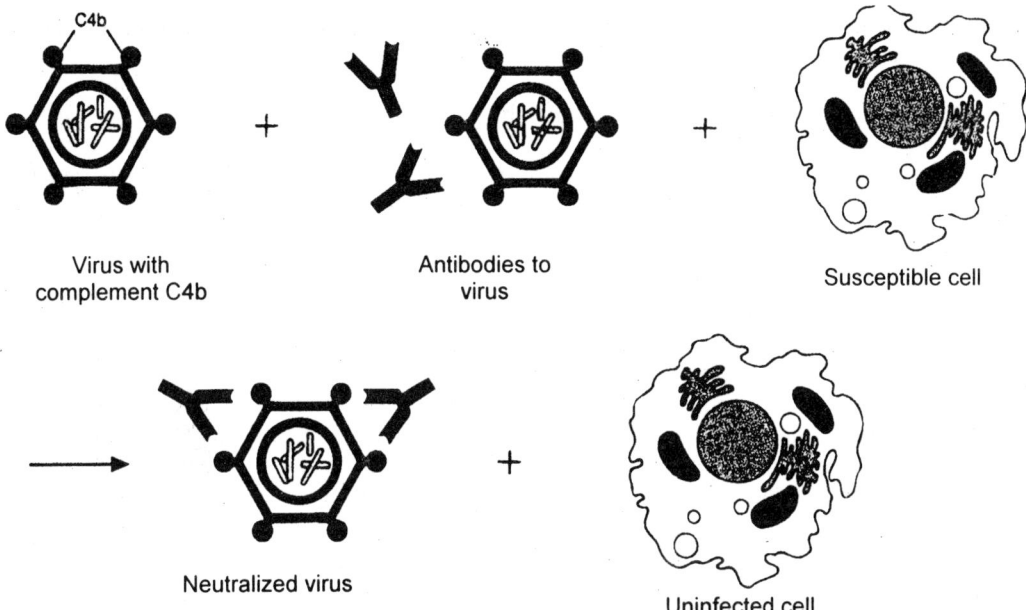

Fig. 12.28 : Diagrammatic presentation of viral neutralization: specific antibodies neutralize the virus and prevent it from attaching tot he susceptible cell

12.24. IMMUNOFLUORESCENCE

Fluorescent dye or fluorochrome can be used in the estimation of antibody or antigen binding to a cell. The antibody or antigen molecule can be tagged with a fluorescent dye and the light emitted by the dye at longer wave length serves as a measure of the amount of antibody bound (Fig.12.29).

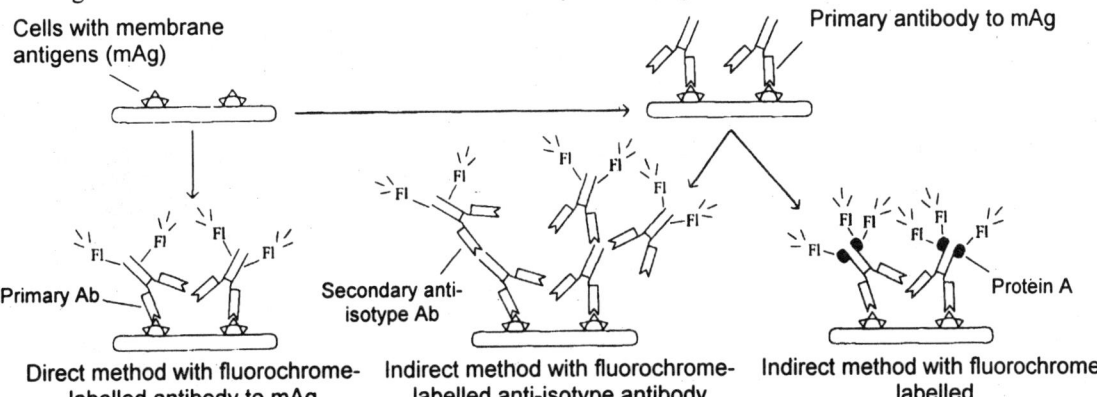

Fig. 12.29 : Schematic representation of immunofluorescence technique

The most commonly used dyes are fluorescein and rhodamine. Both the dyes can be conjugated to the Fc portion of the antibody molecule. Fluorescein absorbs blue light at 490 nm and emits an intense yellow-green fluorsecene at 517 nm, while rhodamine absorbs a yellow-green light at 515 nm and emits a deep red fluorescence at 546 nm.

Immunofluroscence has a wide variety of application. Antibody tagged with fluorescent dyes can be used in identifying a number of lymphocyte subpopulation. They are also helpful in identifying bacterial species, antigen-antibody complexes in autoimmune diseases, in detecting complement components in tissues, and to localize hormones and other cellular products stained *in situ*.

Immunofluorescence can be carried out either by **direct** or **indirect method**. In the former method, the fluorochrome is directly bound to the specific antibody (primary antibody) while in the latter the primary antibody is unlabeled and is detected with an additional fluorochrome-labeled reagent. A third method also exists in which biotin-conjugated anti-isotype antibody acts as the second antibody and the fluorochrome-conjugated avidin, a protein that has high affinity and binds to biotin. The indirect method has an edge over the direct method. The first being that the primary antibody need not be conjugated with the label. The second being the sensitivity of the method which is increased because of the multiple fluorochrome reagents that will bind to each primary antibody.

12.25. WESTERN BLOTTING METHOD

Western blotting method is similar to that of Southern blotting method used for detecting DNA fragments and Northern blotting used for detecting mRNAs. The method can be used in identifying a specific protein in a complex mixture of proteins, or antibody to a given protein, by separating the protein electrophoretically on a polyacrylamide slab gel in the presence of sodium dodecyl sulfate (SDS) (Fig.12.30). The protein bands are then transferred to a nitro-cellulose membrane by electrophoresis and individual protein bands are identified by flooding the nitro-cellulose membrane with radiolabeled monoclonal or polyclonal antibody. The antigen-antibody complex that is formed can be visualized by autoradiography. In case of non availability of labeled specific antibody, antigen-antibody complex can be detected by adding a secondary anti-isotype antibody which is either radiolabeled or enzyme labeled. Western blotting method has been used in the identification of the envelope and core proteins of HIV and the antibodies of these components in the serum of HIV-infected individuals.

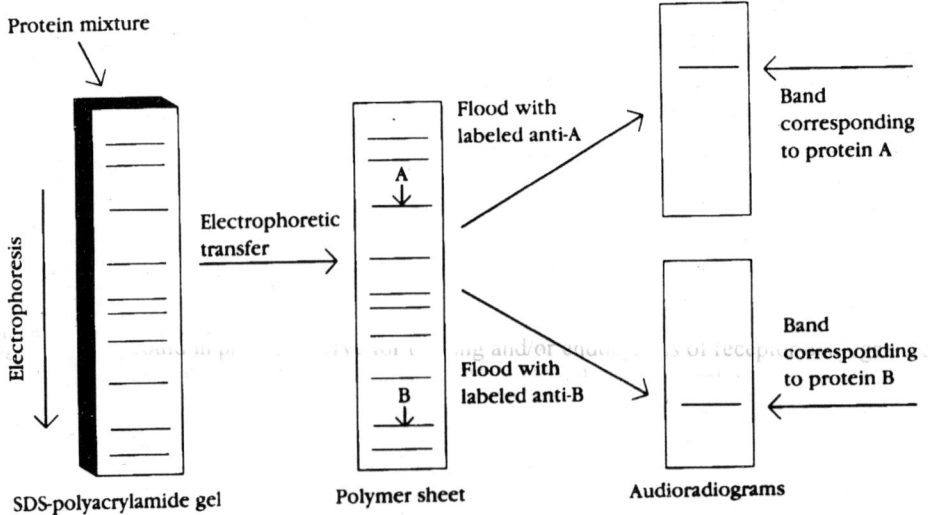

Fig. 12.30 : Schematic presentation of Western blot method

12.26. RADIOIMMUNOASSAY (RIA)

The increasing use of immunologically based methods for the accurate estimation of polypeptide hormones has paved way for development in the estimation methods. One such method where the accuracy is up to the concentration of 0.0001 µg/ml is the radioimmunoassay (RIA). The Nobel prize winning method is now widely used in quantitative estimation of hormones, serum proteins, drugs and vitamins.

The principle of the assay method involves competitive binding of a radiolabeled antigen and unlabelled antigen to a high affinity antibody. Commonly used labeling material is the gamma-emitting isotope such as ^{125}I. The method involves mixing of labeled antigen to antibody at a concentration that just saturates the antigen-binding sites of the antibody molecule. Now, on increasing the amount of unlabelled antigen the bound antigen (labeled) is displaced due to competitive binding between the labeled and unlabelled antigen. By increasing the amount of unlabeled antigen the free but labeled antigen in solution can be estimated and thus it is possible to determine the concentration of antigen, which combines antibody affinity sites.

12.27. ENZYME-LINKED IMMUNOSORBENT ASSAY(ELISA)

Enzyme-linked immunosorbent assay, commonly known as ELISA, is a the latest method. In principle, the method is similar to that of the RIA which involves competitive binding. This method differs from the above that it does not involve in use of any radio-labeled material and the sensitivity of the method is equally good (0.0001-0.001µg/ml). Above all, the method is sage and cheaper as compared to RIA. Here, the enzyme conjugated to an antibody reacts with a colorless substrate to generate a colored reaction product. The color is measured spectrophotometrically. A variety of enzymes such as horseradish peroxidase, alkaline phosphatase, *p*-nitorphenyl phosphatase have been used to link to the antibody or antigen molecule as may be the case. When mixed with a suitable substrate each of these enzymes generates a colored reaction product.

A number of different ELISA methods have been developed which can be used as per the requirement for either determining the antigen or the antibody. First, a standard curve is prepared using known concentrations of antibody or antigens from which the unknown concentration of the sample can be determined.

The various methods include **indirect ELISA** (Fig.12.31a) where the antigen is bound to the plastic plate, the antibody to be assayed constituted the second layer and the enzyme linked to immunoglobulin as the top layer. The enzyme substrate is finally added and the color change is estimated spectrophotometrically. Next falls the **sandwich technique** (Fig.12.31b) where the micro titer well is first coated with an antibody and the sample containing antigen is then added and allowed to react with the bound antibody. Now the well is washed and the second enzyme linked specific antibody is added and allowed to react. Subsequently, the substrate is added and the color produced is measured. Third comes the **competitive ELISA** (Fig.12.31c), which involves the principle similar to RIA. First, incubation of the antibody with the sample containing antigen is allowed. The antigen-antibody mixture is then added to an antigen coated micro titer well. As the antigen concentration increases, the amount of antibody available for binding of the antigen coated well decreases. If a substrate, i.e. enzyme-conjugated secondary antibody specific for the primary antibody is added, the amount of primary antibody bound in the well can be estimated.

12.28. HYPERSENSITIVITY

Not all immune responses against an antigen produce a desirable resistance, when the sensitivity is beyond limits it is termed as **hypersensitivity**. It can be defined as when an adaptive immune response occurs in an exaggerated or inappropriate form causing tissue damage, then the condition is termed as hypersensitivity. Hypersensitivity depends on an individual. It usually occurs to people who have been previously 'sensitized' by exposure to an antigen, i.e., upon second contact with a particular antigen. Hypersensitivity may be broadly classified under two main heads:

1. Immediate or humoral hypersensitivity.
2. Delayed or cell-mediated hypersensitivity.

As the name indicates, immediate hypersensitivity appears rapidly and depends on the production of pharmacologically active mediator substance activated by antigen-antibody interaction. While the delayed hyper-sensitivity appears more slowly (after 24 h) and depends upon immunologically aetivated lymphoid cells which, on reaction with antigen, appear to release substance known as lymphokines having a variety of effects on other cells and effects on blood vessel permeability.

a. Indirect ELISA

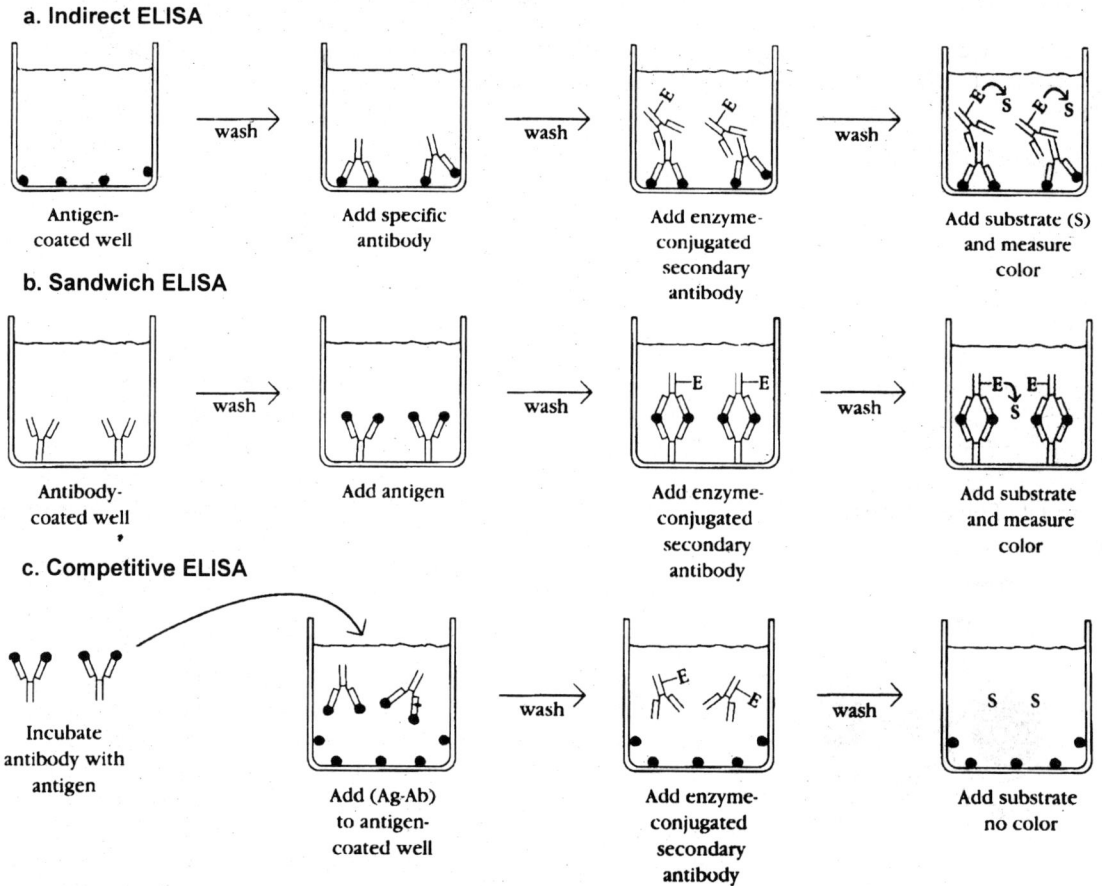

Fig. 12.31 : Schematic representation of ELISA

Hypersensitivity has been classified by many and various classification are available. However, the classification by Gell and Coombs is widely accepted. This has four principal types and are distinguished by difference in effector molecule generated in the course of reaction. In immediate hypersensitive reaction, different antibody isotypes induce different immune effector molecule. A brief about the four types of hypersensitivity is given in the table 12.6.

12.28.1. Type I hypersensitivity IgG-mediated

TypeI hypersensitivity reaction is induced by certain types of antigens, referred to as **allergens**. Allergens refer to non-parasitic antigens capable of stimulating type 1 hypersensitivity in allergic individuals. An allergen induces a humoral antibody response resulting in generation of antibody -secreting plasma cells. The secretion of IgE by plasma cells differs type-1 hypersensitivity from a normal response (Fig.12.32). IgE appears to have four main activities.

a. The capacity to find via its Fc fragment to mast cells in Asophils.

b. Subsequent interaction with antigen that takes place on the cell membrane of the mast cell.

c. Resultant triggering of the release of pharmacological mediators.

d. Attraction of other cell types-eosinophils.

Table 12.6 : Gell and Coomb classification of hypersensitive reactions

Descriptive name	Type	Mechanism
IgE mediated hypersensitivity (Anaphylaxis)	I	Ag induces cross-linkage of IgE bound to mast cells and basophils with release of vasoactive mediators
Antibody-mediated cytoxicity	II	Ab directed against cell surface antigens mediates cell destruction via complement activation or ADCC
Immune complex-mediated hypersensitivity	III	Ag-Ab complexes deposited in various tissues induce complement activation and an ensuing inflammatory response
Cell-mediated hypersensitivity or delayed type hypersensitivity	IV	Sensitized T_{DTH} cells release cytokines that activate macrophages or T_c cells which mediate direct cellular damage

The mechanism of systemic anaphylaxis could be prevented if the parenterally injected antigen is prevented from reaching the tissue-fixed IgE. This can be achieved by the simple expedient of injecting frequent small doses of the antigen to which the patient is sensitized. This induces the formation of increasing levels of IgG antibody, circulating in the blood and tissue fluids, mops up the injected antigen so that it does not reach the tissue-fixed IgE. This IgG antibody has been termed as **blocking antibody**. Some commonly used drugs in the treatment of type I hypersensitivity are antihistamines, cromolyn sodium, theophylline, epinephrine (adrenaline) and cortisone.

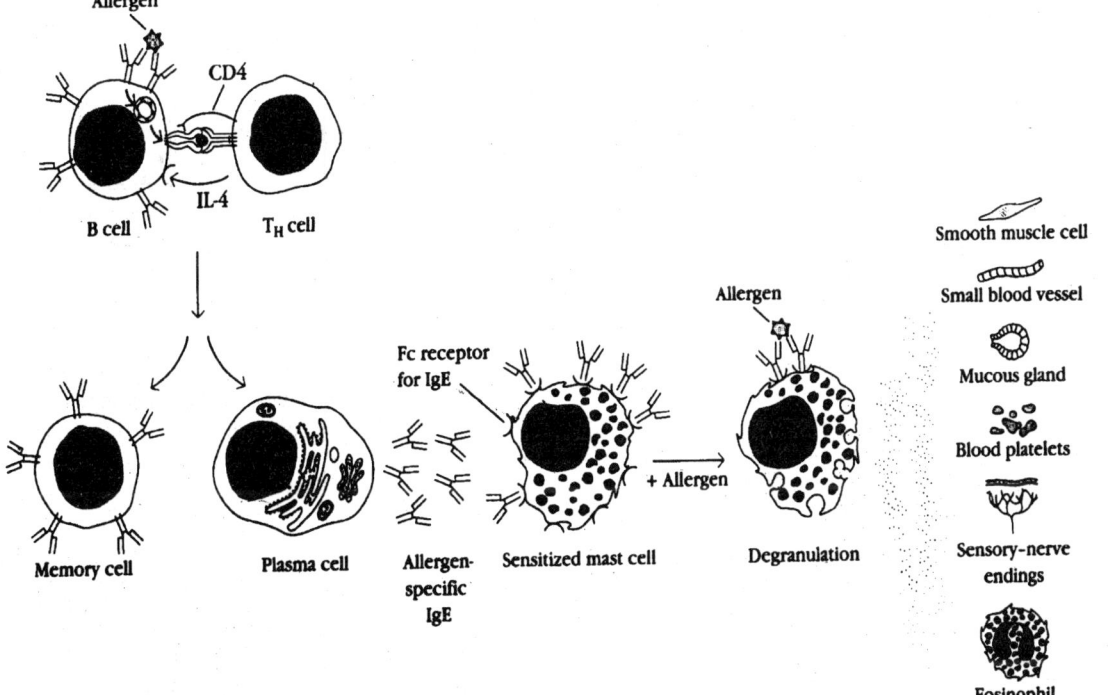

Fig. 12.32 : Mechanism of Type I (Anaphylaxis) hypersensitivity

12.28.2. Type II or antibody-mediated cytotoxic (ADCC) hypersensitivity

This type of reactions are initiated by an antigenic component either part of a tissue cells or closely associated with it. The antibodies directed against such a cell-associated antigen bring about a cytolytic effect usually involving complement. Type II reactions generally involved antibody-mediated destruction of cells (Fig. 12.33). The best examples for this is blood transfusion reactions in which host antibodies react with foreign antigens expressed by the incompatible transfused blood cells and mediate destruction of these cells and hemolytic destruction of new born. Antibody can also mediate cell destruction by antibody-dependent cell-mediated cytotoxicity (ADCC).

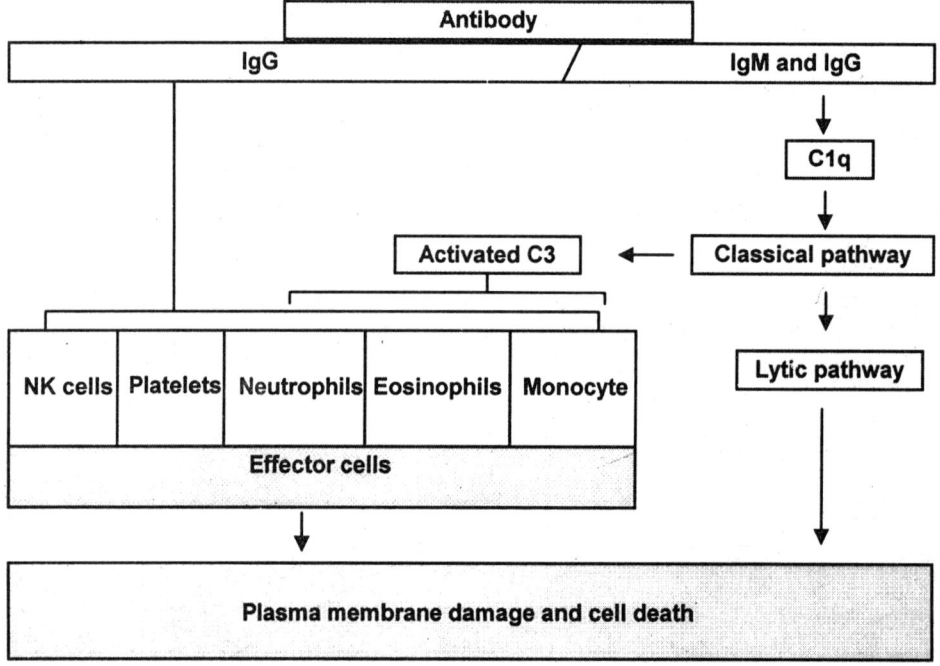

Fig. 12.33 : Mechanism of Type II (Cytotoxic) hypersensitivity

The consequence of the reactions are as follows:
1. Direct lysis of the cells by complement activation.
2. Adherence to phagocytes by the Fc and C3b receptors leading to phagocytosis.
3. Antibody-dependent cell-mediated cytotoxicity (ADCC) by both phagocytic and non-phagocytic cells.
4. IgG bearing cells killing by non-adherent lymphoid K-cells through an extracellular mechanism.

12.28.3. Type III or immune complex mediated hypersensitivity

Type III reactions are due to the combination of antigen with circulating antibody, with the formation of immune complexes. This combination leads to the formation of micro-precipitates in and around small blood vessels which leads to inflammation and sometimes mechanical blockade of these vessels which results in interference with the blood supply to the surrounding tissues. Two types of reactions fall under this category the first is **localized** or **Arthus reaction** and the second is **systemic** or **serum sickness.** Type III hypersensitive reactions develop when immune complexes activate the complement systems array of immune effector molecules. Much of the tissue damage in this type of reaction is due to the release of lytic enzymes by neutrophils as they attempt to phagocytose immune complexes (Fig. 12.34).

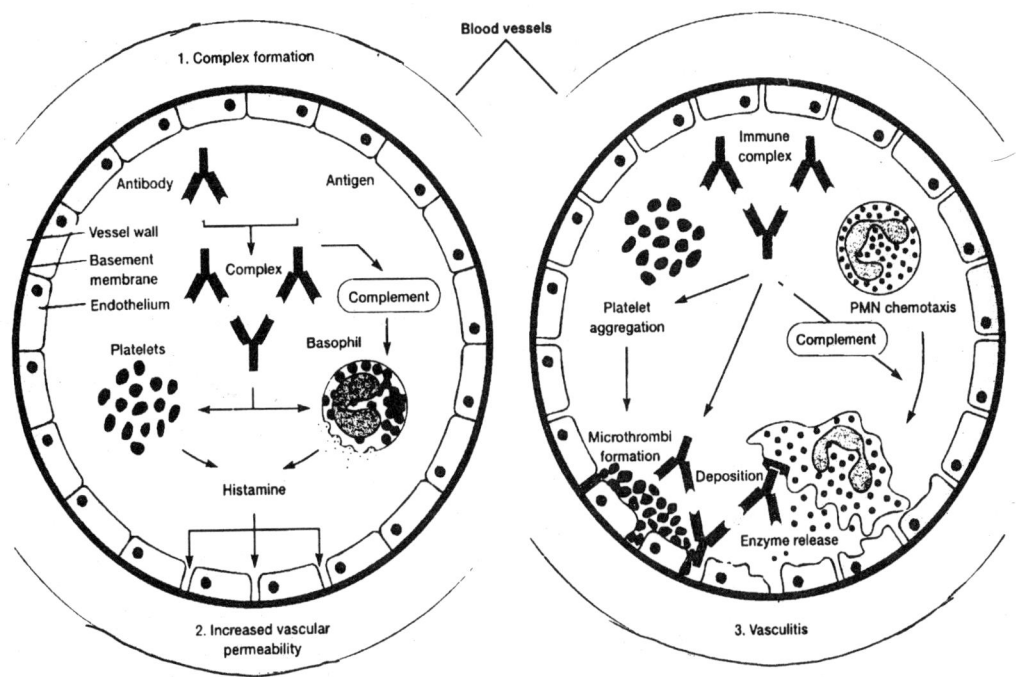

Fig. 12.34 : Mechanism of Type III (Immune complex) hypersensitivity

12.28.3.1. Arthus or localized reaction

Injection of an antigen intradermally or subcutaneously into an animal that has high levels of circulating antibody specific for that antigen leads to formation of localized immune complexes. This reaction generally occurs in walls of small blood vessels in the presence of large quantities of IgG antibody forming micro-precipitates with antigen, which mediates acute Arthus reaction within 4-12 h. In this reaction, there is the activation of the vasoactive amines such as histamine, with resulting increase in vascular permeability and consequent edema. These reactions may occur in diabetics who have received many injections of insulin and have developed high levels of IgG antibody to antigenic constituents contained in the insulin preparation.

12.28.3.2. Serum sickness or systemic reaction

Serum sickness, as the name suggests, occurs following injection of foreign serum to any individual for therapeutic purpose. Antigens other that serum proteins can also cause serum sickness. Among them the most likely candidates are drugs such as penicillin and sulfonamides. The susceptible patient will develop rashes, pyrexia, arthralgia, lymphadenopathy and perhaps nephritis. Even certain bacterial and viral infection may lead to hypersensitivity of this type.

12.28.4. Type IV or cell-mediated hypersensitivity

Cell-mediated or type IV hypersensitivity reactions is developed when an antigen activates and sensitized T_{DTH} cells (delayed type hypersensitivity cells) (Fig.12.35). It is well known that type IV reaction is important in host defense against parasites and bacteria that can live intracellularly. The pathogenic organisms, in this case is inside the cell and thus not available for the antibodies to reach them. However, the phagocytic activity and lytic enzymes leads to destruction of the cells in a non-specific way and thus destroy the intracellular pathogen. If this defensive mechanism is not effective the continued presence of the pathogenic antigen can provoke a chronic DTH reaction, which is characterized by excessive numbers of macrophages, continual release of lytic enzymes, and consequent tissue destruction. Examples of such cases are the skin lesions seen with *Mycobacterium leprae* and lung cavitation seen with *Mycobacterium tuberculosis*.

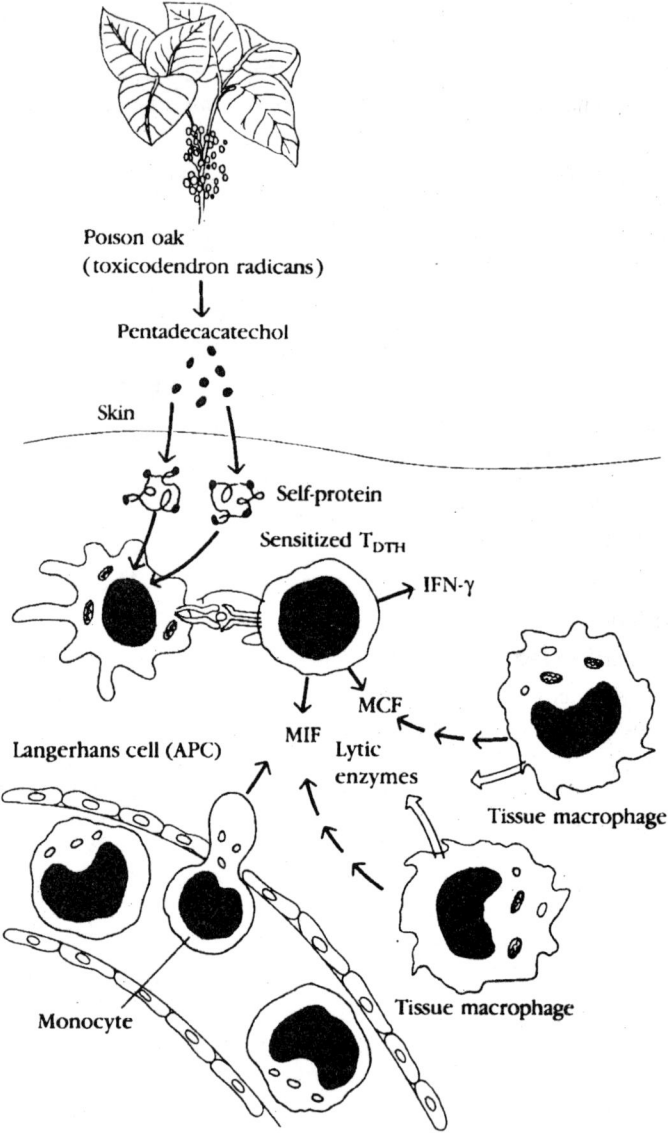

Fig. 12.35 : Mechanism of Type IV (Cell-mediated) hypersensitivity

Many contact dermatits reactions including those of the response to nitrophenol, nickel, turpentine, various cosmetics, poison ivy, poison oak, and hair dyes are mediated by T_{DTH} cells. Most of these substances are small molecules capable of forming complex with the skin proteins. This complex is internalized by the APC present in the skin and is then processed and presented by the class II MHC molecules, causing activation. Approximately after 48 h of exposure, activation of the macrophages and release of their lytic enzymes results in the redness (Fig. 12.35).

SUGGESTED READINGS

Bck, G. and Habicht, G.S., (1996) **Scientific Am.**, 275(5), 60.

Bellanti, J.A., (1985) **Immunology III**, 3 rd ed., W.B. Saunder, Philadelphia.

Bier, D.G., daSliva, W.D., Gotze, D., Mota, I., (1981) **Fundamentals of Immunology**, Springer-Verlag, New York.

Braciale, T.J. and Trowsdale, J., (1993) **Current Opinions Immunol.**, 5, 1-55.

Coleman, R.M., Lombard, M. and Sicard, R., (1992) **Fundamental Immunology**, 2 ed, Wm. C. Brown Publishers, USA.

Desowitz, R.S., (1987) **The thorn in the starfish: How the human immune system works**, Norton, New York.

Hood, L.E., Weissman, I.L., Wood,W.B. and Wilson, J.H., (1984) **Immunology**, Benjamin/Cumming Publishing Company Inc. California.

Hudson, L. and Hay, F.C., (1980) **Practical Immunology**, Blackwell Scientific Publications, Australia.

Janeway, C.A. and Travers, P. **Immunology: The immune system in health and disease**, Blackwell Scientific.

Kuby, J., (1994) **Immunology**, W.H. Freeman and Company, USA.

Litman, G.W., (1996) **Scientific Am.**, 275(5), 67.

Paul, W.E., (1990) **Fundamental Immunology**, 2nd ed., Raven Press, New York.

Prescott, L.M., Harly, J.P. and Klein, D.A., (1993) **Microbiology**, 2 nd ed., Wm. C. Brown Publishers, USA.

Rath, S. and Bal, V., (1997) **Resonance**, 2, 90-93.

Roit, I.M., Brostoff, J. and Male, D.K., (1989) **Immunology**, 2 nd ed., C.V. Mosby, St. Louis.

Roitt,I., (1986) **Essential Immunology**, Blackwell Scientific Publications, Australia.

Stites, D.P., Stobo, J.D., Fudenberg, and Wells, J.V., (1984) **Basic and Clinical Immunology**, 5 th edition, Lange Medical Publications.

Tizard, I.R., (1988) **Immunology: An introduction**, 2 nd ed., W.B. Saunders, Philadelphia.

Weir, D.M., (1979) **Handbook of Experimental Immunology**, Blackwell Scientific Publications, Australia.

BIOTECH IN NEWS . . . .

Cloned animals to provide organs for humans?

Cloning or copying humans is theoretically possible but may not be desirable ethically and from a religious standpoint, say experts. "Clonning humans is illegal already in England," says Dr. Ian Wilmut, the embryologist who cloned sheep at the Roslin Institute in Edinburg. He said that he is more interested in producing genetically altered pigs whose organs can be transplanted on humans than in cloning humans. The Roslin Institute of Edinburg has revealed that the institute and its collaborators have cloned not one sheep, as originally announced, but seven from three different breeds from three different cell types.

. . . . . *from Express Pharma Pulse, Mar 6, 1997.*

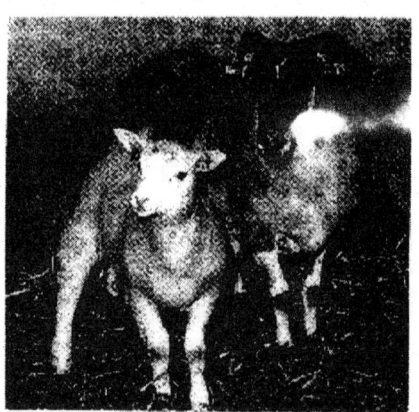

This Century Wonder: 'DOLLY'

MONOCLONAL ANTIBODIES AND HYBRIDOMA TECHNOLOGY

13.1. INTRODUCTION AND HISTORICAL BACKGROUND

Antibodies are glycoprotein molecules present in the serum. They are produced in response to antigens, which are either protein or polysaccharide molecules which may be foreign to the body. They may be a component of invading organisms such as bacteria or virus, or environmental agents which enter the organism accidentally. Antibodies are secreted by a class of blood cells known as **B-lymphocytes**. These B lymphocytes form a clone of cells called plasma cells. The plasma cells produce proteinaceous molecules called antibodies. Antibodies are produced when body comes in contact and is invaded by a foreign particle or organism as a result, the system continues to produce proteinaceous molecules until the stimulation persists. A person can synthesize different types of antibodies depending upon the type of stimulant involved. Each antibody produced is specific to that particular antigen which has stimulated its production. The elicited antibody reacts with the specific antigen by binding non-covalently to it.

Antibodies are composed of two identical heavy chains and two identical light chains (for further details refer chapter 12). Antibodies may be classified under five major classes which are IgG, IgA, IgM, IgE and IgD. The antibodies produced in response to an antigen are heterogeneous in nature because of the multiple epitopes on the antigen which could induce proliferation and differentiation of a variety of B cell clones. The heterogeneity of antibodies that increases immune protection *in vivo* often reduces the efficacy of an antiserum for various *in vitro* uses. Conventional heterogeneous antisera vary from animal to animal and contains undesirable non-specific or cross-reacting antibodies. Removal of antibodies with unwanted specification from a polyclonal antibody preparation is a time consuming task involving repeated adsorption techniques. These methods often result in the loss of much of the desired antibody and are seldom effective in reducing the heterogeneity of an antiserum.

An alternative approach is to generate pure (monospecific) clones of plasma cells *in vitro* from which monoclonal antibody (MAb) with a single antigenic specificity can be isolated. Monoclonal antibody technology is considered to be the second of the two major revolutionary landmarks in biotechnology. Kohler and Milstein in 1975 were the first to report on the production of monoclonal antibodies. The development of monoclonal antibodies production technology is the cumulation of many years of basic research in immunology and in cell-culture methodologies.

The first production of monoclonal antibodies represents the convergence of three areas of basic medical research: immunochemistry, the *in vitro* **cultivation of cancer cells** and the molecular biology of **malignant transformations**. For many years this approach was not technically feasible because plasma cells have a short life span and can not be maintained in tissue culture. In 1975, Georges Kohler and Cesar Milstein devised a solution to this problem by fusing a normal B cell (plasma cell) with a myeloma cell (a cancerous plasma cell), called a **hybridoma** or **heterokaryons**, that possessed the proliferating growth properties of the myeloma cells but secreted the antibody product of the B cell. The fusion was initially accomplished with Sendai virus, but later polyethylene glycol (PEG) was found to be a much more effective fusogenic agent.

13.2. FORMATION AND SELECTION OF HYBRID CELLS

The most important aspect of heterokaryon research is the ability to select hybrids of the two parent cell lines. Littlefield devised an indigenous method of ensuring that all other cells would die by exploiting the redundant nature of nucleic acid biosynthesis.

After fusion the hybrid cells must be separated from intact parent cells. When Sendai virus or polyethylene glycol is used as the fusing agent, only a small percentage of the cell actually fuse, and some of the fused cells are homogeneous, i.e. A-A or B-B cells rather than the desired A-B hybrid. In order to select for the hybrid cells; a selective medium called HAT medium is used. This selection depends upon the synthesis of nucleotides by mammalian cells. Mammalian cells can synthesize nucleotide by two different pathways. The *de novo* and the salvage pathways.

The *de novo* synthesis of nucleotides required **tetrahydrofolate** derivatives in three places. Two of the carbons in the purine ring, which is the central structure of adenine and guanine are provided by N^{10}-formyl-tetrahydrofolate, while the methylation of deoxyuridine monophosphate (dUMP) to form thymidine monophosphate (TMP) requires N^5,N^{10}-methylene tetrahydrofolate. The folic acid analogue **aminopterin** inhibits the **enzymes dihydrofolate reductase**, which is needed to provide tetrahydrofolate.

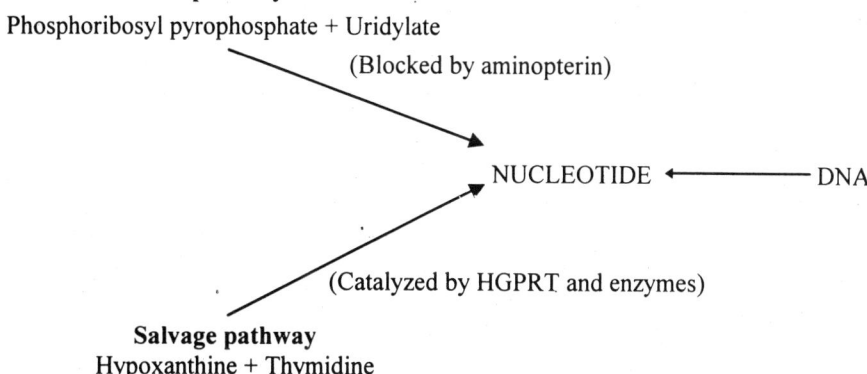

De novo pathway

Phosphoribosyl pyrophosphate + Uridylate

(Blocked by aminopterin)

NUCLEOTIDE ← DNA

(Catalyzed by HGPRT and enzymes)

Salvage pathway
Hypoxanthine + Thymidine

When the *de novo* pathway is blocked, cells utilize the salvage pathway, which bypasses the aminopterin poisoning by converting purines and pyrimidines directly into DNA. The enzymes catalyzing the salvage pathway include hypoxanthine guanine phosphoribosyl transferase (HGPRT), that catalyzes the conversion of guanine to guanosine monophosphate (GMP) and hypoxanthine to inosine monophosphate (IMP) and thymidine kinase (TK), that catalyses the conversion of thymidine to thymidine monophosphate (TMP). A mutation in either of these two enzymes blocks the salvage pathway.

Littlefield screened cells of a given line that were deficient in HGPRT by adding 8-azaguanine or 6-thioguanine to the culture medium. Conversion of these bases to their corresponding nucleotides by HGPRT caused the incorporation of guanine analog into nucleic acid, resulting in cell death. Cells that do not possess a functional HGPRT gene could avoid this poisoning and survive. These HGPRT deficient cells when cultured in a medium containing hypoxanthine, aminopterin and thymidine (HAT medium) would not survive since they could not overcome inhibition of nucleotide synthesis by the aminopterin. Only hybrids formed by fusion of HGPRT deficient cells with cells possessing a functional HGPRT gene would produce the enzyme and proliferate in HAT medium.

13.3. PRODUCTION OF MONOCLONAL ANTIBODIES

Four basic steps are involved in the production of a given monoclonal antibody:

1. Immunization
2. Generation of B cell hybridomas by fusing primed B cells and myeloma cells
3. Selection and the screening of the resulting clones for those that secrete antibody with the desired specificity.
4. Cloning by propagating the desired hybridomas.

This process is summarized in figure 13.1.

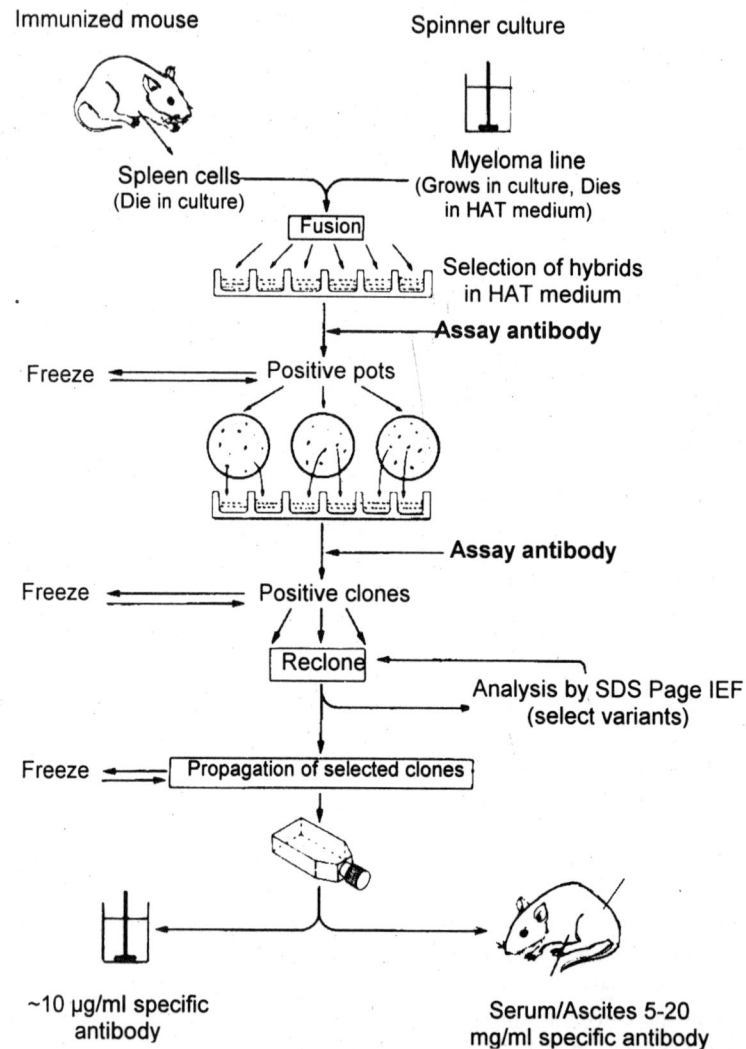

Fig. 13.1: The major stages of monoclonal antibody production ; ELISA: enzyme linked immunosorbent assay; HAT: hypoxanthine-aminopterine-thymidine; PEG: polyethylene glycol

13.3.1. Immunization

Immunization of animals with immunogens is performed by injecting microgram or milligram quantities of immunogen mixed with an adjuvant (aluminum salts, Freund's complete or incomplete adjuvant), intradermally or subcutaneously at multiple sites repeatedly at different times. The serum of animal is assayed for the relative concentration of antibodies of desired specificity at various time intervals. When the concentration of antibodies is found to be nearly optimal, the animal is sacrificed and the spleen, which contains a large number of plasma cells, is dissociated into single splenocytes by mechanical and/or enzymatic method.

13.3.2. Cell fusion

Splenocytes are then mixed with plasmocytoma cells in an appropriate medium. This mixture is exposed to a high concentration (e.g. 50%) of PEG for short period of time and fusion is allowed to proceed over a period of time. Mouse has been used in the production of monoclonal antibody secreting hybridoma with splenocytes, because these animals are inexpensive and several billion cells can be obtained from a mouse spleen. In contrast, mice are rarely used for the production of polyclonal antisera, because of their very low blood volume (≈ 2 ml).

The use of HGPRT cells (that cannot grow in HAT medium) assured that only hybridomas (hybrid myeloma-spleen cells) are selected. After 7-10 days of culture in the HAT medium most of the wells contain dead cells, but a few wells contain small clusters of viable cells. Each cluster represents clonal expansion of a hybridoma. After HAT selection, single cells are transferred and cultured in separate wells to ensure the monoclonality of the secreted antibody. Wells containing viable clusters are then screened for antibody production and antibody positive clones are subcultured at low cell densities, again to ensure clonal purity in each microwell.

The first hybridoma obtained by Kohler and Milstein secreted not only antibody from the spleen B cell but also unwanted antibody from the myeloma cell as well as one hybrid antibody containing heavy or light chains from both original parent cells. To avoid this difficulty a HGRPT, Ab⁻ myeloma cell was chosen as ideal fusion partner. This fusion partner has the immortal properties of a cancer cell but does not secrete its own antibody or gene product. Hybridomas generated with this fusion partner thus secrete only the antibody from the B cell partner. These hybridomas can be propagated in tissue culture to give rise to large clones secreting homogeneous monoclonal antibody.

13.3.3. Selection and screening of the clones for monoclonal antibody specificity

Once pure clones of antibody-secreting hybridomas are obtained, they must be screened for the desired antibody specificity. Selection of hybridoma cells in HAT medium is usually followed by screening of hybridomas for secretion of antibodies of the desired specificity. After fusion, the cells may be transferred to HAT medium in tissue culture flasks. After an appropriate incubation time, all viable cells will be hybridomas. They are removed from the flasks, transferred to regular culture medium and aliquots are distributed among the well of 96-well plastic culture plates. The supernatant of each hybridoma culture can be assayed for a particular antigen specificity in various ways. Two methods are frequently used (a) ELISA and (b) RIA. Both are easily adapted to mass screening with 96-well plastic culture plates. In both assays, antigen that reacts with the desired antibody is bound to the bottom of 96-well plates, and washed to remove unbound antigen. Supernatant from each hybridoma well is added to separate well and incubated for an appropriate period of time. If a sample of supernatant contains the desired antibody it will bind to the antigen and will remain associated with the well as unbound material is washed off.

In ELISA, this antibody is then detected by an immunoconjugate consisting of two components covalently linked to each other. One component is an antibody specific for an epitope in the constant domain of the first antibody (e.g., mouse Fc or mouse Y chain). The second component is an enzyme such as alkaline phosphatase or horse radish peroxidase. After another washing step, a colorless substrate that is converted to a colored product by the enzyme of the immuno-conjugate is added. After an appropriate incubation, the enzymatic reaction is stopped and the optical density of each well is determined at the respective λ max. with a specialized colorimeter known as a 'plate reader'. In RIA the anti-isotype antibody is radiolabeled; bound label can be detected by counting the wells individually in a gamma counter or the entire plate can be exposed to X-ray film.

If the desired monoclonal antibody is specific for a cell-membrane molecule, immunofluorescent techniques can be used for screening. In this case, target cells with the particular cell membrane antigen are stained with monoclonal antibody in microliter wells and visualized by the addition of fluorochrome-conjugated anti-isotype antibody.

13.3.4. Cloning of hybridomas secreting specific monoclonal antibody

Single cells secreting the desired antibody are isolated from positive cultures and propagated into cell lines. There are two cloning techniques which are most widely used:

1. Limiting dilution
2. Soft agar.

In limiting dilution, the cells in the culture are enumerated, diluted and aliquoted into new wells so that only one cell found in any well. Cells are allowed to regrow and the procedure is repeated several times to increase the probability that all the cells in a given well are monoclonal. The second method is based on the fact that many malignant cells will proliferate, forming spherical colonies, in a semisolid medium containing low amounts of agar. If the culture can be reliably dispersed into single cells and the cell concentration is such that the colonies will be well spaced, then visible colonies picked out of the agar are likely to be monoclonal.

When a hybridoma is grown in tissue culture flasks, the antibody is secreted into the medium at fairly low concentration (10-100μg/ml). An increase in the yield of monoclonal antibody secreting hybridoma can also be propagated in the peritoneal cavity of histocomplatible mice, where it secretes the monoclonal antibody into the ascites fluid at concentrations of 1-25mg/ml. The antibodies can be purified from the mouse ascites fluid by chromatography.

To meet the increased demand of monoclonal antibodies, biotechnology companies have been developing various techniques to increase yield. **Damon Biotech Company** encapsulates hybridomas in alginate gels, which allow nutrients to flow in and waste products and antibodies to flow out. In these capsules, a much higher concentration of hybridoma cells can be achieved than in tissue culture, as a result 100 fold greater yield of antibody production has been obtained. Another approach has been used by Cell Tech in UK. In this method hybridomas are grown in 100 liter fermenters, which yield 100 gm of monoclonal antibodies in a 2 week period.

13.3.5. Human monoclonal antibody

The homogeneity and specificity of monoclonal antibodies make them particularly suitable for *in vivo* administration in humans for diagnostic or therapeutic purposes. However, a major problem to the clinical use of monoclonal antibodies in human is that they are usually mouse antibodies and therefore are recognized as foreign, including an anti-isotype response. For human clinical trials, the use of human monoclonal antibodies is preferable, thus avoiding any anti-isotype response.

The production of human monoclonal antibody has been hampered by a number of technical difficulties which are as follows :

1. Difficulty in obtaining antigen prone B cell in humans (equivalent to mouse spleen);
2. One can not immunize a human volunteer with the range of antigens that can be given to mice or other animals;
3. Another major difficulty in producing human monoclonal antibodies has been finding partner for the B cell.

To overcome these difficulties normal human B lymphocytes can be transformed with Epstein Barr Virus (EBV). When lymphocytes are cultured with antigen in the presence of EBV, some of the B cells acquire the immortal-growth properties of the transformed cell while continuing to secrete the desired antibody. Cloning of such primed, transformed cells has permitted production of human monoclonal antibodies.

EBV is a lymphotrophic DNA herpes virus which is capable of converting normal human and mouse B-lymphocytes into cancer cell lines that proliferate indefinitely *in vitro*. The major difficulty with the method is the danger of the presence of the virus and the loss of antibody production with time. EBV transformation can be brought about by many ways e.g., (i) isolate the peripheral blood lymphocytes and culture them *in vitro* with antigen and EBV or (ii) first select the isolated peripheral blood lymphocytes for a specific antigen and these selected cells are then used for EBV transformation.

Human myeloma cell fusion is another method by which human hybridomas can be produced. The technique proposed by Kohler and Milstein involves the availability of a suitable HAT (a selective biochemical killer) for sensitive myeloma cell line. However, the success in fusing mouse x human cells using this technique is limited. Olsson and Kaplan in the year 1980 produced the first human-human myeloma (SKO-007), against the hapten 2,4-dinitrophenyl (DNP). Similarly, IgG secreting myeloma have been studied.

The major drawback in producing human hybridomas is the limitation for its production only at *in vitro* conditions. This is because of the need of human volunteers for *in vivo* cultivation.

13.4. ADVANTAGES OF MONOCLONAL ANTIBODIES

Monoclonal antibodies are of exceptionally high quality; represents only one molecular species and which may be obtained virtually in a homogeneous state. Conventional antiserums possess certain disadvantages, for e.g., they consist of a mixture of antibodies and a major portion of the sample contain irrelevant immunoglobulin. These properties of conventional antiserum lead to cross reactions with other antigens. A summary of the advantages of MAbs over conventional antisera is listed below.

1. Pure one molecular species only.
2. Specificity for one antigenic determinant.
3. Cross reaction means shared determinants.
4. Antiserum titer values obtained are very high.
5. Antibodies with high avidity can be produced.
6. Immure immunogen can be used.
7. *In vitro* or *in vivo* production is possible with high production rate.
8. Maintenance of farm/animals is not required for immunization and bleeding.
9. Immortal cell lines.
10. Antiserum having identical antibody with an identical specificity and constant property can be obtained world wide.
11. High reproducibility with respect to specificity and avidity.
12. Production of cell lines to individual components of a mixture is possible.
13. Radiolabelling and fluorescent conjugation or enzyme marking of MAbs are easy.

13.5. LIMITATIONS OF MONOCLONAL ANTIBODIES

The first and foremost limitation is the initial cost involved in the technique. However, on continues production, the cost is less as compared to conventional antiserum production. The method is time consuming and has its own drawbacks.

13.5.1. Precipitate formation

In general, MAbs do not form a precipitate in a standard double-immuno diffusion method. This leads to the necessity to produce a lattice framework for precipitation in tests like Ouchterlony assays (refer chapter 12).

13.5.2. Complement fixation

Conventional antiserum possesses better complement fixing capabilities than do MAbs. For an efficient complement fixation, binding of C1q component to two antibody, the molecules (Fc regions) are required either adjacent to them or nearby to the determinants. IgM and IgG are the classes of antibody which fix complement easily. Among them IgM is the best. MAbs produced via cell fusion contain mainly IgG class. Yet, they show poor complement fixing capabilities. The reason given is related to the population density of antigenic determinants present. Henceforth, a blend of MAbs required to produce the necessary synergism.

13.5.3. Antibody specificity

Production of MAbs is against a single antigenic determinant principally incorporates high level of selective specificity in to the MAbs thus rendering them incapable to distinguish between a groups of different molecules, cells bearing the chemical structure or determinants except one against which they are raised. A conventional antiserum contains antibodies to all the determinants on an antigen and can be precisely used as 'fingerprint' identification for that antigen. However, complete cross reactions can occur for MAbs and may pose problems in assays where one molecular species amongst several very similar molecular entities is to be detected. The well identified problem of cross reactivity could effectively be addressed by production of determinants specific antibody clone. The approached adds to the precision and efficiency of MAbs based analytical techniques.

13.5.4. Antibody avidity

The energy of binding to an antigen is 'precise' in case of MAb whereas it is 'average' in case of conventional antiserum. The high antibody avidity of a MAb has advantages as well as disadvantages. It is advantageous in case of immunoassay methods and undesirable for purification process (affinity chromatography).

13.6. CHARACTERIZATION AND STORAGE OF MONOCLONAL ANTIBODIES

The final determination of monoclonality requires biochemical and biophysical characterization of the immunoglobulin. Spectrophotometric, electrophoretic and chromatographic methods which can detect multiple molecular populations are frequently used for this purpose. It is also characterized immunochemically to defined its affinity for antigen, its immunoglobulin subclass, the epitopes for which it is specific and the effective number of binding site that it possesses.

Genetic stability of the cell lines can be determined by monitoring its properties during serial passage of the cells through culture. The properties include the number, shape and size of the chromosome, biochemical properties of the immunoglobulin product and other proteins, and various metabolic and growth characteristics. Finally, the physical and chemical stability of the antibody itself during different conditions of storage and use especially for its intended purpose must be determined.

Samples of incipient cell lines secreting antibodies of the desired specificity should be frozen in liquid nitrogen at several stages of cloning and culture seed stocks should also contain maximum number of clones, secreting antibodies for the desired specificity so that alternatives are available, as intended applications of the antibody.

13.7. COMMERCIAL PRODUCTION OF MONOCLONAL ANTIBODIES

Commercially monoclonal antibodies are produced by two methods:

a. Ascites production in mice, or
b. *In vitro* fermentation.

13.7.1. Ascites production in mice

In this method hybridoma cells are injected into the peritoneal cavity of histocompatible mice. The mice are pretreated by i.p. injection of pristane to irritate the peritoneal cavity and to establish a conditioned environment that facilitates the growth of ascitic tumor. The fluid produced can contain a high concentration of secreted monoclonal antibodies 3 to 15 mg/ml, and 3 to 5 ml or more can be harvested per mouse. Many pharmaceutical grade monoclonal antibodies have been produced using this technique especially for initial clinical trials. The first monoclonal antibodies approved by FDA for therapeutic use OKTS, is produced by ascites. The method has the following drawbacks:

1. It is very costly.
2. It is not reliable, product is contaminated with low levels of normal mouse immunoglobulin as well as other mouse protein.
3. Viruses can be introduced.

4. Human monoclonal antibodies are very difficult and expensive to produce as ascites in mice.

5. The human hybridomas may require special immunodeficient mice.

6. The antibody yield in ascites is often lower than murine hybridomas.

13.7.2. *In vitro* fermentation

Fermentation is a widely accepted method for the production of monoclonal antibodies because of the problems associated with ascites produced monoclonal antibodies. Potent steps of fermentation based manufacturing process are presented in table 13.1.

This method has offered certain advantages:

1. There is no contamination with normal mouse immunoglobulin.
2. The process can be cost effective especially as serum requirements in the culture medium are reduced.
3. It is reliable.
4. It can be directly scaled up from small pilot bioreactors to very large production scale.
5. There is very less contamination by adventitious agent.
6. Human monoclonal antibodies can be produced but at lower level (0.1 to 0.5 mg/ml).

The major problem in this method is the contamination of product with serum or protein based growth factors and other constituents.

Table 13.1: Outline of potential steps used in fermentation-based manufacturing

1.	**Preparation of cell banks**	
	a)	Master cell banks
	b)	Manufacturer's work cell banks (MWCB)
2.	**Fermentation**	
	a)	Preculture of MWCB
	b)	Fermentation
	c)	Harvest of culture medium
	d)	Clarification and concentration
3.	**Downstream processing**	
	a)	Initial purification
	b)	Digestion of fragments (pepsin, papain)
	c)	Further purification
	d)	Conjugation (radioisotopes chelator, toxin, drugs)
	e)	Final purification
4.	**Pharmaceutical manufacturing**	
	a)	Formulation
	b)	Vialating
	c)	Lyophilization

The stirred tank and airlift systems are used for the production because they can be readily scaled up to very large size (>1000L). The harvested culture broth containing the monoclonal antibody product requires the separation of cells and cell debris. This clarification step can be accomplished by centrifugation or filtration. The product is then concentrated (10 to 20 fold) by ultrafiltration to reduce volume prior to subsequent downstream processing.

13.7.3. Processing

The purification of monoclonal antibodies from ascites or fermentation production is done to remove contaminants from the production process such as proteins, nucleic acids, endotoxins and adventitious agents and other process additives such as enzyme for digestion and reagent for producing conjugates. The removal process must reproducibly remove contaminants to very low levels to meet the FDA requirements, while maintaining the immunogenicity of the monoclonal antibodies.

13.7.4. Chromatographic purification

Various chromatographic methods are available for purification of monoclonal antibodies. The initial purification is often performed by affinity chromatography which enables high degree of purification in a single step for IgG monoclonal antibodies, this step utilizes protein A, agarose. Subsequent processing may involve ion exchange, gel filtration and hydrophobic interaction chromatography. Endotoxins and DNA are removed by anion exchange chromatography. Gel filtration chromatography is used to remove both high and low molecular forms of monoclonal antibodies such as aggregates and small fragments.

13.7.5. Fragmentation

Fragments of IgG monoclonal antibodies such as F(ab')$_2$, Fab and Fab', produced by enzymatic digestion are often used for the final clinical product. IgG molecules are digested with immobilized papain. After digestion, the fragments are purified on an immobilized protein column (Fig.13.2).

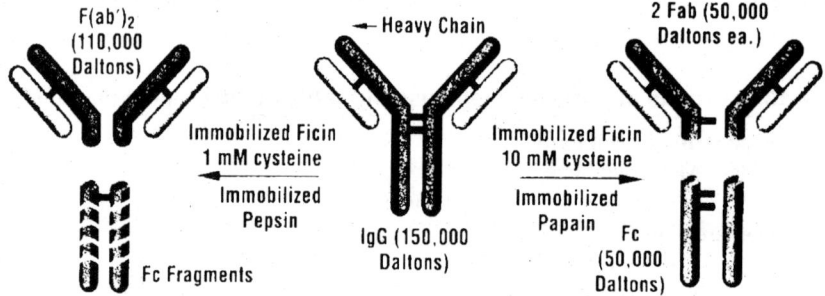

Fig. 13.2: Fragmentation of IgG

The fragmentation of IgM is necessary because intact IgM does not effectively penetrate tissues and its large molecular size creates difficulties in applications *in vitro*. Fragmentation of IgM is brought about by digestion with immobilized trypsin and pepsin. Immobilized trypsin can generate F(ab')$_2$, Fab, "IgG-type" and Fc (5μ) fragments from IgM. Immobilized pepsin can generate F(ab')$_2$, Fab, and Fv fragments (Fig. 13.3).

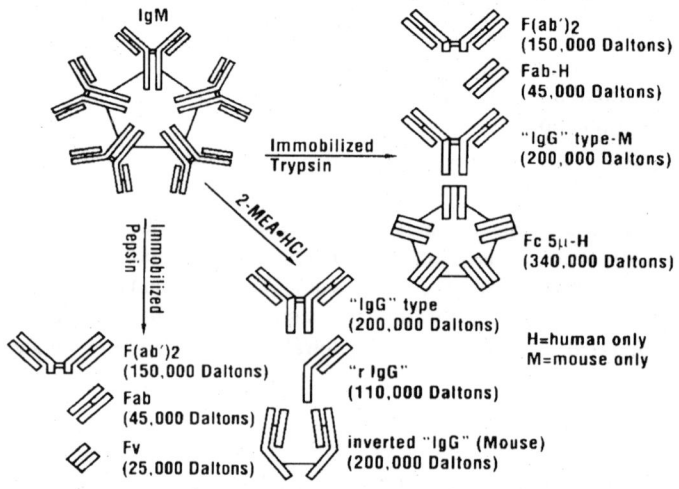

Fig. 13.3 : Fragmentation of IgM

13.7.6. Conjugation

The monoclonal antibodies are presented intact or fragmented, which may be conjugated with a variety of agents. These agents may be chelates which allow the product to form a stable bond with radioisotopes and cytotoxic agents such as toxins and chemotherapeutic agents. It is very important that conjugation must not damage the binding ability of the monoclonal antibody and by-products of the reaction must be removed using subsequent purification step.

13.7.7. Miscellaneous processing techniques

Controlled precipitation with certain salts and other agents may be used to purify and concentrate the product. Ultrafiltration can also be utilized to concentrate monoclonal antibodies and dialysis via ultrafiltration, i.e. diafiltration is used to remove low molecular weight elements. Special treatment may be added to the process in order to remove or inactivate the adventitious agents such as viruses. Sterilization filtration through 0.2 μm filters is normally performed at the end of all processing steps.

13.8. FORMULATION

The formulation is referred to as pharmaceutical manufacturing. It involves formulation, vial filling, stoppering and lyophilization (if necessary). The formulation process consists of concentrating the product by ultrafiltration, buffer exchange into the final filtration and then dilution to the required protein concentration. Radiolabelled products require additional steps for the blending of specialized ingredients and may need special precautions such as anaerobic conditions to preserve the sulfhydryls of Fab' products.

Before filling, the product is passed through a final sterile filter. Generally, the filling is done by using standard automated pharmaceutical filling machine, but may require specialized conditions such as filling under an inert gas to preserve Fab' sulfhydryls. Lyophilization is frequently applied for MAb products especially when shelf-life stability of liquid formulations is a problem.

13.9. QUALITY CONTROL

Since MAbs are produced from living cells in animals or by *in vitro* fermentation, quality control of these products is designed to assess residual impurities from the production sources, as well as contamination with adventitious agents. Extensive testing must be performed at every stage of the manufacturing process to determine that known impurities are removed and that potential adventitious agents are inactivated or removed. Quality control tests are performed on following stages:

1. At the cell bank stage to determine the cell line stability, identity and the presence of adventitious agents such as viruses and mycoplasma.
2. Testing during downstream processing focuses on the removal of impurities derived from the cell line and fermentation medium, with a particular attention on the ability to remove or inactivate adventitious viruses and to reduce levels of DNA released from hybridoma cells during the production process.
3. Testing of the final product is performed to check the sterility, safety, apyrogenicity and biochemical or immunological characterization of MAb for identity, purity and potency.

13.10. MISCELLANEOUS APPROACHES OF MAb PRODUCTION

13.10.1. Engineered monoclonal antibodies

Mouse monoclonal antibodies when used as immunotoxin in high concentration (which is required to bind sufficient amounts of antibody to tumor) are recognized as foreign and evoke antibody response. The induced human anti-mouse antibodies reduce effectiveness of immunotoxin by clearing it from blood stream. Circulating complexes of mouse and human antibodies can cause allergic reactions also. Sometimes build up of these complexes in organs such as kidney can cause serious and even life threatening reactions. Use of human monoclonal antibodies can be a solution to the above problem but development of human monoclonal antibodies has been hampered by technical difficulties. Researchers have began engineering monoclonal antibodies using recombinant DNA technology to avoid above difficulties and complications.

13.10.1.1. Chimeric monoclonal antibodies

In this approach an antibody is engineered by cloning recombinant DNA containing the promoter, leader and variable regions sequences from a mouse antibody gene and the constant region exons from human antibody gene. The antibody encoded by such a recombinant gene is a mouse-human chimera and commonly known as humanized antibody. Antigen specificity determining variable region is derived from mouse DNA while its isotope which is determined by constant region is derived from human DNA. These chimeric antibodies have fewer mouse antigenic determinants as their constant regions are encoded by human genes therefore they are far less immunogenic than mouse monoclonal antibodies. Chimeric antibody has another advantage of retaining biological effector functions of human antibody and therefore they may trigger complement activation of Fc receptor binding.

Mouse variable region in these humanized antibodies can also induce an antibody response in humans therefore chimeric antibodies containing only mouse CDRs of mouse antibody together with human framework regions could be produced so that the antibodies retain human B-strand framework with only the hyper variable loops of mouse origin.

These antibodies are less immunogenic in humans than humanized antibodies containing the entire mouse variable region. Since hypervariable loops constitute the antigen binding site sometimes CDR grafted antibodies retain antigen binding ability. But often CDR-grafted antibodies exhibit reduced binding affinity. The latter can be corrected in some cases by introducing small changes in the frame work region that induces and incorporates small changes in the three dimensional configuration of the CDRs thus resulting into improved antibody affinity. Complete remission of non Hodgkin's lymphoma has been obtained by injection of CDR grafted monoclonal antibody specific for a cell membrane antigen on lymphoma cells. Table 13.2 illustrates some of CDR grafted monoclonal antibodies that are presently being assessed for clinical applicability.

Table 13.2. : Therapeutic uses for CDR-grafted antibodies

Target antigen	Clinical potential
CDW52 (surface molecule on leukocytes)	Lymphomas; systemic; vasculitis; rheumatoid arthritis
CD3 (T cell marker)	Organ transplantation
CD4 (T cell marker)	Organ transplantation; rheumatoid arthritis; Crohn's disease
Receptor for interleukin 2	Leukemia and lymphomas; organ transplantation; graft-versus-host disease
HIV	AIDS
Herpes simplex virus	Neonatal; ocular and genital herpes infection
Tumor necrosis factor α	Septic shock
Receptor for human epidermal growth factor (EGF)	Cancer
Placental alkaline phosphatase	Cancer
Carcinoembryonic antigen (CEA)	Cancer

An antibody with a constant region possessing a given biological effector function can also be engineered using chimera approach. For example, the γ' constant region in humans is very effective in mediating complement lysis by engineering anti tumor antibody with γ' constant region and complement mediated destruction of tumor cells has been proposed. In another approach terminal constant region domain has been replaced with a toxin where resulting antibodies serve as immunotoxins, and as they lack the terminal domain of the Fc, they are not able to bind to cells bearing Fc receptors and thus remain in circulation.

13.10.2. Monoclonal antibody heteroconjugates

The hybrids of two different antibody molecules known as heteroconjugates have been designed. In some of such heteroconjugates one half of antibody has specificity for the tumor while the other half has specificity for a surface molecule on an immune effector cell such as NK cell, an activated macrophage, or a cytotoxic T lymphocyte (CTL). The heteroconjugates thus serves to cross link the immune effector cell to the tumor.

Some heteroconjugates have been designed to activate the immune effector cell when it is cross linked to tumor cell. For example, T cell receptor is always expressed as a complex with the associated membrane molecule CD3 which is involved in signal transduction. Heteroconjugates consisting of anti CD3 and an antitumor monoclonal antibody have been shown to cross link CTs to tumor cells. heteroconjugates also appear to activate the CTL so that it begins to initiate and mediate the destruction of tumor cells.

13.10.3. Monoclonal antibodies constructed from immunoglobulin gene-libraries

In this approach, DNA from hybridoma or plasma cells encoding for heavy chain and light chain fragments is amplified by polymerase chain reaction (PCR) and separate heavy and light chain libraries are constructed in bacteriophage λ. Each inserted gene contains an Eco RI restriction site, down stream of the heavy chain genes and upstream of light chain gene. Cleavage with Eco RI and joining of the heavy and light chain genes yields numerous random heavy and light chain based constructs (Fig. 13.4).

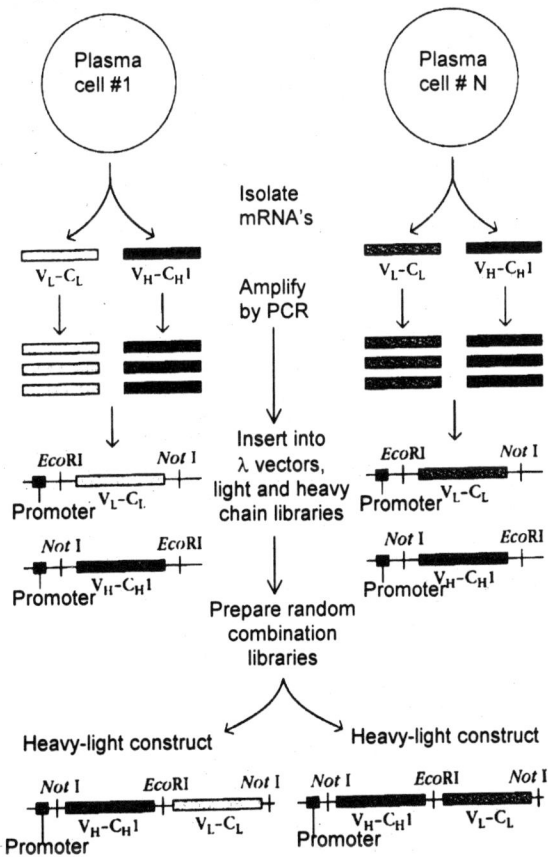

Fig. 13.4 : Procedure for production of gene libraries encoding Fab' fragments

Thus, enormous diversities of antibody combinations could be generated and clones containing their random combinations can be screened for those secreting antibody to a particular antigen.

There is a great potential of producing enormous repertoire of antibody specificity's without employing antigen priming, immunization or hybridoma technology which could to complicate the production of monoclonal antibody.

13.10.4. Anti-idiotype

It was proposed by NielsJerne in 1973 that the immune systems in its process of recognition of self antigen may present a set of consequences and referred them to be as network theory. Theoretically, an antibody is produced as a response to an antigen which in turn may induce the formation of antibodies to its unique variable regions. The individual antigenic determinants of variable region has been referred as an **idiotope**. Obviously each antibody could contain multiple idiotopes and some of them is called **idiotype** of the antibody in reference. In some of the cases idiotopes and actual antigen combining sites may be identical and referred as paratope. While in other cases idiotopes are consist of variable region sequences outside the antigen binding sites. It was proposed that during antibody response the antibodies formed in response to the antigen may in turn induce the formation of secondary antibodies to the individual idiotopes of the first antibody. The idiotype of primary antibody thus activates the proliferation network of B cells, whose receptors recognize the individual antibody, i.e. AB1. These B-cells then differentiate in plasma cells which effectively secrete anti-idiotype antibody (AB2). The individual idiotopes of AB2 can further extend the network by inducing production of anti-anti-idiotype (AB3). This typically resembles idiotypes of AB1 and network begins to limit them self as decreased level of antibody is produced during each successive activation event. In nutshell, it can be appreciated that some anti-idiotype antibody are directed against the paratope thus emerge as the internal image of the original epitope on the original. This anti-paratope antibody thus mimics the original. In fact this mimicking is evidenced by ability of anti-paratope antibody to bind to the antigen receptor (Fig. 13.5).

Anti-idiotype antibody which are internal image of the original antigen can serve as a **vaccine** so as to induce an immune response to a pathogenic antigen thus at large avoiding immunization with the pathogen. anti-idiotype vaccines have been shown to induce protective immunity in mice against hepatitis B, rabbis, sendai, *Streptococcous pneumoniae*, *Listeria monocytogenes*, *trypanosoma rhodesiense* and *Schistosoma mansoni*.

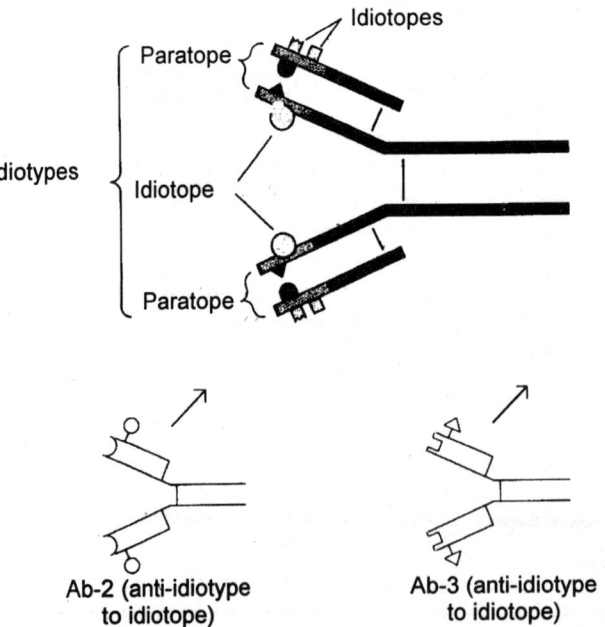

Fig. 13.5 : Schematic representation of the network theory

13.10.5. T cell hybridomas (Thymomas)

T cells hybridomas can be produced by fusing primed T cells with cancerous T cells called **thymoma cells** by a procedure similar to that used for fusion of primed B cells with cancerous plasma cells. T cells hybridoma do not secrete antibody, but rather possess other immunologic functions, e.g. secretion of cytokines and expression of T cell receptors specific for a particular antigen MHC molecules.

Antigen specific T helper and T cytotoxic hybridomas have been cloned. The technique has facilitated the identification of various T cell specific molecules. For example, an ovalbumin specific class II MHC restricted T cell thymoma. The resulting hybridoma, which displayed the antigenic specificity and MHC restriction of the parent TH cell, could be assayed for TH function by its capacity to secrete interleukin-2 in response to ovalbumin on an appropriate antigen presenting cell. As T cell hybridomas grow as tumors, large number of cells can be obtained within a short period of time. This property has been utilized in biochemical isolation and purification of various T cell products as T cell cytokines.

13.11. APPLICATIONS OF MONOCLONAL ANTIBODIES

Monoclonal antibodies are having a remarkable range of applications. The following criteria are helpful to understand the areas of MAbs application.

1. Antibodies against a range of molecules including those on cell surface and microorganisms are possible.
2. The ability of antibodies to lyse target cells in the presence of complement.
3. Hybridoma technology can produce a range of hybridoma cell line secreting antibodies against an antigenic determinant.
4. In affinity chromatography a powerful purification technique wherein antibody bound in solid systems are used to separate specific antigen from crude material.
5. MAbs have the ability to behave in its normal physiological way to attack foreign material, thus finding place in defense against infection.

Monoclonal antibody based products are covered by a number of recent compendia. The *in vivo* application of MAbs is based on critical factors listed in table 13.3

Table 13.3 : Critical factors for monoclonal antibodies used *in vivo*

Antibody related	Target related
Affinity	Vascularity
Specificity	Distribution of antigens
Class and subclass	Antigenic heterogeneity
Murine vs. human	Antigenic modulation
Intact vs. fragments	Circulating antigen
Dose	
Route of administration	
Immunogenicity	

For effective localization, the monoclonal antibodies should have high affinity for the target antigen. Cross-sensitivity with non target tissue should be minimal. The class and subclass of the immunoglobulin affect both biodistribution and blood clearance as well as interaction with immune mechanisms of the host. Blood clearance and catabolism are generally faster with heterologous murine immunoglobulins as compared to homologous human MAbs.

The lower the molecular weight of the antibody, the faster the blood clearance. Intact murine IgG has a blood half life of approximately 30h. and is catabolized in liver and spleen, as well as other sites in the body. F(ab')$_2$ and Fab/Fab' have half lives of approximately 20 h. and 2 h., respectively, and tend to accumulate in kidney. Due to their smaller molecular size, fragments are better able to diffuse out of capillaries and onto target tissue. However, for interaction with immune effector functions of the host, intact immunoglobulin with the Fc portion is required. Antibody dose also has an effect on blood clearance and biodistribution. Higher dose generally at

10mg or above, appears to saturate non-specific sites in the liver and other organs, as a consequence, more antibodies remain in the blood and clearance is slower. Routes of injection other than intravenous have also been shown to alter biodistribution. Intralymphatic and intraperitoneal administrations tend to concentrate and prolong the dose at these sites and lead to lower systemic levels.

Characteristics of target tissue are also important in MAb localization. The tissue should be well vascularized or directly exposed to the blood system. This is often a problem with solid tumors, which are poorly vascularized. The antigen in the target tissue should be densely and uniformly expressed and accessible to antibody binding. Viable cells must express target antigen on the cell surface, whereas MAbs that localize dead cells may depend on reactivity with intracellular antigens. Tumor cells often demonstrate antigenic heterogeneity. In some cases antigenic modulation has also been demonstrated, whereby the process of antibody binding to cell-surface antigen causes the complex to be shed or internalized, rendering the cell devoid of expressed antigen. Cross reactive target antigen may also be found in the circulation, often as a consequence of tumor cell shedding. This circulating antigen could complex with the injected MAb and block it from binding to the target site.

The applications of monoclonal antibodies can therefore be classified as:

A. Diagnostic uses

  1. Diagnostic reagents
  2. Diagnostic imaging

   a) Cardiovascular diseases
   b) Sites of bacterial infection
   c) Cell surface markers
   d) Detection of circulating antigens
   d) Cancer
   e) Hormones
   f) Immunometric assay procedures

B. Therapeutic application

  1. General

   a) MAb itself
   b) Radioisotope immunoconjugates
   c) Toxin drug conjugates

  2. Transplantation

   a) Organ
   b) Bone marrow

  3. *Infectious diseases*

   a) Micro-organisms
   b) Parasites

  4. Enzyme and proteins
  5. Cardiovascular diseases
  6. Autoimmune disease
  7. Cancer
  8. Antidotes

C. Investigational and analytical application

  1. Lymphocyte phenotyping
  2. Purification of proteins
  3. Radioimmunoassays

D. Drug Targeting

  1.Immunotoxins
  2.Suppresser deletion
  3.Site specific modification

4.Antibody enzyme conjugates
E. Miscellaneous
1. Abzymes
2. Autoantibody fingerprinting

13.11.1. Diagnostic application of monoclonal antibodies
13.11.1.1. Diagnostic reagents

Monoclonal antibody based diagnostic reagents include products for detecting pregnancy, diagnosing infectious protozoan, bacterial and viral pathogens; monitoring therapeutic drug levels, detecting heart damage; matching histocompatibility antigens; detecting diabetes and detecting tumor cells.

Many of these test kits utilize strips of paper impregnated with an appropriate monoclonal antibody. Diagnostic products are relatively inexpensive to produce and are projected to have growing markets.

13.11.1.2. Diagnostic imaging

Diagnostic imaging with radiolabelled MAbs has also been referred to as immunoscintiography. It employs the use of planar gamma camera to detect the two dimensional distribution in the body of the gamma emitting radioisotopes conjugated to MAbs. Recently camera utilizing single photon emission computed tomography (SPECT) has been used to give more sensitive three dimensional evaluations (Fig. 13.6). Certain critical factors specific to imaging MAbs are presented in table13.3. Radioisotope commonly used in imaging with MAbs along with their half lives and gamma emission have been listed in table 13.4. Application of diagnostic imaging is discussed here.

This is also known as immunoscintography using a planar gamma camera to detect the two dimensional distribution in the body of gamma-emitting radioisotopes conjugated to MAbs. Various imaging applications of MAbs are given below:

1. Cardiovascular disease
   a) Myocardial infarction
   b) Deep-vein thrombosis
   c) Atherosclerosis
2. Sites of bacterial infections
3. Cancer
   a) Solid tumor (antitumor associated antigen)
   b) Locating and sizing
   c) Detection of occult tumors
   d) Determining suitability of MAbs
   e) Monitoring response in therapy

13.11.2. Cardiovascular disease
13.11.2.1. Myocardial infarction

The antimyosin MAb is specific for human myosin and binds to intracellular myosin exposed as a consequence of myocardial necrosis. Myosin™ is the antimyosin containing MAb product approved by the Committee for Proprietary Medicinal Products of the European Economic Community. The product consists of a kit containing 0.5 mg of antimyosin Fab fragment conjugated with the chelator DTPA (diethylene triaminepenta acetic acid). The liquid formulated Fab-DTPA is labelled by mixing with approximately 2mCi of ^{111}In chloride. After incubation for about 1.0 minutes, the ^{111}In-labelled MAb is ready for IV injection. Imaging is performed after 24 to 48 h. using either a planner gamma camera or single photon emission computed tomography (SPECT). The product has shown a high degree of sensitivity for detecting infarction and specificity excluding a recent ischemic event in patients with chest pain syndrome. Indium antimyosin is able to detect the location and extent of necrotic heart tissue and should be useful in the diagnosis of heart attack and in the early risk stratification of patients demonstrated to have myocardial damage.

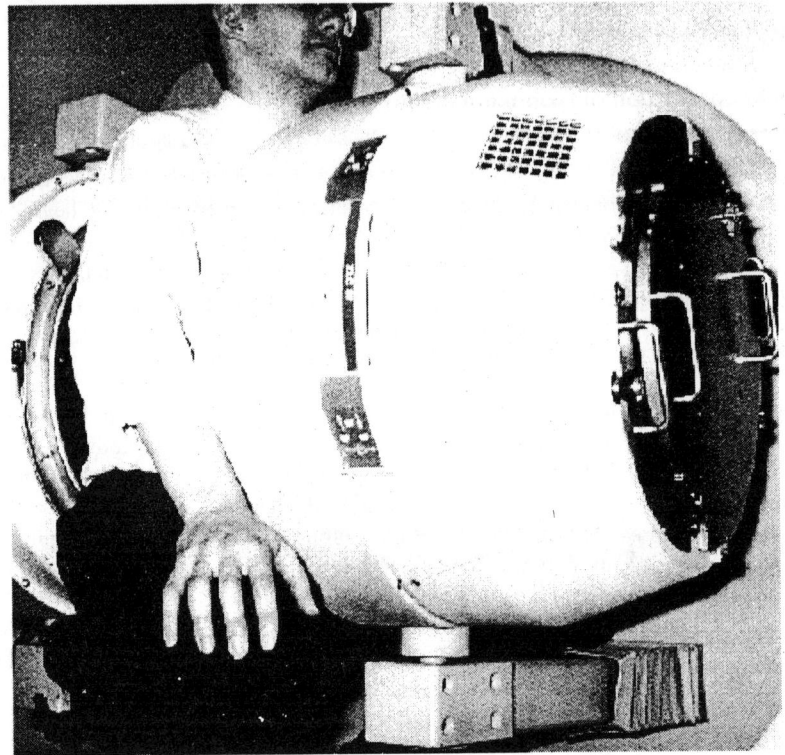

Fig. 13.6 : Photograph of a patient undergoing examination by a gamma camera

13.11.2.2. Deep vein thrombosis

Deep vein thrombosis (DVT) is an ideal disease for imaging applications due to the following reasons:

1. The target clots within the blood, which has direct access to i.v administered MAb.
2. DVT is located primarily in the lower extremities and thus well away from nonspecific uptake in the blood pool and organs of the central body.

The approaches have been divided into use of labelled MAbs directed against platelets, which are components of actively developing thrombi, and against fibrin. This technique is useful during the acute phase of thrombogenesis but may not be effective with clots older than 24 to 48 h. ^{111}In-labelled Fab-DTPA showed a sensitivity of 86-100 % in directing thrombi in the extremities of the patients. Imaging is performed after 4 h. of injection. The general critical factors which are to be considered in imaging applications are shown in table13.4.

Table 13.4 : Critical factors specific to imaging MAbs

Radioisotope	Pharmacokinetics	Target
Energy	Blood clearance	Size
Half life	Uptake in normal tissue	Attenuation
Labelling chemistry	Dosimetry	Target to non target ratio
Stability of linkage		
Availability and cost		

The choice of radioisotope is an important step. The selected isotope must have following properties:

1. It should have a gamma emission energy suitable for patient safety and current gamma camera technology.
2. The half life must be long enough to allow time for MAb localization, at the same time should be short enough not to pose a safety issue.
3. The labelling chemistry must be practical and yield a stable linkage.
4. The isotope should be relatively inexpensive and readily available.

Table 13.5 lists the isotope commonly used in imaging applications.

Table 13.5 : Radioisotopes used in imaging

Isotope(s)	Half life	Gamma Emission(κ_εV)
^{123}I	13 h.	159
^{125}I	60 days	35
^{131}I	8 days	364
^{111}In	2.8 days	173
^{99m}Tc	6 h.	140

The pharmacokinetic aspects are also critical to imaging application. The labelled antibody must be cleared from the blood at sufficiently faster rate so that target uptake is not obscured.

Certain membrane proteins are present on the tumor cells but are absent from the normal cells (or present at much lower levels). Monoclonal antibodies specific for these tumors associated membrane proteins can be produced and used in tumor detection and imaging. Production of MAbs specific for these membrane proteins involves screening of large numbers of hybridomas to identify clones secreting antibody specific for the tumor associated antigens.

Minna and coworkers immunized mice with human lung cancer cells and fused the immunized spleen cells with mouse, myeloma cells to generate hybridomas secreting monoclonal antibody to human lung cancer cells. They screened 20,000 hybridoma clones and could identify 80 clones those were specific for various lung cancer cells and did not react against normal lung cells. Monoclonal antibodies with such tumor specificity can be used either to detect the spread of tumor or to kill tumor cells.

13.11.3. Diagnosis of sites of bacterial infections and sexually transmitted diseases(STDs)

The sexually transmitted diseases are now a days becoming more popular and popular. Most common pathogens for STDs are *Neisseria gonorrhoeae, Chlamydia trachomatis, H*erpse simplex virus. The diagnosis of these organisms is accomplished using the following classical methods:

(i) Microscopic examination of tissue specimens and exudates for identification of the bacterium, fungi or virus infected cells using staining process.
(ii) Culture methods in which the micro-organisms are specifically cultured and grown in a specific growth medium permitting multiplication of some micro-organisms, which could then be identified and checked for susceptibility against antibiotics.
(iii) Immunological methods where the antigens associated with the pathogen are identified in the tissue or body fluids.
(iv) Measurement of antibodies produced in the patient as a result of infection with an organism.

Under general conditions the pathology laboratories used at least two of the methods for gaining surety in diagnosis, which sometimes are not full proof. However, the hybridoma technology has revolutionized the field. Specific testing kits are now available for testing of these disorders.

The cell hybrids are first prepared as discussed earlier in the hybridoma technology. The screening of the cell lines is accomplished by replica plating techniques, due to random loss of chromosomes in the cell hybrids.

These cell hybrids are then placed in 96 well microtest plates. Small samples of the culture fluid from each well is placed in the replica plates, each of which is impregnated with a specific antigen. The immune reaction is detected through radio-immunoassay in which ^{125}I-labelled protein A which binds to a Fc protein of human IgG in the immune complex. The positive reactions can be traced back to original wells and the cell lines then multiplied for production of specific antibodies. The method could successfully be utilized in the preparation of antibodies so as to specifically distinguish *N. gonorrhoeae, C. trachomatis*, and HSV. For example a mixture of three antibodies (4-G5, 2-H1 and 3-C8) identified 99.6% of 719 isolates of *N. gonorrhoeae* and these never reacted with other species of *Neisseria*.

The same technology has been extended for the identification and diagnosis of *Chlamydia* and HSV. *Chlamydia* infections (from elementary body) enter the cells within 48-72 h from large inclusion body containing several elementary bodies, which on release causes infections in neighboring cells. These cells could be fixed in ethanol and stained with fluorescence-conjugated antibodies, characteristic inclusion bodies could be detected as early as 18h. after infection by immunofluorescence. In the case of HSV, a panel of four different monoclonal antibodies allowed distinction between type I and II of HSV. Such tests are named as typing of HSV.

13.11.4. Cell surface markers

Monoclonal antibodies have found an important place in cell surface diagnosis thereby paving way to direct detection of diseases which was previously impossible.

13.11.4.1. ABD and rare blood groups

Anti-ABD, anti (rare blood groups) and anti-HLA monoclonal antibodies produced by immunizing mouse with human cells are practically useful in blood grouping. Monoclonal antibodies have been produced against group A erythrocytes. Monoclonal antibodies against membrane glycoproteins of the human erythrocytes especially glycophorin A at different sites as well as antibodies which bind to other erythrocyte surface molecules have been developed. Thus, it is possible to use these antibodies to detect similar determinants on other cells as well as to isolate and purify the cell surface molecules.

13.11.4.2. HLA antigens and tissue typing

The human major histocompatability complex (MHC) is involved in a number of important immuunological events, e.g. graft rejection, graft-versus-host reactions, cellular co-operation and cytotoxic reactions, etc., The human leukocytes in the above mentioned immunological phenomena are being detected (HLA tissue typing) using the antisera obtained from multiparous women. The disadvantage with the present system is that such antisera are not available against some rare HLA-antigens. This makes one to turn towards hybridoma technique to elicit monoclonal against the rare HLA antigens.

13.11.4.3. Classification of cells, cell-cell interactions

Specific monoclonal antibodies against all cell surface antigenic determinants enable one to select antibodies which are specific only to a given cell line. This can be explained with the following example. Monoclonal antibodies with clinical application in immunosuppression and in depletion of T cells are to cite a few. This is brought about by raising monoclonal antibodies against human T- and B cell population. It has been shown that specific monoclonal antibodies against various T cell antigens have brought about substantial changes in T cell population in a variety of diseases such as systemic lupus erythroematosus, multiple sclerosis, rheumatoid arthritis and a number of infectious diseases.

Hybridoma technology helps in the identification of new and previously unknown cell surface differentiation antigens. It is also now possible to study cell-cell interactions. because changes in cell surfaces can potentially be monitored with the help of monoclonal antibodies.

13.11.4.4. Cell separation

Cell sub-populations belonging to the liver, lung, kidney, central nervous system, sperm cells, macrophage and monocytes have can be separated using labelled antibodies and reisolating as 'pure' cells. Separation can be achieved using FITC techniques (readers may refer chapter 8), Where the antibody will bind to only one cell sub-population and then the separation is achieved using fluorescent-activated cell sorter (FACS). An alternative method is to separate cell sub-populations using solid-phase affinity chromatography (refer chapter 4 for details).

13.11.4.5. Cell surface biochemistry

Understanding cell surface biochemistry is important. However, determining it is difficult. To overcome such difficulties, monoclonal antibodies which can distinguish between different cell types can be developed. These antibodies bind to a certain specific chemical structure and therefore help in elucidation of the structures of cell surface molecules. This helps in revelation of the exact surface biochemical changes associated with cellular differentiation, cellular communication, special physiological functions, the vast range of diseased and deficient cells, carcinogenesis and its effect on different cell types.

13.11.5. Detection from antigens circulating in blood

Monoclonal antibodies can also be used in the detection of tumors which shed tumor specific antigens into the blood. This type of detection is highly useful and has great potential. For example, a monoclonal antibody has been developed, which detects a shed pancreatic tumor antigen. This is of considerable diagnostic value since the level of pancreatic tumor antigen in blood indicates the stage of tumor pancreatic cancer, which usually can not be diagnosed until an advanced stage is arrived. However, it now may be detected early utilizing ability of monoclonal antibody to detect even low levels of this shed tumor antigen. Similarly monoclonal antibody to a glycolipid antigen shed by colorectal tumor has been developed.

13.11.5.1. Location of primary or metastatic tumors

Primary and metastatic tumors can be located in patients by using radiolabelled monoclonal antibodies specific to tumor associated membrane proteins. Monoclonal antibody specific to breast cancer cells labelled with iodine 131 when introduced into blood, detects tumor spread to regional lymph nodes. This radiolabelled monoclonal antibody based imaging technique successfully detects breast cancer metastases that otherwise stands to be undetectable by other scanning techniques.

Similarly, monoclonal antibody to breast cancer cells labelled with the metal gadolinium Gd can be detected by magnetic resonance imaging (MRI). By this method even pin head size metastases located in regional lymph nodes could be visualized.

In spite of the potential of these approaches, there are several of obstacles to the wide detection and imaging. Major problem is that many tumors of a given type do not share common tumors specific membrane proteins. Investigations in diagnostic imaging of all major types of solid tumors including melanoma, colorectal carcinoma, ovarian carcinoma, sarcoma, lung carcinoma have been conducted The tumor markers used in diagnostic imaging using MAb are given table 13.6.

Table 13.6 : Tumor markers used in MAb imaging

Carcinoembryonic antigen	Transferrin receptor
α-Fetoprotein	Epidermal growth factor receptor
Human chorionic gonadotropin	Oncogene products
Human milk fat globule	Tumor-associated cell surface antigens
Prostatic acid phosphatase	Gangliosides
Ferritin	Necrosis-associated intracellular antigens

Imaging after tumor therapy can be used to monitor therapeutic responses, detect reoccurrence and guide subsequent clinical decisions. An initial evaluation using scintillation counter with the same MAb for its selective localization may help to determine its suitability for therapy. The mixtures of MAbs (termed cocktails) directed against different antigens have been applied with some success in colorectal carcinoma and may address the central problem of antigenic heterogeneity.

13.11.5.2. Tumor immunotherapy

Treatment of tumor has been an exciting and important field. Monoclonal antibodies have appreciated for their pivotal role in the chemotherapy of neoplasia. A number of reports have claimed suppression of human colorectal tumors in mice following the injection of tumor specific monoclonal antibodies. A monoclonal anti-mouse T cell antibody when added *in vitro* to a leukemia cell lines demonstrated a halt of cell proliferation.

Monoclonal antibodies have been tested experimentally as immunotherapeutic agents for cancer. For example, Levy & coworkers successfully treated a patient with B-cell lymphomas with anti-idiotype MAbs. Since the cancer was related with B cell, the membrane bound antibody on all the cancerous cells were evaluated to possess the same idiotype (Fig. 13.7). These researches produced mouse monoclonal antibody specific for the B-lymphoma idiotype. This anti-idiotype MAb when injected into the patient, was found to bind specifically to the B-lymphoma cells. This in turn activated the complement systems and entailed the lysis of the B-lymphoma cells without harming other cells.

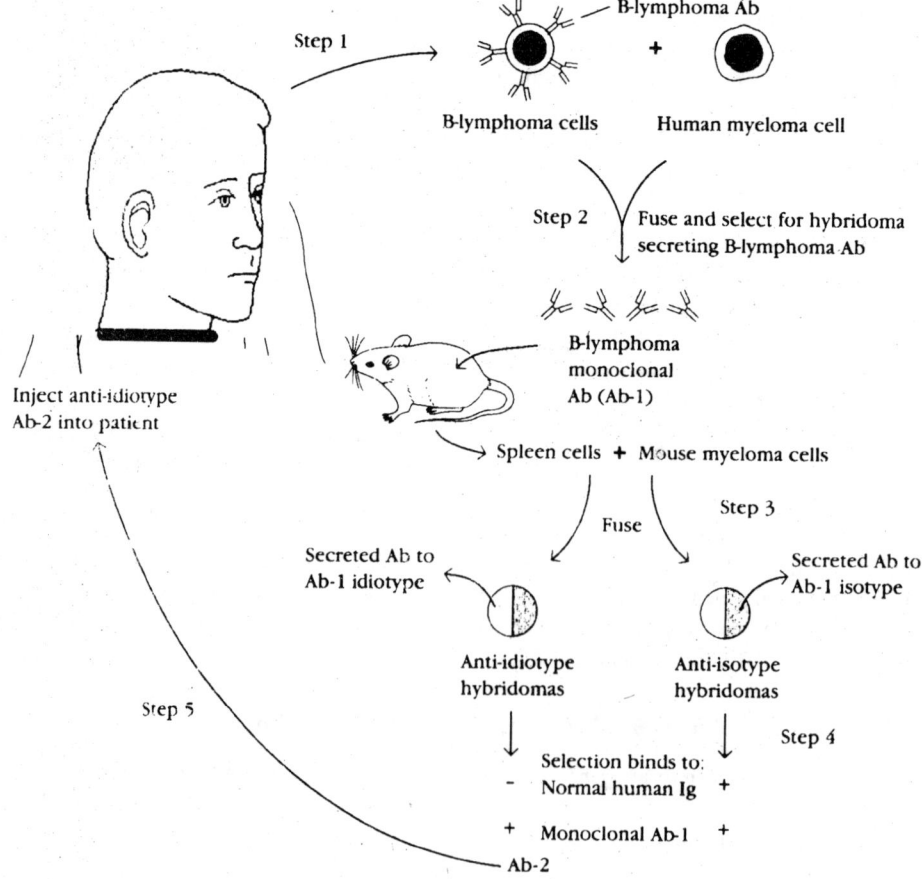

Fig. 13.7 : Treatment man with B-cell lymphomas with monoclonal antibody specific for idiotypic determinants on the B-lymphoma cells

Monoclonal antibodies have also been used to prepare tumor-specific immunotoxins. These agents consist of the inhibitor chain of a toxin linked to an antibody against a specific tumors.

In another approach, an effort was made to induce nonspecific T cell activation *in vivo* by administering monoclonal antibody specific to CD3 which is known to activate T cells in *in-vitro*. Monoclonal antibodies can also be used to bridge activated T cells directly to a tumor. Here, two different monoclonal antibodies are produced; one specific for a tumor-cell membrane molecule and one specific for the CD3 membrane molecule of the TCR complex. A hybrid monoclonal antibody, or heteroconjugate is then prepared with specificity for the tumor antigen and for CD3.

13.11.5.3. Immunosuppressive therapy

The major limitation with the conventional immunosuppressive treatments is that they lack specificity, thus producing a generalized immunosuppression and thereby increasing the risk of infection. An ideal immunosuppressive agent therefore should be antigen-specific wherein they have reduced immune response to alloantigens of the graft while they are active against unrelated antigens.

Monoclonal antibodies have been so far successfully used to suppress T cell activity or its subpopulations. Injection of such monoclonal antibodies results in a rapid depletion of T cells from the circulation. This is caused by binding of antibody-coated T cells to Fc receptors on phagocytic cells, which then phagocytose and clear the T cells from circulation. Monoclonal antibodies specific for the high-affinity IL-2 receptor (anti-TAC) also have been used successfully to increase graft survival. The disadvantage with the monoclonal antibodies preparation, is that these antibodies are generally of mouse origin. Hence, the recipient often develops an antibody response to the mouse monoclonal antibody, rapidly clearing it from the body. To overcome this, human monoclonal antibodies and mouse-human chimeric monoclonal antibodies are being evaluated.

The use of toxins bound to monoclonal antibody in tumor destruction has gained wide attention. Toxins could be of bacterial and plant origin. Bacterial toxins such as diphtheria toxin and *Pseudomonas aeruginosa* toxin A and the plant toxins ricin, abrin and modecin are some representative examples of toxin. Therapy for gliomas form of brain therapy is achieved by fusing lymphocytes extracted from gliomas with a human myeloma line to produce human hybridomas secreting antiglioma antibodies. The isolation of these antibodies indicates that patients with gliomas do produce antibodies against their own tumors and these are secreted by lymphocytes within the tumor. These human antibodies may be isotope labelled and used for the localization of intracerebral disease by brain scanning as well as being used as a immunotoxin for the tumor cells.

13.11.6. Hormones

Conventional antisera used in immunoassay procedure have been replaced by monoclonal antibodies produced against hormones. They are also being explored;
- to study the antigenic determinants present.
- with the aim of the isolation and purification of the material.
- in certain cases to study the physiology/pathophysiology of the hormone.
- purely as a method for detection and localization of the substance.

Substance P was one of the earliest small molecules to be investigated in this field (Table 13.7). Radioimmunoassays for the polypeptide human growth hormone and a sensitive solid phase chemiluminescence immunoassay for urinary pregnanediol-3α-glucoronide has been established using monoclonal antibodies.

13.11.7. Pregnancy testing kits

The agglutination reaction is defined as the formation of an immune complex by the cross linking of cells or particles (acting as antigens) with specific antibodies (refer Chap12). These agglutination reactions form visible aggregates or clumps (agglutinins) that can be seen by the naked eyes also. These direct agglutination reactions could be effectively utilized for the detection of a number of substances. For example, Widal's test is the reaction involving the agglutination of the typhoid bacillus when mixed with serum containing typhoid antibodies from an individual having typhoid.

Table 13.7 : Monoclonal antibodies made against hormones

S. No.	Hormone	S.No.	Hormone
1	Human chorionic gonadotropin (hCG)	2	Thyroxine and Triiodothyronine (T_4 and T_3)
3	Human growth hormone (hGH)	4	Human Thyroid Stimulating Hormone (TSH)
5	Pregnanediol-3α-glucoronide	6	Renin
7	Insulin	8	Gastrin
9	Progesterone	10	Substance P

Recently the technique has been developed that employs microscopic synthetic latex spheres coated with the antigens. These coated microspheres are extremely useful in the diagnosis of various reactions. The modern pregnancy testing kits detect the elevation in the levels of the human chorionic gonadotropin (HCG), hormone which occurs in the female urine and the blood in the early phase of the pregnancy. The principle for the testing is schematically represented in figure 13.8.

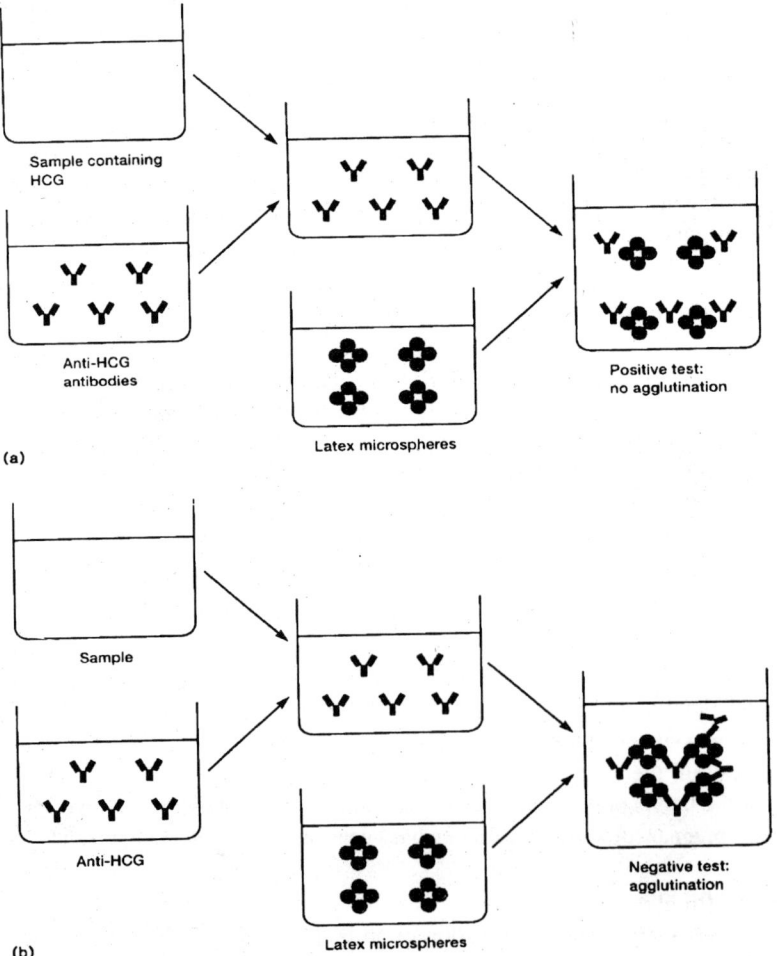

Fig. 13.8 : Principle of pregnancy testing based on specific antibodies for HCG tagged to latex microspheres; (a) positive test (b) negative test

In a positive test, urine from the female containing HCG is mixed with a solution of antibody specific for HCG. In the second step latex microspheres coated with HCG are added. If the HCG is present, it binds to the HCG specific antibodies thereby preventing them from agglutinating the microspheres. In an negative test, the microspheres coated with antigen are agglutinated by HCG specific antibodies which favors detection. Many rapid pregnancy testing kits are now available in the world market. Most of them are disposable home use kits based on color detection using sticks. These kits allow the successful testing for the presence of pregnancy even after one day of conception.

13.11.8. Rapid detection of drugs in urine

The screening of the drugs in the urine is undertaken by the use of some classical techniques like thin layer chromatography (TLC), liquid chromatography (LC) which are quite laborious procedures. With the requirement of the massive drug testing in sports, federal civilian employment, military and the fields when, rapid procedures are needed.

The best and the one of the most rapidly applicable procedures in the testing is based on the latex sphere agglutination immunoassay for the detection of cocaine, morphine, barbiturates, THC (marijuana), methadone, phencyclidine and amphetamine. This method provides accuracy of the immunoassay approach with the requirement of expensive chemicals and equipment.

The latex agglutination-inhibition test relies on the competition for the antibody between a latex drug conjugate and any drug that may be present in the urine. A urine sample is placed in the mixing well of the slide containing antibody reagent, buffer, and latex reagent. If the drug is absent, the latex drug conjugate binds to the antibody and forms a larger particles that agglutinate (Fig. 13.9). Therefore the agglutination is the evidence for the absence of the drug in the urine specimen. However, the positive urine sample does not change the smooth milky appearance of the test mixture.

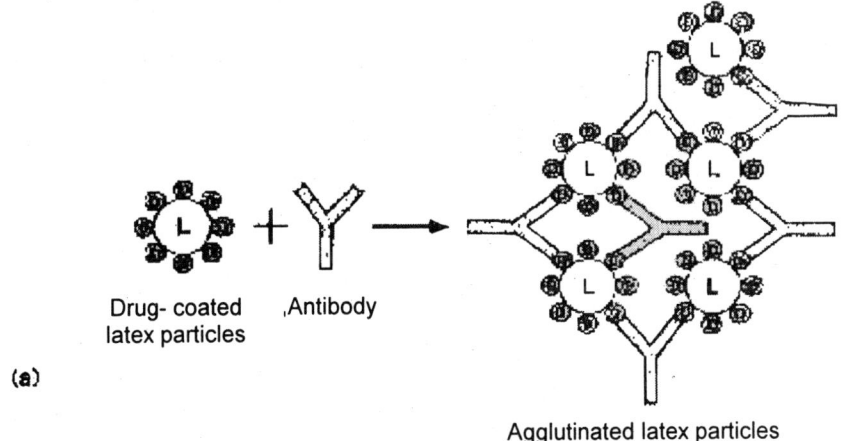

Drug- coated latex particles , Antibody   Agglutinated latex particles

(a)

Drug- coated latex particles   Antibody   Drug   No agglutination

(b)

Fig. 13.9 : Schematic representation of principle of rapid drug kits (a) Agglutination for negative test (b) Non-agglutination for positive test

13.11.9. Antenatal diagnosis of congenital diseases

In some cases pregnant women could have the chances of baring a baby having some genetic defects. It is required that a proper diagnosis should be undertaken in the fetal sages itself. The diagnosis is accomplished by withdrawing small quantities of amniotic fluids containing fetal cells using a hypodermic needle. The free cells could be further collected and cultured and tested in various ways e.g. karyotype enzyme production and restriction fragment length analysis of its DNA. At least 35 diseases which can be identified by this technique are known. If the disease could be detected form such a antenatal diagnosis, abortion of the fetus could be recommended.

The advancement in the biotech process have made it possible to detect the disorders within 2 months of the pregnancy unlike 4 1/2 months required with the conventional procedures. The number of disease specific DNA probes are also increasing at a faster rate, so that the antenatal diagnosis of DNA analysis or 'enzyme linked immunosorbant assay [ELISA], should be possible for a single gene defects. In the recent years, the incidences of the disease thalassaemia, in Cyproit community in Britain has fallen from 30-20 per year due to the use of antenatal diagnosis.

13.11.10. Immunometric assays

The use of polyclonal antisera in immunometric assays pose numerous disadvantages. Among them is the purity problem associated with polyclonal antisera. To overcome this, MAbs which can be obtained in a pure state in large quantities can be used. MAbs have the advantage that they can appropriately be selected for bridging ability to a particular determinant on the antigen. These antibodies will allow increased sensitivity, specificity and reproducibility in immunoassays. Among the variety of assay methods available for labelled MAbs in immunometric assays, the two-site sandwich immunometric assay is of particular importance offering a number of advantages especially that of increased specificity (Fig. 13.10).

13.11.10.1. Enzyme immune filtration assay

The class, concentration and specificity of the monoclonal by a highly efficient method of enzyme immune-filtration assay (EIFA). Immunofiltration was first described by Cleveland in 1979 to immobilize antisera. The technique is more versatile and easy than ELISA or RIA. In principle the technique is quite similar to EIA and RIA. It is performed in two ways direct and indirect. In direct EIFA enzyme is covalently conjugated to the MAb itself for detecting reactivity to its antigen whereas in the indirect EIFA an enzyme conjugated Ig class specific antiglobulin is used to react with the test MAb already bound to its antigen . Modification by computer based equipment from signal (color) to noise (background) could be quantified for assay purposes.

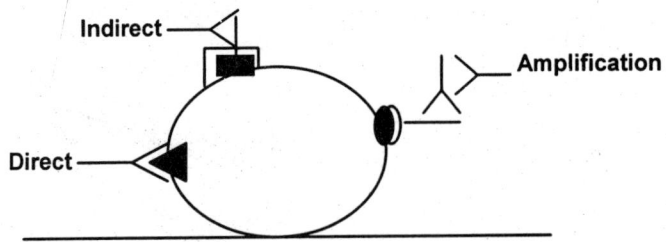

EIFA protocol with monoclonal antibodies

In the direct type enzymes or some other chromophores or fluorophores are conjugated to test MAbs however, in the indirect type of assay an Ig class specific affinity purified antisera conjugated to an enzyme such as horseradish peroxidase is used; which could be further amplified by addition of anti-peroxidase to greatly boasting of signals to noise ratios. Enzyme assay offers the added advantage of longer shelf-life of reagents, the elimination of radioactive waste and comparable scientific results. EIFA has the added feature in that it utilizes the principle of liquid surface tension to provide an incubation chamber that acts both as a solid phase reactionsite and a filtration device. EIFA's do this by utilizing a 96 well microtiter plate modified with small holes in the bottom of each well. Over each hole the filter paper is placed which acts as a surface for reaction. The filters are available in either glass fibber, cotton lentil, nitrocellulose or polycarbonate form.

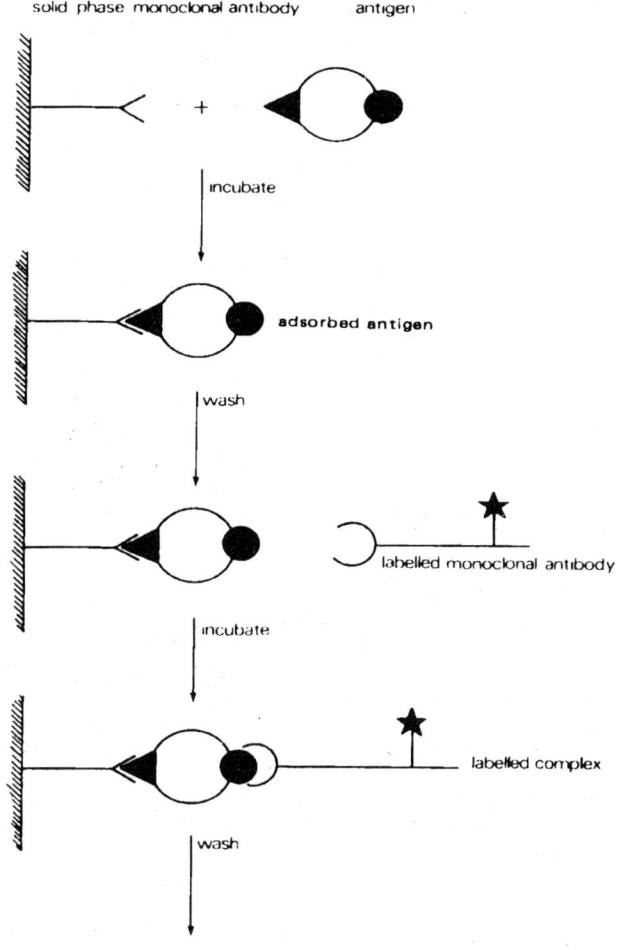

solid phase monoclonal antibody   antigen

incubate

adsorbed antigen

wash

labelled monoclonal antibody

incubate

labelled complex

wash

Quantitate label and antigen

Fig. 13.10 : Immunometric assay procedure

13.11.11. Therapeutic applications

13.11.11.1. General therapeutic mechanisms

13.11.11.1.1. MAbs alone

MAbs when used intact however free i.e., without attachment to cytotoxic agents have therapeutic activity in certain cases. By binding to an antigen, its biological effects may be neutralized or activity of growth factor receptor may be blocked by MAb.

Intact MAbs bearing Fc portion are capable of recruiting the immune effector functions of the host. Circulating antigens and antigen bearing cells of RES complement dependent cytotoxicity and antibody dependent cytotoxicity involving host cytotoxic lymphocytes and monocytes may also be equally functional operative in the destruction of target cells. The species sources of the MAb and its immunoglobulin class and subclass are critical for successful interaction with host immune function. Most important advantage of using MAbs alone is that they produce or cause minimal to no toxicity to non-target tissues.

13.11.11.1.2. Radioisotope immunoconjugates

These MAbs conjugates deliver cytotoxic doses of radioactivity to target cells. Critical factors for imaging MAbs also apply to radio therapy. The choice of isotopes and energy of emission is critical, some of the isotopes currently being evaluated are listed in the table 13.8.

Table 13.8: Some potential radioisotopes for therapy

Isotope	Half-life	Emission
^{125}I	60 days	Auger election
^{131}I	8 days	β (0.6 MeV)
^{186}Re	3.5 days	β (1.1 MeV)
^{188}Re	17 h.	β (2.1 MeV)
^{90}Y	2.5 days	β (2.3 MeV)
^{211}At	7 h.	α (5.9, 7.5 MeV)

Most studies have used β emitters which are medium energy particles able to penetrate multiple cell diameters in thickness. Thus MAbs carrying these emitters are able to kill nearby Stauder's cells also, which is useful when antigenic heterogeneity of tumor cell is not only a problem but troublesome also as it causes damage to surrounding non-target cells. High energy emitters which are more dangerous and difficult to work with are also being evaluated. The chemistry of conjugation is a critical factor in using radioisotope immunoconjugates.

13.11.11.1.3. Toxin and drug immunoconjugates

MAbs are being evaluated for the delivery of potent toxin and drugs to target cells while reducing toxicity to non-target tissues. The principle involved in these construct is an exclusion of intrinsic infectivity (undefined) and incorporation of selectively for presentation to target cells.

Toxins: Toxins include ricin, abrin, pokeweed antiviral protein, gelonin, diphtheria toxin and pseudomonas endotoxin. Chemotherapeutic agents have included doxorubicin, daunorubicin, methotrexate, melphalan, chlorambucil, vinca alkaloids and mitomycin C. Conjugation chemistry is one of the major critical factors here also. After binding of the MAbs to the cell surface, the toxin or drug must be internalized and be made available for damaging cell. It is observed that some but not all antigens internalize after antibody is bound. Often the conjugation chemistry involves a labile bond that is cleaved intracellularly, releasing free toxin or drug. MAbs directed against ricin A and B subunits can be noncovalently bind to the whole toxin or its toxic unit A. The combination of these antibodies with a cell directing antibody can give a unique hybrid with dual binding specificity. Thus capable of carrying toxin subunit A into and kill target cells (Fig. 13.11) .

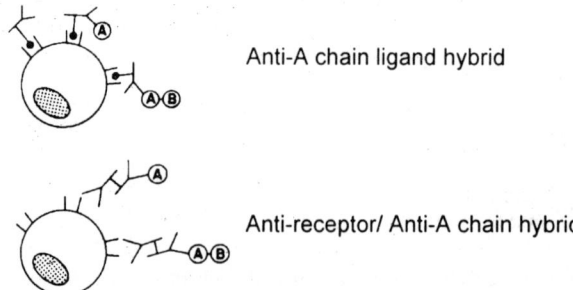

Anti-A chain ligand hybrid

Anti-receptor/ Anti-A chain hybrid

Fig. 13.11 : Modes of hybrid delivery of ricin A chain

The construction of this typical hybrid conjugate is presented schematically in (Fig. 13.12). The bond however must remain relatively stable in blood. MAb conjugates spare toxicity to normal tissues because relatively low dose reaches these sites as compared against free drug administration, thus improving therapeutic index. A potential problem with toxins is that they are relatively large, foreign protein capable of inducing strong immune response. Alternatively, four different modes have been suggested through which antiricin A and antiricin B chain antibodies may be used in combination with a cell reactive carrier antibody (ligand). As shown in figure 13.13 anti-A chain antibodies used with carrier can deliver free A chain which has no affinity as such for cells, or whole ricin in the presence of lactose to block the binding rate of its B chain. Similarly, anti-B chain antibodies can deliver whole ricin in the presence of lactose.

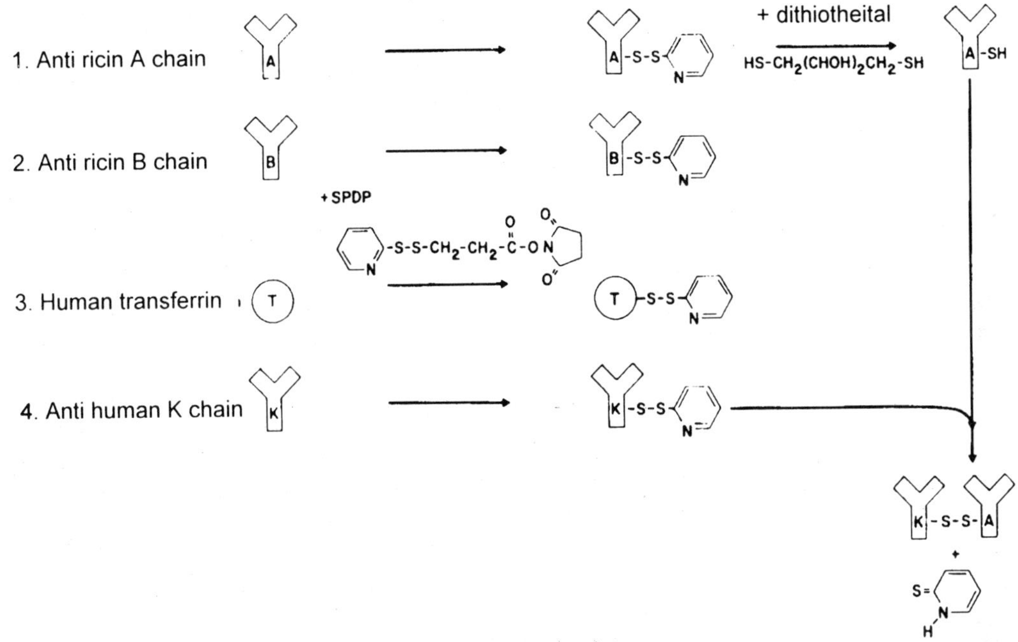

Fig. 13.12 : Disulfide linked hybrid reagents

Drug immunoconjugates: Based on a similar principle target specific immuno-drug conjugates of daunomycin has been prepared and found to be potentially cytocidal. Prototype drug conjugates as target specific carrier have been reported directed towards haptens or other immunogens. Another interesting example is of cytotoxic immunoconjugates which are capable of selective elimination of lymphocyte sub-population. Unlike antigen containing immunoconjugates, Ig specific cytotoxin immunoconjugate could eliminate almost all immuno-globulin receptor bearing B-lymphocyte. Apparently the system is based on immunoglobulin receptor recognition by drug-immunoglobulin conjugate and the strategy explicitly speaks the of potential of monoclonal antibody post for selective sequestering of such cells which express class II receptor i.e., lymphocytes.

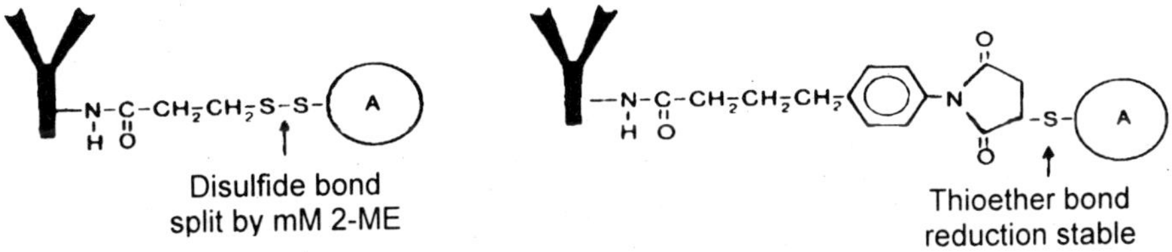

Fig. 13.13 : Chemical linkage of antibody-ricin A chain conjugate

Similarly, anthracycline antibody complexes have been reported for antitumor activity where adriamycin, a cytotoxic drug has been coupled to monoclonal antibodies. In this strategy typical anti-ly-2,1, monoclonal antibodies were used. An interesting report utilizes Ks1/4-DAVLV monoclonal antibody-vinca alkaloid conjugate for directed chemotherapy to the epithelial malignancies. Conventional hybridoma technology was adopted to generate monoclonal antibody for human tumor cells. Some drug-antibody conjugates are reported which employ an antibodies where receptor of later is expressed excessively on the surface of highly proliferating cancerous cell, for the maximum utilization of folic acid for their growth requirement, the schematic presentation of such construct development essentially involves activation and generation of aldehyde groups from carbohydrate moieties of immunoglobulins and their subsequent conversion into hydrazones is followed by stabilization via reduction of imino bond. The process is schematically represented in figure 13.14.

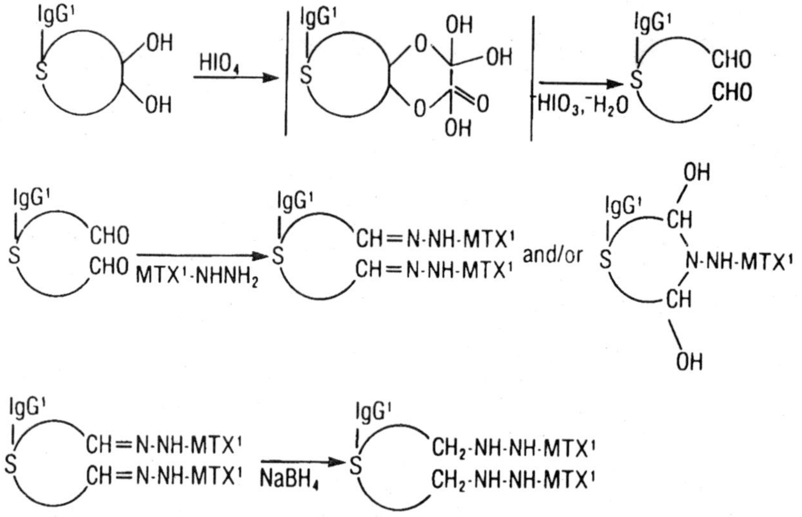

where IgG¹...polypetide portion of IgG
S...carbohydrate moiety of IgG
MTX¹...remainder of MTX molecule

Fig. 13.14 : Schematic representation of linkage of antifolate hydrazides to carbohydrate moieties of immunoglobulins

Recently reported applications of monoclonal antibodies specifically plunge upon the concept of selective cell sorting followed by deletion as in most of the immunological events, T cell suppression is a normal consequence which regulates the fate of monoclonal antibody under immunogenic situation as per requirement. However, where T cells are effectively damaged being harboring tropic of pathogen, it is desirable that such T cells at one hand should be prevented from utilization by pathogen and at the same time much more T cells be recruited or supplemented to meet out the requirement. This highly considered compromisable situation could be arrived at via deletion of suppresser T cell, thus, allowing continual proliferation. Suppresser T cell deletion has been reported by employing targeted immunotherapy. The approach is seemingly distinct in comparison to other from more traditional methods. In this method T suppresser cells are identified as target and the goal of treatment is immune modulation, so that tumor bearing animals could reject their own tumors. The approach is novel. It is generally assumed that by and large tumor cells do not differ antigenically, as compared against their normal counter parts except for cryptic carbohydrate antigens, which may be expressed differentially. In the reported approach B-cell hybridomas, were isolated to generate population T suppresser cells and obviously the constant of region of TSF (T suppresser cell factor) secreted by them. This monoclonal antibody B-16-G, was used subsequently to screen T cell hybridomas which express B-16G reactive molecule (TSF). So isolated hybridoma have been found to be selective and could bind antigen associated membrane of P-815 cells. The administration of such specific sequestering cell could effectively interrupt and delete T-suppresser cells and hence leading to tumor cell rejections by the animal itself. A simple mechanism depicting principles involved in drug immunoconjugate is shown in figure 13.15.

Monoclonal antibodies have been generated against cobra venom and subsequently conjugated with venom neutralizing factor to modulate the targeted biological response. A modification of strategy presents a unique approach towards metal toxicity, Fe^{+++} portions of immunoglobin–G conjugated with proliferation which could effectively chelate and remove accumulated metal in liver hepatocytes as FC-porphyrins-C4 conjugate chelate B subsequently filtered through urine, thus could effectively be removed resulting in inversion of metal toxicity (Fig. 13.16)

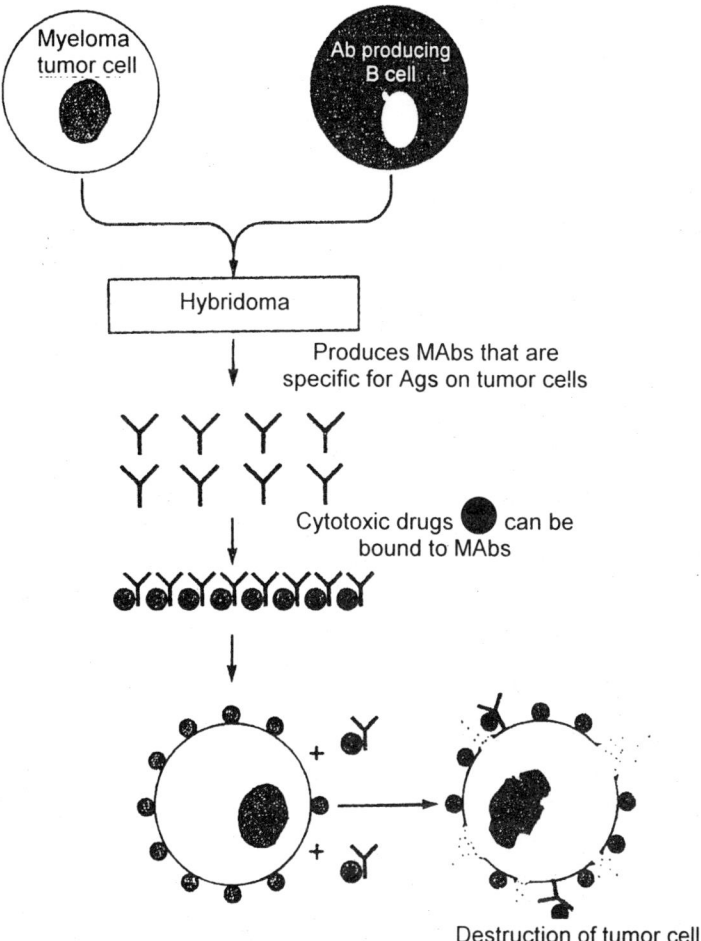

Fig. 13.15 : Schematic representation of use of immunotoxin in tumor targeting

13.11.11.2. Transplantations

13.11.11.2.1. Organ transplantation

For the treatment of solid organ transplant rejection, several MAbs against T cell antigens have been evaluated. The most successful of these is orthrochrome **OKT3** which was first MAb to be licensed for human use. The murine intact IgG antibody, directed against CD3 antigen or T lymphocytes, is used unconjugated to effectively reverse acute rejection episodes with renal, hepatic, cardiac and combined kidney pancreas transplants.

MAb binding blocks T cell functions, in part by opsonization and removal of T cells by reticulo-endothelial system (RES). OKT3 may also be useful prophylactic during post transplantation period. Acute side effects such as fever and chills are common and probably may be as a consequence of T cell damage.

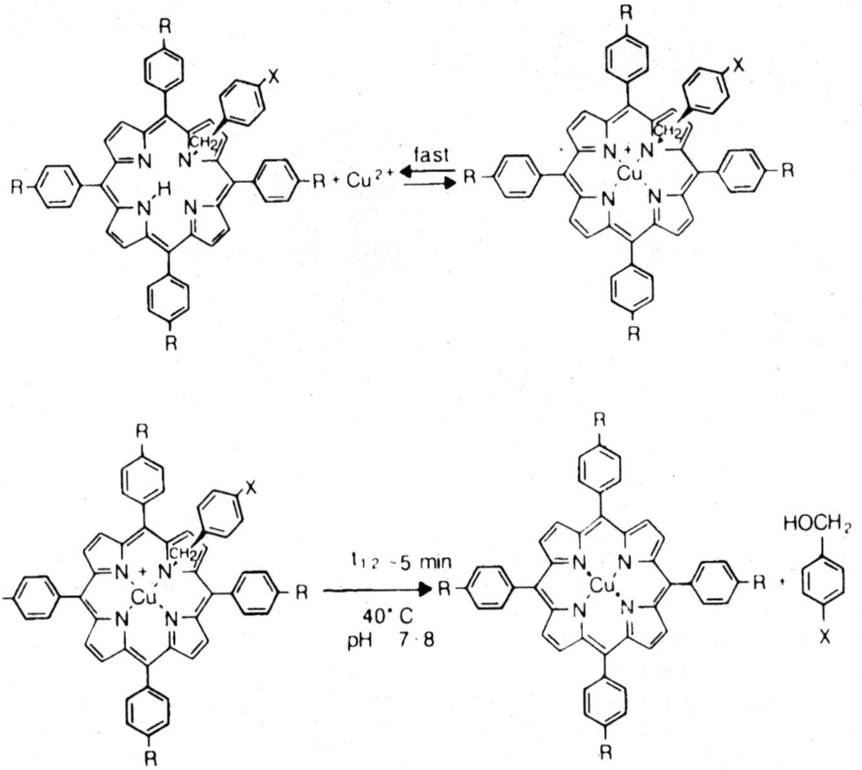

Fig. 13.16 : Mechanism of the metalation reaction of N-benzyl in porphyrin (R-represents for antibody Ig G)

13.11.11.2.2. Bone marrow transplantation

MAbs are being evaluated for graft versus host disease in bone marrow transplantation. A ricin toxin immuno conjugate directed against CD5 antigen of T lymphocyte is effective both in the treatment and prevention of graft-versus host disease with histocompatible marrow grafts. OKT3 has also shown promise in the management of immune related graft rejection events.

13.11.11.3. Infectious diseases

MAbs against endotoxin have been evaluated as aids in antibiotic therapy of bacteria and sepsis. A human IgM, MAb, HA1A, directed against the lipid component of endotoxin has been developed by Centocor. The MAb has been shown to reduce the lethal effects of gram negative bacteria in animal models. HA-1A is the first human MAb taken up for clinical studies. The MAb was found to be well tolerated in patients. HA-1A has been hypothesized to block toxic effects of circulating endotoxin, which include induction and release of mediators of shock and tissue damage although exact mechanism is still to be establishied.

Monoclonal antibodies against viruses have also been developed. A classical example of this type of antibodies is the antibody which has been cloned, developed against *Cytomegalo* virus. They are in early clinical trials.

13.11.11.4. Microorganisms

Monoclonal antibodies against micro-organisms can be readily made. These MAbs can be used in the isolation, identification, detection, structural investigation, genetic variation and classification of the micro-organisms (Table 13.9). It is very helpful in antigenic mapping of viral proteins and antigenic drift in viruses or bacteria.

For example, new strains of influenza virus differ from each other by several amino acid substitutions in the viral haemagglutinin and/or neuraminidase antigens.

1. The isolation of the critical immunogenic determinants on the micro-organism will allow the production of subunit vaccines.

2. Useful in immunopathology wherein significance and recognition of the antigens and their effects on the host can be known.

3. To study the properties of antiviral or antibacterial antibodies *in-vitro* and *in vivo*.

Table 13.9 : Monoclonal antibodies made against microoragnisms

Viruses	Bacteria
Influenza	*Streptococci A*
Rabies	*Streptococci B*
Hepatitis B	*Neisseria gonorrhoeae*
Epstein-Barr	*M. tuberculosis*
Herpes Simplex	*Pseudomonas aeruginosa*
Measles	
Mumps	
Choriomeningitis	
Murine leukaemia	

13.11.11.5. Parasites

The role of monoclonal antibody technology in immunoparasitology and in parasite immunodiagnosis has gained wide publicity. Parasitic diseases are of late gaining importance. The most important among this class is the malarial parasite. Vaccination against this widespread disease is difficult due to the complex life cycle of these organisms. Monoclonal antibodies offer better scope for the reason that they may be screened to ascertain which one can offer protection and then the surface antigens responsible can be purified and used as vaccines,. Monoclonal antibodies can be used for exact parasite identification and diagnosis. Specific human monoclonal antibodies when available will help in the treatment, interception and inactivation at certain stages of the parasite life cycle and therefore can be used for passive immunization when vaccination is not satisfactory. Table 13.10 shows a list of MAbs against parasites.

Table 13.10 : Monoclonal antibodies against parasites

Malaria (Plasmodium)
Sporozoite
Merozoite
Schistosoma
Toxoplasma gondii
Leishmania enrittii
Trypanosoma cruzi
T. rhodesiense
T. brucei

13.11.11.6. Enzymes, proteins and receptors

The application of monoclonal antibodies in this area has been made with the aim to specifically measure or locate the enzyme/proteins, to isolate, purify and characterize the substance and to show and study the antigenic differences in respect of distinct enzymes or isoenzymes. These monoclonal antibodies which are specific for a particular enzyme receptor is of potential use in the study of physiological and pathological mechanisms. They are also useful in activating or turning off the receptor triggered responses. Monoclonal antibodies have been developed against cytochrome P-450. These antibodies have been proven to be valuable tool for the investigation of different forms of cytochrome P-450 and for molecular studies of enzyme structure and function and role then in carcinogenesis and drug metabolism.

13.11.11.7. Cardiovascular diseases

A murine MAb, 7E3, specific for glycoprotien IIb/IIa fibrinogen receptor of platelets has been evaluated by Centocor. The F(ab')2 and Fab fragments alone, by binding to the receptor are potent inhibitors of *in vitro* platelet thrombus formation in animal studies. It is interesting that haemorrhagic toxicity has not been noted

13.11.11.8. Autoimmune diseases

MAbs directed against B and T lymphocytes are currently being evaluated for therapy of autoimmune diseases such as rheumatoid arthritis and multiple sclerosis. Initial clinical trials have demonstrated significant therapeutic effects.

13.11.11.9. Cancer

Main obstacles in the treatment of cancer by MAbs are antigenic heterogeneity, lack of cytotoxicity of MAbs used alone and as conjugates, chemistry of conjugation, proper dosage form and dose regimens and the immune response to mouse antibodies.

Tumor cells can be killed by MAb directly through complement-mediated lysis in some cases or by conjugating monoclonal antibody to a lethal toxin or radioisotope or drug. In other cases, tumor cells were resistant to complement mediated lysis. Unconjugated MAbs have been used with some success in treating human B cell lymphomas and T cell leukemias. The approach suggested by Ronald Levy and his colleagues that claims for complete remission of terminal B-lymphomas, principally based on anti-idiotype monoclonal antibodies has been discussed in this chapter under 13.10.1.6.

Large number of tumor cells are resistant to complement mediated lysis. But tumor specific monoclonal antibody can be conjugated to lethal toxin or radioisotope to form an immunotoxin capable of killing tumor cells. Several toxins such as *Shigella* toxin, diphtheria toxin, ricin can be used, all of which inhibit protein synthesis and are so potent that a single molecule has been shown to kill a cell. Each of these toxins consists of two or more distinct polypeptide components, one the toxin itself and other serves as a ligand that binds to receptor on cell surfaces. Without binding to receptor the toxin cannot get into cells and therefore is harmless. This binding polypeptide can be replaced with a monoclonal antibody having specificity for a particular tumor cell, and could target the toxin selectively to tumor cells, causing cell death by inhibiting protein synthesis (Fig. 13.17). Since very few molecules of immunotoxin actually make contact with the tumor mass, therefore humoral high toxicity of toxin should be considered. Various ongoing clinical trials include immunotoxins directed against cell-membrane antigens of melanoma, colorectal carcinoma, metastatic breast carcinoma, various lymphomas and leukemias, and graft versus host diseases.

This approach has been limited by disappointing responses in patients with large tumor masses which may be due to inaccessibility of the immunotoxin to most tumor cells.

13.11.11.10. Antidotes

Murine MAbs have been produced which react with digoxin and tetanus toxins. Previously rabbit antibodies reacting with digoxin were used. However, these antibodies suffer from the disadvantage of limited supply and variability of antiserum produced in different rabbits. MAbs are free from these disadvantages, being homogeneous in nature and can be produced in unlimited quantities.

These antibodies couple with digoxin to form a complex that is inactive and cleared in urine. They also remove digoxin from receptor sites and reverse potentially the fatal cardiac arrhythmias induced by overdoses of this drug. Similarly murine MAbs and human MAbs are reported to react with tetanus toxin have also been generated.

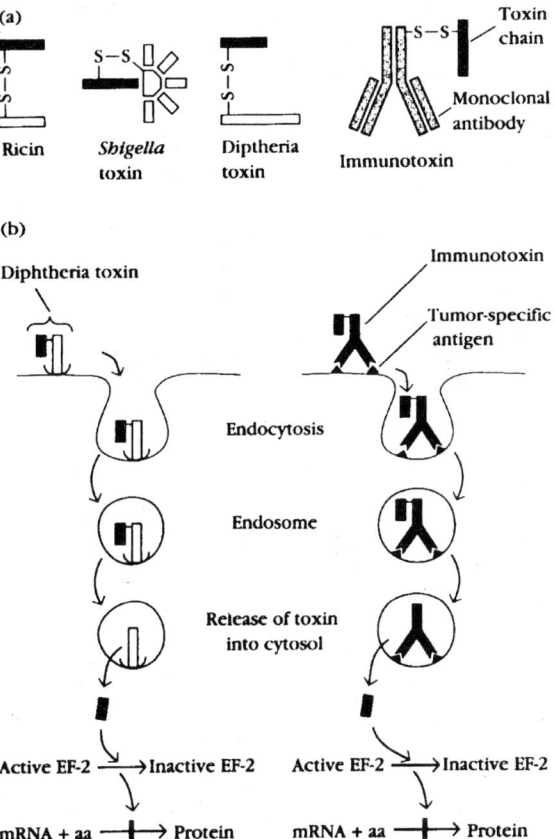

Fig. 13.17 : (a) Toxins used to prepare immunotoxins include ricin, *Shigella* toxin and diphtheria toxin; (b) Binding of diphtheria toxin to the receptor present on the cell membrane (left) and binding of diphtheria-immunotoxin to a tumor associated antigen (right)

13.11.12. Investigational and analytical applications

13.11.12.1. Identification and isolation of lymphocytes subpopulation and clones

Various lymphocyte subpopulations express characteristic patterns of membrane proteins depending on the cells state of differentiation. Monoclonal antibodies specific for each of these membrane proteins can be applied to identify various stages of lymphocyte differentiation. For example, T helper cells express CD8 membrane proteins in both human and mice. By incubating a lymphocyte preparation with monoclonal antibodies to CD4 and CD8 labelled with two different fluorochromes, the T_H cells and T_C cells can be separated in a fluorescence activated cell sorter (Fig. 13.18).

A given subpopulation can be removed from a preparation by treating the preparation with monoclonal antibody and complement, causing lysis of cells for which the monoclonal antibody is specific.

13.11.12.2. Purification of proteins

Minor protein components from a complex mixture of proteins require numerous chromatographic steps and generally have low yield before the advent of the monoclonal antibodies. Monoclonal antibodies can be made to any minor protein (P) in a complex mixture since any hybridoma clone that secretes antibody to proteins other than P are eliminated during the screening phase of monoclonal production. This monoclonal antibody to a particular protein can be used for its purification.

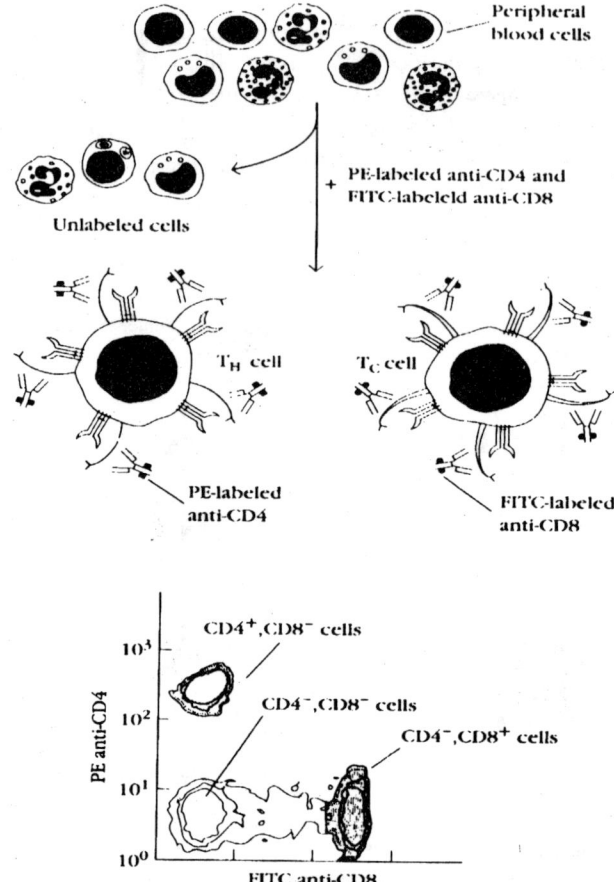

Fig. 13.18 : Separation of T_H cells and T_C cells from human peripheral blood lymphocytes

Secher and Burke obtained highly purified sample of interferon using this approach from white blood cells. They produced monoclonal antibody to interferon (IFN) using a partially purified preparation for immunization of mice. Then they formed an immunoadsorbent column based on anti-IFN monoclonal antibody immobilized on beads. When a crude IFN preparation was passed through this column, a 5000 fold increase in interferon purity was obtained (Fig. 13.19).

13.11.12.3. Radioimmunoassays

MAbs have the potential to replace or supplement conventional antibodies in a series of assays. In particular, availability of more than one monoclonal antibody reacting with different sites of single molecules allows investigators to produce highly specific radioassays in which one of the monoclonal antibodies is labelled rather than the antigen. A number of antibodies generated have the requisite specificity and sensitivity for use in radioassays.

13.11.13. Miscellaneous applications

13.11.13.1. Catalytic monoclonal antibodies (Abzymes)

The binding of antibody to its antigen and binding of enzyme to its substrate both involves weak, non covalent interactions and exhibits high specificity and often high affinity. But an antigen is not altered by antibody, where as an enzyme alters the substrate and as a result the binding by catalyzing a chemical change. The enzyme uses it binding energy to stabilize the transition state of substrate, thus reducing activation energy for chemical modification of bound substrate. Similarities between antigen-antibody interaction and enzyme-substrate interaction have led Lerner and his colleagues to explore the probability of enzyme like action of some antibodies.

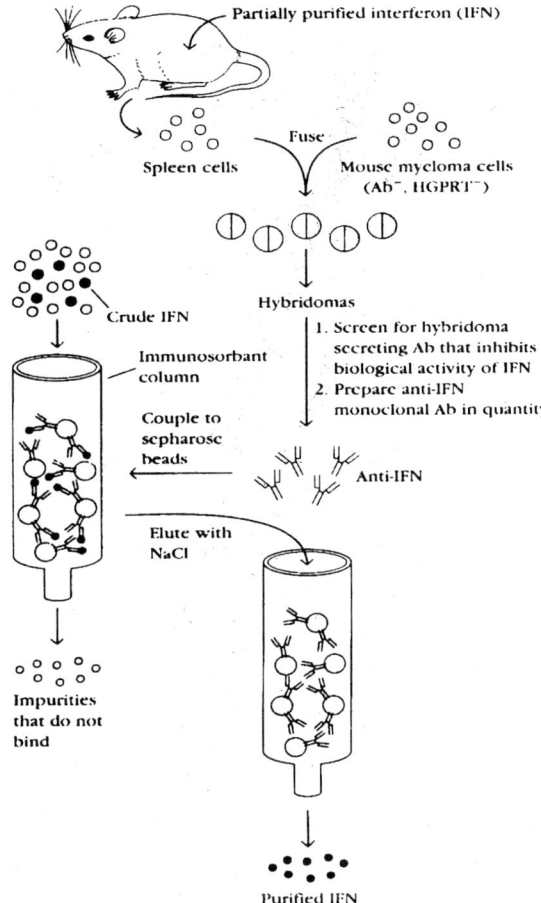

Fig. 13.19 : Purification of interferons by using a immunosorbent column

They produced a **hapten-carrier** complex in which the hapten structurally resembled the transition state of an ester under going hydrolysis. Using this conjugate they generated **antihapten monoclonal antibodies**. When these monoclonal antibodies were incubated with an ester substrate, some of them accelerated hydrolysis by about 1000 fold. The catalytic activity of these antibodies was highly specific towards the esters whose transition state structure closely resembles that of the hapten in the immunizing conjugate (Fig. 13.20).

Similarly catalytic monoclonal antibodies catalyzing ester hydrolysis and carbonate hydrolysis have been also generated. These have been named as abzymes in reference to their dual role as antibody and enzyme.

Lerner pioneered the development of immunoglobulin-gene libraries to produce an enormous antibody replication without the requirement of antigen priming, so that large numbers of antibodies could be screened for their catalytic activity. Generation of more and more abzymes by this method may make it possible to produce a battery of abzymes that cut peptides at specific amino acid residues, much as restriction enzymes cut DNA at specific sites. Such abzymes would be invaluable tools in facilitating structural and functional analysis of proteins. It may also be possible to generate abzymes with the ability to dissolve blood clots or to cleave viral glycoproteins at specific sites, thus blocking viral infectivity. Abzymes are likely to represent a major technological advance that will affect various branches of science in the coming years.

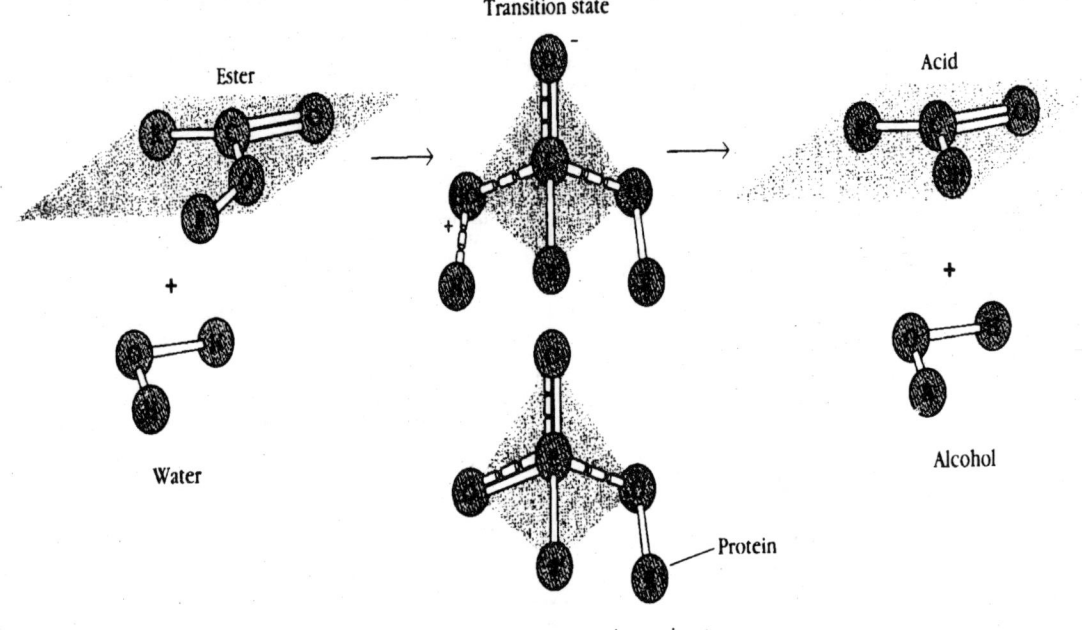

Fig. 13.20 : Schematic representation of the action of Abzymes in ester hydrolysis

13.11.13.2. Autoantibody fingerprinting using dipsticks

The patients suffering from rheumatic diseases are found to have autoantibodies that react to cellular components. Recently a newer class of autoantibodies have been identified in normal humans which reacts with cellular components. Unlike the diseases associated autoantibodies which are restricted in number, these autoantibodies increase in number after birth up to two years and then remain constant for decades. These antibodies have unique complement which differ from person to person and hence referred to as individual specific (IS) autoantibodies. These IS autoantibodies could be physically separated comprising of an antibody fingerprinting that could serve in the identification of an individual. The autoantibodies could be collected from blood, saliva, tears perspiration etc. and examined for crime detection.

13.11.14. Monoclonal antibodies in drug targeting

The concept of using specific antibodies conjugated with toxic or isotopically labelled materials for specific sites and drug localization is not new. This concept with the development of MAbs and hybridoma technology have gained wide appreciation in their use. The use of monoclonal antibodies to target drugs to specific cell types is a promising approach. Drugs are coupled to an antibody, thereby creating a hybrid molecule with the specificity of the immunological ligand as well as retaining the therapeutic activity of the drug.

13.11.14.1. Antibody and antibody conjugates

Antibodies or their fragments are the ideal modules to augment the association of drug carrier with macrophages (Mφ) because of their ability to interact with the Fc/C3b receptors, in a manner similar to the way as bacteria. The latter are cleared from the system in the presence of antibodies, which enhance their uptake by Fc receptor bearing cells. It has shown that for heat aggregated antibodies and for haptens expressed on the surface bound antibodies, the process of opsonization followed by endocytic internalization by macrophages, have been mediated by the Fc regions of specific antibodies of IgG class, as one of the manifestations of the antigen-antibody interaction. No binding was seen to cells lacking the Fc receptors or when opsonization was mediated through $F(ab')_2$ or IgA antibodies, confirming the specificity for the Fc portion of IgG.

On the other hand, there appears to be no receptor port for IgM antibody on macrophages. However, galactosyl ceramide bearing systems have been observed to be taken up by peritoneal macrophages in the presence of IgM, antigalactosyl antibodies and complement. Therefore uptake was established to be mediated through complement receptor. The access of MAbs to receptor bearing cells can be improved by employing immunologically active fragments $[F(ab')_2$ and Fab'] instead of complete IgG portion. It has been shown recently that MAbs directed to cell surface molecule, encoded by murine/human MHC can be internalized specifically by T-lymphocytes (Class I MHC molecules) and by B-lymphocytes (Class II MHC molecules), as these molecules are expressed by T and B cells respectively. The same phenomenon has been observed by immunotoxins directed to different cell-surface determinants (Table 13.11).

Table 13.11 : Antibody-receptor interaction

Hapten/Antibodies	Target cell(s) & determinants
Antibodies (opsonized)	Fc/C3b receptor bearing on liver endothelial cells
MAbs encoded by MHC (murine/human)	Activated human T-lymphocytes
Anti-MHC MAbs	Recombinant neoplastic cells
MAbs coded by protein A	Lymphoid tumor cells
Hapten bearing colloids	
DNP-cap-PE	Fc-receptor bearing & other murine tumor cell lines
DNP-cap-PC	Fc receptor bearing peritoneal macrophages
Nitroxide phospatidyl ethanolamine	Human macrophages/murine macrophages
Gangliosides, Sulfatides and cerebrosides	Murine peritoneal macrophages in presence of antibodies to their lipids

Closky and Peacock (1989), incorporated palmitate derivatized antibody molecules on to the cell membranes, where they function as "surrogates receptors"(SR) for facilitating specific cellular interaction. Therefore, the palmitate anchor, bypasses the requirement of FcR or other endogenous membrane proteins, in antibody dependent cellular conjugation. Since this mode of attachment is similar to that of PI anchored proteins, SR-mediated cellular interactions are likely to be reminiscent of native receptor induced cellular conjugation, enabling SR to cooperate with endogenous target recognition process, that is pivotal in 'receptor-ligand interaction' at the cell-cell interface. The selective targeting of the drug carrier using MAbs is discussed in detail in chapter 16. Interested readers may refer the same.

13.11.14.2. Suppresser deletion therapy

In this approach, targeted immunotherapy concept has been utilized. The target in this case is T suppresser cells wherein immune modulation takes place and the tumor-bearing animal rejects their own tumors The T suppresser cells have been deleted by conjugating antibodies with hematoporphyrin which can be targeted towards specific tumor cells. Conjugation is brought about by using carbodiimide as a coupling agent. Carbodiimide serves as a condensing agent, bringing about the formation of a peptide bond between ligands as described in the figure 13.21.

The first step involves protonation of carbodiimide to yield an intermediate which is attached by a carboxylate anion to produce the O-acylurea. This O-acylurea in turn conjugates with the amino groups on carrier protein molecules to form a stable peptide bond.

R : CH_3CH_2-

R' : $(CH_3)_2NCH_2CH_2CH_2$-

Ab : Antibody

R' : Hematoporphyrin

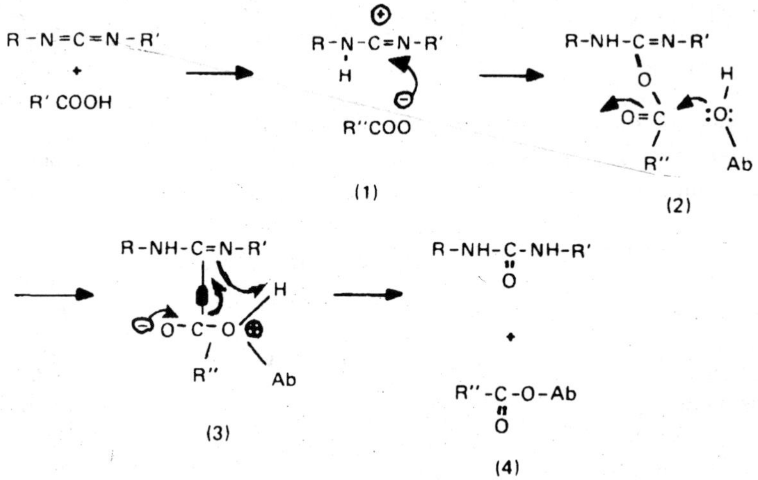

Fig. 13.21 : Mechanism of carbodiimide conjugation. Initial protonation of carbodiimide leads intermediate (1), which is attacked by a corboxylate anion to produce the O-acylurea (2) which participates in conjugation

13.11.14.3. Site-specific modification of MAbs

Site-specific modification refers to covalent chemical modification at a specific site on an antibody molecule. Modification of MAbs either by direct labelling with isotopes or conjugation to drugs, chelators or toxins can severely hamper the immunoreactivity of the antibody. The site-specific modification of MAbs makes use of the complex carbohydrate, found on the heavy chains, normally at sites far from the antigen combining site. This paves way for modification of antibodies by oxidation of the sugar residues to aldehydes followed by reaction with appropriate aldehyde reactive groups such as amines, hydrazides or hydrazines.

13.11.14.4. Antibody-enzyme conjugates

A novel strategy for the delivery of drugs to tumor specific sites or to specific infected cells has been reported. The strategy namely **antibody-directed enzyme prodrug therapy (ADEPT)**, targets the enzyme to the tumor site using a monoclonal antibody followed by administration of a non-toxic prodrug which can be converted by the enzyme to a potent anti-tumor agent. The enzymes to be targeted are chosen for their ability to convert a relatively non-toxic prodrug precursors into their active form. Using monoclonal coupled to enzymes, they can be delivered specifically to the cell type that expresses the antigenic determinant. Once the antibody enzyme conjugate reaches the site, a non-toxic prodrug which can be converted into a potent anti-tumor agent or anti-viral agent by the enzyme is administered. This now gets converted only at the site where the enzyme is present and hence the toxicity is limited only to the tumor cells while the systemic level of the drug remains very low.

Enzymes that have been studied so far includes:

- alkaline phosphatase (for the conversion of phosphate prodrug);
- carboxypeptidase (an enzyme converting inactive carboxyl compounds into their active carboxylic counter parts);

- glucoronidase;
- lactamase (hydrolyse various β-lactam ring containing antibiotics);
- penicillin V/G amidase (to active p-hydroxy acetic acid bearing moiety);
- nitroreductase;
- cytosine deaminase (converts 5-fluorocytosin to 5-fluorouracil);

Drugs which can be used for ADEPT strategy should be those which can be converted into a prodrug easily. Ideally, the drug should be of low molecular weight and relatively lipophilic. The most important criteria in selection of a drug is its specificity to the chosen enzyme Readers may refer chapter 16 for more details on ADEPT.

13.11.14.5. Antibodies as receptor surrogates for mediating cell-cell interaction

The underspinning and mysteries of immunological competence are intimately tied to accomplish network of exquisitely specific intercellular encounter. Through these interactions host defense could mediate adverse spectrum of immune functions. The derivatized antibodies could serve as surrogate receptors where derivative forming ligand mediates cell-cell interaction. In an interesting report palmitate derivatized antibody molecules have been incorporated onto cell membranes where they function as surrogate receptors to initiate and mediate specific cell interaction. In general surrogate receptors are anchored to the plasma membrane by insertion of palmitate hydrocarbon chain into the outer leaflet of phospholipid bilayer. Therefore the palmitate anchor by passes the requirement of endogenous membrane proteins (MHC I and MHC II) in antibody dependent cellular conjugation. Due to this mode of attachment which is quite similar to phosphatidylinositol anchored proteins the surrogate receptors mediate cellular interaction may be considered to be reminiscent of native receptor induced cellular conjugation. This provides for possible application of so modified cellular systems to elucidate and establish. The after consequences could be physiological and biochemical in nature of cell-cell interaction.

13.11.14.6. Immunoliposomes based diagnostic kit

Liposomes the artificially created microscopic spherical vesicles consisted of phospholipid have recently been reported as an addition to new immunological techniques. These microvesicle typically contains concentric rings of intercalated water within artificially created lipid bilayers. The liposomes are prepared encapsulating colored dye into their aqueous domains. Subsequently, dye loaded liposomes are sensitized by immobilizing specific antigen or antibody on their surface. Antibodies specific for target pathogen(s) are immobilized on nitrocellulose membrane in a particular shape i.e., like a triangle as shown in figure 13.22a. The analyte with pathogenic antigen load on addition to such membrane selectively coats/binds to the immobilized antigen or antibody of the cellulose nitrate membrane. Thus, the analyte gets linked immobilized. On addition of dye filled liposomes to such a test sample a triangle is generated indicative of positive reactions. However, the sample is negative if contains no target analyte as no binding or reaction is visualized in the test area even on addition of sensitized lipsomes. Liposomes based diagnostic kits are now available for a group of *Streptococci* and respiratory syncytial virus.

Diagnostic kits are getting importance as a result for prompt diagnosis of various diseases. The diagnostic immuno kits are available in the market. Some of them are listed in table 13.12.

13.12. IMMUNOGENICITY AND SIDE EFFECTS OF MAbs

The most often reported side-effects with MAbs administration are fever and chills, some of which may be the consequence of MAb reactivity with target cells. Mild allergic reactions have occurred in10% of patients receiving mouse MAbs. However, less than 1% of these patients developed anaphylactic shock mediated by IgE antibodies. Steroids and epinephrine treatments have allowed repeated MAb administration in anaphylactic patients.

In more than 50% of the patients treated, human antimouse antibodies (HAMA) of the IgG and IgM classes have been shown to develop low levels of allergic and anaphylactic reaction. The antibodies complex with administered MAb and prevent them from reaching target site. Thus effectiveness of MAb may be compromised, to be prolonged over a period of time.

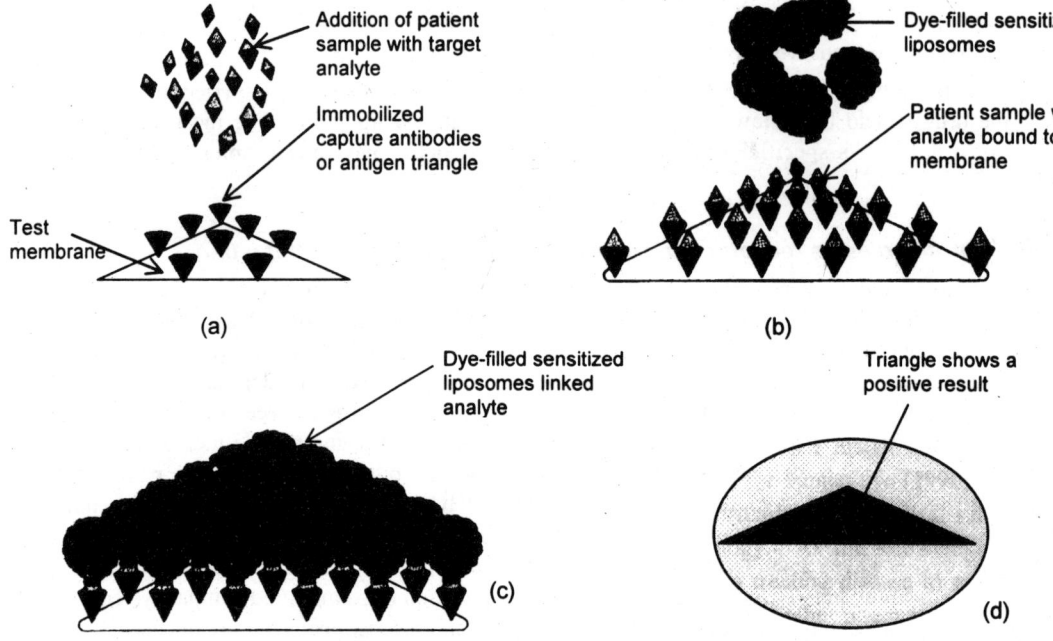

Fig. 13.22 : The liposome based diagnostic kit

Table 13.12 : Rapid Immunologic test kits for detection of bacteria and virus in clinical specimens

Trade Name	Company	Use
Bactigen	Wampole Laboratories, Ranburg N.J.	Detection of *Streptococcus pneumoniae, Haemophilus influenzae* type b, *Neisseria meningitidis*
Cutturete Group A Streo ID kit	Morion Scientific, Kansas city, Mo.	*Streptococci* group A
Directigen	Hynson, Wescott and Dunning, Boltimore MD	*H. influenzae* type b, *S. pneumoniae, M.meningitidis*
Fluortec-F and -M	General Diagnostic, Morris Plaius, N.J	Two kits are used for detection *Bacteroside fragilis* and *B. melaninogenicus*
Gono-Gen	Micro-Media System, San Jose, Calif	*N. gonorrhoeae*
Quick Vue *H. Pylori* test	Quidel, San Diego, CA	Detecting antibody (IgG) against *H. pylori* in serum or plasma.
Staphaurex	Wellcome Diagnostics Nostrus, Research Triangle Park, N.C	Screening and confirmation *S. aureus* in 30 S.
Surecell Herpes (HSV) test	Kodak, Rochester, NY.	Details the herpes (HSV) 1&2 viruses in minutes
SUDS HIV-1 Test	Murex Corporation Norcross, C.A.	Detect antibodies to HIV-1 antigens in 10 min.

HAMA derived allergic reactions can be minimized by using lower doses and non repeated doses. Antibody fragment lacking Fc portion and clearing rapidly from blood also minimizes impact of HAMA. Persisting HAMA has also been removed by plasma phererin prior to reinjection. Use of immunosuppressant drugs for example cyclosporin-A has also been found effective. Mouse-human MAbs may be rendered to be non immunogenic as has been shown in the case of by HA-1A, still there are possibilities for anti-idiotypic response to occur.

SUGGESTIVE READINGS

Beverley, P.C.L., (1986) **Monoclonal antibodies**, Churchill Livingstone, New York.

Bier, D.J., Dias-de-Silva, W., Gotze, D. and Mota, I., (1981) **Fundamentals of Immunology**, Springer-Verlag, New York.

Campbell, A.M., (1984) **Monoclonal Antibody Technology**, Elsevier, Amsterdam.

Coleman, R., Lombards, M. and Sicard, R., (1992) **Fundamental Immunology**, Wm.C.Brown Publishers, Dubuque.

Figuroa, J.E. and Densen, P., (1991) *Infections associated with complement deficiencies*, **Clin. Microbiol. Rev.**, 4, 359-395.

Goding, J.W., (1983) **Monoclonal antibodies: Principle and Practice**, Academic Press, London.

Hermann, J.E., (1986) *Enzyme linked immunoassay for the detection of microbial antigen and their antibodies*, **Adv. Appl. Microbiol.**, 31, 271-289.

Kennedy, R.C., Melinick, J.L. and Dressman, G.R., (1986) *Antiidiotype and immunity*, **Sci. Am.**, 255, 48-56.

Kuby, J., (1991) **Immunology**, W.H. Freeman and Company, New York, Second edition.

Lenner, R.A. and Belkoric, S.J., (1988) *Principle of Antibody catalysis*, **Bio Essay**, 9, 107.

Manser, T., Hung, S.Y. and Gefter, M.L., (1984) *Influence of clonal selection and expression of immuno-globulin variable gene regions*, **Science**, 266, 1236-1288.

McIntosh, D. and Thorpe, P., (1983) *Roll of B chain in cytotoxic action of antibody ricin and antibody abrin conjugates.* In G. Gregoriadis, G. Post, J. Senior and A. Trouet (Eds.), **Receptor Mediated Targeting of Drugs**, Plenum Press, London, 105-119.

Payne, W.J.(Jr.), Marshall, D.L., Shockley, R.K. and Martin, W.J., (1988) *Clinical laboratory applications of monoclonal antibodies*, **Clin. Microbiol. Rev.**, 1, 331-329.

Pezuto, J. M., Johnson, M.E. and Manasse, H.R.(Jr.), (1988) **Biotechnology and Pharmacy**, Chapman and Hall, New York, 39-53.

Prescott, L.N., Harley, J.P., Klein, D.A., (1990) **Microbiology**, Wm.C.Brown Publishers, Dubuque, 606-646.

Raso, V. and Basala, M., (1983) *Monoclonal antibodies as cell targeted carriers of covalently and noncovalently attached toxins.* In: G. Gregoriadis, G. Post, J. Senior and A. Trouet (Eds.), **Receptor Mediated Targeting of Drugs**, Plenum Press, London, 125-129.

Rodwel, J.D., (1988) **Antibody Mediated Drug Delivery Systems**, Marcel Dekker Inc., New York.

Seaver, S.S., **Commercial Production of Monoclonal Antibodies**, Marcel Dekker Inc. New York.

Thompson, K.M., (1988) *Human monoclonal antibodies*, **Immunol. Today**, 9, 113-117.

Vaccine to fight diabetes...

Type I diabetes, an auto-immune disease, is due to the destruction of insulin-producing B cells in the pancreas by the immune system. The only treatment that is currently available is regular insulin injection.

Strategies being developed to fight this disease include protection of B cells through a sort of 'immune counter-attack'. Oral administration of insulin has a vaccine-like effect which causes an immune reaction when it comes into contact with cells of the intestinal mucosa.

Activated lymphocytes trigger the production of anti-inflammatory cytokins that protect pancreatic B cell. The underlying mechanisms are unclear and clinical trials are underway. One of the main problems is that large quantities of insulin have to be administered orally for several years. Now a French scientist has found a solution to this problem. He combined insulin with CTB, the non-toxic B subunit of the cholera toxin. The aim was to amplify the immune reaction and thereby obtain similar efficacy with a much lower dose of insulin, reports CEDUST. He first tried this on mice. After 15 weeks of treatment, only two of the 17 animals in the group treated with insulin and CTB had developed diabetes, compared to even and 16 control animals treated with CTB alone. According to him, these results are similar to those obtained with other studies in which milligram doses of insulin were given for several weeks, whereas he administered micrograms of insulin in a single intake.

. . . . The Hindu, 18/09/'97.

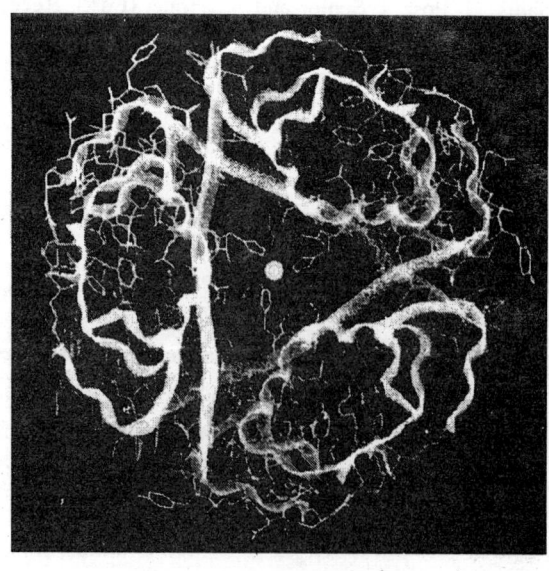

Insulin-Dextran complex

CURRENT TRENDS IN VACCINES

14.1. INTRODUCTION

The increasing cost of modern health care, that relies heavily on the direct treatment of on-going disease, is leading to a need to reappraise current medical practice. It is becoming highly desirable to place more emphasis on preventive medicine. An attractive and highly cost-effective preventive approach is the use of vaccines. Numerous vaccines are known today to protect mankind. Once inside the body, the vaccines in general, create a state that alarms the host in the same way as in the case of a particular pathogen attacking the body. Thus, vaccines activates the body's defense mechanism thereby alerting a brigade of special white blood cells that play a phenomenal role in killing any invading foreign organism. Traditionally, vaccination has been focused on immunization of infants against infectious diseases. To make vaccination an even more cost-effective option, we could develop a vaccination policy aiming at the introduction of safe and efficacious vaccines against a broader range of diseases in all age groups is to developed.

New advances in immunology, molecular biology, and biotechnology allow us now to realistically approach diseases for which vaccines were previously unfeasible. The advances have already led to the improvement of existing vaccines such as those against hepatitis B and the replacement of reactogenic Pw vaccines by fully defined, safer acellular vaccines. In addition, some vaccines may prevent or stop the development of cancers and there is a real potential for preventive and therapeutic vaccination against tumors, auto-immune and allergic diseases. One can also exploit new technologies to improve the delivery and immunogenicity of vaccines. The nature of the immune response can be influenced to elicit specific protective mechanisms needed for specific diseases.

The recent commercialization of new vaccines such as those against *Haemophilus influenzae* type b, hepatitis B and A, and our steadily increasing interest and concern to develop novel vaccines will make it necessary to take into account not only the presently available vaccines but also those that are likely to come in the future. New developments in biotechnology applied to vaccine research are likely to provide us with new powerful ways to present antigens in individual or combined forms for the induction of the highest levels of immune protection for the longest duration. Several approaches are workable, such as the development of live attenuated bacteria and viruses, nucleic acid vaccines, semi-synthetic vaccines, microencapsulation, new adjuvants, and new delivery systems including mucosal administration of vaccines.

An ideal vaccine should provide effective protection against disease and possibly against infection. The most successful vaccine would also allow the eradication of the disease. Although this is not feasible with most vaccines available or under development, the ultimate goal of an ideal vaccine should be to induce long-term protection even after a single dose. Vaccines should only induce protective immune responses with no side-effects. They should be easy and safe to administer, and be available for every individual in every walk of life.

The routes by which vaccines can effectively be administered need also to be carefully evaluated. At present the choice of several possible routes are available. Classically, there are injections and mucosal administrations. Mucosal vaccines can be administered by the oral, nasal, respiratory, rectal or vaginal route. To have an effective vaccination, one has to work on the most appropriate route of administration. It is desirable to revise in brief as to how our immune system works and what facets of it provide us the basis for development of immune accessories or vaccines. Some important components are dealt in the chapter.

14.2. IMMUNE RESPONSE INDUCTION

The cascade of events taking place following the invasion of body by a foreign antigen or immunogen can be sequenced and described as follows.

14.2.1. Macrophage: The antigen presenting cells (APC)

Most invading organisms are first phagocytosed and partially digested by macrophages, as a result the antigenic products are liberated into the macrophage cytosol. These antigens are then passed on to lymphocytes and bind to the antigen receptor molecules present on the surface of B-and T-cells resulting in the activation of B-and T-cells. Macrophages, thus work as APC.

14.2.2. Role of major histocompatible complex molecules/antigens (MHC)

Histocompatibility antigens are normally present on the surface of many mammalian cells and strongly influence regulatory T-cell responses. These antigens are of two types :

Class I histocompatibility complex : are found on all nucleated host cells and stimulate antibody production when injected into a host with different class I antigens.

Class II histocompatibility complex : occur on lymphocytes and macrophages and cells bearing these receptors have the potential to act as APC. Antigens are presented on the surface of these cells in association with class II MHC which are recognized by T-cells in order to activate antigen-specific T-cell help through lymphokine secretion.

14.2.3. Humoral immunity

Activated B-lymphocytes (specific for the antigen) enlarge to become lymphoblasts which, in turn, differentiate and proliferate to form plasma cells and memory cells. Mature plasma cells then produce antibodies at a very high rate, while memory cells remain dormant until activated once again by the same antigen. Lymphokines released by helper T-cells, also contribute to a greater extent, to the stimulation of B-cell growth and differentiation to form plasma cells and antibodies.

14.2.4. Cell mediated immunity

On exposure to the appropriate antigen, T-lymphocytes of lymphoid tissue proliferate to form activated T-cells which are of three types -

(a) Helper T-cells (T_H-cells) - release lymphokines which stimulate :

- growth and differentiation of activated B-cells to form plasma cells and antibodies;
- the growth and proliferation of cytotoxic T-cells and suppresser T-cells;
- the macrophages to cause far more efficient phagocytosis of invading microorganisms;
- activation of T-cells by direct positive feedback effect.

Thus, lymphokines play an important role in overall immunity. In the absence of lymphokines from the T-helper cells, the immune system is almost paralyzed (e.g., destruction of T-cells by AIDS virus which leaves the body almost totally unprotected against infectious diseases) and the antibodies formed by B-lymphocytes are usually limited and insufficient.

(b) Cytotoxic T-cells - bind tightly to those organisms or cells that contain their binding specific antigen and thereafter secrete pore forming proteins (perforins) that punch round holes in membrane of attacked cell. Then the cytotoxic T-cells release cytotoxic substances directly into the attacked cell to cause lysis of the cell.

(c) Suppresser T-cells - they are believed to inhibit the conversion of B-cells into plasma cells. They also suppress the activity of some other T-cells and thus immune responses are not developed against host antigens.

14.3. VACCINES

Recent advances in immunology has led to the development of new and promising vaccine strategies. Knowledge of the differences in epitopes recognized by T cells and B cells have enabled immunologists to begin to design vaccines to maximize activation of the humoral or cell-mediated branch of the immune system. Genetic engineering techniques can be used to develop vaccines to maximize the immune response to selected epitopes. This chapter focuses on some of the existing vaccine strategies as well as some experimental designs that may become the vaccines of the future. Table 14.1 indicates some of the commonly used vaccines currently in use.

Table 14.1 : Classification of common vaccines in use

Disease	Type of vaccine
Whole organism	
Bacterial cells	
Tuberculosis	Attenuated
Cholera	Inactivated
Pertussis	Inactivated
Plague	Inactivated
Viral particles	
Polio (Sabin)	Attenuated
Polio (Salk)	Inactivated
Influenza	Inactivated
Mumps	Attenuated
Measles	Attenuated
Yellow fever	Attenuated
Purified Macromolecules	
Toxoids	
Diphtheria	Inactivated exotoxin
Tetanus	Inactivated exotoxin
Capsular polysaccharide	
H. influenza type b	Polysaccharide + protein
S. pneumoniae	23 distinct capsular polysaccharides
N. meningitis	Polysaccharide

Improved and novel strategies involved in the development and designing of new generation vaccines can be classified as

1. Multivalent subunit vaccines
   a. SMAA complexes
   b. Liposomes
   c. ISCOMS
   d. Micelles
2. Purified macromolecules
3. Synthetic peptides as vaccines
4. Immunoadhesion(s)
5. Antigen vaccines
   a. Recombinant antigen vaccines

b. Adjuvant independent immunotargeted vaccines

c. Class II MHC target antigen

6. Vector vaccines

a. Recombinant vector vaccines

b. Minicells as vaccines

7. Anti-idiotype vaccines

8. Targeted immune stimulants

9. Miscellaneous

a. Antisense oligonucleotides

b. Competitive inhibition of ribosome binding to 5' unsaturated region (5'-UTR)

14.4. MULTIVALENT SUBUNIT VACCINES

Synthetic peptide vaccines and recombinant protein based vaccines are poorly immunogenic. Additionally, they also tend to induce humoral antibody production but are less able to induce a cell-mediated response. These limitations call for a method of structuring a vaccine to contain immunodominant B-cell and T-cell epitopes. Also, if a CTL response is required, the vaccine should be delivered intracellularly so that the peptides can be processed and presented together with class I MHC molecules. Multivalent vaccines represent an approach that presents multiple copies of peptide or a mixture of peptides to the immune system. Some of the techniques for developing multivalent subunit vaccines are discussed below:

1. Solid matrix-antibody-antigen (SMAA) complexes

2. Liposomes

3. Immunostimulating complexes (ISCOMS)

4. Micelles

14.4.1. SMAA complexes

SMAA complexes are prepared by coupling monoclonal antibodies to solid particulate matrices and then the antibodies are saturated with the desired antigen. These complexes are then utilized as vaccines. A variety of monoclonal antibodies can be attached to the solid matrix (Fig. 14.1).

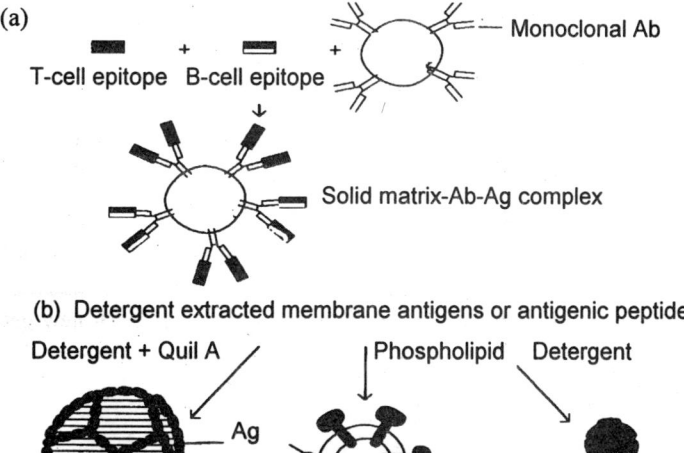

Fig. 14.1 : Multivalent subunit vaccines (a) solid matrix-antibody complexes; (b) ISCOM, liposomes and protein micelles prepared with extracted with antigens or antigenic peptides

This property can be exploited to bind a mixture of peptides/proteins to the solid matrix. Thereby, immunodominant epitopes for both T cells and B cells can be composed. These multivalent complex vaccines are reported to induce vigorous humoral and cell-mediated responses. Their particulate disposition facilitates phagocytosis by phagocytic cells which play an important role in augmenting their immunogenicity.

14.4.2. Liposomes

Another approach of obtaining a multivalent vaccine is utilization of detergent to incorporate peptide/protein antigens into lipid vesicle called liposomes. Pharmaceutical research in the field of drug delivery systems has grown to a far extent with the help of medical research. Novel drug delivery systems have attained utmost attention in delivering the drug to the target site in a targeted or controlled manner, etc. They have also been tried as vaccines and vaccine adjuvants. This has opened the door in the development of vaccines against newly emerging pathogens that cause infectious diseases.

The liposome based vaccines are an attractive choice as they are biocompatible, biodegradable and composed of natural products that are non-toxic and immunologically inert. Besides, they can be frozen and freeze-dried without any deleterious effects. The classical DRVs and emulsion reverse phase evaporation technique(s) have been discussed for successful incorporation or encapsulation of antigen(s), microbes, etc., to present them immobilized. The methods are discussed in chapter 3.

Protein antigens associated with or encapsulated within liposomes are converted from soluble antigens to particulate antigens. Thus, by association of small soluble antigens with liposomes they can be targeted to macrophages. The toxicity of some antigens may be reduced by their incorporation in liposome and at the same time their immunogenicity is increased by several fold by this procedure. Immunopotentiation has been established both for antigens encapsulated within the liposomes and for antigens exposed on to the liposomal surfaces. Liposome encapsulated antigens are masked and prevented from recognition by surface receptors present on lymphoid cells. Thereby, the liposomes are phagocytosed by macrophages. Thus, phagocytosis of liposomes followed by unmasking of the encapsulated antigens appears to be a logical first step in the induction of an immune response. It has been reported that macrophages are necessary and sufficient for presentation of antigens encapsulated in liposomes to T-cells, whereas B-cells by themselves are incapable of presenting the same. Similar to B cells, dendritic cells have only a limited activity of phagocytosis and are not expected to take up any appreciable amount of liposomes. Also, the macrophages that had been fed liposome encapsulated antigen in culture could have enhanced the immune response.

The liposomes have a unique structural versatility and now it is possible to manipulate their membrane fluidity, size, surface charge and phospholipid to antigen mass ratio so that optimal adjuvanticity can be achieved for a number of antigens. An amplification in adjuvanticity has been observed by receptor-mediated targeting to antigen presenting cells and the co-entrapment of IL-2 with the antigen.

14.4.2.1. Cloned gp120 liposomal vaccines

The strategy is based on cloning **gp120** soluble HIV virus envelope protein. The recombinant gp120 protein is non virulent and induces significant $CD8^+CTL$ response. However, to evoke $CD8^+CTL$ response at significant level it is desirable that the gp120 antigen(s) must be processed and presented by MHC class I molecules. Liposomal immobilization of gp120 antigen presents them to MHC class I molecules. Thus, enabling contained gp120 to be processed by class I MHC via endogenous pathway. Further, the system, i.e. recombinant gp120 antigen (envelope protein) could be administered in the form of a ISCOMS (particles with mean diameter 35-40nm), carrying antigen in adjuvant based micelles. Moreover, concerns regarding gp120 originated **syncytia** formation leading to $CD4^+$ T cell depletion are yet to be evaluated.

14.4.3. Immunostimulating complexes (ISCOMS)

The ISCOMS comprise of a carrier structure and antigens which are incorporated into this matrix through hydrophobic interactions. The building blocks of the ISCOMS are triterpenoids. Some of these triterpenoids on association with cholesterol and phosphatidylcholine form a typical 40nm size cage-like structure. Other terpenoids in the Quil A mixture have adjuvant activity, some cause side effects in higher doses whereas others give rise to none or negligible side effects. Recently, structure forming triterpenoids giving rise to ISCOM-like particles which are virtually non-toxic for mice have been isolated.

For adjuvants like aluminum hydroxide or oil, the important immunopotentiating factor is the depot effect at the site of injection. On the contrary, antigens in ISCOMS are rapidly transported from the site of injection to the draining lymphatic organ. Therefore, in comparison to aluminum hydroxide and oil adjuvants negligible local inflammatory reaction and no granulomas are observed with ISCOMS. Following subcutaneous injection of high doses of ISCOMS only a transient redness is observed. After intraperitoneal immunization with radiolabelled antigens contained in ISCOMS, a comparatively high proportion of the antigens becomes cell associated and transported to the spleen. It localizes there for a longer period of time than the same antigen when administered in micellar form.

Studies have indicated that macrophages internalize ISCOM borne antigen more efficiently than native B cells or monocytes. Splenic dendritic cells are less efficient than macrophages but more active than monocytes or native B cells in taking up ISCOM borne antigen. Cytokine studies have indicated that ISCOMS and the matrix of the ISCOMS could induce macrophages to produce IL-1 and IL-6.

The ISCOMS have the unique property of having the ability to induce immune response via both MHC class I and class II pathways and this occurs in spite of the fact that it does not replicate as involvement of these pathways is generally observed with replicative proteinaceous system like viruses.

The prospectives for future development of ISCOM as an immunological carrier system are bright. They are useful for defined antigens produced by any means, i.e., by chemical synthesis, gene technology techniques or in conventional microorganism. ISCOMS can be formulated for parenteral as well as mucosal administration. Formulation with purified components from Quil A can be carried out which has been proved to be innocuous in toxicological studies.

14.4.4. Micelles

Micelles are formed by mixing proteins in detergent and then removing the detergent employing dialysis technique. The individual proteins orient themselves with the hydrophobic residues packed towards the center thereby at large, excluding their interaction with the outer aqueous environment towards which the hydrophilic residues are oriented. The antigen may be incorporated in micelles and could be used as an adjuvant for improved immunogenicity.

14.5. PURIFIED MACROMOLECULES

The risk involved in vaccines that are based on attenuated or killed microorganisms can be avoided with vaccines that comprise of specific purified molecules. For instance, the vaccines for *Meningococcal meningitis* and *Pneumococcal pneumonia* consist of a mixture of purified capsular polysaccharides as the immunogen. Polysaccharide vaccines are unable to activate T_H cells and this is considered as a serious limitation in their utility. They activate B cells in a thymus-independent manner, resulting only in the production of IgM and not IgG. There is also hardly any development of memory cells. Several methods have been tried as an attempt to circumvent this limitation. One such technique is the conjugation of the polysaccharide antigen to some sort of protein carrier. The vaccine for *Haemophilus influenza* type b (Hib), for example, is the major cause of bacterial meningitis in children under 5 years of age. It consists of type b capsular polysaccharide covalently linked to tetanus toxoid, a protein carrier. In comparison to polysaccharide alone, the polysaccharide-protein conjugate is relatively more immunogenic and as it activates T_H cells, it enables class switching from IgM to IgG. This type of vaccine can only induce memory B cells but not memory T cells specific for the pathogen. In the case of the Hib vaccine, it appears that the memory B cells can be activated to some extent in the absence of a memory T_H-cell population and in all probabilities this accounts for the efficacy of this vaccine.

One of the problems associated with the vaccines containing purified surface macromolecules is the difficulty of obtaining the purified component. This limitation can be overcome with recombinant DNA techniques whereby a gene encoding an immunogenic protein is expressed in bacterial, yeast or insect cells. For example, diphtheria and tetanus vaccines can be made by purifying the recombinant bacterial exotoxin and then inactivating the toxin with formaldehyde to form a toxoid. Vaccination with the toxoid induces antitoxoid antibodies, which are also capable of binding to the toxin and neutralizing its toxic effect. In production of toxoid vaccines the conditions demand close control so that detoxification can be achieved without excessive modification of the epitope structure.

14.6. SYNTHETIC PEPTIDE VACCINES

Developments, in the recent past, in the methods for identifying and synthesizing specific B-and T-cell epitopes offer the potential to induce disease neutralizing immune response with completely synthetic structures. Now, it is well established that short chain peptides can be used to mimic antigenic sites of viruses and thus can be used as the basis for vaccine development. Therefore, attempts have been made to synthesize such peptides, which act as surrogate immunogens, as an alternative to the existing conventional vaccines, i.e. chemically modified toxins, attenuated strains of microbes and killed but antigenic microbes. There are various reasons responsible for motivating the interest of researchers to develop synthetic peptides and they are as following :

- relatively easy and cheap to produce;
- stable for longer periods of time without the need for refrigeration; and
- scale-up to production and purification is easy in contrast to conventional vaccines.

Various considerations and approaches pertaining to the development of synthetic peptide based vaccines have been dealt in this chapter. In order to fall in with the concept, a brief review on generalized mechanism involved in the immunity development is presented so as to have a better understanding of the approach.

To synthesize a peptide which can induce production of antibodies reacting with the coat proteins of viruses, it is necessary to identify the critical epitopes involved in providing protective immunity and determining the sequence of amino acids that constitute an epitope.

14.6.1. B- and T-cell epitopes : A pre-requisite for antigenicity of peptides

There are a number of predictive approaches and experimental approaches which can be used to identify potential immunogenic determinants. In the past it was believed that owing to relatively smaller molecular size, synthetic peptides behave like haptens and are necessarily poor immunogens requiring some means of enhancing their immunogenicity (e.g., coupling to carrier proteins). However, it is now clear that synthetic peptides, like any other antigen, must contain appropriate B-cell epitopes (antibody recognition sites) and T_H-cell epitopes (site capable of eliciting help for antibody production), in order to evoke antibody responses. These T_H-cell epitopes must be capable of binding class-II MHC molecules on the surface of host APC and B-cells and subsequently interacting with the T-cell receptor in the form of a trimolecular complex so that the differentiation and proliferation by B-cells can be induced.

Identification of potential B-cell epitopes of a protein antigen can be carried out by examining its structure for peptide sequences representing sites that are accessible, hydrophilic and mobile. Generally, B-cell epitopes are chosen by identifying strongly hydrophilic sequences. This is based on the assumption that strongly hydrophilic sequences are most likely to represent accessible surface regions that constitute B-cell epitopes. For induction of humoral immunity, vaccine, should include peptides composing immunodominant B-cell epitopes. Such epitopes can be identified by determining the dominant antibody in the sera of individuals recovering from a disease. This is to be followed by testing peptides for their ability to react with that antibody with a high affinity.

A vaccine must also include immunodominant T-cell epitopes, since an effective memory response for both humoral and cell-mediated immunity requires generation of a population of memory T_H cells. Owing to the unpredictable role played by MHC in influencing immunodominance for the T-cell system, it is very difficult to identify those epitopes with synthetic peptide vaccines. In the majority of cases T cells recognize processed peptides that appear to represent internal amphipathic peptides. These peptides should possess a site (the agretope) that enables them to interact with MHC molecules and a site (the epitope) that enables them to interact with the T-cell receptor. MHC molecules have differences in their ability for peptide presentation. Thus, MHC polymorphism within a species therefore influences the level of T cell responsiveness by different individuals to different peptides. Also, different sub-populations of T cells recognize different epitopes. Studies have identified some peptides that induce immunologic suppression and other peptides that induce a strong helper response. Generally, these helper and suppresser peptides represent different, non-overlapping amino acid sequences. For instance, immunization with the amino terminal residues (1-17) of hen egg-white lysozyme suppressed the response to native lysozyme. Immunity can be enhanced by the identification and thereby elimination of the suppressing peptides. These suppressing peptides can also be exploited in cases where the immune response is to be decreased, as in the treatment of autoimmune diseases.

The current approach in designing synthetic peptide vaccines against viruses involves location of invariant regions, whose amino acid sequence is highly conserved. For example, some regions of the hemagglutinin (HA) molecule of influenza virus display high levels of amino acid variation. This generates the type and subtype differences which enables the virus to escape the immune system. But invariant regions mediating essential biological functions are also present in the HA molecule. For instance, the sialic acid-binding site on HA allows the virus to bind to sialic acid residues on cell surfaces. Normally, this region on the intact viral particle does not induce antibody formation but still the synthetic peptide vaccines of this conserved region have been found to neutralize viral infectivity against a number of different influenza types and sub-types. However, if a peptide is a poor immunogen or non-immunogenic, as in the case of peptides which contain only a B-cell epitope, they can be rendered immunogenic by :

a) coupling to a large carrier protein (that contains many T_H-cell epitopes);
b) polymeric presentation of such peptides;
c) incorporating an identified T_H-cell epitope into the peptide.

14.6.2. Synthetic peptides and T-helper cell determinants

It is relevant to understand the role of T_H cell determinants in designing synthetic immunogens, by now it is established that synthetic peptides can be highly immunogenic in their soluble form (free form) provided they carry appropriate antibodies recognition sites what we refer as B cell epitopes should also carry sites capable of eliciting help for antibody production via T_H cell epitopes. The latter in turn must bind to class II MHC molecule on the surface of host antigen presenting cells and B cells and subsequently should interact with T cell receptor via trimolecular complex orientation which could induce B cell to differentiate and proliferate. If however, a peptide in its free form turns to be a poor immunogen or produce cells an immune response that is genetically restricted then in such cases an appropriate T_H cell epitopes may be added. This wide spread concept of combination of B cell and T cell epitopes introduces an important class of vaccines of interest.

The combination could be brought about by the process of B and T cell epitopes co-polymerized by employing a number of chemical means. A typical case is exemplified where Chedid and his colleagues used glutaraldehyde to polymerize four peptides from two bacteria antigens, i.e. *S. pyrogen* M and protein and diphtheria toxoid or HBsAg and proteinoid *Plasmodium knowlensii*. The approach exhibited enhanced immunogenetics as compared to their homopolymers. The concept of immunization employing this approach is schematically presented in figure 14.2.

14.6.3. Carrier coupling

A foreign substance with low molecular weight (hapten) is often not antigenic unless it is made larger by attachment to a carrier molecule. Once an antibody against the hapten is formed, however, the hapten alone reacts with antibodies (Fig.14.3) e.g., penicillin is not antigenic by itself, but it combines with serum proteins of some persons and the resulting molecule initiates an immune response. The same approach, i.e., coupling to large carrier proteins is the most convenient and straight forward approach to enhance the immunogenicity of a poor/non-immunogenic synthetic peptide. The carrier proteins provide T-cell help for B-cell antibody production to poor/non-immunogenic peptides. The results of different studies indicate that the protective immunity can be induced in experimental animals with synthetic peptides coupled to carrier proteins. Full protection of animals against foot and mouth disease virus (FMDV) and hepatitis-B virus (HBV) has been demonstrated.

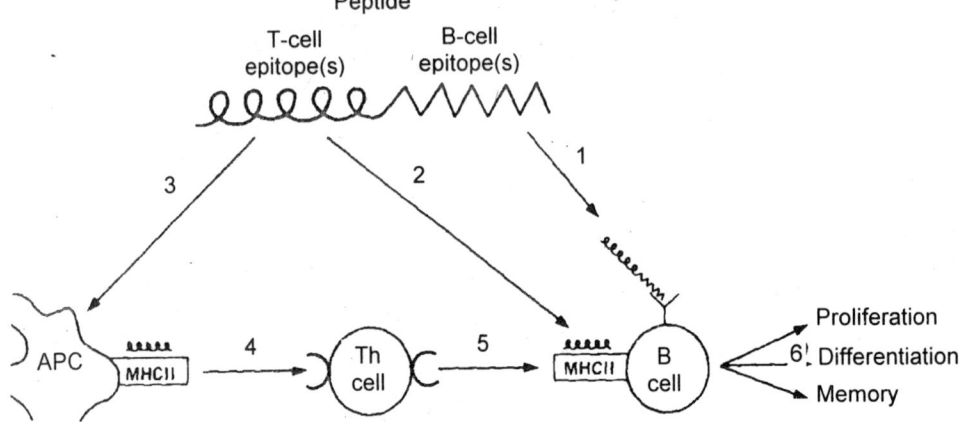

Fig. 14.2 : T-cell help for B-cell antibody production to uncoupled peptides. (1) B-cell epitopes are recognized by immunoglobulin receptors on B-cells; (2) the T-cell epitopes within the same peptide are presented on the surface of B-cells in association with class II MHC; (3) the same T-cell epitopes are presented on the surface of APC in association with MHC II; (4) T_H –cells recognize the peptide-MHC II complex; and (5) the B-cells proliferate and differentiate into antibody-secreting plasma cells.

14.6.3.1. Mechanism of immunogenicity

There may be more than one different mechanisms involved in the immunogenicity enhancement effect of carrier peptides:

- The coupling of small synthetic peptides to carrier proteins increases the molecular mass of peptide and thereby improves the uptake by APC.
- Biological half life of small peptides may be increased via their linkage to carrier proteins.
- If the synthetic peptide itself is immunogenic (as in case of peptides having B- and T-cell epitopes), the carrier protein merely functions as a polymeric delivery system.

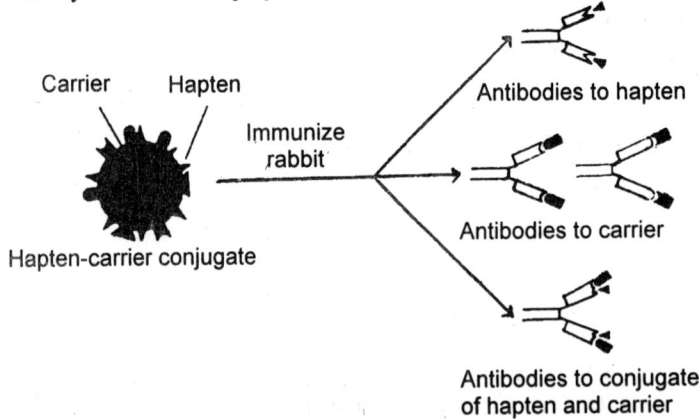

Fig.14.3 : Attachment of hapten to the carrier molecules to form antigenic molecules

14.6.3.2. Commonly used carriers and selection of a suitable carrier

The carrier proteins which are commonly used for synthetic peptides include:

(a) Keyhole limpet hemocyanin (KLH) and sperm whale myoglobin (SWM).

(b) Albumins (bovine serum albumin, ovalbumin).

(c) Bacterial toxoids (tetanus toxoid, diphtheria toxoid) and other bacterial proteins used in vaccines such as PPD from BCG.

KLH and SWM are the traditional carrier proteins and offer a number of distinctive advantages such as -

- likely to be highly foreign to species to be immunized;
- unlikely to elicit cross-reactive or interfering antibodies;
- are well established model immunogens;
- SWM is extensively characterized;
- when used in man, KLH does not produce any obvious side effects.

While albumins offer the advantage of free availability but the anti-carrier antibodies generated with these carriers is a drawback. Bacterial toxoids and bacterial proteins have also been used as carriers believing that a pre-primed human population exists which may produce an enhanced response to the peptide linked to these carriers. However, it has been a subject of argument as some researchers observed that no pre-priming occurs or even active suppression does take place. Various factors that must be considered while selecting a carrier are identified and presented below:

- Purpose of coupling - to immunize an animal against infection or to elicit high titer antipeptide antibodies.
- Nature of the peptide - hydrophilic or hydrophobic, effect of carrier coupling on the residues important for its antigenicity, presence of cysteine residues that may form disulfide bridges.
- Choice of carrier - natural or artificial carrier, common protein or an unusual protein, risk of eliciting hypersensitivity or auto immunity, possibility to elicit cross-reactive or interfering antibodies, possibility of occurrence of prepriming against carrier.
- Method of conjugation - effect of method on antigenicity of peptide as well as peptide to carrier ratio.
- Method of immunization - route, dose, choice of adjuvant, frequency, age, sex, interval between primary and subsequent booster inoculations, difference in responses between laboratory animals and target species.

14.6.3.3. Coupling methods

The carrier proteins require some form of chemical coupling to the synthetic peptide molecules to enhance their immunogenicity. Various methods and reagents can be used for this purpose. Some of the important chemical agents employed for coupling are listed in table14.2.

Glutaraldehyde is the most commonly used reagent. However, the reaction is relatively uncontrolled and may deleteriously affect antigenic sites on the peptide. The problem can be overcome by use of heterobifunctional cross-linking agents which, unlike glutaraldehyde, facilitate specific linkages.

Table 14.2: Chemical agents employed and the functional groups involved in coupling reaction

Reagents	Functional groups involved in the coupling reaction
Glutaraldehyde	amino,imidazole,phenolic hydroxyl, sulfhydryl
Carbodiimides	amino, carboxyl,phenolic hydroxyl, sulfhydryl
Bis-imido esters	amino
Heterobifunctional cross linkers	amino, sulfhydryl
Homobifunctional NHS esters	amino

14.6.3.4. Potential drawbacks

While the method of chemical coupling of carrier proteins to synthetic peptides offers the advantage of being a quick simple and convenient method, it inherits certain drawbacks which include -

- poor batch-to-batch reproducibility as the coupling reaction is poorly defined and is difficult to control.
- carrier induced suppression and hypersensitivity to the carrier.

- adverse effect of the coupling method on the antigenicity of the peptide, i.e. masking or modification of important antigenic sites on the peptide.

14.6.4. Polymeric presentation of peptides

The polymeric presentation of peptides is a viable approach which improves the immunogenicity of synthetic peptides significantly. Various researchers have conducted different studies in the direction of establishing such presentation systems as commercially viable wholly synthetic vaccines. Francis prepared a number of synthetic forms of 141-160 peptide from VPI of FMDV and subsequently tested for their immunogenicity. Various forms that were prepared are presented in figure 14.4

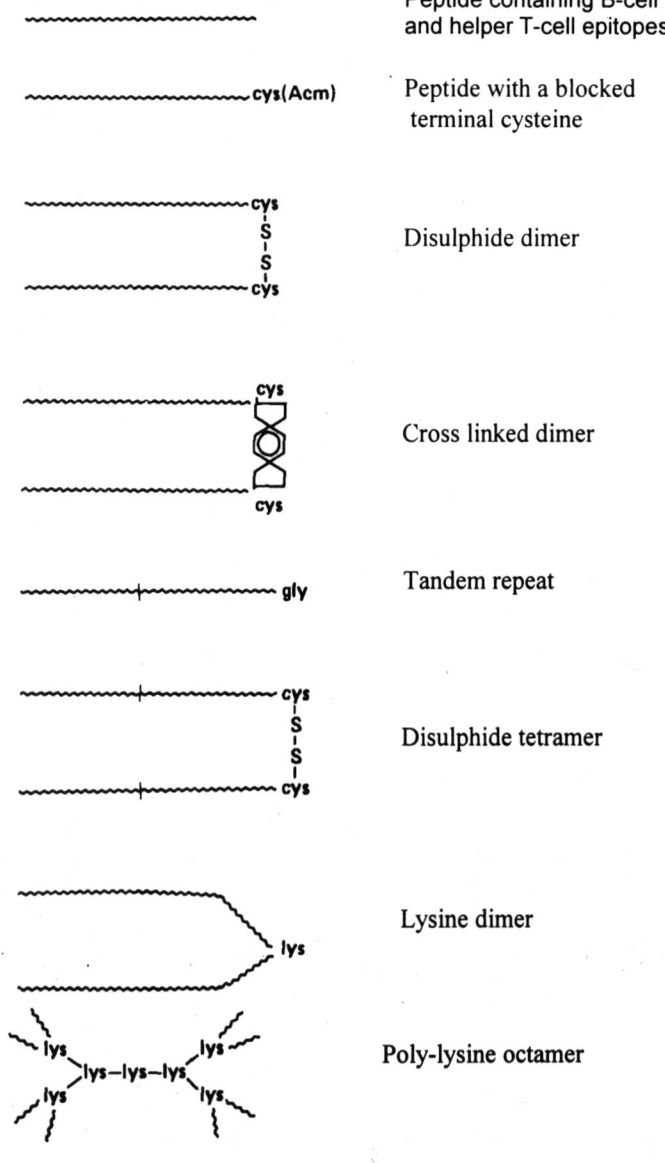

Fig.14.4 : Various forms of uncoupled synthetic peptides used for comparative immunogenicity studies

The role of non natural terminal free thiol cysteine residue in the enhancement of immunogenicity of free FMDV peptide has been examined and reported by many workers. The presence of free thiol cysteine residue results in the formation of peptide dimers responsible for its increased immunogenicity. Similarly, tandem repeats of FMDV VP1 137-162, with or without terminal cysteine residue, have been shown to produce higher titer value of neutralizing antibodies in guinea pigs as compared to single copy peptides. In addition, polylysine octamer based constructs have been produced by utilizing multiple antigenic peptide (MAP) system. This system provides an effective method for direct solid phase synthesis of a peptide antigen onto a branching lysine backbone. It has been shown that presentation of peptide in the form of octamer or tetramer induces higher neutralizing antibody titer values than those produced by lysine dimeric forms. Therefore, it is now very much clear from various reports that effective quantitative and qualitative immune response can be produced by polymeric form of the synthetic peptides.

Using recombinant DNA technology, small peptide sequences have been fused to the genes encoding larger proteins in order to produce a novel construct. The use of peptidal sequences fused to bacterial proteins as immunogens has the potential advantage of being uniform with a defined structure as compared to the uncharacterized peptide/carrier conjugates.

In an interesting work to express foot-and-mouth-disease virus (FMDV) peptides, were fused to the N-terminus of β-galactosidase in *E. coli* cells. Preliminary studies revealed that multiple copies of the inserted peptide sequence may be beneficial. Similarly, in an other development, the fusion protein concept for multiple peptide presentation has led to the production of particulate structures with epitopes repeated over their entire surface. The work has been mainly concentrated on hepatitis B surface antigen, hepatitis B core antigen (HBcAg) and yeast Ty protein, which spontaneously self assemble into 22, 27 and 60 nm particles respectively (Fig.14.5).

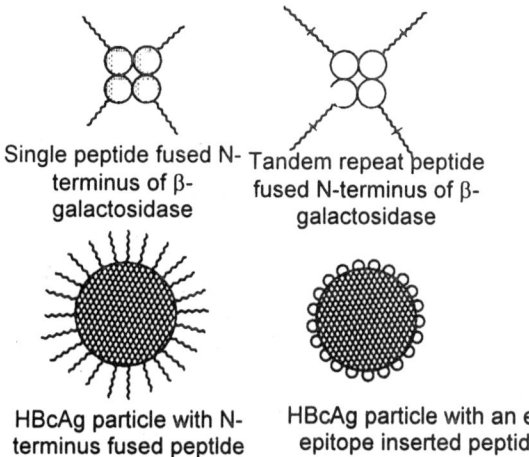

Single peptide fused N-terminus of β-galactosidase

Tandem repeat peptide fused N-terminus of β-galactosidase

HBcAg particle with N-terminus fused peptide

HBcAg particle with an e1-epitope inserted peptide

Fig.14.5 : Schematic presentation of various forms of recombinant peptide/protein fusion molecules

14.6.5. Incorporation of identified T_H- cell epitopes into the peptide

As already described, synthetic peptides must contain appropriate B-and T_H-cell epitopes in order to be immunogenic in their free form. Peptides that contain only B-cell epitope are non-immunogenic. Incorporation of appropriate T_H-cell epitopes into such peptides is another approach to render them immunogenic. Different methods of generating such combinations of B- and T_H-cell epitopes are:

(1) Polymerization of B- and T-cell peptides.
(2) Chemical linkage
(3) Co-linear synthesis.

14.6.5.1. Polymerization of B- and T-cell peptides

This is the simplest method of combining B- and T-cell epitopes. In this method co-polymers of a number of individual peptides are produced by chemical means.

Some limitations of this approach are -

- uncontrolled nature of polymerization reaction.
- risk of affecting antigenic properties of peptides.

14.6.5.2. Chemical linkage

This is more controlled method of chemical linkage which utilizes a heterobifunctional cross-linking reagent, such as M-maleimidobenzoyl-N-hydroxysuccinimide ester (MBS). This compound has an amino-reactive NHS-ester as one functional group and a sulfhydryl reactive group as the other. Amino groups on one peptide (e.g. B-cell epitope) are acylated with the NHS-ester via the hydroxysuccinimide group. This is followed by the introduction of a second peptide (e.g. T_H-cell epitope) having a free sulfhydryl group that can react with the maleimide group of the coupling reagent. Good et. al, have used this method to link the malaria-encoded sequence $(NANP)_n$ from the circumsporozoite (CS) protein to another peptide from the CS protein. However, this technique may require the synthesis of a specific peptide with a non-natural cysteine residue added to its carboxy terminal. Also, the presence of essential natural cysteine or lysine residues within either peptides may ultimately affect the nature and final antigenicity of the conjugated produced (Fig. 14.6).

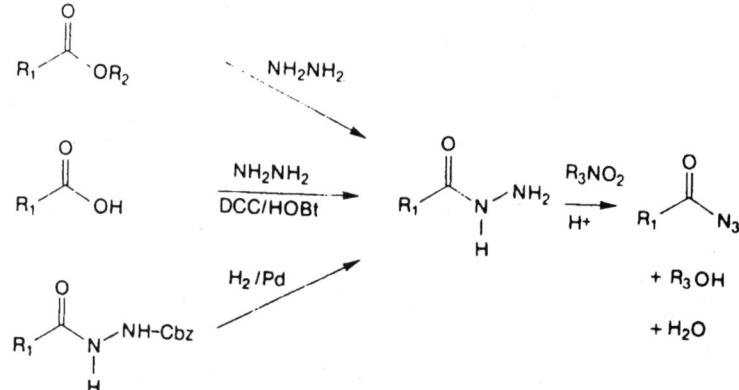

Fig. 14.6 : Preparation of peptide azides from esters, acids and protected azides

14.6.5.3. Co-linear synthesis

This technique overcomes the limitations associated with the first two methods. A peptide with known immunological properties can be synthesized utilizing this approach. The method offers the flexibility to alter the position of one epitope in relation to other and to synthesize peptides containing a number of B-and/or T-cell epitopes. B-cell epitope/T-cell epitope co-linear peptides have been successfully used as synthetic vaccines.

A brief review of the works in the direction of producing B-and T-cell epitope combinations for enhancing their immunogenicity is summarized and presented in table14.3.

The conventional types of vaccines, though widely used right now, have certain restrictive limitations :

- batch to batch reproducibility is difficult to attain as they usually consist of live (attenuated) or killed strains of microbes,
- production involves sophisticated technology and therefore relatively expensive,
- purification is rather difficult,
- stringent storage conditions are necessary to maintain in order to keep them stable at their optimum activity level.

Table 14.3: A brief review of work done in the direction of producing B-cell and T-cell epitopes combinations

Researchers	Work
Francis, 1990	Demonstrated the importance of location of the T-cell epitope in relation to B-cell epitope using FMDV system.
Borras-Cuesta et al. 1987	Synthesized two peptides from major coat protein VPG of bovine rotavirus (which contained non-immunogenic B-cell epitopes) and a peptide from influenza virus (which contained T-cell epitope). Both the peptides were shown to induce anti-rotavirus responses in mice greater than those produced by the same rotavirus sequences conjugated to bovine serum albumin.
Good et al. 1987	Linked the malaria-encoded sequence $(NANP)_n$ from circumsporozoite (CS) protein to another peptide from the CS protein. The resultant conjugate raised anti $(NANP)_n$ antibodies in mice which were non-responders to $(NANP)_n$ antibodies sequence alone.
Francis et al. 1987	140-160 peptide from VP1 of FMDV (which contained B-cell epitope and H-k T-cell epitope) was co-synthesized with three different sequences containing H-2^d and T-cell epitopes, one from ovalbumin and two from sperm whale myoglobin. The resultant three peptides produced anti-FMDV peptide antibodies in both H-2^k and H-2^d haplotype mice.
Chedid et al. 1984	Polymerized four peptides from two bacterial antigens, one viral antigen and one parasitic antigen using glutaraldehyde. Workers showed that association of peptides enhanced their respective immunogenicities.
Leclerc et al 1987	Co-polymerized a streptococcal protein peptide (which contained B-&T-cell epitopes) with a hepatitis-B virus surface antigen peptide (containing B-cell epitope)
Francis et al. 1989	Five predicted ten amino acid T_h cell epitopes (T1 to T5) from HRV (human rhinovirus) were used to improve the performance of a non-immunogenic B-cell epitope peptide from the same virus.
Jolivet et al. 1990	Showed the importance of T-cell epitopes in the polymers.
Ho et al. 1990 Pollur et al. 1988, Rusche et al. 1988, Goudssmit et al. 1988	Succeeded in raising virus neutralizing antibodies with synthetic peptides for a linear B-cell epitope of human immunodeficiency virus (HIV). These antibodies neutralized HIV *in-vitro*.

Development of fully synthetic peptides with suitable groups and structure offers an alternative to conventional vaccines. These synthetic peptides mimic the antigenic sites of the microbes and thus could induce immunological responses. By proper structural design and presentation the peptides can be made to provide immunological response as effective vaccines and could be used to provide a cover against a particular type of antigen or microbe. The concept is still in its infancy and lot of experiments are in progress to render the synthetic peptides effective and acceptable.

14.7. IMMUNOADHESION(S)

The major problem with CD4 clone prophylaxis is fast clearance of these molecules. In the case of CD4 vaccines biological half-life recorded to be 30-120 minutes in serum. Therefore, frequent injections are required. Immunoadhesion gene strategy reported by Capon and colleagues is principally based on recombinant technology where CD4 gene is linked with constant region gene of IgG1. So formed immunoglobulin-CD4 gene hybrid is referred as immunoadhesive which exhibited high affinity to gp120 (typical characteristics of CD4) and longer biological half-life that corresponds to IgG1. The biological half-life of CD-IgG1 has been reported to be 200 fold longer than soluble CD4; expected half-life in human of this systems as about 21 days. This opens up vistas for diverse immunoadhesive expressions, thus various associated factor and functions like opsonization or complement activation.

14.8. RECOMBINANT ANTIGEN VACCINES

14.8.1. rDNA vaccines - The rationale

During the last two decades, recombinant DNA (rDNA) technology has revolutionized basic and applied biomedical research. It has brought about a great change in the view of biomedical research and overcoming research associated problems. A wide range of impressive new products have been developed by using recombinant techniques which are available in the market. These products range from biologicals such as insulin and tissue plasminogen activator (TPA), to genetically engineered organisms that can be used to protect valuable fruit crops to enzymes utilized in the manufacture of foods to new generation vaccines. They have also played an important role in developing diagnostic kits helping to detect infections at a very early stage and in crime laboratories for "finger printing" tests on blood and semen samples. In the preceding few paragraphs, focus will be on the use of recombinant technology in development of new generation vaccines. However, comprehensive details of the vaccines developed till date or in progress will not be discussed. Certain vaccines currently available in market are efficacious and cost effective, however, they are still being developed using age old techniques. The rDNA technique effectively and successfully could be used to incorporate safety in the products as well as lend them to be cost effective.

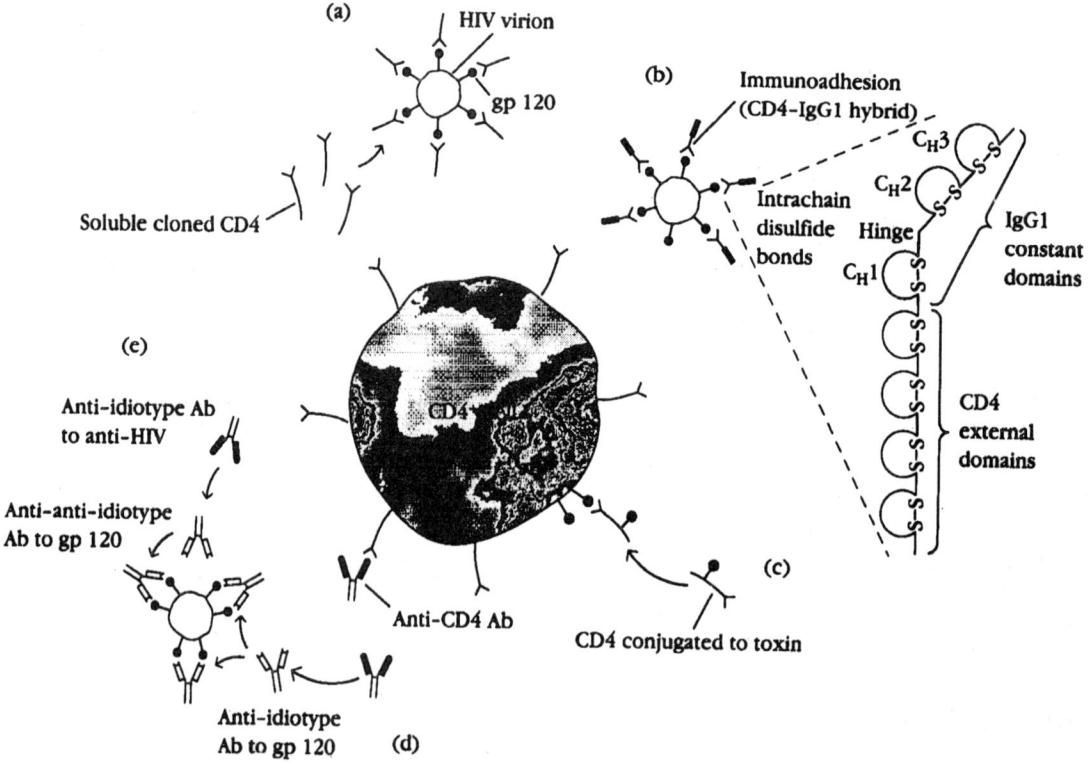

Fig. 14.7 : Mechanismss by which various reagents can interfere with the gp120-CD4 interaction, which is necessary for HIV to infect T cell. (a) Soluble cloned CD4 binds to gp120 on HIV virions. (b) An immunoadhesion formed from the external domains of CD4 and the constant region of IgG1 also binds to gp120 virions. (c) Binding of CD4 linked to a toxin to viral gp120 on HIV-infected cells leads to death of the cell. (d) anti-CD4 antibody, anti-idiotype antibody specific for the paratope on anti-HIV antibody (e) can induce production of antibodies that bind to gp120 without exposing the individual to HIV or to HIV components

However, there are varying problems like handling infectious agents and the safety concern of the personnel handling the same. Since vaccines are developed to prevent infectious diseases, it is apparent that traditional approaches of vaccine development are attended with a variety of concerns about safety. rDNA vaccines have clear advantages over those where the organism are used to produce the vaccine. The disadvantages associated with traditional micro-organism based vaccine systems are mentioned below:

a. it is dangerous to handle;
b. it could produce disease in vaccinated hosts;
c. it needs to be attenuated, and/or; and
d. it could produce toxic end products.

Using organisms that are highly virulent pose an obvious problem in developing, producing and using the vaccine. This is one of the reason for the failure of the conventional technique in developing a vaccine for hepatitis B. Applying rDNA technique successful development of hepatitis B vaccine (HBV) has been possible which has now flooded the market. By cloning the genes required to produce HBV-soluble antigen (the protective antigen) in a bacterial host, it was possible to create a nonvirulent, recombinant organism capable of synthesizing large amounts of the protective antigens of HBV.

Using rDNA technology, the amount of antigen produced by an organism can be increased. Isolation and cloning of DNA encoding for antigenic determinants can be carried out in yeast, bacteria or mammalian cells. A number of genes from viral, bacterial, and protozoan pathogens have been successfully cloned and attempts are being made to develop them as vaccines. The DNA encoding the relevant antigen can be cloned in bacterial, yeast, insect, or mammalian expression systems. The first recombinant vaccine was developed successfully for the major antigen (VP1) of the foot-and-mouth disease viruses. Here, viral RNA encoding the VP1 surface antigen was transcribed into cDNA using **reverse transcriptase**. The VP1 cDNA was then inserted into an *Escherichia coli* plasmid and cloned in *E. coli* (Fig. 10.15). With this procedure production of large quantities of the VP1 antigen is possible, which could then be purified and used as a vaccine in animals.

Hepatitis B vaccine was the first recombinant antigen vaccine approved for human use. The vaccine was developed by cloning the gene for the major surface antigen of hepatitis B virus (HBsAg) in yeast cells. The recombinant yeast cells are grown in fermenters and accumulation of HBsAg occurs intracellularly in the cells. The yeast cells are harvested and disrupted by high pressure thereby releasing the recombinant HBsAg which is then purified by conventional biochemical techniques. The recombinant hepatitis B vaccine has been tested successfully and has immense potential for exploitation.

Studies are presently being carried out for development of recombinant vaccines for human immuno-deficiency virus. Other recombinant vaccines are being developed in animal models and these include the **circumsporozoite protein** of the malaria parasite, the B subunit of cholera toxin, a glycoprotein membrane antigen from Epstein-Barr virus and the enterotoxin of *E. coli*. In some cases promising results have been obtained with a protective immune response to a subsequent challenge. The prominent limitation of recombinant protein or glycoprotein vaccines is that they are processed as exogenous antigens and therefore fail to induce much activation of class I MHC-restricted T_C cells.

For recombinant proteins which are weakly immunogenic, some safe and powerful adjuvants are designed so that their immune response can be augmented. One of the approaches utilizes genetic grafting of immuno-stimulatory lymphokines, such as IL-1 or TNFα into a recombinant protein. However, their practical application is strongly limited in humans due to their toxic, proinflammatory and pleiotropic effects. For example, IL-1 is an important modulatory molecule of the immune system and also induces *in vivo* after administration of several adjuvant molecules, such as bacterial products. But, IL-1 cannot be used as such because it is also a potent pyrogen and proinflammatory agent. To alleviate this problem, the **163-171 sequence** of human IL-1β has been proposed as adjuvant for poorly immunogenic vaccines. This non peptide was found to be the minimal structure responsible for the immunostimulatory properties of the entire molecule. It was also devoid of many undesired *in vivo* and *in vitro* pro-inflammatory activities of IL-1. In addition, it can stimulate the immune response to both T-dependent and T-independent antigens. So this technique of using recombinant antigens with 'built-in' adjuvanticity opens up new vistas in designing vaccines in which poorly immunogenic proteins are coupled to domains endowed with immunostimulatory properties.

14.8.2. Adjuvant independent immunotargeted vaccines

The approach involves antigen-antibody conjugation. The complex is presented to the determinant expressed *in vivo* on the surface of cells of immune system. The immunization as such a parenteral preparation administered intravenously with saline have referred as antigen independent. Thus, physical properties and passivasion for disposition of conjugate itself, presumably dominated the event via antibody specific binding affinity of the conjugate thus antigen is presented and in turn localized at the surface of specific preidentified target cells.

14.8.3. Class II MHC targeted antigen

In a classical strategy using avidin as a model antigenic protein which has affinity to MAb specific for class II MHC, a target oriented immunization system has been developed. It is reported and accepted that in order to have an appreciable immune response as well as priming for secondary antibody response both B-cells and T-cell recognition are needed. Class II MHC bearing cells therefore have been appreciated to be a target cell line. The immunogenic responses of anti avidin IgG was compared with avidin-anti-I-A MAbs in mice. Avidin bound to the anticlass II MAbs was found to be approximately 40 fold more immunogenic than avidin conjugated to the anti-NP MAb (a control antibody non reactive). Thus, it was inferred that ligand specific to receptor port could have brought by the improvised activity profile.

The results indicate an early immunoglobulin response which peaked after 10 days of immunization. A strong memory response to the initial priming with immunoconjugate could be induced by avidin-plain. It has also been proved experimentally that the targeted immunization is able to restore long lived memory response. This is in accordance with very important and desirable feature of immunization strategy particularly of significant in vaccine design. It is noted that immunotargeting could establish immune system related manipulation even in the absence of adjuvants. Furthermore, with recent speculation concerning to molecular basis of immunological memory, the anti-class II MHC immunoconjugates seem able to deliver antigen to the cellular level selectively where the maintenance of long term memory is desirable.

Figure 14.8 schematically represents the events involved in the enhancement of immunogenicity via immuno targeting.

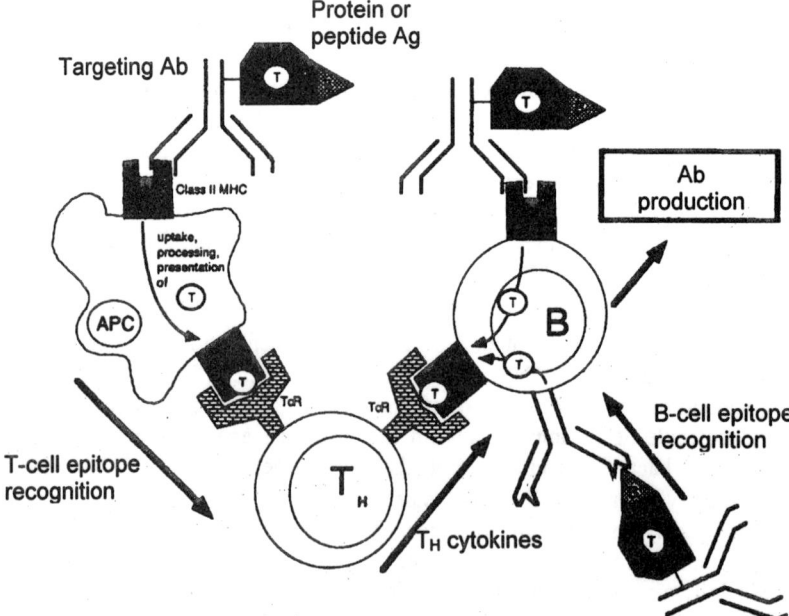

Fig. 14.8 : Schematic presentation of the proposed mechanism for the enhancement of immunogenicity by immunotargeting. T: T-helper cell epitope ; B : B-cell epitope; TcR : T cell receptor ; APC : antigen presenting cell; TH : T-helper cell

Cells bearing class II MHC possess potential for antigen presentation, employing that beginning with a uptake followed by proteolytic processing and in turn the association of released T-cell epitopes (peptides) together with class II MHC can result in the activation of T-cell help. It is likely that following subcutaneous immunization anti-class II MHC immunoconjugates could encounter class II specific determinants present on specialized antigen presenting cells such as dendritics, interact with class II MHC on B cells. The antigen specific T cells determinants are presented following their processing by the cascade of events described above, as a result it leads to activation of class II MHC restricted T helper (T_H) cells capable of signaling through cytokine(s) regulation necessary for B cell differentiation and proliferation. However, only B cells which had already received traditional signal shall be capable of responding to this "help". The traditional signals are originated or induced by engagement of antigen specific receptors with B cell epitopes on the antigen. Thus the process favors enhanced uptake of class II MHC specific antigens by APC hence could serve to augment the immunogenicity of antigens via their targeted presentation.

14.9. VECTOR VACCINES

14.9.1. Recombinant vector vaccines

Genes encoding for major antigens of especially virulent pathogens can be introduced into attenuated viruses or bacteria. The attenuated organism serves as a vector, which replicates within the host and expresses the gene product of the pathogen. Various organisms have been utilized for vector vaccines and include adenoviruses, attenuated poliovirus, vaccinia virus, BCG strain of *Mycobacterium bovis* and attenuated strains of *Salmonella.*

Vaccinia virus, which has been used to eradicate smallpox is widely employed as a vector vaccine. This large and complex virus containing a genome of about 200 genes, can be manipulated to carry scores of foreign genes without any impairment in its capacity to infect host cells and replicates. The gene encoding for desired antigen is inserted into a plasmid vector adjacent to a vaccinia promoter and is flanked on the two sides by vaccinia thymidine kinase sequences. Simultaneously, tissue culture cells are infected with vaccinia virus and transfected with the recombinant plasmid. The desired gene and promoter are inserted into the vaccinia virus genome by homologous recombination at the site of the non-essential vaccinia thymidine kinase gene. This results in a thymidine kinase-negative recombinant virus. Selection of tissue culture cells infected with recombinant (thymidine kinase-negative) vaccinia viruses are then carried out by adding bromodeoxyuridine (Budr), a thymidine analog which kills all thymidine kinase-positive cells (Fig. 14.9).

The genetically engineered vaccinia expresses high levels of the inserted gene product, which can later serve as a potent immunogen in an inoculated host. Attempts have been made to insert genes from hepatitis B virus, influenza and herpes simplex viruses into vaccinia virus. It was observed that this engineered vaccinia induces antibodies to all three engineered gene products. As with small pox vaccine, genetically engineered vaccinia can be administered simply by dermal scratching. Thus, a limited localized infection is caused in host cells. If the foreign gene product expressed by the vaccinia is a viral envelope protein, it is inserted into the membrane of the infected host cell, inducing development of both T-cell-mediated immunity and antibody-mediated immunity.

Vaccinia virus engineered with the glycoprotein envelope of the human immunodeficiency virus (HIV) is being examined as a potential vaccine for AIDS. However, the vaccinia vector vaccine may not be suitable for individual with AIDS, because in immunity deficient individuals even an attenuated vaccine can be fatal.

Various other attenuated vector vaccines safer than the vaccinia virus have been tried. An attenuated strain of *Salmonella typhimurium* has been engineered with genes from the bacterium that causes cholera. This vector vaccine is advantageous in that Salmonella infects cells of the mucosal lining of the gut and thereby inducing secretory IgA production. For various diseases like cholera and gonorrhea, an increased level of secretory IgA at mucous membrane surfaces is required for immunity. Another potential candidate for a safe and effective vector vaccine is the **sabin vaccine** strain of **poliovirus**. Here the poliovirus vector is genetically engineered to replace a portion of the gene encoding the outer capsid protein of poliovirus by DNA encoding the epitope of choice. The resulting poliovirus chimera expresses the desired epitope(s) in a highly accessible presentation protruding from the poliovirus nucleocapsid. In animal models a chimeric poliovirus vector vaccine expressing epitopes from the envelope glycoproteins of HIV has shown to induce high levels of neutralizing antibodies specific for HIV.

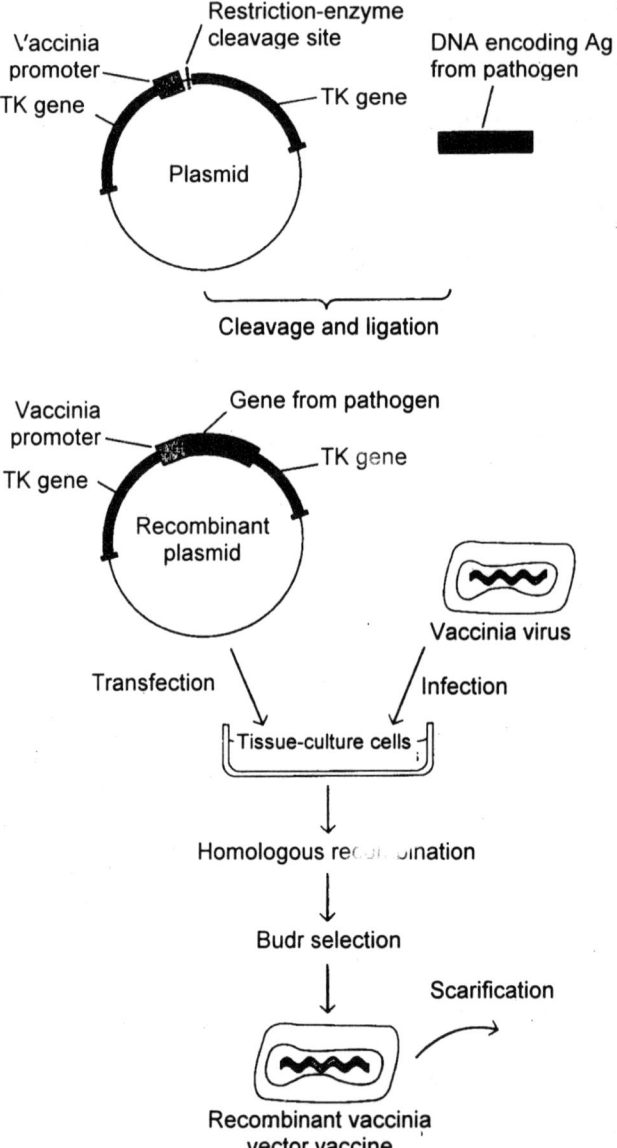

Fig. 14.9 : Production of vaccinia vector vaccine containing a gene encoding an antigen from a pathogen

14.9.2. Minicells as vaccines

The use of whole cell organism has the disadvantage that once they enter the GALT they produce antibodies. However, they create their own environmental challenges and problems. To overcome such regeneration problem, a non-regenerating vaccine carrier such as minicells can be used. Strains of *E. coli* (minicell-producing) and *S. typhimurium* have been reported. Minicells are non-regenerating vaccine carriers containing somatic and surface antigens. They possess the advantage that they do not express any pathogenic activity and are capable of eliciting both humoral and cellular immune responses.

14.9.2.1. The concept

When a rod-shaped bacterium undergoes cell division at the midcellular axis, it generates two daughter cells, each containing not only the cellular constituents of the mother cell but also a full complement of the genetic material. Chromosomal genes responsible for the replication of the chromosome (genophore) and its partitioning between the two daughter cells ensure the preservation of the cell size and the inheritance of a genophore. Under most normal growth conditions, some variations in the distribution of daughter cell sizes are observed. On the other hand, under some special physiological conditions, such as aged culture or in cells treated with antibiotics, anomalous cell division leads to asymmetrical cells, that is the formation of daughter cells of unequal sizes.

Figure 14.10 illustrates the normal cell growth, elongation and division of a typical rod shaped bacteria. The daughter cells which are resulting from cell division, perpetuate the cell cycle and formation of progeny cells. The formation of daughter cells is controlled both physiologically and genetically. Once, there is an intervention with the normal process of cell division in rod-shaped bacteria through antibiotics, or mutation or metabolic disorders, it yields daughter cells of unequal size called **anucleated minicells** (AMCs) (Fig. 14.11).

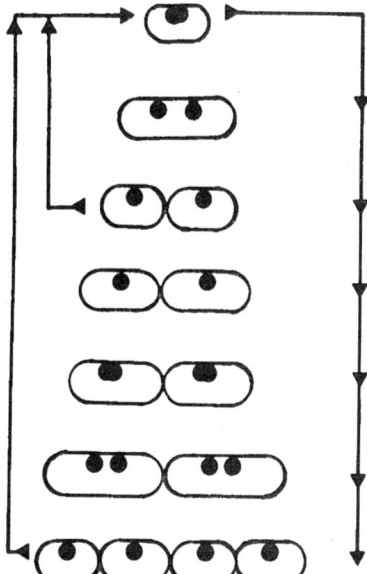

Fig. 14.10 : Schematic presentation of cell growth and division in a typical rod-shaped bacterium. The arrows on the left show re-entry of each daughter cell into the cell cycle

The term minicells implies to small daughter cell of an unequally divided rod-shaped bacterial cell. These minicells can be produced after subjecting the growing cultures to a number of physiological treatments. The principal chromosomal lesion responsible for the production of a minicell in *E. coli* is in the *min* B gene. The other species of minicell producing rod-shaped bacteria includes, *Salmonella, Haemophilus, Bacillus, Shigella, Pseudomonas, Erwinia*. The genetic event takes place due to multiple mutations. The size of minicell obtained from *E. coli* is 1/5 to 1/10 the size of the parent cell. They contain most of the cellular contents which helps them in carrying out the physiological activity. Minicells can be produced using continuous or batch fermentation. The so produced minicells are stored at lower temperature (+4 to -70°C) until used.

Tankersly and Woodward in the 1974 were the first to demonstrate the potential use of minicells as vaccines. They used a strain of *S. typhimurium* obtained from a clinical specimen and treated it with triethylene melamine. They recovered the minicell producing derivative and cultured it. Minicells which were obtained were purified and then injected into adult rabbits. After the completion of the immunization regimen the rabbits were bled and the sera collected which was found to contain antibodies against group B *Salmonella*.

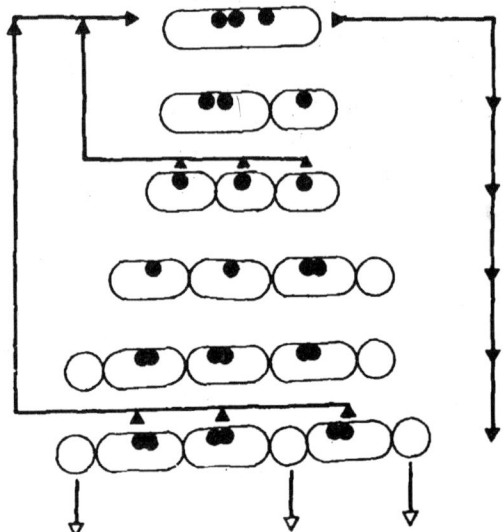

Fig. 14.11 : Schematic presentation of cell growth, division and anucleated mini cell (AMC) production in typical rod shaped bacteria. It can be noted that AMCs do not re-enter cell cycle as shown in figure 14.10

14.9.2.2. Nucleic acid vaccines

Immunization using nucleic acid is becoming a promising new field. Immunization is achieved by directly administering plasmid DNA containing genes encoding antigen. The plasmid DNA enters cells and the antigen is expressed via normal cellular mechanisms. These nucleic acid vaccines act by delivering the antigen for presentation via MHC class I and class II mechanisms. Similar to live-attenuated vaccines, immunization using nucleic acid are capable of inducing both antibody and MHC class I restricted $CD8^+$ cytotoxic T lymphocyte (CTL) responses. Presently, clinical trials of DNA vaccines against HIV-I have been initiated.

14.10. ANTI-IDIOTYPE VACCINES

Anti-idiotype antibody specific for the antigen-binding site (the paratope) on anti-pathogen antibody can potentially serve as a vaccine. This approach holds promise since effective immune response to pathogenic antigen is generated without exposure of the vaccinated individual to any form of pathogen, i.e. attenuated or killed whole-pathogen vaccine. This facilitates in avoiding any undesirable or uncontrollable side effects. When anti-idiotype antibody specific for the paratope is administered, an animal makes antibody to the binding site on the anti-idiotype antibody, and this antibody (called anti-anti-idiotype antibody) will also bind to the original antigen (Fig.14.12). In this manner an animal can become immune to an antigen without having seen the antigen itself, but instead it is exposed to anti-idiotype antibody. For example, if animals are immunized with anti-idiotype antibody specific for the binding site of TEPC-15, they will be immune when they are later challenged with live pneumococci.

Anti-idiotype antibody to HIV antigens have been produced which were then injected into animals to produce anti-anti-idiotype antibody (Fig.14.7e) that binds to HIV antigens as well. Thus immunizing with the virus or viral components can be precisely avoided. Following the same principle, vaccines have been designed to bind to a conserved region on the gp 120 envelope glycoprotein that is required for binding to the CD4 membrane molecule on host cells. Anti-idiotype vaccines have been reported to induce protective immunity in mice against hepatitis B virus, Sendai virus, rabies virus, *Listeria monocytogenes*, *Schistosoma mansoni*, *Streptococcus pneumoniae* and *Trypanosoma rhodesiense*. The development of anti-idiotype vaccine for humans would be a reality in the near future and it holds much promise in avoiding the unacceptable risks involved with a killed or attenuated virus.

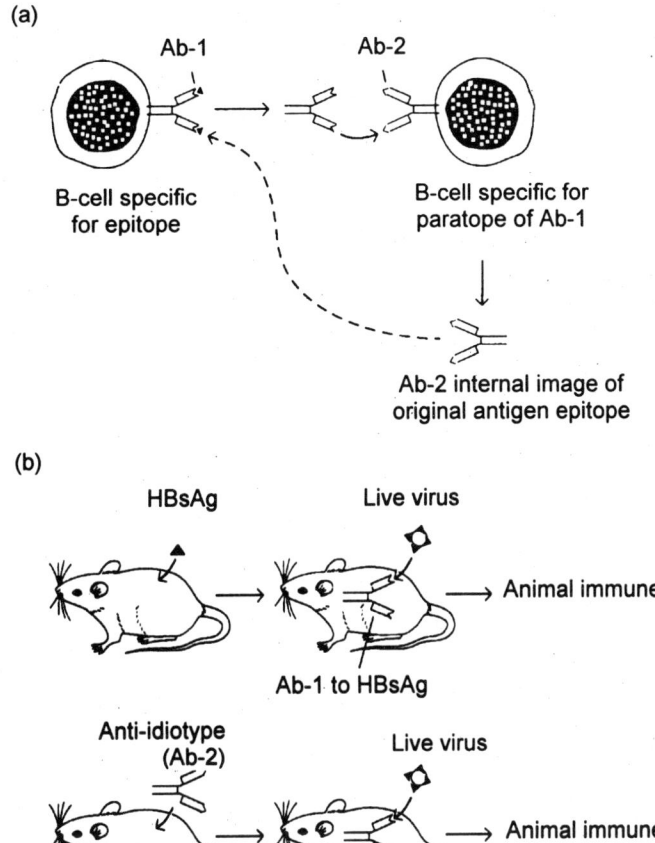

Fig.14.12 : Use of anti-idiotype antibody as a vaccine. (a) The binding site on some anti-idiotype antibodies. (b) Immunization with anti-idiotype antibody

14.11. TARGETED IMMUNE STIMULANTS

Bacillus Calmette Guerin (BCG) has recently been recognized as general immunostimulant and has been introduced into clinical practice as a mode of treatment for superficial blood tumors. The mode of action of BCG particularly against tumors can be broadly be divided into three phases. Beginning with organ targeting to superficial tumor cells. Secondly stimulation of immune response and finally phagocytosis of tumor cells.

Targeting : Fibronectin receptor and fibronectin interaction has been accounted for targeted delivery of BCG cells to the super bladder tumor by Ratllief and co-workers in 1987. It appears that fibronectin is excreted in very close proximity of tumor cell surface. It has been observed when BCG administered to normal intact urothelium virtually no BCG is found to be associated suggestive for a little evidence that there was direct contact between BCG and urothelial cell. However, with strong evidences it was determined that human T24 carcinoma cell line has been capable of capturing, adhering and ingesting BCG. BCG fibronectin receptor i virtually a member of the group of antigens 85 protein complexes which are the major components of protein excreted by BCG in culture and have molecular weights of order 30-32 kDa. However, even larger size range proteins may be responsible for actual attachments to the cell wall. Thus, via receptor ligand mediation tumor site is approached, where necrotin receptor as approached by BCG surface associated antigen protein complexes.

Immunological response : Truly speaking BCG evoked immunoresponse is local in nature and interesting a delayed hypersensitivity, or undoubtedly the phagocytes stimulation involving partially a phagocytic response followed by a granulomatous reaction generated and localized in bladder wall. The immunological studies have demonstrated that T-lymphocytes, monocytes, macro and leukocytes are the prime infiltrating cells responding to intravesicle BCG treatment. The expression of class II MHC has also been observed on urothelial tumor cell wall which may result into the alteration of the phenotype with implications for at least one of the possibilities of BCG being antitumor in activity. Thus, local response is of great importance in overall antitumor activity.

Phagocytosis: It has been reported by Becich et al., that BCG cells are internalized and digested by both human bladder tumor and murine bladder tumor cell lines which could be a possible situation clinically or well of non-phagocytic cell lines are capable of digesting bacteria *in vitro* and *M. leprae* cells by schwan cells both *in vitro* and *in vivo*. It has been observed that after getting internalized BCG cells kill murine sarcoma cells. The possibility persists that BCG may contain a stable cytotoxic component like lipopolysaccharide which has chemical affinity to lipoarabinomannan (LAMP) identified as toxic composed from *M. tuberculosis*. It is inferred that possibly with defined mode and mechanism of new generation of targeted drug delivery in immunization, it could be a vaccination system of choice with promises to treat diseases in total.

14.12. MISCELLANEOUS APPROACHES

14.12.1. Antisense oligonucleotides

Antisense refers for single stranded, synthetic oligonucleotide(s) which could be used to inhibit gene expression. The compounds are judiciously designed to have anticodon or complementary codon sequence to RNA. Therefore, they via complementary pairing hybridize the target sequence, resulting into translation arrest following some suitable putative mode. Ribosomal blockade is one of them where antisense molecule hybridizes to the sense sequence thus interfere the ribosomal reading of mRNA code, resulting into production of non-functional protein. Another mode of action is specific cleavage of RNA strand by activated RNase H following RNH-ON hybridization. The cleavage causes destruction of coding sequence or (sense region) leading to inhibition of protein synthesis (Fig. 14.13).

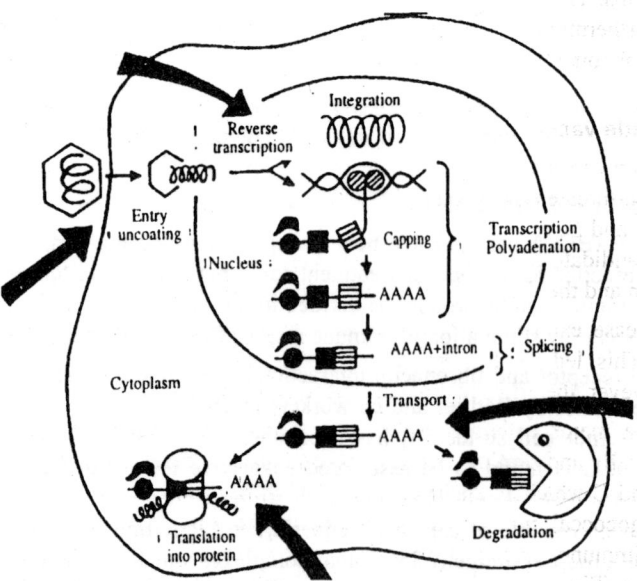

Fig. 14.13 : Antisense oligonucleotide

14.12.2. Competitive inhibition of ribosome binding to 5' unsaturated region (5'-UTR)

Antisense may competitively inhibit the binding of ribosomes to 5' unsaturated region (5'UTR) of RNA. This subsequently lead to activation of RNase H. However, synthesis of mature mRNA in cytosol is prevented at RNA transcription, splicing, processing and trans nuclear membrane diffusion levels. ON can bind complementary sequence of DNA forming triplex DNA, leading to inhibition of DNA transcription.

Oligonucleotides are sensitive to nucleases, therefore may be degraded, beside this they have poor cellular uptake and capacity to hybridize to their DNA or RNA target(s). Nucleases borne degradation to a major extent has been circumvented via chemical modifications of phosphodiester oligonucleotides. Some strategies include modified cations on to methyl phosphorate, phosphorothoacte and C-5 propyne. Lipophilic groups such as cholesterol, vitamin E and tri/tetra/hexaethyleneglycol chains have been incorporated at 5' and 3'-positions either directly or through spacer groups. These modified oligonucleotides containing lipophilic functionalities were reported to show in increased cellular uptake without any alteration in their antisense effect (Fig. 14.14).

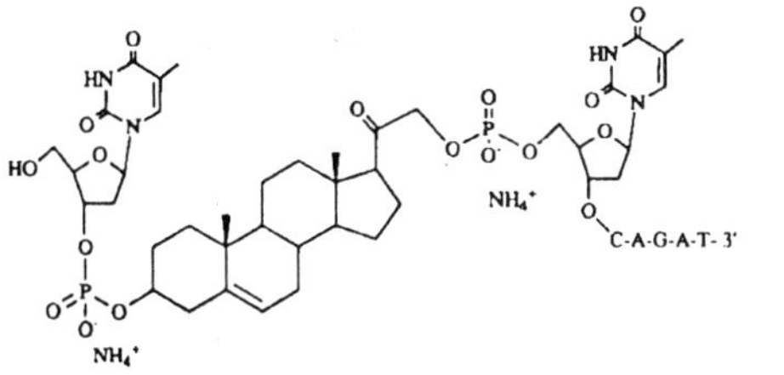

Fig. 14.14 : Structure of an oligonucleotide

Antisense as discussed, act by different mechanisms; hence may exhibit sequence dependent pharmacology (Fig. 14.13). Once hybridized to target RNA or DNA oligonucleotides impose physical blockage of the site as a result access or binding of various factors like ribosomes spliceosomes or other activation factor(s) to the expression gene may be prevented. Additionally, resultant heteroduplex formed by ONs and target is recognized by RNase H which selectively degrades target RNA.

ONs, are relatively large moles (15-28 mers) hydrophilic in nature with MW ranging 5000-10,000 therefore cannot diffuse passively across cell membranes. This, necessitates for strategies to circumvent stability, uptake and accessibility problems. The problems has been resolved to a considerable extent using liposomes (cationic) as carrier for them. Furthermore, the system may be endowed with specific cellular targeting potential using monoclonal antibodies or some surgical ligands.

14.12.3. Polysaccharide vaccines

The focus of attention on capsular polysaccharides as attractive vaccine candidate is from the fact that most of the bacteria causing life-threatening diseases in humans have polysaccharide capsules. *Neisseria meningitidis*, *Haemophilus influenza* and *Streptococcus pneumoniae* are to cite a few. Polysaccharide vaccines turned to be an attractive vaccine candidate for their surface location on the organism, resulting in their direct interaction with the immune system and the discovery of the presence of anti-capsular antibodies.

H. influenzae a disease exclusively confined to children under 5 years, is virtually caused by the type b encapsulated strains. This led to the evaluation of the purified type b polysaccharide polysibosyltribitol-phosphate (PRP). However, the efficacy trials produced controversial results.

N. meningitidis is a major pathogen world wide causing meningitis and septicaemia. The organism is subdivided into structurally and serologically distinct serogroups, defined by the capsular polysaccharide. They are serogroups A, B and C which account for more than 90% of the disease. The first purified polysaccharide vaccine against meningococcal disease was developed in late '60s. However, the immunity produced was not long lasting. The poor immunogenicity of B polysaccharide was found to be that at pH 6, the polymer underwent an internal lactonisation (Fig. 14.15) involving the carboxyl group of one residue and the OH-9 group of an adjacent residue.

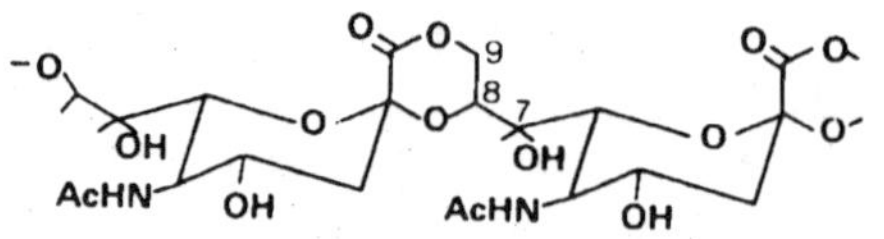

Fig.14.15 : Lactonisation of *N. meningitidis* group polysaccharide at low pH

14.12.4. Glycoconjugates as vaccines

Saccharide-protein conjugates are a class of new generation vaccines. They are of specific use against bacterial diseases caused by *Streptococcus pneumoniae*, *Neisieria meningiditis*, group B *Streptococcus* and others. Saccharides are considered to be T-independent antigens capable of directly stimulating B cells to produce primarily an IgM response to T-independent antigens and are not (usually) capable of boosting or existing at a very low level in infants. To overcome this, saccharides when covalently is conjugated with proteins, converts the saccharides to T-dependent antigens capable of eliciting memory B-cells and achieve a boostable response.

14.13. NEW GENERATION VACCINES

14.13.1. Hepatitis B vaccine (HBV)

Numerous hepatitis B vaccines (HBV) are available today in the market. They can broadly be classified as hepatitis B surface antigen (HBsAg) and recombinant HBV. The drawbacks of HBsAg particles are its low efficacy, in none or low response and low stability during freezing as well as at high temperature. This led investigators to sort out the problem. One such way was by incorporating it into liposomes and there by producing a liposomal vaccine.

14.13.1.1. Liposomal vaccine

HBsAg particle contains three peptides: Small (S), middle (M) and long (L) peptides and lipids. The particle on encapsulation into liposomes serves as an adjuvant-carrier. The three peptides have been coded by ORF Pre-S/S genes. The S-peptide corresponds to the 3' region of the ORF. The M peptide includes the pre-S2 region and the S peptide. The L peptide contains amino acid sequences of Pre-S1, Pre-S2 and S peptides. It has been shown that the Pre-S1 and Pre-S2 amino acid sequences have antigenic determinants independent of the S proteins. The presence of the Pre-S1 region induces specific T cell response which can bypass non-responsiveness to the Pre-S2 and S regions of HBsAg.

Liposomal vaccines were prepared using dimyristoyl phosphatidylcholine (DMPC) and dimyristoyl phosphatidylglycerol (DMPG). The negative charge of DMPG results in the enlargement of the aqueous volume entrapped in the liposomes by electrostatic repulsion between the bilayer leaflets.

HBsAg particles were obtained by isolating HBV DNA and transfecting them into Chinese hamster ovary (CHO) cells. Following selection and cloning, these cells secreted 22-nm HBsAg particles. The efficiency of the vaccine is examined by vaccination of BALB/c mice with different doses of HBsAg entrapped in liposomes.

14.13.1.2. Adenovirus vectored hepatitis B vaccines

Presently, immunization against one of the major infectious liver diseases, hepatitis, caused by hepatitis B virus is done either using an HBsAg or recombinant hepatitis vaccine derived from yeast. The preparation is too expensive that lend it to be difficult to bring it under the World Health Organisation's (WHO) immunization scheme. Thereby, the vaccine is available only to the creamy layer of the society. Live recombinant hepatitis vaccines using adenovirus vectors pose to be an alternative which offers the advantage of cheapness and ease of administration. Considerable progress in the direction of construction of recombinant adenoviruses that express large amounts of HBsAg *in vitro* has been achieved. *In vivo* studies in cotton rat hamster, dog and chimpanzee have been encouraging.

14.13.2. Contraceptive vaccines

Fertility control by immunological approach has become a reality today. Birth control vaccines for human use has reached the stage of clinical trials both in India and abroad. Need for birth control vaccine was identified in 70s. Today, vaccines against three hormones, viz. leuteinizing hormone releasing hormone (LHRH), follicle stimulating hormone (FSH) and human chorionic gonadotropin hormone (HCG) have passed through phase I clinical trials.

14.13.2.1. Human chorionic gonadotropin vaccine (HCG)

Human chorionic gonadotropin is the early signal of pregnancy and is essential for establishment and maintenance of pregnancy during the first seven week period. This hormone is normally responsible for missing of the menstrual period, which by its action on corpus luteum continuous the production of progesterone. This hormone was the target choice for devising a birth control vaccine. HCG neutralizes the hormonal signal by neutralizing the circulating antibodies and thus blocking the HCG support to corpus luteum which leads to continual menstrual cycle (Fig.14.16).

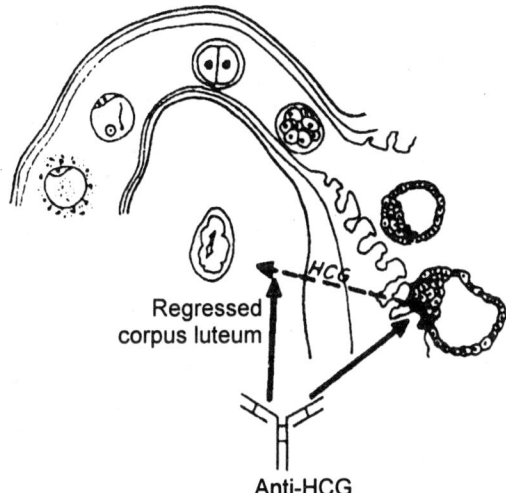

Regressed corpus luteum

Anti-HCG

Fig. 14.16 : Mechanism by which HCG vaccine acts

The strategy behind targeting HCG hormone can well be documented by its need by corpus luteum which brings in continual synthesis of progesterone by ovaries which in turn is responsible for the preparation of endometrium which will receive the embryo. Thus, by blocking the HCG by anti-HCG antibodies, support by corpus luteum is denied and thus intervenes at a point which is post-ovulatory but prior to -the onset of pregnancy. However, the immunological sequence does not interfere with normal physiological functions such as ovulation and secretion of normal steroidal sex hormones. The vaccine approach has an edge over contraceptives which normally acts by blocking ovulating and stops secretion of normal steroidal sex hormones. Above all, the source of HCG is from a natural source and the primary structure of the subunit and its composition is well known.

HCG is composed of two subunits, α and β. The α-subunit is common in three other pituitary hormones. Therefore, the β-subunit or the part their of is chosen. Based on the selection, two types of vaccines were made. first, the 37 amino acids carboxy terminal peptide (CTP) of β-HCG. Second, entire β-HCG was employed. CTP was chosen as it does not exist in β-HLH, thus preventing the antibodies from cross-reacting with HLH. However, it was found that CTP-induced antibodies react with somatostatin-producing cells of the pancreas. Use of entire β-subunit of HCG has the advantage that they are more immunogenic than CTP and the antibodies have better capacity. However, cross reactivity with HLH was observed which did not deplete the monthly LH surge below the amount necessary for ovulation.

β-HCG and CTP are 'self' molecules and thus cannot elicit an antibody response on themselves. Therefore, they are either hapten-modified or linked to a carrier. The first prototype vaccine, linked β-HCG with tetanus toxoid (TT). This vaccine was found to evoke antibodies against both HCG and TT. Linking HCG with TT has the added advantage that immunoprophylaxis against tetanus infection is achieved. It was also observed that HCG did not act as a booster on itself. In order to improve the immunogenicity of β-HCG-TT vaccine, steps have been taken. They are as given below.

1. Sodium phthalyl derivative of lipopolysaccharide (SPLPS) from *Salmonella enteritidis* was included as an adjuvant in the first injection.
2. Diphtherial toxoid (DT) was selected as a carrier in addition to TT.
3. The intrinsic immunogenicity of β-HCG was augmented by associating it with a heterospecies α-subunit of bovine origin.

14.13.2.2. Recombinant products

The genes for β-HCG and α-oLH have been cloned and expressed in vaccinia virus and baculovirus. It was observed that the vaccinia-expressed products are fully glycosylated and identical to the native hormonal subunits. However, baculovirus expression system showed better yield but the products were partially glycosylated. It was observed that in both the cases, the β-HCG is immunoreactive. It was also found that the β-subunit could bind with the α-subunit to generate bioactive hormone. Recently, β-HCG have been expressed in *E. coli* which produced higher yield and the amino acid composition was the same as that of the human β-HCG and the product was not glycosylated.

A live recombinant vaccine has been developed by inserting β-HCG in vaccinia virus along with a transmembrane 48 amino acid fragment. This vaccine when tested in rodents, was found to be highly immunogenic.

14.13.2.3. LHRH vaccine

Luteinizing hormone releasing hormone (LHRH) or gonadotropin releasing hormone (GRH) a decapeptide, controls the secretion of luteinizing hormone (LH) and follicle stimulating hormone (FSH) from the pituitary. These in turn act on the gonads, male or female to generate sperms or egg and also steroidal sex hormones. Activation of LHRH leads to impairment of fertility and fails to produce steroidal sex hormones. In addition to fertility control in human, they are also useful in animal fertility control. This is possible because of the conserved sequence of the hormone in mammals. Immunization against LHRH is also useful in animals which are grown for the purpose of meat. Here, the suppression of the hormone, androgen will have an impact on the quality of the meat. Immunization can be brought about both by active and passive immunization. Passive immunization is brought about by parenteral administration of monoclonal antibodies.

LHRH of natural origin has neither an amino terminal nor carboxy terminal for carrier-linkage. Hence forth, chemically, molecules can be synthesized to have one or the other group. It has been reported that TT linked at the N-terminal amino position produces higher immunogenicity than the one produced with an carboxyl end linked. The vaccine was designed by substituting a D-lysine at position 6 for glycine, thereby producing an analogue, resistant to metabolic degradation with an additional spacer group for linkage. The so obtained vaccine was found to be with higher immunogenicity.

14.13.2.4. Paraneem vaccine

Research, in the field of fertility control has led to a natural source for vaccination. It was observed that a single instillation of purified neem seed extract (Paraneem) into the uterus, prevents pregnancy without impairing ovulation. Paraneem vaccine induces a local cell-mediated immunity. This leads to immunosuppression at the genital tract which reacts against the sperm, which is foreign to the women's immune system. Following the immunological response, activated by the sperm, it turns into local production of cytokines, such as γ-interferon, IL_2 and TNF, that reject implantation.

14.13.2.5. *Male fertility control*

Male fertility control is brought about by using FSH vaccine. An alternate approach is to exploit the in-build developmental potential of selective immunosuppression of spermatogenesis by cell-mediated immune response. At the age of puberty, many proteins, whose ontogenesis takes place, are 'foreign' to the body's immune system. Whereas Leydig cells producing testosterone is recognized as 'self ', as they are present and functioning from the fetal stage. When a suspension of BCG vaccine was injected, it was observed that aspermatogenesis without decline of testosterone was induced. The effect was observed in every mammal that was subjected for investigation. However, the effect was reversible and spermatogenesis was regained with time. Recent studies reveal that by injecting purified neem seed extract into the vas deferens, aspermatogenesis can be brought about without any significant reduction in testosterone.

14.13.3. Anti-sepsis vaccine

Septic shock is the result of consequences which take place after the introduction of a pathogen into a sterile tissue which leads to a battle between the pathogen and the host. In order to design a vaccine against septic shock, one should be well versed with the strategy of the disease at each stage. This in brief is discussed here. The entire act begins with the replication of a pathogenic bacteria or fungi in the tissue. This septic shock is usually caused by gram negative bacteria. Research has led to the development of a vaccine against sepsis resulting from gram negative bacteria. Lipopolysaccharide (LPS), a complex molecule is shed by gram negative bacteria when they replicate. The vaccine targets the important component of this LPS, namely the lipid A portion. LPS is a potent stimulant of immune reaction and is the major contributor in the lethal consequences of septic shock. The anti-sepsis vaccine comprises of lipid A in lipid vesicle (liposomes), where by the inherent toxicity of lipid A is masked, while the adjuvanticity property through which an immunologic reaction is stimulated is retained. This liposome bearing lipid A acts as the antigen stimulating an immune response.

14.13.4. Live recombinant vaccinia-rabies vaccine

Rabies is a viral disease which affects all-warm-blooded animals and is widespread throughout the world. Dogs represent the major vector in our country. The disease is transmitted through the bite of an infected animal whose saliva contains large amount of virus. As rabies is nearly always fatal, immune populations do not exist. Rabies virus (RV), a rhabdovirus, is an enveloped negative single-stranded RNA virus related to vesicular stomatitis virus. The glycoprotein (G), present on the exterior surface of the virion is the only protein capable of inducing or reacting with virus-neutralizing antibody (VNA) and appears to be the main viral protein capable of eliciting protection.

Oral administration is the only appropriate route for vaccination of a large number of animals. Live attenuated rabies virus have been used for vaccination. However, attenuated viruses remain pathogenic and may revert to virulence. It can be noted that inactivated rabies virus is ineffective when administered orally.

Vaccinia virus (VV), a large (180 kb) double-stranded DNA orthopox virus, has been used extensively to control and eradicate smallpox in man. Off-late, they are being studied as live vector for viral antigens and derivatives their of.

A recombinant vaccinia virus (VVTGgRAB) bearing the rabies G coding sequence and expressing the rabies surface antigen was developed by Kieny and co-workers. This was carried out by inserting the rabies G cDNA in to a plasmid vector downstream of the vaccinia virus p7.5K promoter into the non-essential vaccinia TK gene. Double reciprocal recombination *in vivo* between this plasmid the vaccinia virus genome allows integration of the DNA inset into the viral genome. Infection of cell cultures with VVTGgRAB elicited the production of a correctly processed rabies G which was found to react strongly with rabies neutralizing antibodies.

14.13.5. Acquired immunodeficiency syndrome (AIDS)

AIDS was first reported in the year 1981 in the *New England Journal of Medicine*. The report indicated that the victims had decreased counts of $CD4^+$ T cells, confirming the suspected linkage to a compromised immune system. It was in 1982, the Centers for Disease Control (CDC), the agency of the U.S. Public Health Services suggested that this distinct new disorder be called **acquired immunodeficiency syndrome**, now commonly known **AIDS**. Although the disease was first reported and identified in homosexual man in the United States, it was soon observed in other groups including hemophiliacs, blood-transfusion recipients, intravenous drug users, sexual partners of AIDS patients, and eventually in infants of mothers with the disease.

Luc Montaginer's group at the Pasteur Institute in the year 1983 isolated a retrovirus from a lymph node biopsy of an AIDS patient. It was in 1986, the retrovirus was named **human immunodeficiency virus or HIV**. It was also observed that there existed an antigenic variation in the virus. Thus, the original virus was designated HIV-1 and the variant HIV-2. Both were found to be genetically related to the simian immunodeficiency virus (SIVs), found in African primates. Recently, a new variant, designated HIV-O was identified in Cameroon.

Development of a vaccine, for disease of this nature, requires a thorough knowledge about the infectious agent, characterization of the immune response to the agent, and determination of what type of immune response is protective. Going into all these details is beyond the scope of this book. However, the structure of the HIV will be discussed in brief so as to understand the concept leading to the design of an AIDS vaccine.

14.13.5.1. Structure of HIV

All members of the lentivirus family of retroviruses, including the three types of HIV and various SIVs share numerous structural and molecular similarity. The viruses have a RNA genome and two associated molecules of **reverse transcriptase**, which catalyzes the "reverse transcription" of viral RNA into DNA. Other nucleoid proteins include the p10 protease and p32 integrase. Surrounding the viral genome and nucleoid proteins are two layers of core proteins; in HIV these core proteins are designated by p17 and p24 (Fig. 14.17). The viral core, or nucleocapsid, is surrounded by an envelope derived from the host-cell membrane, which is modified by the insertion of two HIV glycoproteins, **gp120** and **gp41**. The gp41 glycoprotein spans the membrane; gp120 is noncovalently associated with gp41 but extends beyond the membrane. Both gp120 and gp41 have important roles in the binding of HIV to cells in the process of infection. Studies have revealed that the HIV envelope is studded with human proteins (including class I and class II MHC molecules) acquired by the virus as it buds from the human cell membrane.

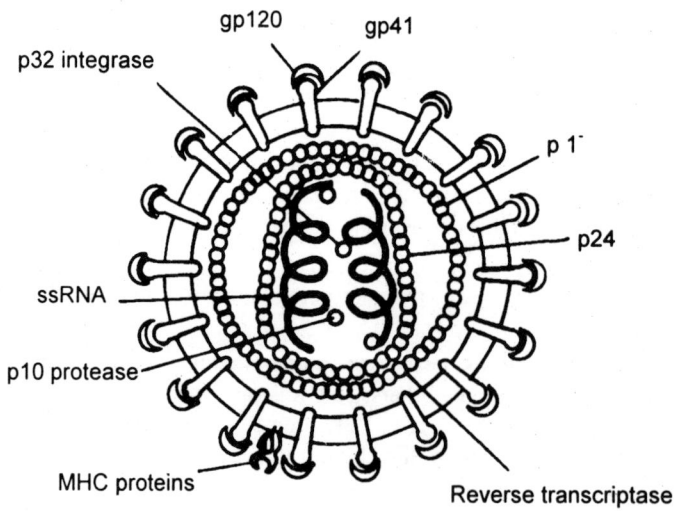

Fig.14.17 : Structure of HIV virus

Entry of the HIV into the target cells involves two steps: **binding** of virions to receptors on target cell is followed by **fusion** of the viral envelope with the plasma membrane of the target cells. The two glycoproteins gp120 and gp41 play vital roles in these steps: gp120 in binding and gp41 in fusion. Once entering into the target cell, the viral RNA is copied into DNA. The viral DNA then integrates into the host-cell DNA, forming a **provirus**, which may remain in a latent state or may be activated and transcribed into viral proteins.

14.13.6. Development of an AIDS vaccine

The time from when HIV was identified as the causative agent of AIDS, enormous efforts have been made to develop a safe and effective vaccine. Among the several types of vaccines designed, includes inactivated whole virus, live recombinant viruses, attenuated virus, synthetic peptides, anti-idiotype antibodies, recombinant DNA products.

14.13.6.1. Inactivated whole viruses

The procedure involved is similar to the one used in developing the Salk polio vaccine. Here, preparations of HIV-1 and SIV have been produced by irradiating the virus followed by formaldehyde treatment. This leads to the inactivation of the retroviral genome and releases much of the gp120 from the envelope. The resultant, noninfectious SIV or HIV preparations then used as a vaccine. Initial trials in animals looked promising. However, the results were challenged as the SIV vaccine was prepared by growing SIV in human T-cell cultures

14.13.6.2. Attenuated viruses

This method of vaccine development also involves the use of the method similar to Sabin polio vaccine, where in, live polio virus is grown in monkey kidney. When a live virus is grown under unusual culture conditions, the viruses are forced to mutate to survive in the new growing conditions.

The majority of viral vaccines used today are attenuated vaccines. As the vaccine is live, it is able to infect cells and grow for a limited amount of time before the immune response eliminates the virus. However, during this time period, the attenuated virus is able to induce a potent immune response, often including generation of cell-mediated cytotoxic T-lymphocytes (CTLs) specific for the endogenously produced viral antigens. In addition, they have an added advantage that these attenuated viral vaccines tend to induce a good memory cell response, which accounts for the life-long immunity developed by these vaccines.

HIV being a highly mutant virus, using attenuated strains were considered to be too dangerous. Desrosiers and his co-workers, in the year 1992 developed an attenuated strain of SIV by eliminating the regulatory gene *nef* from a highly virulent strain of SIV. When this *nef* deleted strain of SIV was injected into six macaques, the animal did not develop symptoms to SAIDS. When the animal was challenged with huge doses of infectious SIV, they remained to be healthy. However, the blow came when it was found that the attenuated strain caused SAIDS in the newborn macques.

14.13.6.3. Cloned envelope glycoproteins

The first cloned gp160 vaccine was produced by MicroGeneSys, Inc. in the year 1987. So far, several groups have applied gene-engineering techniques to clone the gp120 gene or the entire gp160 gene in order to produce large quantities of gp120 or gp160 for immunization. The cloned gp160 vaccine when administered by large induced humoral immunity. The antibodies elicited in the volunteers were shown to inhibit viral replication *in vitro*, but the inhibition being always strain specific.

14.13.6.4. Recombinant viruses carrying HIV genes

An another effective AIDS vaccine development depends on the use of recombinant vectors. Vaccinia virus and the Sabin polio virus are both live attenuated vaccines used effectively as vaccines. These viruses can be engineered to carry genes from HIV-1, and the recombinant virus can then be used as an vaccine. As the recombinant virus is attenuated and not inactivated, it is capable of infecting host cells and is therefore expected to induce CTL activity. Vaccinia virus, a large virus, can be engineered to carry several dozen foreign genes without impairing its capacity to infect host cells and to replicate in them. The administration of the engineered vaccinia virus is also easy, i.e. simply by dermal scratching. The virus causes a limited localized infection in the host cells. The foreign, genes are expressed by the vaccinia, and if the foreign gene product is a viral envelope protein, it is inserted in to the membrane of the infected host cell and there stimulates the development of T-cell mediated immunity. Vaccinia virus carrying gp160 has been shown to infect host cells at the site of scarification; the gp160 is glycosylated, cleaved into gp120 and gp41, and inserted into the plasma membrane of the infected host cells. A number of HIV genes have been engineered into vaccinia virus, including *enve, tat, pol* and *gag*.

14.13.6.5. Synthetic crown-sequence peptides

Synthetic peptides of different HIV crown sequences, including the MN sequence, have been prepared and tested for their ability to activate T-cell proliferation and cytotoxicity *in vitro*. The principal neutralizing epitope of HIV overlaps with V3loop of gp120, and antibodies to the V3 loop have been shown to protect chimpanzees from HIV infection. Because of the high level of variation in the V3 loop, antibody neutralization is always strain specific. However, the so-called crown sequence in the V3 loop is conserved to a considerable degree. These synthetic peptides appear to activate a population of T_H cells and to induce some cytotoxic activity, however, because these peptides are processed as exogenous antigens, the cytotoxic cells induced were all $CD4^+$, class II restricted. These studies suggest that cocktails of synthetic peptides, representing the crown sequences of the predominant HIV isolates, might induce protective antibody or $CD4^+$ T cytotoxic cells.

14.13.7. Malaria vaccine

Malaria, a protozoan disease is a serious disease responsible for 1-2 million deaths every year and infecting about 600 million people around the world. Malaria is caused by various species of the genus *Plasmodium* of which *P. falciparum* is the most virulent and prevalent. The alarming rise in resistance developed by *Plasmodium* to multiple drug therapy has led to the development of new strategies to control the spread of malaria. One such development is the designing of a vaccine.

Keeping in view the present situation in developing countries, an effective malaria vaccine is of utmost importance. The vaccine should be designed to maximize the most effective immune defense mechanisms. Unfortunately, little is known of the roles that humoral and cell-mediated responses play in the development of protective immunity to this disease.

Current vaccine strategies are aimed at producing synthetic subunit vaccines consisting of epitopes that can be recognized by T cells and B cells. One such vaccine, designated SPf66, consists of three epitopes from merozoite proteins together with a conserved domain from the circumsporozoite protein. Present approaches to design a malaria vaccine largely focus on the sporozoite stage. However, the results are not encouraging as the life span of this stage in blood is only 30 minutes which is a short period for a vaccine to be effective.

14.14. NOVEL VACCINE DELIVERY SYSTEMS

Vaccination has proven to be the most efficient, cost-effective means for the prevention of a wide variety of infectious diseases. Concerted immunization programs have resulted in the eradication of smallpox. With few exceptions, most vaccines are administered as part of routine childhood immunization programs. Perhaps the greatest problem faced in effect deliver of such vaccines is that multiple dose primary immunization regimens are essential. In addition, periodic boosters are required throughout life to maintain immunity. In both developed and developing countries, the number of recommended doses of vaccine leading to incomplete immunity. Ease of administration greatly facilitates vaccine uptake.

New vaccine delivery technologies are clearly needed both to remedy the limitations of existing immunization regimens and to allow for the development of new or improved vaccines. Novel vaccine delivery systems, distinct from classical adjuvants, are now being investigated as means to modulate the immune response following vaccination. Several such systems have undergone clinical evaluation with promising results. These systems are discussed here in brief. These systems have gained wide acclaim due to their ability to present antigens in a better way.

Processing and presentation of antigens by antigen presenting cells (APCs) is critical to the recruitment and activation of T cells. Uptake of exogenous antigens generally leads to presentation in association with class II MHC molecules. Cytolytic T lymphocytes (CTLs) are normally CD8+ , and recognize peptides in association with class I MHC molecules. Presentation of antigen by class I or class II MHC proteins is thus dependent upon its route of introduction into the cell and its susceptibility to degradation. These factors can be influenced by the use of specific delivery systems, which are therefore important determinants of the immune response arising for vaccination, which should endeavor to direct the immune response into activation of cells and processes appropriate for each pathogen.

14.14.1. Particulate delivery systems

It is now well appreciated that non-living vaccine delivery systems can play an important role in the development of new strategies for improved vaccine delivery and that such systems could have the major benefit of ease of preparation. The particulate systems presently studied include liposomes, emulsions, ISCOMS, and microspheres.

14.14.1.1. Liposomes

The ability of liposomes to act as a potent and non-toxic immunological adjuvant was first observed in 1974 by Allison and Gregoriadis using diphtheria toxoid as a model antigen. Both humoral and cell-mediated immunity was observed to be induced. This was attributed to the ability of liposomes to slowly release antigens at the site of injection, to migrate to the lymphatics as well as to their avid uptake by antigen presenting cells, usually macrophages. Liposomes have the versatility in terms of structural characteristics, mode of antigen localization within the vesicles, and options in the route of administration. Recently, the first liposome-based vaccine **Epaxal Berna®** against hepatitis A has been licensed for use in Switzerland.

Recent studies have shown that liposomes containing antigens are capable of inducing systemic and mucosal immune responses following intranasal administration. The effectiveness of rectal administration of liposomes has been recently reported.

14.14.1.2. Emulsions

Emulsion as carrier systems was popular in the past. Recently they have gained attention not only in delivery of vaccines but also in other formulations especially in controlled and novel drug delivery. Various systems, including water in oil emulsions and multiple emulsion have been described for delivery of vaccines. However, these systems could not induce sufficient antibody titers or a required CMI effect.

14.14.1.3. Microspheres

Microparticles based on polylactide, co-glycolide have gained much attention as carriers for antigens. Impressive results have been attained for both humoral and cell mediated effects. PLGA has the advantage that the polymer has already been approved for human use and is biodegradable and biocompatible. They have the advantage that they can be freeze dried and therefore avoid the need for cold storage. The incorporation of antigens into biodegradable microspheres has several advantages including the protection of antigen from proteolysis and possible co-incorporation of immunological adjuvants that may further enhance the immune response.

Most of the microspheres evaluation for vaccination has been focused on oral route. Induction of mucosal and systemic responses by the oral route where shown to be influenced by the size of the microsphere; microspheres < 5µm in diameter are not retained in the Peyer's patches but fond int he spleen and in lymph nodes where they induce systemic immunity while those with the size range 5-10 µm remain in the Peyer's patches and induce mucosal immunity. Microspheres other than PLGA have also been studied for immunization. These include alginate, albumin and gelatin microspheres.

14.14.2. Cochleates

Fusogenic proteoliposomes, prepared by the protein cochleate method have been recently developed and tested for their immunogenicity after oral or parenteral administration. Cochleates consists of stable protein-phospholipid-calcium precipitates. Antigens like glycoproteins from influenza or parainfluenza virus or a 12 amino acid peptide from SIV *gag* protein that contains an epitope for cytotoxic T lymphocytes have been incorporated in such structures. A strong and prolonged immune response was observed after oral administration drinking water or as parenteral injection. This can be manifested to the presence of mucosal and systemic antibodies and cytotoxic T cells.

14.14.3. Mucoadhesive polymers

Mucoadhesive and other bioadhesive polymers have been used for drug delivery, particularly in transdermal and buccal devices. Other than this mucoadhesive polymers have many pharmaceutical applications. Some muco-adhesives have adjuvant properties when injected, notably sodium alginate, and others such as carboxymethyl cellulose have been selected for their viscosity to be used a depot agents. Mucoadhesives have been tested for nasal immunization and are being studied for oral drug delivery. Recent experiments have demonstrated oral administration of influenza vaccine in mucoadhesive polymers. They observed a high antibody titer value and was found to be promising.

14.14.4. DNA vaccination

DNA vaccination can serve as an alternative to immunization with purified protein and is effective in generating antibody, helper and cytotoxic responses, and protective immunity. In the case of viral antigens, the immunity generated by DNA vaccination may be at least as protective as that induced by live attenuated viruses. Vaccination with DNA encoding circumsporozoite antigen of the rodent malaria parasite *Plasmodium yoelii* was found to protect mice against subsequent challenge with the parasite.

Vaccine DNAs are constructed using regulatory sequences which function in mammalian cells. Immune response can be generated when the DNA is given in saline intramuscularly, intravenously, intranasally, intradermally and subcutaneously. However, the most widely used method involves intramuscular injection. Using reported genes it has been shown that gene expression following intramuscular injection after 60 days produced significant proteins 18 months after immunization. It was observed that vaccination of mice with DNA coding for the secreted 85A and 85B antigens of *M. tuberculosis* has provided protection equal to live BCG. DNA vaccination may be particularly a valuable approach to screen a large number of genes encoding proteins for their protective efficacy.

Introduction of DNA vaccines into animals has been primarily achieved by intramuscular injection or gene gun delivery. Although protective immune responses have been demonstrated in animals, only a low antibody level was observed. The effect of mucosal administration of DNA has not been extensively investigated, and uptake of DNA from epithelial surface may not be as effective as direct injection of DNA into muscle cells. However, it should be possible to enhance the uptake of DNA by using specific delivery systems.

14.14.5.Transgenic plants an edible immunogen concept

Introduction of genes encoding microbial antigens in plants, represents a novel and potentially important approach in vaccine administration. Manson and co-workers developed a recombinant bacterial vector *Agrobacterium tumefaciens* with a gene for the surface antigen of hepatitis B virus and infected tobacco plants which subsequently expressed this antigen. An alternative approach to deliver the gene is by infecting the plant with *Clavibacter*, tobacco mosaic virus, or by using gene gun. Antigens of hepatitis B virus, rotavirus, Norwalk virus and B subunit of *E. coli* heat-labile enterotoxin (LT-B) have been expressed in such plants. Haq and co-workers have immunized mice with partially purified LT-B produced in tobacco and potato plants, or with raw transgenic potatoes and observed that both systemic and mucosal anti-LT-B neutralizing antibodies were secreted. Using this technique inexpensive edible immunogens suitable for immunization of large populations particularly in developing countries can be produced.

SUGGESTED READINGS

Allison, A.C. and Gregoriadis, G., (1974) **Nature**, 252, 252.

Gregoriadis, G, Allison, A.C. and Poste, G. (Eds.), (1991) **Vaccines: Recent Trends and Progress**, Plenum Publishing Corp., NY.

Gregoriadis, G., (1990) **Immunology Today**, 11, 89.

Gregoriadis, G., Allison, A.C. and Poste, G. (Eds.), (1989) **Immunological Adjuvants and Vaccines**, Plenum Publishing Corp., NY.

Gregoriadis, G., McCormack, B., Allison, A.C. and Poste, G. (Eds.)(1987). **New generation vaccines: The Role of Basic Immunology**, Plenum Publishing Corp., NY.

Hoglund, S., Dalsgaard, K., Lovgren, K., Sundquist, B., Osterhaus, A. and Morein, B., (1989) *ISCOMS and immunostimulation with viral antigens* In: **Subcellular biochemistry**, J.R. Harris (Ed.), Plenum Publishing Co. ,15, 39-68.

Lerner, R., Cnanock, R. and Brown, F. (Eds.), (1985) **Vaccine**, Cold-Spring Harbor Laboratory , NY.

Zanetti, M., Sercarz, E. and Salk, J., (1987) **Immunology Today**, 8, 18.

Zuckerman, A.J. (Ed.), (1989) *Recent Developments in prophylactic immunization* In: **Immunology and Medicine Series,** Vol.12, Kluwer Academic Publishers.

BIOTECH IN NEWS . . . .

There is optimism that gene transfer could help neurosurgeons treat neuromuscular diseases such as Duchenne dystrophy. It could however take place only in the distant future. It has been found that over 90% patients with hereditary neuromuscular disease and over 50% of those with other inherited neurological disorders suffer from the same genetic defect. Nuclear defects were discovered by the process known as reverse genetics in the illness known as Duchenne dystrophy, a progressive disease affecting boys between 2 and 3 years, resulting in death between the ages of 15 to 20 years.

This was the first human illness discovered by the process, which presumed that the defective gene lay in the X-chromosome, since the disease affect boys.

. . . . from *Express Pharma Pulse*, Mar 6,1997.

DELIVERY CONSIDERATIONS OF BIOTECHNOLOGICAL PRODUCTS

15.1. INTRODUCTION

In the recent years therapeutic peptides and proteins have risen to prominence as potential drugs of the future. Management of illness through this class of pharmaceuticals has entered an era of rapid growth. Biotechnology has played a key role in the development of peptide and protein drugs. A new series of peptide based and protein based pharmaceuticals have made their presence felt with the advent of recombinant DNA and hybridoma techniques and with the recent advances in large-scale fermentation and purification processes. These entities are now available in a much purer form in significant quantities, at a reasonable cost. The problem of immunogenicity and antigenicity has also been considerably reduced. Simultaneously, great advances have been made in the understanding of the physiologic and pharmacologic behavior of these biologic response modifiers and regulatory agents. Ailments that might be treated more effectively with this class of therapeutics include autoimmune diseases, cancer, mental disorders, hypertension and certain cardiovascular and metabolic diseases (Table 15.1).

The peptide and protein drugs produced by recombinant DNA technology are the exact replicas of that obtained from natural sources. In spite of their potency and specificity in physiologic functions, a majority of these therapeutics are difficult to administer clinically. The chemical and structural complexities involved demand an effective delivery system so that the physicochemical and biological properties, including molecular size, conformational stability, biological half-life, immunogenicity, dose requirements, complex feedback control mechanisms, susceptibility to break down in both physical and biological environments, requirement for specialized mechanisms for transport across biological membranes are duly considered.

Table 15.1 : Some representative peptidal and proteinaceous drugs with their potential functions and /or biomedical applications

Peptidal/Proteinaceous Drug(s)	Function(s) and/or biomedical application(s)
Cardiovascular-active	
Angiotensin II antagonist	Lowering blood pressure
Bradykinin	Improving peripheral circulation
Captopril	Heart failure management
Tissue plasminogen activator	Dissolution of blood clots
CNS-active	
Cholecystokinin	Suppressing appetite
β-Endorphin	Relieving pain
Neuropeptide γ	Controlling feeding and drinking behaviour
Nerve growth factor	Stimulating nerve growth and repair
GI-active	
Gastrin antagonist	Reducing secretion of gastric acid
Pancreatic enzymes	Digestive supplement
Somatostatin	Reducing bleeding of gastric ulcers
Immunomodulating	
Bursin	Selective B-cell differentiating hormone
Cyclosporin	Inhibiting functions of T-lymphocyte
Enkephalins	Stimulating lymphocyte blastogenesis
Interferon	Enhancing activity of killer cells
Tumor necrosis factor	Controlling polymorphonuclear functions
Metabolism-modulating	
Human growth hormone	Treating hypopituitary dwarfism
Insulin	Treating diabetes mellitus
Luteinizing hormone	Inducing ovulation in women with hypothalamic amenorrhea
Vasopressin	Treating diabetes insipidus

In majority of the cases chronic therapy of these peptides and proteins is warranted. Generally, they have an extremely short biological half-life. This trait precludes the parenteral delivery, as daily multiple injections would be required to maintain the therapeutic levels of drug which has its inherent drawbacks. Oral administration is limited due to enzymatic degradation. Only after the development of viable novel delivery systems to improve their systemic bioavailability, these peptide and protein drugs can be of therapeutic importance. There is an urgent need to develop alternative non-parenteral routes of administration like buccal, nasal, pulmonary, ophthalmic, rectal, vaginal and transdermal routes. Alternatively other approaches such as implants, self-regulatory delivery systems can be exploited. However, the transmucosal route mentioned in the preceding lines may impose additional biological barriers to this class of 'difficult' drugs in terms of tissue permeability, protease activity, etc.

15.2. PEPTIDE AND PROTEIN STRUCTURE

The peptide chains in peptides and proteins are seldom linear and adapt a variety of specific folded three-dimensional patterns or conformations. Conformation of the peptide chain is determined by the covalently bonded amino acid sequence, by disulfide bridges between cysteine residues, and by total conformational energy (the sum of electrostatic energy, hydrogen-bonded energy, non-bonded energy and torsional energy). The properties that are affected by conformation include:

1. Physical properties such as solubility, and spectral properties, such as circular dichroism.
2. Chemical properties, since folding may stabilize reactive groups by hydrogen bonding or sterically shield them from reagents.
3. Biological properties, as the three-dimensional structure places catalytic groups into proper orientation for enzymatic activity or places backbone and side-chain groups into proper orientation for hormone-receptor interaction.
4. Stability to enzymatic cleavage since some of the amide groups susceptible to proteolysis may be sterically shielded in a folded peptide chain orientation.

15.2.1. Levels of protein structure

All peptides and proteins are polymers of amino acids connected via amide linkages referred to as peptide bonds. The **primary structure** of a peptide or protein is the sequence of amino acids in the same. This structure is determined genetically by the sequence of nucleotides in DNA. The other form or conformation is the **secondary structure**. This is the respective arrangement of individual amino acids along the polypeptide backbone. At times, this results in a very specific and well-ordered structures as helices, loops, β-strands and β-turns. **Tertiary structure** is the three-dimensional arrangement of a single protein molecule. It refers to the way that specific secondary structural elements interact with each other as well as with random portions of the molecule to form stable domains. And finally, **quaternary structure** is the form of protein as it exists in the solid state or in solution. It refers to the noncovalent interaction or spatial arrangement of individual protein monomers with each other to form oligomers and also the interaction of monomers and oligomers with the solvent and other solute components that affect the molecular weight distribution of protein.

Proteins can be divided into two major classes depending on the conformation: **fibrous** and **globular**. Fibrous proteins are composed of polypeptide chains that are arranged in parallel position along a single axis and thereby yielding long fibres or sheets. These are insoluble in aqueous systems. Keratin, collagen and elastin are representative examples of this class. On the other hand in globular proteins, the polypeptide chains are tightly folded into compact globular or spherical shapes. A majority of these proteins are soluble in water. Most of the peptide/protein therapeutic agents are examples of this class.

15.3. STABILITY PROFILE

One of the primary differences between the conventional drug entities and peptide/protein drugs is their stability profile. The high chemical and physical instability presents peculiar difficulties in the purification, separation, formulation, storage and delivery of these compounds. Physical instability involves alterations in the secondary, tertiary, or quaternary structure of the molecule. These changes are manifested as denaturation, adsorption, aggregation, and precipitation. Chemical instability results in the generation of a new chemical entity, by bond formation or cleavage. Changes brought about by physical and chemical changes almost always lead to a loss of biological activity.

15.3.1. Physical stability

15.3.1.1. Denaturation

Peptides and proteins comprise of both polar amino acid residues and nonpolar amino acid residues. The hydrophobic, nonpolar amino acid residues fold upon themselves in an aqueous environment to form globular molecules. The hydrophilic, polar amino acid residues of these molecules are exposed to the aqueous environment. On changing the aqueous environment to nonaqueous, they start unfolding and thereby exposing their hydrophobic residues to the hydrophobic environment. This leads to rearrangement and loss of quaternary and tertiary structure (Fig.15.1). On unfolding, hydrophobic and hydrogen bonds are broken. The term denaturation is used to describe any nonproteolytic modification of the unique structure of a native protein that gives rise to definite changes in physical, chemical and biological properties. Conditions that denature proteins include:

1. Solvent change from an aqueous to a mixed solvent as alcohol and water.
2. pH change alters the ionization of the carboxylic acid and amino groups and thereby the charges carried by the molecules. With an increase in the number of like charges on an individual molecule, there is a charge repulsion within the molecule and as a consequence it unfolds.
3. Alteration in ionic strength affects the charge carried by molecules as well. The molecule would be surrounded by ions of the opposite charge to that of the molecule itself, thereby leading to a net reduction in its effective charge.
4. Temperature increase leads to an increment in the thermal energy of the molecules, which may suffice to break the hydrogen bonds that stabilise the secondary, tertiary and quaternary structure of these entities. Even chemical bonds may break at very high temperature.
5. With a rearrangement in structure the inherent biological activity may be lost with an emergence of totally new range of activity. This is usually accounted for the concealing of particular residues and exposure of newer ones respectively.

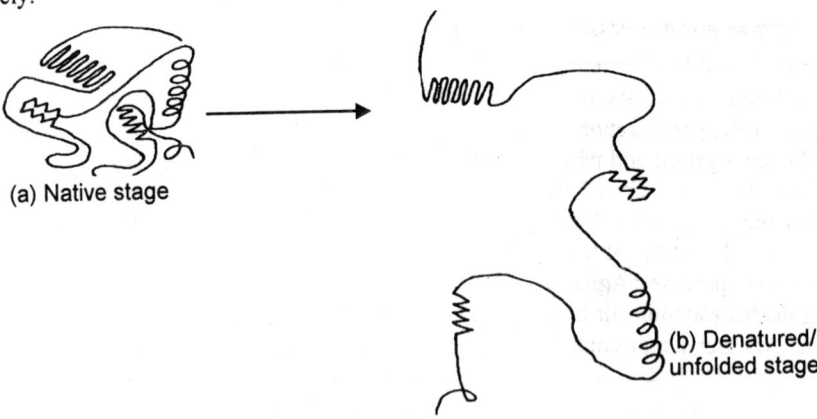

(a) Native stage

(b) Denatured/ unfolded stage

Fig. 15.1 : Schematic representation of polypeptide or protein unfolding

Denaturation can either be reversible or irreversible. In reversible denaturation the conformational changes in the molecules are reversed by coming back to their original state. For example, a protein that has been denatured by temperature increment may revert to its native structure when the temperature is restored. However, in the case of irreversible denaturation, the proteins are unable to restore to their original structure. This may be due to the fact that the protein has undergone some physical or chemical process that inhibits the original pattern of folding, or even the proteins may be misfolded that disallow their proper renaturation.

15.3.1.2. Adsorption

Peptides and proteins possess both polar and nonpolar residues and are thereby amphiphilic in their disposition. This property imparts them the tendency to be adsorbed at interfaces such as air-water and air-solid. True to its nature, polar amino acid residues have the in-built preference for the aqueous environment and the nonpolar ones for the hydrophobic environments on the surface of containers or the air. So, a conformational re-arrangement and denaturation can be induced once they are adsorbed at an interface (Fig.15.2). Once the protein molecules are adsorbed, they are capable of forming short-range bonds (van der Waals, hydrophobic, electrostatic, hydrogen, ion-pair bonds) with the surface and this may lead to further denaturation of proteinaceous moieties. Despite the rapid adsorption of peptides and proteins at the interfaces, the rates of conformational changes are relatively much slower. It is unlikely that the surface proteins may disrobe in their original state. Rather they will disrobe with their hydrophobic residues exposed and in all probability this triggers off unfavorable interactions with water and formation of aggregates and precipitates.

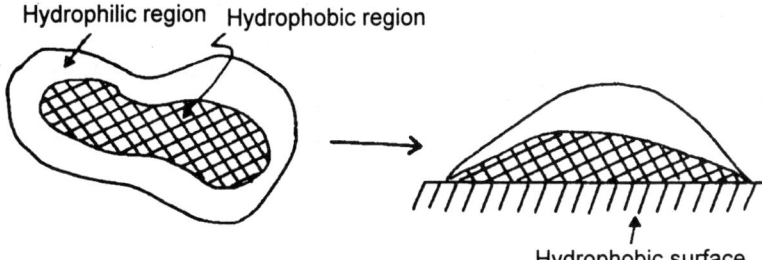

Fig. 15.2 : Schematic representation of protein adsorption at a hydrophobic surface

On adsorption there may be a loss or change in biological activity as the molecular structure is rearranged. For instance, as blood proteins are adsorbed on surface, the antigenic moiety may become exposed. Also, if peptide and protein drug entities are adsorbed at interfaces there may be a reduction in the concentration of drug available to elicit its function. Such loss of these drug moieties may occur during purification, formulation, storage and/or delivery.

15.3.1.3. Aggregation and precipitation

The denatured, unfolded proteins may rearrange in such a manner that hydrophobic amino acid residues of various molecules associate together leading to the formation of aggregates. If the aggregation is on a macroscopic scale, precipitation occurs. As discussed in the preceding paragraphs interfacial adsorption may be followed by aggregation and precipitation. The extent to which aggregation and precipitation occurs is defined by the relative hydrophilicity of the surfaces in contact with the polypeptide/protein solution. The acceleration of aggregation and precipitation by hydrophobic surfaces is a classic example of this. Insulin forms finely divided precipitates on the walls of containers, referred to as frosting. The presence of large air-water interface accelerates this process. Agitation of polypeptide and protein solutions introduces air bubbles, thereby increasing the hydrophobic air interface. In the process, aggregation and precipitation of polypeptides/proteins is augmented. Another factor contributing to this may be the increase in thermal motion of the molecules due to agitation.

15.3.2. Chemical stability

The stability of peptides and proteins against a chemical reagent is decided by temperature, length of exposure, and the amino acid composition, sequence and conformation of the peptide/protein. Conformation of the moiety is of particular importance since the reacting groups may be buried and unavailable for reaction with the reagent. The conformational stability may be vital, for example, chemical reaction may elevate the conformational energy of a peptide in an unstrained conformation or may lower the conformational energy of the peptide in a highly strained conformation. Some of the major reaction mechanisms are discussed in brief below.

15.3.2.1. Deamidation

This reaction involves the hydrolysis of the side chain amide linkage of an amino acid residue leading to the formation of a free carboxylic acid. Asparagine (Asn) and glutamine (Gln) are particularly susceptible to deamidation. *In vivo* deamidation could be enzymatic or nonenzymatic. *In vitro* deamidation is observed with human growth hormone, prolactin and insulin. Factors that favor the rate of deamidation include increased pH, temperature and ionic strength. The tertiary structure of the protein also affects its stability, as observed with trypsin in which the tertiary structure prevents deamidation. Lowering in biological profile after deamidation has been reported with porcine adrenal corticotropic hormone (ACTH).

15.3.2.2. Oxidation and reduction

Oxidation of susceptible amino acids is the major degradation pathway for peptides and proteins that is very common during isolation, synthesis and storage of the same. Oxidation may occur on the side chains of histidine (His), lysine (Lys), methionine (Met), tryptophan (Trp) and thyronine (Tye) residues in proteins. The thioether group of Met is particularly susceptible to oxidation. Under acidic conditions Met residues can be oxidized by atmospheric oxygen. Oxidizing agents like hydrogen peroxide, dimethylsulfoxide and iodine can oxidise Met-to-Met sulfoxides. The thiol group of cysteine can be oxidised to sulfonic acid, oxidation by iodine and hydrogen peroxide is catalysed by metal ions and may occur spontaneously by atmospheric oxygen. These acid or base catalyzed oxidations may be blocked by oxidation scavengers. Air oxidation can be prevented by avoiding vigorous stirring and exclusion of air by degassing solvents.

Usually, the oxidation of amino acid residues is followed by a significant loss in biological activity as observed after oxidation of Met residues in calcitonin, corticotropin and gastrin. Glucagon is an exception as it retains biological activity even after oxidation. Restoration of the lost biological activity can be achieved by reduction. By reduction of Met sulfoxide to Met nearly all the lost biological activity is restored to lysozyme and ribonuclease.

15.3.2.3. Proteolysis

The hydrolysis of peptide bonds within the polypeptide or protein destroys or at least reduces its activity. The vulnerability of peptide bonds to cleavage is dependent on the residues involved. In comparison to other residues, asparagine residues are more unstable and in particular the Asp-Pro bond. Proteolysis may occur on exposing the proteins to harsh conditions, such as prolonged exposure to extremes of pH or high temperature or proteolytic enzymes. Bacterial contamination is the most common source for introduction of proteases. This can be avoided by storing the protein in the cold under sterile conditions. Proteases may also gain access during the isolation, purification and recovery of recombinant proteins from cell extracts or culture fluid. The particular protease co-purified with the recombinant protein decides the fate of proteolysis. This problem can be minimized by the manipulation of the solution conditions during the stage of purification and/or addition of protease inhibitors. Some proteins even have autoproteolytic activity. This property aids in controlling the level or function of protein *in vivo* but is highly unwarranted for a drug moiety if cleavage leads to a loss in biological activity.

15.3.2.4. Disulfide exchange

Disulfide bonds may break and reform incorrectly and thereby an alteration in the three-dimensional structure is followed by change in activity. This reaction can be catalyzed in neutral as well as alkaline media by thiols, which may arise as a result of hydrolytic cleavage of disulfides. In the presence of HSR', a disulfide R-S-S-R, interchanges mercaptan groups to give a mixed disulfide, R-S-S-R'. A peptide chain with more than one disulfide can enter into disulfide exchange reactions, leading to scrambling of disulfide bridges and thereby a change in conformation. Another possibility is the addition of a peptide chain with free cysteine to the disulfide of another peptide chain to give a dimeric disulfide. By analogous reactions, trimers and dimers can be formed. The reaction is concentration dependent, in particular for oligomer formation. These oligomers appear at low R_f value on TLC and are readily removed by gel filtration.

15.3.2.5. Racemization

With the exception of Gly, all the mammalian amino acids are chiral at the carbon bearing side chain and are susceptible to base-catalysed racemization. Racemization is the chemical alteration of L-and D-amino acids. This reaction can be catalyzed in neutral and alkaline media by thiols, which may arise as a result of hydrolytic cleavage of disulfides. The thiolate ions carry out nucleophilic attack on a sulfur atom of the disulfide. Addition of thiol scavengers such as p-mercuribenzoate, N-ethylmaleimide and copper ions, may prevent susceptible sulfur of disulfide.

15.4. BARRIERS TO PEPTIDE AND PROTEIN DELIVERY

15.4.1. Enzymatic barriers

Enzymatic barrier is the most important barrier that limits absorption of protein/peptide drugs from g.i. tract. The enzymatic degradation is brought about mainly in two ways by:

1. Hydrolytic cleavage of peptide bonds by proteases, such as insulin-degrading enzyme, enkephalinase, angiotensin-converting enzyme and renin. Proteolysis is an irreversible reaction and is shorn of absolute specificity thereby potentiating the probabilities of damage of the peptide and protein drug.
2. Chemical modification of protein such as phosphorylation by kinases, oxidation by xanthine oxidase or glucose oxidase, carbamylation by pronase, chymotrypsin and trypsin, denaturation and ubiquitization. These chemical changes in the substrate protein are reported to affect the rate and site of hydrolysis catalyzed by proteases, thus the peptides/proteins become more susceptible to proteolytic attack.

The substrate specificity for several proteolytic enzymes present in the gut is displayed in figure 15.3. The enzymatic barrier predominantly has three essential features:

1. The proteolytic enzymes are ubiquitous and hence the proteins/peptides are prone to degradation in multiple anatomical sites, viz., the site of administration, blood, vascular endothelia, kidney, liver, etc. Thus, they have to be guarded against degradation in all the anatomical sites to ensure their reaching site of action in intact form.
2. The anatomical site where the peptide/protein is located is likely to have the presence of all the proteases capable of degrading the same. Thus, the peptide/protein has to be protected from all the enzymes before it can elicit the pharmacological effect.
3. A particular peptide/protein is prone to degradation at more than one linkage within the backbone, each locus being mediated by a specific protease. Thus, all the vulnerable linkages call for protection or modification.

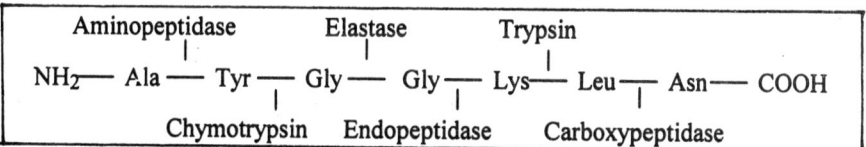

Fig. 15.3. : Substrate specificity for several proteolytic enzymes

15.4.2. Intestinal epithelial barriers

There are several mechanisms that are involved in the transport of peptide/protein drugs across the intestinal epithelium. These are discussed below:

15.4.2.1. Passive and carrier mediated transport

The extensive absorption of di-and tri-peptides from small intestine is well documented. Active transport appears to be the predominant mechanism. Also, there is little evidence that peptides with more than three or four amino acid residues are transported across the intestinal mucosa by the peptide transport system Stereoisomerism, side-chain length, and N- and C-terminal substitution are reported to affect dipeptide absorption. For e.g., L-Ala-L-Phe and L-Leu-L-Leu- were found to be more rapidly absorbed than their D isomers. Likewise, the presence of a larger side chain in either the N-terminal or the C-terminal favors dipeptide absorption. Acidic and basic (Lys-Lys) dipeptides have lower affinity than neutral dipeptides for peptide transport. Methylation and acetylation of N-terminal amino groups, esterification of C-terminal carboxyl groups, presence of ι-linkage and incorporation of β-amino acids are known to decrease the affinity of dipeptides for the peptide transport system.

15.4.2.2. Endocytosis and transcytosis

Cellular internalization of peptides/proteins may occur by endocytosis whereby peptides/proteins which are too large to be absorbed by carrier mediated transport are taken up. The two different pathways of endocytosis are:

15.4.2.2.1. Fluid-phase type (non specific endocytosis, pinocytosis)

In fluid-phase endocytosis (FPE) the macromolecules dissolved in the extracellular fluid are incorporated by bulk transport into the fluid phase of endocytic vesicles (Fig.15.4).

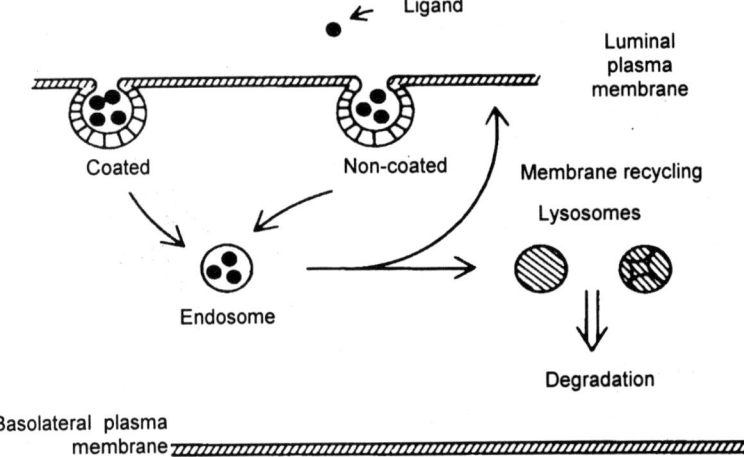

Fig. 15.4 : Cellular uptake by fluid-phase endocytosis

15.4.2.2.2. Adsorptive or receptor-mediated type (specific endocytosis)

In this process the macromolecules are bound to the plasma membrane before they are incorporated into endocytic vesicles. When the membrane binding site is a specific receptor for the macromolecule involved, the process is referred to as receptor-mediated endocytosis (RME) as shown in figure15.5.

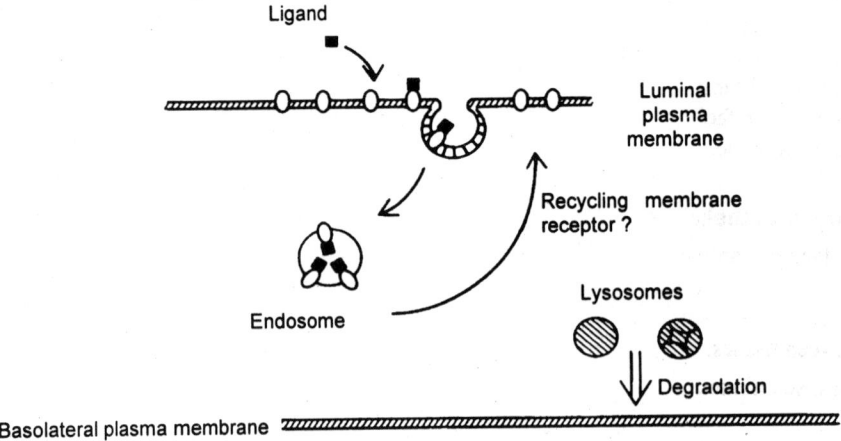

Fig. 15.5 : Cellular uptake by receptor mediated endocytosis

The small intestine epithelial mucosa serves as a barrier to the permeation of macromolecules. However, endocytic uptake provides ways to circumvent this barrier. By RME the absorptive cells of the intestinal epithelium are able to select and transport specific molecules while excluding undesirable/harmful ones like bacterial enterotoxins and endotoxins. Some peptides and proteins that are reported to enter intestinal mucosal cells include, nerve growth factor, epidermal growth factor and IgG.

15.4.2.2.3. Transcytosis

The process of transcytosis combines elements of membrane protein sorting and endocytosis. In polarized cell, such as the intestinal epithelial cells, some endosomes carrying the ligands or the receptor-ligand complex bypass the lysosomes and migrate toward the basolateral membrane. Thereby the ligand is released in the extracellular space bound by the basolateral membrane (Fig. 15.6). This process is known as transcytosis. This pathway presents an important route for mucosal transport of peptides and proteins.

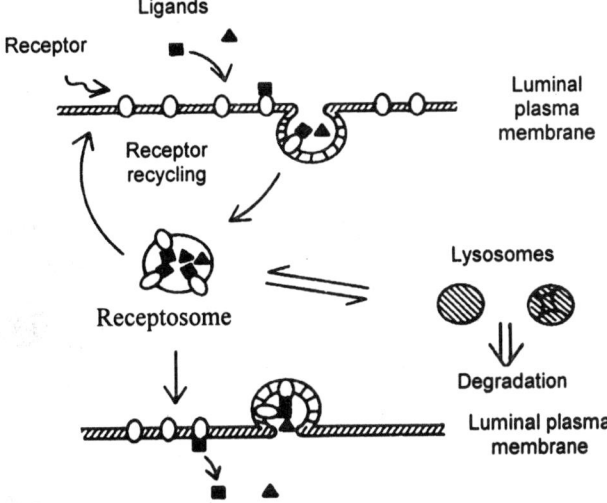

■ - Receptor bound ligand

Fig. 15.6 : Cellular uptake by transcytosis

15.4.2.3. Paracellular movement

This involves the movement between the tight junctions between cells and/or across the spaces formed when cells are extruded into the intestinal lumen. Paracellular movement plays an important role in the absorption of water from the intestinal lumen. Presumably, the passage of water across the tight junction is capable of carrying the dissolved drug(s) or facilitate the transport of macromolecules which are otherwise not capable to travel across the apical membrane.

15.4.3. Capillary endothelial barrier

The luminal surface of capillaries consists of the plasma membrane surface of a monolayer of endothelial cells which are joined together by more or less continuous tight or occluding junctions. The structural features of capillary endothelium are displayed in figure 15.7. The structural and permeability properties of capillaries vary enormously between tissues. Capillaries can be broadly classified into three major classes:

1. Sinusoidal or discontinuous.
2. Fenestrated.
3. Continuous.

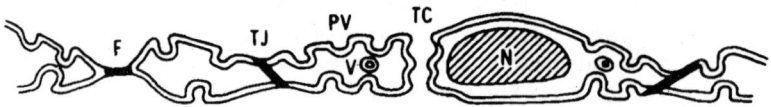

Fig. 15.7 : Structural features of capillary endothelium (F- fenestrated diaphragm; TJ- tight junctions; PV- plasmalemmal vesicles; V- vesicles; TC- transmembrane channel; N- cell nucleus)

To cross the capillary endothelium the peptides/proteins must pass between the cells or alternatively traverse the endothelial cells themselves. Solutes that traverse the endothelial cell membrane may be modified or metabolized by cytoplasmic enzymes. Thus, the endothelial passage poses metabolic or enzymatic barrier to solute passage. The failure of circulating dopamine, ammonia and fatty acids to enter brain can be accounted for by considering the cellular metabolism. Endothelial tight junctions also serve as the major extracellular barrier to solute exchange. The transcapillary movement of macromolecular tracers injected into plasma or interstitial fluid is hampered by these junctions.

15.4.3.1. Mechanisms of solute transit

15.4.3.1.1. Passive, nonfacilitated

Continuous capillaries of the peripheral tissues are permeable to proteins that are <70 kD or even larger. The continuous capillaries contain two sets of rigid water-filled pores: 120Å in diameter and 600Å in diameter, at densities of 12 and 0.05 per square micrometer of capillary surface respectively. The primary mediators of macromolecular exchange between plasma and interstitial fluid are plasmalemmal vesicles. The sequence of events involve the uptake into vesicles at the luminal plasma membrane of the capillary endothelial cells, followed by migration across the endothelial cells and release of the tracer on the albuminal side. This process is referred to as capillary-transcytosis and appears to function bidirectionally unlike other bulk-phase pinocytosis or receptor-mediated endocytosis, transcytosis does not appear to utilize coated pits or culminate in vesicle fusion with lysosomes. Instead, the vesicles appear to be composed of a pool of membrane that does not mix with the plasma membrane pool.

15.4.3.1.2. Carrier-mediated

Specific solute transport pathways allow the movement of solutes across capillary endothelium that otherwise would fail to penetrate. In brain capillary endothelium eight independent nutrient transport systems have been identified. They are:

1. a hexose carrier;
2. a monocarboxylic carrier;
3. a neutral amino acid carrier, which facilitates transport of 14 neutral amino acids;
4. a carrier for lysine, arginine and ornithine;
5. a choline carrier;
6. an adenine/guanine carrier;
7. a porter of purine and uracil nucleosides; and
8. a carrier for aspartic and glutamic acids

Of all the carriers mentioned above, the neutral amino acid carrier holds greatest interest with regard to drug delivery. This carrier holds great similarity to the Na-independent leucine-preferring L system of the peripheral tissues. Its low Km renders it highly sensitive to competition effects.

15.4.3.1.3. Receptor-mediated

Endothelial receptor mediated transcytosis pathways exist for various polypeptides including insulin, transferrin, β-lipotropin and insulin-like growth factor I. The concept of receptor-mediated pathway is discussed in chapter 16.

Basement membrane of the capillaries also imposes a barrier to solute transport. The basement membrane is present everywhere except the sinusoidal gaps of discontinuous endothelium. For instance, in the glomerular capillaries, a thick basement membrane is present and this is reported to limit the capillary permeation by macromolecules like dextrans. The filtration properties are extremely sensitive to charge owing to the anionic disposition of the basement membrane. Basement membranes of the intestinal capillaries are also reported to be limiting barrier.

The endothelial barrier is modulated by several physiological parameters. Some of these are outlined below:

1. Glucocorticoids tighten the blood-brain barrier by decreasing vesicular transport.
2. Angiotensin, bradykinin, histamine and serotonin increase vascular permeability by opening large gaps in the endothelial junctions of post capillary venules.
3. Inflammatory agents, vasopressive agents, certain hormones and hypertension relax the endothelial barrier.

15.4.4. Blood brain barrier (BBB)

The impermeable nature of BBB has been sincerely appreciated and strategies have been evolved to alleviate and obviate the barrier potential to facilitate the targeting of drug to brain compartment. It has been gradually accepted that BBB response particularly in context with permeability as recorded for some vital dyes may not hold the same for bioactive molecules. Recent studies which plunge upon transport kinetics, metabolic, cellular or molecular strategies related to BBB have given major impetus and provided close and better understanding of BBB functioning. It has been demonstrated that various types of metabolic substrates, neuroactive and regulatory peptides and centrally active pharmacotherapeutics could effectively utilize special shuttle services at the BBB. Recently, it has been realized that microvascular endothelium in conjunction with its accessory components, i.e. astrocytes, pericytes and microglia, regulates the homeostasis of neural milieu, rather than simply impeding solute exchange. The neurons, glial cells and brain extracellular fluid are separated from blood by BBB, however, the BBB should not be misconceived as an absolute restriction to blood borne molecular moieties, however, it could be realized as a multiple regulatory unit located at sites within the brain. The morphology of BBB though represented by continuous capillaries of the cerebral micro-circulation, where the endothelial cells are sealed by tight junctions to form a complete composite cellular layer. The functional character of BBB depends upon, geometrical relations amongst the glial and nerve cells and brain extracellular fluid on one hand and cellular fluid as well as humoral extra-brain signals on the other (Fig. 15.8).

The endothelial layer needs to be viewed as two separate membranes, one is referred as luminal located on the inner sides of the vessels and other, abluminal on the outer side of the vessels. These two layers are separated by thick cytoplasm of nearly 300-500nm thickness. Furthermore ,with regard to surface area, it is about 100 cm^2 per gram of brain tissue, in capillary endothelium. Thus total surface area in human brain is about 12 m^2 with the length of capillaries nearly 650 km, the diameter of capillary in human brain 6 µm, where the capillaries are separated apart with a distance of 40 µm. Numerous functional proteins, that are involved in various transports, receptor signal transduction, cell mediated responses of the brain are expressed by the endothelial cells. It appears that different regulatory molecules, many of them being peptidal in nature, mainly control the diversified BBB mechanisms. These peptides could be secreted by astrocytes and some neural endings, acting similar to parachrine, being operative at abluminal site of BBB.

The circulatory molecules could use a number of different mechanism for their transport across BBB. These include:

1. Lipid mediated transport of small but lipophilic molecules.
2. Carrier mediated transport of hydrophilic nutrients and their drug analogues.
3. Plasma protein mediated transport of acidic drugs, peptides and highly lipophilic drugs.
4. Bulk flow transcytosis.

The latter could be pinocytosis or tubulocanalecular transport, independent of molecular size. This transport system however, remains minimal under physiological conditions but may turn out to be significant under certain pathological circumstances.

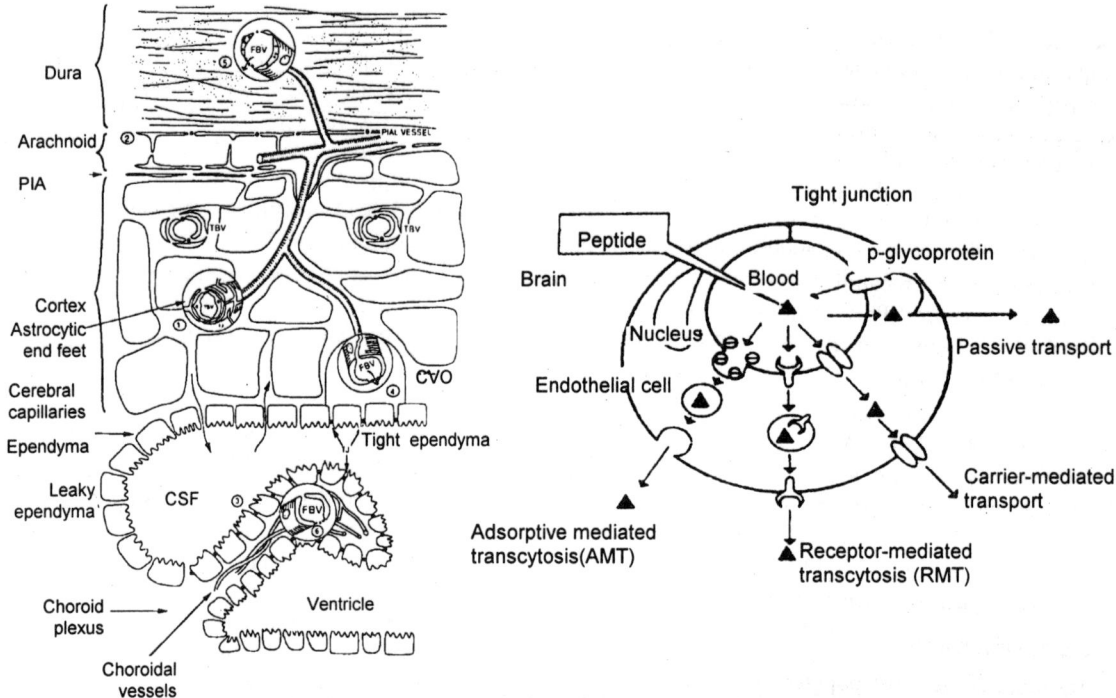

Fig. 15.8 : Schematic presentation of components of blood brain barrier

Peptides which range from 2 amino acid size to a protein of molecular weight of a Lac or more, require special attention when they are considered for permeability across a given barrier. Multiple biologic actions in brain positively suggest about their utility as neuropharmaceuticals in the treatment of diseases of the central nervous system. The role of peptides in the CNS is complex and largely operate at the level of physiologic phenomenon of the brain such as;

1. Neurotransmission.
2. Regulation of neuroendocrine axis.
3. Regulation of cerebral blood flow.
4. Maintenance of integrity of BBB.
5. Permeability to nutrient modulation.
6. Regulation of expression of specific proteins at BBB.

Therefore, peptides register important behavioural effects on higher integrative functions of brain as well as on the vegetative functions of the CNS. For years it was thought that BBB remains, as a composite barrier for peptides and proteins not allowing their access to CNS, however, of late through the set of experiments based on brain perfusion models it has been established that intravenously perfused peptides could be detected in CSF in measurable quantities. It was further propounded that these problem molecules utilise various special transport mechanisms, for their transbarrier localization. It was largely attributed to the passive diffusion of molecules where the concentration obtained in CSF were sub-therapeutic. Barrier factors which have been considered to be responsible for peptide permeability include, lipophilicity, molecular size and charge.

Various strategies which have been suggested for improvisation of permeability profile include:

1. Peptide lipidization.
2. Cationisation.
3. Chimeric protein formation.
4. Antibody mediated transport.
5. Through cytoporter systems. ·

Chemically modified drug could be permeable in brain capillaries, however it may be converted back into an impermeable salt within the brain tissues. Unfortunately, the lipidization approach appears not to be much useful for peptides with molecular weight greater than 1,000 Da. Another approach suggests, inclusion of peptides in detergent based liposomes or poloxomer coated nanoparticles. Specific nutrient transport system could be utilized for brain capillary wall permeation in order to deliver the therapeutic agent selectively to the CNS. Most classical example is the systemic treatment of Parkinson's disease using L-3,4-dihydroxyphenylalanine (L-DOPA), a metabolic precursor of dopamine. This utilizes neutral amino acid transport system. The same system could be utilized wherein phenylalanine and analogues could be utilized as ligand modules. In some cases the permeability of brain capillaries for proteins could be increased. The change in permeability is suggested to be transient in nature. This could be achieved by intra-arterial injection of hyper osmolar solution, which selectively disrupts inter endothelial tight junctions. This approach has been used with success to deliver antibodies to the brain.

Similarly, cationisation using hexamethyldiamine or anionisation by succinylation could enhance the uptake of proteins in the brain. Another interesting strategy describes chemical conjugations of peptides or proteins to antitransferrin receptor antibody as a ligand whereas, transferrin receptor as a shuttle port for permeation enhancement. The approach classically depends upon receptor mediated transcytosis of transferrin receptor complexes by brain endothelial cells.

15.5. DELIVERY OF PROTEIN AND PEPTIDE DRUGS

15.5.1. Oral route

Oral route is the most popular, convenient and acceptable route of delivery from the patients point of view. However, successful oral therapy for peptide and protein drugs has largely eluded solution. Their oral administration is severely prohibited by strong acidic environment, enzymatic and cellular barriers of the intestinal tract. The macromolecular peptide/protein drug(s) also have a low permeability across the gastro-intestinal mucosa. Figure 15.9 illustrates the various barriers to oral absorption. This is the reason why the oral bioavailability of peptide and protein drug is often less than 1%. Molecules that are absorbed via the lumen of the small intestine can either be taken up into a blood capillary or alternatively enter lymphatic lacteal located within the submucosal space. Molecules entering the blood are directed through the hepatic-portal system to the liver and are normally substantially metabolized before they reach the systemic circulation. However, in some cases there is an underlying physiological advantage in directing a peptide or protein to the liver prior to their entry in the systemic circulation. A classic example of such entity is insulin. On referring to its physiology we learn that insulin released from the pancreas travels directly to the liver and first acts on the glucose reserves in respective organ before it acts peripherally.

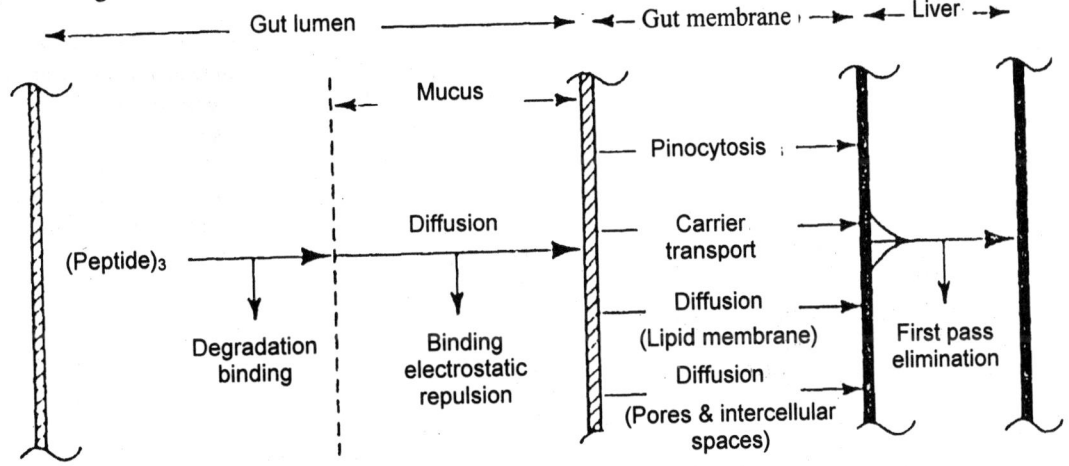

Fig. 15.9 : Various barriers to oral absorption

Uptake from the gut lumen into the lymphatic lacteals offers some advantages:

1. Slower and sustained delivery (3-9 hours for onset of action) in contrast to that observed when molecules are delivered directly into blood capillaries (20-60 minutes for onset of action). The significant difference in blood profiles can be attributed to the fact that lymph moves at 1-2 ml/min while hepatic portal blood at 1,500 ml/min.
2. Drugs can bypass liver which is not the case with molecules entering the blood capillaries. The relative proportion of drug taken up through these two different routes at a particular site within the gut is dependent on hydrophobic nature of the drug and formulation.
3. Finally, it has the potential to target moieties like cytokines and lymphokines to white blood cells present in the lymph system.

To maximize oral absorption of peptide and protein drugs from the gastrointestinal tract, the various components of the penetration and enzymatic barrier should be controlled. The various approaches to achieve the same are outlined in the succeeding paragraphs.

15.5.1.1. *Modifications by chemical synthesis of prodrugs and analogues*

This strategy of chemically altering the peptide/protein structure is aimed to modify physicochemical properties of drugs, such as lipophilicity, charge, molecular size, solubility, configuration, isoelectric point, chemical stability, enzyme lability and affinity to carriers. This modification aids in manipulating the pharmacokinetic parameters and as a result to improve the therapeutic value of the parent drug by facilitating membrane permeation and providing stability against degradation and thereby altering bioavailability. Modification by succinylation, acylation, guanidation and deamination conjugation with polymers such as albumin, dextran, polyvinylpyrrolidone, DL-poly(aminoacid) and poly(ethylene glycol) and lipoamino acids and their homo-oligomers has been tried out to increase lipophilicity, the blood circulating life and/or to reduce immunogenicity.

Some of the enzymes are specifically located at the luminal and subluminal sites of the epithelial cells of the g.i. tract. The strategies interestingly discusses the chemical modification process, where protein is modified to its prodrug. The later serves as substrate with defined propensity for a membrane localized enzyme. The pro-drug is converted into the parent drug via enzymatic reaction and, generated parent drug gets absorbed. The physicochemical characteristics help preventing its possible precipitation at the absorption site. The operational features of the strategy are schematically presented in figure 15.10.

The prodrug synthesis approach has been utilized with success to improvise the absorption of water insoluble peptide renin inhibitor where mucosal membrane peptidases were used as conversion sites. The approach offered better solubility and high permeability. The approach offers an increase in polarity of drug and simulataneously the membrane permeability. As a result of a systematic study conducted with renin inhibitors, it was inferred that substantially improvised delivery of peptidomimetics is possible through structural modification approach. The modification is so carefully conducted that pharmacological effects of the drug remains to be unchanged. It was further proposed that carrier-mediated transport via peptide cytotransporters is one of the important uptake mechanism that operates in the case of brush border membrane. Taken collectively it could be concluded that oral systemic delivery of peptide and peptidomimetics is an achievable aim. It also suggests that nutrient and other natural native cytoportal systems can judiciously be exploited for effective transportation and as a result systemic absorption of protein and peptide drugs. The approach is schematically presented in figure 15.10.

Lipid conjugates by employing phospholipids have been proposed. Phospholipids provide unique interface between lipophilic acyl region and hydrophilic biomolecules. Lipid conjugates have contributed significantly towards promising prodrugs analogues with improved stability, bioavailability and barrier permeation characteristics. Peptides, proteins and carbohydrates are appropriate drug target for conjugation. A variety of approaches including derivatization with phospholipids, fatty acids, cholesterol and long chain alcohols are used to generate pharmaceutical lipid conjugates.

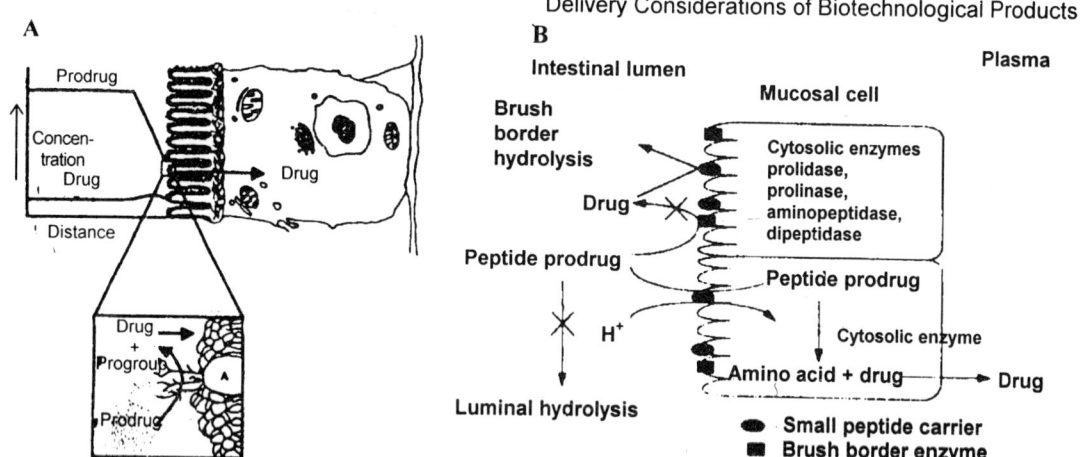

Fig. 15.10 : A. Proposed mechanism for absorption enhancement of water insoluble proteins and peptides. **B.** Schematic illustration of prodrug strategy to improvise absorption of protein and peptide

Conventional methods, i.e. amidation, cross-linking and active anchoring using carbodiimide are utilized for chemical derivatization (Fig. 15.11). The developed prodrugs are amphiphilic thus via supramolecular aggregation state may form lymphotrophic system. The latter has appreciable potential for oral administration of protein and peptide drugs, via lymphatic route.

Thyrotropin-releasing hormone (TRH) is employed clinically to exert control over pituitary functions. However, after oral administration, low levels are observed in the brain. TRH is reported to be resistant to proteolytic degradation in GI tract. The nominal oral activity seems to be due to poor absorption and rapid clearance in the blood stream. To circumvent these problems, analogues have been synthesized. A dimethyl analogue of TRH, p-glu-his-(3,3'-dimethyl-pro-NH$_2$) RX 77368 was synthesized and on clinical examination reported to be long-lasting and more potent. This property was attributed to its stability to protease action. Another analogue MK-771 was synthesized having a sulfur atom in the pyrrolidone ring at position 2 of the proline residue. This analogue was more potent than the parent and also possessed much slower clearance rate but was equipotent in causing the release of TSH. The oral bioavailability of MK-771 was found to be only 2% in humans and 3% in monkeys.

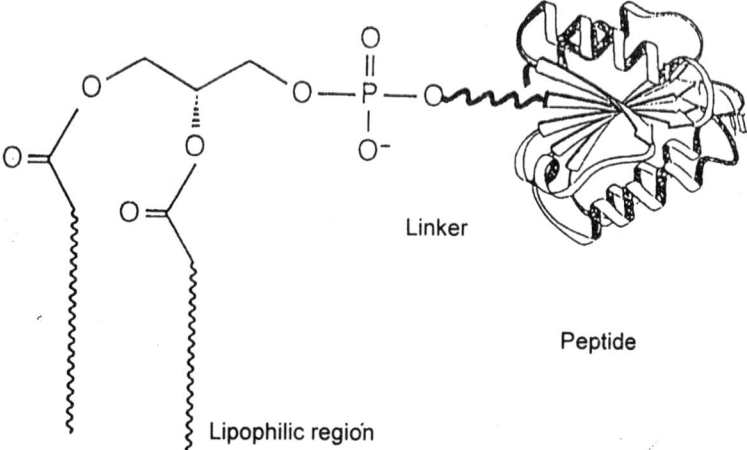

Fig. 15.11 : Schematic illustration of a protein-lipid (unsaturated acid diglyceride) conjugate through a linker

Another approach is that of synthesis of tripeptide TRH and acetylation on the N-terminus. These conjugates were found to have improved oral uptake and stable over a considerable period of time than the native TRH. On the similar lines LHRH has been conjugated to lipoamino acids and lipopeptides, and are reported to give promising results *in vivo*.

Enkephalins, the endogenous pentapeptides, occur naturally in two types, leucine (YGGFL) and methionine (YGGFM) enkephalins. Their oral delivery is precluded due to their susceptibility to hydrolysis by intestinal peptidases. Pentapeptides structurally related to YGGFM have been synthesized by oxidizing YAGFM-ol to sulfoxide[YAGFM(O)-ol] and N-methylating YAGFM(O)-ol [YAGF (Me)M(O)-ol]. These analogues produced significant analgesic activity after oral administration.

Several analogues of vasopressin, the antidiuretic hormone, have been synthesized. These include deamino (4-valine, 8-D-arginine)-vasopressin (DVDAVP), deamino (4-threonine, 8-D-arginine)-vasopressin (DTDAVP), 1-deamino-(8-D-arginine)-vasopressin (desmopressin, DDAVP) and (1-deamino penicillamine, 2-O-methyl-tyrosine)-arginine vasopressin. DDAVP differs structurally from vasopressin in two positions. At position 1, instead of hemicystine, β-mercaptopropionic acid (deaminohemicystine) is present and at position 8 instead of L-arginine, D-arginine is present.

For the oral delivery of the proteins and peptides an interesting approach has been reported based on **protein polymer complex**. In this approach mainly a hydrophobic polymer i.e. co-polystyrene maleic anhydride\maleic acid is conjugated with protein or peptide utilizing their terminal amino active groups. So formed complex is dissolved in triglyceride (medium chain length) containing 5% polyglycerine trioleate. This facilitates solubilization and incorporation of the protein-polymer complex into the fat phase of the emulsion and so formed emulsion could be used for oral administration. Figure 15.12 represents this strategy where NCS (Neocarzinostatin) is complexed with polystyrene co-maleic acid butyryl ester through its N-terminal ε-amino groups (alanine and lysine) and partially hydrolyzed maleic anhydride groups of polymer.

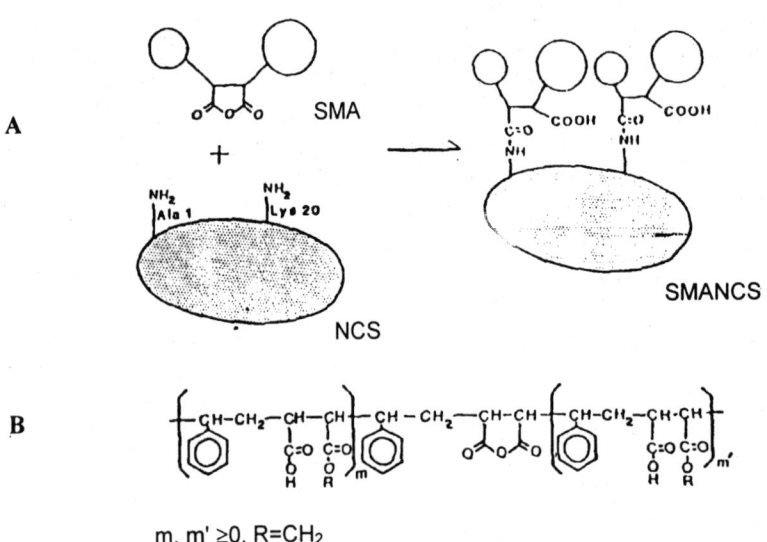

m, m' ≥0, R=CH₂

Fig. 15.12 : A. Poly(styrene co-maleic acid)-neocarzinostatin complex
B. Chemical structure of polystyrene co-maleic acid

15.5.1.2. Site-specific delivery

There are reports that absorption of certain peptides and proteins is limited to a certain specific region within the GI tract, i.e. an optimal site exists for their absorption. For example, dipeptide like angiotensin converting enzyme (ACE) inhibitor is absorbed only from the upper small intestine in humans. The presence of proteolytic enzymes also play a vital role in hampering the favorable absorption of peptides/proteins from GI tract. This is the reason for better absorption of peptides like Met-Met that are better absorbed from jejunum in comparison to otherwise well absorptive ileum.

A number of techniques have been developed for delineating the absorption characteristics of drugs from different regions of the GI tract. Some of the these are discussed below:

15.5.1.2.1. High frequency capsule

The release of contents from this at a predetermined location is achieved by means of an external radio signal. This device thus not only allows for targeting to the possible absorption windows but also offers protection from the enzymatic environments of the GI tract. Theophylline and isosorbide-5-mononitrate absorption have been studied following their administration as high frequency capsules.

15.5.1.2.2. Ileum delivery

The absorption capacity of the ileum is lower than the duodenum but is reported to contain highly specialized mechanisms for absorption of specific macromolecules. For instance, a specialized transport mechanism exists for absorption of bile acids from ileum. For active transport acidic side chain at the 17-position of the ring system of the bile acids is indispensable. C3-derivatives are also reported to undergo active transport. Conjugation of p-toluene-sulfonic acid with cholic acid improved the absorption of the former from the ileum.

Ileum also provides a carrier system for cyanocobalamin (Vitamin B_{12}) that binds with high affinity to three distinct transport proteins viz. transcobalamine II, intrinsic factor (IF) and the nonintrinsic factor cobalamine-binding proteins (R-proteins). Cobalamine analogues have been studied for their binding affinity. It is highly selective and transcobalamine II is moderately selective. On the other hand R proteins are reported to have high affinity for wide range of cobamides and cobinamid. Cobamides are vitamin B_{12} produced by bacteria and differ from cobalamine by the absence of the cyano and the 5,6-dimethylbenzimidazol groups. Studies on similar lines have led to the conclusion that vitamin B_{12} analogues are absorbed from the ileum via a mechanism that is independent of the intrinsic factor. Thus, coupling of macromolecules to cobalamine can give an opportunity for transport into the enterocyte via the receptor-mediated transport process. Promising results have been obtained with LHRH-vitamin B_{12} conjugate.

Peyer's patches are aggregates of lymphoid nodules. Solitary lymphoid nodules are present along the entire intestine but are more numerous and concentrated in the ileum, where they are recognized in aggregate form as Peyer's patches. The migration pathway of Peyer's patch cells have been illustrated in figure15.13.

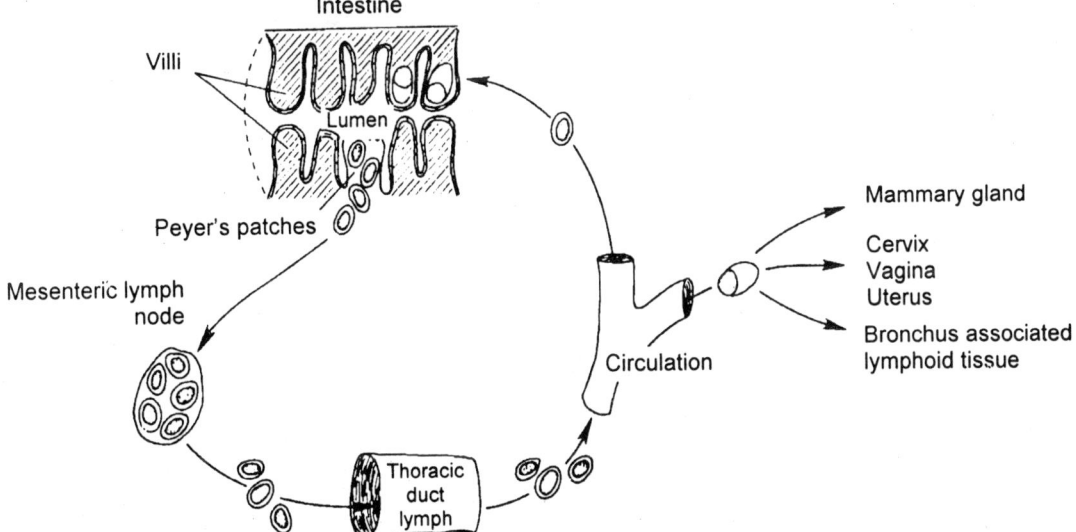

Fig. 15.13 : Schematic presentation of migration pathway of Peyer's patch cells

Studies indicate that particles up to 5μm can be transported within macrophages through Peyer's patches into mesenteric lymph nodes. Accumulation in Peyer's patches is governed not only by the particle size but the surface properties also play a vital role. For instance, better penetration is observed with particles having hydrophobic surfaces. These Peyer's patches (Fig. 15.14) can be exploited as a port for oral immunization. B cells in the Peyer's patches can be induced to develop into IgA plasma cells by subjecting them to antigen challenge and exposure to bacterial lipopolysaccharides. Synthetic fragments of cholera toxin have been administered orally to induce the production of antibodies recognizing the intact toxin. Successful delivery of antigen by liposomes is reported following M-cell uptake. Another approach utilized coated liposomes composed of soya phosphatidylcholine with the reo-virus cell protein, for which receptors exist on the M cells.

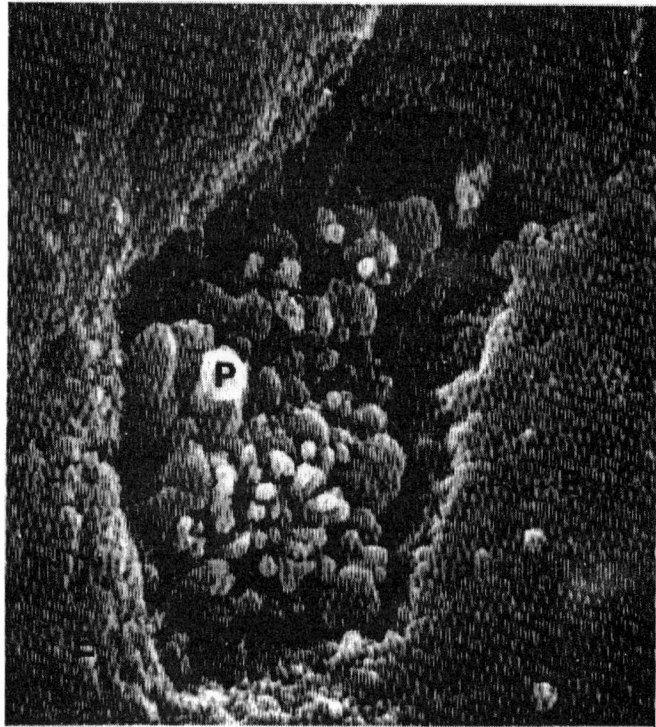

Fig. 15.14 : Photograph showing particulate uptake at Peyer's patches (M-cells)

15.5.1.2.3. Colon Delivery

In comparison to small intestine, the colon has minimal enzyme concentration, especially peptidases and thus may be exploited for systemic peptide absorption. However, this site has several inherent limitations that have been discussed below:

1. Colon has a flat epithelium with a small surface/volume ratio available for absorption, and therefore the permeability of polar compounds is relatively less when a comparison is drawn with the small intestinal epithelium.
2. Longer residence time is supposed to counteract the above mentioned drawback but unpredictable colonic transit jeopardize a predictable absorption.
3. There is a great variation in the colonic pH and this is all the more prominent in the presence of protein rich food, pH can be as high as 8.
4. In the colon, free diffusion of drug across membranes is hampered due to the presence of surrounding solid fecal matter.
5. Presence of higher concentration of bacteria, in particular the anaerobic ones, potentiates the drug degradation.

However, these limitations can be exploited to our advantage by utilizing the microbial enzymes as an aid to targeted delivery to colon. 5-aminosalicylic acid (5-ASA) has been linked to high molecular weight polymers via aromatic azo groups. This conjugate is capable of being absorbed only at the colon where the azo bond is reduced and thereby 5-ASA released. The same conjugation concept can be exploited for colonic delivery of protein or peptide drugs and their absorption thereafter. Another prodrug comprising of two 5-ASA molecules joined by an azo bond has been designed.

An approach that has been used for delivery of insulin involves an azo cross-linked copolymer of styrene and hydroxyethylmethacrylate that coats the insulin. Thus, the drug remains protected from the vagaries of GI tract. The polymer disintegrates only at the ileocecal junction when the azoreductase reduces the $R-C_6H_4-N=N-C_6H_4-R$ bond. Thus, insulin is released at a site where it is least prone to degradation. The same concept has been used for the delivery of vasopressin. A system with Eudragit-S, an acrylic-based resin, coating has been designed. This resin is soluble only at weakly alkaline pH and thereby release of drug is achieved in colon by erosion of the coat.

15.5.1.3. Use of enzyme inhibitors

Enzymatic barriers are the deciding factors for the transport of unstable small peptides that could be effectively transported across the intestinal membrane but for their degradation by various proteases. Majority of the degradation events in the gut revolve around the resident proteases and peptidases. The catabolism of protein and peptide therapeutics can be limited by the use of protease and peptidase inhibitors. Specific catabolic protease and peptidase activities can be identified and a corresponding specific inhibitor can be employed to stabilize the sensitive protein/peptide. Some of the enzymes and their specific inhibitors are listed in table 15.2.

Table 15.2 : Enzymes and their specific inhibitors

Enzyme	Specific inhibitors
Acid protease (e.g. Pepsin; Renin; Cathepsin D;Chymosin)	Diazoacetyl DL-norleucine methyl ester; 1,2-epoxy-3(Q-nitrophenoxy)propane; Pestatine
Aminopeptidases	Bestain
Aminopeptidase B	Arphanamine
Ca^{2+} activated neutral protease	Protease inhibitor
Calpains I and II	Acetyl-leucyl-leucyl norleucinal
Chymotrypsin	Chymostatin; N-Tosyl-L-phenylalanine chloromethyl ketone
Endoprotease	α2-Macroglobulin
Metalloendoproteases	Phosphoramidon
Metalloprotease	Ethylenediamine tetra-acetic acid
Serine proteases (e.g. Elastase; Cathepsin; Trypsin; Thrombin; Kallikrein)	4-Amidinophenyl-methanesulfonyl fluoride Aprotinin 3 4-Dichloroisocoumarine Leupeptin Phenylmethanesulfonyl fluoride
Thiolproteases (e.g. Plasmin; Cathepsin B; Cathepsin L)	Cystain (N-[N(L-3-trans-carboxy-oxiran-2-carbonyl]-L-leucyl-1[-agmatine] Leupeptin
Trypsin	Nα-Q-Tosyl-L-lysine chloromethyl ketone; Trypsin inhibitor

15.5.1.4. Use of absorption enhancers

As discussed earlier, the major pathways available for transport across membrane are the transcellular and the paracellular routes. The transport across this pathway is dependent on the lipophilicity of the membrane and molecule, the molecular and particular size and charge.

Mechanisms involved in the improvement of intestinal membrane permeation through transcellular route by absorption enhancers are presented in figure 15.15 and enumerated below:

1. Interaction of absorption enhancers with membrane lipid protein leads to membrane perturbation followed by an increase in permeability, e.g. mixed micelles, salicylic acid, acyl carnitine, middle chain fatty acids, enhance membrane permeability via membrane perturbation.
2. Disorder of membrane status by decrease in membrane nonprotein thiol, e.g. diethyl maleate, salicylic acid. The mechanisms involved in the improvement of intestinal membrane permeation by absorption enhancers through paracellular route include:

   a. Chelation between enhancer and Ca^{++}/Mg^{++} around tight junctions which force water through by osmosis, enhancing paracellular absorption of water-soluble drugs, e.g., EDTA/bile acids, middle chain fatty acids.
   b. Activation of junctional actomyosin contraction, e.g. glucose, amino acids, decanoyl carnitine, capric acid, mixed micelles.

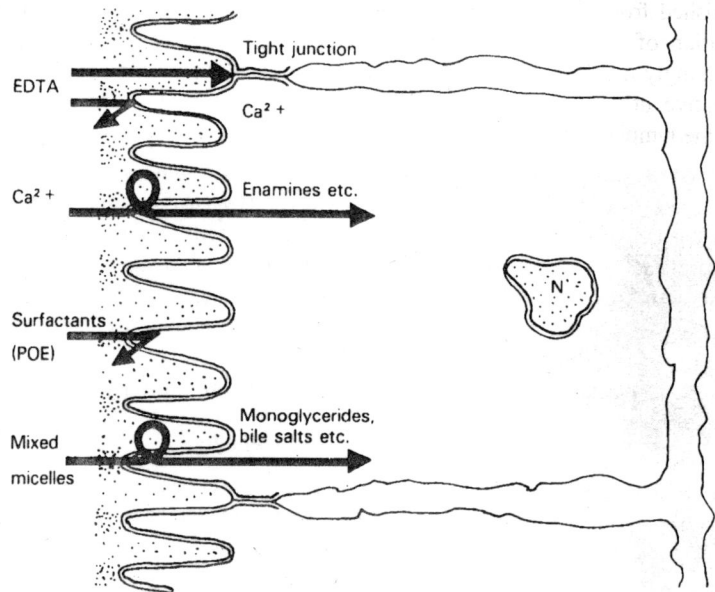

Fig. 15.15 : Schematic presentation of absorption enhancement strategies

15.5.1.5. Dosage form modifications

This strategy is particularly applicable in the case of poorly absorbed peptides and proteins that are unstable in the g.i. lumen where their targeting to a specific tissue or organ is to be affected. The proper designing of the delivery system not only protects the drug from g.i. degrading components but also releases the drug at the site favorable for absorption, whether it is due to low protease content or enhanced permeability characteristics. Some of the delivery systems that have been explored include:

15.5.1.5.1. Lipid vesicles and emulsions

These dosage forms have shown great potential in the delivery of proteins and peptides. Before a drug can exert its therapeutic effects, its penetration through the plasma membrane (a lipoid bilayer) or its uptake through carrier systems is a mandatory step. The use of lipid vesicular carrier systems and emulsions have paved the way to circumvent membrane barriers and thereby promoting the uptake of this 'difficult' class of therapeutics. Solid nanospheres and fat emulsions have also been suggested as lymphotrophs to traffic 'problem' molecules effectively through lymphatic circulation utilizing typical endogenous lipid digestion and assimilation system specially the chylomicrons. Insulin delivered in liposomes produced better hypoglycaemic effects than the free insulin following oral administration. Water-in-oil-in-water (w/o/w) emulsion also exhibited significant delivery potential when compared with the plain aqueous solutions.

15.5.1.5.2. Emulsomes

The emulsome drug delivery system as reported represents a new generation of colloidal drug carrier units. It is typically a lipoidal drug delivery vehicle which could be prepared using relatively higher concentration of lecithin (5-10%). The interesting feature of the system is that unlike oil phase of an emulsion (O/W), the internal phase in the case of emulsomes remains to be in solid or quasi solid state at ambient temperature. Its preparation technique typically employs adequate emulsification at elevated temperature where an ordered bi-phasic dispersion is stabilized through the addition of lectin in higher quantity. The internal phase may contain entrapped macromolecules which are proteinaceous in nature and could be cultivated as nanospheres typically surface stabilized resembling chylomicrons, the endogenous lymphotrophic system. It follows that the system on oral administration could affect the translocation of its content via lymphatic route. The emulsomes can explicitly be distinguished from fat emulsions or lipid microspheres as they are distinctively sphere vesicular system due to utilization of higher quantities of phosphatidylcholine both as emulsifying agent as well as surface modifier. Seemingly it forms phospholipid bilayer onto the surface of lipid solid core. The system holds promises for its effective utilization of oral administration of proteinaceous drug(s)(Fig. 15.16). The basic principle involved in the lymphotrophic uptake is discussed later in the chapter under 15.6.

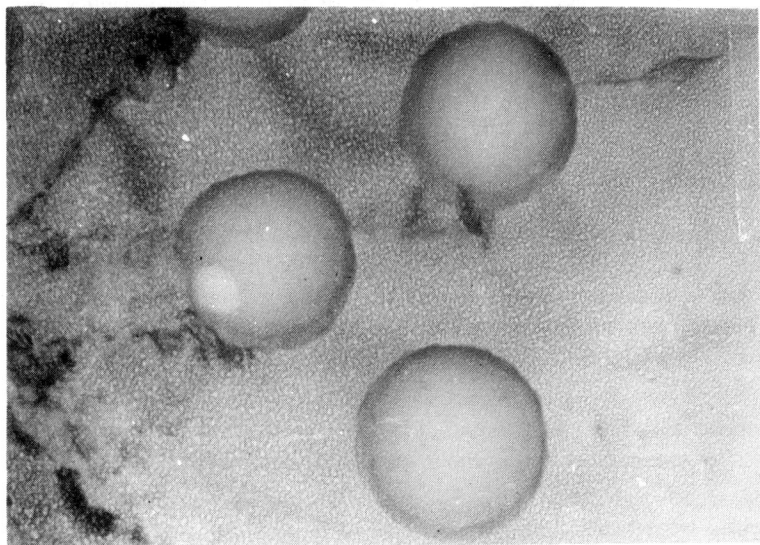

Fig. 15.16 : Photomicrograph (SEM) of emulsomes

15.5.1.5.3. Particulate carriers

Nano and microparticles can be employed as oral carriers for peptide and protein delivery. Intact uptake of particles up to 10 μm from intestinal wall have been reported. Another study claimed that there is no uptake of nanoparticles, but rather the contact time of the drug with the gut wall is increased by the particles and its degradation in the gut lumen alleviated. This unusual approach sounds promising, but it has been observed that the quantitative uptake into general circulation from the g.i. lumen is very small. Native surface properties and chemical composition of the carrier nanoparticles are crucial in determining the extent of uptake. For instance adsorption of poloxamer surfactants are reported to decrease total uptake while covalent attachment of tomato lectin decreases the extent of uptake. Insulin has been administered in 220nm polyalkyl cyanoacrylate nano-particles which resulted in significant reduction in blood glucose level. Luteinizing hormone releasing hormone (LHRH) has also been administered as copolymerized peptide particle with successful results. In this strategy a derivative of LHRH was prepared by conjugating it with vinylacetic acid which was then co-polymerized with n-butylcyanoacrylate (n-BCA) and a radiolable. The reaction conditions were manipulated to exploit the particle forming properties of n-BCA.

It is suggested that the uptake takes place via restricted but specialized mechanism involving the M-cells. This can be exploited in the development of oral vaccines. This strategy can be utilized if low bioavailability of protein/peptidal active species is not a restraint. Uptake also occurs through non-lymphoid epithelial tissues. Poloxamer and tomato lectin increases total uptake through this route only.

Proteinoids are polymeric amino acid aggregation under acidic condition in the form of microspheres. These proteinoids serve to hold a cargo of drug(s) including proteins, peptides and immunogens, which on oral administration set improved absorption of these agents. Characteristically they are quite stable in g.i. tract. However, when discharged into the small intestine, they undergo spontaneous dissociation to release the contents. Apparently, the encapsulated peptides and proteins are protected from enzymatic degradation in stomach. Thus large amount ultimately reaches the absorption site in small intestine. For protein(s) and vaccine on oral administration in proteinoids an improved availability profile has been recorded.

15.5.1.5.4. Bioadhesive systems

Bioadhesive systems are supposed to stick to the intestinal mucosa. This intimate contact between the delivery system and absorbing membrane and or the prolonged residence time at the site of absorption leads to an increment in absorption across the mucosa. Intestinal absorption of 9-desglycinamide 8-arginine vasopressin (DGAVP) with microspheres consisting of p-hydroxyethylmethacrylate having bioadhesive polycarbophil coating have been studied. The absorption of the studied drug has been reported to improve significantly.

15.5.2. Buccal route

For peptide and protein drug delivery buccal route offers some distinct benefits over other mucosal routes like nasal, vaginal, rectal, etc. Although the buccal route displays less efficiency in absorption but it is robust and comparatively much less sensitive even on long term treatment and this is of importance when penetration enhancers are to be employed. Absence of enzymatic barrier to peptide/protein absorption associated with other mucosal sites is an added advantage. Its close resemblance to oral route is expected to well acceptance by patients. Improved patient compliance is anticipated due to the easy accessibility and administration as dosage forms can be attached and removed without any pain or discomfort.

The buccal membrane is linked by a stratified squamous epithelium that are keratinized in some areas. Drug that penetrates this membrane enter the systemic circulation via a network of capillaries and arteries. The lymphatic drainage almost runs parallel to the venous vascularization and ends up in the jugular ducts.

A multitude of dosage forms are available that can be used to deliver peptide/protein. The conventional means include aqueous solutions and buccal or sublingual tablets and capsules. However, the inherent problem with these dosage forms is the risk of drug loss by accidental swallowing or by the salivary washout. To overcome these drawbacks self-adhesive systems have been designed that are capable of being in intimate contact with the mucosa, either buccally, sublingually or on the gingiva. The various adhesive polymers include water-soluble and insoluble hydrocolloid polymers from both the ionic and the nonionic types. Some of the polymers are sodium carbodxymethylcellulose (Sod. CMC), hydroxypropylmethylcellulose (HPMC), polyvinyl pyrrolidone (PVP), acacia, calcium carbophil, gelatin, polyethyleneglycol (PEG). The anionic polyacrylate-type hydrogel is the most commonly used polymer. The adhesion mechanism involves the entanglement and nonspecific or specific interaction between the polymer chains of polymer (used as the dosage form excipient) and the glycoprotein coat of the mucosal membrane. Drug release from soluble polymers is determined by polymer dissolution and drug diffusion. From the non-soluble hydrogels drug release is reported to follow fickian or non-fickian diffusion kinetics.

The designing of dosage forms with different release rates can be performed on the basis of pharmacodynamics of the peptides. When fast and instantaneous release of peptides is warranted highly permeable or rapidly eroding carriers are desired. However, when sustained release is the motive then approaches like matrix diffusion control, polymer erosion control or membrane controlled transport of the peptide can be utilized.

The various adhesive dosage forms are discussed below:

15.5.2.1. Adhesive tablets

Adhesive tablets for buccal administration were designed on the basis of eroding hydrocolloid/filler tablets. Adhesive tablets of nitroglycerin based on hydroxypropylcellulose have been designed and pharmacodynamic effects were observed for up to 5 hours. In stark contrast to conventional tablets, these adhesive tablets allow speaking and drinking without any major discomfort.

15.5.2.2. Adhesive gels

Viscous adhesive gels have been designed for local therapy using polyacrylic acid and polymethacrylate as gel-forming polymers. Gels are reported to prolong residence time on the oral mucosa to a significant level. This not only improves absorption but also allows for sustained release of the active principle.

15.5.2.3. Adhesive patches

Adhesive patches is a relatively new addition to pharmaceutical technology (Fig. 15.17). The various self adhesive set ups are illustrated in figure 15.18. In these approaches the adhesive polymer may act as the drug carrier itself (case-a and -d), act as an adhesive link between a drug loaded layer and the mucosa (case-c). Alternatively a drug containing disk may be fixed to the mucosa by using a self-adhesive shield (case-b). In this approach drug loss to the saliva is decreased and the drug action and the effect of additives is confined to the site of application by creating a local microenvironment.

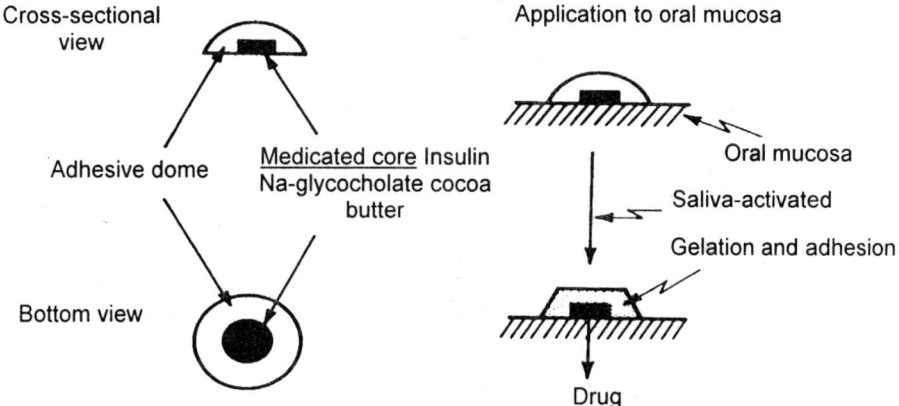

Fig. 15.17 : Diagrammatic illustration of the dome-shaped mucosal adhesive device and its application to oral mucosa

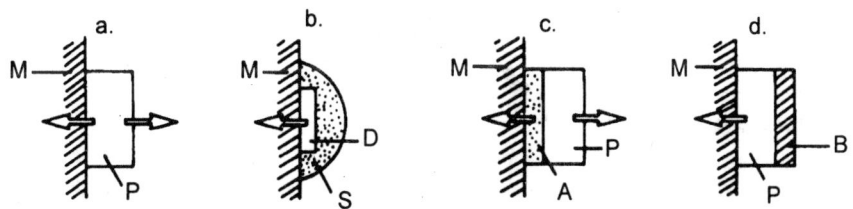

Fig. 15.18 : Schematic representation of various adhesive patches for transmucosal delivery, M - mucosa; P- polymer with peptide; S - adhesive shield; D - drug; A - adhesive layer; B - impermeable back layer

Encouraging results have been obtained with protirelin (a thyrotropin-releasing hormone) and buserelin (a synthetic LHRH derivative). A typical mode of transmucosal patch application is shown in figure 15.19.

15.5.2.4. With the aid of absorption promoters

To augment the efficiency of buccal peptide administration some absorption promoters have been tried. For instance sodium lauryl sulfate, sodium myristate and bile acids have been tried to promote buccal absorption of calcitonin. Enhancement in buccal absorption of insulin was observed when coadministered with sodium glycocholate. Other absorption promoters that have been investigated include sodium 5-methoxysalicylate and citric acid. The challenge with this approach is the need to find biocompatible, non-toxic and effective absorption enhancers.

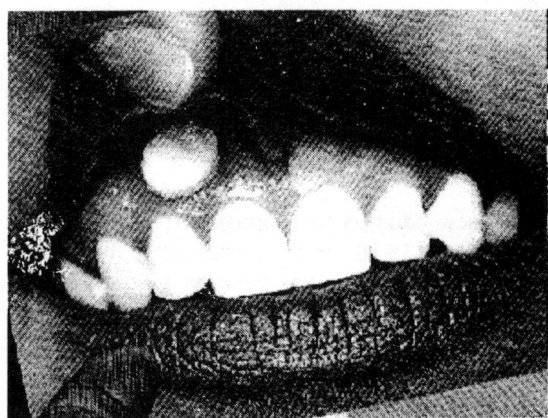

Fig. 15.19 : A patient applying a transmucosal patch

15.5.3. Parenteral route

In the recent times parenteral mode of delivery has been the major route of choice for proteins and peptides, owing to their poor absorption and metabolic instability when given by other alternative routes. This route also offers unique possibility for the targeting of drug moiety.

Potent nature of these peptides/proteins demands their targeting to specific receptors to improve therapeutic index of a drug by optimizing the access, amplitude and nature of interactions and this route precisely aids in achieving this end. There is always the possibility of generation of immune responses and other undesirable and deleterious side effects and interactions, if peptides are present at high dosage levels. Targeting thus protects both the drug and body from these contraindicated manifestations. Targeting may be necessary or desirable event as proteins owing to large size may be unable to leave the drug compartment to their active sites due to their inability to cross various membranes and barriers. Moreover, for these drug moieties pulsed delivery is the preferred mode of delivery rather than the continuous delivery as only then their physiologic delivery pattern is mimicked. This also avoids down-regulation of receptors which generally results due to continuous administration of drug(s). However, all these advantages are overruled by poor acceptance by the patients at large, except those suffering from life-threatening diseases.

15.5.3.1. Parenteral drug delivery systems

These systems include those intended for intravenous, intramuscular, intraarterial, subcutaneous, intraperitoneal and intrathecal use. The drug carrier systems used for defined and controlled delivery of drug through this route can be:

15.5.3.1.1. Particulates

(a) *Microspheres:* These are solid spherical particles in the particle size range of few tenths of a micrometer up to several hundreds micrometer (Fig. 15.20). They contain dispersed drug in either solution or microcrystalline form. They are prepared by various polymerization and encapsulation processes. Microspheres have immense potential in controlled release and targeting of drugs. Biodegradable microspheres of 1:1 copolymer of lactic acid and glycolic acid containing ACTH, poly (d,l-lactide-co-glycolide) microspheres of LHRH,poly (lactide-co-glycolide) microspheres of human serum albumin and poly (d,l-lactide) microspheres of insulin have been tested successfully with promising results. Similar results were obtained with growth hormone and for vaccines based on entrapped antigens and immunomodulators in crystallized carbohydrate spheres.

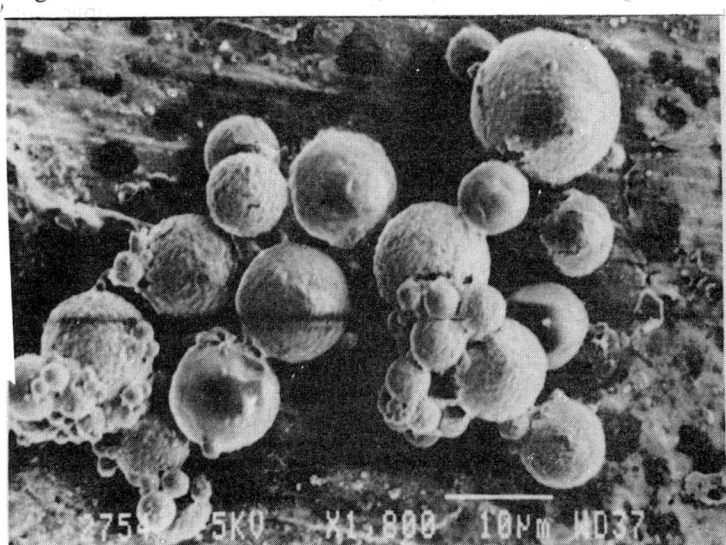

Fig. 15.20 : Photomicrograph (SEM) showing microspheres

Microspheres can be targeted to a particular organ, a specific part of the organ or to a selective intracellular site. Passive targeting can be achieved by occlusion, cellular uptake or local injection. A classical example is targeting of microspheres to the RES (1-7μm particles) and to the lung capillaries (7-12μm particles). The microspheres conjugating receptor specific moieties, such as monoclonal antibodies, (immunomicrospheres) or incorporating magnetic particles, or based on a combination of the two, (magnetic immunomicrospheres) could be used for active peptide(s) or protein targeting. The advantages of microspheres include:

1. can be prepared cheaply if the correct encapsulation method is optimized and chosen, and
2. can be administered subcutaneously, intramuscularly or intraperitoneally and thus implantation is not necessary.

Their disadvantages include:

1. high-molecular weight compounds have limited and restricted loading and their release may be difficult,
2. may successfully pass through biological barriers (like blood, endothelium, RES) and cellular barriers before and they can be effective.
3. may interact or complex with the blood components.

(b) *Microcapsules:* This carrier system holds immense potential for controlled release of peptide moieties from mammalian cells and tissues. The microcapsules are polymeric in nature and prepared employing interfacial polymerization, or interfacial coacervate phase separation of capsule wall forming polymers. The capsule membrane serves as a permeability barrier. The polymers conventionally used include polyvinyl alcohol, polyvinyl acetate, nylon, polyurethane, gelatin, polyacrylonitrile etc. The proteinaceous molecules are effectively entrapped and remain encapsulated within the microcapsules. The capsular system and their application have been discussed in chapter 3 and 4.

(c) *Nanoparticles:* They are very much similar to microspheres but for their particle size which is in the nanometer range (10-1000nm) (Fig. 15.21). They can also be used for targeted delivery. Owing to their small size they can pass through the sinusoidal spaces in the bone-marrow and spleen. Targeting moieties like monoclonal antibodies can be attached to nanoparticles to enhance their specificity. Polycynoacrylate and glycolic acid co-lactate based nanoparticles have been discussed as an effective adjuvant version that demonstrated effective aduvanticity. The immunogenicity of nanoparticulate based antigen(s) was found to be many fold higher than conventional plain form. The better adjuvanticity is attributed to the effective presentation of antigens by nanoparticles. The typical constitutive polymers include cyanoacrylate, polymethacrylate, polystyrene poly co-glyco-lactide, albumin and acrylic resins. The methods employed for preparation are conventional solvation, desolvation, *in situ* micellar polymerization, etc.

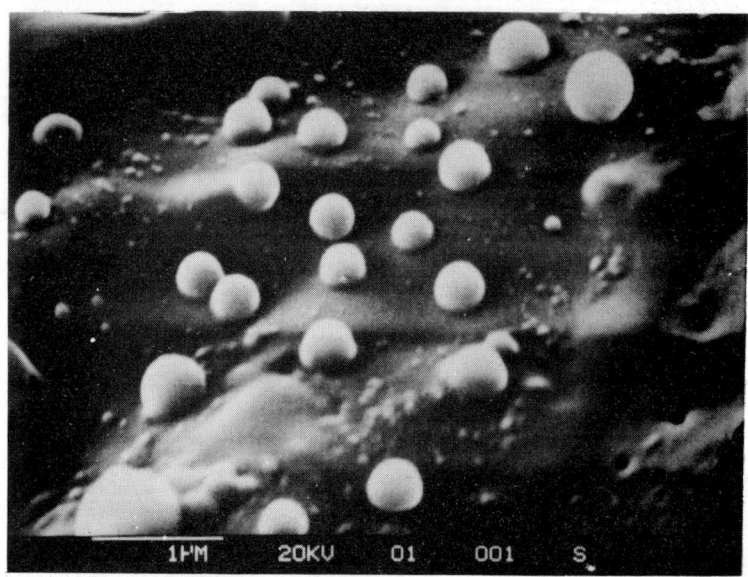

Fig. 15.21 : SEM Photomicrograph of peptide loaded nanoparticles

(d) *Aquasomes :* Aquasomes are self-assembling nanoconstructs comprising of a solid ceramic core and a glassy polyhydroxyl oligomeric surface coating. The system has been studied for the immobilization of various bioactive molecules. These include insulin, antigens for Epstein-Barr virus, HIV, Mussel adhesive protein, hemoglobin, etc.

Water is a vital requirement for maintaining structural conformation of proteins and their biological activities. Nevertheless, it alone cannot sub-serve as a medium which can resist denaturation of the protein molecules. A variety of environment changes such as pH, temperature, tonicity and solvents can cause protein inactivation when in aqueous state leading to irreversible protein inactivation. This has led to the designing of aquasomes which are referred to as **water bodies** being with water-like interactive properties. The latter appear to enable them to preserve biological molecules as well as to act as delivery vehicle.

Proteins are more stable in the solid state, however, dehydration, the loss of water molecules is critical in maintaining the molecular shape and activity. It follows that in order to maintain structural integrity as well as the activity a well balanced mini environment should be contrived so that even on drying a minimum required aqueous domain in immediate vicinity is maintained. Aquasomes, are special systems which while dry and in the solid-state, exhibit water-like properties that enables the molecules to stabilize the 'aqueous conformation' (refer to chapter 3, 4, and 11 for details). Since they are based on ceramic materials coated with polyhydroxyl-oligomeric substances with inherent aqueous properties (bound water) can successfully be utilized for immobilization of susceptible protein and peptide molecules into their well defined interior or through adsorption on to their surface through some keying agent or simple adsorption phenomenon.

Biologically active molecules when adsorbed on to aquasomes and administered intravenously in rabbits, a remarkable *in vivo* activity was observed. For example, aquasome-delivered insulin showed 149.31-156.99 mg/dL fall in blood glucose concentration. This has been attributed to the steric hindrance and hydrodynamic barrier to opsonin which may deter the contents from RES recognition.

(e) *Liposomes*: Liposomes are spherical vesicles formed when phospholipids are allowed to hydrate in an aqueous media. They consist of one or more concentric bilayers surrounding aqueous phases (Fig.15.22). Liposomes are of particular interest since their structure bears great resemblance to that of cell membranes.

Proteins and proteinaceous drug(s) are incorporated in liposomes using dehydration rehydration vesicle (DRV) and reverse phase evaporation methods. Some interesting reports discuss modification of protein in order to lend them an amphiphilic character. The hydrophobic and hydrophilic segment allow them to be intercalated in to the membrane packing. However, the integration could be parallel as shown in figure 15.23 (c) or antiparallel (b) or perpendicular depending on the membrane potential. The membrane potential dependent orientation of α and β helix of a protein is a voltage responsive phenomenon as does operate in the case of natural protein constituents of biomembranes. Nevertheless, antiparallel α and β helix orientation has found to be in a stable state. The protein(s) bearing liposomes can further be surface modified in order to endow them with long circulatory character. The surface modifier(s), i.e., PEG, pullulan coating, Gm coating etc., delay them from their selective RES uptake probably through steric hindrance to opsonin adsorption and as a consequence recognition by reticuloendothelial cells (RES). The modified version has long circulatory half-life thus allowing contained bioactive protein(s) to function as circulatory bioreactive units or slow leaching of therapeutically active protein may result in to its protracted activity profile stretched over a defined period of time segment.

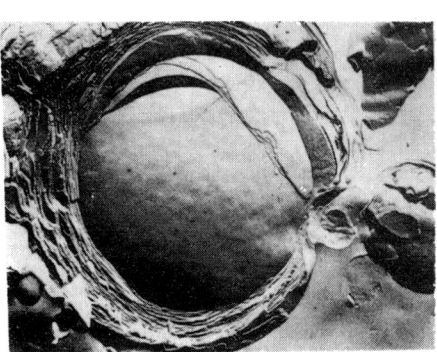 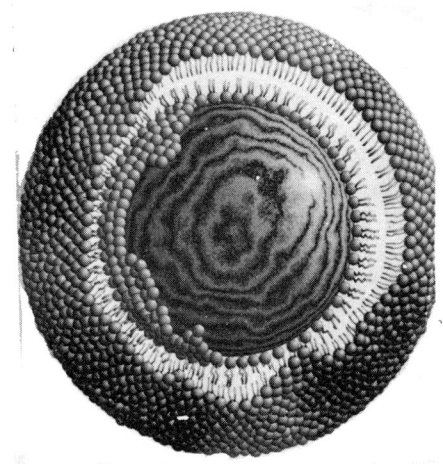

Fig. 15.22 : Freeze fractured SEM photomicrogarph of protein loaded liposomes

Some of the distinct applications of liposomes in parenteral peptide and protein delivery are:

1. After subcutaneous, intramuscular and intraperitoneal injection, liposomes can act as a 'depot', the drug being released slowly with enzymatic degradation and by neutrophils. Intramuscular or subcutaneous administration of liposomes encapsulated insulin and growth hormone immobilized in a collagen matrix resulted in their retention at the site. Similar results were obtained after intramuscular injection of liposomal interferon. Liposomes can be designed to release drug preferentially at a higher temperature attainable by mild local hyperthermia or by application of a magnetic field or by microwave. Various engineered liposomes for selective and programmed delivery of bioactives are discussed in chapter 16.

2. Liposomes protect the entrapped peptides from enzymatic degradation after intravenous administration. Insulin encapsulated in multilamellar liposomes was reported to be more stable against proteolytic enzymes. Cyclosporin entrapped in liposome was observed to be low in nephrotoxicity. Similarly β-fructofuranosidase, amyloglycosidase and neuraminidase have been successfully delivered in liposomes.

3. Liposomes can be exploited for passive targeting of the peptide to a particular site of action. This objective can be achieved by overcoming the two limiting factors, i.e. localizing the liposomes in macrophages and by gaining access to target cells across blood vessel walls. Immunopotentiating agents such as muramyl

dipeptide (MDP) can be delivered to macrophages in liposomes. Calcitonin entrapped in liposome has also been administered successfully. Covalent coupling of antibodies to liposomes can incorporate the specificity to specific cell types or subset of cells within the vascular system.

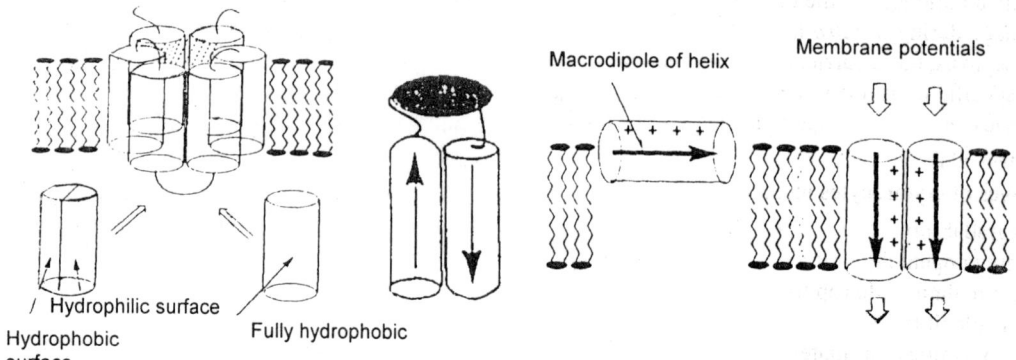

Fig. 15.23 : Topological presentation of protein incorporation into lipid bilayer

Potency of antibody-directed liposomes is proportional to their relative binding and endocytosis by the cells and to the reactivity of the particular antibody with the cell.

The advantages of liposomes include:

1. Flexibility in size, shape and structure.
2. Relatively nontoxic disposition.
3. Ability to encapsulate both hydrophilic and lipophilic peptides and proteins. For instance, the tertiary and quaternary structures of protein can be damaged irreversibly by dehydration. The presence of aqueous phase makes them an excellent delivery system for this class of pharmaceuticals i.e., those soluble in aqueous media.

The drawbacks with particular reference to peptide and protein drug includes:

1. The constituent phospholipids have an inherent tendency to interact with peptides and proteins. This can affect the release kinetics of the peptides/proteins and also the shelf life of the liposomal preparation.
2. Their capacity as adjuvants.
3. Proteins susceptible to aggregation may affect the liposomal stability by initial fusion owing to hydrophobic interaction followed by aggregation.

(f) *Emulsions*: Colloid-sized emulsion droplets can be utilized for parenteral delivery of peptides. This delivery system can be of great significance and utility in protecting hydrophilic or hydrophobic drugs from direct contact with body fluids and also in delivering the drug over a prolonged period of time. Emulsion droplets are usually taken up by the cells of the RES. Multiple emulsion can further prolong the release of drug. After delivery of influenza vaccine and diphtheria toxoid in emulsion, prolonged and higher antibody levels were observed. Subcutaneous administration of muramyl dipeptide in w/o emulsion significantly prolonged the effect. Therapeutic levels of cyclosporin were achieved on its intramuscular administration in intralipid emulsion.

A typically ordered however biphasic emulsion system having one phase as dispersed component where other serves for dispersion vehicle can be a simple, multiple or fat emulsion. The fat emulsion is based on tri-glyceride(s) of unsaturated fatty acid(s) being used as an internal phase. The protein and peptide(s) could be embedded in to the matrix of quasi solidified (viscous) fat droplets. The system offers prolongation of half-life to the contained circulatory protein.

The stability and fate of parentally administered emulsion droplets is decided by the nature of the emulsifying agent used. Drug release from emulsions is controlled by the droplet size of the dispersed phase and the emulsion viscosity. The advantages of emulsion systems are their clinical acceptability and the amenability to large-scale production. The use of this system is rather limited but investigations are in progress to utilize their potential for delivery of peptides.

(g) *Cellular carriers*: Enzymes and/or other proteinaceous pharmaceuticals can be encapsulated in erythrocytes to achieve a prolonged release or targeting of the same. Some of the methods of encapsulation include hemolysis, dialysis, and electric field breakdown. The carrier erythrocytes usually display a bimodal survival curve with a rapid loss of the cells in the first 24 h following injection and a much slower loss of cells afterward. Cell damage during *in vitro* handling is responsible for an early loss. Once damaged erythrocytes are removed by phagocytosis, these carriers can be taken up by spleen or liver. The release of drug occurs by simple diffusion or by a specific transport system following phagocytosis. Some of the enzymes investigated for delivery using erythrocytes include arginase in hyperargineamia L-asparginase for leukemia and aminolevulinic acid dehydratase in prophyrias.

Advantages of erythrocytes include:

1. Biodegradability.
2. Nonimmunogenicity.
3. Large circulation life (up to 4 months).
4. Easy availability.
5. Large quantities of material can be entrapped in small volume of cells (about 20-80%) extracellular concentration.
6. Afford enzymatic and immunological protection.

Drawbacks include:

1. Long-term storage is problematic.
2. Permeable to a large number of drugs .
3. Only those drugs that are not susceptible to irreversible denaturation under hypotonic conditions can be used.

An alternative approach is the utilization of mammalian cells. Ricin toxin has been administered in this delivery vehicle. Immobilized enzymes bound covalently to polymers are reported to have increased stability in circulation and decreased ability to provoke undesirable complications. Another approach that prevents immune rejection of the cells and also aids in controlling the release is to encapsulate the cell within semi-permeable aqueous microcapsule. Microencapsulated pancreatic islet of Langerhans cells are reported to provide a long-term insulin delivery in comparison to pumps. The encapsulated cells as artificial prosthesis have been discussed in detail in chapter 4.

(h) *Replication defective viruses:* Retroviral gene delivery systems have been developed to assist in entry of genes into the cells. This system consists of an RNA copy of a gene package into a viral particle. This is an excellent alternative to physical methods of gene delivery, such as direct injection into the nucleus. The basic concept of gene therapy is that functionally active genes are delivered into the somatic cells of a patient with genetic defect. This mode of treatment can either be gene replacement or gene augmentation. The former involves specific correction of a mutant gene sequence while in the latter a correctly functioning gene is inserted into non-specific sites in a genome and thereby leaving the malfunctioning gene alone.

In a virus, an RNA-protein core is encapsulated in a lipid envelope. The viral glycoproteins bind with specific receptors on target cells, and the viral envelope then fuses with the cell membrane thereby introducing RNA genome into the target cell cytoplasm. Non replicating viral vectors that infect human cells have been developed. An RNA copy of a replacement gene is packed into a nonreplicating viral particle, when the viral gene delivery systems infect target cells, both the viral and exogenous genes are expressed by these cells. However, problems may be posed if sequences are deleted during replication, recombination with endogenous viral sequences occur to produce infectious recombinant viruses, by activation of cellular oncogenes, by introduction of viral oncogenes and by the inactivation of genes.

15.5.3.1.2. Soluble carriers (Macromolecules)

Soluble carrier systems include conjugates, chemically modified drugs and hybrid proteins. The peptide/protein drug can be conjugated with a polymer/macromolecule. This not only decreases immunogenicity, but also improves protease stability and helps in achieving selective or targeted drug delivery. Immunological properties of bovine serum albumin can be reduced by conjugation with polyethylene glycol. Likewise, asparaginase was chemically modified by a DL-alanine-N-carboxyanhyride polymerization technique. The modified enzyme not only retained most of its catalytic activity but also had better protease stability and demonstrated a 7 to 10 fold prolongation in plasma clearance properties. It is hypothesized that polymers serve as a steric barrier (Fig.15.24), which hampers the interaction of macromolecules (antibodies, proteases, immunogenic and/or clearance recognition receptors) with the native enzyme, while macromolecular substances (substrates, products, coenzymes, etc.) can still interact with the enzyme. Polymer modifications bring with it the following changes:

1. Masking of antigenic determinants.
2. Masking of protease-susceptible sites.
3. Masking of immunogenic recognition signals.
4. Masking of clearance recognition signals.
5. Allow free access to low-molecular weight substrates.
6. Alter optimum pH by changing microenvironment.

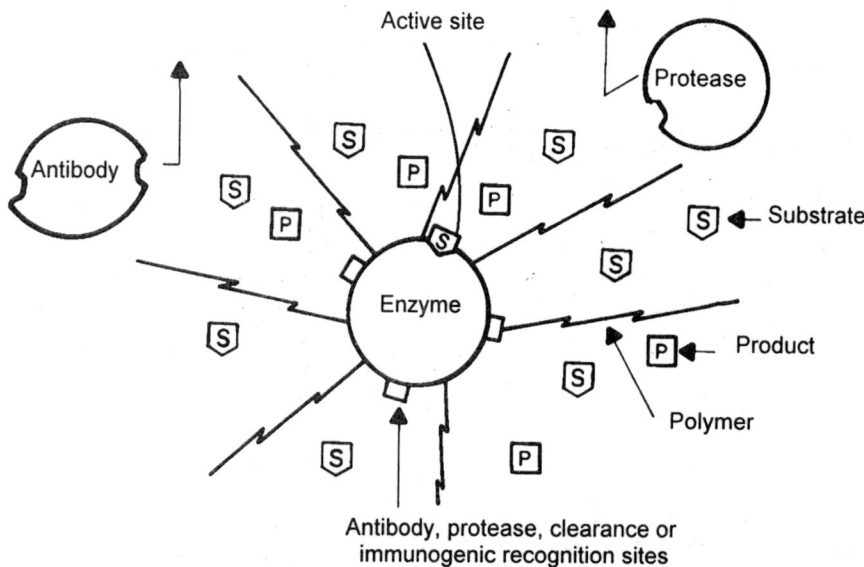

Fig. 15.24 : Model explaining the enzymatic and biological properties of poly-DL-alamylasparaginases

Protein molecules can themselves act as carriers for targeting of other peptides/proteins. The four basic mechanisms involved in targeting are schematically presented in (Fig. 15.25).

1. Interaction with surface receptor.
2. Facilitated uptake and interaction of intact molecules with intracellular target site.
3. Facilitated uptake and intracellular release of warhead moiety.
4. Facilitated uptake and release of a suicide warhead, which is activated only after interacting with its target.

Naturally occurring multi-subunit proteins of toxins also act as conjugates. The subunits of these moieties have different roles. For instance, if one subunit mediates binding, the other is the pharmacologically active entity. A classic example of this type of carriers is the B chain of ricin toxin that has been used with interferon and insulin. The specific binding and the antiviral activity of the conjugate was inhibited in the presence of galactose, an inhibitor of ricin B chain binding.

The ricin A chain can also be conjugated to binding subunit of other proteins or monoclonal antibody to tumor antigen for cytotoxic effect in tumor cells. Synthetic polypeptide carriers have been used as ligands such as muramyl dipeptide. With these carriers the conjugation is multiple and results in to an increased receptor affinity, increased potency, enhanced resistance to enzymatic degradation and prolonged duration of action.

One of the major drawback of this technique is the limited ability of these conjugates to cross capillary endothelium and their susceptibility to removal by the RES.

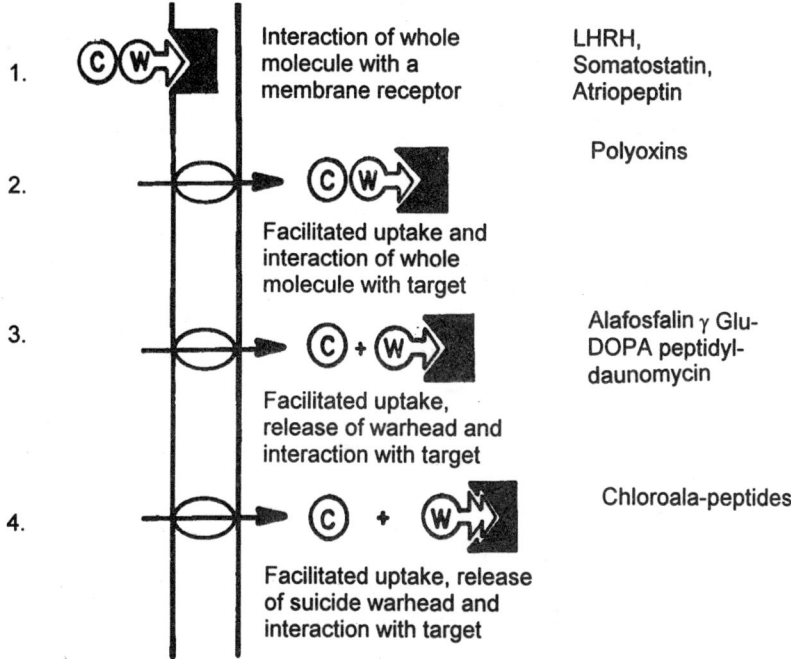

Fig. 15.25 : Schematic representation of mechanisms for targeting peptide drugs

15.5.3.1.3. Others

Some of the other sophisticated systems designed and engineered for parenteral controlled and targeted delivery of proteins and peptides include:

(a) *On-demand systems:* In certain cases it is beneficial to have externally augmented delivery on-demand as in delivery of insulin to patients with diabetes mellitus. Magnetically modulated systems have been designed to achieve this end. The release rate is influenced by the position, orientation and strength of the embedded magnets, the amplitude and frequency of the applied magnetic field and the mechanical properties of polymer matrix. Another approach for external modulation of release is the application of ultrasound (20 kHz for 20 minutes).

(b) *Self-regulated systems:* The self-regulated systems are of great importance to deliver insulin in response to blood glucose concentration for diabetic patients. One of the polymer-based systems utilizes a cationic hydrogel polymer with immobilized glucose oxidase. As glucose diffuses into this glucose-sensitive polymer, the glucose oxidase catalyzes its conversion to gluconic acid. Thereby, the pH of the microenvironment within the membrane is lowered and the amine groups in the membrane are protonated. Due to this, the membrane swells and its permeability to the insulin held in a continuous reservoir increases. However, this approach holds promise only for small peptide molecules. Another approach with a slight modification is based on the increase in solubility of a modified insulin derivative with a decrease in pH in the membrane and corresponding increase in release. A biochemical approach based on competitive binding between glucose and glycosylated insulin (G-insulin) to concanavalin A (lectin) has also been reported. The functioning of system is classically based on affinity binding principle where high affinity ligand occupies the site of binding while low affinity ligand as a consequence released in to the environment where it acts as a therapeutic entity (insulin). The strategy judiciously operates through affinity exclusion as higher affinity ligand that is sequestered and removed from circulation otherwise is a toxic molecule i.e., (glucose). With an increase in glucose level, the influx of the glucose to the pouch increases and thereby G-insulin is displaced from the concanavalin A substrate (Fig. 15.26). The increase in displaced G-insulin in the pouch results in efflux of G-insulin from the system to the body.

(c) Temperature sensitive systems: Some polymers like polyacrylamide derivatives have inherent thermo-sensitive swelling behavior. This leads to a temperature-dependent release pattern that can be exploited in pulsatile delivery of peptides/proteins. It was observed that the temperature sensitivity of insulin permeation through a poly-N-isopropylacrylamide-butylmethacrylate copolymer membrane varies with the hydrophobic component of the copolymer. With increasing hydrophobic co-monomer component in a copolymer, a fractional however gradual drop (37°C to 27°C) in temperature sensitivity was recorded. The sensitivity implies for polymer gate opening character to allow efflux of entrapped protein. The thermosensitive permeation demonstrated reversibility without noticeable lag times. Similar temperature-dependent release pattern due to swelling was observed for myoglobin in N-isopropylacrylamide gel and bovine serum albumin in ethylene-vinyl acetate matrix .

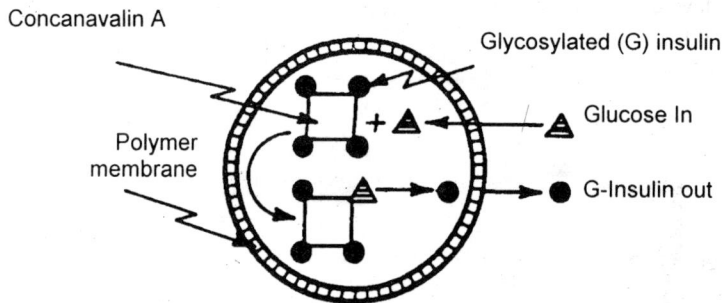

Fig. 15.26 : Schematic diagram of a self-regulating insulin delivery system

(d) Pumps: A pump is different from other diffusion-based system in that the primary driving force for delivery by a pump is pressure difference and not the concentration difference of the drug between the formulation and the surroundings. The pressure difference can be generated by pressurizing a drug reservoir, by osmotic action or by direct mechanical actuation. The pump can either be implantable or externally portable.

(i) Mechanical pumps: Most of the portable pumps for insulin delivery are syringe driven, either lead screw or direct drive. Another widely used principle is roller peristaltic. This utilizes a disposable bag and silicone outlet tube. The tube is stretched around the roller mechanism, and as the roller turns, the contents of the tube are expelled from the cannula. However, this type of drive requires careful filling to avoid air inclusion. Infusaid® implantable pumps sensitive to ambient temperature and pressure have been developed. Portable infusion devices for open-loop insulin delivery and for pulsatile therapy of LHRH have also been designed and developed. For practical reason, the use of infusion pump is restricted to subcutaneous insulin delivery as the routine use of the intravenous and intraperitoneal routes is too hazardous. Infusion pumps have also been used for growth hormone, vasopressin, calcitonin, glucagon and somatostatin.

The advantages of infusion pumps include:

- More flexibility and freedom for the patient.
- The potential for achieving physiological levels of the drug.

The disadvantages of pump therapy may or may not be pump-specific. They are:

- Possibility for mechanical or electrical failure.
- Inconvenient and difficult to use.
- Costly.
- Chances of dermatological complications.
- Aggregation of peptide/protein drug may be problematic since many of the pumps rely on a linear relationship between volumetric flow rate and actual drug delivery rate.

(ii) Osmotic Pumps: Osmotic pumps have been used extensively for delivery of a large number of peptides and protein drugs in animals. Some of the representative examples include insulin, ACTH, calcitonin, LHRH, growth hormone, neutrotensin, vasopressin. Osmotic pumps are simple in principle, small and reliable. The critical features of this pump are stability of the drug at 37°C within the pump for the entire infusion period and the compatibility of the drug with the internal pump components. The osmoregulatory mini pump is structurally consisted of a central drug and osmogen core coated with a semipermeable polymeric rigid lamella. The osmogen facilitates the penetration of biofluid(s) into the pump however the dimensional variation in pump is not allowed thus forcing out drug solution under osmotic gradient through appropriates openings or orifices. There is less flexibility in the delivery program and reservoir volume is low, and hence requires for frequent replacement.

(iii) Controlled-release micropumps: This is a novel addition to the implantable pumps (Fig.15.27). The concentration difference between the drug reservoir and the delivery site causes diffusion of the drug to the delivery site to provide basal delivery. Thus, no external power source is required. A piezoelectric controlled micropump has also been developed. This comprises of piezoelectric disk bender and a cellulose acetate microporous membrane located at the opposite sides of the insulin reservoir. A considerable augmentation in delivery was obtained on applying a square-wave voltage (100 to 1000 Hz, 20 to 90 Vdc) to the piezoelectric bender.

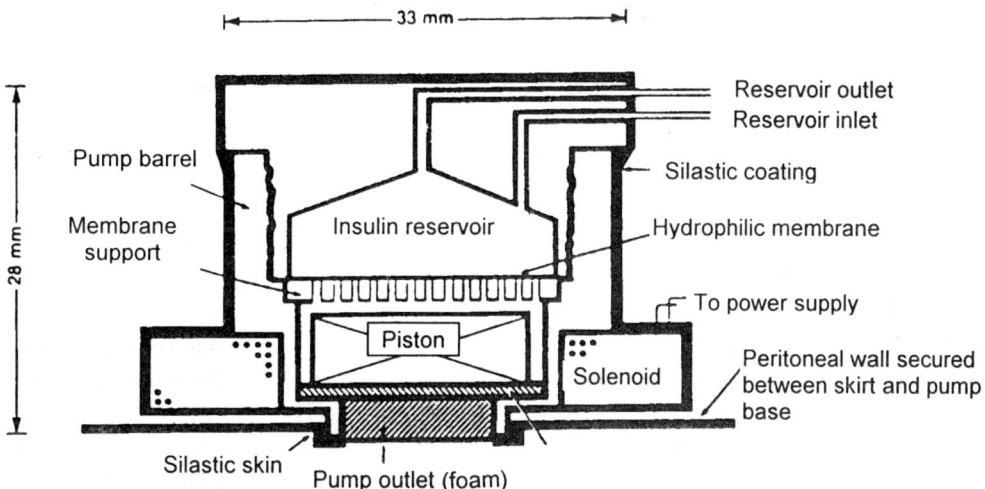

Fig. 15.27 : Schematic illustration of prototype VIII of controlled-release micropump

The exceptional advantages of controlled-release micropumps include:

1. Less susceptible to limiting problems such as catheter blockage and mechanical failure due to absence of an outlet catheter, valves and motors.
2. In case of failure no chances of accidental overdosage due to presence of the membrane and lack of a valve system.

Some of the limitations are:

1. Long term stability of the membrane to repeated compression is to be considered.
2. The location of implant is limited by the need to minimize diffusion resistance and the biocompatibility of the pump exterior plays an important role in this.

Some approaches based on electrochemical principles have been proposed for implantable pumps. One such technique is electroosmosis through a cation-exchange membrane. The membrane is placed between two Ag/AgCl electrodes and an aqueous NaCl solution. On application of electric potential, hydrated Na^+ ions pass through the membrane accompanied by the movement of volume of fluid. A to-and-fro transport of fluid through the membrane was effected due to the reversing of the direction of the current.

Some of the identified advantages of this pump are:

1. Low power requirement.
2. High reliability.
3. Very low flow rates (in µl/day).

Drawbacks include:

1. Possibility of the consumption of electrodes.
2. Necessary valve and reservoir arrangements have not yet been devised.

15.5.4. Rectal route

The large intestine is drained by the hepatic portal vein as well as by the lymphatics. It has been demonstrated that in the lower colon the drainage is mostly lymphatic. With an increase in the molecular weight of a compound, its lymphatic uptake is also augmented. Compounds with molecular weight greater than 2,000 predominantly make an entry into the lymphatic fluid. Thus rectal delivery of peptides and proteins avoids not only the presystemic or first-pass metabolism but also the g.i. tract peptidases. The bypass of hepatic portal system is attributed to the fact that the lower hemorrhoidal veins do not enter the hepatic portal system (Fig. 15.28). Thus, a considerable portion of the rectally absorbed drug enters the general circulation directly. Tight intercellular junctions of the columnar epithelium of the rectal mucosa limits the bioavailability of peptides and proteins.

Rectal absorption of peptides and proteins has been reported. The literature is replete with examples of rectal delivery of insulin. Even relatively large polypeptides like lysozyme have been reported to be absorbed from rectum. Encouraging results have been obtained with calcitonin, gastrin, pentagastrin and tetragastrin.

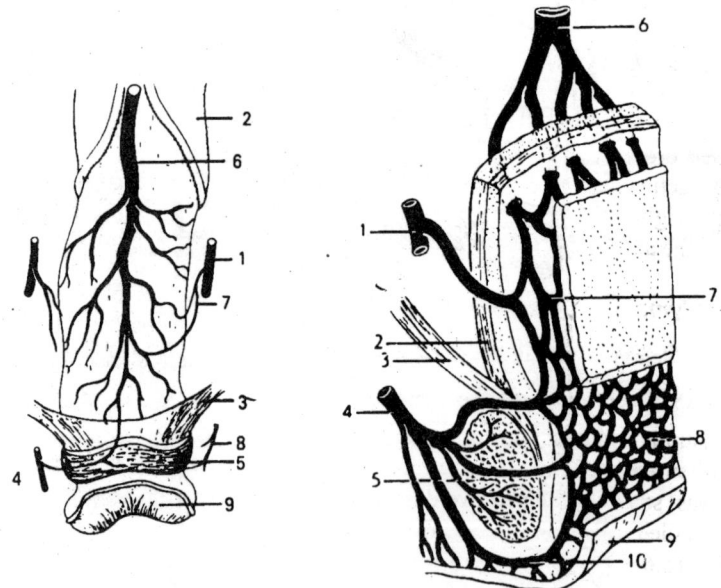

Fig. 15.28 : The venous drainage of human rectum : 1. Middle rectal vein, 2. Tunica muscularis; Stratum longitudinal, 3. Levator ani, 4. Inferior rectal vein, 5. External anal sphincter, 6. Superior rectal vein, 7 and 8. Submucus venous plexus, 9. Skin, 10. Marginal vein and subcutaneous plexus.

15.5.4.1. Adjuvants to enhance the absorption

Most of the peptide/protein drugs require absorption enhancers to obtain reasonable extent of drug absorption. These include surface-active agents, bile acids, saponins, phospholipids, organic alcohols, acids, salts, amines and fats.

Surfactants: Several surfactants including Tween 40, 60 and 61, Span 40, Cetomacrogol, various poly-oxyethylene ethers and esters, glycerylmonostearate, sodiumlaurylsulfate and dioctylsulfosuccinate are reported to enhance absorption. It appears that surfactants interact with the lipoidal fraction of the membrane and in short term the effect is irreversible. It is postulated that surface-active agents enhance drug absorption through damage to the rectal mucosa.

Salicylates: Sodium salicylate, 3-methoxysalicylate, 5-methoxysalicylate and homovanilate were found to be effective in enhancing the rectal absorption of a number of drugs. The effectiveness of sodium salicylate was augmented in the presence of sodium chloride and reduced in the presence of inhibitors like phlorizin and 4, 4'-diisothiocyano-stilbene-2,2'-disulfonic acid (DIDS). Small amounts (<0.5 mg/ml) of N-ethylamaleimide (NEM) or sodium p-chloromercuriphenylsulfonic acid (p-CMP) on concurrent administration reduce the effectiveness of sodium salicylate. However, higher absorption of cefoxitin was observed with higher concentration of (>1 mg/ml) of the same. Ouabain and 2,4-dinitrophenol (DNP) are also reported to inhibit the effectiveness of salicylate as an absorption enhancer. It has been hypothesized that the effects of salicylate occur through a saturable process at the protein fraction of the rectal mucosa.

Ethylenediamine tetra acetic acid (EDTA): EDTA has been reported to enhance the rectal absorption of salicylate and decrease the absorption of m-and p-hydroxybenzoic acids. It has been found to enhance the absorption of sodium cefoxitin. Oubain and DNP suppressed the enhancing effects of EDTA when EDTA was administered at low doses. At higher concentrations of EDTA, DNP had little effect and the effects of EDTA were partially suppressed by ouabain.

Fatty acid enhancers: A number of studies have been carried out with fatty and carboxylic acids as enhancers. It is reported that the effectiveness of the carboxylic acid sodium salts for the rectal absorption of several β-lactam antibiotics is parabolically related to their partition coefficient on a logarithmic basis. Carboxylic acids having metal ion chelating ability enhance the rectal absorption of poorly absorbed drugs including the water-soluble antibiotics. It was suggested that carboxylic acids may serve to make the intercellular space more accessible by temporary removal of calcium ions from the rectal mucosa. With the removal of calcium ions the integrity of the tight junctions is lost. Sodium cefoxitin administered in a triglyceride based suppository form to the small intestine showed promising results. This was supposed to be because of the generation of fatty acids from triglycerides by the action of lipase. In their ionized forms these act as surfactants in the luminal fluid. However, when the same triglyceride suppositories are administered in rectum no increment in absorption was observed, possibly due to the absence of lipase activity in the rectum.

15.5.4.2. Importance of lymphatic uptake

As discussed above, drug on rectal administration bypasses the hepatic portal system and makes direct entry to the general circulation. Lymphatic absorption of drugs also account for delivery of drugs directly to the general circulation, especially the water soluble ones. There are reports indicating the uptake of lymphatic uptake of drugs after rectal administration. They concluded that insulin primarily transported via the lymphatic system to the general circulation when administered in the presence of 5-methoxysalicylate. Also, the peak appearance of insulin in the lymph was somewhat earlier than that in the plasma. In the absence of adjuvants rectal administration of insulin failed to produce appreciable concentrations in the plasma and lymph. The concept is further detailed in section 15.6.

15.5.5. Nasal Route

Until recently, the nasal route was limited to producing local action on the mucosa. But this route appears to hold immense promise for the delivery of peptides and proteins and has lately received considerable attention. This route is not only convenient but also has a large surface area available for absorption, the mucosa is highly vascularized and first-pass metabolism can be avoided. Anatomically the length of nasal cavity is approximately 12 cm with a total volume of 15 ml. It covers about 150 cm^2 area divided into olfactory and vestibule regions. Most of the area is accounted for respiratory region. Major of nasal cavity is covered by epithelium line with microvilli and cilia forming a dense carpet like structure. Functionally, cilia removes mucus and deposited particles from nasal cavity. The main contributory factors towards physiological environments include change in mucus secretion, pH and viscosity and ciliary motility and viability. These factors are mainly affected by the presence of foreign substances and appreciated to have an impact on drug absorption through this route. Figure 15.29 gives the cross-sectional view of the nasal cavity. The nasal mucosa is relatively more permeable to peptides as compared against routes like oral and transdermal. The bioavailability of peptides through this route is reported to be of the order of 1 to 20%. This depends on the physical properties and molecular weight of the peptide but can be extremely variable.

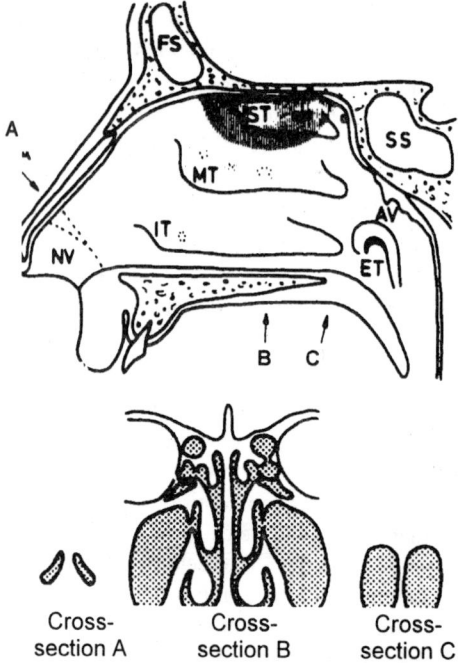

Fig. 15.29 : Lateral view and cross-sections of the nasal cavity through : A - internal ostium; B - middle of the nasal cavity; C - choanae; NV - nasal vestibule; IT - inferior turbinate; MT - middle turbinate; ST - superior turbinate; FS - frontal sinus; SS - sphenoidal sinus; AV - adenoid vegetations; ET - orifice of eustachain tube

Some of the disadvantages of the nasal route include:

1. Extent of absorption varies with the mucous secretion and turnover
2. Mucociliary clearance represents a physical and temporal barrier
3. Peptidase present in the nasal membrane serves as an enzymatic barrier in absorption
4. Alteration in absorption profile in diseased conditions like allergic and chronic rhinitis and upper respiratory tract infections.
5. Penetration enhancers and preservatives may damage mucosal cell membrane and may even be ciliotoxic.

Peptidal and proteinaceous moieties like calcitonin, ACTH, insulin and interferon are reported to have appreciable absorption through nasal mucosa. Lypressin, a synthetic analogue of vasopressin has been introduced commercially as an intranasal dosage form following encouraging clinical trials. Encouraging results have also been obtained with GnRH, LHRH, buserelin, enkephalins and GHRF. Pituitary hormones like vasopressin and oxytocin have been administered by the nasal route for many years.

15.5.5.1. Mechanism to facilitate nasal peptide and protein absorption

Nasal absorption of drugs can be via passive diffusion or by special transport mechanisms. Nasal absorption of metkephamid for instance, is by passive diffusion. A prominent example of transport by special mechanism is sodium guaiazulene-3-sulfonate (GAS). It is believed to be absorbed mainly by a carrier-mediated transport mechanism. Large peptides and proteins are unable to cross the nasal membrane as efficiently as smaller peptides, therefore in order to facilitate their absorption usually adjuvants as absorption enhacer are required.

Several approaches have been used to facilitate nasal peptide and protein absorption. They are-

15.5.5.1.1. pH modification

Peptides and proteins usually exhibit the lowest solubility at their isoelectric point. Thus, by adjusting the pH farther away from the isoelectric point of a particular peptide, its solubility can be increased. It has been demonstrated that insulin is capable of crossing the nasal membrane in an acidic medium. At pH 6.1 the nasal absorption recorded for insulin was the least. This pH was close to the isoelectric point of insulin.

15.5.5.1.2. Dissociation of aggregation

Proteins are likely to form higher-order aggregates in solution. For instance, at pH 7.0, insulin exists in solution predominantly as hexameric aggregates. Insulin failed to cross the nasal membrane in the absence of an enhancer in the formulation. However, good nasal absorption of insulin was observed with sodium deoxycholate. Studies have suggested that sodium deoxycholate disrupts the formation of insulin hexamers and higher-order aggregates. On the basis of these reports, it is assumed that dissociation of insulin hexamers to dimers and monomers by sodium deoxycholate is partly responsible for enhancing the transport of insulin across the nasal epithelium.

15.5.5.1.3. Reverse micelle formation

Bile salts are known to promote the transmembrane movement of endogenous and exogenous lipids, and other polar substances within the g.i. tract by the virtue of their ability to affect the micellar properties of biomembranes. For this very reason, the bile salts present a lucrative option as an adjuvant for transmucosal delivery of drugs. It is reported that with an increase in the hydrophobicity of bile salts its adjuvant activity correspondingly increased. The adjuvant potency for nasal absorption of insulin correlates positively with increasing hydrophobicity of the bile salts. On the basis of the data it was concluded that the hydrophobicity of the steroid nucleus is the major determinant of adjuvant activity. This study also suggested that the insulin absorption commences at the critical micelle concentration of the bile salts and attains a maximal level when micelle formation approaches a well established level. In reverse micelles, the hydrophilic surfaces of the molecules face inward and the hydrophobic ones face outward from the lipid environment. Thus, reverse micelles can be utilized as transmembrane channels or mobile carriers for insulin to move down an aqueous concentration gradient through the nasal mucosal cells, into the intercellular space and finally into the blood stream.

15.5.5.1.4. Membrane transport and enzyme inhibition

Penetration enhancers like bile salts, surface active agents and chelating agents are reported to increase nasal absorption of peptides and proteins. They increase the fluidity of the lipid bilayer membrane and open up aqueous pores as a result of calcium ion chelation. Peptidase inhibitors enhance the absorption of peptide/ protein by depressing peptidase activity in both the mucus and mucosal cells.

Studies have been carried out to study the relationship between the absorption-promoting effect of surfactants like sodium lauryl sulfate and their effect on biomembrane in terms of hemolytic activity and protein releasing effect on the nasal mucosa. It was concluded that the effect of these surfactants on the permeability of the nasal mucosa to insulin may be due to the disturbance of the structural integrity of the nasal mucosa. However, bile salts exhibited less effect on biomembranes in comparison to other surfactants, in terms of hemolytic profile and protein release from the nasal mucosa.

The addition of bile salts is reported to inhibit the enzymatic activity of leucine aminopeptidase and the enzymatic degradation of insulin. Thus, bile salts affect both the permeability of the nasal mucosa and the activity of proteolytic enzymes, and thereby enhance the absorption as a whole.

However, reports indicate that penetration enhancers can damage the nasal mucosa. The membrane damage may be in terms of cell erosion, cell to cell separation and loss of cilia. Laureth-9 is one such surfactant.

Absorption promoters like linoleic acid and oleic acid seem to enhance absorption safely. The effect of these agents are readily reversible within 15-20 minutes after washing. For instance, sodium taurodihydrofusidate serves as an excellent nasal absorption enhancer of insulin and is nontoxic both systemically and locally.

15.5.5.1.5. Increased nasal blood flow

With an increase in local nasal blood flow an enhancement in nasal peptide absorption has been reported. This can be attributed to an increase in the concentration gradient for passive peptide diffusion. Vasoactive agents which are known to enhance nasal blood flow include histamine, prostaglandin E_1 and beta-adrenergic agonists. Studies indicate that in comparison to control, the combination of histamine and desmopressin, an antidiuretic, led to an increase in nasal blood flow and a corresponding increase in antidiuretic activity. The increase in duration of activity of desmopressin was found to be in line with the increased nasal absorption of the peptide.

In practice, considering the long term use of nasal route, it appears to rank low due to the possible toxicity in mucosa and cilia. Alterations in the nasal environment during disease states also limits its application. However, it appears to hold immense potential for short-term delivery of peptides/proteins, small molecular-weight peptides in particular.

15.5.6. Transdermal route

In contemporary therapeutics, oral route is the most preferred route of administration. However, there lies numerous barriers in administering a peptide/protein drug. Secondly, a programmed drug delivery system for the delivery of peptide and protein was of utmost importance in order to have a constant and continual therapeutic level of the drug in the systemic circulation. This necessitated for the search of an alternative route other than oral, vaginal, intravenous or mucoadhesive routes. The site of application/administration that was then exploited for this reason was the **'skin'**. Skin has been used as the site for topical administration of dermatological drugs to achieve localized pharmacological activity. This mode of drug administration was named as **transdermal drug delivery** since the skin serves as the site for administration of the drug.

Until recently, the utility of intact skin as a port for continuous transdermal delivery of drugs was confined to topical medication. With an insight into the anatomy and physiology of the skin and percutaneous absorption it is now evident that through this route benefits of i.v. drug infusion (i.e., direct entry into the systemic circulation and control over drug levels) can be closely duplicated without its inherent hazards. The schematic cross-section of skin is presented in figure 15.30.

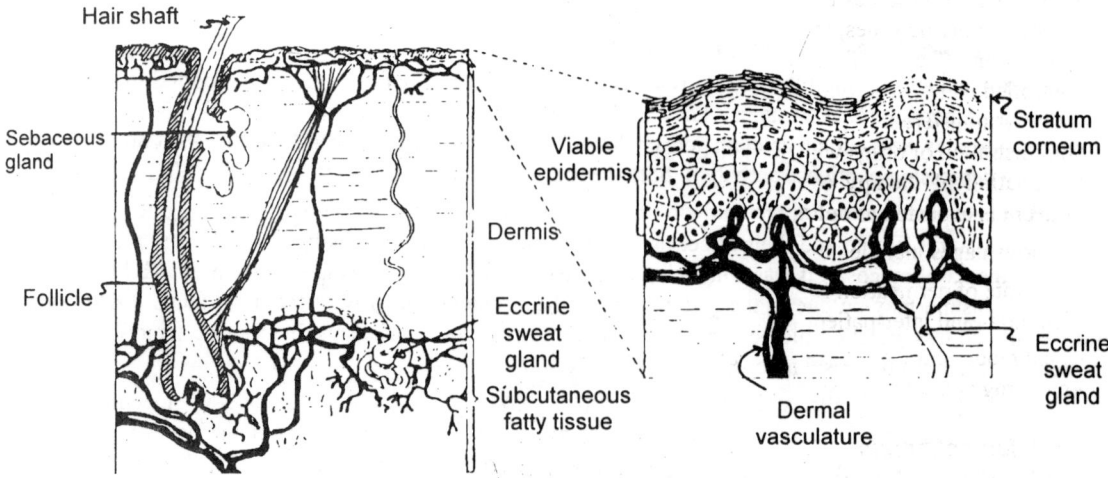

Fig. 15.30 : Schematic cross-section of the skin

Transdermal drug delivery, serves as the site for administration of systemically active drugs. However, the topically applied drug must be distributed following skin permeation, first into the systemic circulation and then transported to the target tissues, which could be distantly located in the body. Skin which lacks in proteolytic enzymes offers the major advantage for the administration of peptides and proteins.

Several transdermal drug delivery systems (TDDS) have recently been developed. These systems can be classified, according to the technological basis involved in their construction, into four categories (Fig.15.31).

1. Membrane permeation-controlled,
2. Adhesive dispersion-type,
3. Matrix diffusion-controlled and
4. Microreservoir dissolution-controlled.

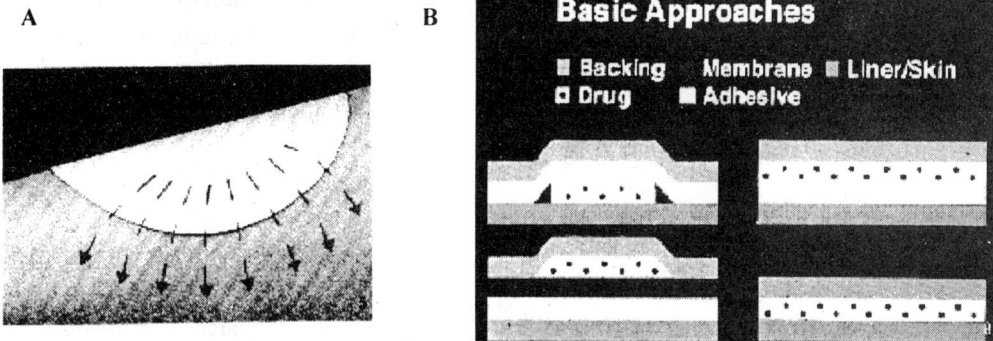

Fig. 15.31 : A. Schematic representation of active drug zone and its release from a TDDS. **B.** Cross-sectional view showing structural components of a TDDS

Although these systems have demonstrated usefulness in affording transdermal controlled delivery of pharmaceuticals that are somewhat lipophilic and relatively small in molecular size, they are having certain limitations in the delivery of peptides and protein drugs. Biological molecules greater than 1000 kDa are not favorable candidates for delivery through TDDS as their structural dimensions do not allow them to permeate across the stratum corneum. However, low molecular weight peptides and peptidomimetics may successfully be administered using various TDDS in along with some well identified permeation enhancers.

Thus, this route not only has improved patient compliance but also offers the following advantages.

1. Elimination of variables that affect g.i. absorption, like pH changes, presence of enzymes, food variations in stomach emptying times, intestinal motilities.
2. Elimination of hepatic first-pass phenomenon
3. Controlled administration is possible and thereby avoidance of toxic effects. Also drugs with shorter half-life can be administered.
4. Administration of drugs with low therapeutic indices are possible.
5. Termination of therapy can be achieved by simply removing the topical device. However, the stratum corneum is expected to deliver drug moieties for some time after removal of delivery system.

The disadvantages include:

1. A low rate of permeation for most protein drugs due to their large molecular weight and hydrophilicity
2. High intra- and inter-patient variability.

A typical mode of transdermal patch application is shown in figure 15.32. Various approaches have been used to improve drug penetration. Some of these are discussed below:

15.5.6.1. Iontophoresis

Iontophoresis is a method that induces migration of ions or charged molecules when an electric current is allowed to flow through an electrolyte medium. In addition to electrophoresis, it serves as a promising strategy to facilitate the membrane transport of charged molecules depending on their ionic characteristics. It is evident that to undergo iontophoresis the peptide and protein molecules must carry a charge. This can be achieved by controlling the pH and ionic strength of the solution. Usually, the drug containing in gauze pad is applied to the skin under an electrode of the same charge as the drug. The other electrode bearing the opposite charge is placed on the gauze pad soaked in saline at a distal location of the body. A small current corresponding to that below the patient pain threshold is applied for a sufficient period of time.

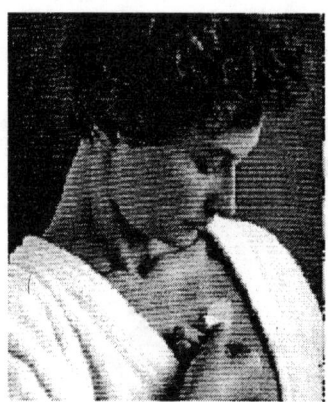 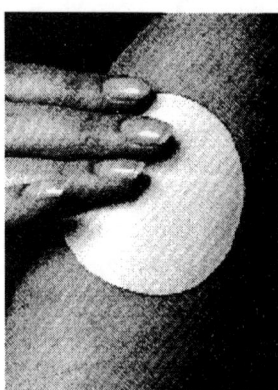

Fig. 15.32 : Application of transdermal patch

Attempts have been made to administer insulin and TRH through transdermal iontophoretic delivery. Delivery of insulin as a highly ionized monomeric form in the presence of iontophoresis produced promising results. Studies with TRH also indicated improvement in delivery. Figure 15.33 illustrates the mechanism of the transdermal iontophoretic delivery of peptide and protein drugs for systemic administration.

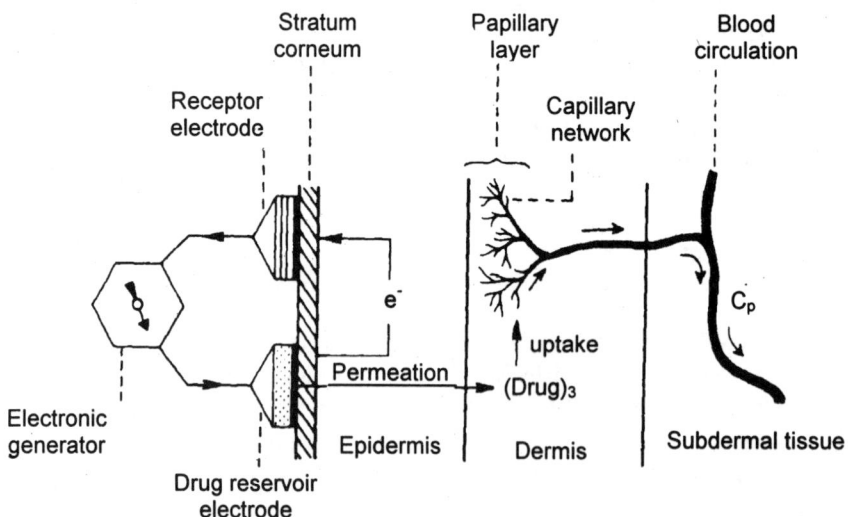

Fig. 15.33 : Diagrammatic illustration of the transdermal iontophoretic delivery of peptide and protein drugs across the skin

The disadvantages associated with this strategy are manifold. There is always the possibility of burning the skin even at low voltages. Denaturation of the peptides and proteins at the pH required to achieve a suitable charge for iontophoresis may be manifested as loss in quaternary, tertiary and secondary structures. The heat generated during the process of iontophoresis can also lead to denaturation.

15.5.6.2. Phonophoresis

Another strategy that has been exploited to enhance transdermal delivery is phonophoresis. In this method ultrasound is applied via a coupling-contact agent to the skin. The drug absorption is enhanced via thermal effect of ultrasonic waves and subsequent temporary alterations in the physical structure of the skin. The limitation posed by denaturation of protein following heat generation during the process is disturbing.

15.5.6.3. Penetration enhancers

Use of penetration enhancers hold promise in delivery of proteins and peptides through transdermal route. For this purpose penetration enhancers like oleic acid and azone has been used. These agents fluidize the inter-cellular lipid lamellae of the stratum corneum. 3% azone improved the absorption of vasopressin across the skin. Fatty acids are reported to disrupt the packed structure of the lipids in the extracellular spaces. However, considerable skin irritation is reported with penetration enhancers and is thus likely to limit its utility.

15.5.6.4. Prodrugs

Another strategy that has shown promising results especially with small peptides is production of prodrugs. The enzymes present in the skin are exploited to regenerate the active drug. The terminal pyroglutamyl residue of LHRH, TRH and neurotensin can be readily derivatized to produce prodrugs. These prodrugs have enhanced transdermal permeability and are capable of undergoing spontaneous hydrolysis at physiological pH, in order to regenerate the active drug.

15.5.7. Pulmonary route

The lungs offer an alternative site for systemic delivery of peptides and proteins. They provide larger surface area (70 m^2) as compared to other mucosal sites such as nasal, buccal, rectal and vaginal. Some of the macromolecules have been extensively studied for their absorption from lungs. They include leuprolide, insulin and albumin. The aerosolized administration of insulin in rabbit, resulted into 40% absorption of the administered dose. This was relatively better than absorption recorded in healthy human subjects (7-16%) receiving aerosolized insulin through nebulizer. A significant increase in absorption with some penetration enhancers such as 1% azone, 1% fuscidic acid or 1% glycerol. Albumin in particular was found to be absorbed largely perhaps via pinocytosis process. In order to appreciate the potential of pulmonary route in systemic administration of proteins and peptides it seems necessary to understand the permeability characteristics of lungs, absorption mechanism in the lungs, lung metabolizing capacity, factors controlling dose deposition and safety consideration with regard to permeation. About 90% of the absorptive surface area of lungs is represented by the alveoli which is comprised of heterogeneous population of epithelial cells. Out of these cells, a small group of cells called type III cells are present as free alveolar macrophages. The epithelial cells remain in intimate contact with the vasculature. The distance between air and blood is much less than 1μm. However, due to its involvement in free exchange of gases it becomes a major barrier to the large molecule, for example, horse-radish peroxidase with a molecular weight of 40,000 deposited on air side fails to reach the interstitium. The principal resistance is offered by alveolar epithelium where the cells are tightly intercalated. The pore size of 6-10 Å in alveolar membrane and 40-50 Å in pulmonary capillary membrane has been established by Taylor and Gar.

15.5.7.1. Absorption mechanism through lungs

Similar to the intestine there operates both simple diffusion and carrier mediated transport mechanism in lungs. The diffusion is involved with the absorption of drug molecules ranging up to a molecular size of 75,000. These molecules include neutral molecules such as urea, mannitol, sucrose, ouagine, dihydroougine, cyanocobalamine and insulin as well as anionic compounds, i.e. carboxyfluorescein, heparin, sulfanilic acid, etc. The absorption rates have been recorded to be related to molecular size as the half-life of absorption from the alveolar region ranges from 0.25 minutes for antipyrine to 26.5 minutes for mannitol.

The active transport involving carrier in the pulmonary absorption of peptides however is yet to be determined, carriers are known to be present in several animal species and they participate in the absorption. 1-aminocyclopentane carboxylic acid, α-methyl-D glucose pyranoside and organic anions such as sodium chromoglycate and phenol red. Carrier mediated transport is usually inferred on the basis of several evidences available as in the case of α-methyl-D-glucose puranoside. The involvement of the carrier is indicated by the sensitivity of the process to inhibition by 0.5 mM phlorizin, 5 mM glucose, 0.5 mM ouabain and Na^+ depletion.

The various factors which play major challenges in pulmonary drug delivery are:

1. Reproducibility in dose deposition.
2. Site of dose deposition.
3. Variation in absorption rates due to variation in epithelial line thickness under physiological conditions.
4. Aerodynamics of aerosolized particles.

The safety issue pertaining to the pulmonary route for protein and peptide administration should be considered with regard to immunogenicity. The responses related to later in turn affect the thickness of pulmonary epithelium and so the permeability or the absorption barrier on receiving antigen challenges, a marked response in tight junction as well as bronchial permeability has been frequently recorded. The alteration in permeability of alveolar epithelium may in turn lead to the complication such as lungs edema. Another possibility is change in degree and volume of movement of fluids across the alveolar epithelium. Another safety issue appreciated with pulmonary administration of proteins and peptides is the unlikely event of destabilization of the surfactant film that coats the alveolar surface specially by proteins and peptides. Thus, the full potential of pulmonary route cannot be realized with full justification unless the various cell types in the conduction and non-conducting air ways are characterized for their absorption capacity and mechanism, types and population of proteases and immunological capabilities.

15.6. LYMPHATIC TRANSPORTATION OF PROTEINS

Proteins and peptides on fatty acylation may form a chylomicron like supramolecular assemblage which as a whole could passively be taken up by the enterocytes of Peyer's patches and transported to the lymphatic lacteals. Similarly proteins and peptides contained in colloidal dosage form with exterior lipophilic character could be absorbed following oral administration. Some typical examples of lymphotrophic carrier include w/o/w multiple emulsions, fat ultra emulsion, emulsomes and supramolecular biovectors. The absorbed carrier or drug entity typically follows the way as it is established for dietary lipids. Orally ingested lymphotrophs are solubilized or taken up by lecithin/bile salt(s) mixed micelles and passively absorbed into the enterocytes, then at the level of RER (rough endoplasmic reticulum) and golgi bodies the apoprotein(s) as targeting ligands absorbed protein coated lymphotrophs are exocytosed from enterocytes slowly. The latter has been recorded as a rate limiting step. The carrier then joins blood stream/circulation at thoracic duct.

For peptide delivery the lymphatics are assumed to be of prime importance due to the following reasons:

1. Lymphatic route being a vital route in some metastatic cancers, lymph nodes lend themselves as a potential target for chemotherapy.
2. Circulation antibodies produced by thymus-dependent small lymphocytes, large lymphocytes and macrophages are reported to be implicated in immunological reactions.

Lymphatic system transports slowly large proteins, antibodies and lymphocytes and then they return to the vascular system. The lymphatic capillary network take up the large particles and molecular complexes that enter the tissue-fluid. After passing through lymph nodes, lymph is transported to the great vein at the base of the neck. The characteristic feature of lymph flow is that it is usually a one-way transport (Fig. 15.34).

For successful lymphatic delivery of peptidal moieties, following approaches can be utilized :

1. For smaller moieties, lympho-selective delivery can be achieved by employing carriers like soluble macromolecules, microparticles, etc. of appropriate sizes (Table 15.3).
2. Bioavailability of peptides at site of action is to be improved.
3. An increment in residence time of peptidal moieties in lymph circulation.

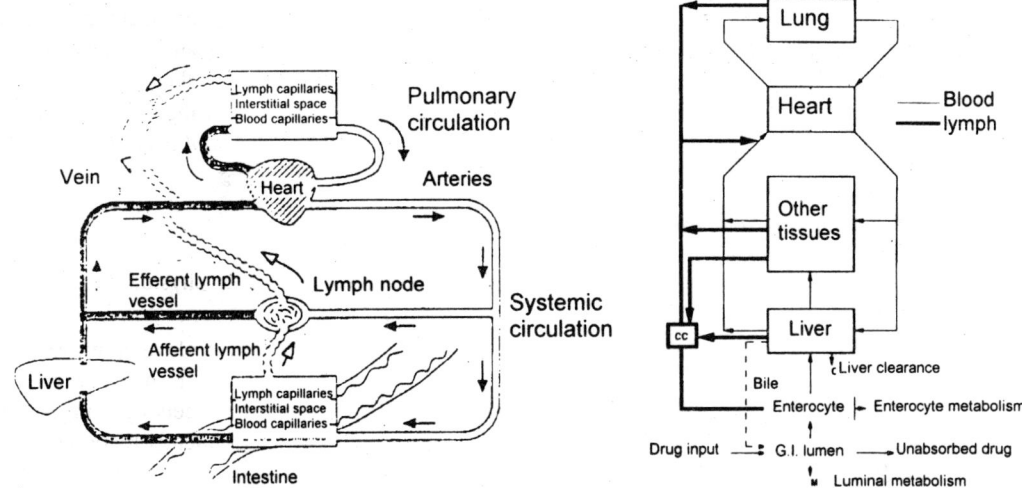

Fig. 15.34 : (a) Schematic representation of the lymph-blood circulation in the body
(b) Physiological pharmacokinetic model depicting the relationship
of venous and arterial blood flow to lymph flow after oral drug input

Transport of drugs through lymphatic pathway is to a large extent affected by the site of administration. For instance, dextran after intravenous administration shows poor lymph levels in comparison to blood levels. However, better lymph levels were observed after interstitial administration. Still better results have been observed with microparticles injected into tissues like stomach wall and subcutaneous areas. This preferential delivery to lymphatics is attributed to the ability of large molecules to penetrate through intracellular gaps of the lymph capillaries. The g.i. tract is a promising port for peptide administration. The transfer into lymph vessels via absorptive epithelial cells can occur through two pathways.

1. **Transcellular lipid pathway:** Here chylomicrons are formed in the cells and transferred into lymph capillaries.
2. **Paracellular pathway:** This plays a negligible role but is reported to operate by the addition of absorption enhancers.

Another important route is transcytosis through Peyer's patches and is believed to be suitable for highly potent moieties like lymphokines and vaccines.

Table 15.3 : Some of the lymphotrophic carriers for lymph targeting

Lyphotrophic carrier	Drug	Force or type of interaction
Carbon colloid	Mitomycin C	Hydrophobic interaction
Chylomicron; LDL	Cyclosporin A	Incorporation
Dextran	Mitomycin C	Covalent binding
Dextran sulfate	Bleomycin	Ion-pair
Intrinsic protein complex	Vitamin B_{12}	Complex
L-lactic acid oligomer microsphere	Cisplatin	Incorporation
Lipid mixed micelle	3',5'-O-dipalm-FUdR	Hydrophobic binding
Mixed micelle (Proliposome)	Interferon	Hydrophobic binding
W/O emulsion	5-Fluorouracil	Encapsulation
Styrene-maleic acid anhydride co-polymer	Neocarzinostatin	Covalent binding

The g.i. epithelial barrier allows easy permeation of lipophilic and small molecules. The limitation that restrains the absorption of peptides and proteins following oral administration has already being discussed. In the case of peptides it has been observed that if the molecule could cross epithelial barrier it may be traced back in systemic circulation. Cyclosporin A is a unique peptide with extra lipophilicity, soluble in lipoidal adjuvants and exhibits good absorption characteristics. When the drug was solubilized in lipoidal micellar solutions, higher lymph levels were obtained following intragastric and rectal administration, since CIA binds to chylomicrons in lymphatic components. Therefore, being related to chylomicron and lipoprotein it is found to be better absorbed following intragastric administration as compared to the rectal. With respect to oral administration endocytotic lymph targeting via non-lymphoid tissue of intestine does not seem to be an approach of potentials. Most of mammalian intestinal cells have capacity to endocytose macromolecules. The process has especially been observed related to mast cells of Peyer's patches so called gut-associated lymph tissues (GALT) consisting of aggregated lymphoid follicles. The Peyer's patches are a standard through luminal-epithelia, lamina propria and lamina submucosa. The size of microparticles may have decisive fate of micro-particles and as a result their peptidal load particles less than 5μm in diameter localize within mesenteric lymph nodes following their transport through Peyer's patches.

15.6.1. Colorectal transport

The colorectal area as well as small intestine region is predominantly supplied with blood and lymph capillaries and vessels. The colorectal mucosa imposes a barrier that is usually tighter in paracellular transport. However, the route of transport could be improved by addition of permeation enhancers like oleic acid and linoleic acid. Bleomycin (BLM) is a cationic glycopeptide that binds to anionic macromolecules, thus it results into the formation of ion-pair in addition with dextran sulfate. Both BLM and dextran sulfate possess a hydrophilic surface, thus, do not qualify for permeation individually. The macromolecular ion-pair complex being relatively apolar in nature could serve as a lymphotroph leading to lymphoselective delivery.

15.6.2. Pulmonary transport

The lung lymphatics are considered significant in the chemotherapy of cancer of lung origin and in the diseases related to pulmonary lymph nodes. Macromolecules were passed through lung epithelium and were transferred from interstitial space into the lymphatic pathway and subsequently blood circulation (Fig.15.35). FITC labelled dextrans of different molecular weights could successfully investigate size related lymph transport of protein molecules.

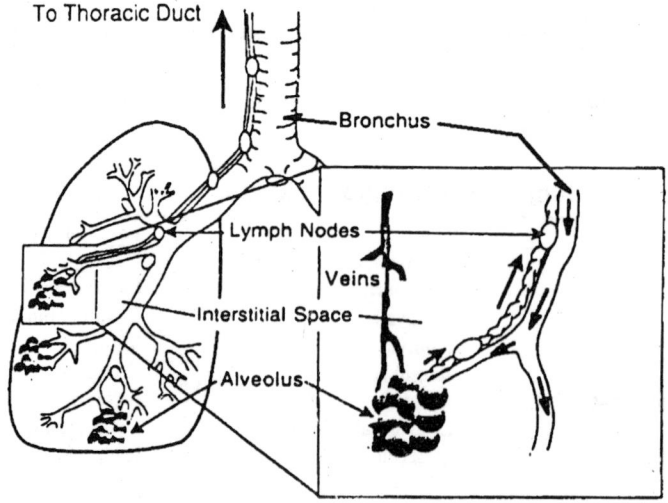

Fig. 15.35 : Schematic representation of macromolecular behavior in the lung interstitial spaces and lymphatics after intrapulmonary administration

Hence it follows that trafficking and targeting through lymphatics could be adopted as a strategy for lymphoselective delivery of peptides where different types of lymphotrophs could be used as carrier units. Furthermore, contribution of aggregated lymphoid tissues such as Peyer's patches, appendix and tonsils is yet to be explored as portal units for successful delivery.

15.7. SITE-SPECIFIC PROTEIN MODIFICATION (PROTEIN ENGINEERING)

This approach is being used to improve the stability and specificity of endogenous proteins, in addition, they improve the selectivity and have a prolonged delivery at the active site. One such approach is **deletion mutants**. The approach has extensively been studied by genetic engineering and cloning of tPA gene and its subsequent expression in eukaryotic cells. An altered pharmacokinetic and thrombolytic property of deletion mutations of human tPA was observed. Using a series of deletion mutants, it has been demonstrated that regions within tPA responsible for liver clearance, fibrin affinity and fibrin specificity are not localized in the same structure.

One another approach towards site-specific protein modification is the **hybrid proteins**. Hybrid proteins have the combination or re-ordered features of one or more proteins as well as their effector functions, protection and recognition properties. These site-specific hybrid proteins can be produced by synthetically linking protein fragments or by using ligated gene fusion processes. A list of hybrid proteins is given in table 15.4.

Table 15.4 : Hybrid protein delivery systems

Fragments of recognition portion	Effector portion
GENE FUSION PRODUCTS	
Interleukin 2	Diphtheria toxin
Growth factor	Toxin (e.g. ricin A)
Cell-specific polypeptide (α/β MSH; substrate P)	Restructured diphtheria toxin
Antitumor Fab immunoglobulin	Fragment A of diphtheria toxin
CD4	*Pseudomonas exotoxin*
	γ-interferon and β-tumor necrosis factor
CHEMICAL LINKAGE OF FRAGMENTS/PROTEINS	
Human placental lactogen hormone	Diphtheria toxin A chain
β chain of *h* chorionic gonadotropin hormone	Ricin A chain
Insulin	Diphtheria A
Epidermal growth factor	Ricin A
Antibody fragments	Deglycosylated ricin A
IgG (2a) fragments	Gelonin
	Diphtheria toxin
	Pseudomonas toxin
Anti-collagen antibody	Toxin
HIV-specific Ab	Ricin A
Antifibrin Ab	Tissue plasminogen activator
Anti-T-cell antibody	Ricin A chain
Antibody fragments	Gelonin toxin
Anti-endothelia IgG	Glucose oxidase
Anti-epithelia Ig/fragments	Ricin and other toxins
Anti-sIgM-IgM	Saporin-6

Ligated gene fusion is an approach by which hybrid proteins can be brought about. Gene fusion techniques are used to produce proteins with special but specific properties which vary from the parent protein. This can be well understood by looking into the examples of targeting bacterial and plant toxins to specific cells using hybrids created by ligating toxin and growth factor genes. The approach basically relies upon the deletion of the toxin gene sequence encoding the cell-binding site and allows the hybrid-fusion protein to display the cell specificity of the growth factor. One such example is the CD4-*Pseudomonas* exotoxin hybrid protein which show selective toxicity towards cells expressing the HIV envelope glycoprotein. An increased antiproliferative activity has been recently reported by a hybrid protein of interferon-γ and tumor necrosis factor-β as compared to either interferon-γ or tumor necrosis factor-β.

Synthetically linked hybrid conjugates constitute another approach by which site specific protein modification can be brought about. The concept is based on the biological disposition of protein after their chemical linkage to other protein fragments. For example, the toxin gleonin with a circulation half-life of 3.5 minutes in mice when conjugated with immunoglobulin fragments, increased to days.

15.7.1. Enzyme-PEG conjugates

Polyethylene glycol derivatives of L-asparaginase have been prepared and were observed to have considerably improved properties over the native enzyme. The PEG conjugates were resistant to proteolytic degradation and were non-immunogenic in nature. However, its catalytic properties were reduced to 52%. Similar approach has been used to prepare PEG conjugates of other enzymes like uricase, catalase, adenosine deamainase, etc. (Fig. 15.36).

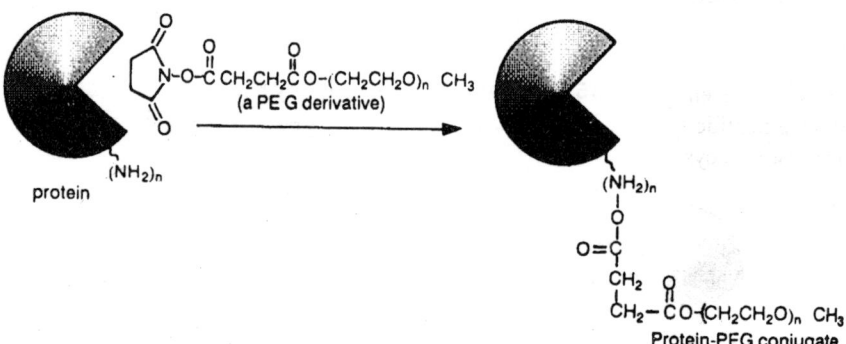

Fig. 15.36 : Schematic representation of formation of protein PEG conjugate

15.7.2. Protein glycosylation

The size, surface character and chemical reactivity mainly control pharmacodisposition of proteins and peptides. It has been identified that most of the endocytosis of glycoproteins are through their specific carbohydrate residues which complex with oligosaccharide specific recognition systems contained on plasma surface of target cell. Therefore, glycosylation pattern could be considered as signals which are used by the body for disposition and regaining of its own glycoproteins. This is largely implicated for enzymes, hormones and immune surveillance. One of the classical example describes translocation of lysosomal enzymes to the lysosomes wherein the process of translocation is mediated by phospho-D-mannopyranosyl moiety of lysosomal enzymes and phosphorylation of D-mannose residues. Acyloglycoproteins having biantennary and triantennary oligosaccharides are preferably absorbed by leukocyte lectins whereas triantennary and tetrantennary oligosaccharides are found to rapidly bind to the plasma membrane of hepatocytes in liver. Galactose specific recognition system for D-galactose and N-acetyl-D-galactosamine have been identified in hepatocytes, lymphocytes and on macrophages. Similarly mannose containing oligosaccharide are intercepted by the endothelial cells and Kupffer cells. Apparently, reductive mannosamination may provide an effective strategy for directing their protein to such cells. Carbohydrates as such play no direct role in the biological activity of glycoproteins. Nevertheless, they may influence the stability and conformation of glycoproteins. They may also impart aqueous affinity to the glycoproteins through their hydrophilic character.

The well identified biological property (circulation half-life) of glycoprotein may be diversified by altering the distribution of carbohydrates on their surface. Likewise immunogenicity and accessibility to the cellular site of action may be affected. In contrast, to the possible changes in the amino acid composition of a protein through sugar coupling, numerous variations are possible which could be glycoproteins and almost limitless variability and diversity in structure could be imparted.

The incorporation of oligosaccharide as affinity handle into macromolecular drug carrier could be utilized effectively for the targeting of small molecules. Various examples have been cited elsewhere in this book. The conjugation of fragment A of diphtheria toxin to galactose containing oligosaccharide such as asilofutein or asilo or orsomucoid interestingly resulted into targeting of diphtheria components to the hepatocytes. The uptake of such systems has been found to be nonlinear. This is an indicative of ligand mediated endocytosis.

15.7.2.1. Expression cell processing

Protein glycosylation is a rare event in prokaryotic cells such as *E. coli*. However, some glycosylation have been reported in eukaryotes such as yeast and mammalian cells with different resultant glycosylation patterns. Although recombination technology in bacteria can produce large amount of protein, this is often changed by bacterial proteases and within expression cells. Mammalian cell is adaptively suitable for proteins with complex modification such as γ-carboxylation of glutanyl residue and for obtaining homologus human glycosyl pattern with marked effect in biological utilization and therapeutic efficacy of proteins.

15.7.3. Modification of proteases into peptide ligases

Peptide ligation of native enzymes tends to high specificity and stereoselectivity. Synthesis of any enzyme capable of catalyzing peptide ligation is advantageous. For example, **"subtilisin"** a protease has been modified by converting a serine into cysteine or seleno-cysteine which can catalyze peptide ligation (Fig. 15.37).

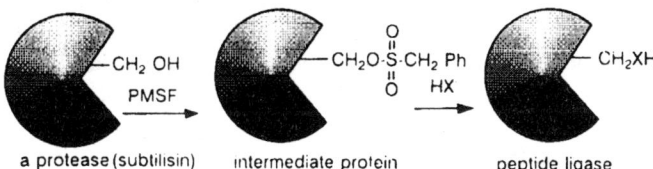

a protease (subtilisin) intermediate protein peptide ligase

Fig. 15.37 : Chemical modification of a protease by phenylmethyl sulfonyl fluoride to produce a peptide ligase

15.7.4. Production of site specific nucleases

The binding properties and DNA recognition properties can be combined using chemical cleavage agent (Fig. 15.38). Cys of *E. coli* CAP protein has been modified using 5-iodoacetamide-1,10-phenanthroline yielding a DNA cleaving agent, that recognized and cleaved DNA at the centre of the recognition site (22 bp) for CAP. This gives restriction enzymes which are capable of recognizing upto 20 bases instead of 6 or 8 bases and are therefore useful in isolating long DNA fragments needed for sequencing and mapping.

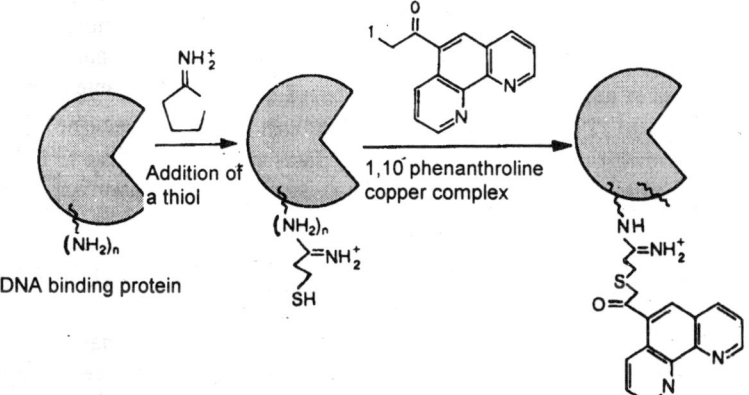

Fig. 15.38 : Method for producing a nuclease from a DNA binding protein

Specific nucleases can also be produced by fusion of nonspecific phosphodiesterases to oligonucleotides of defined sequence (Fig.15.39). This approach can also be used for developing artificial restriction enzymes.

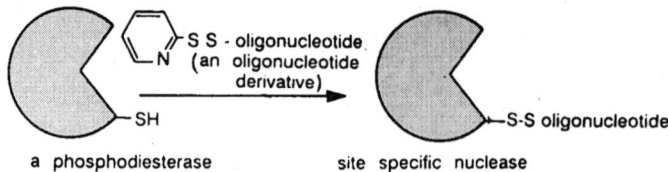

Fig. 15.39 : Generation of a site-specific nucleus from non-specific phosphodiesterase

15.7.5. Production of artificial semisynthetic oxido-reductase (Flavo enzymes)

This can be prepared by incorporating redox-active prosthetic group covalently to the existing sites. In this method a redox-active group, 10-methyliso-alloxazine derivatives is linked to specific sites of several proteins. The efficiency of these semisynthetic enzymes is comparable with that of naturally occurring flavo enzymes.

15.8. TOXICITY PROFILE CHARACTERIZATION

The available literature often lacks data suggesting the possible mechanism(s) of pharmacological and/or toxicological actions of peptide and protein therapeutics in intact mammalian systems. These data are required:-

1. To determine the maximal tolerated dose by a given route of administration.
2. To have an insight into the dose-limiting toxicity and the target organs involved.
3. To confirm the intrinsic and interactive safety of the proposed formulation to be used.
4. To ensure that the manufacturing and formulation processes will provide biologically active and stable material free from contaminating substances that might increase toxicity and/or decrease efficacy.

15.8.1. Classes of toxicity of proteins and peptides

15.8.1.1. Exuberant pharmacologic responses

The dose-related toxicity is the most commonly encountered toxic manifestation of peptides and proteins. The toxicity of this type includes the arteriospasm and hypertension after an overdose of angiotensin II and the profound hypertension and the resultant convulsions after large doses of insulin. To some extent the doses of various fibrinolytic proteins like tissue-type plasminogen activator, urokinase used in thrombolytic disorders are prone to elicit exuberant pharmacologic response.

15.8.1.2. Generic toxicity

Generic toxicity is an adverse reaction which is exhibited by most, if not all, members of a class of proteins. For instance, fever, chill and diaphoresis are observed when monoclonal antibodies are infused that react with circulating cells. Also, fever, fatigue, arthralgias, myalgias, and malaise develop after administration of interferons. Immunogenicity is perhaps the most distinguishing generic toxicity of the peptide and protein drug moieties. This feature has been exploited for therapeutic needs in development of vaccines. Immunogenic behavior of proteins is largely attributed to their molecular weight, extent of structural complexity and hydrophobicity, propensity to aggregate, aromatic amine content and sequence homology to the native protein in the test species.

The general pathogenic mechanisms involved in immunologic injury include (in addition, the readers may refer chapter 12):

Type I reaction: This mechanism involves the release of active mediators (e.g. bradykinin, histamine, serotonin and numerous arachidonic acid metabolites) from mast cells through an antibody-based mechanism. The spectrum of responses observed is wide and includes allergic dermatitis, allergic rhinitis, asthma, urticaria, oesophageal varices, g.i. hypermotility and acute hypotension.

Type II reaction: This mechanism is mediated through the interaction between antibody and antigenic sites at the cell surface. These cells are usually present within the vascular bed but extravascular cells may be targeted as well. Cytotoxicity and cell lysis are the manifestations of this type of reaction. Cytotoxicity mechanisms usually lead to anemias, hemorrhagic conditions, neutropenias and related secondary disorders. Natural activities of a cell may be stimulated or inhibited through receptor binding. They may not be cytotoxic themselves but are capable of leading to disease. For example, long-acting thyroid stimulator (LATS), an antibody to the thyroid cell, brings about increased production of thyroid hormone.

Type III reaction: This reaction is mediated through preformed antigen-antibody complexes, usually in antibody excess, which produce damage if they are deposited on the walls of the blood vessel or in the interstitium of vital organs. This mechanism is proposed to be responsible for immunologic injury following protein administration.

Type IV reaction: This mechanism of immunologic injury occurs in the absence of antibody and complement. It is mediated by sensitized T lymphocytes. The damage is mediated through direct T-cell cytotoxicity and/or cytokine release, which leads to mobilization and attraction of monocytes, other lymphocytes and neutrophils, leading to augmentation in tissue injury. The examples include cell-mediated lympholysis, allograft rejection, tuberculin skin reaction, skin reactions to poison injections and diphtheria toxoid.

15.8.1.3. Idiopathic toxicity

This is an unexpected toxicity and is elicited only by some members of a protein therapeutic class. Generally, these toxic reactions are unrelated to the mechanism of action of the protein. Examples, include the 'vascular leak syndrome' associated with long term IL-2 infusion, hypotension observed with TNF-α administration etc.

SUGGESTED READINGS

Boheim, G., hanke, W. and Jung, G., (1983) **Biophys. Struct. Mech.,** 9, 181.

Bornstein, P. and Traub, W., (1979) **The Proteins,** Vol.4, Academic Press, New York.

Chein, Y.W. (Ed.), (1985), **Transdermal Systemic Medications,** Elsevier, Amsterdam.

Couvreur, P. and Prisieux, F., (1993), **Adv. Drug Deliv. Rev.,** 10, 141-162.

Davis, S.S., (1986) *Advanced Devliery Systems for Peptides and Proteins-Pharmaceutical considerations.* In : **Delivery Systems for Peptide Drugs,** S.S. Davis, L. Illum and E. Tomlinson, (Eds.), Plenum Press, New York, p 1-21.

Davis, S.S., Illum, L. and Tomlinson, E., (Eds.), (1986) **Delivery Systems for Peptide Drugs,** Plenum Press, New York.

Dickerson, R.F. and Gesis, I., (1969) **The Structure and Action of Proteins,** Harper and Row, New York.

Florence, A.T., Hillery, A.M., Hussain, N. and Jani, P.U., (1995) **J. Control. Rel.,** 36, 39-46.

Harris, A.S., (1993) **J. Drug Targ.,** 1, 101-106.

Humphry, M.J. and Ringrose, P.S., (1986) **Dr. Metab. Rev.** 17, 283-310.

Johnson, K.A., (1997) **Adv. Drug Deliv. Rev.,** 26, 3-15.

Langer, R., (1989) **Pharm. Tech.,** 13, 18-30.

Latorre, R. and Alvarez, O., (1981) **Physiol. Rev.,** 61, 77.

Lee, V.H.L., (1991) **Peptide and Protein Drug Delivery,** Marcel Dekker, New York.

Lipka, E., Crison, J. and Amidon, G.L., (1996) **Adv. Drug Deliv. Rev.,** 39,121-129.

Manning, M.C., Patel, K. and Borchardt, R.J., (1989) **Pharm. Res.,** 6, 903-918.

Marshak, D. and Liu, D. (Eds.), (1989) **Therapeutic Peptides and Proteins: Formulation, Delivery, Targeting**, Cold Spring Harbor Laboratory, Cold Spring Harbor, New York.

Mathew, M.K. and Balaram, P., (1983) **FEBS Lett.**, 157,1.

Monsigny, M., Roche, A.C., Midoux, P. and Mayer, R., (1994) **Adv. Drug Deliv. Rev.**, 14, 1-24.

Muranishi, M., Murakami, M., Hashidume, M., Yamada, K., Tajima, S. and Kiso, Y., (1992) **J. Control. Rel.**, 179-188.

O'Hagan, D.T., (1990) **Adv. Drug Deliv. Rev.**, 5, 265-285.

Samanen, J. (1985), **Bioactive Polymeric Systems**, C.G. Gebelein, and C.E. Carraher, (Eds.), Plenum Press, New York p279-344.

Schulz, G.E. and Shirmir, R.H., (1979) **Principles of Protein Structure**, Springer-Verlag, New York.

Tomlinson, E. and Livingston, C., (1989) **Pharm. J.**, 243, 646-648.

MOLECULAR PRINCIPLES OF DRUG TARGETING AND LIPOSOMES

16.1. INTRODUCTION

Selective drug delivery and targeting seeks to improve on the risk/benefit ratio associated with drugs. Ideally, a drug intended for clinical use should have a high therapeutic index, which is a ratio of drug efficacy (therapeutic effect) and the drug toxicity (side effects). Many drugs, particularly chemotherapeutic agents have narrow therapeutic window (low therapeutic indices) and their clinical use is limited and compromised by dose limiting toxic side effects. Approaches are being adapted either to control the distribution of drug by incorporating it in a carrier system or by altering the structure of the drug at the molecular level, or to control the input of the drug into the bioenvironment to ensure an appropriate profile of biodistribution. Rapid applications of the recent developments in molecular genetics are enabling both, the diagnosis of pathogenesis involved with the disease to its highest precision, as well as the design of novel drugs and delivery systems for its radical cure.

The efforts to improve drug effectiveness in therapeutics have been assisted by parallel developments in molecular and cell biology. On one hand, hybridoma and recombinant DNA technology have come to be of age, and on the other, a number of cell membrane receptors and their interactions with respective ligands have been reported for many cell related biological functions. Such developments led to the concept of conferring selectivity to drugs through targeted delivery. Currently, drug delivery technology has infused new interest in seemingly ineffective or inefficient drugs by targeting them specifically to the desired site of action. Also by millennium end, target oriented drug administration systems with improvement in therapeutic efficacy, reduction in side effects and compliance in dosing regimen, shall be the leading trends in the area of therapeutics. The contents of this chapter concern primarily with the concepts and various aspects of the target oriented site specific delivery systems.

16.2. HISTORICAL PERSPECTIVES

The concept of designing specified delivery system to achieve selective drug targeting has been originated from the perception of Paul Ehrlich, who imagined drug delivery as a **'magic bullet'**. It was the very first report to be published on targeting (Paul Ehrlich, 1902) describing targeted drug delivery system as an event where, a drug carrier complex, delivers drug(s) exclusively to the preselected target cells in a specific manner. Bangham's (1965) observation on phospholipid hexagonal liquid crystals, that they are permselective to the ions in a manner similar to biomembrane led to the discovery of artificial somatic system based on phospholipid amphiphiles. Gregoriadis (1972), described targeting with the help of novel drug delivery systems as **'old drugs in new cloths'**.

Targeted therapy, as Ehrlich (1902) imagined remains an unachieved goal as hitherto, however the idea stimulated a long series of experiments that propounded the philosophy of targeting of drugs and genes and attracted present generation of researchers to deal with many of the problems associated with the concept.

16.3. DRUG TARGETING

It is pertinent to discuss the concept and components which are utilized in the targeting of drug(s). A number of essential aspects which should be considered for the designing of drug delivery systems to achieve this goal include target, carrier, ligand(s) and physically modulated components.

16.3.1. Targeting

Targeted drug delivery implies for selective and effective localization of pharmacologically active moiety into the vicinity of preidentified (preselected) target(s) in therapeutic concentration, restricting its access to non target normal cellular linings, thus minimizing toxic effects and maximizing therapeutic index (Gregoriadis,1993).

16.3.2. Target

Target could be described as a cell or group of cells in minority, identified to be in the need of treatment. Two distinctive cellular elements present on the surface of the target cell(s) are considered in designing of carriers for targeting viz.:

1. Cell surface antigens, exploited in generating cell specific, and non cross-selective antibodies (Connor and Huang,1986); and
2. Cell surface receptors which recognize and internalize the macromolecular ligands and associated carrier (Jones,1994).

16.3.2.1. Various types of targets

The appropriate targets for carrier mediate interactions are (Ostro,1987):

(i) Cells *in vitro* for genome grafting or manipulation of DNA (genetic materials).

(ii) Accessible anatomical compartments, i.e. peritoneal cavity, cerebral ventricles, plural cavity, lungs, lymphatics, etc.

(iii) Macrophages and other phagocytic cells including Kupffer satellite cells, tissue macrophages and the blood macrophage or monocytes of MPS.

(iv) Nonphagocytic cells of RES including the liver endothelial cells, endocytic in nature.

(v) Lymphocytes and antigen presenting cells.

16.3.3. Carriers

Carrier is one of the most important entity essentially required for effective transportation of the loaded drug(s). They are vectors which sequester, transport and retain drug en route, while elute or deliver it into the vicinity of target. Carriers can do so either through an ability, inherent or acquired (through structural modification), to interact selectively with biological targets, or otherwise they are engineered to release the drug in the proximity of target cell lines, that demand optimal pharmacological action (therapeutic index). Characteristics of an ideal drug carrier, which can be exploited in drug delivery designing are (Meijer,1992):

(i) it must be able to cross anatomical barriers;

(ii) it must be recognized specifically and selectively by the target cells;

(iii) the linkage of the drug and the directing unit should be stable in plasma, interstitial and other bio-fluids.

(iv) after recognition, and internalization, the carrier system should release the drug moiety inside the target organs, tissues or cells; and

(v) carrier should be non-toxic, non-immunogenic and biodegradable particulate.

16.3.4. Ligands

Ligands are surface appended group(s), which can selectively steerup the carrier to the prespecified cellular lining(s) equipped with the desired receptor units. The carrier systems serve to present the ligands to their respective receptors localized on the cellular surface. The various ligands exploited for selective drug targeting include antibodies, polypeptides, oligo-saccharides, viral proteins, endogenous hormones and fusogenic residues etc. (Ostro,1987). The ligands confer recognition and specificity upon carrier/vector and lend them to approach the respective target and deliver the drug.

16.3.5. Rationale of drug targeting

The rationale for site specific targeted delivery may be appreciated as a set of desirable events including an exclusive delivery to specific pre-identified compartments with maximum potential intrinsic activity of drugs and concomitantly reduced access of drug to irrelevant non-target cells. The targeted delivery to previously inaccessible domains, e.g., intracellular sites, virus, bacteria and parasites offers distinctive therapeutic benefits. The controlled rate and mode of drug delivery to pharmacological receptor and specific binding with target cells; as well as bioenvironmental protection of the drug en route to the site of action are specific features of targeting. Invariably, every event stated leads to higher drug concentration at the site of action combined with lower concentration at non-target tissue where toxicity might crop-up (Gregoriadis, 1983). The high drug concentration in the target site is a result of the relative cellular uptake of the drug vehicle, liberation of drug and efflux of free drug from the target site.

Targeting is only significant if the target compartment is distinguished from the other compartments, where toxicity may occur, and also if the active drug is placed predominantly in the proximity of target site (Goldberg, 1983). The small distribution of the parent drug to the non-target site(s) with more efficient access to the target site(s) could maximize the benefits of targeted drug delivery (Fig. 16.1).

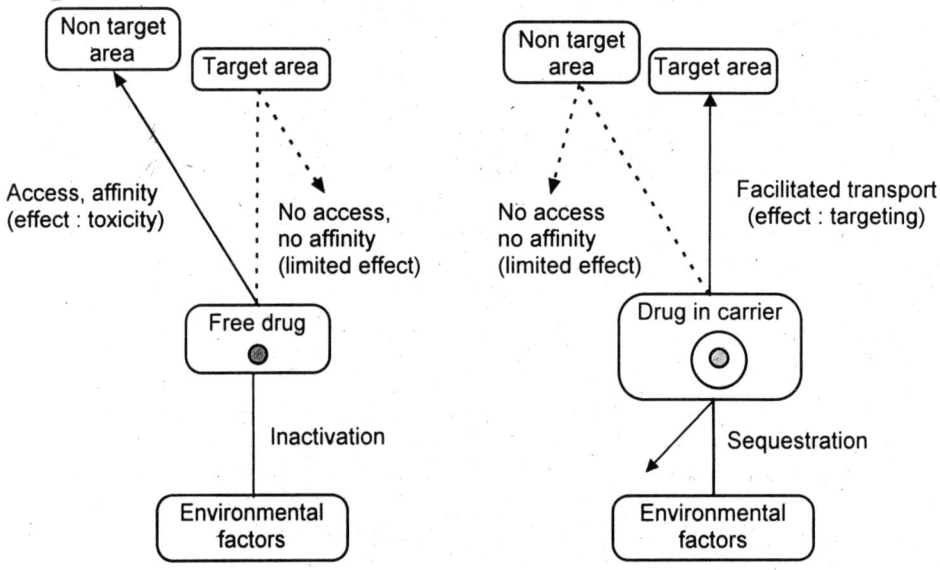

Fig. 16.1 : Principle of drug targeting (Gregoriadis, 1983)

16.3.6. Categorization at various levels

Targeted drug delivery may be achieved by using carrier systems, where reliance is placed on exploiting both, the intrinsic their pathway(s) that these carriers follow, and the bioprotection that they can offer to drugs during transit through the body. The various approaches of vectoring the drug to the target site can be broadly classified as (Widder,1979; Illum,1989; Weinstein,1979; Torchilin,1987; Jansen,1991):

1. Passive targeting

2. Active targeting

3. Inverse targeting

4. Physical targeting

5. Dual targeting

16.3.6.1. Passive targeting

It is a sort of passive process which utilizes the natural course of (attributed to inherent characteristics) 'homing' of the carrier system, through which it finally identifies and eventually approaches the intended cell lines. The ability of some colloids to be taken up by the RES especially in liver and spleen has made them as ideal vectors for passive hepatic targeting of drugs to these compartments. Passive targetability of the colloidal carriers provides therapeutic opportunities for the delivery of anti-infectives for disease conditions that involve macrophage cells of the RES, e.g., leishmaniasis, brucellosis and candidiasis (Croft, 1986). Delivery into lysosomal compartment can also be affected for the treatment of certain lysosomal storage diseases as well as for macrophage neoplasms and macrophage activation (Gregoriadis, 1981).

16.3.6.2. Active targeting

The process of active targeting exploits modification or manipulation of the natural distribution pattern of the drug carrier using some exogenous means, so that it can be identified by a particular cell lines. It is generally achieved by using specific uptake mechanisms such as receptor dependent uptake of natural low density lipoproteins (LDL) particles and synthetic lipid microemulsions from partially reconstituted LDL particles, coated with the apoproteins. The apoprotein coat serves as a ligand for the receptors. The ability of an immunoglobulin coated carrier to promote its accelerated interception by the liver and spleen, possibly via pathways involving Fc or C3B receptor mediated uptake, is one of the approach that exemplifies and signifies active targeting (Wolff et al.1984). Widdar and co-workers (1979), have further classified it into three different levels of targeting: first order targeting (organ compartmentalization), second order targeting (cellular targeting) and third order targeting (intracellular targeting) .

16.3.6.2.1. First order targeting

It refers to restricted distribution of the drug-carrier system to the capillary bed of a predetermined target site, organ or tissue. Compartmental targeting in lymphatics, peritoneal cavity, plural cavity, cerebral ventricles, lungs, joints, eyes, etc., represents first order targeting.

16.3.6.2.2. Second order targeting

The selective delivery of drugs to a specific cell type such as tumor cells and not to the normal cells is referred as second order drug targeting. The selective drug delivery to the Kupffer cells in the liver exemplifies this approach.

16.3.6.2.3.Third order targeting

The third order targeting implies to drug delivery specifically to the internal (intracellular) site of target cells. An example of third order targeting is the receptor mediated entry of a drug complex into a cell by endocytosis, lysosomal degradation of carrier followed by the release of drug intracellularly.

16.3.6.3. Inverse targeting

It is essentially based on successful attempts to circumvent and avoid passive uptake of colloidal carriers by reticuloendothelial system (RES). This effectively implies for reversion of bio-homing trend of the carrier, hence the process is referred to as **inverse targeting** (Lazo and Hacker 1985). One strategy applied to achieve inverse targeting is to suppress the function of RES by a preinjection of a large amount of blank colloidal carriers (Illum et al. 1986) or macromolecules like dextran sulphate (Patel et al. 1983). This approach can lead to RES blockade and as a consequence impairment of host defense system. Alternative strategies include modification of the size, surface charge, composition, surface rigidity and hydrophilicity of the carriers

Recently available literature suggests modification of the surface by imparting distinctive hydrophilicity to the carrier particles, as an effective mode of targeting of drug(s) to non RES organs. Davis and Hansrani (1985) reported that phospholipid microspheres emulsified with Polaxamer 338 showed the slowest RES uptake in mouse peritoneal macrophages *in vitro*. Illum et al. (1987,1989) reported that Poloxamine 908, is another hydrophilic nonionic surfactant which diverts normal RES uptake of coated emulsion and coated nanoparticles (polystyrene microsphere) to inflammatory sites in rabbits. Recently, Lee et al. (1995), suggested inverse targeting of drugs to the sites other than RES rich organs by coating the lipid micro-emulsion (LM) with polaxamer 308. It has been suggested that surface hydrophilicity may reduce or even eliminate the adhesion of opsonin materials/HDL on to the surface of LM, which is believed to be an essential component involved in phagocytosis and sequential uptake of LM by RES system.

16.3.6.4. Physical targeting

The selective drug delivery programmed and monitored at the external level (*ex-vivo*) with the help of physical means is referred to as physical targeting. In this mode of targeting, some characteristics of the environment are used either to direct the carrier to a particular location or to cause selective release of its contents. The first approach is represented by the temperature sensitive liposomes, which were developed and applied to tumor by Weistein et al. (1979). The release of drug from temperature sensitive liposomes in the vicinity of a tumor, that has temperature status higher or equal to the phase transition temperature of constitutive lipid(s), is brought about by serum components mostly the lipoproteins, which at phase transition induce temperature released from rapid release of entrapped drug.

It has been suggested that weakly anionic drugs, e.g. methotrexate, released from liposomes preferentially at low pH regions of tumors. Yatwin and coworkers (1980) have reported pH sensitive liposomes for selective release at low pH. In another physical approach, the application of external magnetic field has been exploited for localization of magno-responsive liposomes and microspheres within a preselected capillary bed.

16.3.6.5. Dual targeting

This classical approach of the drug targeting employs carrier molecules having their own intrinsic antiviral effect thus synergise the antiviral effect of the loaded active drug. Based on this approach, drug conjugates can be prepared with a fortified activity profile against the viral replication process (Jansen et al. 1991). A major advantage is that the virus replication process can be attacked at multiple points, excluding the possibilities of resistant viral strain development.

16.4. CELLULAR LEVEL EVENTS IN TARGETING

Design and development of potential carriers for cell specific delivery of therapeutics are immensely dependent on the selectivity of the carrier to the cellular receptors distributed variably intracellular and on the surface of cellular systems of the body. Other crucial factors include the anatomical and pathological barriers which have to be crossed, en route before these recognition site(s) are arrived as well intracellular mesogenic constrains as well as physiologic constraints which are encountered following receptor recognition and cellular internalization, these constraints are critical for intracellular routing, degradation and release of carrier contents.

16.4.1. Endocytosis

Endocytosis is a main cellular activity involved in the internalization of the colloidal and macromolecular carriers, summing the two processes of 'phagocytosis' and 'pinocytosis'(Cohn et al. 1977). Endocytosis has been defined as the internalization of plasma membrane with concomitant engulfment of extracellular material and extracellular fluid. Phagocytosis is the engulfment of the endogenous and exogenous particulate materials, such as bacteria, erythrocytes, latex beads and colloidal particles and is performed by the phagocytic cells of the RES including the Kupffer cells of the hepatic sinusoids, the tissue fixed macrophages (histocytes) and the blood macrophages or monocytes. The process involves sequential steps of **recognition** (mediated by coating of blood components, mainly opsonin and high density lipoproteins), **adhesion** (attachment of the particle to the macrophage cells of the RES) and **digestion** (whereby the particles are transferred to phagosome, phago-lysosome and finally to digestive vacuoles). Multiple attachment of particle associated ligands with membrane receptors is an essential stimulus for phagocytic capture of particles (Zippering).

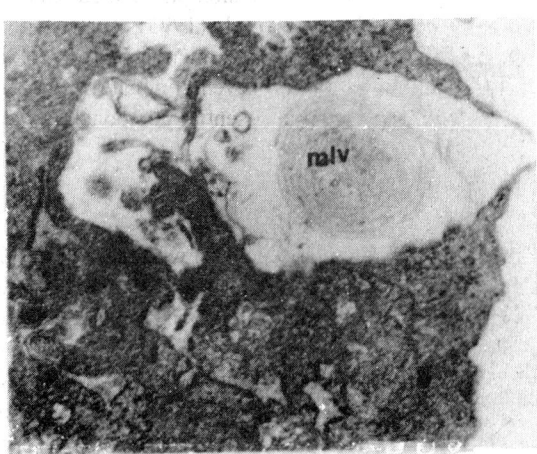
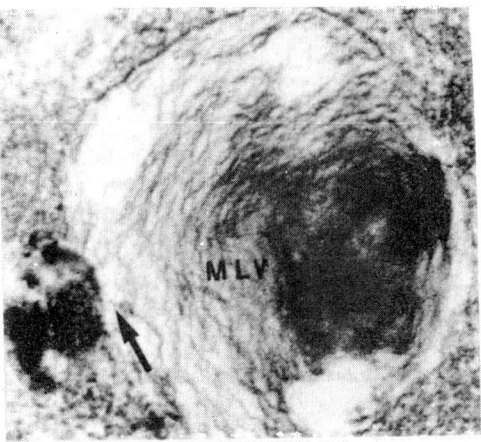

Photomicrograph (TEM) showing internalization of liposomes

On the other hand, pinocytosis is the uptake of small solutes and small droplets of extracellular fluid, the process is also known as 'cell drinking'. It is similar in many ways to phagocytosis. It too involves the formation of intracellular vesicles from the plasma membrane, like 'phagosome' these 'pinosomes' which can carry extracellular materials for digestion by the lysosome. It is performed by most, if not all, nucleated cells. Based on the kinetics and other biochemical characteristics three internalization mechanisms have been proposed. (a) Fluid phase pinocytosis; (b) Adsorptive, receptor mediated pinocytosis, and (c) Adsorptive, non receptor mediated pinocytosis (Fig. 16.2).

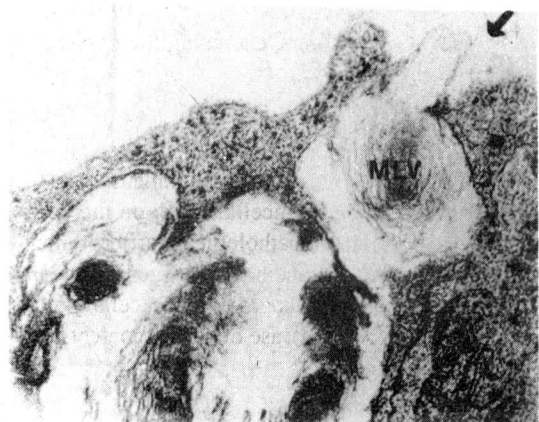
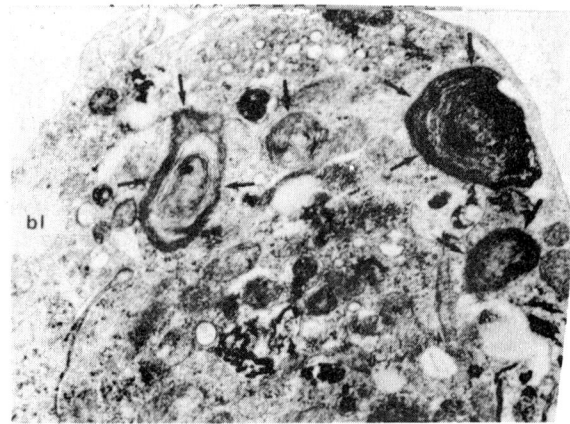

Photomicrograph showing recognition of liposomes   Photomicrograph showing digestion of liposomes

As already noted, pinosomes only capture liquid and the contained solute(s), present in the extracellular fluid surrounding a cell (fluid phase pinocytosis), but differential uptake is also a prominent feature. This is possible by adsorptive pinocytosis, in which a solute binds to an external phase of the plasma membrane and drawn into the cell interior forming pinosome with solute concentration higher than that in the ambient liquid. This process can be highly efficient and could facilitate higher uptake rate as compared to substrate captured through fluid phase. Further, adsorptive pinocytosis can be categorized as: substrate specific (receptor mediated) and non specific. In the former, the cell surface recognizes and internalizes a liquid of narrowly defined structural composition, whereas in the latter substrate specificity is much broader, and vague.

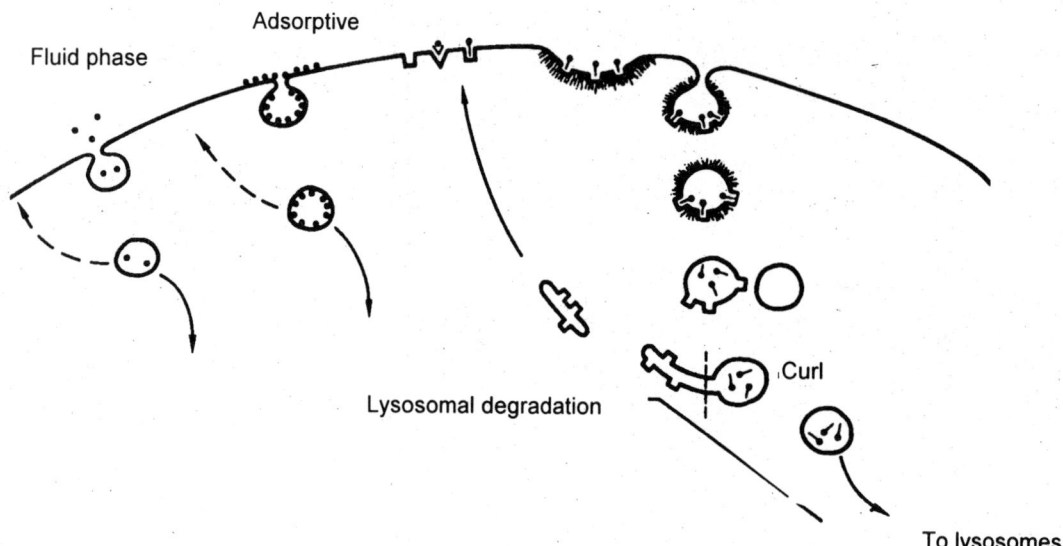

Fig. 16.2 : Diagrammatic presentation of cellular uptake mechanism

Substrate specific adsorptive pinocytosis has been described for several classes of proteins, glycoproteins, lipoproteins and for a range of growth receptors. It has been realized that the fluid phase and receptor mediated pinocytosis are not separate cellular events, but they are different facets of the same event. Non-specific adsorption pinocytosis is responsible for the uptake of many non-glycosylated proteins particularly following damage or denaturation. Exogenous particulate material is also taken up by adsorptive non receptor mediated endocytosis.

16.4.2. Ligand mediated transcytosis

Transcytosis is the principle mechanism involved in the receptor mediated uptake of ligand(s). Ligand transcytosis suggests that exclusive localization of particulates does not occur necessarily within sinusoidal cells, but the particulate ligands may also end up in hepatocytes (in case, if hepatocyte is not capable to endocytose initially). VanBarkel et al., (1985) explored that colloidal gold particles coated with either lactosylated serum albumin or mannan are taken up initially by liver macrophages and endothelial cells, however subsequent redistribution to hepatocytes, confirms ligand transcytosis to be operative *in vivo*. Seemingly, these cellular uptake characteristics constitute central dogma for ligand-receptor mediated drug targeting.

16.4.3. Receptor recognition

Receptor recognition is a prerequisite for the ligand mediated targeting. The concept assumes cell specific recognition of the carrier, internalization or binding of the drug conjugate, intracellular release and cellular retention of the active drug.

These recognition sites could in principle serve for binding and/or endocytosis of receptor conjugated carriers for the intracellular delivery of drugs and genetic materials. Although such receptors often provide help for internalization followed by intracellular transport to degradative compartments, the relative rates of these processes in various cell types can be markedly different. In some cases only external binding occurs. In the latter case, local release of drug from carrier in the micro-bioenvironment of the cell membrane should then provide a sufficient driving force for uptake by target cells. Both receptor and its density and affinity for a given substrate as well as the presence of competing endogenous ligands determine the extent of carrier receptor occupation and as a result the extraction of the carrier drug complex by the target tissue(s).

16.5. LIGANDS AS MEANS OF TARGETING

Targeting components, which have been studied and exploited are pilot molecules themselves or anchored as ligands on some delivery vehicle (drug-carrier system). All the carrier systems, explored so far, in general, are colloidal in nature, which can be utilized as a platform for the presentation of various biologically relevant molecular ligands including antibodies, polypeptides, oligosaccharides (carbohydrates), viral proteins and fusogenic residues. The ligands afford specific avidity to drug carrier or vector systems and lend them to selectively deliver the drug to the cell or group of cells, generally referred as target. The cascade of events involved in ligand affinity driven specific drug delivery is termed as *ligand mediated targeting*.

16.5.1. Conceptual aspect of ligand induced targeting

16.5.1.1. Definition

A ligand is neither, a shield, nor a motor. Ligands can be either covalently or noncovalently associated with the surface of the carrier in such a way that carrier tends to approach the accessible cells, those expressing surface receptor, with an affinity to the ligand. Carrier target recognition is a prerequisite for ligand mediated targeting and provides a basis for using cell specific (receptor specific) ligands, attached to the colloidal surface as a means of promoting recognition and conferring specificity.

16.5.1.2. Types

Different ligands have been reported so far in the pursuit to provide optimal targeting. An attempt is made here to categorize them on the following lines:

i. Antibodies and antibody-conjugates: Polyclonal (heat aggregated) antibodies, monoclonal antibodies (MAbs), haptens, radiolabelled antibodies, antibody-enzyme conjugates, bispecific antibodies, immuno-toxins.
ii. Glycoconjugates: Lectins, glycolipids, glycoproteins, glyocosides, viroproteins, polysaccharides and lipo-polysaccharides.
iii. Endogenous ligands: Interleukins, macroglobulins, transferrins, interferons, α-fetoprotein, CD4 toxins, advanced glycation end products (AGE) and major histocompatibility complex (MHC) classes.

16.5.1.3. Receptors as ports for drug targeting

The approach of cellular drug targeting with ligand appended carriers is intimately dependent upon the selectivity and the distribution of the receptor equipped cellular targets in the body, followed by their recognition and ligand-receptor interaction, for intracellular routing of the drug-carrier complex. Table 16.1 lists a number of receptors for macromolecular ligands which are more or less specific for the cell type indicated. These blood cell specific receptors may serve as a port and may offer the fundamental principle of cellular drug targeting.

16.6. BLOOD CELL RECEPTORS FOR ENDOGENOUS COMPOUNDS/LIGANDS

Membrane lectins and endogenous ligand receptors have been investigated in relation to drug targeting.

16.6.1. Lectins as glyco-conjugate receptors

The existence of membrane lectins, as carbohydrate specific receptors, which recognize carbohydrate epitopes also present on membrane glycolipids and glycoproteins, suggest their distinctive role in cellular adhesion and recognition process. Furthermore it provides the basis of several delivery systems based on carbohydrate mediated interactions (Weir,1980). Lectins are sugar specific proteins which agglutinate cells and/or precipitate as glyco-conjugates. They are found in a wide variety of bacteria, plants, invertebrates and vertebrates. Table 16.2 enlists lectins with their sugar affinities and specificity's. Various kinds of extracellular ligands, such as hormones, growth factors, antibodies, viruses and toxins are taken up into cells by lectin-receptor mediated endocytosis (Monsigny et al.,1989).

Table 16.1: Cell specific receptors expressed by various cell types in the bio-environment

Cell types	Receptor(S)
Monocytes	Mannose 6-phosphate - t(n)GP, β-glucan
Hepatocytes	Galactose -t(n)GP (high-density), HDL, LDL, EGF, IgA, transferrin
Enterocytes	Maternal IgG, dimeric IgG, transcobalmin II
Macrophages	Mannose-6-phosphatet (n)GP, galactose -t(n)GP, manGlcNAct (n)GP, fucosyl-glycoconjugates, AMPC
Kupffer cells	Mannose -t(n)GP, galactose-particles, polymeric negative charged proteins, complement factors, fucose, LDL, AMPC, fucosyl-glycoconjugates
T4cells	Galactose -t(n)GP (low-density), interleukin, transferrin, CD4
Fibroblasts	Mannose-6-phosphate-t(n)GP, transferrin, transcobalminII, LDL, EGF, AMPC
Endothelial cells	
i. Liver	Monomeric negatively charged proteins, manGlcNAc--t(n)GP, Fc receptors
ii. Blood brain	Transferrin, insulin
iii. Lung, diaphragm and heart	Albumin
Mammary acinar cells	Growth factor
Renal tubular cells	Low molecular weight proteins (cationic)

16.6.1.1. Lectins of human origin

Human mononuclear phagocytes express a cell surface lectin receptor that specifically recognizes glyco-conjugates bearing terminal mannose, mannose 6 phosphate (Man6P) fucose and GlcNAc residues. Receptor expression changes according to macrophage type and down regulation occurs upon activation of macrophages.

Table 16.2 : Lectin receptors on various blood cell types with their sugar affinities and specificities

Species	Cell type	Sugar specificity
Human	Lymphocytes	Mannose, galactose, glucose and fucose
	Macrophages	Galactose, Mannose and Mannose-6-phosphate
	Monocytes	Mannose-6-phosphate
	Mono-nuclear phagocytes	Mannose, fucose and GlucNAc
	Granulocytes	Rhamnose
	B-lymphocytes	Mannose
	Promyelocytic cell HL60	Mannose
Mouse	Lymphocytes, splenic	Mannose
	Lymphocytes, thymic	Galactose, GalNAc
	Lymphocytes	Sulfated polysaccharides
	Macrophages	Mannose, mannose-6-phosphate, galactose, heparin, fucoidan and k-carrageenan
	Monocytes	Mannose-6-phosphate
	Mast cells	Galactose
	L-1210 leukemia cells	Fucose
Rat	Lymphocytes	Fucose
	Macrophage, alveolar	L-fucose, mannose, glucose and GlucNAc
	Macrophage, preitoneal	Galactose
Pig	Lymphocytes	Galactose
	Mononuclear cells	Galactose

Adapted from Molema and Meijer, 1994.

In monocyte derived macrophages of human origin mannose receptor and mannose 6-phosphate receptor, both are expressed that bind the ligands followed by receptor mediated internalization. Human B and T lymphoblastoid cells also express mannose, glucose, GlcNAc, GalNAc, xylose and β-lactose specific lectins. Some of these receptors have been recorded to bind IgE (Ralpati et al.,1985).

16.6.1.2. Lymphocyte homing.receptors

Lymphocyte homing.receptors are believed to belong proteinaceous lectins, which include the serum mannose binding protein and mannose receptor on various tissue macrophages. These are lectin like receptors present on the cell membrane of various lymphocyte subsets, functionally indispensible to the recirculation of lymphocytes from the blood to lymphoid organs. Determinants specifically recognized by these lectins consist of a mannose, phosphomannan, fucose and fructose groups with their negative charged moieties (Jutila et al.,1990). Homing receptor lectins (mainly mannose) on lymphocytes may serve to mediate the extracellular release of drugs bound to suitable carriers.

16.6.1.3. Leukocyte adhesion molecules

Leukocyte adhesion molecules are intercellular immune adhesion molecules, which express leucocyte receptors for ligands (Steinhoff et al.,1993). These include members of

1. Immunoglobulin super family, includes MHC Class I & II, CD2, CD4, CD8 and also ICAM, VCAM, NCAM and PECAM (standing for intracellular, vascular, neural cell and platelet/endothelial cell adhesion molecules respectively). CD4 molecules bind to the anionic hyaluronic acid, similarly, CD22 is a sialic acid binding lectin receptor expressed on β-lymphocytes.

2. Integrin family includes lymphocytes fusion associated antigen (LFA1) and very late antigens (VLA) that have laminine, collagen and fibronectin as ligands.

3. Selectin family includes LECAM and ELAM adhesion factors (respectively leukocytes/endothelial and endothelial/leukocytes adhesion molecules that have the carbohydrate sialyl lewis^x and heparin as counter receptors).

The families of selectins and integrins on lymphocytes may contain binding sites for sulfated glycoconjugates and polyanionic compounds, different from above mentioned polyanionic binding sites on CD lectin receptors. By virtue of these anionic binding sites polyanionic carriers could be targeted to these blood cells.

16.6.2. Receptors for endogenous ligands

Various blood cells, through their adhesion molecules and receptors are capable of specifically recognizing the ligands. Here a brief account of various blood cell receptors with their preferred ligands is reviewed and presented.

16.6.2.1. Endogenous cytokines and lymphokines

Antigens and MHC encoded molecules can be presented on the surface of B-cells and macrophages, resulting in the activation of T-lymphocytes mediated by interleukin-1 (IL1). Activated T-cells produce IL2, with simultaneous expression of high affinity IL2 receptors. In the tumor T-cell lines, IL2 was constantly internalized by receptor mediated endocytosis (RME). IL4 is secreted by activated T-lymphocytes. Human monocytes and acute myeloblastic leukemic cells express high affinity IL4 receptors. IL6 is a cytokine which is able to induce protein synthesis by the liver and augments the cytotoxic T-cell generation and B-cell immunoglobulin secretion. IL6 is drawn processed fast by human T-cells and monocytes/macrophages, followed by intracellular transport and presentation to degradative compartments i.e., cellular targets (Mancilla et al.,1990). Human and mouse T-lymphocytes contain carbohydrates, usually expressed as gangliosides, that can act as cell surface receptors for regulatory molecules like interferons and human growth hormones (Barclay et al.,1993).

16.6.2.2. Endogenous proteins and glycoconjugates

These includes macroglobulin, transferrins, α-fetoproteins, advanced glycation end (AGE) proteins and other proteins.

1. Macroglobulins: Human monocytes and macrophages express a membrane receptor with high affinity for macroglobulin-proteinase complex, followed by RME and lysosoaml degradation (Moestrup et al.,1990).

2. Transferrins: Transferrins receptors are present on actively dividing cell types for cellular growth and differentiation. T-cells internalize and recycle their Tf receptors. The receptor is essentially utilized by the growing cells for the uptake of ferritin protein for nutrient iron (Perrins, 1985).

3. α-fetoproteins (AFP) : Mitogen stimulated normal human lymphocytes bind and internalize AFP. They are also expressed by human T- and B-neoplastic lymphoid cells (Torres et al., 1991).

4. AGE proteins : AGE modified bovine serum albumin specifically bind to mouse peritoneal macrophages. AGE protein binding proteins are also expressed on rat monocytes and resident peritoneal macrophages (Vlassara et al.,1986)

16.6.2.3. Immunoregulatory molecules

These include factors mediating help and suppression of antibody formation, viz., insulin like growth factors (IGF I & II), major histocompatibility complex classes (MHC class I & II), β-glucanes and glycoprotein 120 (gp120).

1. IGF : Human monocytes and alveolar macrophages express insulin like growth factor II/Man 6P receptors. Human peripheral blood T-cells upon anti CD3 activation express receptor for IGFI, IGFII and insulin in a sequential manner (Rom, 1991).

2. MHC : Receptors for MHC classes are expressed by blood T-lymphocytes and monocytes/macrophages. MHC I molecule functions as transport module and internalized by coated pits. Class II MHC molecules carry a sulfated glycosamino-glycan (anionic polysaccharide) that is essential for antigen presentation (Pernis, 1985).

3. β-glucans : Receptors for these particular immune activators are present on human monocytes and initiate phagocytosis of glucan, production of leukotrienes and release of lysosoaml enzymes (Czop et al.,1990).

4. gp120 : MHC class II positive T-lymphocytes are capable of internalizing, processing and presenting this antigen. The HIV virus infected cells shed it abundantly (Lanzavecchia et al.,1988).

16.6.3. Ligand receptor interaction

Cell surface receptors are excellent ports which may be effectively used in selective targeting of drugs, oligonucleotides or even genes by making use of their specific affinity ligands. Ligand-receptor interaction at the cellular level leads to the consequences of site specific delivery through uptake of carried contents. Various ligands (Fig. 16.3) have been identified and used as novel navigators for selective delivery of drug(s). Table 16.3 summarizes various ligands with their specific receptor present in the bio-cells.

16.7. CARRIER SYSTEMS FOR TARGETING

In order to achieve specific targeting, it is required that there should be some specific carrier molecule to carry the drug. A carrier itself in some cases acts as a pilot molecule due to some of its inherent characteristics. It follows that with the intended target cells in RES predominant organs, the only criteria for successful delivery is that the carrier systems should quantitatively retain their load while they are in circulation.

The distinctive and defined intrinsic passivity of carrier at large decide its ultimate localization. However, to promote its selective and intended association with any fixed cells which are anatomically accessible to the carrier; the carrier must be able to recognize the cell(s) target; should bind to them and if necessary, penetrate into their interior. Similarly, tailoring the structural components of carrier systems (to take advantage of, or tackling bioenvironmental properties) has led to the development of carrier systems of diversified nature and ultimately action specific. Some surface modifications of the carrier systems with particular ligands like sugars or Abs could impart a specific targeting potential to the carrier. Hence, in essence to deliver drug selectively to a target we should have specific carriers and a specific ligands.

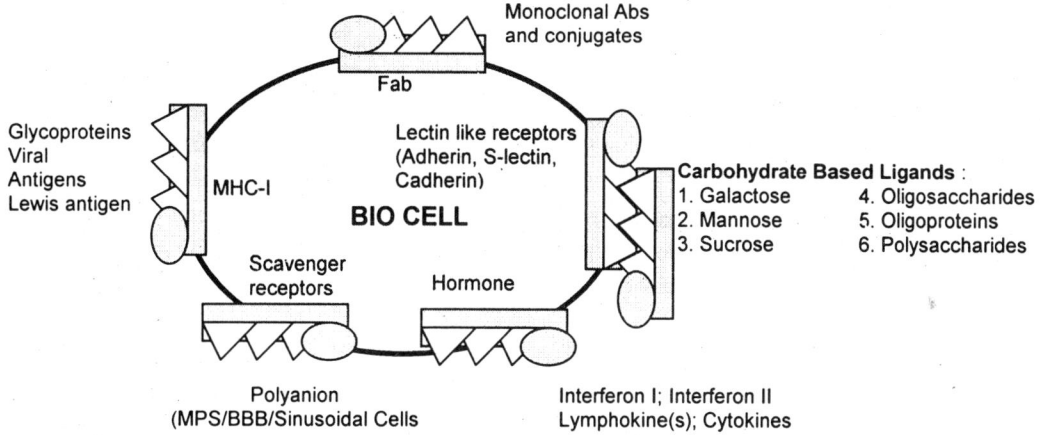

Fig. 16.3 : Distribution of receptors on bio-cell surface

Table 16.3 : Cell specific receptors expressed by various biocells with their preferred ligands

Ligands	Receptors	Expression by various biocells
1. Antibody and its conjugates		
(a). Immunoglobulin IgG class (polyclonal or MoAb); Haptens; Fab' or F(ab)$_2$ immunological fragments	Fc/C3b.receptors	Human/murine macrophages; peritoneal macrophages; Fc receptor bearing tumor cell lines
(b). IgM class	complement receptor	Peritoneal macrophages
(c). Palmitate derivatized IgG	surrogate receptors	Macrophage cell lines
2. Endogenous ligands		
(a). Endogenous cytokines & lymphokines	Interferons (ganglioside expressing receptors); interleukin- I, II, IV,VI receptors	T-lymphocytes; hepatocytes; macrophages; tumor T-cell lines
(b). MHC classes	MHC class I & II	Resting & activated human T cell lines
(c). Lectins & other protein receptor based ligands	Insulin growth-factor (IGFII/Man 6P); Transferrin (Tf); r-T cell (rCD4) receptor; α_2 macroglobulin; gp120; complement receptors	Human monocytes; alveolar macrophages; proliferating cell lines; T4 cells; macrophages; monocytes; Kupffer cells
3. Glyco-conjugates		
(a). Glycosylated carrier	Galactose specific; 4GalNaC; asialoglycoprotein receptors	Kupffer cells; liver endothelial cells
(b). Negative charged particles	Scavenger receptors	Liver endothelia (monomeric); Kupffer cells (polymeric)
(c). Glyco-conjugates based on galactose; mannose; fucose; β-glucan; biantennary glycans & oligosaccharide with terminal reduciblegalactose residue; etc.	lectin receptors (galactose specific; ASGP; mannosylated; mannose 6P fucosyl; and β-glucan) lympho-cyte homing receptors	Macrophage hepatic endothelium; macrophage leukocytes; lymphocytes, rat kupffer cells; proliferating cell lines

*Adopted & modified from Ostro et al., 1987; Molema et al., 1994; and Monsigny et al., 1994

Several carriers appended with the pilot molecules to selectively deliver the drug to the intended cell lines have been reported. Based on the nature of their origin they are categorized as endogenous (low density lipoprotein, high density lipoprotein, chylomicrons, serum albumin, erythrocytes, etc.) and exogenous (microparticulate, soluble polymeric and biodegradable polymeric drug carriers). Based on the above considerations, a variety of site specific and target oriented drug delivery systems have been developed. Table 16.4 provides a categorical presentation of these potential targetable systems.

Table 16.4 : Various carrier systems investigated for their targeting potential (classified)

Carrier systems	References
1. Colloidal carriers	
a) Vesicular systems	
Liposomes; Niosomes; Pharmacosomes; Virosomes; Immunoliposomes	Bangham et al., 1965; Handjani-villa et al.,1979; Vizaglou et al.,1988; Al - Ahdal et al., 1986; Gregoriadis, 1993; Zelphati et al., 1996
b) Microparticulate systems	
Microparticles; Nanoparticles; Magnetic microspheres; Albumin microspheres; serum albumin microbeads; nanocapsules; albumin nanospheres; solid lipid nanoparticles (SLN)	Sjoholm & Edman, 1978; Marty et al., 1978; Widder et al., 1979; Tomlinson et al., 1983; Ammoury, 1989; Karajigi et al., 1993; Maliya & Vyas, 1988; Muller et al.,1996; 1997
2. Cellular carriers	
Resealed erythrocytes; serum albumin; antibodies; platelets; leukocytes	Ihler et al., 1973; Ahn et al., 1978; Segal 1979; Jain and Vyas 1993; Vyas et al., 1993
3. Supramolecular delivery systems	
a) Low aggregation number	
Micelles; reverse; mixed micelles; polymeric micelles	Kumar 1986; Turoo 1984; Dangi et al., 1996
b) Intermediate aggregation number	
Liquid crystals	Ringsdorf et al., 1988; Jaitely and Vyas,1997
c) High aggregation number	
i) Lipoproteins (Chylomicrons; VLDL; LDL)	Demant et al.,1988; Bijsterbosch et al., 1990
ii) Modified semisynthetic lipoproteins	VanBerkel 1990
iii) Synthetic LDL mimicking particles (SMBV)	Samain et al., 1989; Jaitely et al., 1997
4. Polymer based systems	
Signal sensitive; Mucoadhesive; Biodegradable; Bioerodible; Soluble synthetic polymeric carriers	Hutchinson 1985; Kopecek 1990
5. Macromolecular carriers	
a) Proteins	
Serum albumin (human and bovine); glycoproteins; neo glycoproteins and artificial viral envelopes (AVE)	Baurain et al., 1983; Steer et al., 1986; Molema et al., 1990; Scherier et al., 1995
b) Glycosylated water soluble polymers (poly-L-lysine)	Midoux et al.,1989
c) *MAb*: immunological Fab fragments; antibody-enzyme complex & bispecific Abs	Vitetta et al., 1985; Haisma et al., 1992; Fanger et al., 1992
d) *Toxins,* immunotoxin & rCD4 toxin conjugates	Kim et al., 1996; Till et al., 1988
e) *Lectins* (Con A) & polysaccharides	Kitao & Hatta 1977; Reemen et al., 1984

Microparticulates have been investigated intensively during the last decade to explore and exploit intrinsic targeting potential of the plain or surface manipulated carriers. Nanotechnology has infused new dimensions into the site directed target oriented drug delivery through self assembling supramolecules based nanostructures. **Starburst dendrimers** (polyamidoamine cascade polymers) have been recently identified for the delivery of anti-infective drugs and for the expression of encoding genes (Service et al., 1995). Surface modified nanocrystalline ceramics offer an exciting approach that circumvents challenges encountered in drug delivery. While the ceramics provide the structural stability of a largely immutable solid, the surface modification creates a glassy molecular stabilization film to which pharmacologic agents may be bound non-covalently to an aqueous phase with minimum structural denaturation, as a consequence, drug activity following surface immobilization is detered and retained (**aquasomes**). Kossovsky et al., (1994), successfully developed surface modified nanocrystalline ceramics to deliver viral antigens for the purpose of evoking an immune response, oxygenated hemoglobin for cell respiration and insulin for carbohydrate metabolism.

16.7.1. The colloidal carriers

This category of targetable devices include drug bearing bilayer vesicular systems as well cellular carriers in the micron or submicron size range. The passive targetability attributed to the microparticulate drug carriers is due to the recognition of these exogenous particulates either in the intact or in the opsonised form, by the phagocytic cells of the **reticulo-endothelial system** (RES) and this sensing behavior is exploited to target MPS associated diseased cell lines (Table 16.5).

Table 16.5 : Passive hepatic targeting concept exploited in the treatment of macrophage associated diseases

Macrophage associated infected cell lines	Drugs proposed for encapsulation
Intracellular parasites	
Leishmaniasis; brucellosis; candidiasis	Antimalarial & anti-infective
Intracellular fungal infections	
Histoplosmosis; systemic mycoses	Antifungal (Amphotericin B)
Neoplasms	
Histiocytes medullar reticulosis; monocyte & hairy cell lukemia;	Cytotoxic drugs
Hodgkin's disease	
Viral infected diseases	Anti-viral drugs
Hepatitis	
Enzyme storage diseases	
Gaucher's disease, mucoliposes type II & III	Glucocerebroside & other enzymes

A major disadvantage of microparticulates is that they cannot pass the endothelial cell lines, as a result extroversion is generally poor. Although some investigations claim that slow transcellular (vesicular) transport of liposomes and microspheres is possible through endothelia. The practical applications of microparticulate carriers are largely restricted to intravascular targets. Attempts have been made for targeting them to intravesicular non-RES cell lines and to increase circulation half-life by exploiting strategies that involve modification of size, surface charge, composition, surface rigidity and surface hydrophilicity. These long circulatory modules, can then be relied as carrier base. However, to endow them with target specificity some site directing ligands could be appended on their surface site specific ligands can be immobilized with optimal targeting efficiency. Recent literature is exhaustively dedicated towards the pilot molecules (ligands) appended microparticles in general and liposomal systems in particular.

16.8. VESICULAR SYSTEMS FOR LIGAND MEDIATED DRUG TARGETING

The vesicular systems are highly ordered assemblies of one or several concentric lipid bilayers formed when certain amphipathic building blocks are confronted with water . Various polar drugs can be accommodated in the aqueous domains and nonpolar drugs within the lipid domains respectively . Vesicles can be formed from a diverse range of amphiphilic building blocks, the terms such as synthetic bilayers allude to the non-biological origin of such vesiculogens. Biological origin of these vesicles was first reported in 1965 by Bangham and were given the name 'Bangham bodies'. Liposomes, (lipid hollow sphere) as they are know today, can be defined as spherical concentric 'fluid mosaic' generated due to highly precise self assembly of phospholipid molecules (having zwitterionic amphiphilic structure) on confrontation with aqueous buffer. The building blocks of these bilayered vesicles are glycerol based amphiphilic phospholipids (mainly lecithin). Steroids mainly cholesterol and its derivatives, are included to increase the rigidity or microviscosity of the bilayer (fluidity buffer) and also to stabilize the bilayer membrane in the presence of biological fluids. Non biological origin of such components has been considered to improve the *in vivo* and *in vitro* stability as compared to the natural lecithin based bilayer vesicles. In order to alleviate and improve the thermodynamic stability problems confined to natural phospholipid based vesicles, several modified versions of liposomes, have been reported for their *in vitro* stability nevertheless their targeting potential is hampered due to immunogenic and nonbiodegradable nature of the constitutive lipids. Several other nonbiological synthetic vesiculagous have been investigated which are able to impart *in vitro* stability to the liposomes, simultaneously projecting some targeting potential; however synthetic origin limits their *in vivo* applicability. Bilayer vesicular systems of biological origin and non biological origins reported in the literature are summarized in table 16.6.

Antibody mediated or ligand mediated targeting of liposomes has been reported in the literature (Ostro,1987), but a direct correlation of *in vitro-in vivo* performance still remains to be the aim of targeted drug therapy. Still many of the new approaches are discussed in the latter part of this chapter, they would be the subjects of future research.

Table 16.6 : Various vesicular systems from biological and non-biological origin, reported in the literature

Origin	Building blocks	References
1. Biological origin		
Liposomes	Natural zwitterionic phospholipids	Bangham et al., 1965; Gregoriadis 1972
	Synthetic saturated phospholipids	Chiang &Weiner, 1987
Polymerizable liposomes	Diacetylenic lipids; methacryloyl lipids; Dienoyl lipids	Regen et al., 1980 Fendler 1982
Polymer capped liposomes	Cationic phospholipids polymerized with polymerizable anion like methacrylate	Regen et al., 1984
Polymerized phospholipid liposomes	Phospholipids polymerized with 1,2-bis-(2-mercapto-hexadecanoyl)Sn glycero-3-phosphocholine	Weber et al., 1987
Redox liposomes	Vesicles based on thiol-disulfide redox cycle	Samvel et al., 1985
Virosomes	Reconsituted viral spiked glycoproteins	Al-Ahdal et al., 1986
Polymer grafted liposomes	Nature synthetic phospholipids with covalently linked PEG polymer	Allen et al., 1991
Emulsomes	Phospholipids of high concentration along with high molecular weight fatty acids	Amselem et al., 1994
2. Nonbiological origin		
Niosomes	Single chain non-ionic surfactant of low HLB values	Handjani-Villa et al., 1979
Discomes	Solubilization of niosomes with a non-ionic surfactant solulan (polyoxyethylene cetyl ether class)	Kim and Kim., 1991; Vyas et al., 1997
Pharmacosomes	Mesogenic drug itself as a building block in combination with a lipid	Vizagolu et al., 1986
Ufasomes	Single chain unsaturated fatty acids	Gebicki et al., 1973
Cryptosomes	Natural phospholipids in combination with suitable poly-oxythylene derivatives of PE	Blume et al., 1990

A number of developments in liposome technology have been instrumental in helping to make *in vivo* targeting of liposomes a reality. Various strategies have been adopted to engineer liposomes as a vector anchored with pilot molecules/ ligands. Some of them are categorized as follows;

1. engineered liposomal construct;
2. engineered for steric stabilization and long circulation; and
3. engineered for anchoring ligands/ pilot molecules.

16.8.1. Engineered liposomal constructs

Liposomal constructs can be engineered in order to facilitate their access to other vascular or extravascular targets by manipulating lipid composition, vesicle size and drug loading techniques.

The role of lipid composition on liposome clearance is well established. The liposomes composed of phospholipids with high phase transition temperature (T°C) based acyl moieties (rigidized bilayer) were found to exhibit relatively prolonged circulation, offering the probability of interacting with target cells other than MPS. Distearoylphosphatidylcholine (DSPC) or distearoylphosphatidylethanolamine (DSPE) or sphingomyelin (SM) mixed with cholesterol in different molar ratios have been examined for their rigidization effect on the bilayers. The sphingomyelin can form additional hydrogen bonds, whereas distearoyl and dipalmitoyl derivatives of constituent lipids have a high T°C. These features confer prolonged circulation behavior to the liposomal formulations.

The ability of liposomes to extravasate and penetrate into diseased states other than MPS is directly related to their size. Large liposomes (5μ or above) are rapidly removed via mechanical filtration of lungs and from this size range down upto 150 nm are removed by tissue macrophages originated in the liver and spleen, which are the natural target for these vesicles. In order to achieve significant levels in other tissues, liposomes of smaller size (≤100 nm) with a homogeneous distribution have been developed. They could penetrate into either normal tissue having sinusoidal or fenestrated epithelium or otherwise into diseased tissue having altered capillary permeability. This has in turn increased the chances of achieving targeting *in vivo* to non-MPS cell linings.

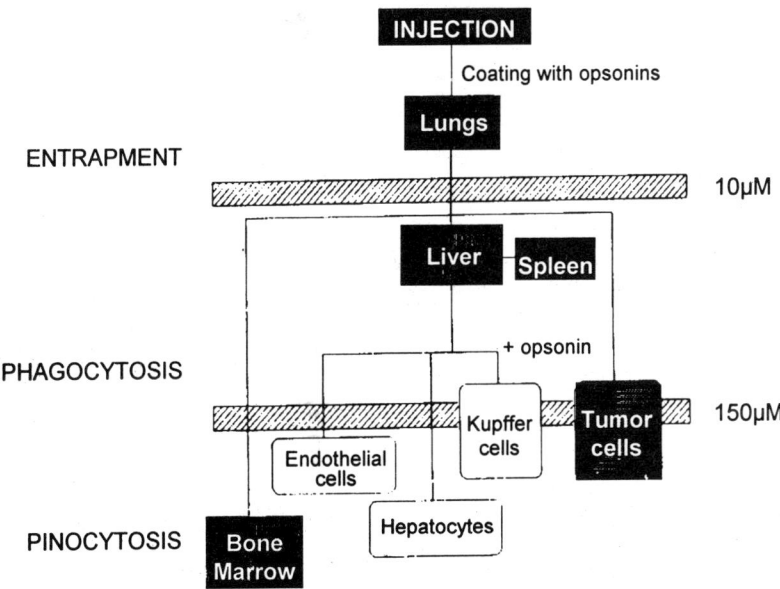

Fig.: 16.4 : Schematic diagram of bio-fate of colloidal particles *in vivo*

Some significant advances have been made in the development of technology for efficient drug entrapment in liposomes. Passive loading techniques have now been replaced by active loading strategies, especially for weakly acidic/basic drugs. These compounds can be actively loaded into liposomes (**remote loading**) with an efficiency of approximately 90 % by establishing a pH or chemical gradient across the bilayer membrane. The liposome composition, the internal pH or presence of counter ions can be manipulated to obviate the leakage of drugs from liposomes which ought to be tailored to suit the specific applications, being pursued. These technologies have been important preludes to the development of targeted liposomes.

16.8.2. Steric stabilization for long circulation

Surface modified liposomes have been developed to provide a long circulatory 'sterically stabilized' module on which pilot molecules/ligands can be successfully anchored. The attempts to target plain 'classical' liposomes have at large been disappointing due to their very short blood circulation half-life, their preferential accumulation in liver and spleen (RES uptake) and their dose dependent pharmacokinetics. Long circulatory sterically stabilized liposomes (SSL) however may now assist successful implementation of the targeting strategies (Allen,1989). Major aims of SSL can be accounted on the following lines:

1. Making liposomal system more stable in normal biological surroundings.

2. Making them long circulatory (i.e., less opsonizable and hence less recognizable by phaogocytic cells of RES).

3. Making them targeted with or without anchoring pilot ligands.

4. Making them more sensitive towards some external stimuli, such as pH, substrate or temperature.

Some of the earliest attempts include **coating** liposomes with proteins and macromolecules (serum albumin), glycoproteins (sialoglycoprotein fetuin) and polysaccharides (pullulan). Recently, non-ionic surfactants coated liposomes have been reported by Khattab et al., (1995), with the sorption of silicone-glycol co-polymers onto the surface of SUVs. The highest retention was obtained with SUVs coated with the silicone polymer possessing the highest glycol content and the longest ethylene oxide chains. Silicone glyco-copolymer coated liposomes (sterically stabilized vesicles) showed longer half life comparable to that of polaxamer 338 coated. In contrast to coatings, methods of **doping** involving the mixing of amphipathic molecules with special polar heads at low molar ratios in the lipid bilayers, have been reported with glycolipds (GM$_1$, monosialoganglioside) and hydrated phosphatidyl-inositol. Recently, a number of investigations have been conducted with the incorporation of glycolipids/glycoproteins or other glyco-conjugates for prolonging the circulation time and to avoid or reduce RES uptake of liposomes. Yamauchi et al., (1995), reported a novel synthetic sialic acid derivative (sialo-glycolipid) as a mimic of GM$_1$, having a sialic acid group (Neu5Ac) at the terminal position of the glycolipid. Long circulatory behavior of these surface modified liposomes could be ascribed to three different strategies:

1. Glycocalyx similar to RBC, which is instrumental to provide an ability to surface modified liposomes to mimic the outer monolayer of RBC.

2. Hypothesis of shielded negative charge, that proposes existence of screened negative charge; that increases the surface hydrophilicity of the liposomes without imparting a negatively charge binding site at the surface of the liposome for scavenging system.

3. Hypothesis of dysopsonin, proposes specific recognition of GM$_1$, by a serum protein (i.e., a dysopsonin), which prevents the attack and recognition by opsonin.

Most of the recent literature concentrates and discusses the PEG-ylated liposomes (or, polymer grafted liposomes), obtainable with both fluid or rigidized bilayer combinations. The developments of sterically stabilized liposomes (SSL), in which hydrophilic polymer, such as polyethylene glycol (PEG) is **covalently coupled** to the surface group of a lipid i.e., PE (phosphatidylethanolamine) or DSPE (distearoyl PE), have been reported (PEG-PE or PEG-DSPE) for their relatively low level of MPS uptake, therefore resulting in long circulation half life and dose-independent pharmacokinetics (Papahadjopoulos et al., 1991). Zalipsky et al. (1996) recently evaluated blood clearance rates and biodistribution of poly (2-oxazoline) grafted liposomes in which DSPE was covalently coupled to the carboxylic groups of the polymers namely, PMOZ [Poly(2-methyl-2-oxazoline)] and PEOZ [poly{2-ethyl-2-oxazoline)], resulting in conjugates which incorporate readily in liposomes providing than a long circulatory nature. Furthermore, three different mechanisms have been proposed for polymer grafted systems (Fig. 16.5).

1. Hypothesis of steric barrier, that proposes steric stabilization (polymer brush surface hydrophilicity) by the grafted polymer.

2. Inhibition of the nonspecific adsorption of plasma proteins and lipoproteins.

3. Inhibition of specific opsonization of the lipid surface by immunoglobulin.

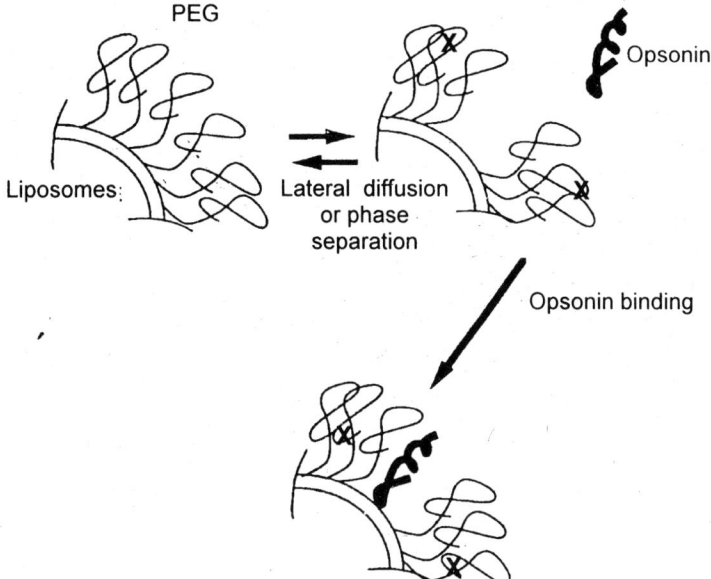

$X \Rightarrow$ 1. Polyethylene glycol conjugates   2. Sialic acid conjugates   3. Pullulan   4. Stearlyamine derivatized dextrans
5. Polyoxazoline DSPE conjugates (Glutrate interlinked G type conjugates or propionates interlinked P type conjugates)
6. Monosialoganglioside 'GM1   7. Inosterols   8. Sphingomyelins

Fig. 16.5 : Various approaches reported to confer long circulatory nature to SSL

16.8.3. Anchoring of ligands/Abs

Once long-circulatory liposomes are developed, it seems appropriate to examine approaches for the efficient anchoring of ligands/Ab through PEG at the liposome surface. The PEG however could interfere with the process in either of two ways; the PEG could provide a steric hindrance to the access of Abs or ligands to the liposomal surface and decrease the coupling efficiency, or otherwise, once the Abs are attached to the liposomal surface, PEG could interfere with the recognition of the Ab/ligand by its target. Table 16.7 enlists various covalent and non-covalent techniques conventionally used for anchoring Abs/ligands to liposomal surface. These techniques are pivotal in providing long circulatory nature to SSL along with targeting potential imparted by anchoring ligands (Fig. 16.6).

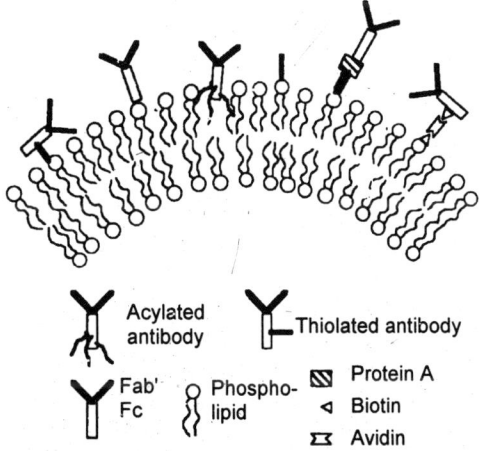

Fig. 16.6 : Schematic representation of conjugation of antibodies/ligands to the liposomal surface

Table 16.7 : Various covalent and noncovalent techniques
for anchoring Ab/ligands to liposomal surface

Techniques	Reference
I . Noncovalent coupling technique	
1. Biotin-Avidin conjugates (Ab/ligand-biotin + avidin + biotinylated-liposomes)	Loughrey et al., 1987
2. Biotin-Streptividin coupling (Streptividin lipid derivative + liposome + biotinylated ligand)	Loughrey et al., 1990
II. Covalent coupling techniques	
1. Coupling reagent methods	
a. Carbodiimide coupling (DSPE-PEG-COOH + carbodiimide reagent + glu-plasminogen)	Blume et al., 1988
b. Thioether coupling (Maleimide derivatized phospholipid + thiolated ligand)	Martin & Papahadjopoulous 1982
c. Modified thioether coupling	
i. Maleimide derivatized phospholipid (MPB- DOPE/MCC-DOPE) + thiolated ligand (SPDP)	Hansen et al., 1995
ii. Thiol derivatized phospholipid (PDP-DOPE) + maleimide derivatized ligand (SMPB-ligand))	Hansen et al., 1985
iii. Maleimide-derivatized PEG-liposomes + thiolated ligand (SPDP-ligand)	Kirpotin et al., 1996
iv. Thiol-derivatized PEG liposomes (PDP-PEG-DSPE) + maleimide derivatized ligand (MPB-ligand)	Allen et al., 1995
d. Hydrazone bond coupling (Hydrazide-PEG-DSPE + periodate treated ligand)	Hansch et al., 1995
2. Post coating method (Ab/ligand + liposome + PEG succinyl cysteine)	Suzuki et al., 1995
3. Detergent dialysis method (Ab-NGPE+ S-liposome + detergent octylglucoside)	Kilbanov & Huang 1992

MCC: n-(Maleimidomethylcyclohexane)1-carboxylate; MPB: N-(4'(-4''-Maleimidophenyl)butyroyl); DOPE: Dioleoylphosphatidyl ethanolamine; SPDP: N-succinimidyl-3-(2-pyridyl-thio)propionate; SMPB: (H-succinimidyl-4-(p-maleimidophenyl)butyrate), PDP: N-(3'-(pridyl dithio)propionyl); NGPE: N-glutaryl-PE

16.9. SPECIALIZED LIPOSOMES FOR CELLULAR DRUG TARGETING

Novel drug delivery systems in general and liposomal technology in particular have provided the opportunities for designing and practicing the site specific targeted drug therapy with added dimensions. Retrospecting the conceptual aspect and relevant features of liposomal system, it could be presented as a construct which is further engineered and structured with maximum therapeutic benefits. With this perspective an attempt is made to categorize various targeting strategies appreciated to be adoptable or proposed with various promises particularly relating to liposomal constructs.

16.9.1. Glycoprotein bearing liposomes

The incorporation of glycoproteins onto the liposomal surface has been employed as an approach for targeting to sendai virus (Sarkar et al.,1987), macrophages (Russel et al.,1986) and amoebae/traphozoites (Bailey et al.,1990). The major glycoprotein, **the glycophorins** of the human erythrocyte plasma membrane, has been incorporated into liposomes, and the potential of glycophorin based liposomes has been discussed.

The glycophorins carry numerous blood group antigens, but as site directing molecules for liposomes, it is the sialic acid (N-acetyl-nuraminic acid) present at the termini of the oligoasccharide side chains. It is utilized at large to target liposomes to the lectin receptors. Sialic acid has been thought to play a key role in prolonging the circulation time of serum proteins (Morell et al., 1968). Since then, sialic acid residues on the liposomal surface have been incorporated and appreciated for their biodistribution and cell recognizability. The sialo-conjugates include **sialo-glycoprotein** of human erythrocytes as glycophorin reconstituted liposomes (Utsumi et al., 1983), **monosialoganglioside GM$_1$** (Allen and Chonn, 1987), sialoglycopeptide derived **fetuin** (Saito et al.,1988), **sialic acid** conjugated, cholesterol substituted polysaccharide (Sunamoto et al., 1988) and **sialoglycolipid**, a novel synthetic sialic acid derivative (Yamauchi et al., 1995).

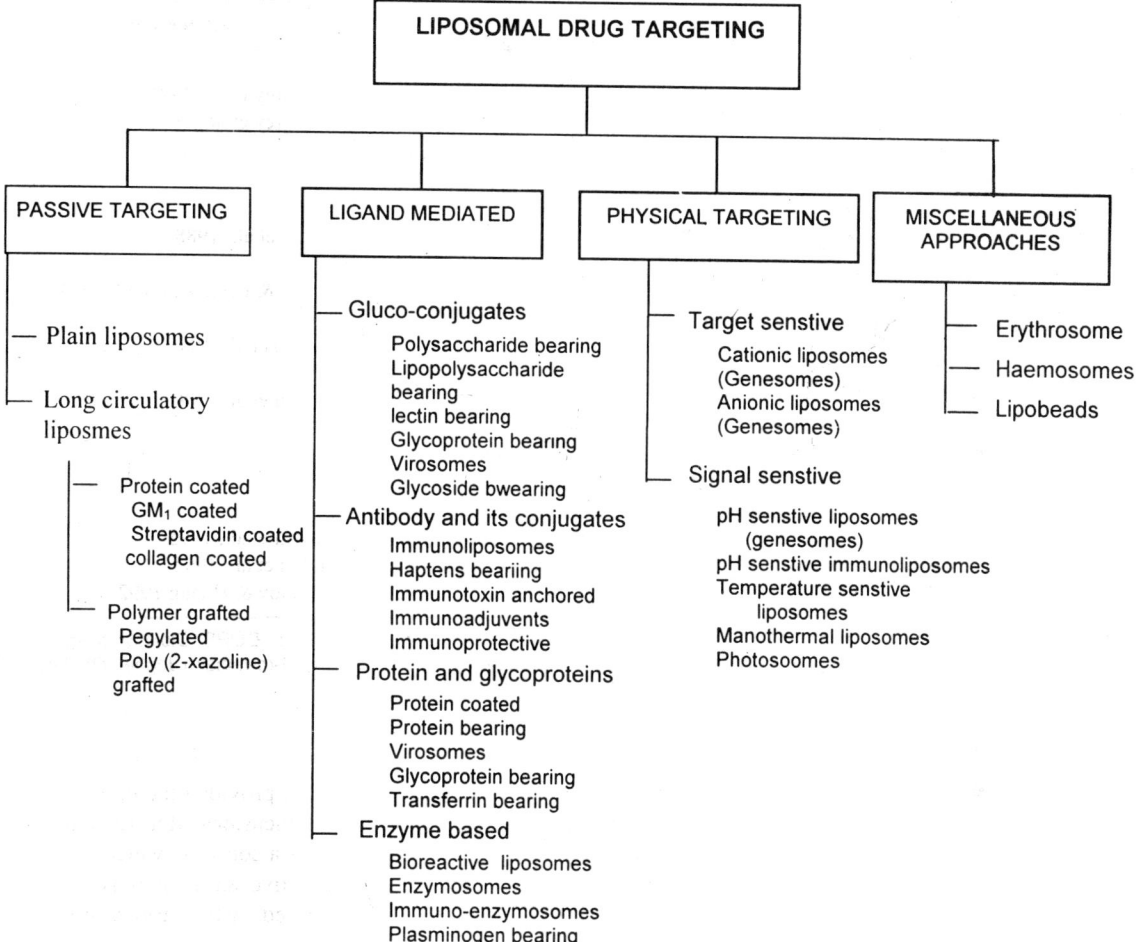

An interesting approach which exploits glycoproteins in liposomal drug targeting and subsequently delivers drugs to the intended cell lines, could be the use of synthetic glycoproteins that are based on **serum albumins** (neoglycoproteins). The synthesized glycoproteins are immobilized on the liposomal system (Gabius et al., 1987; Yamazaki et al., 1992). The high affinity binding of immobilized (neoglycoprotein coupled) liposomes bearing **mannose** and **melibiose residues** has been established *in vitro* with human adenocarcinoma cells, suggesting targeting applicability of these novel liposomes to tumor cell lines. Similarly, neoglycoprotein coupled liposomes are found to be potential immunological adjuvants. Dehydration-rehydration vesicles (DRVs) with surface bound mannosylated albumin as ligand and containing immunopurified tetanus toxoid as active moiety have been found to bind selectively to mouse peritoneal macrophages and able to evoke a stronger immune response than either naked or albumin coated liposomes.

16.9.2. Virosomes

Virosomes are liposomes spiked with virus glycoproteins, incorporated into the liposomal bilayers based on retroviruses derived lipids (generally murine/avion). Reconstitution of a number of spike glycoproteins including those of sendai virus (Al-Ahdal et al.,1986), rabies virus (Perrin et al.,1985), influenza virus (Sizer et al.,1987), herpes virus (Ho et al.,1990), HIV- I (Thibodeau et al.,1989) and vesicular stomatis virus (Nagato et al.,1991) into liposomes has been described. The virosomal constructs have been developed and used as a means of targeting to hamster hybridoma cells (Nagato et al.,1991), murine lymph node T-cells (Garnier et al.,1991), to elicit immune response in animals (Perrin et al.,1985) and in the mice and guinea pig (Ho et al.,1992).

Commonly encountered problem with conventional liposomes is their internalization via endocytic compartment into the lysosomal system. To directly introduce molecules into the cytoplasm, liposomes that merge with cell membranes have been developed. The principle mimics the natural way by which several viruses bind and merge with cell membrane at neutral pH releasing their genome into the cytoplasm. Development of virosomes exploits the ability of spike glycoprotein to undergo a conformational change at the endosomal pH, resulting in exposure of their hydrophobic residues to initiate fusion with plasma membrane of the cell or in case of small liposomes, fusion with endocytic vacuoles. An alternative strategy to the reconstitution of virus spike glycoprotein in liposomes, involves the reconstitution of the virus receptor of the target cell contained in the liposomes. Fusion between the receptor bearing liposomes and the target cell is then brought about by the virus particle. The virosomes may be target oriented and their fusogenic characteristics could be exploited in genome grafting and cellular microinjection. Proteoliposomes have been reported to deliver gene expression systems to cells (Fogerite et al.,1989). Liposomes prepared with fusogens (F) of sendai virus, incorporated into lipid bilayers (reconstituted fusogenic viral membrane) acquires character to merge with cell membrane. Molecules with poor cellular membrane permeability [like the RNA duplex poly (rl).poly(rc)] have been very efficiently delivered to the cells with the help of fusogenic virosomes (Compagnon et al., 1990). Virosomes are recently reported as a carrier for intracellular delivery of antisense oligonucleotides (Zelphati et al.,1996). Morishita et al.(1993), have encapsulated oligonucleotides into negatively charged liposomes complexed to the protein core of an inactivated sendai virus. The approach exhibited a more rapid cellular uptake and higher transfection efficiency of oligonucleotides or plasmid DNA as compared to Lipofectin (discussed elsewhere in the article) or passive uptake. Virosomes have exhibited potential as immunological adjuvants and as a result subsequent studies are directed towards their exploration and exploitation in immunological manipulations (Gregoriadis, 1990).

16.9.3. Glycolipid bearing liposomes

Glycolipids have been used extensively as site directing molecules for targeting to a wide range of target sites including lymphocytes (Sharom et al,1986), ricin (Utsumi et al.,1987), sendai virus (Tsao et al.,1986), antibodies (Clausen et al.,1988), Fab fragments (Rock et al.,1990) and vesicular stomatis virus (Sinibadi et al.,1985).

Glycolipids (mainly monosialo-ganglioside) appended liposomes are expected to participate in interactions such as cellular recognition and fusion and can function as receptors for viruses, antibodies and lectins. The interaction of glycolipid bearing liposomes with lectins demonstrated that galactosylated liposomes are preferentially taken up by the liver parenchymatous cells whereas mannosylated liposomes were mainly localized in non parenchymatous cells (Ghosh and Bachhawat,1992). Shen in the year 1987, reported the above approach by entrapping I(125) labelled β-glucocerebrosidase in glycolipid coated liposomes for the treatment of Gaucher's disease, proposing potential use of liposomes in enzyme replacement therapy. Further studies were carried out with lactosyl ceramide and Tris-Gal-Chol which were employed to target small liposomes to hepatocytes and the larger ones to Kuppfer cells (Spanjer and Scherphof,1983; Spanjer et al.,1985). It has been demonstrated that the cetyl-mannosylated liposomes are selectively delivered to blood monocytes whereas galactosylated liposomes to peritoneal macrophages (Ghosh and Bachhawat,1992).

Haensler et al., (1988) proposed liposomes appended with synthetic galactolipids, in order to target vesicles to galactose receptor expressing target cells. Neo-galactosylated liposomes have been proposed by covalent coupling of β-D-1-thiogalacto-pyranoside residues, substituted with a hydrophilic spacer-arm and functionalized with a sulfhydryl group, to preformed large unilamellar vesicles (LUV) containing 4-(p-maleimido-phenyl)-butyryl PE. Compared to the control vesicles, the neo-galactosylated liposomes demonstrated an increased binding to cells *in vitro* possessing a β-D-galactose specific receptor, i.e. resident mouse peritoneal macrophages.

Liposomes coated with natural gangliosides GM₁ (monosialoganglioside) possess steric stabilization and prolonged circulation potential (Stealth liposomes™), which is a prerequisite in targeting tissues other than liver and spleen. Recently, a theoretical model has been proposed demonstrating the interaction of the surface polymers (polyolphosphate polymer) of the bacterial glycocalyx with liposomes, incorporating lipids with poly-hydroxy head groups such as phosphatidylinositol (PI). Jones (1994), proposed this model (PI-Liposomal system) to a range of biofilms of oral and skin associated bacteria. Glycolipids have considerable potential as immunomodulators and glycolipid bearing liposomes demonstrated appreciable potentials as adjuvants in vaccines (Wang et al., 1987).

16.9.4. Glycoside bearing liposomes

Liposomal preparations guarded, tracked and drived by suitable glycoside(s) based pilot molecules have been developed against macrophage associated disorders involving *Mycobacterium leprae* and *M.tuberculosis* (Medda et al., 1995).

Plant glycosides, **asiaticoside** and **corchorusin D**, having rhamnose and glucose as terminal sugar respectively, have been grafted on to the liposomal surface. Liposomal asiaticoside demonstrated better microbiological property against *M. leprae* and *M. tuberculosis*, as compared to that of free asiaticoside. The liposomes containing asiaticoside and corchorusin D, however, were found to be equally or more active as compared to liposomal asiaticoside alone. It is inferred that appropriate glycosides, could direct and target the liposomes selectively therefore, could be used for chemotherapeutic control of several other diseases.

16.9.5. Protein coated liposomes

Liposomes with proteins immobilized on their surface were investigated for increased passive targeting to extravascular spaces. Longaman and co-workers (1995) reported an *in vivo* liposomal targeting approach that involves bindings SA-LUVs (**streptavidin liposomes**) to target cells, prelabelled with surface associated **biotinylated antibody**. Opsonin and RES scavenge hydrophobic surfaces and hence biotin-PE containing liposomes show higher agglutination with streptividin *in vitro* in the presence of PEG-PE (Fig.16.7). Results have shown that this double step targeting strategy was as efficient as approaches involving antibody coated liposomes for labelling cells *in vitro*.

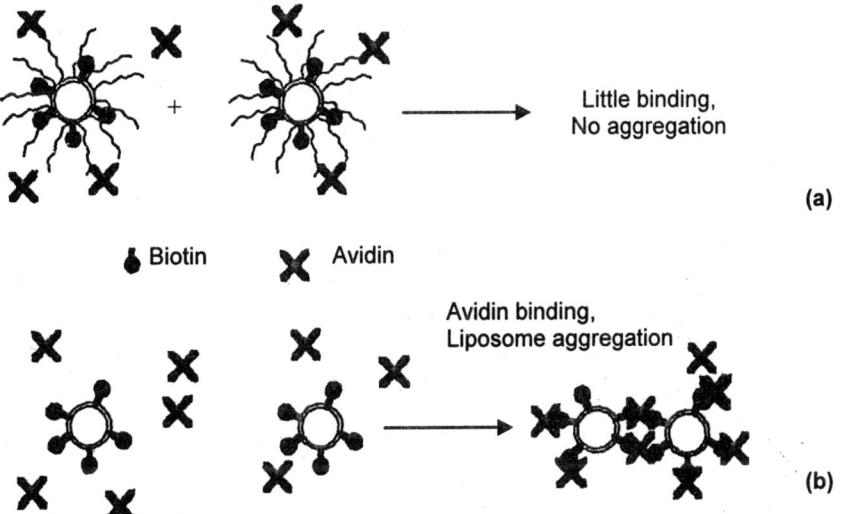

Fig. 16.7: Mechanistic presentation of biotin-PE liposomal agglutination *in vitro* with strptividin in (a) absense, and (b) in presence of a hydrophilic surface (PEG-PE)

Fonseca et al., 1996 reported collagen coated vesicles for increased uptake in liver. Two hydrophobic (hexyl and lauryl residues) derivatives of collagens (Mw 50,000) were incubated with preformed vesicles. Coated vesicles were found to be more stable *in vitro* and their clearance from circulation was faster. The *in vivo* tissue distribution (liver uptake) of these liposomes was higher than plain liposomes. Tetsui et al., (1996) proposed a multivalent ligand in which enkephalin/ phospholoipid conjugates were immobilized on polymerized liposomes. A hydrophilic spacer chain was introduced between enkephalin and phospholipid parts to alleviate steric hindrance due to liposomes against receptor binding of the enkephalin unit. The affinity of the immobilized enkephalin conjugate for opioid receptor was dependent on the density of enkephalin unit on the surface of polymerized liposomes.

16.9.6. Peptide carrying liposomes

The PEGylated liposomes offer opportunities by functioning as long circulatory platforms presenting biologically relevant ligands to their respective receptors. Liposomal conjugates of γIGSR were prepared by mild-periodate oxidation of TγIGSR-NH$_2$ and incubation of the product with hydrazide-PEG-(DSPE) capped liposomes (Zalipsky et al., 1995). Therlaminine pentapeptide capped liposomes, with 555 γIGSR residues per vesicle despite exhibiting faster blood clearance rates than the plain liposomes in rats, remained in circulation for extended period of time. The concept promises important implications for systemic delivery of peptides and for their use as targeting moieties.

16.9.7. Polysaccharide bearing liposomes

Lipopolysaccharide and polysaccharide coated liposomes have been used as a means of targeting to *Legionella pneumophilia* infected human monocytes and guinea pigs (Sunamoto et al.,1984), phagocytic cells (Sunamoto et al., 1988), lung and liver macrophages (Kohno et al.,1988). Naturally occurring polysaccharide, which when employed to coat the outermost surface of liposomes as an artificial cell wall, were found to behave as a sensory device towards specific cells and specific tissues. Polysaccharides used for capping liposomes include pullulan, mannan and amylopectin. Mainly palmitoylated polysaccharides anchored onto the bilayer sheet.

Sunamoto and Evamoto (1987) identified following attributes of polysaccharide capped liposomes and justified their use in drug delivery:

1. Reduced permeability of encapsulated materials in the presence of plasma components.
2. Increased stability against enzyme attack and protection of liposomal phospholipids from the action of lipases.
3. Mechanical stability towards biochemical and physico-chemical stimuli such as pH, osmotic challenges, ionic strength and challenges of bio-fluids.

Liposomes bearing O-palmitoyl pullulan (OPP) and O-palmitoyl amylopectin (OPA) are mainly localized in organs like liver and spleen. However, OPA coated liposomes have been reported to be retained selectively in lungs by anionic scavenging receptors. **Sismosin** loaded OPA liposomes are reported to be active significantly against treatment of *Legionella pneumophilia*. Cell wall protein polysaccharide conjugates associated with the liposomal surface exhibit better immunological adjuvanticity. Recently, the biodistribution of liposomes modified by mannobiose residues, and their targeting potential to Kupffer cells and other macrophages, have been reported (Yachi et al., 1995). Mannobiose mono-arachidic acid esters (MAEs) were synthesized and used to modify the surface of liposomes. Mannobiose modified liposomes eliminate from the systemic circulation rapidly than plain liposomes, establishing the role of mannobiose ligands in mediating macrophage targeting.

16.9.8. Lectin bearing liposomes (bacteriosomes, proteoliposomes)

Lectinized liposomes have been used for targeting to HeLa cells (Liautard, et al., 1985), glycophorin-A biofilms (Hutchinson, 1988), mouse embryo and transformed fibroblast (Bogdanor, et al., 1989), chicken erythrocytes (Carpenter et al., 1983) and *Streptococcus* infections (Kaszuba, et al., 1991)

Among the lectins that have been incorporated onto the surface of the liposomes, a few are listed below.

- Wheat germ agglutinin (WGA), specific for N-acetyl nuraminic acid
- Concanavalin A (ConA), specific for glucose and mannose residues.
- *Ricinus communis* agglutinin (RCA), specific for galactose residues.

Lectin appended liposomes interact selectively with the sugars expressed on cell surface as glycoconjugates. The specificity of the lectins for binding to a particular sugar type has led to their appreciation as site directing molecules. The targeting could be negotiated via carbohydrate mediated interactions. Binding of a multivalent ligand, such as the liposome bound WGA to cells, is expected to induce efficient clustering of receptors. Receptor clustering is an essential step in ligand induced cellular responses. Potential application of the liposome bound lectin is in the utilization of this system as a vehicle to introduce macromolecules into cells via liposome-cell fusion process. Liposomes with covalently associated WGA were preferred. It has been shown that liposomes with noncovalently associated ConA bind specifically to the lense capsule, when injected intraocularly (Holmes et al., 1985).

The proteoliposomes have also been used as a means of targeting to a range of oral and skin associated bacteria. Succinylated ConA (S ConA) is very effective in targeting liposomes to skin associated bacteria, viz, *S. triptococcus, S. sanguis and S. mutants* (Jones et al.,1994). S ConA bearing liposomes have been evaluated to be effective for the delivery of bactericide (Triclosan) to the biofilm of the oral bacteria (Jones et al.,1994). Figure 16.8 presents schematic mode of SConA mediated liposomal targeting to bacterial films. Lectinized liposomes are reported to have considerable potential as a delivery system for the control of dental plague and gingivitis (Marsh et al, 1990). Recently, Chen and co-workers (1996), examined the retention potential of lectin modified polymerized liposomes as a vehicle for oral delivery. Surface immobilized lectins exhibit their carbohydrate binding activities and specificities. These group of workers established that lectin bearing polymerized liposome can promote binding to Peyer's patches, providing opportunities for targeted delivery on these cell lines. It was also proposed that these lectinized liposomes are novel vehicles for oral vaccination.

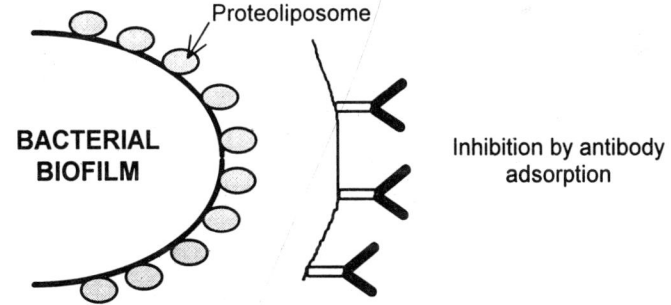

Fig. 16.8 : Lectin appended liposomes (proteosomes) for bacterial cell specific targeting
[Lectins like WGA Wheat germ agglutinins, S.Con A Concanavalin A, having specificity for sugars N-acetylnuramenic acid and glucose and mannose respectively which are found on the bactrerial cells leads to cell specific delivery. The concept has been used to deliver Triclosan for gingivitis and dental plague]

16.9.9. Bioreactive liposomes

Liposomes with encapsulated macro-molecular catalysts, represent a model for primitive cellular systems, in which a biocatalyst is entrapped within a protected micro-environment. These, so called bioreactive liposomal systems, may have either an encapsulated or immobilized biocatalyst in the aqueous or lipid domains respectively. Gregoriadis et al. (1983), described the encapsulation of enzymes for lysosomal storage disorders. Nguyen and co-workers (1990), suggested a thrombolytics therapy for acute myocardial infarction with **streptokinase** as plasminogen activator. The streptokinase was encapsulated in large unilamellar phospholipid vesicles (liposome encapsulated streptokinase, LESK). In view of the critical role played by phagocytic cells in both, induction and maintenance of inflammation, liposomes containing anti-inflammatory drugs (**superoxide**

dismutase, SO) may be an appropriate tool for targeting to inflamed tissues. Turrens et al.(1984), and Axelsson et al.(1989), reported liposome encapsulated antioxidant enzymes, superoxide dismutase and catalase. Recently, Chakrabarti et al. (1994) reported production of RNA by a polymerase protein encapsulated within phospholipid vesicles. It has been further described that a template-independent RNA polymerase (polynucleotide phosphorylase) can be encapsulated in dimyristoyl PC based vesicles without substrate. When the substrate **adenosine diphosphate** (ADP) is provided externally, long chain **RNA polymers** are synthesized within the vesicles. Substrate flux was maximized by maintaining the vesicles at the phase transition temperature of the constituent lipid (Fig. 16.9).

Sun et al., (1996) reported an immobilized bioreactive liposomal system by immobilizing **chymotrypsin** on reversibly precipitable polymerized liposomes (PLS). Polymerized liposome was prepared using synthesized PE with **di-acetylenic moiety**, with intrinsic precipitable property on addition and removal of salt. To prepare a soluble-insoluble immobilized enzyme, chymotrypsin was covalently immobilized on the outer surface of the PLS. This immobilized enzyme reactor was interestingly found to be reusable and more stable at varied temperature and environmental conditions.

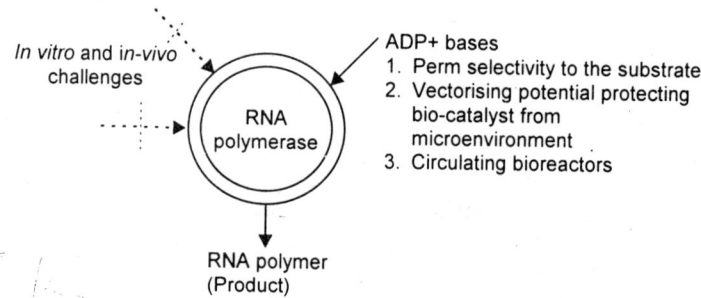

Fig. 16.9 : Schematic representation of bioreactive liposomes

16.9.9.1. Plasminogen bearing liposomes

Glu-plasminogen (thrombolytic enzyme) immobilized on the surface of liposomes, serves as an active entity to specifically target thrombolytic agents, for the treatment of acute myocardial infarction (Storm et al.,1995).The immobilized bioreactive liposomal system could produce localized delivery of thrombolytic, tissue plasminogen activator (tPA) at the site of **thrombus**. The therapeutic action of current thrombolytics is attributed to their catalytic effect on the conversion of the human **zymogen plasminogen** into plasmin (enzyme), which subsequently lyses the thrombus. The proposed approach is presented schematically in figure 16.10.

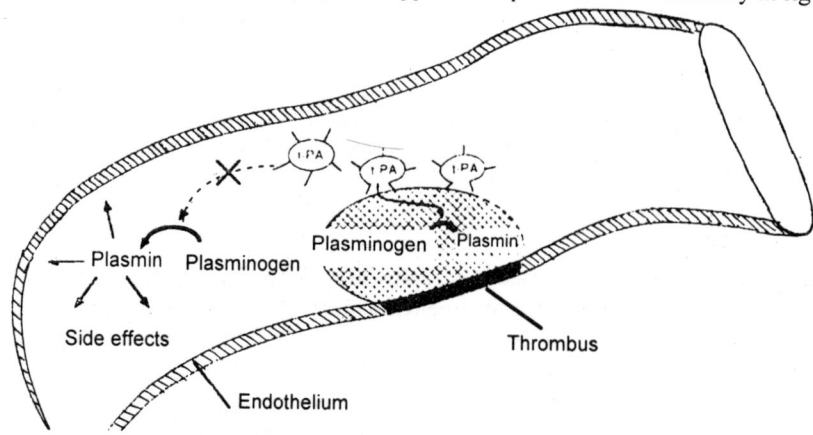

Fig. 16.10 : Schematic representation of the concept of targeted delivery of t-PA immobilized with liposomes

Specific targeting of tPA to thrombi is persuaded by encapsulation of tPA into liposomes, equipped with homing device with affinity to clots i.e., glu-plasminogen. The procedure for covalent binding of anchor molecule to liposomes with preservation of fibrin binding capacity is reported (Heeremans et al 1992). Release of encapsulated tPA takes place upon reaching the clot, and thereby produced a lytic effect. tPA encapsulated plasminogen bearing liposomes have been reported to produce an improvement in the therapeutic index at both qualitative and quantitative levels (Storm et al.,1995).

16.9.10. Immunosomes

Immunosomes are liposomal constructs engineered by employing immunoglobulins as pilot molecules anchored on or as a structural part of vesicles to confer specificity to a wide range of target sites. Immunosomes could be broadly grouped into the following classes:

- Immuno-liposomes
- Haptenated Liposomes
- Immunotoxin anchored liposomes
- Immunoprotective liposomes
- Immunoadjuvant liposomes

16.9.10.1. Immunoliposomes

Liposomes appended with antibodies or their fragments, as target oriented moieties are known as immunoliposomes. It is a well established strategy with functional cellular targeting competence. Many approaches have been attempted in order to attain quantitative targetability through immunoliposomes in drug delivery (antimicrobial and cancer therapy), enzyme delivery (lysosomal storage therapy) and gene delivery (gene transfection therapy). These include heat aggregated cell specific antibodies and covalently or noncovalently associated polyclonal or monoclonal antibodies, which are used as site directing endogenous ligands.

Liposomes coated with heat aggregated isologous IgM containing enzyme horse-raddish peroxidase (HRP) have been efficiently taken up by lysosomes of peroxidase deficient phagocytes (Weissmann et al.,1975). Gregoriadis (1977), has reported the use of liposomes coated with polyclonal antibodies against a variety of tumor cell lines. Recent developments in liposome technology make it possible to explore therapeutic applications involving site specific delivery mediated through MAbs. Liposomes anchored with anti-target monoclonal antibody having specific avidity to target (immuno-liposomes) could direct liposomes to carbohydrate antigens. This approach has been investigated to deliver drugs like IUDR/ACV (iodoxyuridine/acyclovir) in the treatment of herps simplex virus (HSV) infected cell lines (Norley et al., 1986). Monoclonal antibodies raised against glycoprotein D of HSV could deliver carrier contents selectively and transclusively to the site of infection (Norley et al.,1986). Instead of using complete IgG portion, immunologically active fragments [F(ab)$_2$ and Fab'] could be used to improve accessibility of MAbs to the receptor bearing cells (Roerdink et al., 1983) (Fig.16.11)

An improved methodology for safe binding of the sensory device, i.e., MAb fragments as site directing module anchored on the liposomes for providing an element of selectivity has been proposed (Sunamato et al., 1987). Recently designed immunoliposomes have been ameliorated by coating the outermost surface of large oligolamellar vesicles of egg PC with the polysaccharide pullulan, to carry both cholesterol as the hydrophobic anchor and the monoclonal antibodies fragment (anti-sialosyl Lewis x : IgMs) as a sensory device. The system showed better *in vivo* targetablity.

Antibody-associated liposomes containing antisense oligomers would provide dual specificity i.e., the antibody mediated selection of the particular cell lines selectivity of the target mRNA sequence followed by oligomer delivery (Leonetti et al.,1991). Zelphati and co-workers (1994), reported immunoliposomes as carrier for intracellular delivery of antisense oligonucleotides. Khaw and co-workers (1996), have envisioned a novel approach to seal the membrane lesions associated with acute myocardial infarction, using antimyosin MAb directed, immunoliposomes. Here, an antigen to intracellular cytoskeletal myosin in hypoxic. embryonic cardiocytes is used as an anchoring site, and a specific antibody on immunoliposomes as sensing ligand to **'plug and seal'** the membrane lesions. The group of workers indicated that cell death in hypoxic cardiocytes can be prevented by targeted cell membrane sealing. The concept holds exploitable promises in different immunological consequences.

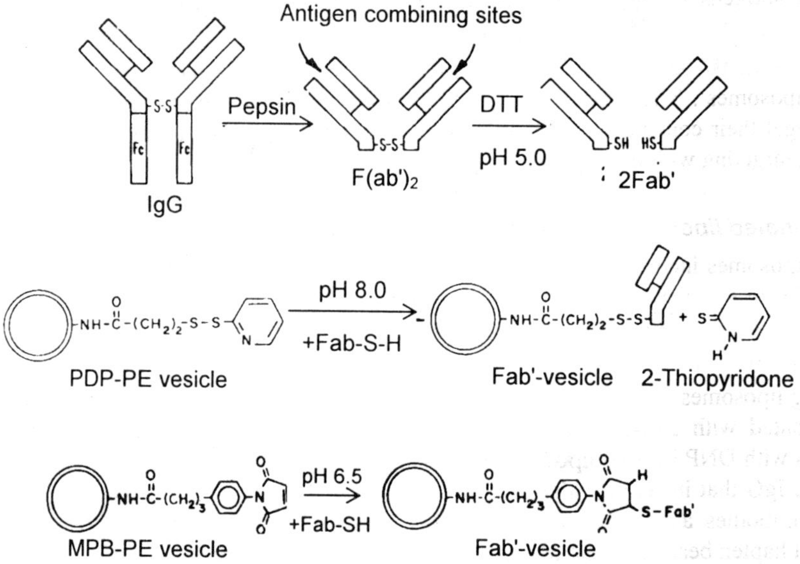

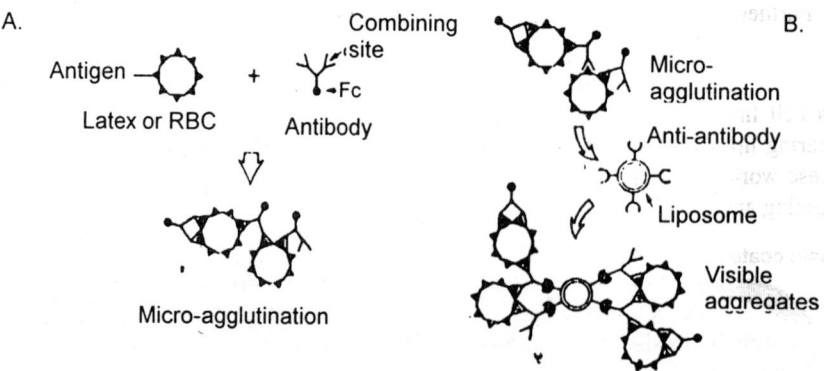

Fig. 16.11 : Immunoliposomes with Fab' fragments as targeting ligands (a) Conversion of IgG to Fab' fragments containing free endogenous thiol groups, and (b)Fab' fragments with free sulfhydryl groups react with liposomes containing PDP-PE/MPB-PE

The concept of bivalent antibodies immobilized on the liposomal surface has been proposed and could be exploited in various micro-agglutination studies as a tool to measure antibody titer and eventually the performance and degree of chemotherapeutics (Martha,1987) (Fig.16.12).

Fig. 16.12 : Liposomes bearing bivalent antibody

Recent developments of sterically stabilized liposomes (SSL), renewed interest in systemic application of immunoliposomes due to low RES uptake and long circulation half life as a result of their hydrophilic, opsonin repelling and sterically stabilized surface; these include liposomes that incorporate GM_1 ganglioside or that coated with PEG polymers (protein pegylation), i.e. polymer grafted immunoliposomes. The development of new technologies for incorporation of MAb at the surface of PEG containing liposomes permits the resulting sterically stabilized immunoliposomes (SSLs) not only to exhibit greater recognition and target binding but also allows them to remain longer in circulation as compared to classical immunoliposomes. SSL mediated targeting of anticancer drug doxorubicin has been reported in the treatment of murine solid tumors, human solid tumor xenografts and human haematological cancers. The surface immobilized MAb directs the liposomal carrier to tumor associated antigens for immunospecific binding and reduces the level of non-specific distribution to nontarget cells (Allen, et al., 1994; Emanuel, et al., 1996).

One of the future goals, as suggested by some of the authors would be the development of 'target triggered release immunoliposomes'. These are highly specialized immunoliposomes evolving with a triggered release mechanism to target their contents at the cellular level. These are discussed in detail in the section of physical strategies of drug targeting with liposomal system.

16.9.10.2. Haptenated liposomes

The haptenated liposomes incorporate biological target sensor and pilot module. The vesicular constructs were developed using PE lipids, containing the hapten linked via carbon spacers of various lengths, in the presence of to specific antibody. It can be exploited for the fixation to target cells that express surface immunoglobulin with specified affinity for the hapten.

Hapten-bearing liposomes were pioneered by Kinsky et al.(1977), PE was modified by dinitrophenyl hapten (DNP) and incubated with anti-DNP antibody. Weinstein et al.(1977), reported that rabbit antinitrophenyl antibody interacts with DNP bearing liposomes in the similar way as e murine myeloma cells, which are known to express surface IgG that interacts with nitrophenyl hapten. Liposomes present haptens to the cells equipped with surfacial antibodies as well as antibody sequestering receptor(s). The concept has been effectively exploited to direct hapten bearing liposomes to Fc receptor bearing tumor and/or normal cells. The DNP bearing liposomes, opsonized by rabbit anti-nitrophenyl antibodies, bind to cells of the murine macrophage (tumor cell lines) that express Fc receptor for IgG. No binding was evident to the cells lacking the macrophage Fc receptor or when liposomes were opsonized by F(ab)₂ or IgA antibodies, confirming their specificity to the Fc portion of IgG. Lewis et al.(1980), reported haptenated liposomes containing PE modified with a nitroxide spin-labelled hapten and studied the interaction of liposomes with Fc receptor bearing cells in the presence of antibody to hapten. It should be emphasized that not necessarily all antibody classes bound to liposomes direct the carrier towards eventual cellular uptake via Fc receptors. However, galactosyl ceramide bearing liposomes are intercepted and taken up by peritoneal macrophages in the presence of IgM anti-galactosyl antibodies together with complement. Furthermore, subsequent uptake, via complement receptor mediation was recorded (Roerdink, 1983).

Recently, Avrilionis et al.(1996), reported specific targeting of phototoxic haptenated liposomes to a hapten specific B lymphoma cell lines. The photosensitizer coupled to a phospholipid was incorporated into tri-nitrophenol (TNP) bearing lipid vesicles in order to target the photosensitizer to B-lymphoma IgM receptors *in vitro* (Fig.16.13). These workers demonstrated the potential use of antigen-bearing liposomal phototoxic drugs for the purpose of targeting and selective elimination of B cells with antigen-specific surface Ig receptors.

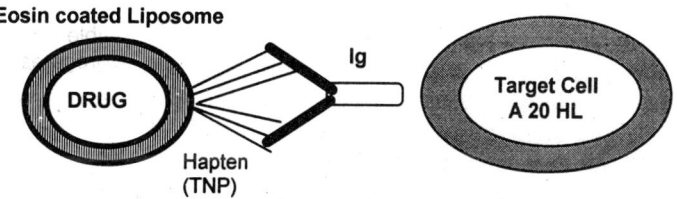

Fig. 16.13 : Photoxic haptenated liposomes

[Eosin, the phototoxic material, coated liposomes, which on photo-irradiation emit O₂ signals leading to the expression of methylated trinitro phenol (TNP) whose receptor is present at 20 HL B cell (lymphoma)]

16.9.10.3. Immunoconjugate anchored liposome

Liposomes equipped with immunotoxins were developed for their possible use in the treatment of various tumors, the concept is documented for antiviral therapy (Vitetta, 1990). Immunotoxins (ITs) are conjugates of antibodies (MAb) and toxins (ricin) in which the cell binding moieties of the toxins are replaced by the binding specific chain of Ab. Ricin toxin consists of two chains, the A- and B-chain. The A-chain is responsible for the cellular activity, whereas the B-chain (a galactose specific lectin), is responsible for binding to cells. Replacement of the B chain of toxin with a MAb, imparts specific and improved cell selectivity hence targeting competence. Cytotoxic chain of ricin can be covalently linked to receptor specific F(ab)$_2$ portion of MAb. Being specific, they act as piloting appendages. These F(ab)$_2$ handled immunotoxins are anchored on the liposomal surface, which provides avidity to them and effectively present and place them to recognition sites, leading to receptor mediated endocytosis, eventually killing cells which express F(ab)$_2$.

For treatment of HIV infections, IT composed of anti-CD4$^+$ MAb directed against HIV-1 envelop gp120 has been engineered which targets at CD4$^+$ cells (expressed on T4 lymphocytes or other cells).The developed system has been recorded to possess specific targeting potential (Till et al. 1989) (Fig. 16.14).

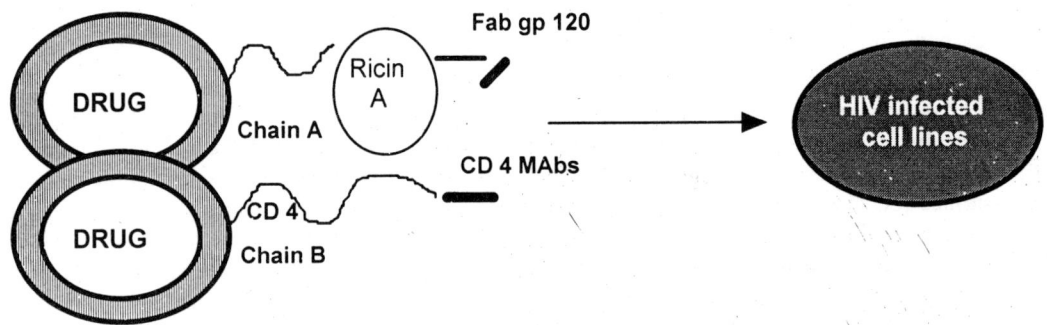

Fig. 16.14 : Immunocojugate anchored liposomes
[Toxins, the natural cell killers, with Chain A are responsible for ribonuclease inhibition and Chain B that is galactose specific is replaced by MAbs]

16.9.10.4. Diphtheria toxin immunosomes

Diphtheria toxin is a potent cytotoxic, however its selective and effective delivery has been a stigma. Liposomes have been appreciated to be a vector for diphtheria toxin to deter them from immunoglobulins pool and present them to the site of action . Diphtheria toxin inactivates vital cytosolic components of the protein synthesis machinery and can effectively used in selective killing of target cell lines. However, due to diphtheria toxin anti-MAbs pool encountered *in vivo* (generated through immunization), diphtheria toxins are sequestered and thus obstructed for their access to the cytosol of the target cell lines (Nassander et al. 1992). The immobilization of liposomal DPT could deter them from anti-DTP-MAbs and present them safely to the tumor cell lines, thus, so engineered *diphtheriosomes* may be utilized as a potential future strategy in **pick and hit therapy** (Fig. 16.15).

16.9.10.5. Immunoadjuvant liposomes

Liposomes as an artificial cellular system can be appreciated and used as a vaccine carrier or as an adjuvant. Several strategies of vaccine delivery system relying upon immobilized cellular systems have been described, including incorporation of particulates (killed *Bacillus subtilis* and killed Bacillus Calmette-Guerin) and soluble antigens (tetanus toxoid) in giant DRVs prepared by double emulsion technique. The other modifications combine two technologies, the encapsulation of antigens within liposomes and liposomes within hydrogels, to protect them from a rapid degradation *in vivo*. The technology has been adopted to increase the immunogenicity of poorly immunogenic peptides and protein vaccines.

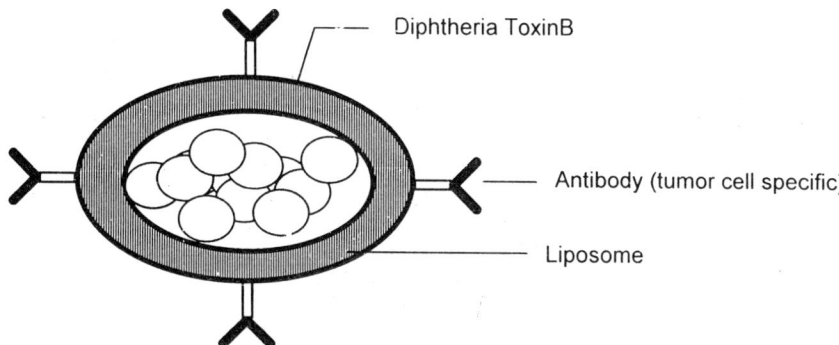

Fig. 16.15 : Diphtheria toxin immunosomes a cytotoxic construct

Since, liposomes are known to act as immunological adjuvants and vaccine carrier, giant vesicles containing microbes (live or attenuated) and soluble antigens have been reported as multiple vaccine system to ensure simultaneous presentation of antigens to immunocompetent cells. It is now known that **antigens**, presented or constituted in liposomes, can promote **humoral** and **cellular** immune responses, the concept provides basis for new generation **vaccines** (Alving, 1991). Liposomes interact efficiently with macrophages, thus macrophages may serve as antigen presenting cells for liposomal antigens (Szoka,1992).

Immunoadjuvant properties of liposomes are now well established with the first IRIV (Immuno Reconstituted Influenza Vaccine) liposomal vaccine (against hepatitis A) being licensed for use in humans. Vaccines based on **Novasomes** (nonphospholipid, biodegradable, plausilamellar vesicle formed from single chain amphiphiles, with or without other lipids) have also been investigated (Gupta et al., 1996). In the case of liposomes, further improvement of adjuvanticity has been reported to be possible by the use of immobilized co-adjuvants such as "endogenous cytokines", namely, interleukines IL-2 and IL-6, interferons (IFN) and tissue necrosis factor (TNF). Some "exogenous products" namely, muramyldipeptide (MDP, immuno-modulator) and derivatives, lipopolysaccharide (LPS) and O-polysaccharide (OPS) and positively charged lipids; have also been successfully delivered to "antigen presenting cells" to elicit and modulate immune response (Gregoriadis et al.,1993).

Microencapsulated liposomes (MEL): Liposome associated vaccine against malaria has been found safe and appreciably immunogenic (Wassef et al. 1994), however exhibited inability to provide and maintain a long term immune response against the antigen probably due to liposomal destabilization *in vivo*. This has switched interest to microencapsulated liposomal systems (MLS) to control the delivery of liposome associated macromolecules, in *in vitro* and *in vivo* (Cohen et al. 1991). The microencapsulated liposomes are engineered lipid vesicles (MEL), encapsulated within polymeric embryonic cell or sphere which is tailored to be permselective to provide controlled release of antigens. Microencapsulated liposomal systems coated with nylon (Yeung and Nixon,1988), nylon-gelatin and nylon-gelatin-acacia (Nixon and Yeung, 1989) were proposed for the controlled delivery of proteins and macromolecules. Machluf et al. (1996), reported that the liposome associated macromolecules are released in a controlled and well defined manner when liposomes are administered combined in some appropriate polymeric gel, i.e., MELS. Thus liposome-polymer based system serves as an excelled adjuvant vehicle for vaccine delivery. The liposomes have been encapsulated within microspheres of calcium crosslinked alginate, with an additional membrane of alginate-poly-L-lysine (PLL). They inferred from findings that *in vivo* presentation of model antigen ^{3}H-labelled BSA could be accomplished successfully, and proposed the potential applicability of MELs for hepatitis B vaccination.

16.9.11. Transferrin based liposomes

Liposomes coated with transferrin could selectively approach the proliferating neoplastic cell lines, which especially express receptor modules for transferrin which is uptake via receptor mediated endocytosis, thus delivering the contents intracellularly.

Transferrin is a major serum glycoprotein, transporting iron through specific cell surface receptors and delivers Fe^{3+} across plasma membrane. The transferrin investigated for its possible targeting profile is structurally bilobal (80,000 mw) which can carry two ferric ions in nonidentical binding sites. The membrane receptor for transferrin (Tf) is a dimeric glycoprotein (1,80,000 mw) with apparently identical binding units, each could bind one transferrin. The transferrin receptor is frequently expressed by T4 cells and tumor cell lines. Upon binding transferrin relinquishes its iron content, while other conjugated component, i.e., liposomes may remain associated with receptor or may be endocytosed to release the drug to the cell(s) target thus leading to cell specific targeting (Fig.16.16). Wagner et al. (1994), reported delivery of drugs, proteins and genes into cells using transferrin as a sire directing ligand.

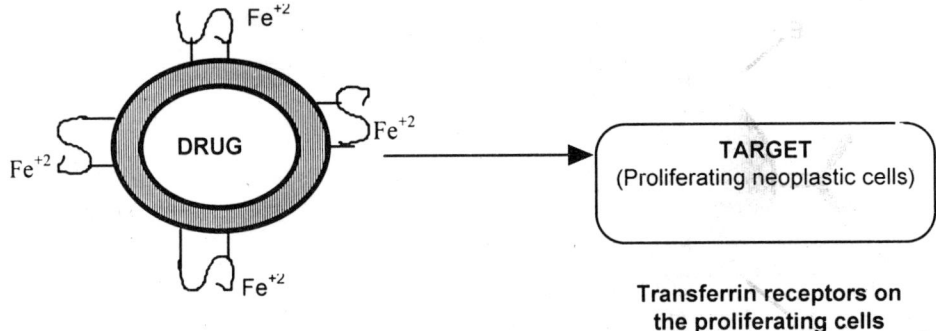

Fig. 16.16 : Transferrin appended liposomes

(Transferrin, a major serum glycoprotein transporting iron from the sites of absorption to the cells could be appended onto the liposomal1 surface and cell specific targeting, i.e., delivery of entrapped drug to the proliferating neoplastic cells containing the transferrin specific receptors could be negotiated.)

16.9.12. Enzymosomes

An interesting strategy towards selective and specific chemotherapeutics has been developed and proposed namely enzymosomes. Enzymosomes are liposomal constructs engineered to provide a *mini* bioenvironment. Enzymes are covalently immobilized or coupled to the surface of liposomes, therefore, when a nontoxic prodrug is administered simultaneously, is converted by the immobilized enzyme to a potent antitumor agent in the vicinity of tumor cell lines. The specificity of enzyme reaction provides the means to limit prodrug activation at the tumor site, through prior enzyme targeting by using liposomes, or via enzyme expressing gene delivery into the tumor cells (VDEPT). Figure 16.17 provides a schematic of the concept of targeted delivery of anticancer prodrug activating enzymes with immunoliposomes (ADEPT based liposomal system), also known as immuno-enzymosomes (Vingerhoeds et al.,1996).

The enzyme bearing immunoliposomes, are first targeted to tumor cell lines with the help of appropriate MAbs. After binding of the immunoenzymes to target, a prodrug is administered, which is activated by cell bound immunoenzymes in the close proximity of the tumor cells. Vingerboeds and co-workers in 1993 reported the coupling of the enzyme β-glucouronidase, capable of activating the prodrug epirubicin-glucouronide, to epirubicin. It was found that pretreatment with enzymosomes (bearing no specific antitumor antibodies) or immunoliposomes (bearing no enzymes) were ineffective, but preincubation with immunozymes (enzymosomes) resulted in an enhanced antitumor activity of the prodrug.

It is the flexibility provided by the choice of enzymes for ADEPT/VDEPT (Antibody/Gene directed enzyme prodrug therapy), the range of tumor antigen-targets and the prodrug chemistry make these enzyme/prodrug/carrier seemingly a complex concept exploitable in cancer chemotherapy and furthermore can be extended to clinical gene therapy in the near future. There is a wide selection of antigen specific targets available, which provide the opportunities of targeting a range of tumors with MAb-enzyme conjugates (ADEPT) and a range of antigen markers are also available which might be used for selective expression of prodrug activating enzymes coded by genes in GDEPT. Sherwood et al. (1996), reported several enzyme-prodrug systems and proposed carboxy-peptidase G2 enzyme and a nitrogen mustard prodrug based enzymosomes for further clinical trials. Herpes simplex virus-thymidine kinase (HSV-tk) has been a leading candidate conceivably suitable for VDEPT (virus directed EPT), based on large differential insensitivity to GCV (Gancyclovir) between cells expressing HSV-tk and parental cells.

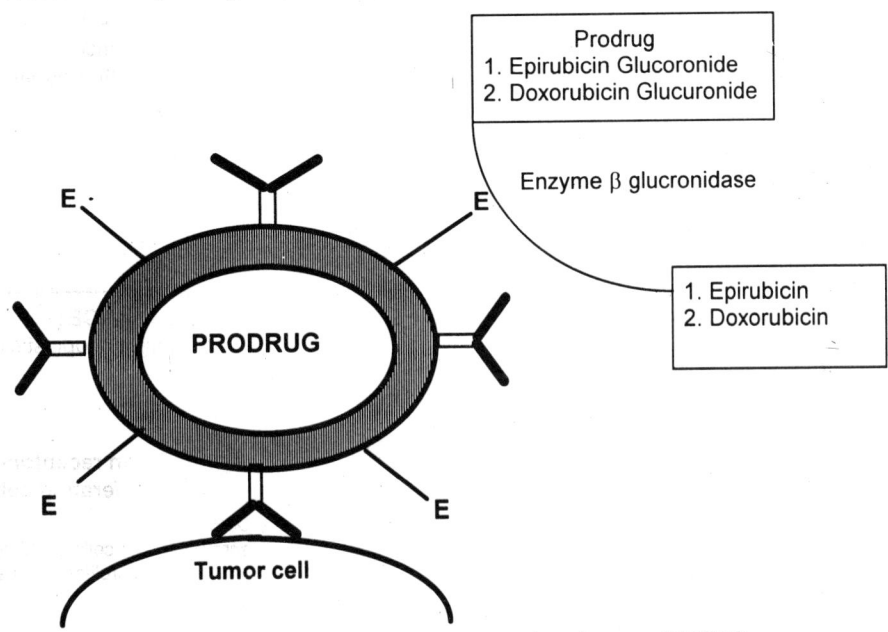

Fig. 16.17 : Antibody directed enzyme prodrug therapy (ADEPT)

In recent studies, full range of gene delivery techniques have been exploited (adenoviral, retroviral and naked DNA) to ascertain *in vivo* tumor cell lining regression in a wide range of model systems of murine myeloma, human lung cancer , human gastric carcinoma, human pancreatic adenocarcinoma, hepatic metastases of colon carcinoma and brain tumor (Sherwood et al.,1996).

16.9.13. Physical targeting based approaches (triggered release liposomes)

1. Target sensitive liposomes
   - Target sensitive immunoliposomes
   - Cationic liposomes
   - Anionic liposomes

2. Signal sensitive liposomes
   - Thermo sensitive liposomes
   - Temperature sensitive immunoliposomes
   - Magnothermal sensitive liposomes
   - pH sensitive liposomes
   - pH sensitive immuno-liposomes
   - Stimuli responsive liposomes
   - Photoactivated liposomes

16.9.13.1. Target sensitive liposomes

Liposomes which could bind to the target cell via bilayer destabilization are based on phosphatidyl-ethonolamine (PE) lipids. Liposomal constitutive lipids used in this system cannot form gelled bilayers and are not stable in the bilayer state. However incorporation of palmitoylated MAbs stabilizes the bilayers. As the system approaches its target the MAbs specific to target get separated leaving vesicles unstable. Thus, receptor ligand interaction of these constructs leads to their conversion to liquid crystal (mesophages), resulting into the burst or triggered release of the liposomal contents (Bentz et al. 1987).

16.9.13.1.1. Target sensitive immunoliposomes

Target sensitive immunoliposomes (Ho et al., 1986) have been designed to release their contents upon binding to the target cell(s) via bilayer destabilization. Among the strategies which could be adopted, is the use of phosphatidylethanolamine (PE) as a lipoidal component which is not stable in bilayer state, or otherwise, one can adopt bilayer state in the presence of acylated antibody. Binding of antibodies to the target site(s) results into the redistribution of acylated antibodies, whereas PE reverts to its hexagonal phase (inverted micelles) with the release of entrapped drug. Ho et al.(1986), proposed the design of target sensitive immunoliposomes, based on palmitoylated antibody stabilized PE bilayers which get destabilized on binding to an antigen present on the target cell, leading to a local release of loaded drugs into the cytoplasm of the target cells (Fig.16.18). This target selectivity and sensitivity has been reported to build a 1000-fold increase in the uptake of ACV (acyclovir), *in vitro*, as compared with the level achieved on free drug administration. Target sensitive immunoliposomes incorporating the mouse monoclonal IgG_{2a}, (antibody against antigen glycoprotein D of the HSV) were used to deliver the cytotoxic drugs, Ara C (cytosine-β-D-arabinoside) and ACV (acyclovir) to mouse fibroblasts to the tropics of herpes virus (Ho et al., 1987).

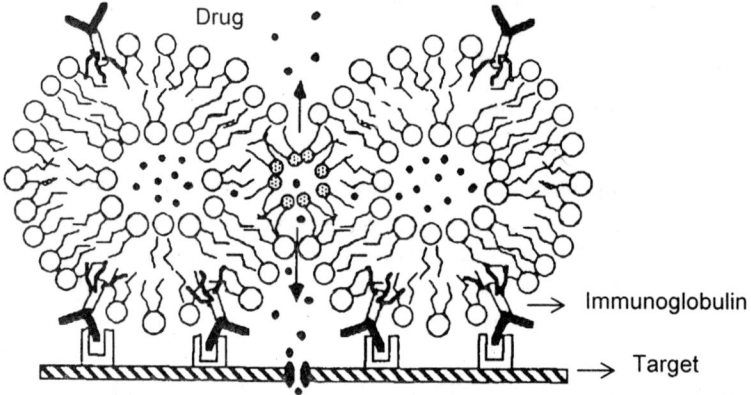

Fig. 16.18 : Mechanistic representation of drug release from target sensitive immunoliposomes

16.9.13.1.2. Genosomes

Liposomes as a carrier, for therapeutic agent, directed at genomes with an expectation of exquisite selectivity, have been considered recently in two forms:

1. Plasmids for transportation, transfection and supplementation of new gene expression to cells, and

2. Small oligonucleotides for inhibition of selected gene function (antisense, ribozyme and triplex oligos).

Genosomes represent a range of phospholipid based liposomes which act as non-viral gene vector for controlling the intracellular trafficking of DNA following liposome endocytosis by cells (Fig. 16.19).

The release of a gene expressing system from endosomal compartment is a limiting step in the transfer of encapsulated plasmid DNA to the nucleus of the target cells. A review of the literature proposes pH sensitive liposomes (Wang and Huang, 1987), immunoliposomes (Leonetti et al. 1991), pH sensitive immunoliposomes (Wang and Huang, 1989) and fusogenic liposomes (Fogerite et al. 1989), as potential vectors for cell specific gene transfer. These systems are discussed elsewhere in this chapter. They are also reported as suitable carriers for intracellular delivery of antisense oligonucleotides.

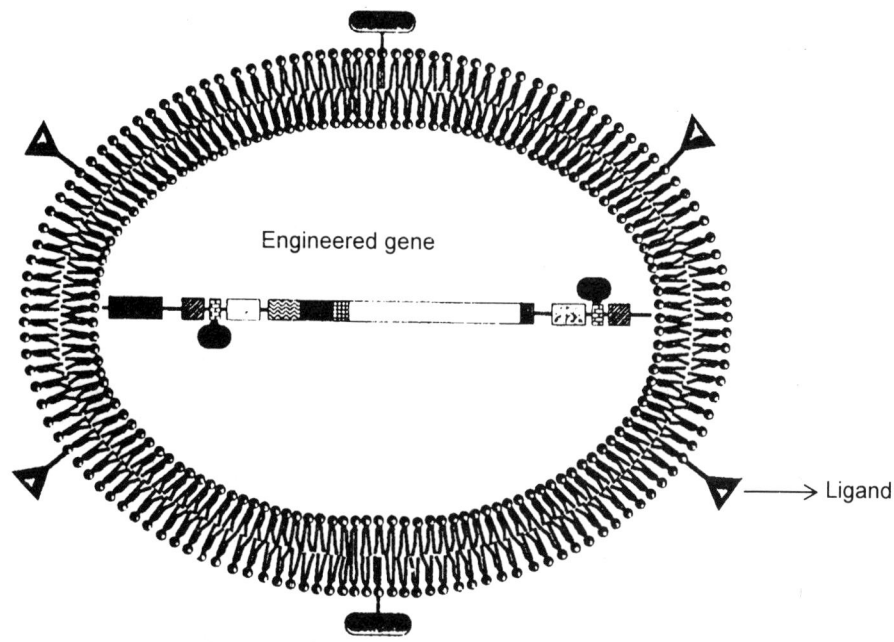

Engineered gene

Ligand

Fig. 16.19 : Schematic of non-viral liposomal gene vector system, genosome

In the same context, the delivery of gene expression plasmid vectors in different mammalian cell lines has also been evaluated by exploiting either cationic/anionic/pH sensitive (anionic/cationic) liposomal systems. Another major focus in gene therapy vector development has been tissue specific targeting. A variety of targeting ligands have been examined for liposome targeting, including folate targeted, anionic/cationic liposomes containing polylysine condensed DNA for tumor cell specific gene transfer (Fig.16.20).

16.9.13.1.3. Delivery of DNA using cationic liposomes

Cationic liposomes, first developed by Felgner et al.,(1987), reduce the net negative surface charge on DNA plasmid based gene expression systems, in attempts to reduce charge-charge repulsion (electrostatic interaction) at the surface of biological membranes, (Fig.16.20).

Cationic liposomes based on DOTMA (dioleoyl-oxypropyl-trimethyl-ammonium chloride) with or without fusogenic component (1:1 w/w DOTMA: DOPE liposomes correspond to transfection reagent, Lipofectin), have been used exclusively *in vitro* and *in vivo* as vectors for gene expression and as a carrier for intracellular delivery of antisense oligo-nucleotides. DOTAP{N-1(2,3-dioleoyloxy) propyl}N,N,N-trimethylammonium chloride and DOGS (dioctadecylamidoglycyl spermine),associated with DOPE could also be used for gene delivery. As DOPE (dioleoyl PE) can fuse with endosomal membrane, it is generally included in such complexes to bring about the endosomal release of a gene expression system.

It has been suggested that cationic liposomes are superior to pH-sensitive liposomes for transfection of gene expressions for two reasons:

1. They achieve a higher cell associated level of high molecular weight plasmid DNA, and
2. They follow a different or parallel pathway for DNA/ oligonuclotide delivery into the cell.

Gao and Huang (1996), recently designed a cationic liposome - polylysine - DNA ternary complex **(LPDI)** consisting of a condensed polylysine/DNA core and a cationic lipid envelope. The same group of workers further developed poly-lysine conjugated with antibody which delivered plasmid DNA to cells in a target specific manner with a three component system, i.e., DNA vector containing a targeting ligand, a polycation and a lipophilic moiety. However, Budker et al., (1996), described the use of cationic, pH sensitive liposomes to mediate efficient transfer of DNA into a variety of cells in culture. Cationic lipids, containing an amine group with a pKa corresponding to physiological fluid(s) ranging 4.5 to 8.0, were synthesized and incorporated with DOPE into liposomes. Acidic conditions promoted DNA-binding, DNA-incorporation, and DNA induced fusion of these cationic, pH sensitive liposomes.

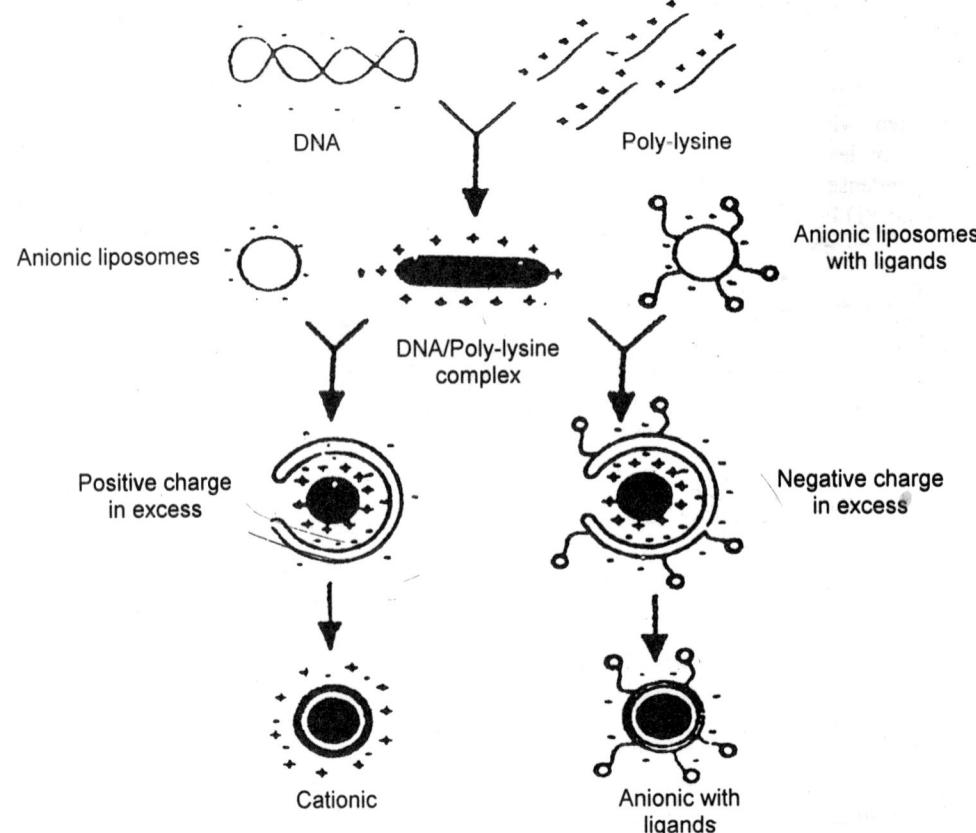

Fig. 16.20 : Anionic /cationic DNA-lysine conjugates for liposomal cytosolic delivery

16.9.13.1.4. Anionic liposomes as a gene or oligonucleotide vector

Anionic liposomes from phosphatidylserine were first reported to deliver oligonucleotides into cells (Loke et al.,1988). This technique was reportedly relevant to circumvent problems due to repulsion of the negative charge of oligonucletides. The charge bound repulsion results in low encapsulation efficiency, as reported with DNA and RNA. Phosphorothioate antisense oligonucleotides based genosomes could be exploited to target the c-myc, an oncogene of the human or mRNA of the mouse. Interleukin (IL) receptors were encapsulated in anionic liposomes which may become potential tools for anti-viral therapeutics (Loke et al. 1988). An anionic liposome composed of DPDG phospholipids for the delivery of anti HIV ribozymes to HIV-infected cells has also been reported (Rossi et al. 1992).

Reports on DNA vectoring potential of anionic liposomes are not encouraging due to poor encapsulation efficiency resulted from the large size and negative charge of the uncondensed DNA. Anionic, pH sensitive liposomes have been designed to destabilize or fuse with the endosomal membrane at acidic pH. All the anionic, pH sensitive liposomes reported so far are constructed as PE bilayers that are stable at nonacidic pH by the addition of lipids that contain a carboxylic acid group. However, at acidic pH within endosomes, the uncharged or reduced charge species are unable to stabilize the PE-rich bilayers (Fig.16.21). The negative charge of these pH sensitive anionic liposomes prevents efficient entrapment of the DNA and interaction with cells, thus decreasing their transfection competency. Recently, in order to endow liposomes with tissue specificity, targeting ligands are coupled to the surface of charged liposomes. A variety of targeting ligands have been examined to place liposome selectively. Folate has its recognition site as a tumor marker, especially among ovarian carcinomas, where it is exclusively expressed. Folic acid, as a low molecular weight ligand, has the advantage of being nonimmunogenic compared to MAbs, and still possesses high receptor affinity. First successful reports of folate targeted liposomes pertains to its use in the tumor cell specific delivery of anticancer drugs and antisense oligonucleotides *in vitro* (Wang et al., 1995). Folate derivatized **polylysine-DNA complexes**, combined with inactivated adenoviruses have been shown to mediate tumor cell specific transfection. In a recent development, Lee and Huang (1996) reported a lipidic vector **(LPD II)** for gene transfer where polylysine condensed DNA is entrapped into folate targeted anionic liposomes via charge interaction (LPD II differs from LPD I in that anionic lipids instead of cationic lipids are used).

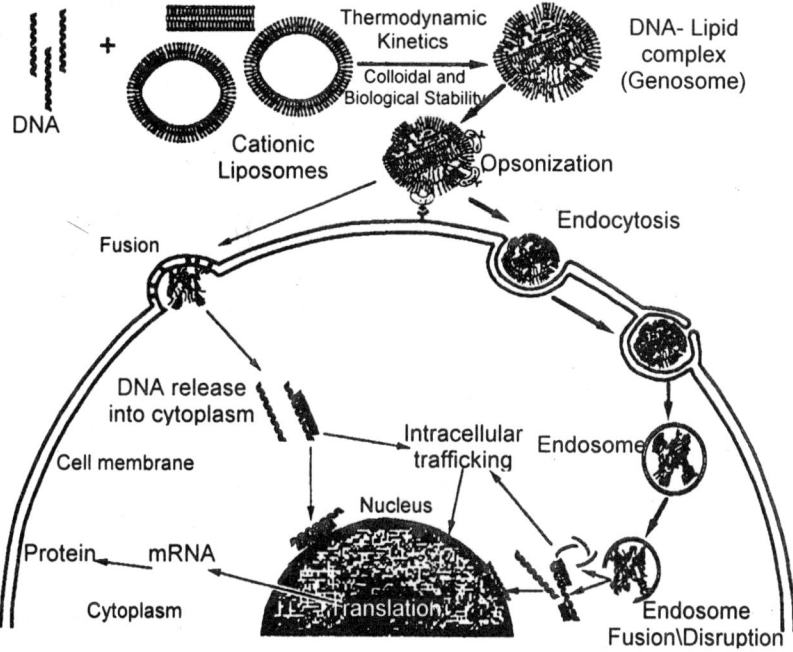

Fig. 16.21 : Uptake pathways and intracellular trafficking mechanisms of various engineered genosomes

16.9.13.2. Signal sensitive liposomes

Signal sensitive liposomes belong to a class of ligand appended liposomal constructs which are responsive to bio-signals and environmentally modulated by physical means to program and monitor selective release of contents.

16.9.13.2.1. Temperature sensitive liposomes

Temperature sensitive liposomes take the advantage of the fact that liposomes tend to be leaky enough at the phase transition temperature (Tc) of their membrane forming lipids. These liposomes are designed to be stable upto 37°C, however the contents tend to release as they pass through an area of the body where they are exposed to a temperature higher than physiological temperature (e.g. within a tumor, or an area subjected to local external heating) (Fig. 16.22).

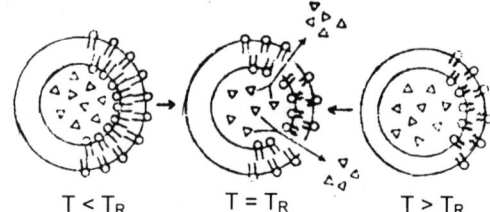

$$T < T_R \qquad T = T_R \qquad T > T_R$$

Fig. 16.22 : Schematic representation of temperature sensitive liposomes where T is the phase transition temperature and Tr is the release temperature

Liposomal constructs based on synthetic lipids, DPPC:DSPC (dipalmitoyl PC: distearoyl PC) have been used very often, with locally applied hyperthermia and the system is receiving attention as a valuable therapeutic tool, and gathering appreciation for chemotherapy. Yatvin et al., (1981), have reported that uptake of cisplatin from temperature sensitive liposomes coupled with local hyperthermia at sarcoma-180 tumors, reduced tumor growth, several times as compared to plain liposomes. Weinstein et al., (1979), also described higher uptake, under local hyperthermia when MTX (methotrexate) containing SUV liposomes were administered for Lewis lung tumors. Combinations of thermosensitive liposomes and localized hyperthermia in brain tumor treatment have been reported as an effective mode of targeted chemotherapy (Kalinuma et al., 1996).

Hayashi et al. (1996), discussed DOPE vesicles bearing a thermosensitive polymer, poly (N-isopropyl acryl amide) which show a lower critical solution temperature (LCST) and a better release of the drug calcein. The temperature controlled release property of the polymer coated DOPE vesicles was attributed to stabilization and destabilization of the vesicle membranes modulated through copolymer, incorporated into vesicle membrane below and above the LCST, respectively. Recently, Chelvi et al., (1995), reported thermosensitive liposomal system engineered using natural lipids, egg PC: Chol. (7:1 molar ratio) and ethanol 6% v/v, having a phase transition temperature of 43°C, treatment has been reported to be clinically attainable and practicable under local hyperthermia. These natural lipid derived thermosensitive liposomes were found to be biodegradable, nontoxic and more cost effective in comparison to liposomes prepared from synthetic lipids for use in multimodulous cancer therapeutics.

16.9.13.2.2.. Temperature sensitive immunoliposomes

Temperature sensitive immunoliposomes (Sullivan and Huang, 1986) are designed to release their contents at the cells surface (target) upon heating to their intrinsic transition temperature. Devanathan et al., 1990, proposed the design of heat sensitive immunoliposomes containing phototoxic drugs. The liposome could be activated through irradiation after they arrive at the target tissue, offering a second degree of targeting (Fig. 16.23).

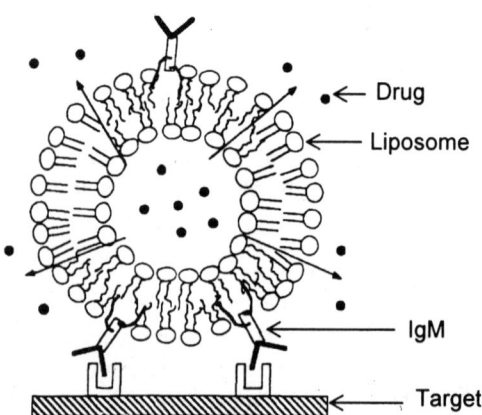

Fig. 16.23 : Schematic representation of drug release from thermosensitive immunoliposomes

16.9.13.2.3. *Magnoresponsive-thermo sensitive liposome*

Liposomal system can be contrived as being thermosensitive and at the same time magnoresponsive too. The system offers opportunities of active targeting under the guidance of external magnetic field of appropriate strength, and utilizes physical means for auto-destruction of liposomes in the target vicinity in response to local hyperthermia, negotiating a triggered delivery of the liposomal contents. The liposomal constructs based on DPPC/DSPC (dipalmitoyl/distearoyl PC) with optimum molar ratio of cholesterol to optimize phase transformation above the physiological temperature, and dextran magnetite was incorporated to endow them with thermosensitivity and magnetic responsiveness. Based on the discussed principle, a DPPC based liposomal surface modified by Me-PEG-PE have been reported for the selective doxorubicin chemotherapy (Sato et al., 1995). Virooenchatapan and co-workers (1996), have reported dextran magnetite in targeting of thermosensitive magnetoliposomes to mouse livers in an *in situ* on-line perfusion system (Fig. 16.24). The group established an efficient targeting of thermosensitive magneto-liposomes in RES blocked livers with a targeting advantage index (TAI) of 1.6-3.1 (compared to TAI in normal liver of 1.1-1.4) revealing a critical role of RES uptake in the physically modulated systems.

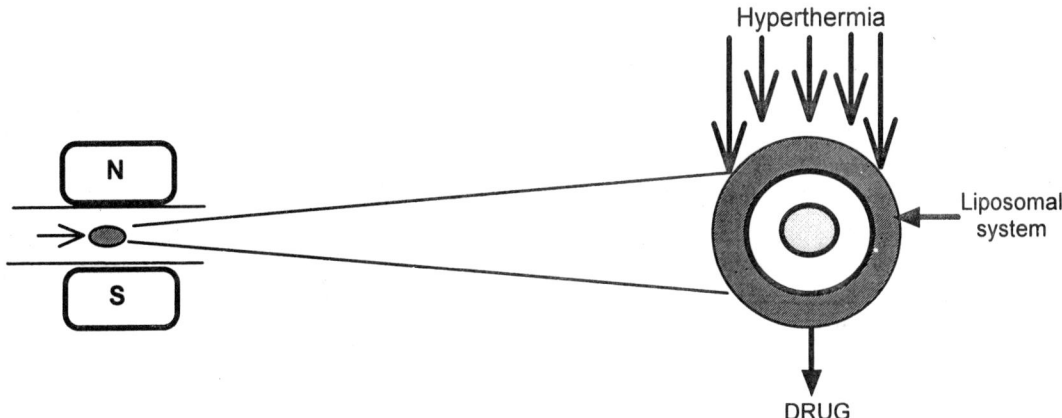

Fig. 16.24 : Dextran magnetite based thermosensitive magneto-liposomes

16.9.13.2.4. pH sensitive liposomes

pH sensitive liposomes are designed with an aim to circumvent the problems associated with plain liposomes (e.g., lysosomal enzymatic degradation), and to deliver their contents directly to cytoplasm. The lipid composition of pH-sensitive liposomes, of which commonly used lipid is DOPE (dioleoyl PE), determines the membrane stability at neutral pH and the sensitivity to destabilize the membrane to be fusogenic at acidic pH of endosomal system. In the event of pH change, pH sensitive liposomes are converted into a form which prefers to adopt an inverted hexagonal phase rather than the conventional bilayer sheet of the lipoidal membrane. Thus, delivery is based on acid-triggered events within an acidic endosome following endocytosis. The pH sensitive liposomes have been reported as plasmid expression vectors for the delivery of DNA (Wang and Huang, 1987a). Zelphati et al., (1996), reported them to be effective carriers for intracellular trafficking of antisense oligonucleotides. Diphtheria toxin, radiolabeled albumin and pH sensitive fluorescent dyes (Chu et al. 1990), and calcein and chloroquine (Connor and Huang, 1985), have also been selectively targeted using pH sensitive liposomes.

16.9.13.2.5. pH sensitive immunoliposomes

pH sensitive immuno-liposomes (Conor and Huang 1986; Wang and Huang, 1987b) have been developed to release their contents in response to an acid triggering machinery within endosomal system following receptor mediated endocytosis (RME). They undergo transient destabilization at a mildly acidic pH as found in the endosomes thus they could selectively deliver the contents to cellular components (Fig. 16.25).

Incorporation of the antitarget MAbs on pH sensitive liposome surface, allows selective delivery to the respective target cells. Recently, pH-sensitive immunoliposomes mediated delivery and subsequent expression of exogenous genes in target cells have been reported. Some workers have also compared pH sensitive immunoliposomes to both, non pH-sensitive immunoliposomes and pH-sensitive liposomes for their efficiency in tranfecting the HSV-tk gene into the mouse lymphoma cells *in vitro*. Immunoliposomes were shown to adsorb DNA non specifically on their surface and to transfer it directly into the cytoplasm, without being presented to lysosomes for degradation (Fig. 16.25). pH sensitive immunoliposomes guided by MAbs against a surface antigen on mouse L cells, were observed to fuse with endosomal membrane in response to acidic pH of the endosome. Specific gene delivery via this latter mode was found to express TK (thymidine kinase) genes at a statistically significant level as compared to pH sensitive plain liposomes (without immunological targeting ligand).

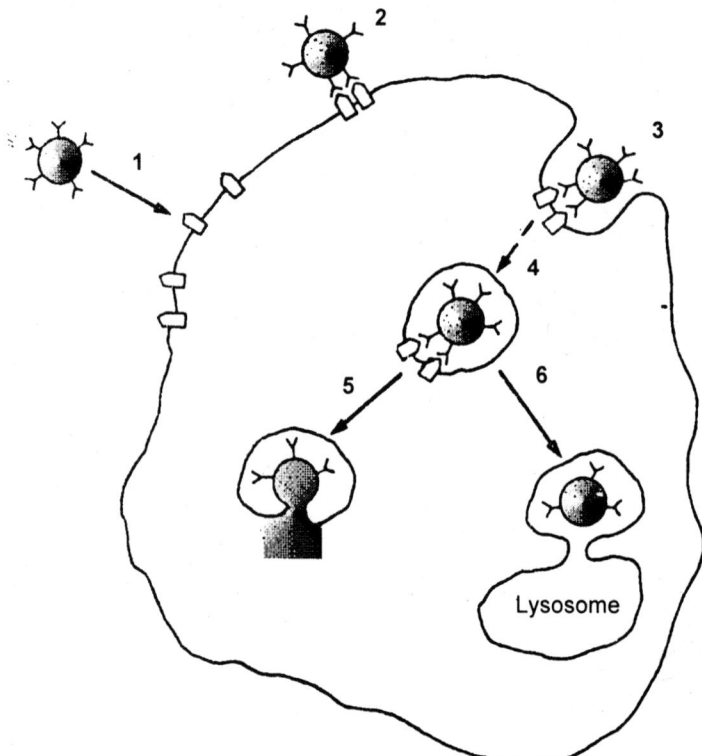

Fig. 16.25 : Schematic representation of interaction of immunoliposomes with target cells
1. Immunoliposomes bearing antibody are incubated with target cells expressing antigen; 2. Binding to cell surface antigen; 3. Receptor mediated endocytosis; 4.. Internalization into acidic endosomes; 5. Fusion of pH sensitive immunoliposomes with endosomes and release of contents into cytoplasm; 6. Fusion of endosome with lysosome and delivery of pH insensitive module into lysosome.

16.9.13.2.6. Stimuli sensitive liposomes

Stimuli sensitive liposomes are classically designed systems responsive to biosignals, i.e., physiological pH, substrate or light. The engineered constructs are based on PC appended with polyamine, polyethylacrylamide in the protonated state. Adsorptive aggregation leads to reorientation in lipid bilayers thus allowing release of liposomal contents. The basis of this approach has been the environmentally sensitive association of hydrophobic polyelectrolytes, the latter are integrated into the liposomal membrane. In particular poly(2-ethyl)acrylic acid (PEAA) that is adsorbed strongly on the liposomal surface at low pH (pH<7), but only weakly in basic solutions. The pH sensitive adsorption leads to important changes in the membrane structure accompanied with the loss of the barrier properties of the membrane. Liposomes suspended in dilute aqueous solutions of PEAA are stable above pH 7 but release their contents rapidly upon acidification. The incorporation of glucose oxidase into suspending medium, renders the liposomal membrane sensitive to glucose concentration. The pH responsiveness of the liposomal suspension similarly can be tuned finally via copolymerization of 2-methylacrylic acids, so that the release may be triggered essentially at the desired pH.

Modification of PEAA is brought about by attachment of appropriate chemophores (e.g., axobenzenes or spirobenzopyran) to the photosensitive systems (Photosomes). Photosomes engineered using light sensitive lipids, for example retinoid lipids also reported to release the contents upon irradiation. Figure 16.26 explains various ligands (x) conferring responsiveness to the liposomal systems towards bio-signals.

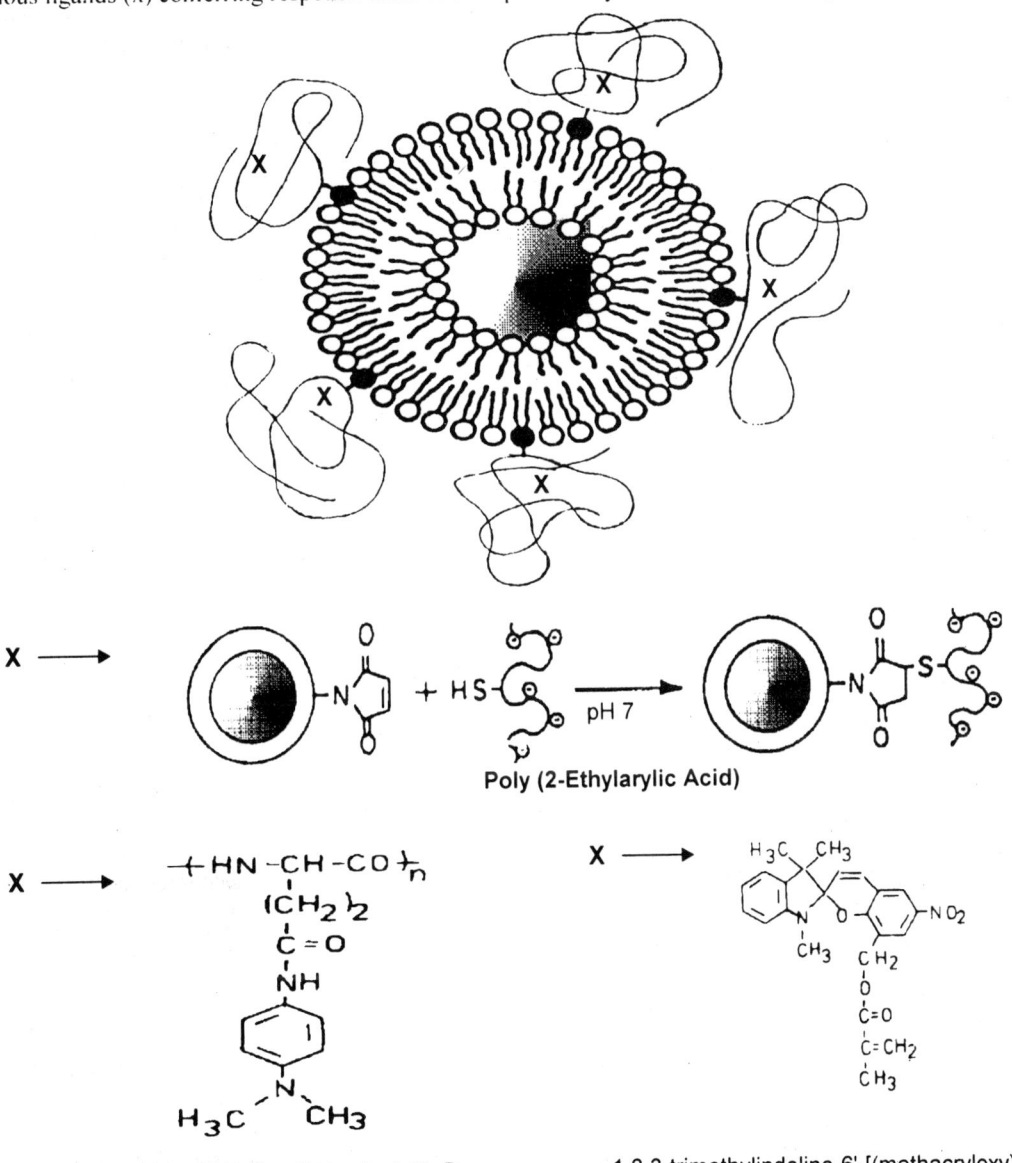

X ⟶

Poly (2-Ethylarylic Acid)

X ⟶

Poly [p-(N,N-dimethylamino)-Nγ-D-Glutamanilide]

X ⟶

1,3,3-trimethylindolino-6'-[(methacryloxy) methyl] spirobenzopyran

Fig. 16.26 : Signal responsive liposomes. Liposomal constructs appended with signal sensitive modules (X) X = pH sensitive (a) and Photosensitive liposomes (b & c)

16.9.13.2.7. Photoactivated liposomes (Photosomes)

Photo-activated liposomes are especially engineered liposomal constructs liable to photo-triggered changes in membrane permeability characteristics and subsequent release of contents. Bennett et al. (1995), reported photo-activated induction of liposomal fusion with the photo-polymerization of two component namely, DOPE and either bis-sorb PC or mono-sorb PC (3:1). Examination of the polymerized and unpolymerized liposomes showed that an enhancement in fusion rate occurred in a particular temperature range accompanied by the formation of activated cubic phase.

Thompson et al. (1996), described photo-activated liposomes which are generally applicable for triggered release of encapsulated hydrophilic materials (Fig. 16.27). The approach of photo-triggered release, is based on the known process of plasmalogen photo-oxidation and its effect on membrane permeability in whole cells and model membrane systems. The photoresponsive orientation relies on a lamellar phase change or increase in permeability due to transformation of constitutive lipids to single chain mesogens on exposure to 630-820 nm light. The light sensitizes the photo-oxidation of the plasmalogen vinyl-ether linkage. The capacity of photolyzed plasmenylcholine liposomes to undergo membrane fusion makes photodynamic therapy a possible event with liposome associated sensitizers viz., bacteriochlorophyll, zinc-phthalocyanine or tin-octabutoxy-phthalocyanine

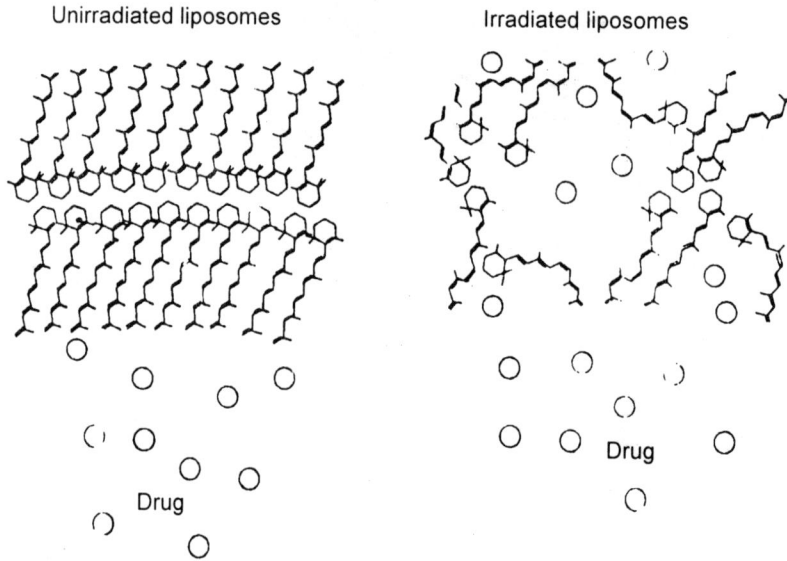

Fig. 16.27 : Schematic representation of liposomes prepared from light sensitive lipid (Photosomes)

16.9.14. Miscellaneous

16.9.14.1. Erythrosomes

Erythrosomes are especially engineered liposomal systems in which chemically crosslinked human erythrocytes cytoskeletons are used as a support upon which a lipid bilayer is coated (Fig. 16.28). This can be achieved by a modified procedure normally adopted for reverse phase evaporation. This is proposed as a useful encapsulation system for drug delivery particularly for effective targeting of macromolecular drugs (Cuppoletti et al.1981; Jung, 1987).

16.9.14.2. Lipobeads

Lipobeads have been introduced recently which are based on hydrogel anchored lipid vesicles (Jin et al., 1996) and combine complementary properties of liposomes and polymeric beads. Lipobeads have been designed using a lipid bilayer shell anchored on the surface of a hydrogel polymer core, which acts like a cyto-skeleton. Anchoring is provided by fatty acids, covalently attached to the surface of the hydrogel. The system has potential application in drug delivery and for functional reconstitution of membrane proteins. Cohen et al., (1994), proposed nearly similar strategy for controlled release vaccine delivery systems. The strategy combines two technologies, the encapsulation of antigen within liposomes and liposome covalent immobilization on hydrogels, to protect them from rapid degradation *in vivo*. This increases the immunogenicity of poorly immunogenic peptides and protein vaccines.

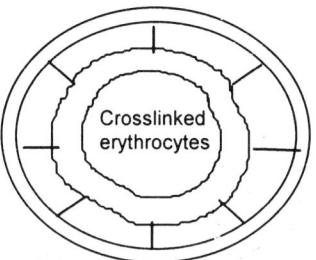

Fig. 16.28 : Schematic representation of erythrosomes

16.9.14.3. Hemosomes

Liposome entrapped haemoglobin (Hemosomes) is a widely investigated system leading to the development of red blood cell substitutes, as a high capacity artificial oxygen carrying system (Farmer and Gaber, 1987)(Fig. 16.29). Haemoglobin immobilized on synthetic membranes permits tailoring of its oxygen-carrying properties and simultaneously provides fine tuning of the oxygen affinity by co-encapsulating natural allosteric effectors. Tsuchida (1994) reported artificial red cells as blood surrogates engineered by immobilizing haemoglobin with a polymerizable phospholipid and found almost the same oxygen transport capacity as of RBCs.

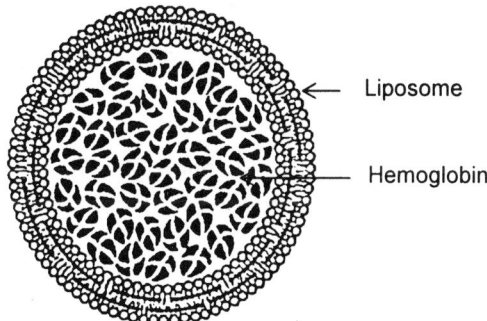

Fig. 16.29 : Liposomes encapsulated hemoglobin

The liposomes and their vital applications have been studied extensively. They have covered a wide spectrum of diversities. The liposomes based systems are highly sophisticated versions of drug carrying units (carriers), which perform drug delivery task in an intended and envisaged manner. The molecular basis of drug targeting seems to be an attainable state with the help of various modules based systems endowed with specificity, affinity and stability. Molecular drug targeting if attained will certainly offer opportunities to correct biological ailments at cellular levels and at the same time will offer possibilities of radical cure. Delivery to molecular target shall further open up the vistas for cellular modification leading to spectacular biotechnological events like gene cloning, gene modification, biocell sensitivity profile tailoring etc. Nevertheless, with the advent of highly putative yet formidable liposomal systems the Paul Elhrich magic bullet concept shall be a practical reality of future.

SUGGESTED READINGS

Ahn, Y.S., Byrnes, J.J, Harrington, W.J., Cayer, M.L., Smith, D.S., Brunskill, D.E., Pall, L.M. (1978) **N. Engl. J. Med.**, 298, 1101-07.

Al-Ahdal, M.N., Abid, T.F., Flanagan, T.D., (19986) **Biochim. Biophys. Acta**, 854, 157-168.

Allen, T.M., Agrawal, A.K., Ahmad, I., Hansen, C.B., Zalipsky, S. (1994) **J. Lip. Res.**, 4, 1-25.

Allen, T.M., Brandeis, E., Hansen, C.B., Karo, G.Y., Zalipsky, S. (1995) **Biochim. Biophys. Acta**, 1237, 99-108.

Allen, T.M., Chonn, A. (1987) **FEBS Lett.**, 223 , 42-46.

Allen, T.M., Hansen, C., Martin, F., Redemann, C., Yau-Young, A. (1991) **Biochim. Biophys. Acta**, 1066, 29.

Allen, T.M., Hansen, C., Rutledge, J. (1989) **Biochim. Biophys. Acta**, 981, 27-35.

Alving, C.R. (1991) **J. Immunol. Methods**, 140, 1-13.

Ammoury, N. (1989) **S.T.P. Pharma.**, 5, 537-540.

Amselem, S. Vogev, A., Zawoznik, E. Frideman, D. (1994) **Proc. Int. Symp. Control Res. Bioact. Mater.**, 21, 1369.

Avrilionis, K., Boggs, J.M. (1996) **Cell. Immunol.**, 168(1), 13-23.

Axelsson, B. (1989) **Adv. Drug Deliv. Rev.**, 3, 391-404.

Bailey, G.B., Gilmour, J.R., McComer, N.E. (1990) **Infect. Immun.** 58, 2389-2391.

Bangham, A.D., Standish, M.M., Watkins, J.C. (1965) **J. Mol. Biol**, 13, 238.

Barclay, A.N., Birkeland, M.L. Brown, M.H., Beyers, A.D., Davis, S.J., Somoza, C., Williams, A.F. (Eds.,) (1993), **The leucocyte antigen facts book**, Academic Press Ltd., London.

Baurain, R., Masquelier, M., Deperez-Decompeneere, D., Trouet, A. (1983) **Drugs Exp. Clin. Res.**, 9, 303.

Bennett, D.E., O'Brien, D.F. (1995) **Biochemistry**, 34(9), 3102-3113.

Bentz, J., Ellens, F.C., Szoka, F. (1987) **Biochemistry**, 26, 2105-2116.

Blume, G., Ceve, G., Crommelin, M.D., Bakker-Woundernberg, T.A., Kluft, C., Storm, G. (1993) **Biochim. Biophys. Acta**, 1149, 180-184.

Blume, G., Levi, G. (1990). **J. Lip. Res.**, 2(3), 355.

Bogdanor, A..A., Gardeeva, L.V., Torchilin, V.P, Margolis, L.B. (1989) **Exp. Cell. Res.**, 181, 362-375.

Budker, V., Gurevich, V., Hagstorm, J.E., Bortzov, F., Wolff, J.A. (1996) **Nature Biotechnology**, *14* (6) , 760-764.

Carpenter, G.S., Huang, L. (1983) **Anal. Biochem.**, 135, 151-155.

Chakrabarti, A.C,. Breaker, R, R., Joyce, G.F., Deamer, D.W.(1994) **J. .Mol. Envol.**, , 39 (6), 555-559.

Chelvi, T.P., Ralhan, R., (1995) **Int. J. Hyperthermia**, 11(5), 685-695.

Chen. H., Torchilin, V., Langer, R. (1996) **Pharma. Res.**, 13, 1378-83.

Chu, C.J., Dijkstra, J. Lai, M.Z., Hong, K., Szoka, F.C. (1990) **Pharm. Res.**, 7, 824-834.

Clausen, H., Stroud, M., Parker, J., Springer, G., Hakomor, S.I. (1988) **Mol. Immunol.**, 25, 199-207.

Cohen, S., Alfonso, M.J., Langer, R.(1994) **Int. J. Technol. Assess. Health Care**, 10(1), 121-130.

Cohen, S., Bernstein, H., Hewes, C., Chow, M. Langer, R. (1991) **Proc. Natl. Acad. Sci. USA**, 88, 10440-10444.

Cohn, A., Silverstein, S.C., Steinman, R.M. (1977) **Annu. Rev. Biochem.**, 46, 669.

Compagnon, B., Milhand, P., Bienvenue, A., Philippot, J.R. (1990) **Exp Cell Res.**, 200, 333-338.

Conor, J., Huang, L. (1985) **J. Cell. Biol.**, 101, 582-589.

Conor,J., Huang, L.(1986), **Cancer Res.**, 461, 3431-3435.

Croft, S.L (1986) **Pharm. Internet.**, 7, 229.

Cuppoletti, J., Mayhew, E., Zobel, C.R., Jung, C.Y. (1981) **Proc. Natl. Acad. Sci. USA**, 78, 2786.

Czop, J.K.., Gurish, M.F., Kadish, J.L.(1990) **J. Immunol.**, 145, 995-1001.

Dangi, J.S., Vyas, S.P. and Dixit, V.K. (1996) **Drug Dev. Ind. Pharm.**, (in press).

Davis, S.S. and Hansrani, P., (1985) **Int. J. Pharm.**, 23, 69-77.

Demant, T., Sheperd, J., Packard, C.J. (1986) **Ubers. Klin. Wochenschr.**, 66, 703-712.

Devanathan,S., Dahl,T.A., Midden,W.R., Neckers,D.S. (1990) **Proc. Natl. Acad. Sci. USA**, 87, 2980-2984.

Ehrilich, P. (1902) *A General review of the recent work in Immunity*, **In: Collected Papers of Paul Ehrlich, Immunology and Cancer Research**, Pergamon press, London (1956), Vol.2, 442.

Emanuel, N., Kedar, E., Bolotin, E.M., Smorodinsky, N., Barenholz, Y. (1996) **Pharm.Res.**, 13(3), 352-359.

Fanger, M.W., Moroganelli, P.M., Guyre, P.M. (1992) **Crit. Rev. Immunol.**, 12, 101-124.

Farmer, M.C., Gaber, B.P. (1987) **Meth. Enzymol.**, 199, 184-200.

Felgner, P.L.. (1987) **Proc. Natl. Acad. Sci. USA**, 84 : 7413-7147.

Fendler, J.H. (1982) **Membrane Mimetic Chemistry**, Wiley Interscience, 158-183.

Fogerite, S.G., Mazurkiewica, J.E., Raska, K., Voelkerding, K., Lehman, J.M., Mannino, R.. (1989) **Gene**, 84,429-438.

Fonesca, M.J., Alsina, M.A., Reig, F. (1996), **Biochim. Biophys. Acta.**, 1279(2), 259-265.

Gabius, H.J., Engelhardt, R., Hellman, T., Midoux, P., Monighy, M., Nagel, G.A., Vehmeyer, K. (1987) **Anticancer Res.**, 7, 109-112.

Gao, X., Huang, L. (1996) **Biochemistry**, 35, 1027-1036.

Garnier, F., Farauet, F., Bertolino, P. and Gerlier, D. (1991) **Vaccine**, 9, 340-345.

Gebicki, J.M., Hicks, M. (1973) **Proc. Aust. Biochem. Soc.**, 6, 45.

Gegoriadis, G., McCormack, B., Allison, A.C., Poste, G., (Eds.) (1993) **New Generation Vaccines, The role of Basic immunology**, Plenum Press , London.

Ghosh, P.C., Bachhawat, B.K. (1992) **J. Lip. Research**, 2(3), 369-382.

Goldberg, E. P., (Ed.) (1983) **Targeted drugs**, John Wiley and Sons, New York.

Gregoriadis, G. (1981). **Lancet**, 2, 241.

Gregoriadis, G. (1983), **Pharmacy international**, 33.

Gregoriadis, G. (1990) **Immunol. Today**, 11, 89-97.

Gregoriadis, G. (Ed.) (1993) **J. Drug. Target.** ,1(1), 3-6.

Gregoriadis, G., Neerunjun D., Hunt, R., (1977) **Life Sci.**, 21, 357-370.

Gregoriadis, G., Ryman, B. (1972) **Boichem. J.**, 129, 123-133.

Gupta, R.K., Varanelli, C.L., Griffin, P., Wallach, D.F.H., Siber, G.R. (1996) **Vaccine**, 14(3), 219-225.

Haensler, J , Schuber, F. (1988) **Biochim. Biophys. Acta.**, 946(1), 9b-10b.

Haisma, H.J., Boven, M., Van Muije, M., De Jong, J., Van der Vijgh, W.J.F., Pinedo, H.M. (1992) **Br. J. Cancer**, 66, 474-478.

Handjani-vila., Ribier, R.M., Rondot, A., Vinterberghe, G. (1979) **Int. J. Cosmetic Sci.**, 1, 303.

Hansen, C.B., Kao, G.Y., Moase, E.H., Zalipsky, S., Allen, T.M. (1995) **Biochim. Biophys. Acta**, 1239, 133-144.

Hayashi, H., Kono, K., Takagishi, T. (1996) **Biochim. Biophys. Acta.**, 1280(1), 127-134.

Heermans, J.L.M., Kraaijenga, J.J., Los, P., Kluff, O., Crommelin, D.J.A. (1992) **Biochim. Biophys. Acta.**, 1117, 258-264.

Ho, R,J.Y., Rouse, B.T., Huang, L.(1986) **Biochemistry**, 25, 5500-5506.

Ho, R.J.Y., Rouse, B.T., Huang, L. (1987) **J. Biol. Chem.**, 262, 13973-13978.

Ho, R.J.Y., Burke, R.L., Merigan, T.C. (1990) **Antiviral Res.**, 13, 187-199.

Holmes, M.J., Mannis, M.J., Lund, J., Jacobes, L. (1985) **Cornea**, 4, 30-34.

Hutchinson, F.G., Furr, B.J.A. (1985) **Biochem. Soc. Trans.**, 13, 520-523.

Hutchinson, F.J., Jones, M.N. (1988) **FEBS Lett.**, 234, 493-496.

Ihler, G.M., Glew, R.H., Schnure, F.W. (1973) **Proc. Natl. Acad. Sci.**, 70, 2663-2666.

Illum, L., Davis, S.S. (1984) **FEBS Lett.**, 167, 79-92.

Illum, L., (1987) G. B. Patent, 2185397 A.

Illum, L., Thomas, N.W., Davis, S.S. (1986) **J. Pharm. Sci.**, 75, 16-22.

Illum, L., Wright, J., Davis, S.S. (1989) **Int. J. Pharm.**, 52, 221-224.

Jain, S.K. and Vyas, S.P. (1993) **J. Microencapsulation**, 11(2), 141-151.

Jaitely, V. and Vyas, S.P. (1997) **J. Drug Targeting** (in press).

Jansen, R.W., Molema, G., Pouwels, R., Schols, R., De Clercq, E., Meijer, D.K.F. (1991) **Mol. Pharmacol.**, 39, 818-823.

Iin, T., Pennefather, P., Lee, P.I. (1996) **FEBS Lett.**, 397(1), 70-74.

Jones, M.N., Kaszuba, M. (1994) **Biochim. Biophys. Acta.**, 1193, 48-54.

Jones, M.N., Kaszuba, M., Lyle, I.G. (1992) Treatment composition, **British patent application** No.9208339-3, field April 15th.

Jung, C.Y.(1987) *Erythrosomes: Erythrocyte cytoskeleton coated with exogenous phospholipid as an encapsulating system.* In : **Drug and Enzyme Targeting, Methods in Enzymology**, Gree, R. and Widder K.J. (Eds.), Vol. 149, Part-B, Academic Press, Inc., California, 217-219.

Jutila, M.A., Kishimoto, T.K., Butcher, E.C. (1990) **Blood**, 76, 178-183.

Kalinuma, K. Tanaka, R., Takahashi, H., Watanable, M., Nagagawa, T. Kuroki, M., (1996) **J. Neurosurg.**, 84(2), 180-184.

Karajigi, J.S., Jain N.K. and Vyas, S.P. (1993) **J. Drug Targeting**, 1, 197-206.

Kaszuba, M., Franklin, M., Hill, K.J., Jones, M.N. (1991) **Biochem. Soc. Trans.**, 19, 4165.

Khattab, M.A., Farr, S.J., Taylor, G., Kellaway, I.W. (1995) **J. Drug Target.**, 3(1), 39, 49.

Khaw, B.A., Torchilin, V.P., Vural, I., Marula, J. (1995) **Nat. Med.**, 1(11), 1195-1198.

Kim, J., Kim, J. (1991) **Biochemistry**, 110, 436.

Kim, Y.W., Fung, M.S.C., Sun, N.C., Sun, C.R.Y., Charg, N.T., Chang, T.W. (1996) **J. Immunol.**, 144, 1257-1262.

Kinsky, S.C., Nicoletti, R.A. (1977) **Ann. Rev. Biochem.**, 46, 49.

Kirpotin, D., Park, J.W., Hong , K., Keller, G., Benz, J., Papahadjopoulous, D. (1996) **Proc. Am. Assoc. Cancer Res.**, 37, 467.

Kitao, T.,Hatto, K. (1977) **Nature**, 81, 265.

Klibanov, A.L., Huang, L. (1992) **J. Liposome Res.**, 2, 321-324.

Kohno, S., Miyazaki, T., Yamaguchi, K., Tanaka, H., Hayashi, T., Hirota, M., Saito, A., Hara, K., Sato, K., Sunanoto, J. (1988) **J. Bioact. Compat. Polym.**, 3, 137-147.

Kossovsky, N., Celman, A., Sponsler, E.E., Hnatyszyn, H.J., Raiguru, S., Torres, M., Pham, M., Crowdei, J., Zemanovich, J., Chuang, A. (1994) **Biomaterials**, 15(15), 1201-1207.

Kumar,V.V., Raghunath, P.(1986) **Lipids**, 21, 764-768.

Lanzavecchia, A., Roosnex, E., Gregory, T., Berman, P., Abrignani, S. (1988) **Nature**, 334, 530-532.

Lazo, J.S., Hacker, M.P. (1985) **Fed. Proc.**, 44, 2335-2338.

Lee, M.J., Lee, M.H., Shim, C.K. (1995) **Int. J. Pharm.**, 113, 175-187.

Lee, R.J, Huang, L. (1996) **The Journal of Biological Chemistry**, 271(14), 8481-8487.

Leonetti, J.P., Meehthi, N., Deglos, G., Gagnor, C., Lebeeu, B., (1991) **Proc. Natl. Acad. Sci. USA**, 88, 2702-2706.

Lewis, J.T., Hafeman, D.G., McConnel, H.M. (1980) **Biochemistry**, 19, 5376.

Liautard, J.P. Vidal, M., Philipott, J.R. (1985) **Biol. Int. Rep.**, 2, 1123-1137.

Loke, S.L., Stein, C.A.., Avigan, M., Cohen, J.J., Neckers, L.M. (1988) **Cur. Top. Microbial. Immunol.**, 141, 282-289.

Longaman, S.A., Tardi, P.G, Parr, M.J., Lewis, C. pieter, R.C. and Marcel, B.B. (1995) **The Journal of Pharmacology and Experimental Therapeutics**, 275,1177-1184.

Loughery, H., Bally, M.B., Cullis, P.R. (1987) **Biochim. Biophys. Acta**, 901,571-160.

Loughery, H.C., Choi, L.S., Cullis, P.R., Bally, M.B. (1990) **J. Immuno. Meth.**, 132, 25-35.

Machluf, M., Regev, O., Peled, Y., Kost, J., Ohen, S. (1996) **J. Control relaease**, 43, 35-45.

Malaiya, A. and Vyas, S.P. (1988) **J. Microencapsulation**, 5, 243-253.

Mancilla, J., Schindler, R.,Dinarello, C.A. (1990) *Importance of glycosylation for receptor binding and biological activity of IL-6,* **In: Molecular and Cellular Biology of Cytokines**, C.A. Dinarello (Ed.), Wiley-Liss, NY, 51-56.

Marsh, P.D. (1990) **J. Clin. Periodontol.**, 18, 462-467.

Martha, C., F. , Gaber, B.P. (1987) *Liposome-encapsulated haemoglobin as an artificial oxygen carrying system,* **In : Method in Enzymology** (Green, R. and widder, K.J., eds.), part B, Volume 149, Academic Press, Inc., London, 185-189.

Martin, F.J., Papahadjopoulos, D. (1982) **J. Biol. Chem.**, 257, 286-288.

Marty, J.J., Oppenheim, R.C., Speiser, P. (1978) **Pharm. Acta. Helv.**, 53, 17-22.

Medda, S., Das, N. Mahato, S.B., Mahaderan, P.R., Basu, M.K. (1995) **Indian J. Biochem. Biophys.**, 32(3), 147-151.

Meijer, D.K.F., Jansem, R.W., Molema, G. (1992) **Antiviral Res.**, 18, 215-258.

Midoux, P., Derrien, D., Petit, C., Negre, E., Mayer, R., Monsigny, M., Roche, A.C. (1989) **Glycoconjugate J.**, 6, 241-255.

Moestrup, S.K., Kaltoft, K., Munck, P.C., Pedersen, S., Gliemann, J., Christensen, E.I. (1990) **Exp. Cell Res.**,190,195-203.

Molema, G., Gansen, R.W., Pauwels, R., De Clercq, E., Meijer, D.K.F. (1990) **Biochem. Pharmacol.**, 40, 2603-2610.

Molema, G., Meijer, D.K.F. (1994) **Adv. Drug Deliv. Rev.**, 14, 25-50.

Monsigny, M., Hubert, J., Obrenovitch, A., Schreves, J. (1989) *Neoglycoproteins as toos to analyze endogenous lectins and glyco-conjugates,* **In: Electron microscopy of subcellular dynamics**, H. Plattner (Ed.,), CRC Press, Inc., Boca Raton, FL, 239-263.

Monsigny, M., Roche, A.C., Bailly, P. (1984) **Biochim. Biophys. Res. Commun.**, 121, 579-584.

Morell, A.G., Irrine, R.A., Sternlieb, I., Schinberg, I.H., Ashwell, G. (1968) **J. Biol. Chem.**, 243, 155-159.

Morishita, R., Gibbons, G.H., Ellison, K.E., Nakajma, M., Zhang, L., Kaneda, Y., Ogihara, T., Dzeau, V.J. (1993) **Proc. Natl. Acad. Sci. USA**, 90, 8474-8478.

Muller, B.G. , Leuenberger, H., Kissel, T. (1996) **Pharm. Res.**, 13(1), 32-37.

Nagato, S., Yamamoto, K., Veno, Y., Kurata, T., Chiba, J. (1991) **Hybridoma**, 10, 317-322.

Nassander, U.K., Steerenberg, P.A., Poppe, H., Storm, G., Jap, P.H.K., Poels, L.G., de Jong W.H., Crommelin, D.J.A. (1992) **Cancer Res.**, 52, 646-653.

Nguyen, P.D., O'Rear, E.A, Johnson, A.E,. Patterson, E., Whitsett, T.L., Bhakta, R. (1990) **Circulation Research**, 66, 875-878.

Nixon, J.R., Yeung, V.W. (1989) **J. Microencapsulation**, 6(1), 43-52.

Norley, S.G., Huang, L., Rouse, B.T. (1986) **J. Immunol.**, 136, 68-685.

Ostro, M.J. (ed.) (1987) **Liposomes : From Biophysics to Therapeutics**, Marcel Dekker Inc., New York.

Papahadjopoulos, D., Allen, T.M., Gabizon, A. Mayhew, E., Huang, S.K., Lee, K.D., Woodle, M.C., Lasic, D.D., Redemann, C., Martin, F.J. (1991) **Proc. Natl. Acad. Sci. USA**, 88, 11460-11464.

Patel, K.R., Li, M.P., Baldeschwieler, J.D. (1983) **Proc. Natl. Acad. Sci. USA**, 80, 6518-6522..

Pernis, B. (1985) **Immunol. Today**, 6, 45-49.

Perrin, P., Thibodeau, L., Surea, P. (1985) **Vaccine**, 3, 325-332.

Ralapati, S., Lee, C.M.J., Teodorescu, M. (1985) *Membrane lectins of human lymphocytes*, **In: Proceedings, 15th International Leukocyte Culture Conference**, Asilomar.

Reemen, J.P., Duncan, R., Schacht, E. (1984) **J. Control. Release**, 1, 47.

Regen, S.L., Czech, B., Singh, A. (1980) **J. Am. Chem. Soc.**, 102, 6638-6640.

Regen, S.L., Shin, J.S., Yamoguchi, K. (1984) **J. Am. Chem. Soc.**, 106, 2446-2247.

Ringsdorf, H., Scharb, B.,Venzymer, J. (1988) **Angewandte Chemie**, 1, 116-118.

Rock, P., Allietta, M., Young, W.W. Jo., Thompson, T.E., Tillack, T.W. (1990) **Biochemistry**, 29, 8484-8490.

Roerdink, F., Wassef, N.M., Richardson, E.C., Alving, C.R. (1983) **Biochim. Biophys. Acta.**, 734, 33.

Rom, W.N.(1991) **Am. J. Respir. Cell Mol. Biol.**, 4, 555-559.

Rossi, J.J., Elkins, D., Zaia, J.A., Sullivan, S. (1992) **AIDS Red. Hum. Retroviruses**, 8, 183-189.

Russel, D.G., Wilhelm, H. (1986) **J. Immunol.**, 136, 2613-2620.

Saito, K., Ando, J., Yoshida, M., Haga, M., Kato, Y. (1988) **Chem. Pharm. Bull.**, 36, 4187-4191.

Samain, D., Bec, J.L., Coben, E., Nguyen, F., Peyrot, M. (1989) **PCT/FR 89/00229**.

Samvel, N.K.P., Singh, M., Yamaguchi, K., Regen, S.L. (1985) **J. Am. Chem. Soc.**, 107, 42-47.

Sarkar, D.P., Blumenthal, R. (1987) **Membr. Biochem.**, 7, 231-247.

Sato, H., Viroonchatapan, E, Isao A., Ueno, M., Nagae, H., Tazawa ,K., Horikoshi,I. (1995) **Pharm. Res.**, 12(8), 1176-1183.

Scherier, S.,Ausborn, M., Gunther, S., Weissig, V., Chander, R. (1995) **J. Mol. Recognit.**, 8 (1-2), 59-62.

Senter, P.D. (1990) **FASEB. J.**, 4, 188-193.

Service, E.F. (1995) **Science**, 267, 458-459.

Shen, T.Y. (1987) **Ann. NY Acad. Sci. USA**, 507, 272-280.

Sherwood, R.F. (1996) **Adv. Drug Deliv. Rev.**, 22, 269-288.

Sinibadi, L., Goldoni P., Seganti, L., Superti, F., Tsiang, H., Orsi, N. (1985) **Microbiologica**, *8,* 355-365.

Sizer, P.J., Miller, A., Watts, A. (1987) **Biochemistry**, 26, 5106-5113.

Sjoholm, I., Edman, B. (1978) **J. Pharm. Sci.**, 67, 693-696.

Spady, D.K., Meddings, J.B., Deitschy, J.M. (1986) **J. Clin. Invest.**, 77, 1474-1481.

Spanjer, H., Scherphof, G., (1983) **Biochim. Biophys. Acta**, 734, 40-47.

Spanjer, H., Van Berkel, T., Scherphof, G., and Kempen, H. (1985) **Biochim. Biophys. Acta**, 816, 396-402.

Steer, C.J., Ashwell, G. (1986), *Hepatic membrane receptors for glycopreteins,* **In : Progress in Liver Diseases**, Popper, H. and Schaffner, F. (Eds.), Vol.VIII, Grune and Stratton, New York, 99-123.

Steinhoff, G., Behrend, M., Schrader, B., Pichlmatr, R. (1993) **Hepatocytology**, 18, 440-453.

Storm, G., Koppenhogen, F., Heeremans, A., Vingerhoeds, M., Woodle, M.C., Crommelin, D.J. (1995) **J. Control. Release**, 36, 19-24.

Sullivan, S.M., Huang, L., (1986) **Proc. Natl. Acad. Sci. USA**, 83, 6117-6121.

Sun, Y., Jin, X.H., Dong , X.Y, Tu, K, Zhou, X.Z. (1996) **Appl. Biochem. Biotechnol.**, 56(3), 331-339.

Sunamato, J., Iwamoto, K. (1987) **CRC Crit. Rev. Ther. Drug Carrier Syst.**, 2, 117-136.

Sunamoto, J., Goto, M., Iida, T., Hara, K. Saito, K., Tomonaga A. (1984) **Receptor Mediated Targeting of Drugs**, NATO ASI Ser. Ser. A 82, 359-371.

Sunamoto, J., Sakai, K., Sato, T., Kondo, H. (1988) **Chem. Lett.**, 10, 1781-1784.

Sunamoto, J., Sato, T., Hirota, M., Fukushima, K., Hiratani, K., Hara, K. (1987) **Biochim. Biophys. Acta.**, 898, 323-330.

Suzuki, SD., Watanabe, S., Masuko, T., Hashimoto, Y. (1995) **Biochim. Biophys. Acta.**, 124, 9-16.

Szoka, F. (1992) **Res. Immunol.**, 143, 186-187.

Tetsui, S., Zhao, J., Kimura, S., Imanishi, Y., (1996) **Int. J. Pept. Protein. Res.**, 48(1), 95-101.

Thibodeau, L., Chagnon, M., Flamand, L., Oth, D., Lachapelle, L., Tremblay, C., Montagnier, L. (1989) **C. R. Acad. Sic.**, 309, 741-747.

Thompson, D.H., Gerasimov, O.V., Wheeler, J.J., Rui, Y., Anderson, V.C. (1996) **Biochim. Biophys. Acta.**, 2(21), 1279(1), 25-34.

Till, M.A,. Zolla-Pazner., S.,Gorny, M.K., Patton, J.S. Uhr, J.W., Vietta, E.S. (1989) **Proc. Natl. Acad. Sci. USA**, 86, 1987-1991.

Till, M.A., Ghetie, V., Gregory, T., Patzer, E.J., Porter, J.P., Ubr, J.W., Capon, D.J. and Viatta, E.S. (1988) **Science**, 272, 1166-1168.

Tomlinson, E. (1983) **Int. J. Pharm. Technol. Prod. Manuf.**, 4, 49-57.

Torchilin, V.P. (1987) **CRC Crit. Rev. Ther. Drug Carrier Systems**, 2, 65-115.

Torres, J.M., Geuskens, M., Uriel, J. (1991) **Int. J. Cancer**, 47, 110-117.

Tsao, Y.S., Huang, L. (1986) **Biochemistry**, 25, 3971-3976.

Tse, D., Pernis, B., (1984) **J. Exp. Med.**, 159, 193.

Tso, P., Balin, J.A. (1986) **Am. J. Physiol.**, 250, 715-726.

Turrens, J.F., Crapo. J.D., Freeman, B.A. (1984) **J. Clin. Invest.**, 73, 87-95.

Turro, N.J., Chung, C. (1984) **Macromolecules**, 17, 2123-2126.

Tuschida, E. (1996) **Artifical Cells Blood Substitute and Immobilization Technology**, 22, 467-477.

Utsumi, S., Shinomiya, H., Minami, J., Sonada, S. (1983) **Immunology**, 49, 113.

Utsumi, T., Aizono, Y., Funatsu, G. (1987) **FEBS Lett.**, 216, 99-103.

Van Berkel, Th.J.C., Kruij, K., Kempen, H. (1985) **J. Biol. Chem.**, 260, 12203.

Vingerhoeds, M.H., Haisma, H.J., Belliot, S.O., Smit, H.P., Crommelin, D.J.A., Storm, G. (1996) **Pharm. Res.**, 13(4), 604-607.

Vingerhoeds, M.H., Haisma, H.J., van Muijen, M., van de Rijt, Crommelin, D.J.A., Storm, G. (1993) **FEBS Lett.**, 336, 485-490.

Viroonchatapan, E., Sato, H., Ueno, M., Adachi, I., Tazawa, K. Horikoshi, I. (1996) **Life Sci.**, 58(24), 2251-2261.

Vitetta, E.S. (1990) **J.Clin. Immunol.**, 10, 515-518.

Vitetta, E.S., Uhr, J.W. (1985) **Annu. Rev. Immunol.**, 3, 197-212.

Vizaglou, M.O., Speizer, P.P. (1988) **Acta. Pharma. Scec.**, 23, 163.

Vlassara, H., Brownlee, M., Cerami, A. (1986) **J. Exp. Med.**, 164, 1301-1309.

Vyas, S.P., Talwar, N., Karajgi, J.S. and Jain, N.K. (1993) **J. Contrl. Rel.**, 23, 231-237.

Vyas, S.P., Jaitely, V., Kanaujia, P. (1997) **Ind. J. Exp. Biology**, 35(3), 212-218.

Vyas, S.P., Mysore, N., Jaitely, V. and Venkatsan, N., (1997) **Die Pharmazie**, (in press).

Wagner, E., Curiel, D., Cotten, M. (1994). **Adv. Drug Deliv. Rev.**, 14, 113-135.

Wang, C.Y., Huang, L. (1987a) **Biochim. Biophys. Res. Commun.**, 147, 980-895.

Wang, C.Y., Huang, L. (1987b) **Proc. Natl Acad Sci. USA**, 84, 7851-7853.

Wang, C.Y., Huang, L. (1989) **Biochemistry**, 28, 9508-9514.

Wang, K.C., Verret, C.R., Yu, R.K., Gershon, R.K., Lee, S. (1987) **Immunobiology**, 174, 139-145.

Wang, S., Lee, R.J., Cauchon, G., Gorenstein, D.G., Low, P.S. (1995) **Proc. Natl. Acad. Sci. U.S.A.**, 92, 3318-3322.

Wassef, N.M., Alving, C.R., Richards, R.L., (1994) **Immunomethods**, 4, 217-222.

Weber, B.A., Border, N., Regen, S.L. (1987) **J.Am. Chem. Soc.**, 119, 4419-4421.

Weinstein, J.N., Magin R.L., Yatvin, M.B., Zaharko, D.S. (1979) **Science**, 204, 188-191.

Weinstein, J.N., Yoshikami, S., Henkart, P. Blumenthal, R., Hagins, W.A. (1977) **Science**, 189, 485.

Weir, D.M. (1980) **Immunol. Today**, 1, 45-51.

Weissmann, G., Bloom garden, D., Kaplan, R., Cohen, C., Hoffstein, S., Collins, T., Gotlieb, A., Nagle, D. (1975) **Proc. Natl. Acad. Sci. USA**, 72(1), 88-92.

Widder, K.J., Senyei, A.E., Ranney, D.F. (1979) **Adv. Pharmacol. Chemother.**, 16, 216.

Wolff, B., Gregoriadis, G. (1984) **Biochim. Biophys. Acta.**, 802, 259-273.

Wright, J.J., Illum, L. (1992) *Active targeting of microcapsules and microspheres to specific regions*, **In: Microcapsules and Nanoparticles in Medicine and Pharmacy**, Donbrow, M. (Ed.) CRC Press, Boca Raton, 281-297.

Yachi, K., Kikuchi, H., Yamauch, H., Hirota, S. Tomikawa, M. (1995) **J. Microencapsulation**, 12(4), 377-388.

Yamauchi, H., Yano, T., Kato, T., Tanaka, I., Nakabayashi, S., Higashi, K., Miyoshi, S., Yamada, H. (1995) **Int. J. Pharm.**, 113, 141-148.

Yamazaki, N., Kojima, S., Gabius, S., Gobius, H.J. (1992) **Int. J. Biochem.**, 24, 99-107.

Yatvin, M.B., Krentz, W., Horwitz, B.A., Shinitzky, M. (1980) **Science**, 210, 1253-1255.

Yatvin, M.B., Muhlensiepen, H., Porschen,w., Weinstein, J.N., Feinendgen, L.E. (1981) **Cancer Reserch**, 41, 1602-1607.

Yeung, V.W., Nixon, J.R. (1988) **J. Microencapsulation**, 5, 331-337.

Zalipsky, S., Puntambekar, B., Boulikas, P., Engbers, C.M., Woodle, M.C. (1995) **Bioconjug. Chem.**, 6(6), 705-708.

Zelphati, O., Francis, C., Szoka, Jr. (1996) **J. Control. Rel.**, 41, 99-119.

INDEX